Masahide Tsutsui
Teruko Tsutsui

Comprehensive Dentistry

Quintessence Publishing Ltd.
London, Berlin, Chicago, Tokyo, Barcelona, Istanbul, Milan, Moscow, New Delhi, Paris, Beijing, Prague, São Paulo, Seoul, and Warsaw

© 2008 Quintessence Publishing Co, Ltd

Quintessence Publishing Co, Ltd
Grafton Road
New Malden
Surrey KT3 3AB
United Kingdom
www.quintpub.co.uk

All rights reserved. This book or any part thereof may not be reproduced, stored in a retrieval system, or transmitted in any form or by any means, electronic, mechanical, photocopying, or otherwise, without prior written permission of the publisher.

ISBN: 978-1-85097-161-0
Printed in Germany

Table of Contents

Foreword

It is with great pleasure and honor that I accepted the invitation to write the foreword to this outstanding text on comprehensive dentistry, which was first published in Japanese. I was so impressed with the case presentations, including the quality of the documentation and illustrated material, that I suggested to Quintessence that the book should be published in English.

In a remarkable paper delivered during the 2003 International Academy of Esthetic Dentistry meeting in Washington, DC, Dr Masahide Tsutsui's lecture was presented in English and astounded dentists from all over the world. To quote Dr Leonard Abrams, "Dr Tsutsui has it all together." This response was typical of those in the audience, which included Drs David Garber, Henry and Maurice Salama, Ronald Goldstein, and Dennis Tarnow, and just about the entire audience was of this caliber. Sadly, with the untimely death of Masahide Tsutsui, this foreword might well serve as a requiem for the life of this outstanding dental practitioner, teacher, human being, and the co-author of this beautiful text.

As indicated by the title *Comprehensive Dentistry*, the Tsutsuis have formulated an approach to the study and practice of the art and science of dentistry that takes into consideration an understanding of all aspects of the many parts of the stomatognathic system as well their relationship to the whole body. For this approach, they started viewing their patients as individuals who may be quite different from each other and, therefore, "statistically insignificant." Hence, they present a significant series of anecdotal (ie, single case) histories that were diagnosed based on careful, critically strict criteria. Their therapeutic intervention with these patients produced respectively similar results, giving birth to evidence-based information. In addition to the exquisite quality of Dr Masahide Tsutsui's restorative dentistry and periodontal therapy as well as Dr Teruko Tsutsui's imaginative and exacting approach to orthodontic diagnosis and therapy, one can be sure of the consistency of their approach to the clinical problem.

The Tsutsuis take us through the complex arena of traditional problems associated with the era of periodontal prosthesis and the increased attention to esthetics, particularly as it relates to the dentogingival complex. These problems presented difficulties when dealing with the restoration of the natural dentition; they presented even more difficulties when dealing with the restoration of anterior implant abutments. Dr Tsutsui competently managed this transition along with the intelligent integration of osseointegrated implants into his treatment plan. I can only give this book my highest recommendation, and I congratulate and thank the publisher for recognizing its need to be translated into English.

Morton Amsterdam, DDS, ScD

Professor Emeritus of Periodontics and Periodontal Prosthesis
Norman Vine Professor of Restorative Dentistry
University of Pennsylvania
School of Dental Medicine

Preface

This book introduces the most important concept in our clinical practice: control of inflammation and forces. Control of inflammation is relatively simple; inflammation can be diagnosed, and its cause and consequences are related to each other. On the other hand, forces are not easy to deal with because forces are invisible.

Clinical incorporation of treatment of forces can be assumed to occur if inflammation is properly controlled and basic procedures are routinely conducted with high precision. The result of these forces is manifested in the "shape" of a total oral system comprising the individual tooth, the dentition, and the arches. To precisely determine change with the passage of time, diagnostic tools such as facial and clinical photographs, probing data, full-mouth radiographs, temporomandibular joint radiographs, cephalograms, and study casts must be available. Adding an analysis of functional jaw movements to this diagnostic material helps to determine what forces will affect the patient.

The decisive role of the clinician comes into play in the thorough examination and analysis of a patient's intraoral and facial conditions, as well as the body as a whole. Review of all the gathered data will allow a better understanding of how forces are incorporated in the patient's overall dental health.

Principles of these approaches to forces are discussed in chapter 2 of this book. The format of this chapter is different from that of other chapters. Many readers may find this chapter less approachable and more difficult to understand. We propose some hypotheses, which are not included in commonly accepted theories, and have tried to prove them through clinical cases. Because clinical practices by their nature do not suit quantitative evaluations nicely, an indisputable demonstration is impossible. Still, the concept of force control described in chapter 2 is the backbone of our current clinical practice.

The objective of our clinical practice is not to prove these hypotheses. In our clinical practice, we are confronted with the results of these hypotheses every day. Even if we were not advocating these hypotheses, we see them in practice every day. We wish to obtain stable treatment results, to maintain beautiful gingiva, to restore natural bone level and a fine arch shape, and to achieve an easily maintainable dentition in a healthy and comfortable way. The hypotheses are continually examined thoroughly as they are routinely utilized in our practice.

In the late 1980s, we started to consider introducing our treatment concepts to others. More than 10 years passed while we developed this project. One difficulty was our ability to articulate our ideas clearly. Incorporation of new technologies into our practice was also a stumbling block to completing this work.

Fortunately, in cooperation with Mr Hidetoshi Akimoto, Editorial House AKI, Ltd, who is a longtime sympathizer and excellent editor, we brought our thoughts together in this book. A large number of patients have taught and encouraged us, helping us to realize our goal. We would like to thank all of those patients, and we sincerely hope this book will be of some help to our colleagues in their daily practice.

Acknowledgments

It has been 27 years since we opened our private practice in Kitakyushu, Japan. We were fortunate to have graduated from dental school when the Japanese dental academy was in its growth period. Flooded with information, we incorporated without hesitation any idea that was said to be "good," and these choices resulted in our present clinical practices.

In our practice, Masahide is responsible for endodontics, periodontics, prosthetics, and implantology, while Teruko is responsible for occlusion, orthodontics, and pedodontics. Our fundamental policy is that both of us should be able to critically evaluate and perform the basics of clinical dentistry, in addition to which we each have our own areas of expertise.

We owe what we are today to our many patients, our respected teachers at the university, our honored mentors in clinical practice, senior clinicians in our study group, colleagues in our community, and clinicians who are students of our Tsutsui Study Club, which started as a lecture course on orthodontics in 1988 and later developed into a course that covers comprehensive dentistry. Because students who complete the lecture course of this study club are allowed to participate in the course as observers, for life, we as instructors always have to be conscious of the graduates' observations. Their questions about how our thinking has advanced or what has happened within a specific clinical case have become the source of our progress.

It is customary in books to list the names of mentors who taught the authors, senior clinicians who influenced the authors, and colleagues who encouraged the authors. Our list of names would be long. Excuse us for refraining from giving the names here, since there are too many to be specific. If asked from whom we have learned the most, starting from the most fundamental ethical issues as health care professionals to clinical issues, we would say that we owe it to our patients. Without fail, it is our patients who have taught us the most.

We would like to thank our staff members who support us in our daily practice. We will continue in our endeavor to improve the health of our patients while searching for further advances in clinical practice. Both of us are grateful for being given the opportunity to work with a wonderful partner within our profession.

Last, but not least, we would like to express our gratitude to Mr Ikko Sasaki of Quintessence Publishing Co, Ltd, who published this book after patiently watching over us as we completed this seemingly endless task.

Chapter 1

Diagnosis in Comprehensive Dentistry

Principles of Comprehensive Dentistry

Diagnosis of force elements

Faced with a patient who complains of a toothache, no dentist would provide treatment without considering its cause. However, if no caries, fracture line, or radiographic change is found, making a diagnosis is difficult. A distinguishing characteristic of stomatognathic diseases or disorders is that force elements, together with inflammation, are involved in a complicated manner. Similarly, if even one tooth shows mobility, it is essential to consider force elements. In this book, the authors emphasize the control of inflammation and forces, which must begin with diagnosis. Although the cause of inflammation is generally clear, elements of forces are very complicated because they are invisible, extended, and change every moment. Because of this, force elements often are overlooked in daily clinical practice.

Diagnosis of force elements requires that the case be viewed from many different perspectives. The authors emphasize the importance of paying attention not only to an affected region but also to a patient's posture, habits, face, occlusion, and form of dental arch. Examination of one tooth alone will never lead to a diagnosis of force elements.

Comprehensive dental care

Comprehensive dental care is often misunderstood to mean full-mouth occlusal reconstruction, making full use of prosthodontics, periodontal surgery, and orthodontics. On the contrary, this approach emphasizes diagnosis based on a complete evaluation of inflammation and force elements in order to achieve maximum therapeutic effect with minimal invasion. In fact, unless force elements are properly diagnosed, treatment results will not be stable and therapy will have to be excessive whether intended or not, possibly including extraction of all teeth with uncertain prognosis, splinting of all teeth with insufficient periodontal support, placement of a number of dental implants to ensure occlusal support, and incorporation of many abutment teeth in prostheses. If, however, a clinician understands forces that are involved in a patient's stomatognathic system, splinting connections can be avoided as much as possible and orthodontics can be kept to a minimum. In order to achieve maximum therapeutic effect with minimal invasion, clinicians need to have various methods for diagnosing and improving force elements. This is the comprehensive dental care that the authors promote, as demonstrated in Case 1-1.

Case 1-1 Rationale for comprehensive dental care

Patient: *22-year-old woman at the time of first visit in 1997*
Chief complaint: *Pain in the left temporomandibular joint during jaw opening, which started 4 to 5 years previously, and disturbance of mouth opening*
Diagnosis: *The three major symptoms of temporomandibular disorder (TMD), trismus or motility disturbance, pain during mandibular opening, and clicking, are confirmed. It was diagnosed as anterior disc displacement with reduction of the left temporomandibular joint.*
If the cause of disharmony of occlusion is detected and rectified, the body will recover good health. This particular condition was diagnosed as anterior disc displacement with reduction of the left temporomandibular joint.
This patient naturally chews using the right anterior area. Because of her habit to bite and fold her lips, the maxillary central incisors have inclined lingually, which has caused retrognathism of the mandible. Although she chews on the both sides, the external force applied to the right is stronger. This force has pushed the mandible to the left, which has resulted in lowering of the left condyle, followed by anterior disc displacement. Bruxism, indicated by attrition of the anterior teeth, occurs with the mandible protruded to the right anterior. The unstable occlusion due to lingual inclination of the maxillary anterior teeth may be one of the causes of bruxism.
Her habits of biting her lips and chewing on the right were cured to recover a healthy condyle-disc relationship. As a result, bruxism was reduced and periodontal tissue was restored to health. Although the therapeutic intervention was extremely limited, the whole stomatognathic system changed dramatically to regain its harmony (Figs 1-1 to 1-12 and Box 1-1).
Although examinations generally begin with the face, the following sequence of figures begins with oral findings because they are most relevant to this clinical case.

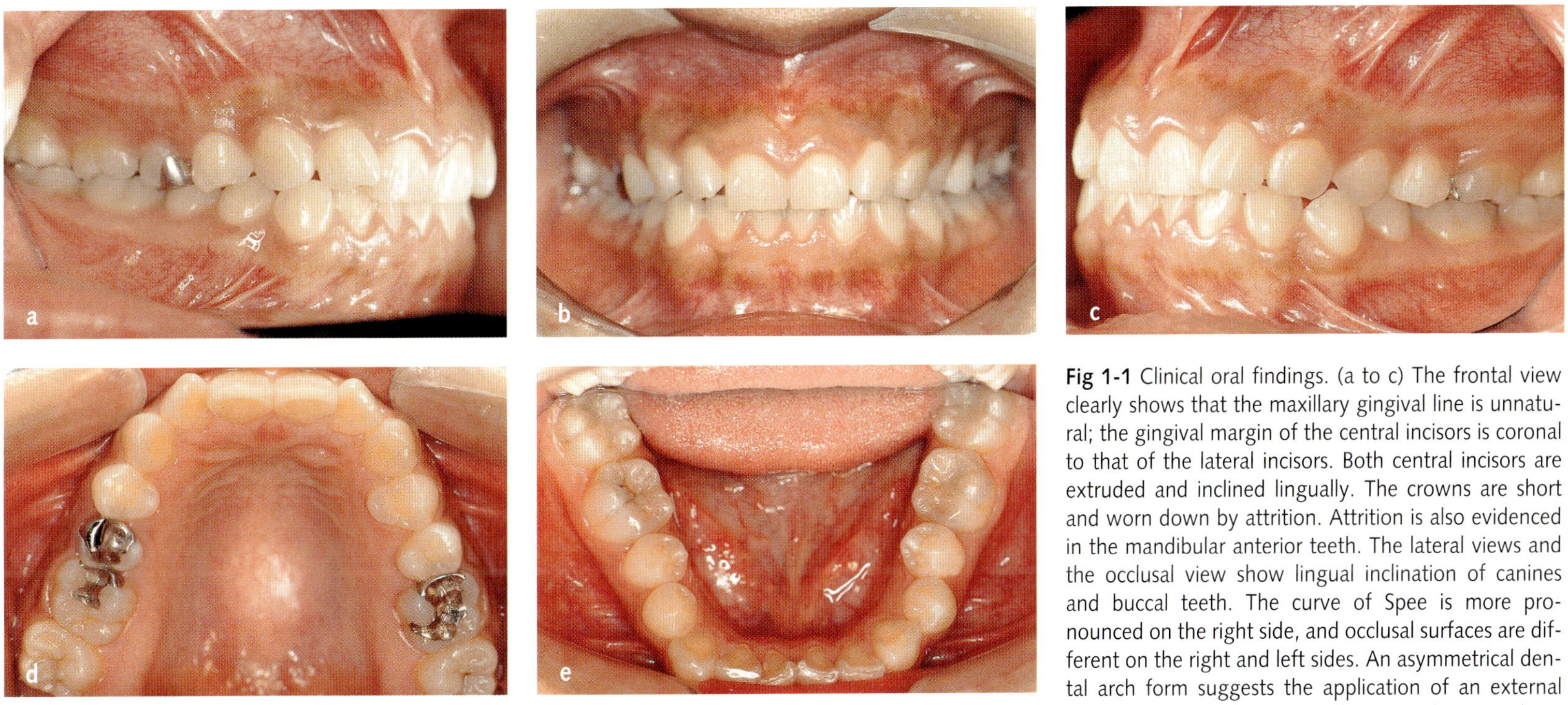

Fig 1-1 Clinical oral findings. (a to c) The frontal view clearly shows that the maxillary gingival line is unnatural; the gingival margin of the central incisors is coronal to that of the lateral incisors. Both central incisors are extruded and inclined lingually. The crowns are short and worn down by attrition. Attrition is also evidenced in the mandibular anterior teeth. The lateral views and the occlusal view show lingual inclination of canines and buccal teeth. The curve of Spee is more pronounced on the right side, and occlusal surfaces are different on the right and left sides. An asymmetrical dental arch form suggests the application of an external force. (d and e) The occlusal view indicates a box-shaped arch form. Since anatomic forms of the tongue, maxilla, and mandible are U shaped, it is essential to the diagnosis to question why the arch would have this unnatural box shape.

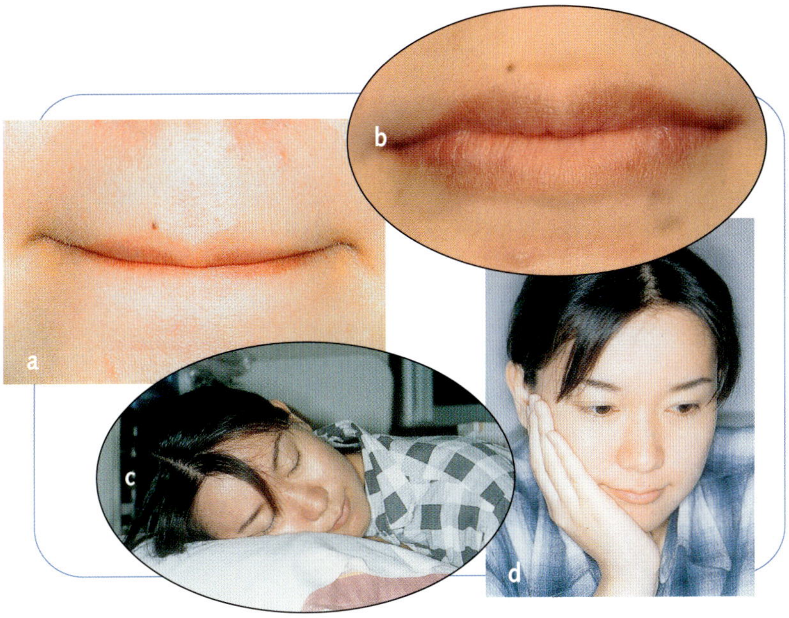

Fig 1-2 External forces that have distorted the dental arch. (a) While in the dental chair, the patient was observed biting her lip. It was surmised that this habit has caused the lingual inclination and extrusion of the maxillary central incisors as well as the box shape of the arch. (b) The brownish change around the lips indicates a habit of folding the lips. (c and d) The curve of Spee and lingual inclination of molars on the right side were attributed to the patient's habits of resting her cheek on her right hand and sleeping on the right side of her face.

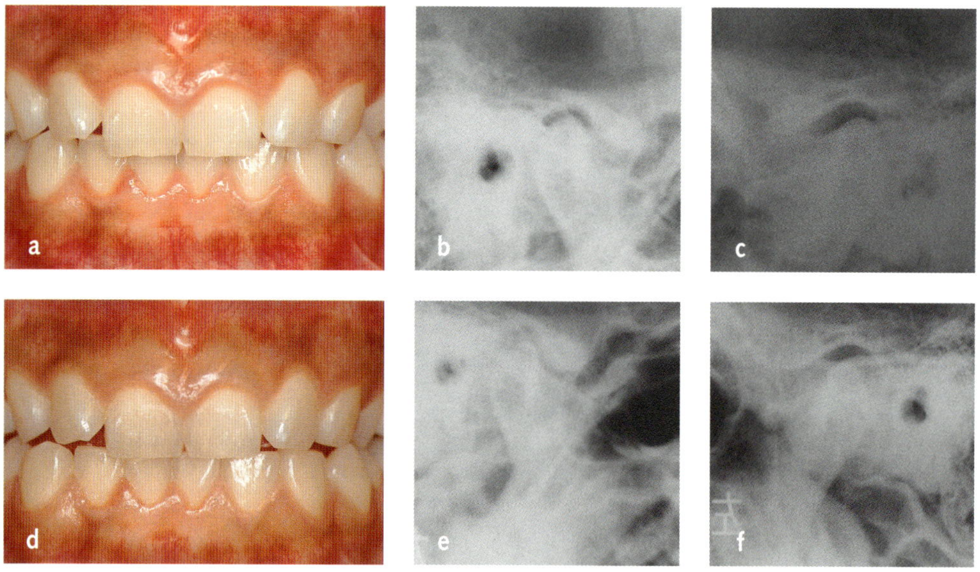

Fig 1-3 Mandibular position and temporomandibular joint (TMJ) at the first visit. (a to c) Intercuspal position (ICP). (a) The left condyle is off the disc with no midline shift. (b) Transcranial radiograph of right TMJ shows the joint space in a normal range. (c) Transcranial radiograph of left TMJ shows the condyle is off the disc and pushed posteriorly.(d to f) Relaxed position (RP). (d) When the patient is allowed to lightly tap the teeth in a relaxed manner, contact occurs at the right anterior area. In this position, the left condyle is on the disc. (e) Transcranial radiograph of right TMJ indicates protrusion of the mandible. (f) Transcranial radiograph of left TMJ shows the left condyle is on the disc, indicating protrusion of the mandible.

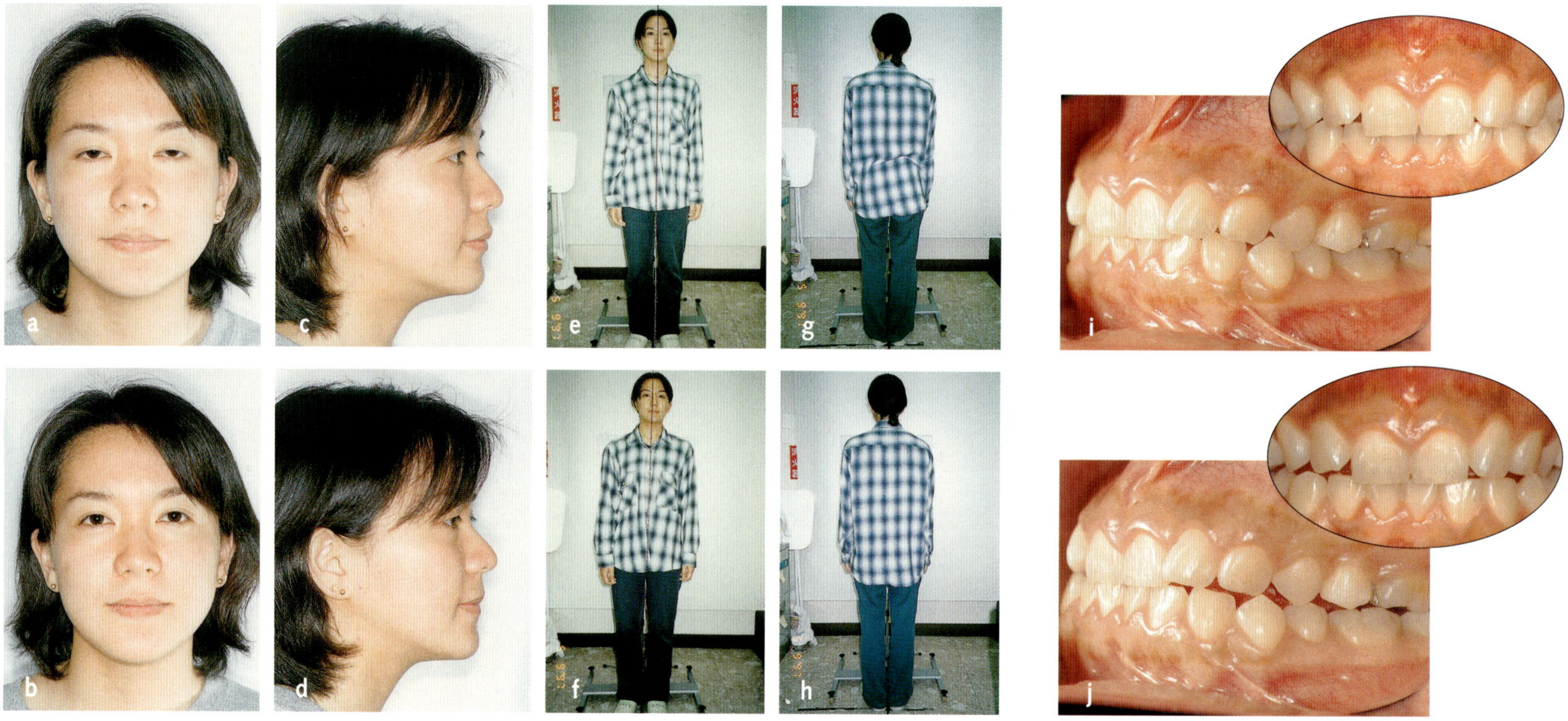

Fig 1-4 ICP (upper row) and RP (bottom row) at the first visit. (a) The patient's face at ICP (with the left condyle off the disc) shows that the left masseter is well developed (suggesting left-side chewing). The mandible is shifted to the left. Her eyes are half open, which may seem accidental; however, patients with jaw position discrepancy seem to have difficulty fully opening their eyes. (b) At RP (with the left condyle on the disc), the mandible is not shifted to the left. (c) The profile at ICP. (d) The profile at RP shows that the mandible is slightly protruded. (e and f) At ICP, the right shoulder is sloping. (g and h) At RP, the right shoulder is less sloping. (i) Occlusion at ICP. (j) Occlusion at RP.

Box 1-1 Correcting bad habits

First, the patient's current conditions and problems, including the dental arch, gingival line, tooth inclination, TMJ, and oral habits, were explained to her. She was encouraged to be aware of and refrain from her habits of biting her lips (which proved to be difficult even with attention), resting her cheek on the right hand, and sleeping on the right side of her face. She was also encouraged to turn her head to the right while chewing and bite on the right side. (To chew facing right facilitates right-side chewing, during which the left [nonworking] condyle will translate to an anterior inferior position.) Also, a mandibular position that did not produce clicking was demonstrated to the patient, helping her to consciously conduct light tapping in the right anterior area and therefore maintain the left condyle on the disc. She was instructed that biting off hard food using the left dentition was most detrimental.

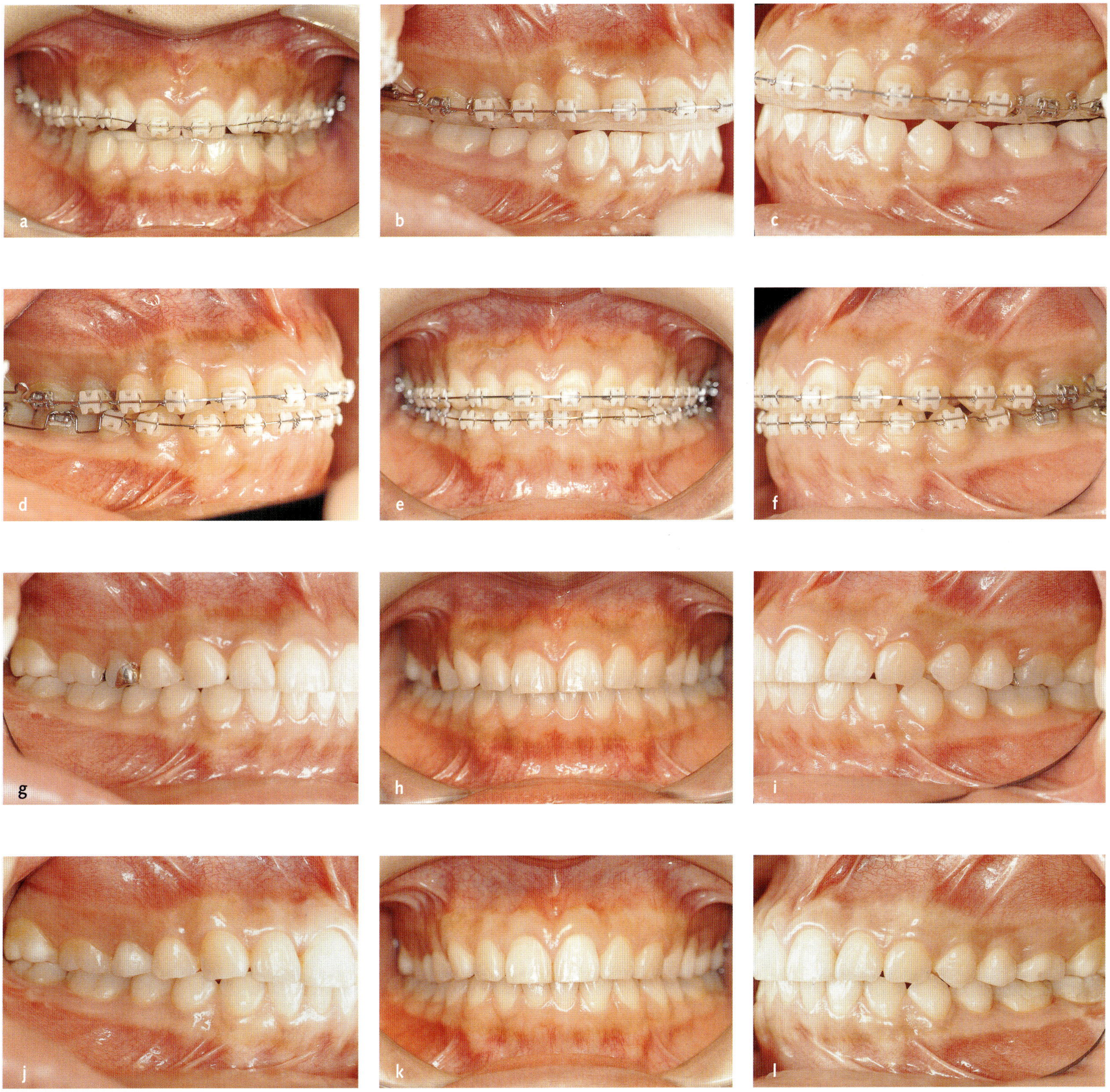

Fig 1-5 Restorative tooth movement. (a) About 1 month after the first visit, full brackets are bonded for the maxilla only to incline the maxillary central incisors labially while a stabilizing splint is used for the mandible. Once the maxillary central incisors have been moved labially, allowing protrusive movement of the mandible, the mandibular teeth will be bonded. The splint is also used to determine a suitable mandibular position. (b and c) After 5 months of continued use of maxillary brackets and mandibular splint. At this point, the mandibular arch received full brackets. (d to f) After 9 months, both maxillary and mandibular teeth have received full brackets. (g to i) After removal of appliances. The maxilla was bonded for 1 year and 4 months, while the mandible was bonded for 2 years. The dental midline is slightly shifted to the right. (j to l) At 2 years and 8 months after the first visit, the posterior teeth have been restored and maxillary gingival depigmentation conducted. Gingival lines were harmonized using only orthodontic treatment in this case. Bruxism was cured, and the left condyle is stable on the disc.

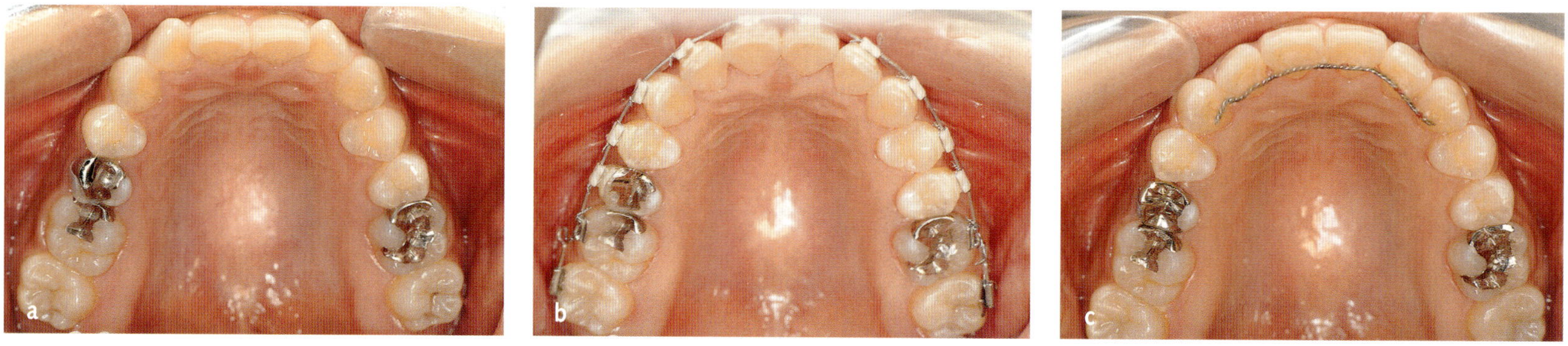

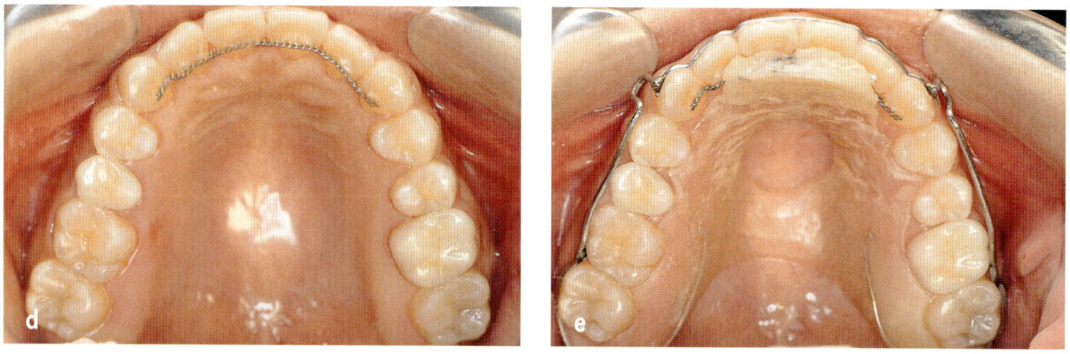

Fig 1-6 Changes in the maxilla and mandible. (a) The box-shaped maxilla at the first visit. (b) Orthodontic treatment is ongoing with full brackets, changing the box shape of the maxilla into a U shape. (c) Maxilla with orthodontic treatment completed (1 year and 6 months). (d) Maxilla after restorative treatments (Empress crowns and porcelain inlays). (e) During maintenance, the patient learned to sleep on her back. A flap was given to her night-use maxillary retainer so that the mandible would not retrude. (f) The box-shaped mandible at the first visit. (g) Orthodontic treatment is ongoing with full brackets, uprighting the axes of the right retroclined

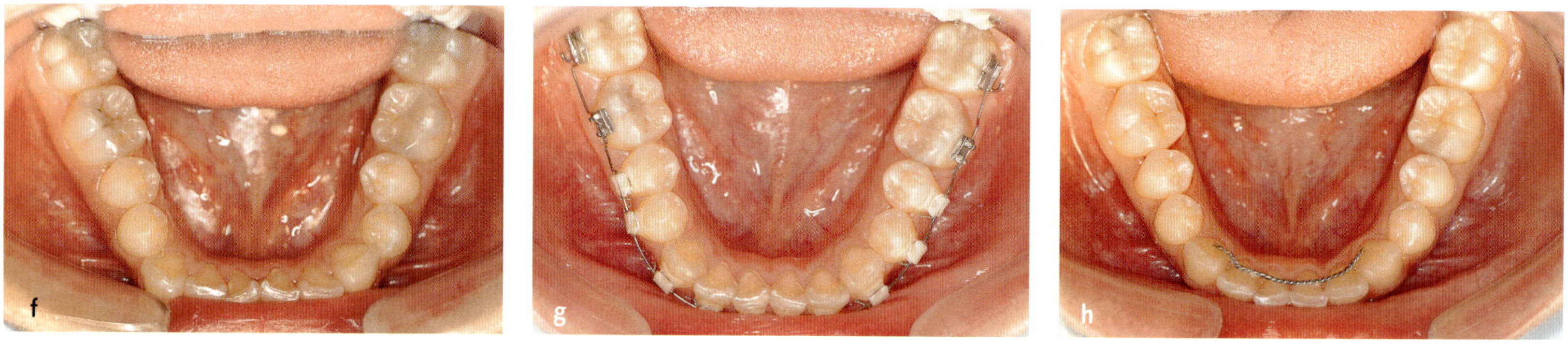

teeth and changing the box shape of the mandible into a U shape. (h) It is difficult for the patient to refrain from the lip-biting habit. The posterior teeth are not sufficiently upright. Porcelain inlays have been delivered to the mandibular first and second molars.

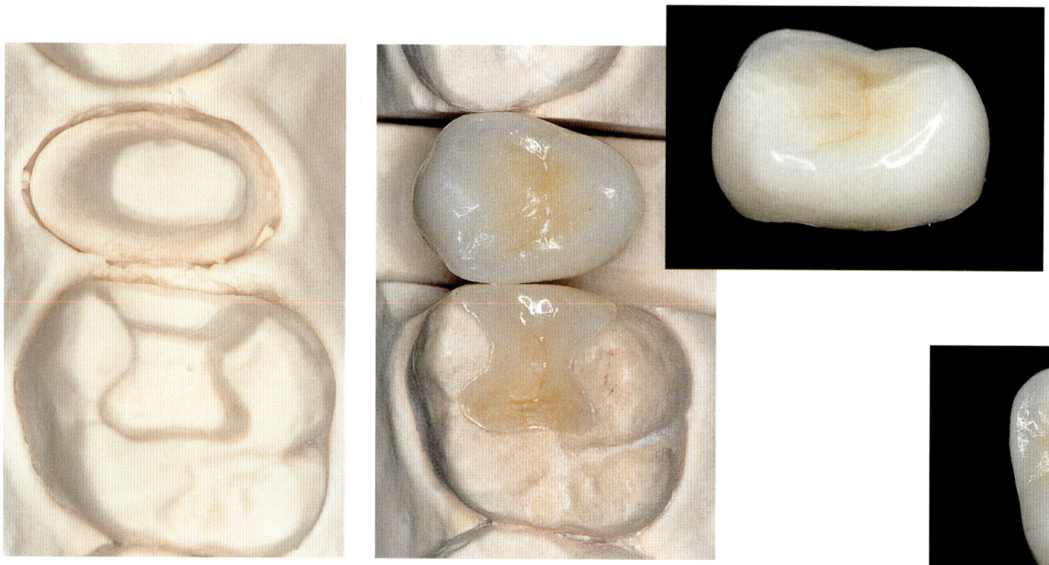

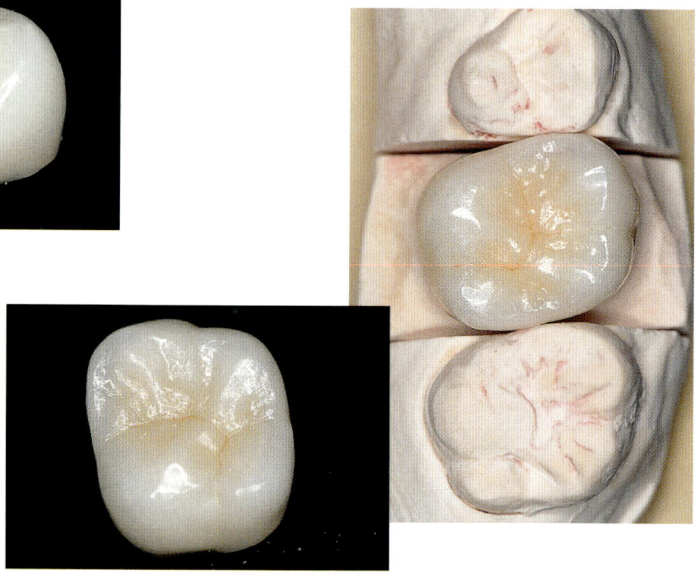

Fig 1-7 Maxillary restorations with Empress crowns and porcelain inlays. As their physical condition and the esthetics of their anterior teeth improve, patients often desire further esthetic improvements.

Fig 1-8 Completion of treatment (2 years and 5 months after the first visit). The left TMJ is on the disc. Her eyes appear larger because she is able to fully open them now that the mandibular position has been corrected. Symptoms such as stiffness in the neck and shoulders, eyestrain, and dizziness upon standing up, which existed at the first visit, have disappeared. The left masseter is still tense; it seems that she still chews on the left side.

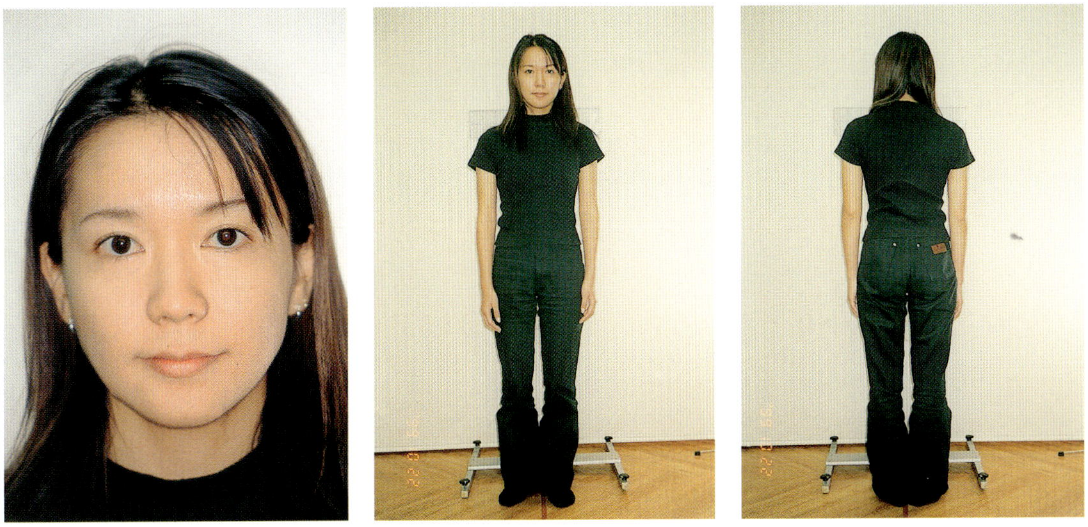

Fig 1-9 Radiographs before and after treatment. (a) Before treatment. (b) After treatment. The comprehensive harmony of the stomatognathic system has been restored.

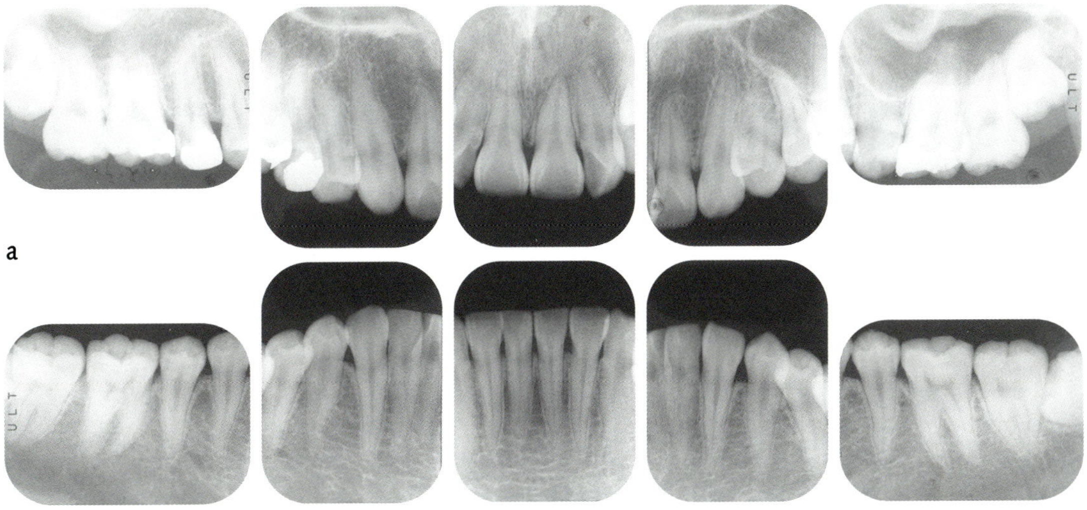

a

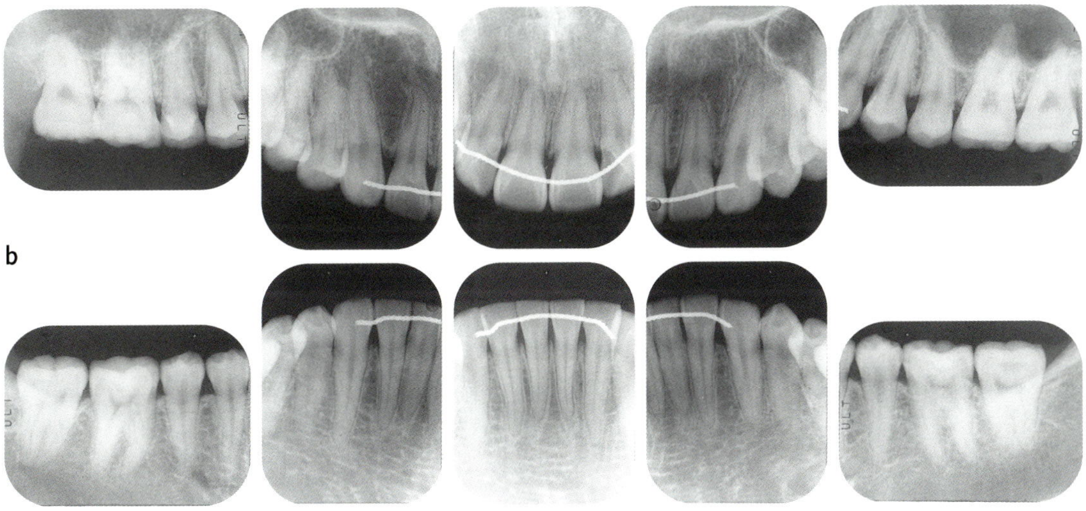

b

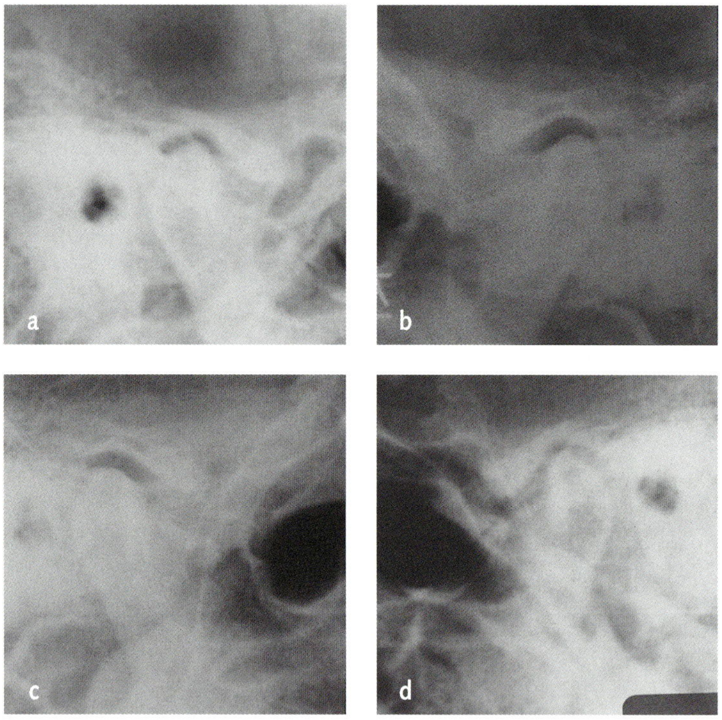

Fig 1-10 Transcranial radiographs of TMJs before and after treatment. (a and b) Before treatment. (a) The right TMJ in maximum intercuspation. (b) The left TMJ in maximum intercuspation (off the disc). (c and d) After treatment. (c) The right TMJ in maximum intercuspation. (d) The left TMJ in maximum intercuspation on the disc. Compared to the conditions at the first visit, the left condyle has moved forward while the right condyle has moved slightly backward. The left clicking has been resolved. As a maintenance therapy, the patient is instructed to turn her head to the right while eating and bite into food using the right side of the dentition, not to chew hard food on the left, and not to bite the lips. However, she tends to bite into food using the left side of the dentition and bite the lips. Her computer is located on the left side of her desk in her office; therefore, she had her head turned to the left for many hours a day.

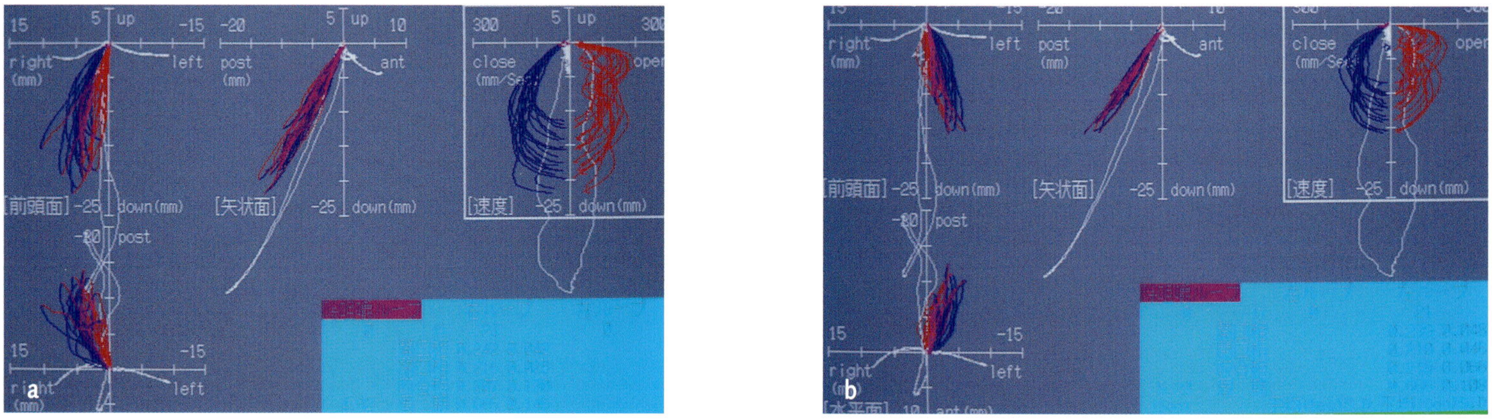

Fig 1-11 Masticatory movement at the first visit. (a) The right chewing path is shown. The maximum opening on the frontal plane indicates that it is pulled to the left at about 20 mm, on the disc at 25 mm and brought back to the midline, shifting to the right due to the force. During usual chewing, the condyles move on and off the discs depending on the way she chews food. (The turning point locations are mixed: It is sometimes on the right and somewhat shifted to the left at other times.) (b) The left chewing path is shown. Chewing takes place while the condyle remains off the disc. The speed, shown in the upper right, is limited.

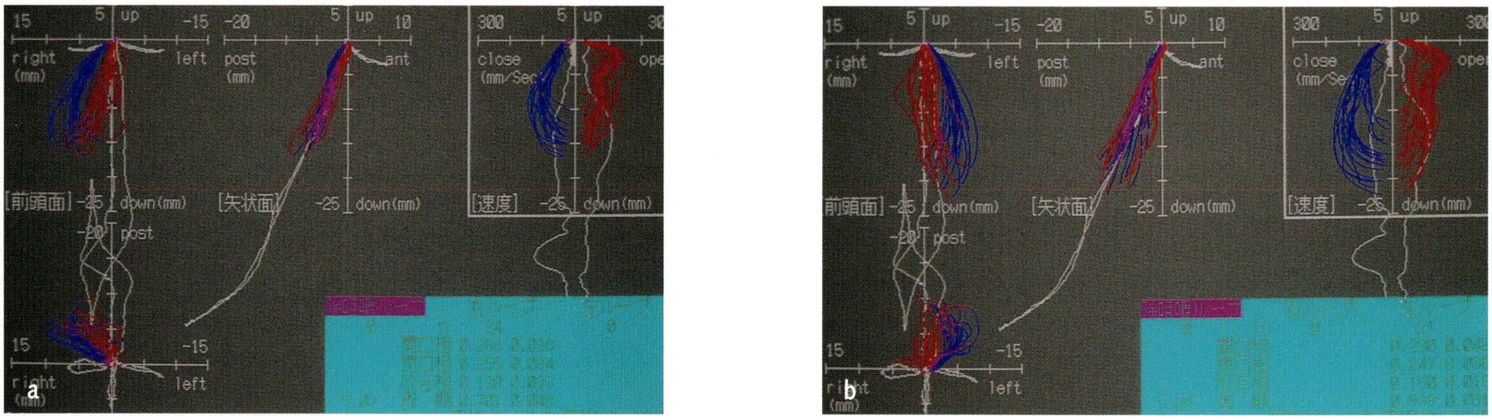

Fig 1-12 Masticatory movement after treatment. (a) The right chewing path is unsatisfactory, showing the turning point on the right. (b) The left chewing path is satisfactory, showing good speed.

Goal of Dental Care and the Systematization of Science of Occlusion

Systematization of science of occlusion

The role of dental care, according to Mitani et al, is to support the development and maintenance of occlusion, which becomes the source of health and vitality with favorable morphology and function throughout the processes of growth, development, maturation, and aging. Namely, the basis of dental clinical practice is to seek maintenance and stabilization of various tissues in the stomatognathic system and to contribute to overall health through such a life cycle. Especially important is to consider maintenance and stabilization of various tissues in the stomatognathic system for the future.

However, dental care in the past was mostly concerned with improvement in morphology. Although it aimed at control of inflammation as well as maintenance and improvement of oral function, dental care previously did not have an effective methodology for evaluation of function or consistent occlusal therapies (Table 1-1). Today it is known that a comprehensive, systematic approach integrating methods of preventive dentistry, orthodontic dentistry, restorative dentistry, and other disciplines is indispensable.

Comprehensive promotion of health

Child rearing, food production, dietary habits, housing environments, transportation systems, and other elements of our environment have changed drastically only in the last one or two generations. Due to these changes, our nutritional conditions and body build have been improved. At the same time, however, a variety of changes are occurring that jeopardize the stability of stomatognathic system, including changes in respiration, mastication, balance of muscle force, posture, bacterial flora of the oral cavity, and allergens. As a result, mouth breathing, underdeveloped masticatory muscles, habits of circumoral muscles including tongue and lip habits, lack of spontaneity for mastication, underdevelopment of mandibular body and condyle, and other problems are widely observed. It is the role of dental care not only to cope with individual diseases or symptoms, but also to consider systematic and comprehensive promotion of health.

The goal of dental care lies in supporting healthy life throughout the patient's life by maintaining and stabilizing homeostasis of stomatognathic functions. Also, it is one of the important roles of a primary care dentist to develop a stable stomatognathic system so that occlusal collapse will not occur in the future. These principles are illustrated in Cases 1-2 to 1-4.

Table 1-1 Outline of the directions and themes of future occlusion studies*

- Consistent occlusal therapies are to be conducted, considering continuity in the processes of growth, development, maturation, and aging.
- During the growth and development period, favorable occlusion is to be developed, achieved through correction, maintained, and/or reconstructed from the viewpoint of lifetime health promotion.
- Attention is to be paid to possible relationships with symptoms and/or diseases in other areas in the body.
- It is expected that, while conventional dental diseases may tend to decrease, more cases will require delicate occlusal therapy, demanding further advanced treatments.

*From the Liaison Committee on Occlusion, Science Council of Japan (1994).

Case 1-2 Improvement of lateral tongue thrusting and development of occlusion

Patient: *7-year-old boy at the time of first visit in 1990 (Fig 1-13)*
Chief complaint: *Anterior crossbite*
The anterior crossbite was more or less corrected after 7 months by the maxillary expansion arch and the chin cap. However, due to the lateral thrusting of the tongue in its lowered position, the bite was open at the premolars on the left side of the mouth (Fig 1-14). This space made it difficult for the patient to keep food in his mouth. In order to correct lateral and frontal tongue thrusting, myofunctional therapy and tongue guard therapy were conducted from the initial stage of the treatment. They were, however, not successful. Because of the tongue thrusting, erupted primary teeth are intruded, aggravating the lateral open bite (Fig 1-15). After the eruption of permanent teeth, when the patient was 11 years old (5 years and 4 months since the first visit), twisted wires were delivered to the permanent teeth to prevent the tongue thrusting. The primary mandibular right second premolar was extracted and the space was maintained until the eruption of the permanent tooth, while the tongue was kept away (Figs 1-16 to 1-19).
It is not rare that existing morphologic problems produce habits that cause additional morphologic disturbances in development.
In clinical dental practice, where we aim to develop a healthy stomatognathic system, it is essential to break this vicious cycle through minimal intervention during growth and development.

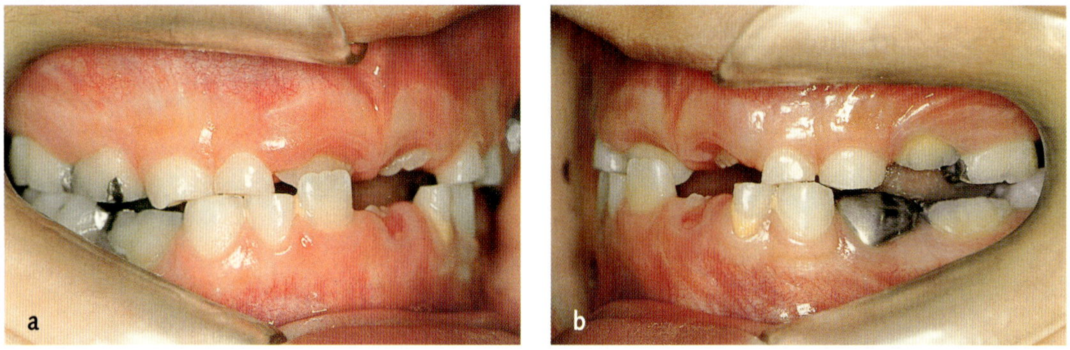

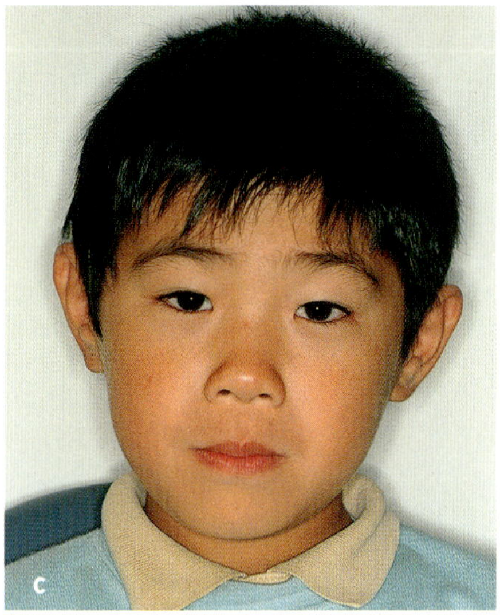

Fig 1-13 (a to c) Photographs taken at the first visit. The patient is 7 years old.

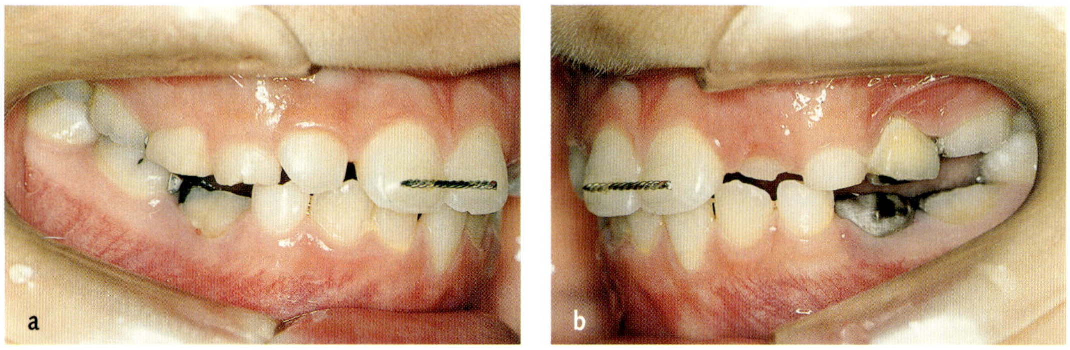

Fig 1-14 (a and b) Photographs taken at the age of 8 years, 3 months.

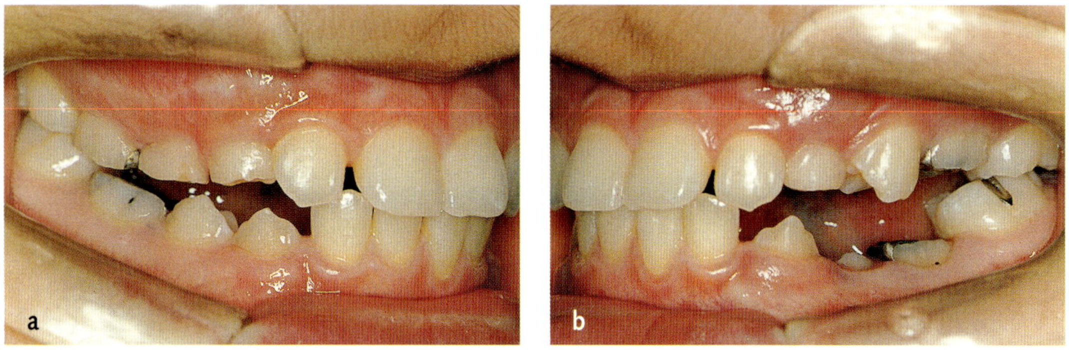

Fig 1-15 (a and b) Photographs taken at the age of 10 years, 2 months.

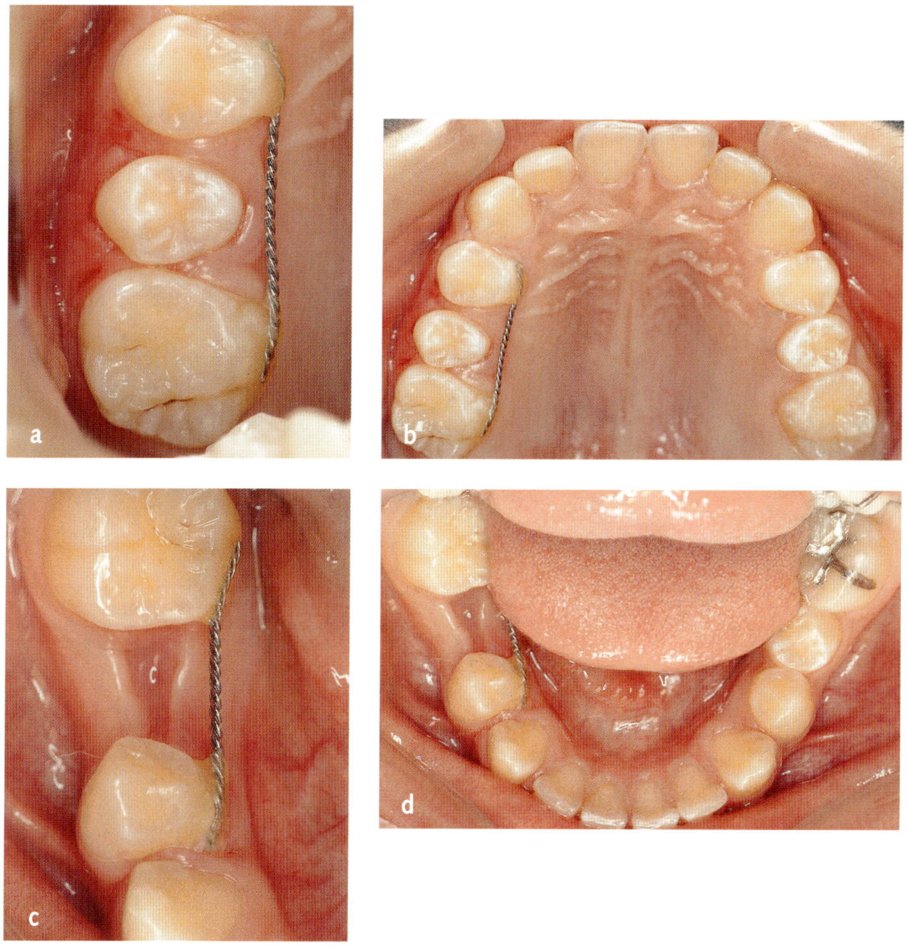

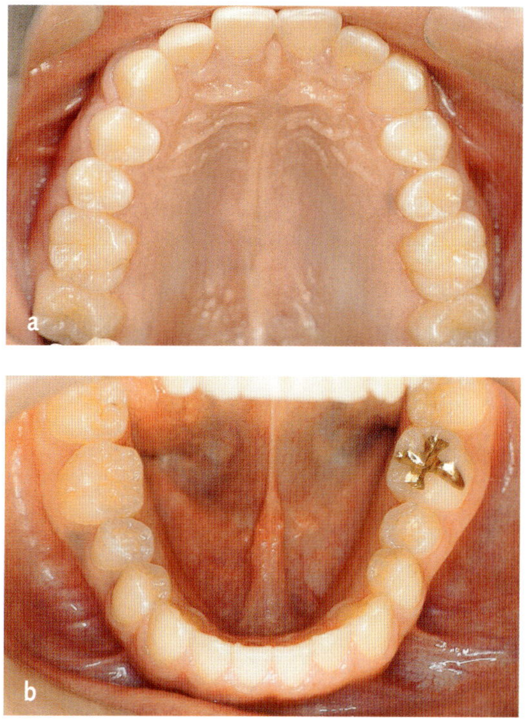

Fig 1-17 (a and b) Photographs taken at the age of 17 years. The teeth in the left arch started to incline lingually due to his habit of resting his cheek on the left hand. Although he was instructed to refrain from the habit, no improvement was seen.

Fig 1-16 (a to d) Photographs taken at the age of 12 years, 4 months. Twisted wires were delivered to the permanent teeth to prevent tongue thrusting in the premolar spaces.

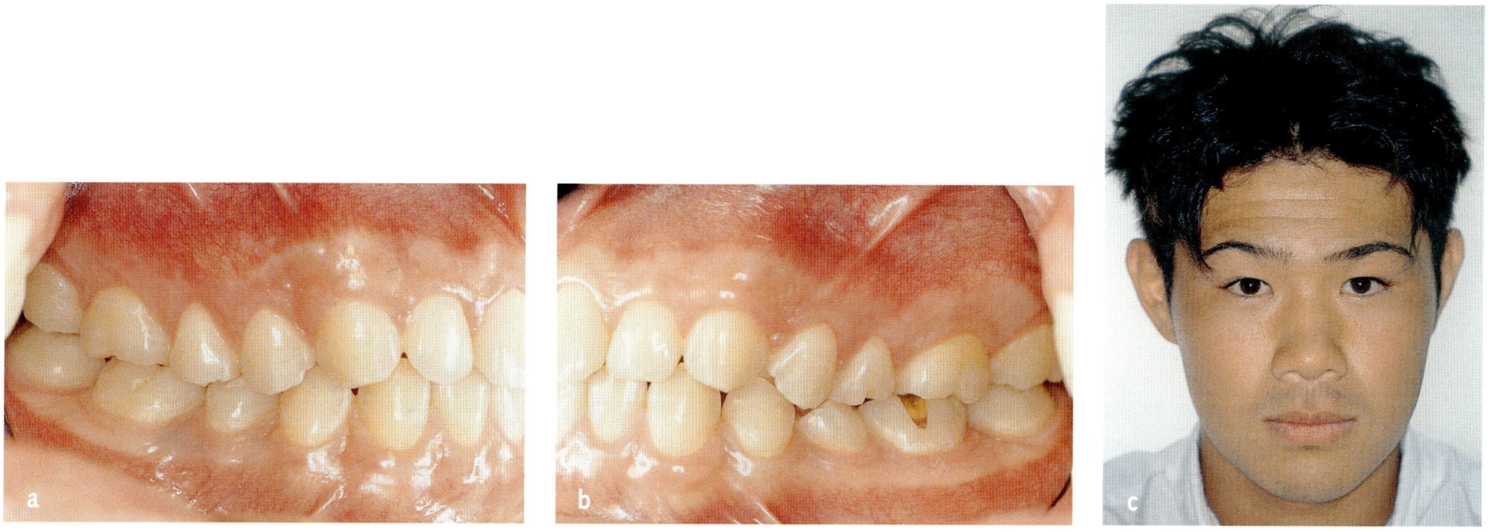

Fig 1-18 (a and b) Intraoral photographs taken at the age of 17 years. The maxillary left premolars are extruded due to the habit, enhancing the lateral curve. (c) Facial photograph.

Fig 1-19 Radiographs.
(a) Patient age: 9 years, 6 months.
(b) Patient age: 10 years, 9 months.
(c) Patient age: 11 years, 2 months.

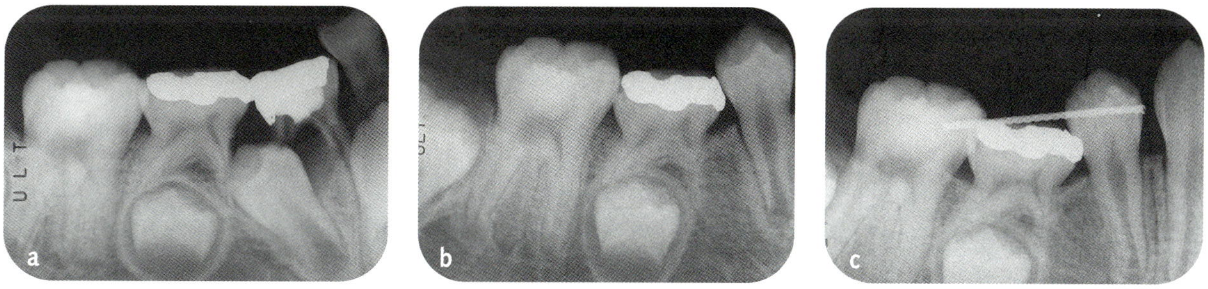

Case 1-3 Habits in the growth period and jaw dysfunction

Patient: *9-year-old girl at the time of first visit in 1997*
Chief complaint: *Sound and pain in the TMJ area*
She had been a regular patient starting at the age of approximately 3 years, but had not visited the clinic for some time. At the first visit after some absence (Fig 1-20), she presented with joint sound in the left TMJ during opening, which had been occurring for about 6 months. Sound in both TMJs developed later, as did occasional pain during opening. Based on various clinical symptoms, it was diagnosed as bilateral anterior disc displacement with reduction (Box 1-2). A plate-type repositioning splint (Figs 1-21 to 1-23) was used with the goal of natural extrusion of the posterior teeth. She had persistent habits of resting her jaw in her hands and biting her lips, which may have caused posterior movement of the mandible. As the mandibular position was improved, her posture also was improved (Figs 1-24 to 1-30).

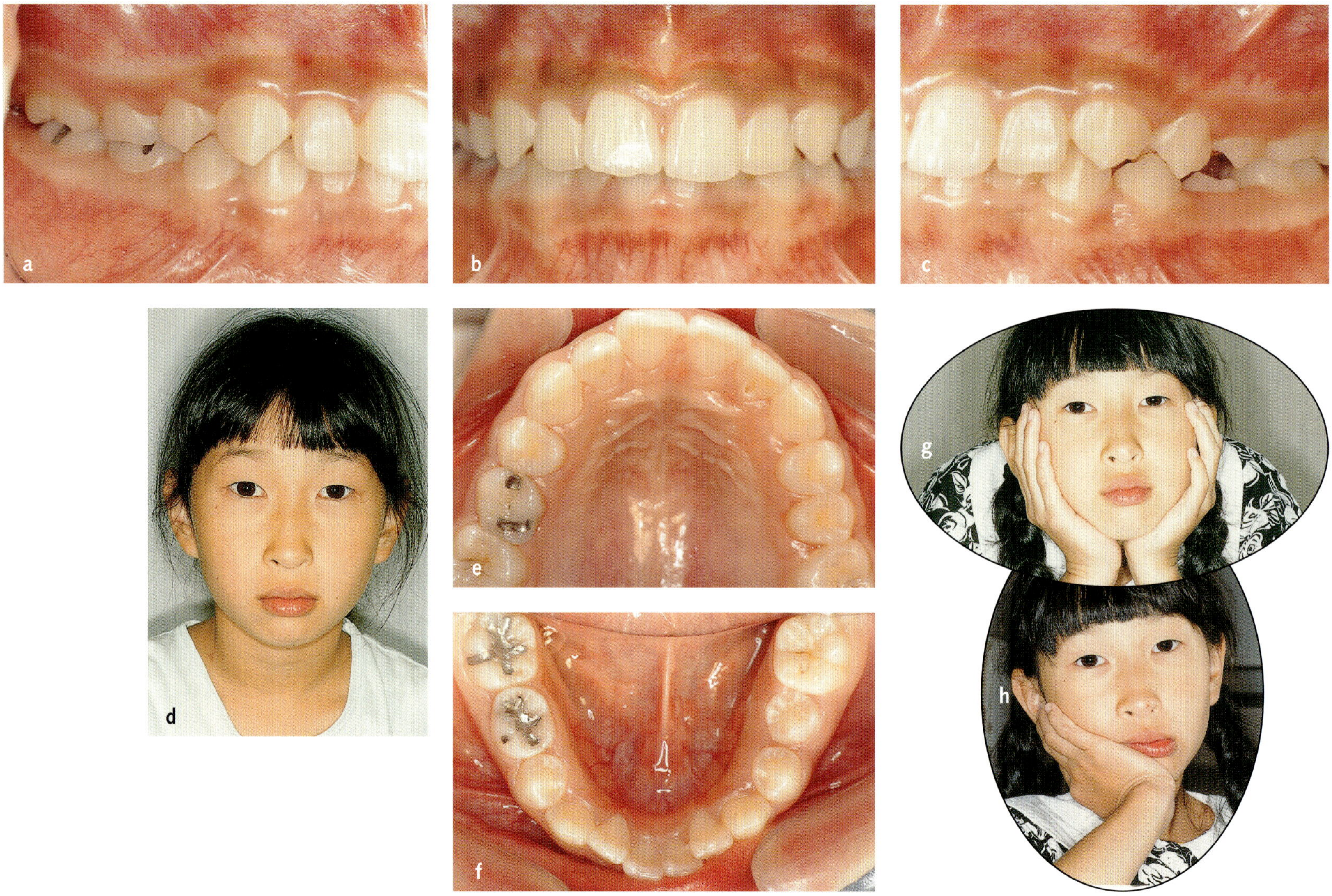

Fig 1-20 Photographs taken at the first visit; patient age: 9 years. (a to c) The gingiva in the mandibular anterior region is thin, and the root forms can be seen through the soft tissue. It seems that the labial bone was thinned by the persistent habits of resting her jaw in her right hand or both hands and biting her lips. The vertical overbite has become deeper. (d) The lip line is slanted so that left side of her mouth is higher than the right. The lower lip is thick and somewhat swollen. The left masseter is tense. The lower face is shifted to the left (indicating left-side chewing). (e to h) The dental arches, which should be U-shaped, are V-shaped, indicating the presence of an external force. During history taking, it was found that she rests her jaw in her hands for long periods of time. For example, when watching television, she laid on the floor and rested her jaw in her hands. This habit pushed both condyles in a posterior and superior direction.

Box 1-2 Signs indicating parafunctions

- V-shaped dental arches
- Thin labial gingiva in the anterior region
- Red and swollen lips
- Slanted lip line
- Mandibular shift
- Asymmetric eyes

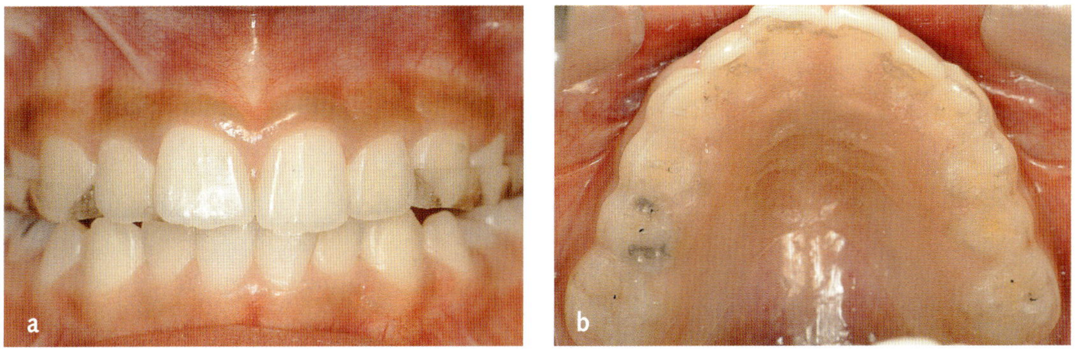

Fig 1-21 (a and b) Photographs taken 1 month after the first visit. A stabilizing splint was delivered to arrest the muscle spasms and determine an appropriate mandibular position. If a condyle has not been off the disc for long, a splint of this kind may suffice to reduce the disc. In this relatively rare case, reduction was not achieved.

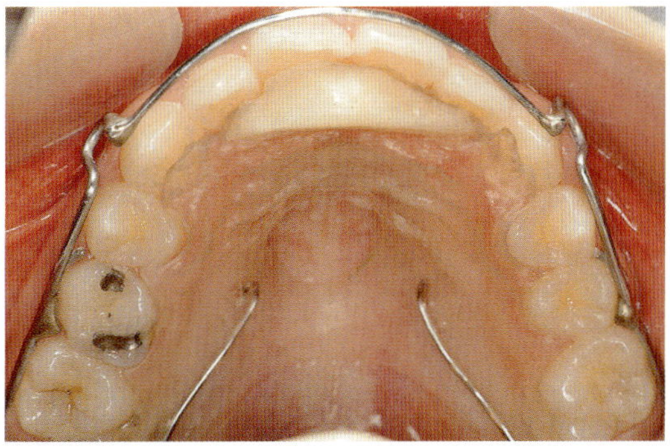

Fig 1-22 Photograph taken 2 months after the first visit. A flap was added to the plate-type repositioning splint to guide the mandible in such a way that the condyles move anteriorly and inferiorly to catch the discs.

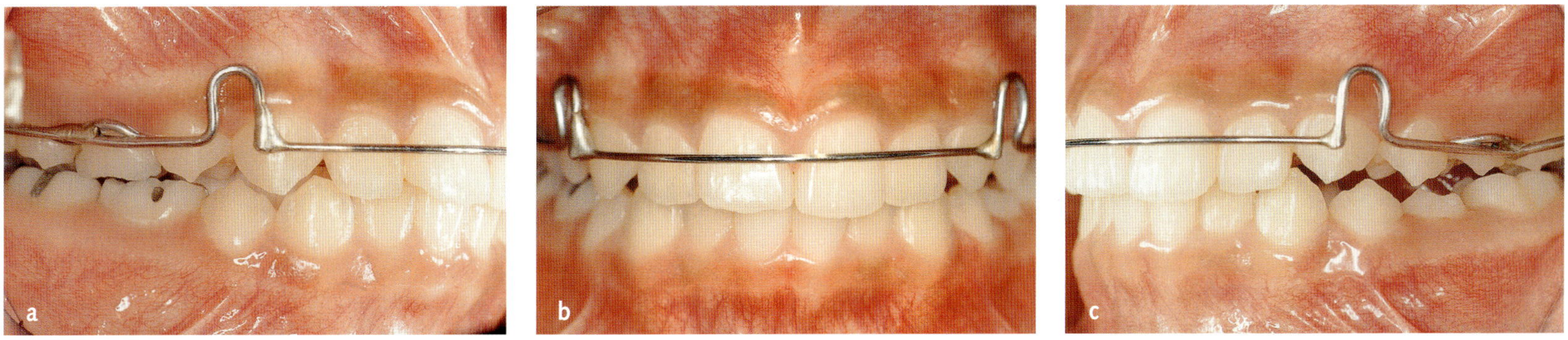

Fig 1-23 (a to c) The flap was provided at a mandibular (anterior) position where no clicking occurred, and the appliance was used all day long. The patient was required to chew in this position throughout the day so that the condyles would adapt to the discs, although an open bite in the posterior region made it difficult for her to chew. Natural extrusion of the posterior teeth was expected.

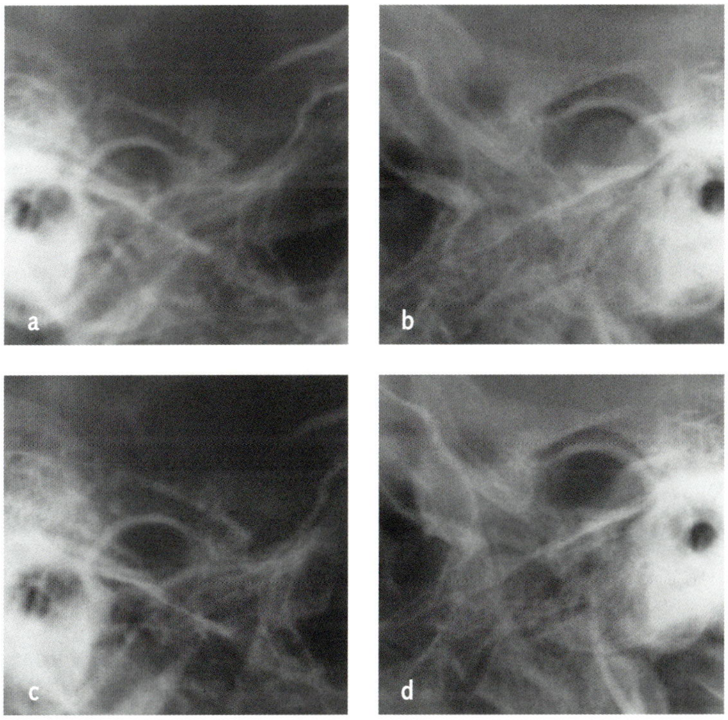

Fig 1-24 Transcranial radiographs at the first visit. At the intercuspal position, the articular space is narrow. (a and b) Right and left TMJs at intercuspal position. (c and d) Right and left TMJs at maximum opening of 4.5 cm.

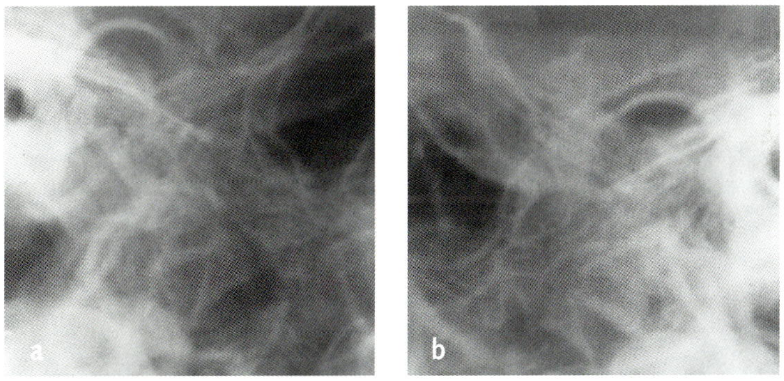

Fig 1-25 (a and b) Radiographs of the right and left TMJs at intercuspal position, 6 months after the delivery of the repositioning splint. These TMJ radiographs were taken when the discs were reduced. The condyles are located anteriorly and the articular spaces are wide. Although the condyles are on the disc, they are not stable and the space may be too wide.

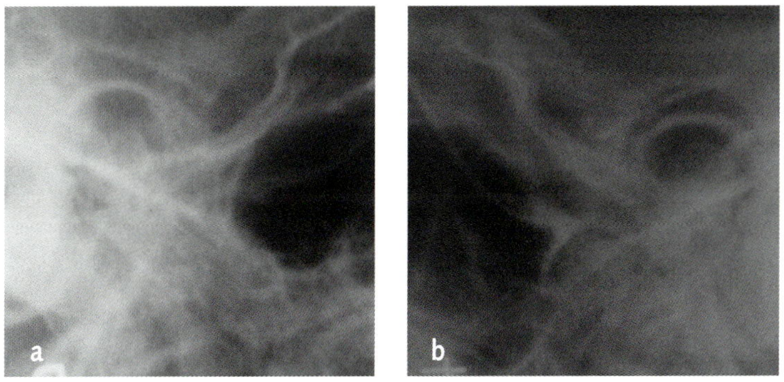

Fig 1-26 (a and b) Radiographs taken 1 year after the first visit, during maintenance therapy. The spaces are now more narrow (with the condyles set back); the condyles are on the disc in the TMJ space and are stabilized.

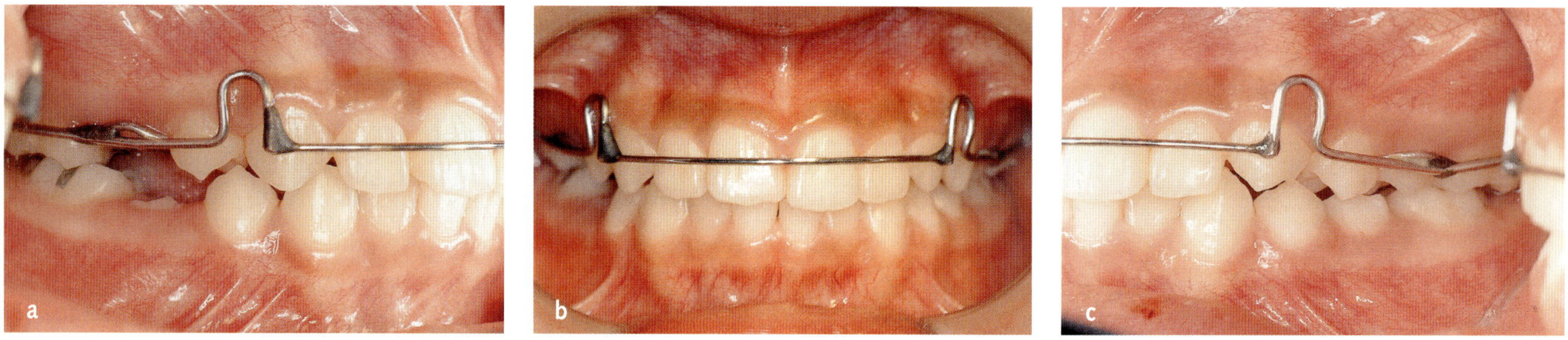

Fig 1-27 (a to c) The posterior teeth started to occlude 3 months after the delivery of the repositioning splint.

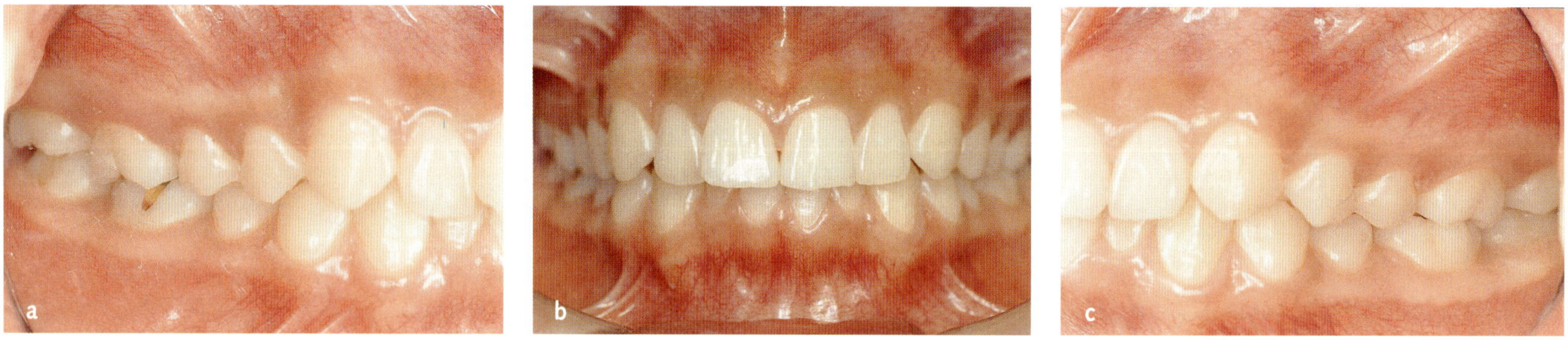

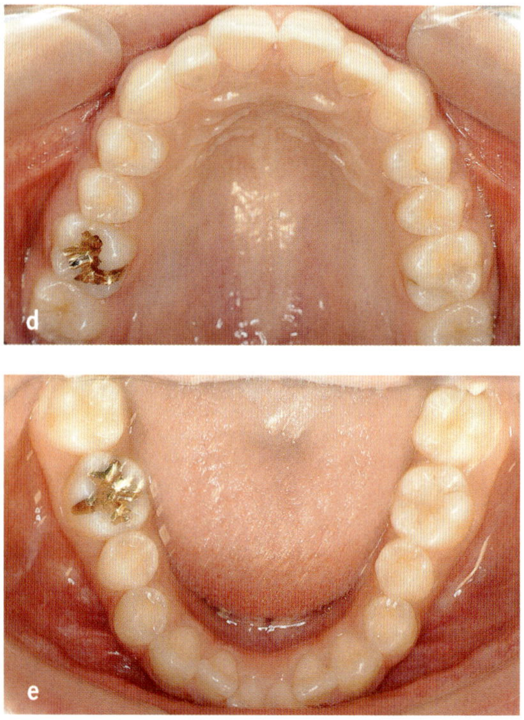

Fig 1-28 (a to e) Photographs taken 3 years and 2 months after the first visit; patient age: 12 years.

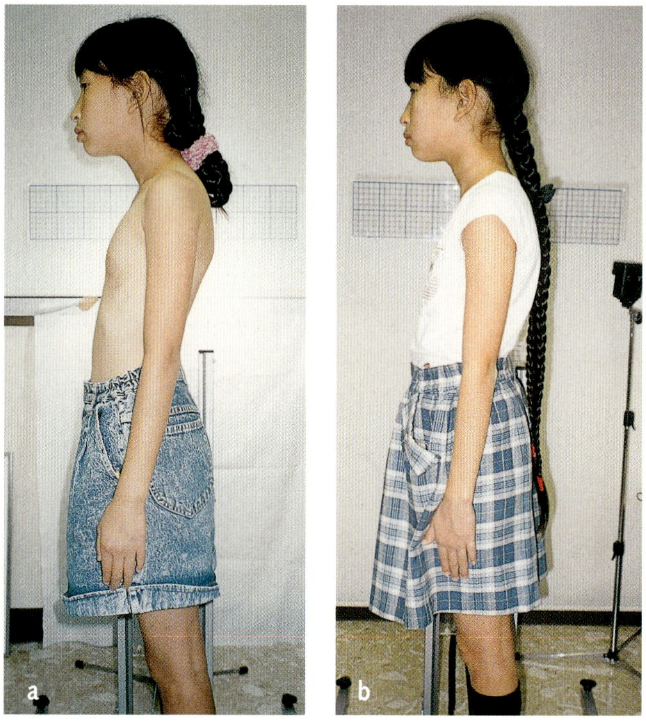

Fig 1-29 (a) Photograph taken at the first visit. A strong S-shaped curvature of the spine is observed. She complained of back pain due to carrying her backpack for school. (b) Photograph taken 4 months after the first visit. The spine curvature is somewhat improved. She has no back pain.

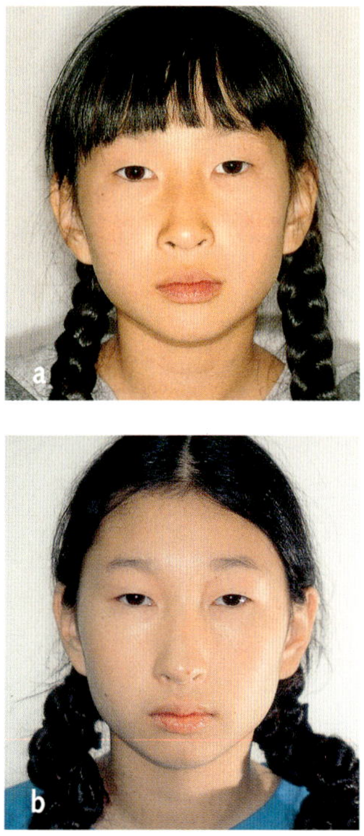

Fig 1-30 (a) Photograph taken 6 months after the first visit. (b) Photograph taken 3 years after the first visit. The left shift of the lower face is improved, and the face is symmetric. She still has a habit of biting her lips, and the lips are red and swollen. She may still have a habit of resting her jaw on her hands.

Case 1-4 Clenching closely related to arch deformation

Patient: *50-year-old woman at the time of first visit in 1998*
Chief complaint: *Irregular teeth (protrusion of maxillary anterior teeth), facial deformation, cheek biting, and difficulty in pronouncing s sound*
Major dental treatment history: *Fixed partial dentures for the maxillary right first premolar to second molar (pontic on the first molar) and the mandibular left second premolar to second molar (two implants for missing first molar), delivered 10 years previously*

When a patient's mouth and/or face are examined, some intuitive questions may arise that should be addressed as therapy progresses. This patient's face suggests complicated shifts, including one to the left from the nose to the philtrum and another to the right from the philtrum to the chin. The right corner of the mouth is higher, the right masseter is tense, and the mandible seems to be shifted to the right (Fig 1-31).
Since the maxilla can be shifted against the cranium, often it is difficult to evaluate mandibular shift by simply observing the frontal view. This patient has severe clenching and a complaint of fatigued jaw muscles, but neither trismus nor symptoms in the joints. It is difficult to determine whether or not the TMD symptoms she reported, such as headache, pain in the neck, shoulder stiffness, and ear discomfort, are related to occlusion. She often bites her tongue (right posterior area) and cheeks (both sides).
The porcelain occlusal surfaces (buccal side) of implant prostheses at the mandibular left second premolar and first molar were fractured. Maxillary anterior teeth were flared out with interdental spaces between all teeth from the maxillary right canine to the left lateral incisor.
Cheek biting is a complaint often observed in a case with decreased occlusal vertical dimension. Biting of the right posterior part of the tongue suggests mandibular shift to the right. It was surmised that the maxilla was shifted to the left. The mandibular dental arch is more significantly V-shaped than the jawbone arch, with linguoversion of the mandibular left canine. The anterior teeth and right molars are lingually inclined, and the tooth axes are generally inclined to the left.

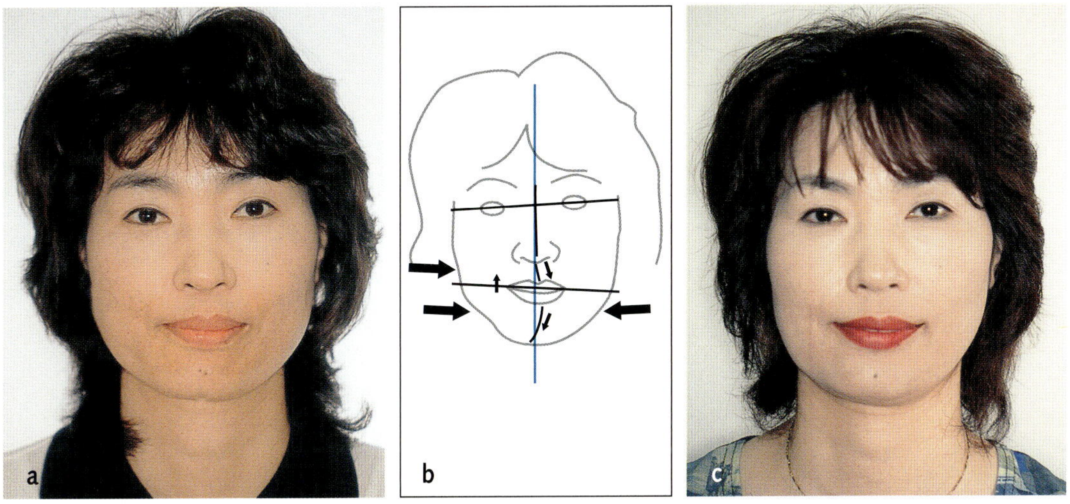

Fig 1-31 Facial view at first visit (a) indicates complicated distortions, as depicted in the illustration (b). If questions arise about the cause, a continuing analysis of the situation should be carried out as therapy progresses. (c) At the completion of prosthetic treatment, much of the facial distortion has disappeared, and the lower facial height has increased. However, there is still asymmetry in the face. The remodeling process seems to continue.

Diagnosis and treatment plan

For patients such as this, with obvious problems in occlusion and complaints of various systemic symptoms at the first visit, clinicians may assume such general symptoms are related to occlusion. However, such a judgment must not be made too lightly and, most importantly, such an explanation should not immediately be given to the patient.
Not all systemic symptoms are caused by occlusal anomalies.
The following treatment plan was developed for this case (Figs 1-32 and 1-33):

1. *Myofunctional therapy and correction of habits are begun.*
2. *Stabilizing splint is used to find an appropriate mandibular position.*
3. *Myofunctional therapy is conducted, the main goal being to keep the tongue in the palatal space. (The patient simply being aware of this goal is beneficial even if sufficient control is not achieved.)*
4. *After existing crowns are removed, provisional resin restorations on a metal framework are provided. During steps 1 through 5, formerly compressed muscles will start to relax, inducing remodeling of the bone, which results in counterclockwise rotation of the mandible and changes in the mandibular position. This will necessitate addition of resin to the occlusal surface. However, provisional restorations with excessive occlusal height should not be provided from the beginning, even if such changes are expected. Light tapping should be performed regularly to determine an appropriate mandibular position, and provisionals should be adjusted.*
5. *Axes of lingually inclined mandibular teeth are uprighted to change the V shape of the arch into a U shape.*
6. *When posterior teeth are stabilized, the interdental spaces in the maxillary anterior teeth are addressed (ie, distalization of anterior teeth, mesial movement of molars, and/or increase of coronal widths).*

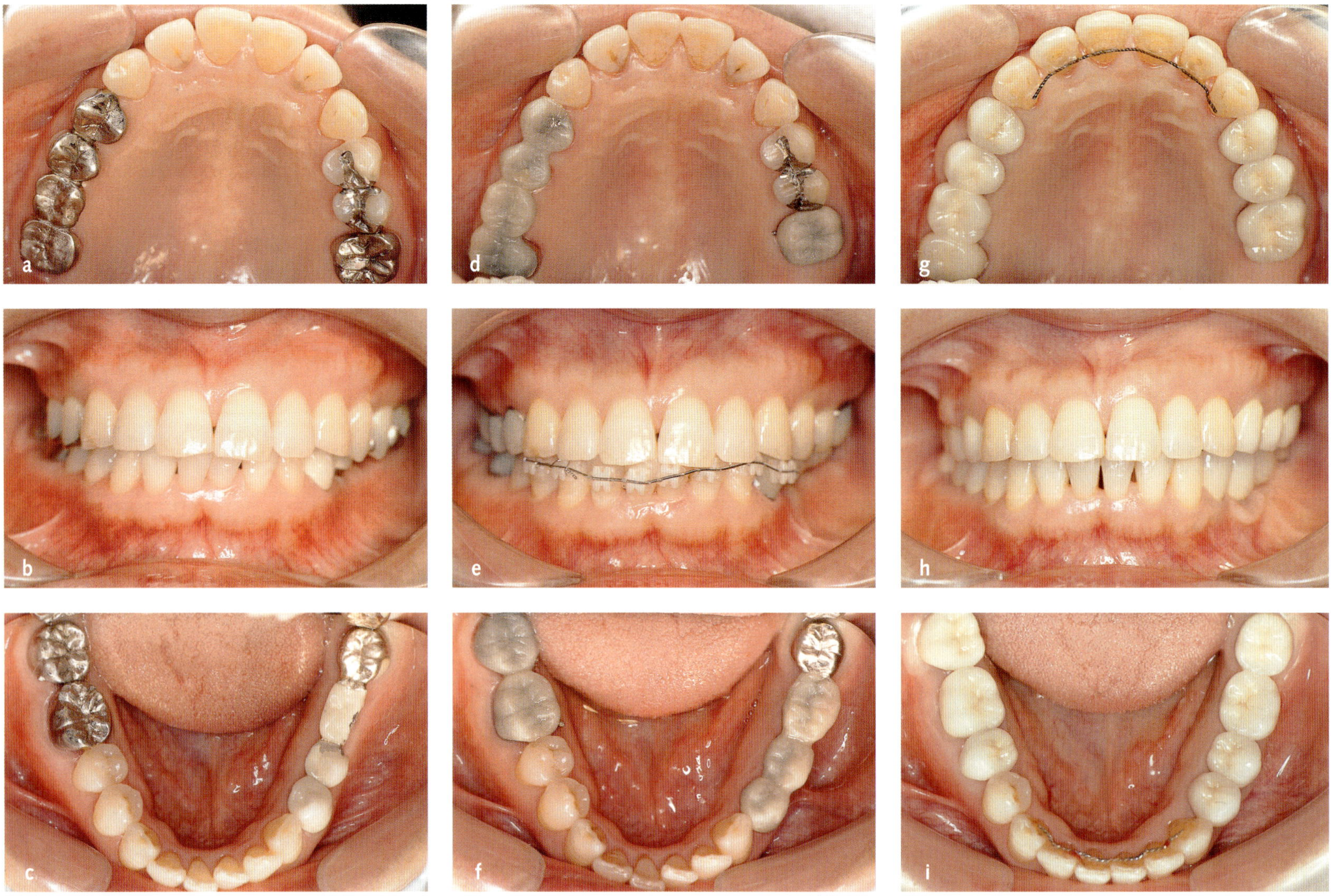

Fig 1-32 Changes in dental arches, occlusal plane, and inclination of tooth axes. (a to c) At the first visit. The patient complained of various TMD symptoms as well as protrusion of anterior teeth and facial deformation. The mandibular dental arch is more significantly V-shaped than the jawbone arch, with linguoversion of the mandibular left canine. The anterior teeth and right molars are lingually inclined, and the tooth axes are generally inclined to the left. (d to f) Seven months after first visit. Existing crowns were removed, and provisional resin restorations on a metal framework were provided. In the mandible, uprighting of lingually inclined teeth was initiated. (g to i) Modification of provisional restorations was repeated as needed, mucogingival surgery was conducted, and implants were placed with provisional restorations about 2 years after the first visit, based on which final prostheses were delivered. Interdental spaces in the anterior segment resolved almost naturally.

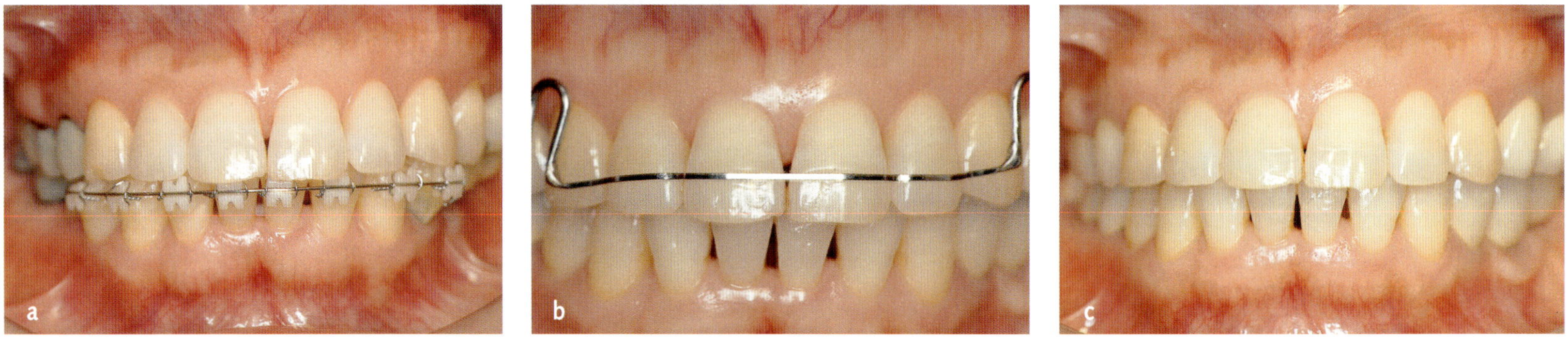

Fig 1-33 Changes in midline and inclination of the tooth axes. (a) At 6 months after delivery of the orthodontic appliance in the mandible, inclination of the tooth axes has improved significantly. The mandibular position is almost determined, and small remaining interdental spaces are tightened using a blade. (b) Eight months after delivery of final prostheses. Because the tongue is still in a low position, a retainer is used only at night. (c) About 2 years after delivery of final prostheses. There is still some distortion remaining when the jaws are in a relaxed position. The remodeling process seems to continue.

Clinical finding

After the stabilizing splint was used, the patient reported that she no longer suffered from shoulder or lower back pain.

At 9 months after the first visit, when the stabilizing splint was removed, she complained that she did not know how to bite. As the occlusion was stabilized, the mandible shifted to the right.

At 10 months after the first visit, she learned to chew equally on the right and left sides.

In the following month, she said the fatigue around her eyes had been relieved. Protrusion of the maxillary anterior teeth was naturally improved to a considerable degree. The patient said she came to feel at ease in the last month. As the tongue space was expanded with increase of vertical dimension, her habit of pushing her tongue against her teeth was resolved. Around this time, she learned to place her tongue against the palate.

In this clinical case, if the premolars had been extracted and the arch narrowed, it is highly likely that severe TMD symptoms would have been induced.

As shown in the clinical photographs, treatment steps 1 through 5 resulted in improvement in posture and facial distortions. Also, vertical dimension was gained in the molar region, lower facial height was increased, and TMD symptoms were mostly resolved (Figs 1-34 to 1-38).

After delivery of the final prostheses, the mandible shifted back to the right and some occlusal contacts were lost on the left side. The patient was instructed to chew on the left side; however, it will take several years to reestablish natural facial morphology after such drastic and systemic distortions. At 4 years after the first visit, she still occasionally complains of pain in the neck and the back of the left eye when there appear to be some strong occlusal contacts. However, the frequency of her complaints of discomfort has decreased significantly. The patient is undergoing a maintenance program as well as inflammation control. Because there is still asymmetry in the face, remodeling seems to be ongoing.

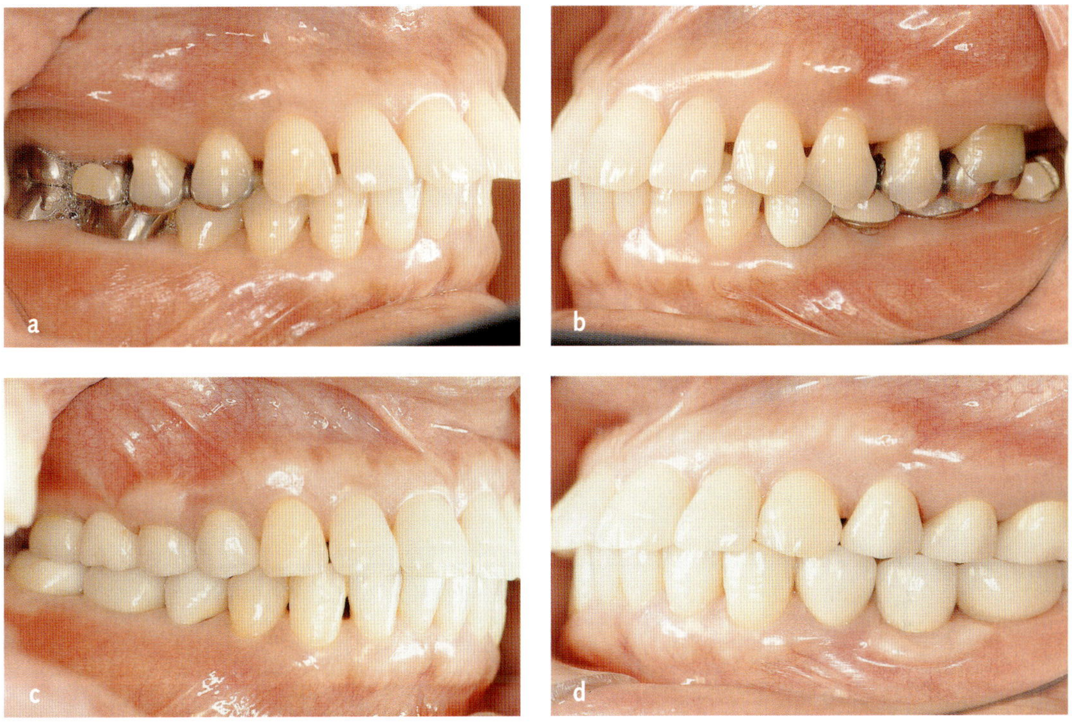

Fig 1-34 Changes in vertical dimension in the molar region. (a and b) At first visit. (c and d) At delivery of final prostheses. Crown-lengthening surgery was conducted for the maxillary right second molar, and implants were placed at the mandibular left second premolar and first molar. Posterior intermaxillary distance has been established through uprighting of the tooth axes together with counterclockwise rotation of the mandible. Note harmony in cervical lines and the well-aligned occlusal plane. Single-crown restorations were provided for the maxillary left premolars and first molar to stabilize occlusion.

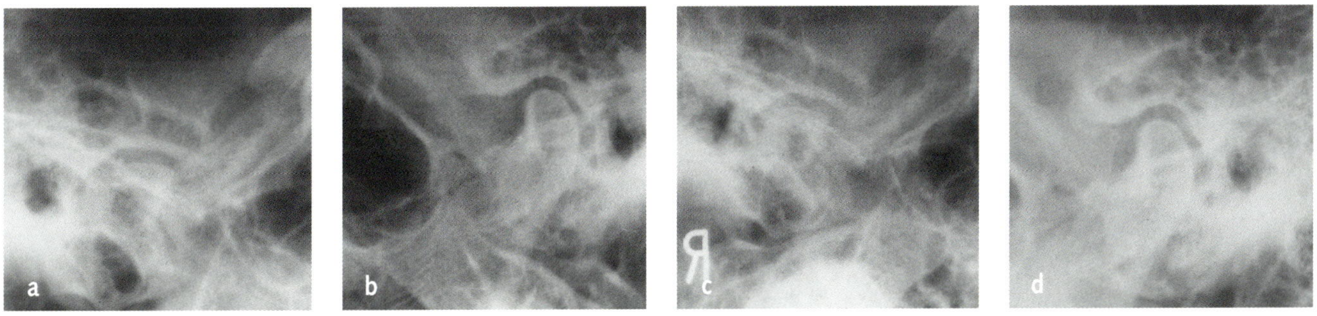

Fig 1-35 Transcranial radiographs of TMJs in intercuspal position. (a and b) At the first visit: (a) right TMJ; (b) left TMJ. (c and d) One month after delivery of the final prostheses: (c) right TMJ; (d) left TMJ.

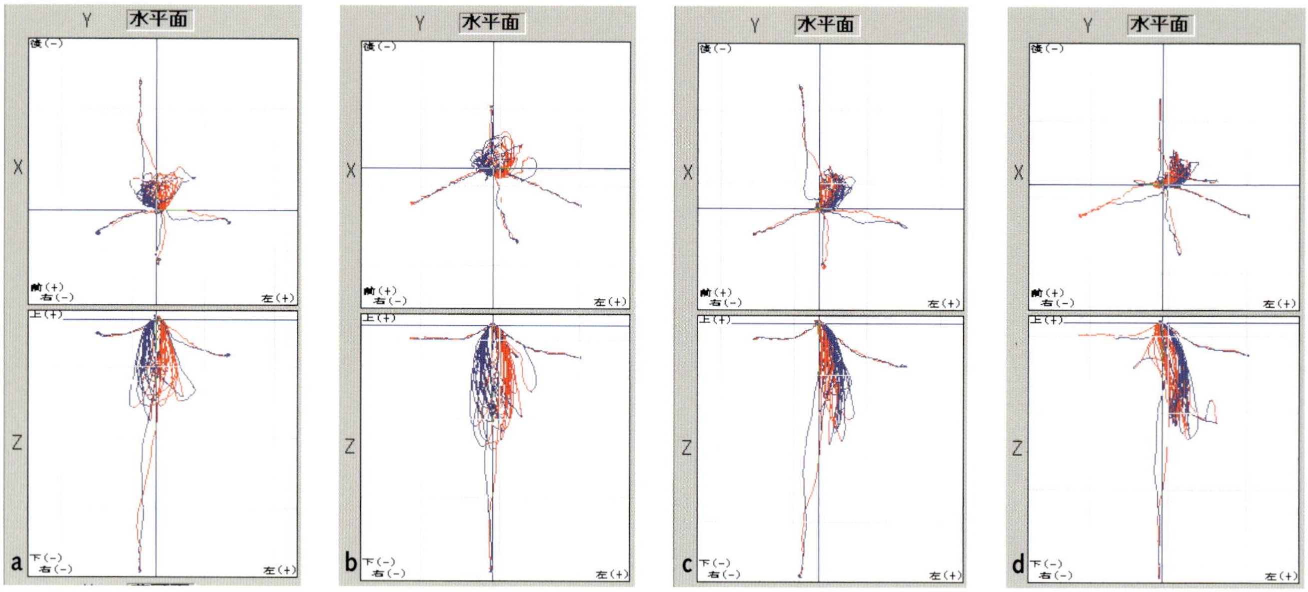

Fig 1-36 Changes in chewing paths, with the transverse plane shown on top and the frontal plane below. (a and b) Right-side chewing at first visit (a) and at 2 months after delivery of final prostheses (b). After treatment turning points are stabilized and chewing cycles are smoother. (c and d) Left-side chewing at first visit (c) and at 2 months after delivery of final prostheses (d). Even after treatment, interference at opening, which had been observed at the first visit, was not sufficiently eliminated.

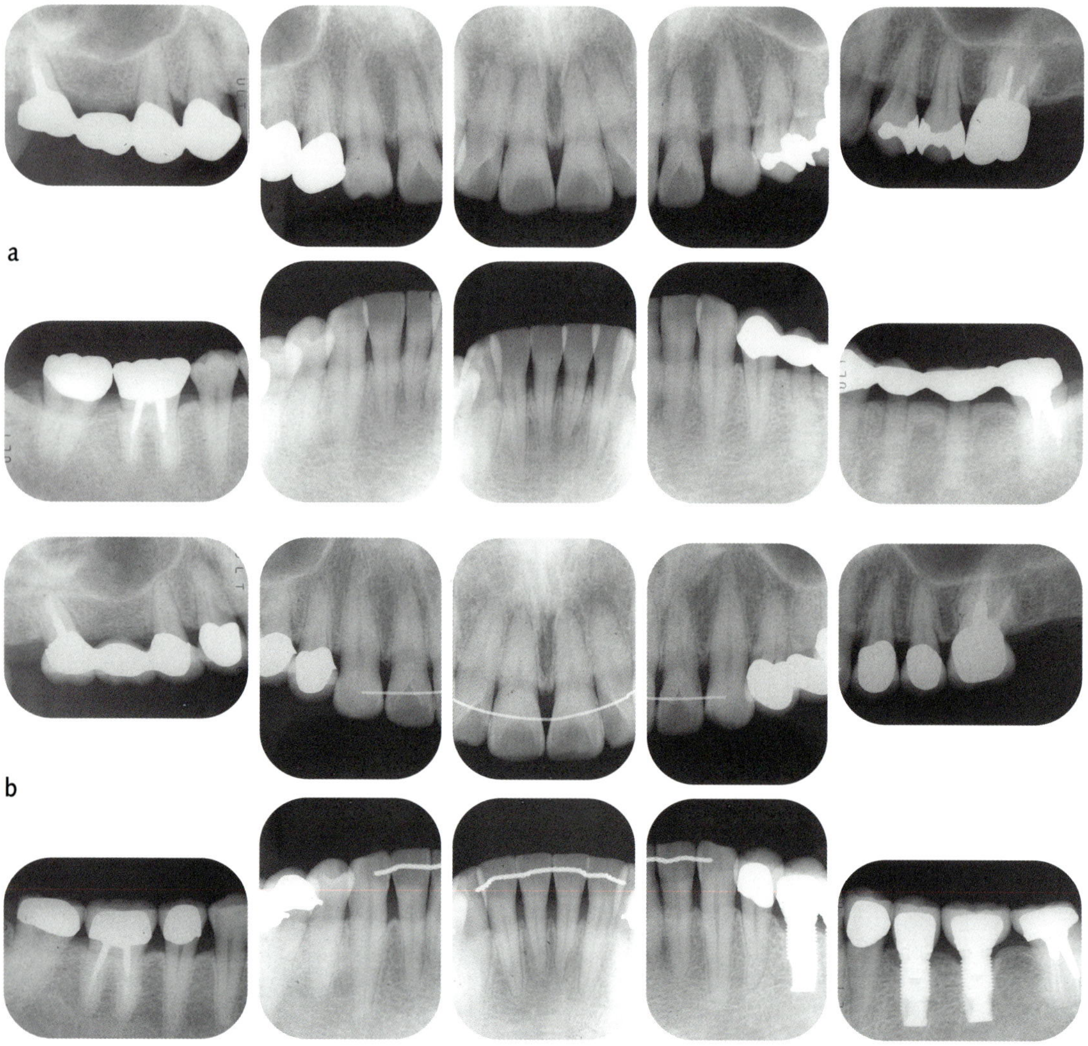

Fig 1-37 Full-mouth radiographs. (a) At first visit. (b) After 4 years, during maintenance. Interdental spacing has been improved, and the conditions are stabilized with lamina dura.

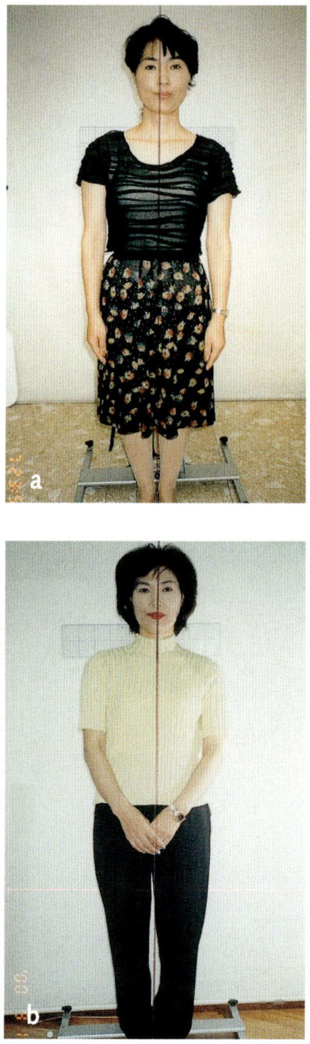

Fig 1-38 Changes in systemic posture and face. The posture at first visit (a) and at completion of prosthetic treatment (b). The patient can now stand straight. Distortions in the body and various systemic symptoms seem to be strongly related.

Comprehensive Diagnosis and Treatment

Comprehensive diagnosis

Comprehensive diagnosis has been discussed for years as patient-centered clinical practice: not examining patients from subdivided viewpoints such as prosthodontics, operative dentistry, and orthodontics, but paying attention to the pains and suffering of the patient, eliminating them, and preventing their recurrence. Certainly, it has become a trend to put prosthodontics in the center of the clinical practice, and multidisciplinary teams of specialists for the treatment of serious disorders are being introduced. Most important, however, is comprehensive diagnosis and treatment, not in the sense of complex treatment approaches for serious disorders, but consideration of background and ancillary factors of the disease and searching for the most natural route to restore homeostasis of the stomatognathic system, even for a minor sign of disease. In keeping with this approach, the authors use the terms *tooth unit, dentition unit*, and *occlusion unit* to specify the area of focus when examining clinical cases.

Treatment goals

Even minor hard tissue destruction should be considered in the context of the anatomical characteristics, saliva, bacterial flora, and masticatory habits that are unique to the oral cavity of a patient with particular living backgrounds or immunologic characteristics. These factors need to be studied comprehensively in making a diagnosis. Contrary to popular belief, restoration of morphology is not the goal in treating missing hard tissue. Instead, the goal is restoration of homeostasis of the functionally stabilized stomatognathic system through minimal therapeutic intervention.

In restoring homeostasis of the stomatognathic system, it is important to select an effective treatment method based on the patient's current pathology and to proceed with the treatment while promoting the patient's healing ability in order to obtain maximal therapeutic effect with minimal therapeutic intervention.

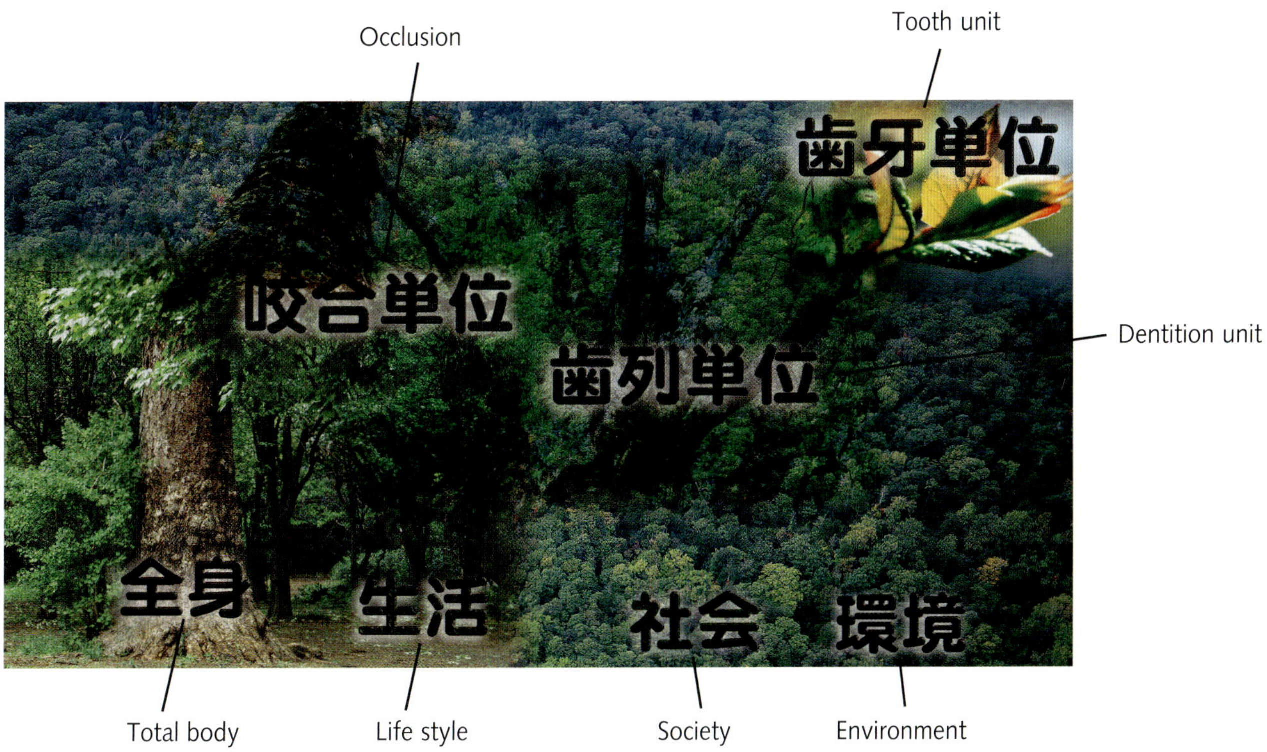

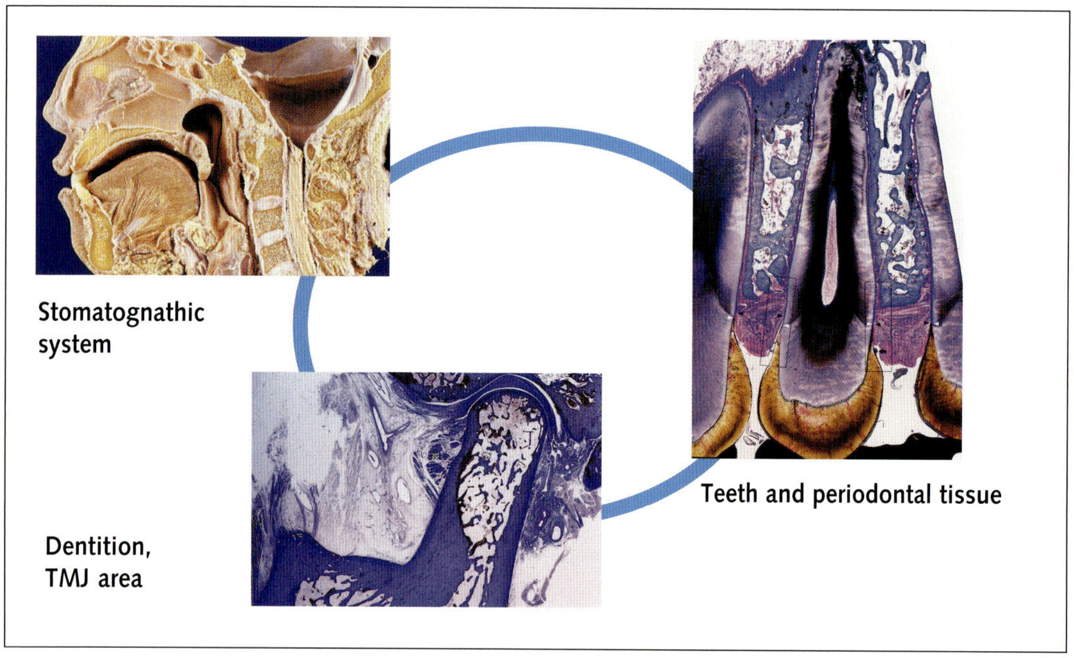

Fig 1-39 Structure of masticatory organs. (Courtesy of Dr A. Urago.)

Table 1-2 Examination of specific areas of focus

- **Tooth-unit examinations**
  Attention is to be paid to the periodontal tissue, tooth mobility, dental caries, root fracture, tooth malposition and malformation, crown-root ratio, premature contact, and occlusal interferences, among other aspects.
- **Dentition-unit examinations**
  Attention is to be paid to contact relationships between the maxilla and mandible, amount of vertical and horizontal overlap, discrepancy in position between opposing teeth/dentition, deformation of dental arches, occlusal plane, vertical dimension, occlusal curve, type of edentulism, pressure exerting/receiving elements, and horizontal and vertical guidance in the anterior and posterior regions.
  It is important to examine chronological changes in the dental arches from the viewpoints of morphology and function, while paying due regard to the relevance to the tooth unit and the occlusion unit. That is, not only static relationships but also dynamic relationships in function are to be examined.
- **Occlusion-unit examinations**
  Attention is to be paid to abnormal mastication pattern or mandibular position, abnormality in TMJ, disharmony in masticatory muscles and circumoral muscles, abnormal habits, clenching, and bruxism, among other aspects.

Viewpoints in clinical case examination

A variety of elements are involved on many different levels in the stomatognathic system (Fig 1-39). The authors classify therapeutic intervention in the stomatognathic system as being at one of four levels: a tooth unit, the smallest unit; a dentition unit, the aggregate of tooth units; an occlusion unit, a comprehensive unit including other elements; and a patient unit that is only occasionally employed (Table 1-2). This approach keeps both the big picture and the details in the forefront when a clinical case is examined. It is important, for example, to bear the dentition unit in mind when examining a tooth, and conversely, not to overlook the tooth-unit problems when studying occlusion (Fig 1-40).

The masticatory organ has a hierarchical structure in which a tooth unit, a dentition unit, and an occlusion unit support and affect each other. In examination and diagnosis, we have to relate macroscopic occlusion to details of the teeth and examine the harmony between the mastication pattern and the teeth and periodontal tissue. The same way of thinking applies to the clinical approach and its goals. In fact, this book is structured to show that details are the whole and the whole is details, which may seem repetitious to the reader, but is indicative of the comprehensive approach promoted by the authors.

Collapse of occlusion

Examinations • Diagnosis • Treatment plan

Initial therapy

Reevaluation

Reevaluation

Definitive therapy

Reevaluation

Reevaluation

Maintenance

Reevaluation

Reevaluation

Flow of periodontal therapy

Inflammation control

Treatment against infection
Tooth-unit treatment

Motivation
Initial therapy
- Plaque control
- Root planing
- Soft curettage

Emergency treatment for pain
Caries control
Removal of failed prostheses
Tooth reshaping, endodontic treatment
Tooth extraction, hemisection
Provisional restoration

Attachment conditions
Bone conditions (infrabony defects)
Gingival conditions, furcation involvement
Subgingival dental caries
Tooth malposition
Natural realignment of teeth (dentition unit)

Periodontal surgery
- Resective therapy
- Conservative therapy
- Regenerative therapy

Periodontal plastic surgery
Orthodontic tooth movement, natural extrusion

Restoration, periodontal prosthesis

Inflammation, morphology, esthetics, function

Plaque, periodontal pockets
Inflammation type, mobility, function, force

Motivation
Plaque control
Tooth cleaning
Root planing

Periodontal surgery
Partial re-treatment

Flow of occlusal therapy

Force (function) control

Occlusion-unit treatment

Motivation
Treatment for habits and muscles
Search for an appropriate mandibular position, stabilization of occlusion
Treatment for malfunction of jaws
- Various splints

Check for cessation of habits and muscle spasms
Confirm appropriate mandibular position
Stabilization of mandibular position and occlusion, appropriate guidance

Tooth-unit treatment

Removal of failed prostheses, simple restoration
Reshaping, therapeutic denture

Verticalization and naturalization of occlusal pattern
Confirm reduction of forces and increased stability of functional axes

Dentition-unit treatment

Reconstruction of occlusal surface
- Provisional restoration
- Placement of crowns

Reconstruction of occlusion
- Orthodontic tooth movement
- Prostheses/implants

Stabilization of mandibular position and occlusion
Vertical occlusal pattern

Gap between mandibular position and ICP, attrition
Periodontal tissue, personal habits, chewing habits
Muscles, TMJ

Motivation
Splinting
Reshaping

Partial re-treatment

Fig 1-40 Flow of treatment in reconstruction of occlusion.

Even in a case of inflammation or hard tissue defect limited to one tooth, the treatment should have extensive, comprehensive goals not only to eliminate pain and prevent its recurrence but also to restore and maintain unity and continuity of the dentition as well as harmony with the opposing teeth, the masticatory system, and the gingiva and periodontal tissue. Comprehensive dental treatment does not merely mean employment of various treatment measures. Rather, it is the most rational treatment for the patient to achieve far-reaching treatment goals.

In dental therapy, including hard tissue restoration and prosthetic procedures, patients or dentists may set different treatment goals. Also, even when two treatment goals are similar, ways to reach the goals are diverse. Still, when the advantages and the disadvantages of a therapeutic intervention for the patient are considered, there is only one best way. Comprehensive dental treatment is also to select the most rational way, making full use of diverse alternatives (Case 1-5).

Case 1-5 Importance of comprehensive diagnosis and its challenges

Exhibited are canine guidance at lateral movements and bilateral abfraction (cervical wedge-shaped defects, root caries, gingival recession, and festoon-like marginal gingiva) observed at the maxillary canines and first premolars (Fig 1-41). The patient complained of hypersensitivity.

In a clinical case like this, even if a Class V cavity is prepared and resin composite restoration is conducted, it is highly likely that microleakage will occur or the restoration will dislodge. If so, what is the appropriate treatment for this case? Today, it may be common sense to conduct risk control based on cariology. However, what is to be done about the hypersensitivity? Should fluoride be applied? What should we do if it is ineffective? Perhaps the first question should be, why is there such an extreme amount of loading in this region?

Patient: *22-year-old woman at the time of first visit in 1986*

Propriety of premolar extraction

Usually excessive lateral guiding force is concerned in a case like this. This patient presented with strong clenching habits (note exostoses on the lingual sides of the posterior mandible) and had all four premolars extracted for the treatment of crowding. After the orthodontic treatment, the arches became slightly smaller, and clenching was not improved (Fig 1-42). (Note the imbalance between the right and left masseter and tension in the chin shown in the facial photographs.)

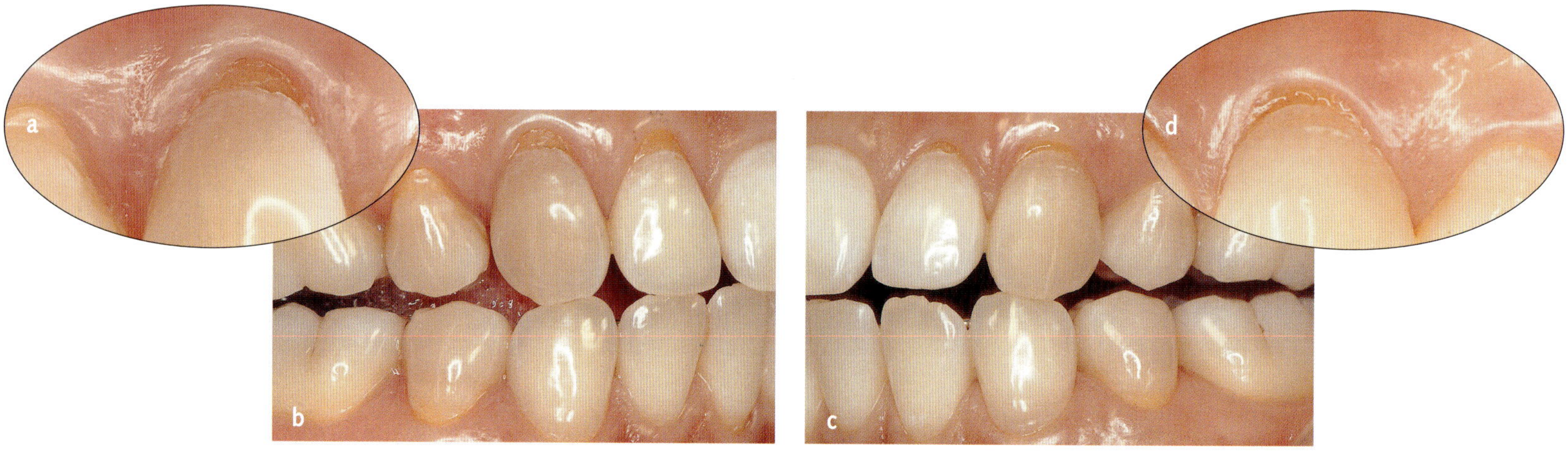

Fig 1-41 (a to d) Guidance at lateral movements and bilateral abfraction (cervical wedge-shaped defects, root caries, gingival recession, and festoon-like marginal gingiva).

Scope of occlusal reshaping

In order to improve clenching, the occlusal morphology of the posterior inlays, which almost locked into each other and did not allow much movement, was corrected. As far as observation of the patient's face is concerned, this improved clenching to a certain degree (Figs 1-43 and 1-44). However, problems still existed. An inlay fracture occurred 2 years and 5 months later as a result of pathologic movement of teeth (Fig 1-45). Reshaping of occlusal surfaces was conducted at the time of crown restoration, which was a challenging task.

Propriety of less invasive root coverage for cervical root caries treatment

For the cervical regions of the maxillary left lateral incisor and canine, a connective tissue graft with collar harvested from the palate was conducted (Figs 1-46 and 1-47). This grafting, however, caused overcontour of the gingiva, and consequently abrasion and cleft-shaped gingiva were not improved as expected.

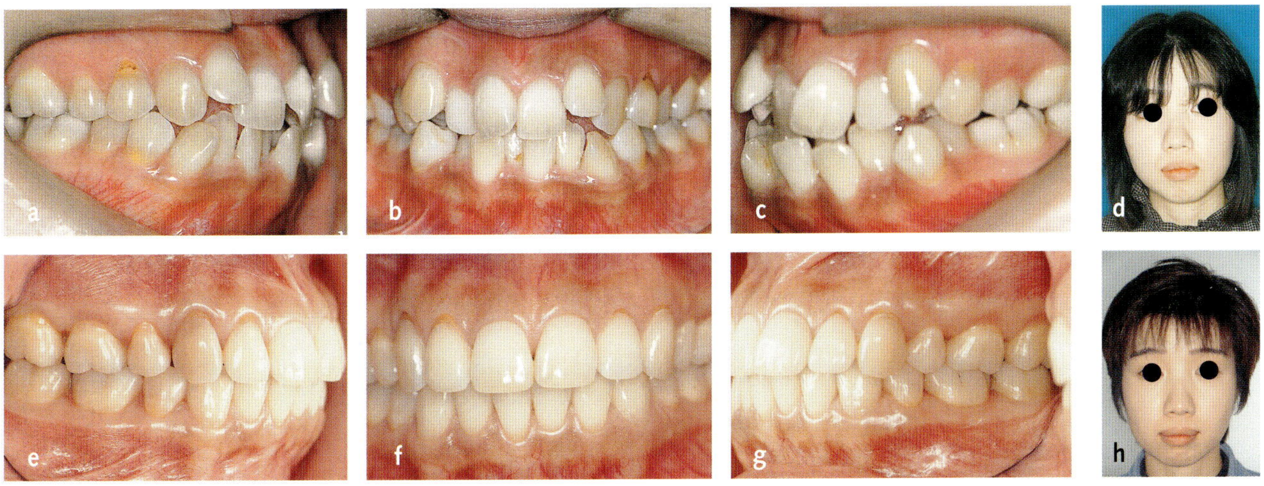

Fig 1-42 (a to d) At the first visit. All four premolars were extracted for the treatment of crowding. Following orthodontic treatment, the arches became slightly smaller. (e to h) Eight years and five months after the first visit. Arch constriction in the posterior region (especially on the left) due to patient habits is observed.

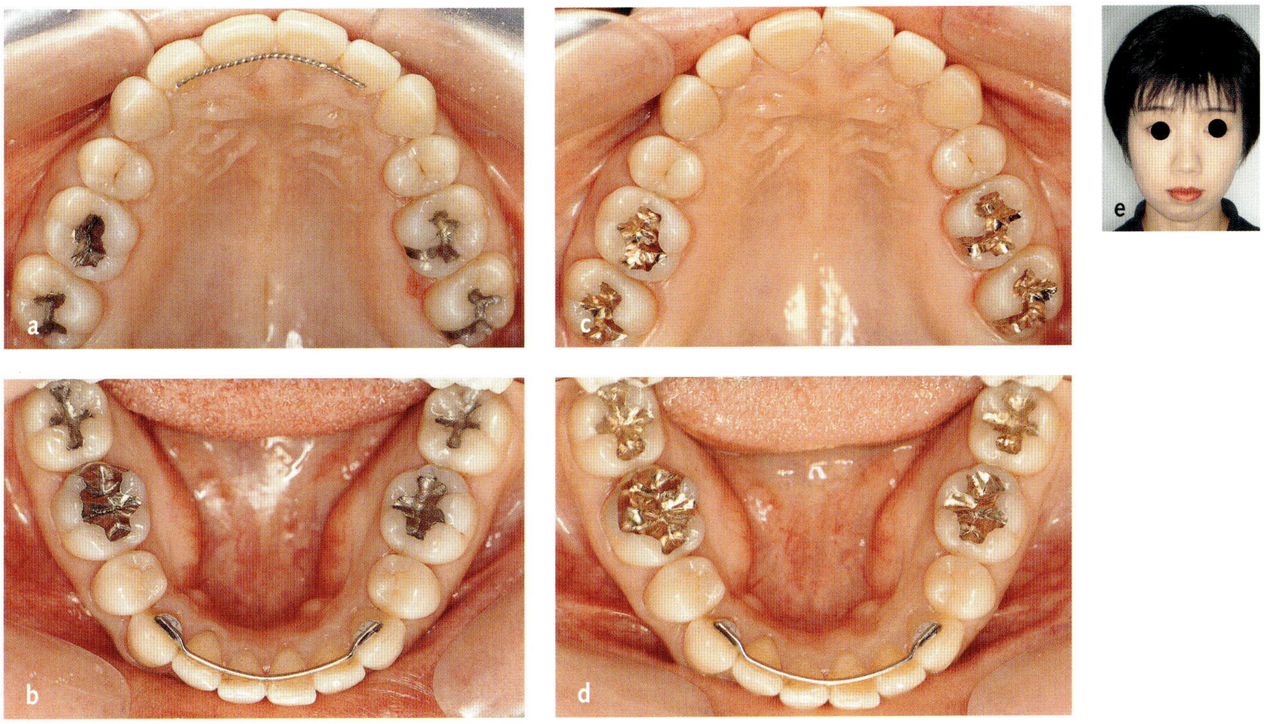

Fig 1-43 (a and b) Eight years and five months after the first visit. (c to e) After correction of posterior occlusal morphology, 9 years after the first visit. Tension around the mouth has been eliminated.

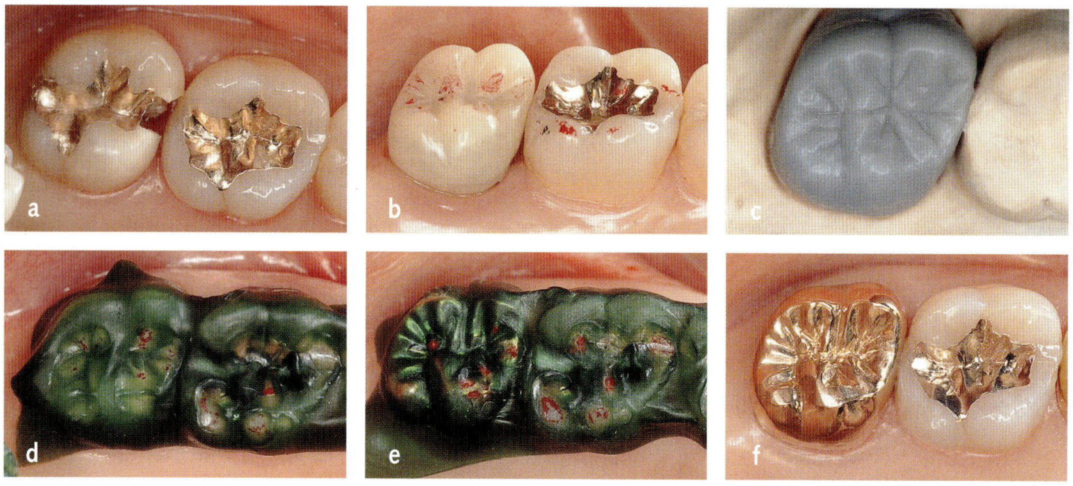

Fig 1-44 Maxillary right molars. (a) Occlusal view of right maxillary molars 10 years and 10 months after the first visit. The first molar was moved buccally, which caused secondary caries on the proximal surface. Pulpectomy was conducted. (b and c) Waxup for provisional restoration. (d) Even for provisional restoration, indicator wax is used to study occlusal contacts to achieve good harmony of morphology and functions. (e) Examination with indicator wax after temporary cementation of final prostheses. (f) Completion of treatment. As a result of correction of tooth malposition using placement of crowns, an environment has been established that facilitates plaque control and mastication. This clinical case demonstrates that the oral environment constantly changes due to force factors.

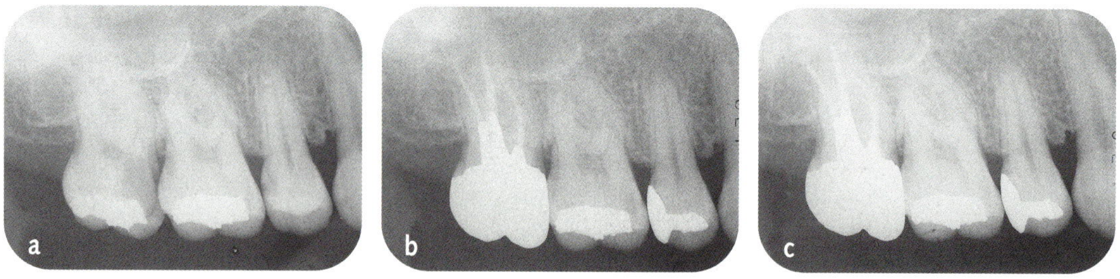

Fig 1-45 An inlay fracture in February 1998 (a). Delivery of a crown in March 1998 (b) and August 1999 (c).

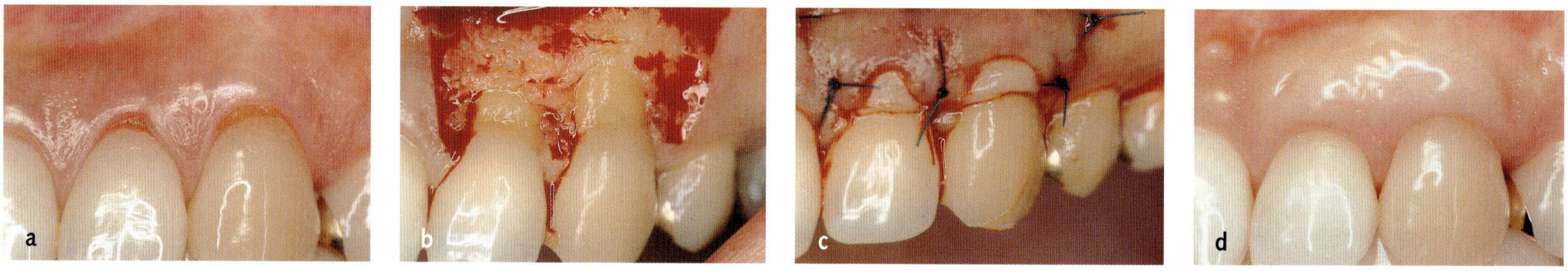

Fig 1-46 Connective tissue graft with collar harvested from the palate was conducted in the cervical regions of the maxillary left lateral incisor and canine. (a) Gingival recession at the maxillary left lateral incisor and canine. (b) Root surface treatment with tetracycline solution. (c) Langer and Langer method. (d) After treatment.

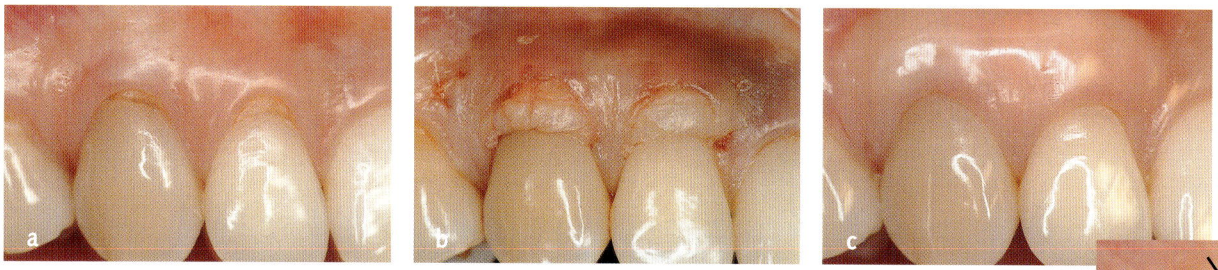

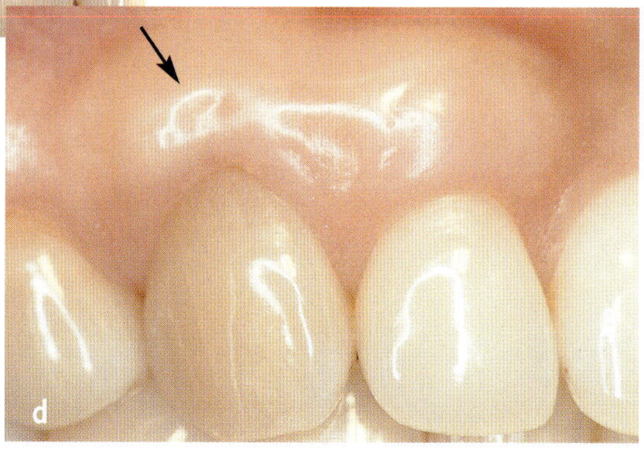

Fig 1-47 The connective tissue graft using an envelope technique at the maxillary right lateral incisor and canine. (a) Gingival recession at the maxillary right lateral incisor and canine. (b) A continuous envelope flap was prepared, root surfaces were treated with enamel matrix derivative, and connective tissue grafting was conducted (June 1998). (c) Overcontour of the gingiva developed, and abrasion and cleft-shaped gingival were not improved (January 1999). (d) Condition 14 years and 7 months after the first visit (May 2001). The root coverage procedure enabled treatment of dental caries and gingival recession, but it also created a maintenance problem. This demonstrates the kinds of difficulty that can arise in clinical practice.

Inflammation Control and Tooth-Unit Diagnosis

Unraveling complicated pathology

Upon initiating comprehensive diagnosis and treatment, it is difficult to know where and how to begin. Now matter how complicated the disease or disorder, making a diagnosis is made possible by untying tangled threads one by one in a certain order.

The first step to unraveling complicated pathology is plaque control. Without fundamental improvement of inflammation through plaque control, making a diagnosis of malposition of a tooth unit or a mandibular position would be misleading if not meaningless. Force elements that act in the masticatory system and are equally important as inflammation can be concealed by bacteria-oriented inflammation. Only after raising the veil of inflammation through plaque control can we detect the influence of force elements in morphologic changes. Inflammation control via removal of inflammatory substances and subsequent reevaluation is the basis of comprehensive diagnosis, allowing the clinician to understand the individual factors involved. Therefore, control of inflammation is a diagnostic procedure as well as a treatment.

Tooth-unit diagnosis

The foundation of understanding and managing tooth-unit diseases or disorders is to determine their relationship with endodontic tissue (root canal–derived periapical inflammation and tissue destruction), periodontal tissue (marginal inflammation and tissue destruction), and occlusion. Specifically, when local inflammation, a bony defect, or pain is observed, it has to be ascertained whether it is due to dental caries or fracture, root canal–derived inflammatory substances, marginal or periodontal pocket–derived bacteria, or abnormal forces, including occlusion.

Although probing to ascertain the conditions of periodontal pockets and soft tissue attachment and intraoral radiographic examination to determine the conditions of tooth roots and alveolar bone are extremely important, clinicians must not fail to document the gingival texture, color, and morphology, and changes in these aspects, as well as tooth attrition and associated changes so that they can detect any subtle signals through inspection and palpation.

Tooth-unit diagnosis also assists in dentition-unit and occlusion-unit diagnosis. Periodontitis is an inflammatory disease of periodontal tissue cased by bacterial plaque. In diagnosing the illness, not only the condition of plaque accumulation but also various risk factors of the patient, including his or her immune response, smoking habits, occlusion, and the morphology of teeth and roots must be taken into consideration. In a therapeutic approach, clinicians must have a comprehensive viewpoint that includes function, esthetics, and prognosis.

Endodontic treatment in infected root canals

Reaming and filing should be performed carefully, using palpation to explore and prepare a main root canal and to remove infected dentin thoroughly. Based on experience, the authors consider it difficult to explore an apical foramen accurately and to obdurate lateral canals with gutta-percha points and therefore routinely use chemical antisepsis. Also, even when it seems possible to obdurate root canals easily and tightly with gutta-percha points, treatment is not completed without reevaluation. Because of this, in most infected canals, the authors make it a rule to fill canals with a paste product principally composed of iodoform and calcium hydroxide and wait for the beginning of radiographic callus formation. The paste provides antibacterial action in the complicated lateral canals and periapical lesions. After radiographic reexamination, master canals are prepared again and obturated with gutta-percha points. Needless to say, technical discipline is required to ensure good prognosis. However, clinicians should not overestimate their own technical abilities and must always perform a reevaluation prior to final treatment. For follow-up purposes, standardized radiographs must be kept (Figs 1-48 to 1-52).

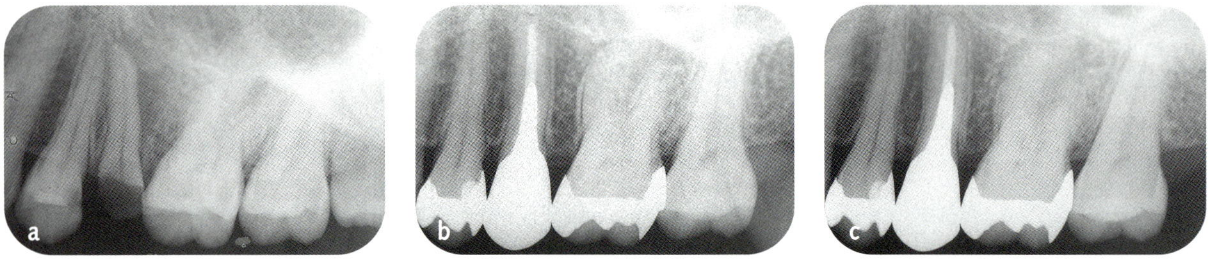

Fig 1-48 Root canal treatment and natural extrusion. (a) The patient was a 34-year-old woman at the first visit in April 1983. The residual root of this maxillary left second premolar had moved mesially as a result of inflammation. Temporary root filling was conducted with Vitapex, and interproximal disking was conducted on the part of the tooth contacting the first molar. A living body has an innate response to eliminate foreign bodies; therefore, time was allowed for natural extrusion and uprighting of the tooth. (b) The obliteration of the root canal was confirmed, and the tooth was built up with a temporary post and core. After uprighting with module and further extrusion with elastic, post-and-core buildup and crown placement were conducted 5 years after the first visit. (c) A radiograph taken 16 years after the first visit (1999). Improvement in traumatic and periapical lesions and uprighting of the tooth are observed.

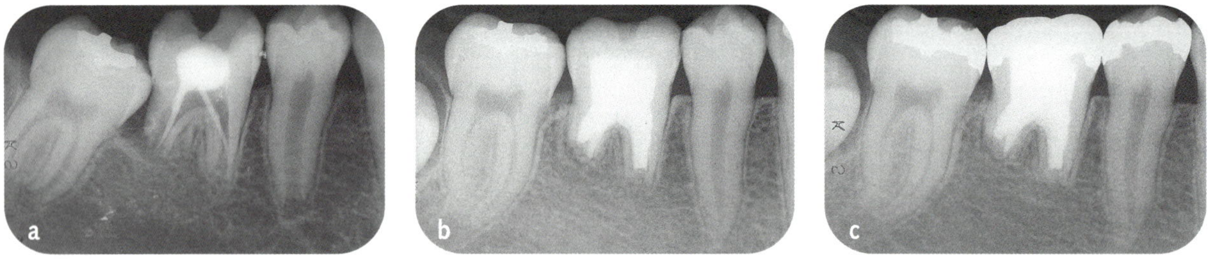

Fig 1-49 Endodontic treatment of infected canals of immature teeth. (a) The patient was an 11-year-old boy at the first visit in September 1982. In treating infected canals of immature permanent teeth, apexification should be conducted after promoting apical closure with a paste product (Vitapex). (b) While orthodontic extrusion of the mandibular right second molar is conducted (coronally repositioning), Vitapex is renewed every 3 to 6 months. After follow-up observation (about 2 years and 6 months), root canal filling was conducted. (c) A radiograph taken 3 years after the first visit (1985). A crown is restored and obliteration of root canals and bone regeneration are observed at the mandibular right first and second molars.

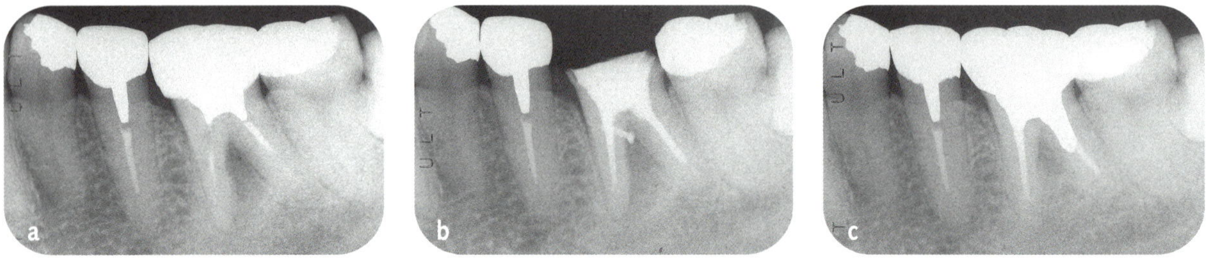

Fig 1-50 Furcation involvement caused by endodontic treatment. (a) A furcation involvement without communication with a periodontal pocket. Presumably, a lateral canal with a foramen in the furcation area was overlooked and root canal filling was conducted. (b) The paste (Vitapex) remains in the lateral canal. Root canal obturation was conducted with gutta-percha points. (c) A radiograph taken 5 years after the first visit.

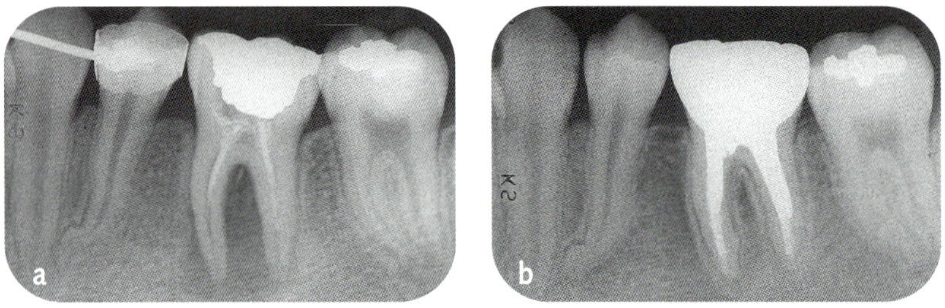

Fig 1-51 Furcation involvement caused by endodontic treatment. (a) A root canal with a foramen in the floor of the pulp chamber was overlooked. If there is no communication between a periodontal pocket and the bony defect, and an apex of the overlooked canal is obturated with certainty, the furcation involvement will be improved. (b) A radiograph taken 5 years after the treatment.

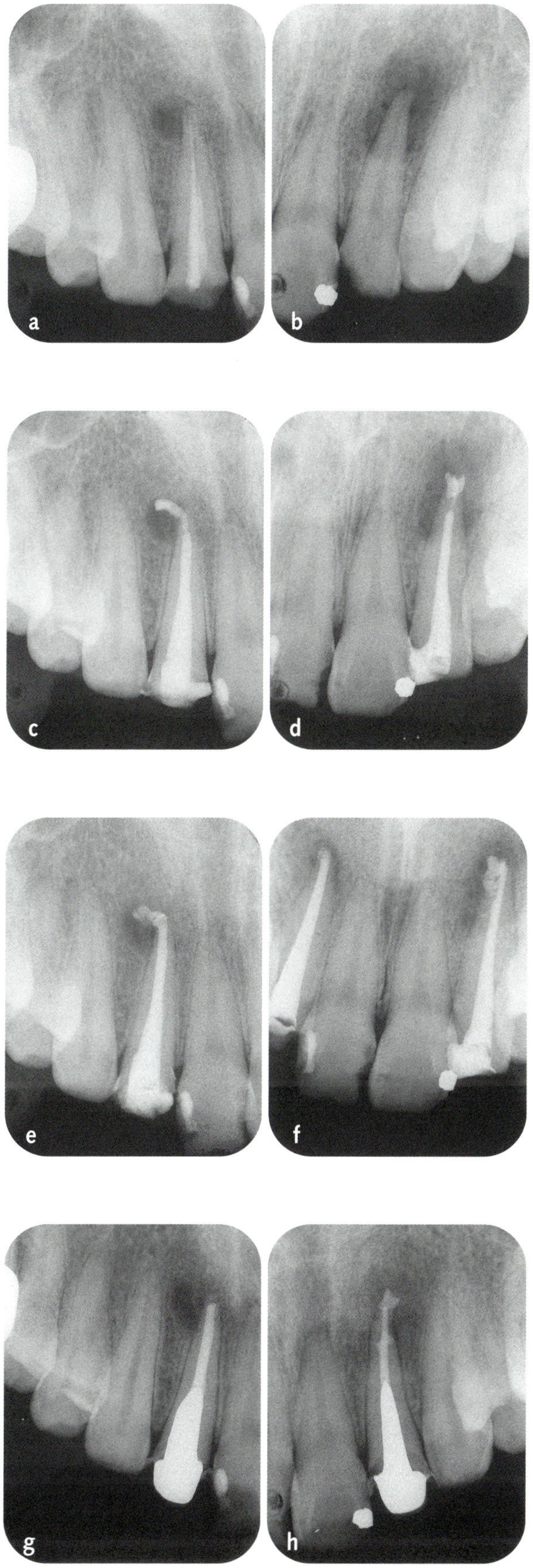

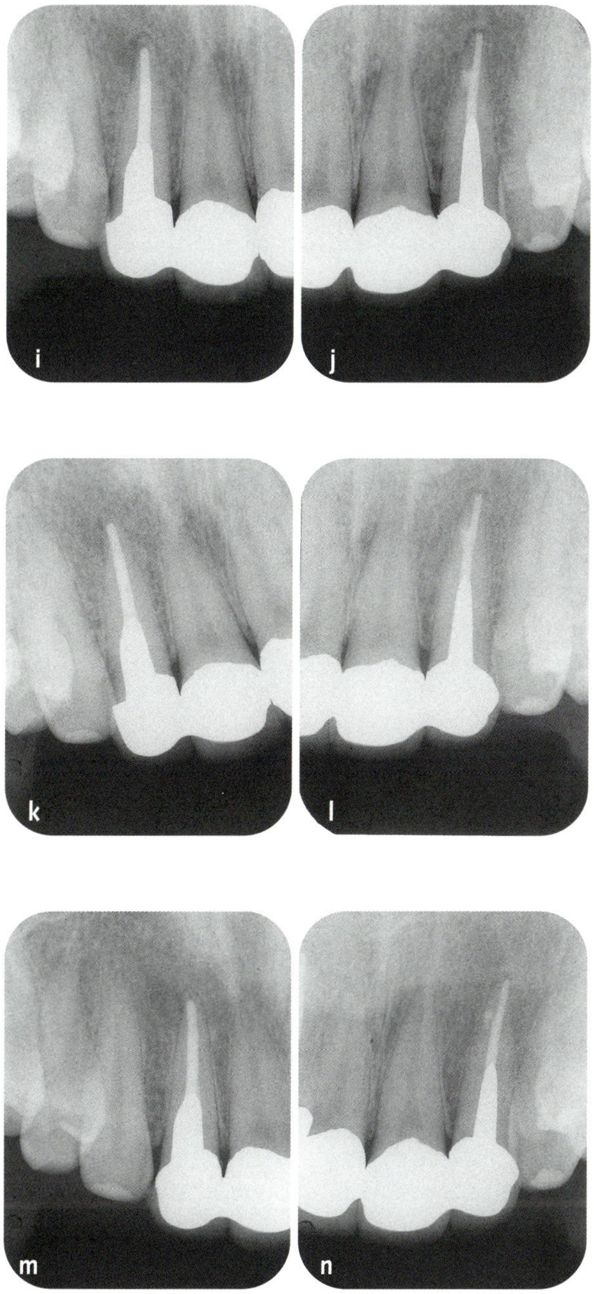

Fig 1-52 Progress in endodontic treatment in infected canals. (a and b) Periapical lesions are observed at the maxillary lateral incisors. (c and d) After infected dentin in the main canal was thoroughly removed, Vitapex paste is used to fill the canal for follow-up observation. (e) Root canal obturation was conducted on the right side with gutta-percha points after about 1.5 months. (f) After 25 days, Vitapex paste spilled out of the apical foramen of the right lateral incisor and was almost completely absorbed. Root canal obturation was conducted on the left lateral incisor with gutta-percha points about 2 months after the first visit. (g and h) Radiographs taken 3 months after the first visit when metal posts and cores were tried. Vitapex paste is observed in a lateral canal of the left lateral incisor. (i and j) Radiographs taken 4 years and 10 months after the first visit (November 1998). The apex of the right lateral incisor, from which Vitapex paste had spilled distally, is covered with cementum, indicating that the primary apical foramen was located distally. The paste spilled out of the apex of the left lateral incisor and is almost completely absorbed. (k and l) Radiographs taken 5 years and 11 months after the first visit (December 1999). Radiolucent areas at the apices have completely disappeared. (m and n) Radiographs taken 6 years and 6 months after the first visit (August 2000). Almost translucent lamina dura is observed.

Evaluation of questionable endodontic cases

When a restoration is dislodged, it should be assumed that root canals are contaminated with saliva. Retreatment of root canals is necessary even if there is no radiolucent finding in the periapical area. However, there are some clinical cases with good prognosis even though a pathologic lesion is suspected. Because of this, clinicians may hesitate to conduct re-treatment in a case where a wide metal post and core has been delivered.

In the case shown in Fig 1-53, the maxillary left lateral incisor had been treated by another dentist 10 years before the patient's first visit in 1985. The authors remade the post and core only. A periapical lesion developed, however, and periapical flap surgery was conducted.

In hindsight, it should have been diagnosed as a traumatic lesion accompanied by external absorption, judging from the disturbance of bone trabeculae. Most likely the seal was not complete because of periapical absorption. It is regrettable that the turbulence of periapical bone trabeculae and shadow-like findings were overlooked. When there is a secondary caries lesion around an existing post and core it is highly likely that root canals are contaminated; therefore the presence or absence of contamination should have been confirmed.

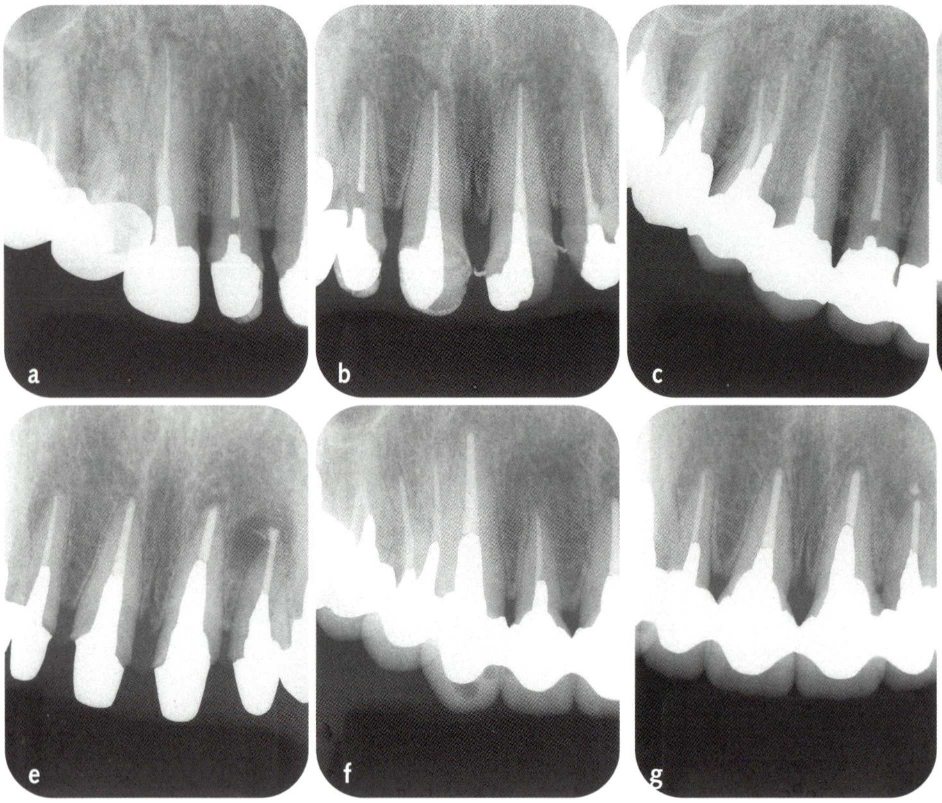

Fig 1-53 (a) The patient was a 37-year-old woman at the first visit in 1985. There is no distinct periapical lesion observed. Root canal treatment was conducted for the maxillary right premolars. For the maxillary lateral and central incisors and right canine, dowel posts and cores were remade because of secondary caries in the left central and lateral incisors. (b) The patient did not return for treatment for 11 years following the delivery of metal-ceramic crowns. At this point, a clear cyst-like lesion at the maxillary left lateral incisor as well as fine shadow-like lesions at the right canine and left central incisor are observed. (c) Root canal treatment was conducted for the infected canals of the central incisors, left lateral incisor, and right canine. After filling the canals with Vitapex paste, follow-up observation was conducted for some time, final root canal obturation was performed, and dowel posts and cores (type III gold) were delivered at the maxillary lateral and central incisors and right canine. However, remarkable improvement was not seen after re-treatment of infected canals. After about 1 year, debridement was conducted in the periapical area of the left lateral incisor, and Emdogain and resorbable membrane were used to improve the conditions. (d) Radiographs taken 2 years after the re-treatment (17 years after the first visit). Periodontal tissue seems stable.

Inflammation and force: Initial therapy against the collapse of occlusion

The clinical case shown in Fig 1-54 has notable inflammation. Also, horizontal bone resorption was radiographically observed in all regions, as were disturbance of bone trabeculae and widening of the periodontal spaces. Cervical wedge-shaped defects were also found, suggesting bruxism. Still, the mandibular arch responded well to tooth-unit inflammation control and reshaping. Treatment was carried out as follows: existing prostheses were removed, root canals were temporarily filled, temporary posts and cores were delivered, and provisional restorations were placed while thorough plaque control was conducted. Because this case responded very well to the initial periodontal therapy, no periodontal surgery was performed, with the exception of prosthodontic-related plastic surgery. Using the labial guiding wire of a plate-type repositioning splint, the flared-out maxillary anterior teeth were moved lingually, and a series of treatments were conducted to secure occlusal support.

Fig 1-54 (a) The patient was a 48-year-old woman at the first visit in 1995. The chief complaint was mobility and occlusal pain of the maxillary first molars and left second molar. The occlusal relationship is Class I on the right and Class II on the left, accompanied by anterior disc displacement of the TMJ. (The patient received only initial periodontal therapy and did not return for subsequent treatment.) (b) Photograph taken 3 years after the first visit. In the maxilla, the palatal root of the left first molar was extracted, and a periodontal prosthesis was delivered, connecting all teeth from the right lateral incisor to the left first molar (pontics: left premolars). The right canine and premolars were connected separately. An implant was placed for the missing right first molar. In the mandible, the distal root of the right first molar was extracted, and the remaining mesial root of that tooth and the adjacent premolar were connected. Two implants were placed in the area of the left first molar, and a fixed partial denture was delivered, connecting these implants and the premolars (pontic: second premolar) to increase the vertical height in the posterior region.

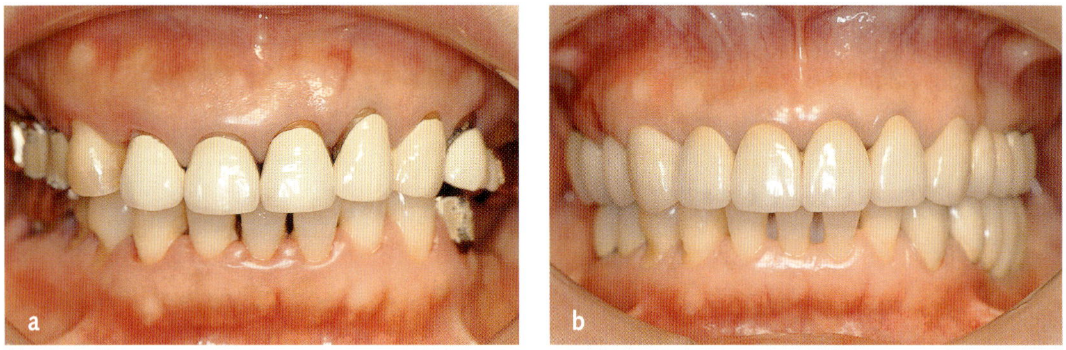

(c) Probing chart at the first visit. The probing depth was around 5 to 7 mm in the maxilla and 4 to 5 mm in the mandible with bleeding in most areas.

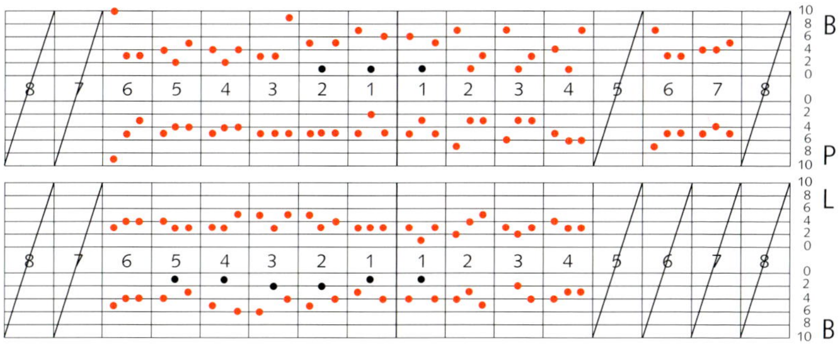

c

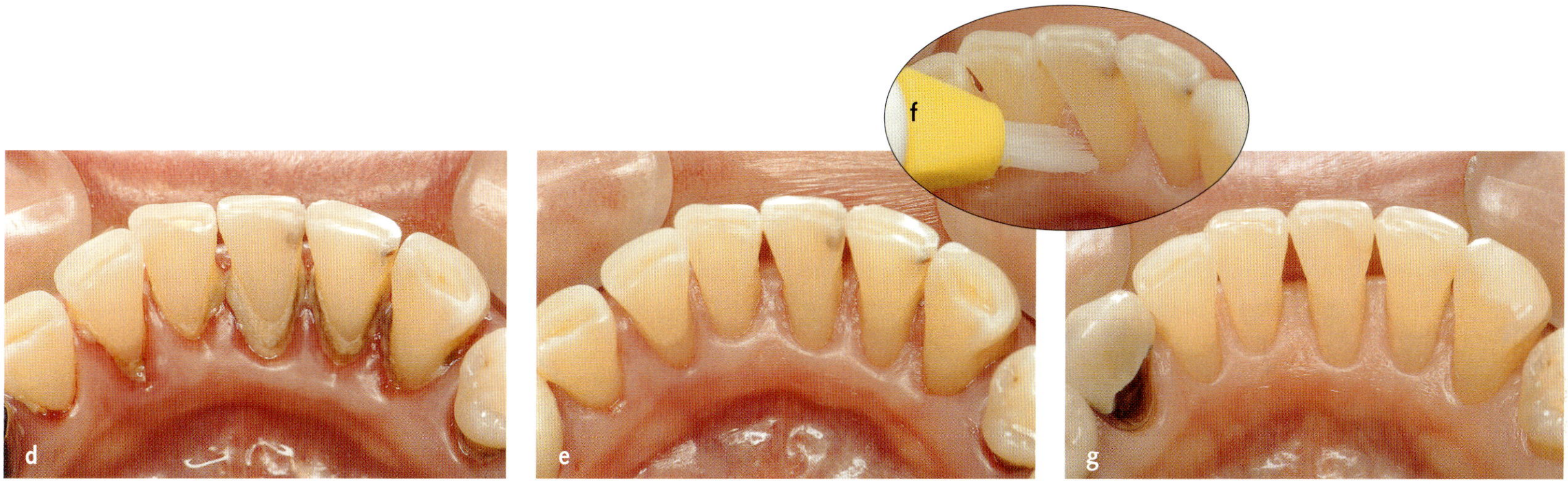

(d) Photograph taken at the first visit. There is noticeable inflammation and attrition due to bruxism. (e) Initial therapy is completed after 6 months. Intrapocket cleaning with Pocket Cleaner brush (Morimura) and modified rolling brushing technique, which does not damage the gingiva, show remarkable effects. (f) Pocket Cleaner brush designed by the authors for cleaning inside a periodontal pocket. (g) Root surface debridement was conducted in a secure and reasonable manner, and worn occlusal surfaces were reshaped (3 years after the first visit). (h to j) Radiographs of the mandible taken at the first visit. Infrabony defects and findings of secondary occlusal trauma are observed. (k to m) Radiographs taken at the completion of final restoration, 2 years and 8 months after the first visit. Left first premolar was connected to retrievable implant-supported partial denture using double crowns. (n to p) Radiographs taken during the maintenance phase, 6 years and 4 months after the first visit. At this time, the maxillary fixed partial denture connecting all teeth from the left canine to the first molar (pontics: premolars) had been fractured and repaired. Plaque control and reshaping has reduced signs of occlusal trauma.

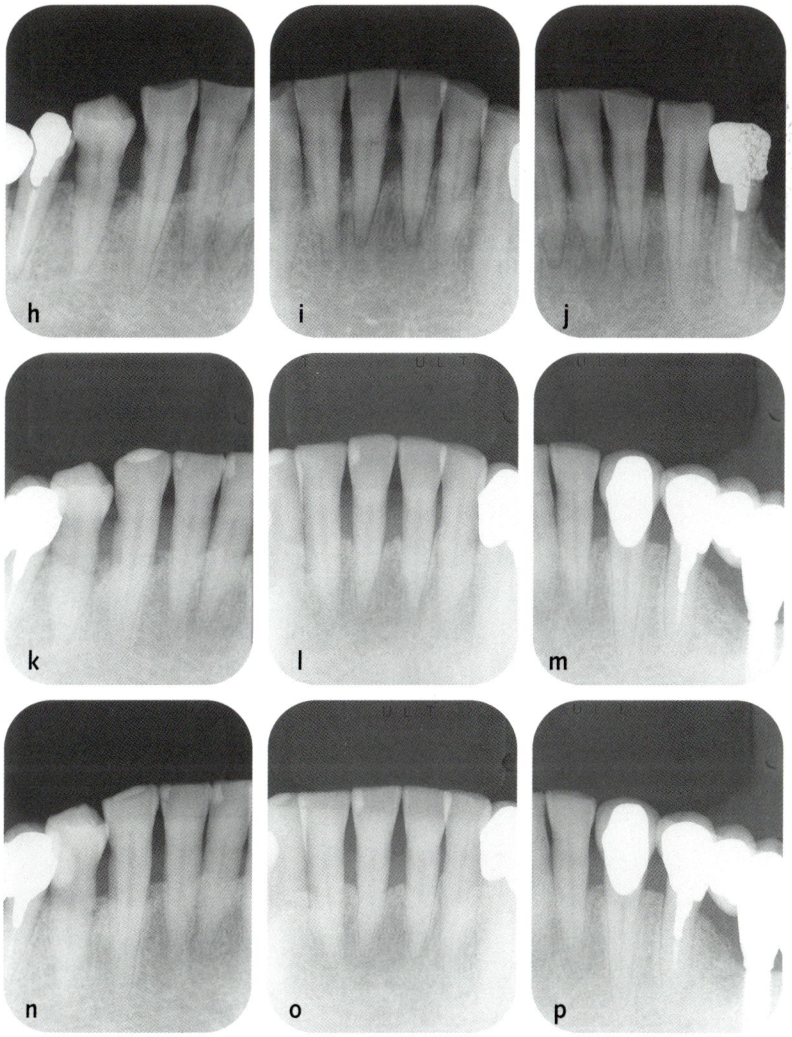

Single-tooth transplantation

In a case with a single missing tooth triggered by dental caries and its treatment (Fig 1-55), the objective of the treatment is to restore the integrity of the dental arches and occlusal relationships. If the missing tooth is the most posterior molar, not replacing it is one alternative. If the missing tooth has an adjacent tooth on both sides, possible treatment is a removable denture, a fixed partial denture, an implant prosthesis, or tooth transplantation. The treatment modality is chosen based on conditions such as occlusal relationships (occlusal support), integrity of the adjacent teeth, bone support of the teeth, esthetic requirements of the patient, the region of the mouth where the tooth is missing, bone conditions in the area, and availability of a tooth to be transplanted. Minimally invasive treatment should be the goal.

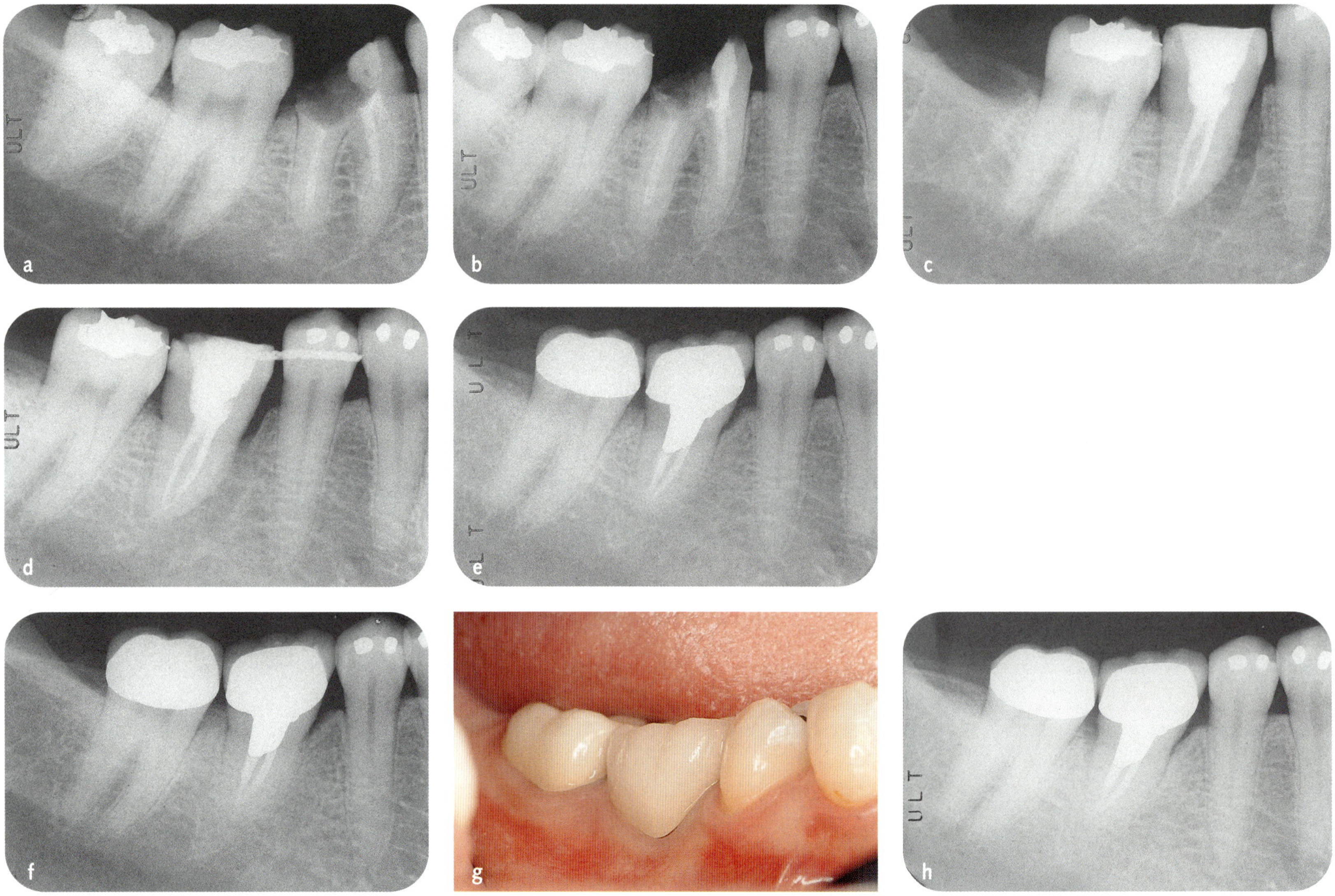

Fig 1-55 (a and b) The patient was a 42-year-old woman at the first visit in April 1992. The mandibular right first molar had dentinal destruction extending to the subgingival area, accompanied by root fracture. The third molar in this quadrant was healthy. (c and d) After extracting the first molar, the third molar was transplanted to the extraction socket. Pulpectomy was conducted in the third molar, followed by temporary root canal filling with Vitapex. The teeth were splinted with twisted wire for 2 months. (e) About 3 years after the transplantation. (f) About 6 years after the transplantation. (g) A clinical photograph taken 7 years and 8 months postoperatively. Although keratinized gingiva is limited, continuity of the dentition is maintained. (h) A radiograph taken 8 years and 4 months postoperatively. There is no external absorption of roots, but slight bone loss is observed distally.

Tooth-unit diagnosis of occlusal pain and a radiolucent lesion

In the case shown in Fig 1-56, the chief complaint was occlusal pain at the mandibular right molars. A fistula was observed on the buccal side of the first molar. Radiographs revealed widening of the periodontal space and a radiolucent lesion in the furcation area of the first molar. Disturbance of bone trabeculae around both molars indicated trauma. For the purpose of differential diagnosis, a radiograph was taken with a gutta-percha point inserted in the fistula. It was determined that the lesion was derived from mesial root canals. Next, a gutta-percha point was inserted in a gingival sulcus in the furcation area to confirm that the point did not reach the base of the bone. From these findings, it was diagnosed as a mesial root-derived fistula and an initial stage of furcation involvement combined with trauma. Based on this tooth-unit diagnosis, treatments were conducted including natural extrusion, root canal treatment, reduction of the periodontal pocket, periodontal surgery aiming at extending the vestibule and increasing attached gingiva, and restoration (Box 1-3).

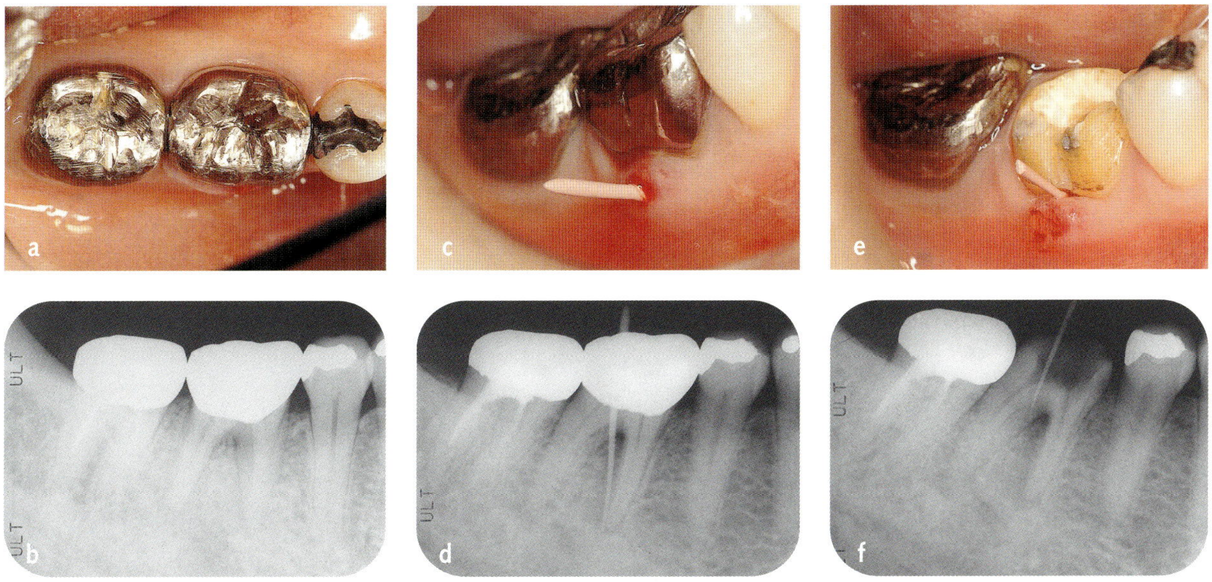

Fig 1-56 Tooth-unit diagnosis of occlusal pain and a radiolucent lesion

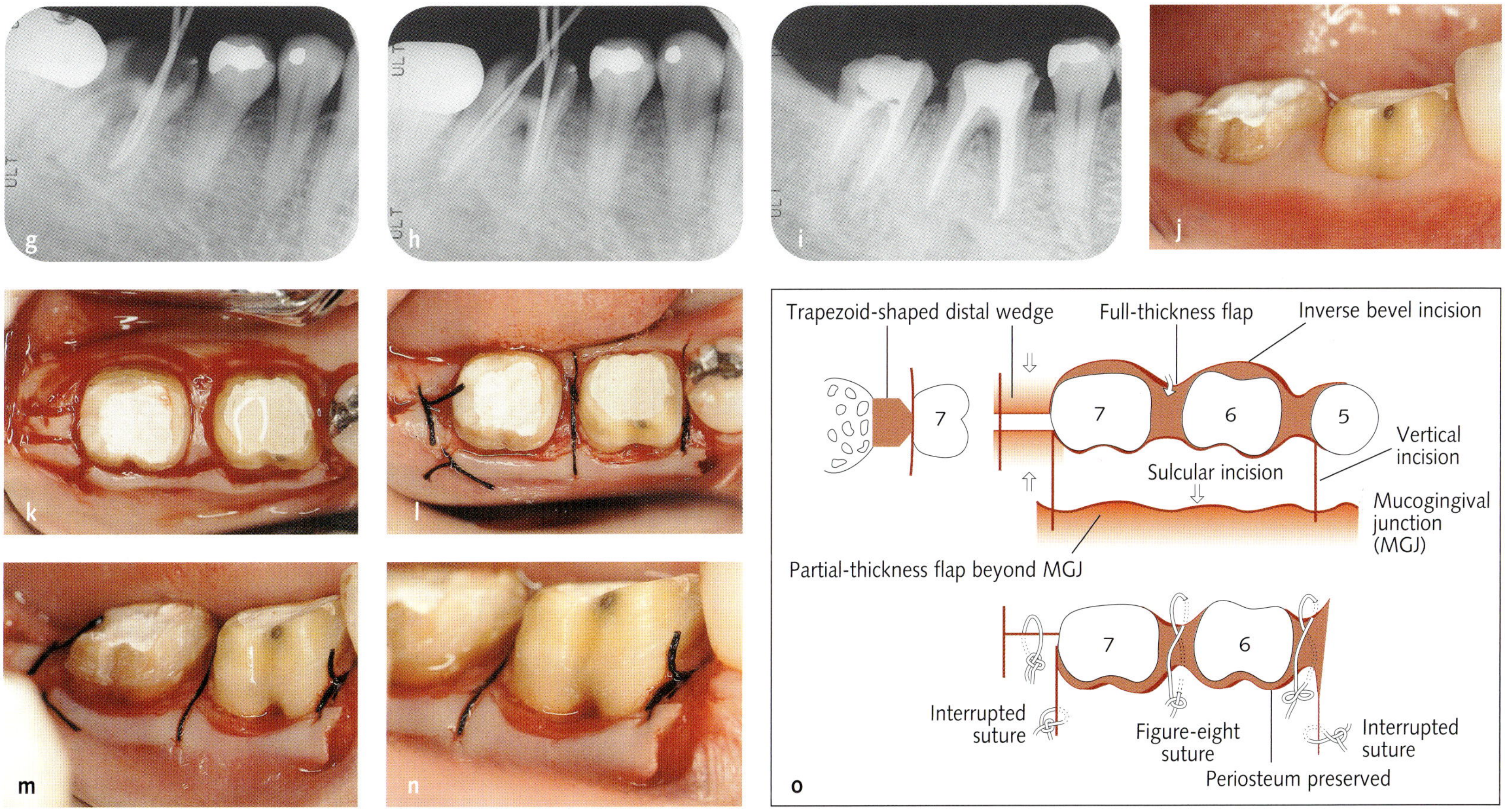

Fig 1-56 (a) At the first visit. The patient, a 44-year-old woman, complained of occlusal pain at the mandibular right molars. Premature contact was observed on both molars. (b) A radiograph shows widening of the periodontal space and bone resorption in the furcation area of the first molar. (c and d) A gutta-percha point was inserted in the fistula. The radiograph showed communication between the apex of the mesial root of the first molar and the fistula. (e and f) To confirm possible communication with a periodontal pocket, another gutta-percha point was inserted in a gingival sulcus in the furcation area. The radiograph showed that the point did not reach the base of the bone. It was diagnosed as an initial stage of furcation involvement (acute phase) combined with trauma. (g) Gutta-percha point trial. Eccentric projection of the mesial root. (h) Gutta-percha point trial. Eccentric projection of the distal root. (i and j) The crown was removed to improve traumatic conditions, promoting natural extrusion. In the meantime, calcium hydroxide paste (Vitapex) was used to fill the root canals for sterilization and recalcification to improve endodontically derived aspects of the lesion. The radiograph and clinical photograph were taken after root canal obturation of the first molar. (k) The vestibule was shallow, and the attached gingiva was limited. Surgery was conducted to reduce periodontal pockets and to increase attached gingiva. Distal to the second molar can be seen a distal wedge of a full-thickness flap. An inverse bevel incision was made on the lingual side to raise a full-thickness flap for periodontal pocket reduction. A sulcular incision was made on the buccal side to raise a partial-thickness flap for attached gingival gain. (l to o) The periosteum was preserved on the buccal side and interdental areas. Figure-eight sutures were placed in the interdental papilla regions, involving periosteal connective tissue.

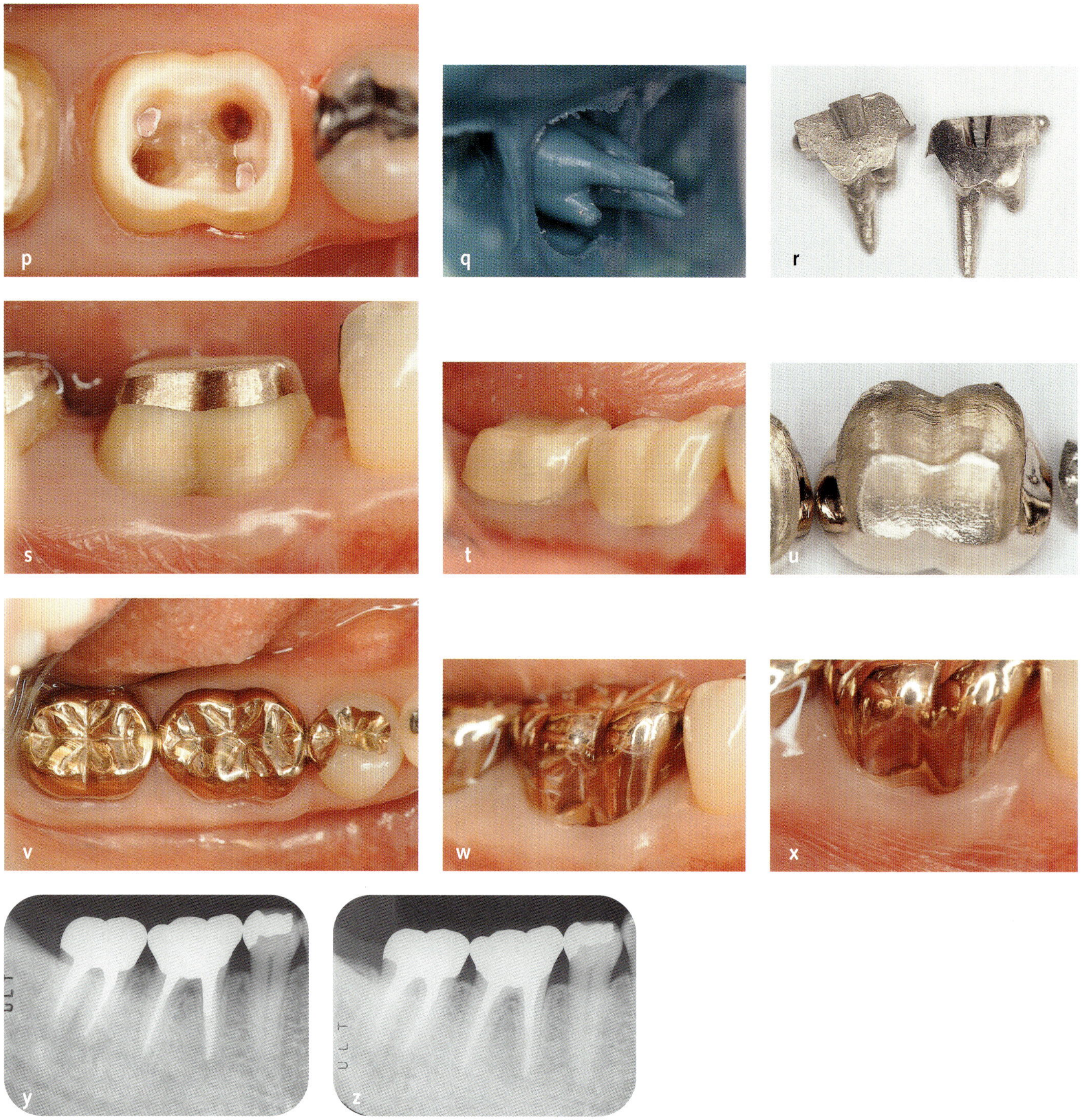

Fig 1-56 (cont) (p) Preparation for a dowel post and core. Minimal tooth reduction were conducted to prevent root damage with a 2-mm female placed to direct occlusal forces inward and vertically. (q) Impression using silicone material. (r) A two-piece post and core with a keyway (type IV gold). Adhesive cement was used. (s) Final preparation is a concentric circle design. Subgingival preparation is limited. (t) With provisional restoration, appropriate harmony with the gingiva and occlusion is sought using trial and error. The design of the furcation area was slightly too straight. (u) Interior of the crown. (v) Attached gingiva was increased. The occlusal surface was designed to facilitate chewing. (w) Clinical photograph 3 months after delivery of the prosthesis. (x) Close-up view 3 years after delivery of the prosthesis. Although the gingiva in the furcation area is thick, the straight emergence profile (poor contour) makes maintenance difficult. (y) Radiograph 1 year after delivery of the prosthesis. (z) Radiograph 4 years after the first visit. Continuity of lamina dura, uniform periodontal space, and distinct bone trabeculae are observed, indicating clinical healing of the lesion.

Box 1-3 Inflammation control and improvement of attachment

1. Initial therapy
2. Periodontal surgery
   - Resective treatment
   - Conservative treatment
   - Regenerative treatment
3. Natural extrusion (reshaping)
4. Orthodontic tooth movement

Comprehensive Diagnosis of Dentition-Unit Pathology and Treatment Goals

Successive changes in dentition

In dentition-unit examination, the relationships among tooth units as well as occlusion units have to be taken into consideration, and successive changes in the dentition have to be examined from the viewpoints of morphology and function.

Dentition-unit examination cannot be conducted without examination of static occlusion, such as the stability of dentition and the overlap between the maxillary and mandibular dentition, as well as examination of dynamic occlusion. Examination of static occlusion looks at mandibular positions as well as the contacts between the maxillary and mandibular dentition, including the stability of the ICP, the propriety of guidances, and occlusal interferences.

Dentition-unit viewpoint

There is a misconception that the stable unity and harmony of the dentition is lost mainly because of attachment loss due to bacterial plaque–derived inflammation. Although inflammation does play a role in the destruction of the dentition, forces are perhaps a greater factor in the process. When inflammation causes attachment loss, secondary occlusal trauma accelerates the destruction of the dentition. Although serious TMJ problems are less likely to occur in patients with considerable periodontal tissue breakdown, secondary occlusal trauma accelerates the periodontal tissue breakdown. The greater effect of occlusal forces on the destruction of the dentition as compared with inflammation is evidenced in the fact that even though excessive forces are exerted on periodontal tissue in bruxism, periodontal tissue breakdown is not so striking in patients with significant horizontal attrition; conversely, in patients with attachment loss and remarkable tooth mobility, attrition does not progress much. Therefore, the importance of restoring mechanical harmony, ie, concentrating on the dentition unit, cannot be overemphasized as a measure against the destruction of the dentition. Cases 1-6 and 1-7 demonstrate the dentition-unit approach.

Measures against destruction of the dentition

When there is an ill-balanced, weak element in teeth, periodontal tissue, temporomandibular joints, or muscles, forces of the masticatory system will destroy the area where the weakness lies in a concentrated manner. Moreover, this destruction will not stop unless therapeutic intervention is made.

Important measures against the destruction of dentition are correction of tongue or lip habits and abnormal postures, rationalization of mandibular positions, reconstruction of an arch form, control of periodontal disease and dental caries, and tooth-unit and occlusion-unit understanding of a clinical case. In comprehensive dentistry, restoration of stable tooth positions or harmony in the dentition as well as inflammation control are important healing goals.

Control of the tongue and circumoral muscles

Abnormal tongue habits exert forces on the teeth. When there is no bacterial plaque–derived inflammation, tissue destruction is reversible. When inflammation is also present, however, attachment loss will result. When supporting tissue is reduced, an abnormal tongue habit or a lip habit can be a main cause of occlusal collapse.

Like plaque control, control of circumoral muscles (see chapter 2) is one of the most important and basic oral health measures.

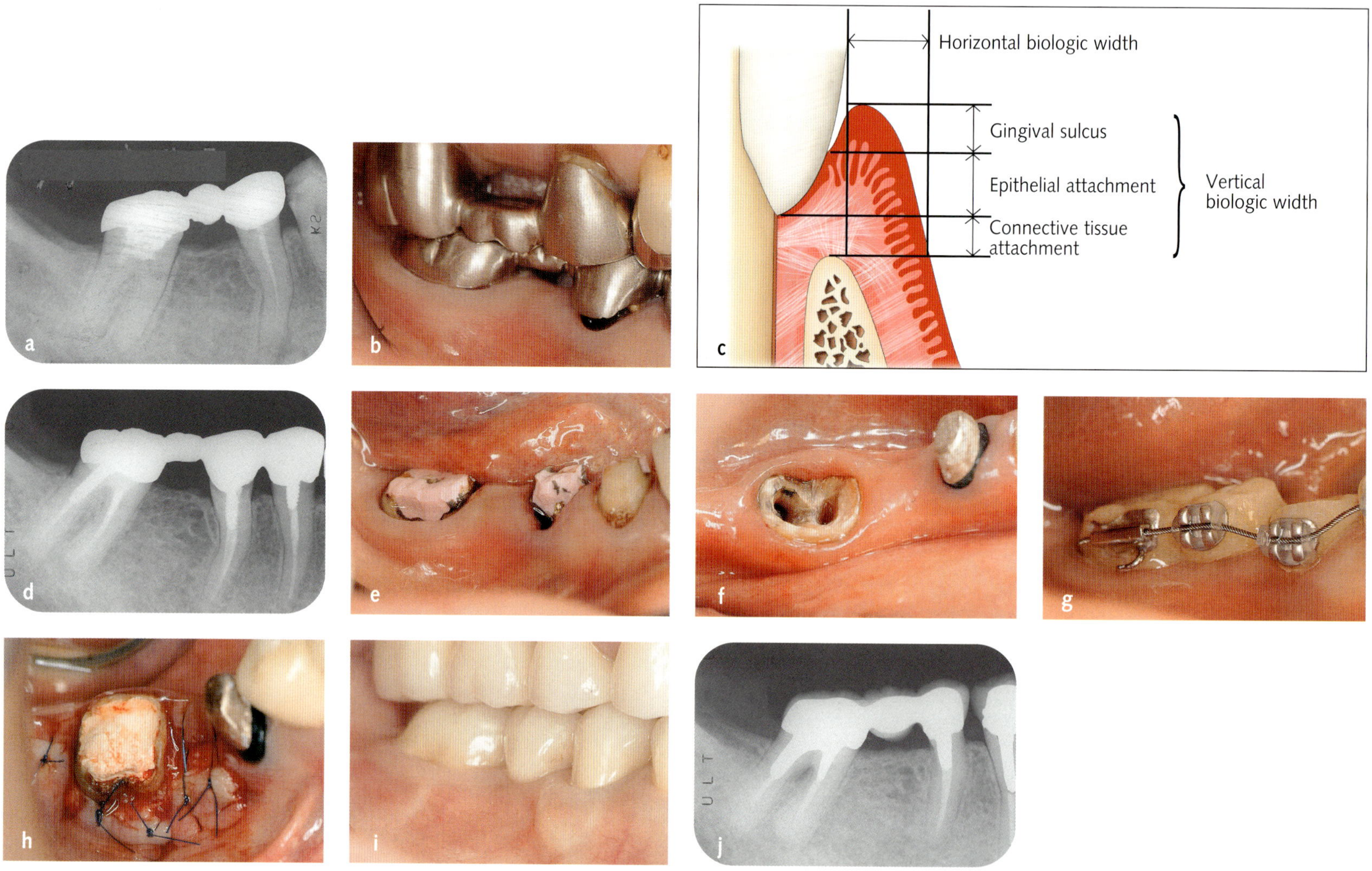

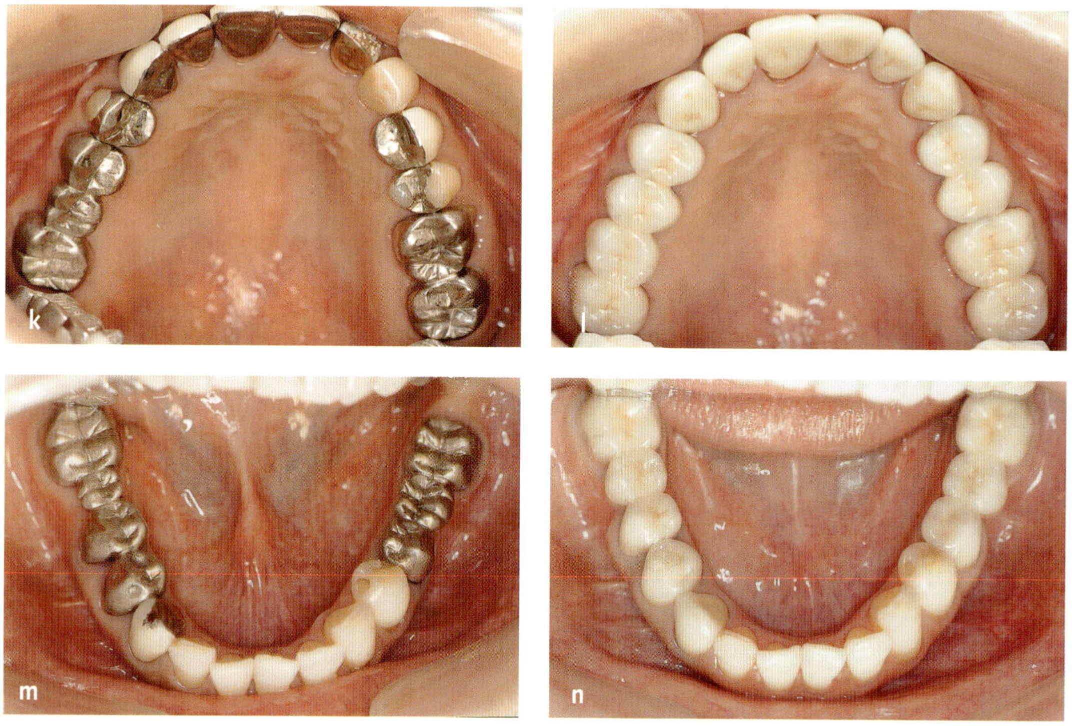

Fig 1-57 Dentition-unit treatment. (a) Radiograph at the first visit in 1979. (b) Subgingival dental caries after 18 years (1997). (c) In a case with subgingival caries, lengthening of the clinical crown is essential to securing biologic width. With regard to the biologic width, attention is generally paid to the distance from the bony crest to the free gingival crest. (d) Radiograph taken 18 years after the first visit. (e) The crowns were removed. The pink material is old resin core. (f) Core material of the mandibular right second molar was removed in preparation for orthodontic extrusion and crown lengthening for subgingival caries. (g) Orthodontic extrusion of the mandibular right second premolar was conducted to obtain sufficient dentin supragingivally, which is required for the biologic width. The provisional restoration of the molars (pontic: first molar) was used as anchorage. (h) Calcium hydroxide paste was used for the second molar for follow-up of the root canal treatment result, while the clinical crown was reduced in anticipation of natural extrusion. The crown-lengthening procedure was then conducted. The roll technique was used buccally and lingually in the missing first molar area. (i and j) Clinical photograph and radiograph 23 years after the first visit. Because of the inadequate treatment and lack of maintenance, extensive re-treatment was required. Still, homeostasis of the dentition is somehow maintained. The first molar is an ovate pontic. (k and l) Clinical photographs 18 years after the first visit. (m and n) Clinical photographs 4 years and 6 months after re-treatment. (Prosthetics by Kiyoharu Takada, RDT.)

Case 1-6 Understanding dentition-unit pathology

Patient: *41-year-old woman at the time of first visit in February 1986*

The patient had strong clenching habits and did not follow a maintenance schedule regularly, visiting our clinic only when conditions worsened. Occlusal balance was improved, interdental spaces were closed, and natural uprighting of inclined teeth was achieved. Although crown morphology was corrected and care was taken to avoid stress concentration, fracture of the key tooth occurred. This clinical case strongly demonstrates the importance of harmony in the dentition (Figs 1-58 to 1-65).

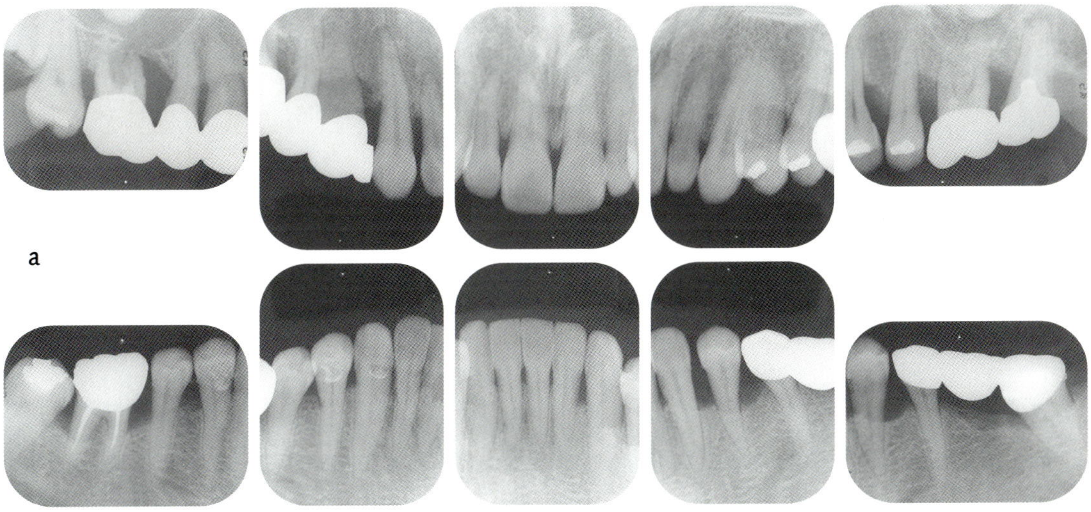
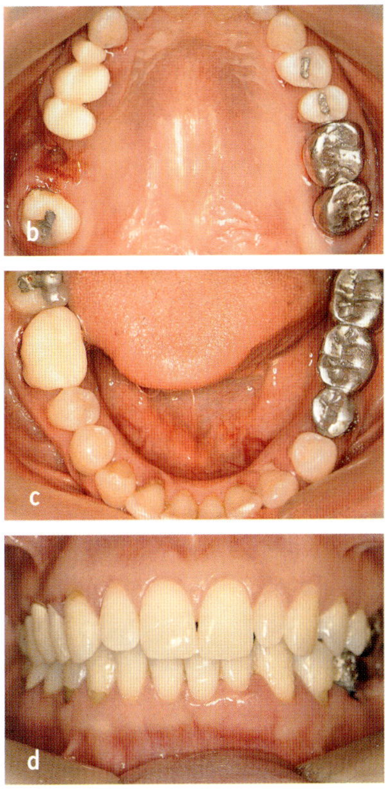

Fig 1-58 (a to d) The patient presented with pain in the molar regions. Severe bony defects were observed at the maxillary right and left and mandibular right first molars. Most likely because sufficient occlusion was not possible in the right and left molar areas, stress was concentrated in the premolar areas, indicated by cervical wedge-shaped defects at the mandibular first premolars and right second premolar, as well as dislodgment of the facing of the left second premolar.

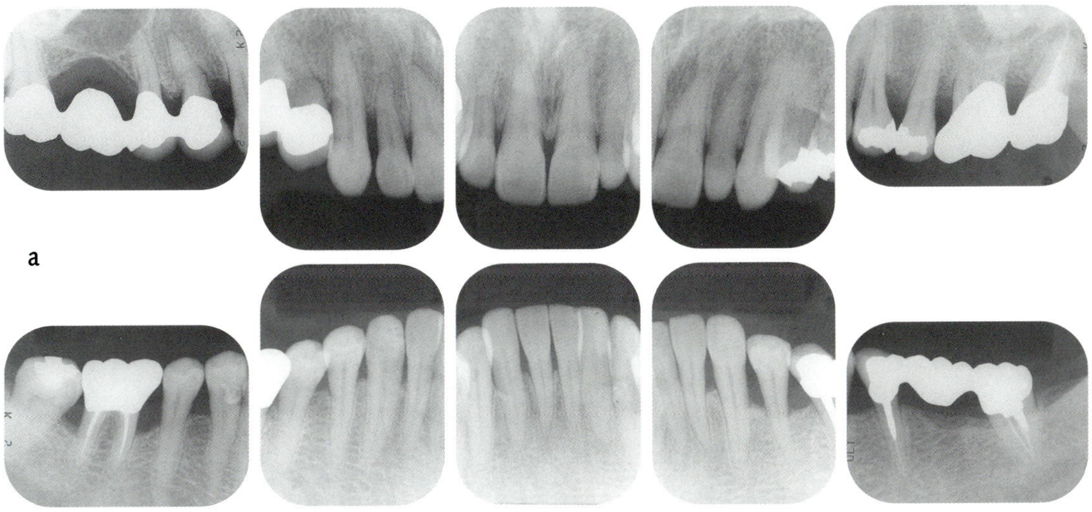
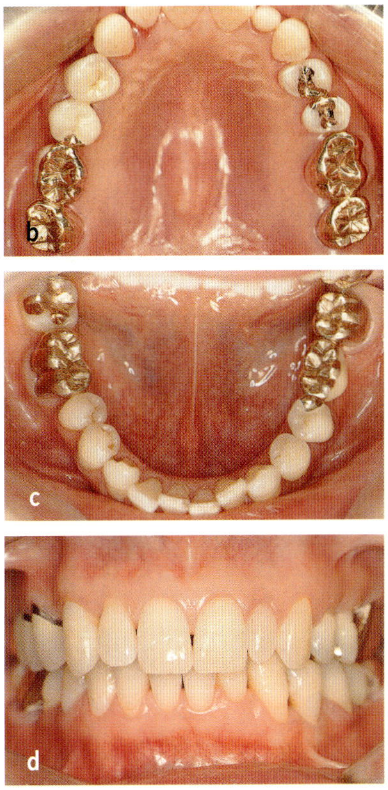

Fig 1-59 (a to d) After 1 year and 10 months. Final prostheses were delivered.

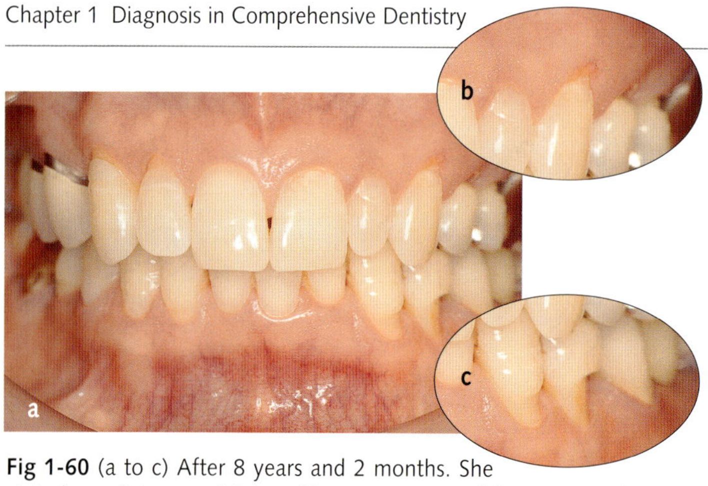

Fig 1-60 (a to c) After 8 years and 2 months. She visited our clinic, complaining of hypersensitivity. Abfraction was observed, including dislodgment of cervical composite fillings at the mandibular left canine and first premolar and significant wedge-shaped defects in the cervical areas of these teeth as well as the adjacent second premolar.

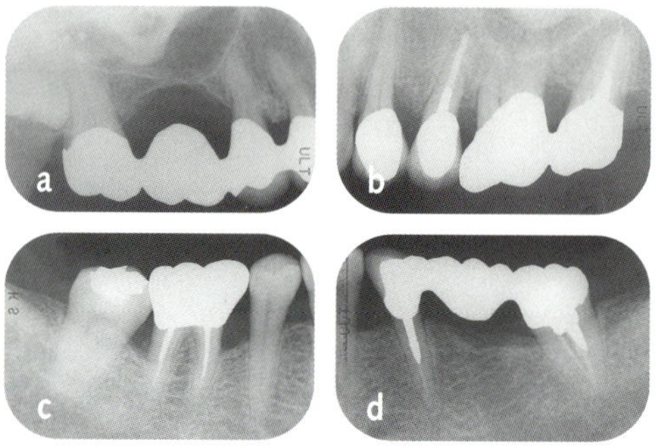

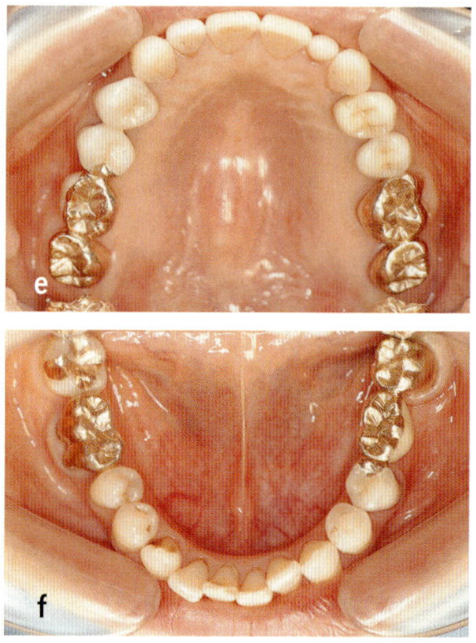

Fig 1-61 (a to f) After 8 years and 10 months. Lateral forces were avoided by placing crowns on the maxillary left premolars. The first premolar was maintained vital and rotated prosthodontically.

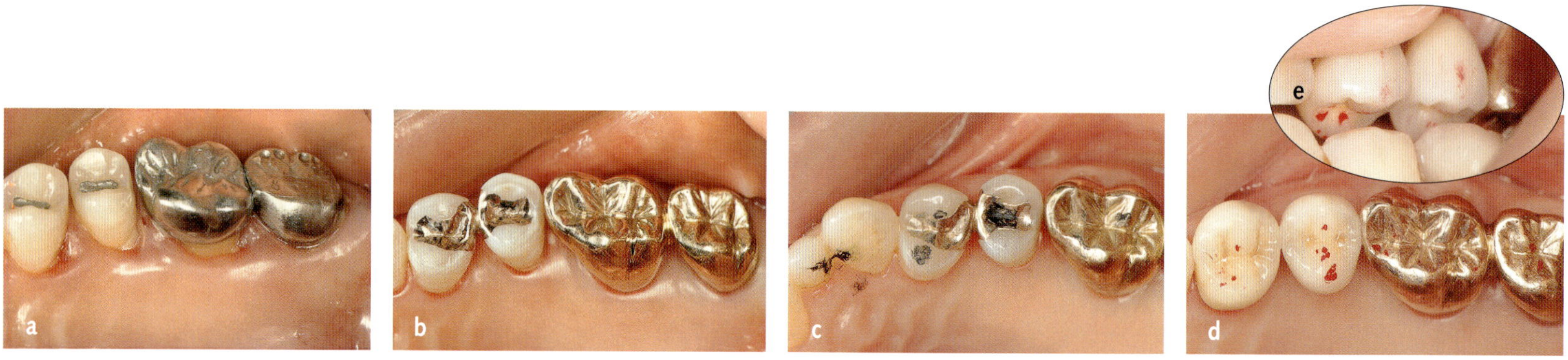

Fig 1-62 The occlusal morphology of the maxillary left premolars and molars has changed in response to abfraction, as shown in: (a) the first visit (February 1986), (b) after periodontal surgery and completion of restoration (December 1987), (c) after 8 years and 4 months, and (d and e) after 8 years and 10 months, when the morphologic correction via crown restoration was completed. Rotation of the tooth axis was corrected prosthodontically to give point contact.

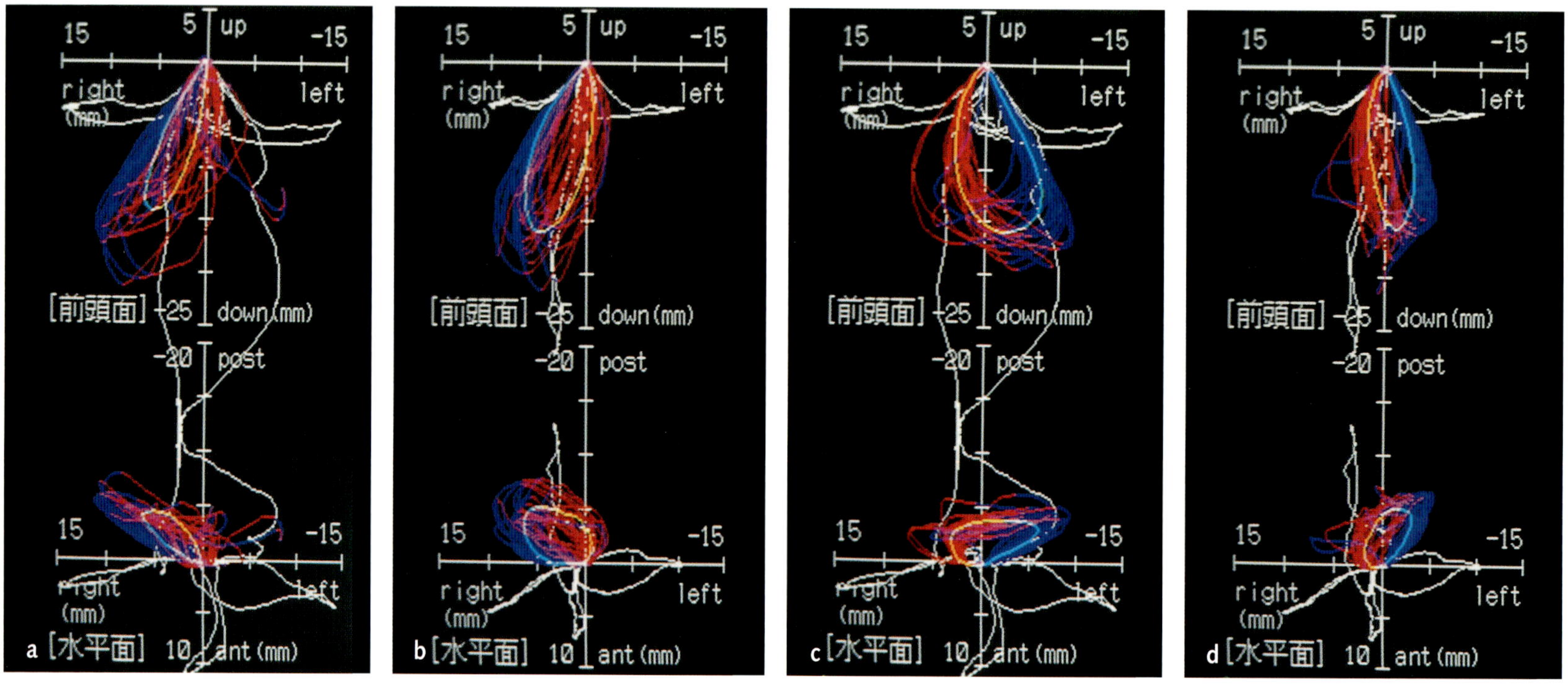

Fig 1-63 Chewing cycles with the frontal plane shown on top and the transverse plane below. (a and b) Incisal path during right-side chewing before (a) and after (b). At this point in time, occlusal surfaces of the left side only were treated. However, right-side chewing is also improved. (c and d) Left-side chewing before (c) and after (d) crown reshaping of the maxillary left premolars. Chewing cycles have become more vertical, with fewer extraneous movements in the path.

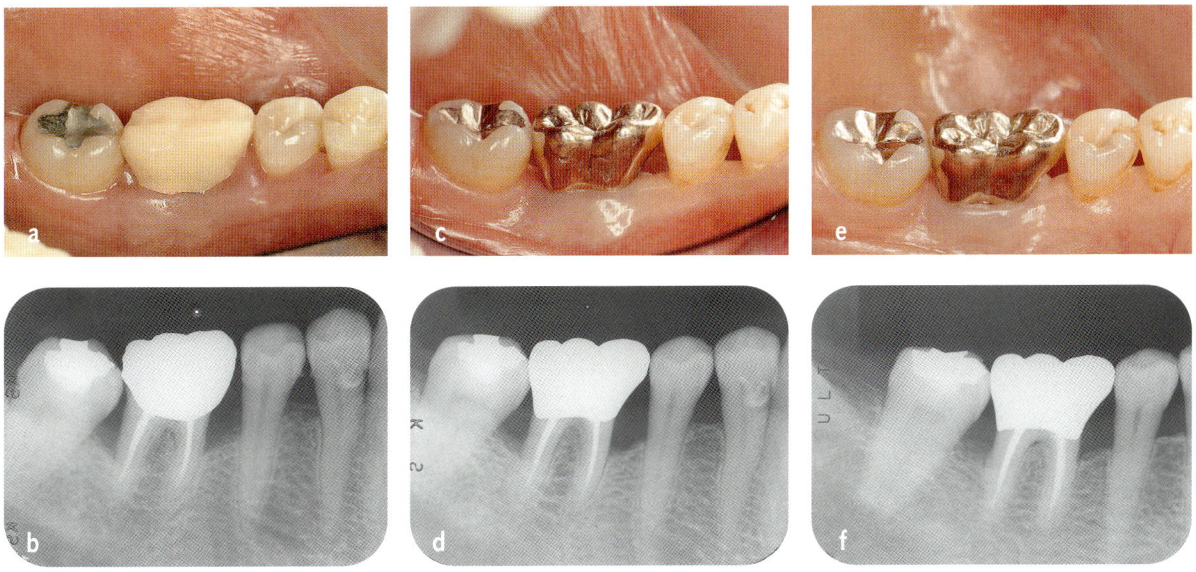

Fig 1-64 The mandibular right first molar was naturally extruded by reducing the occlusal height. By uprighting and natural extrusion of the adjacent second molar, mesial and distal infrabony defects and the traumatic lesion are gradually improved. (a and b) At the first visit; (c and d) after 1 year and 10 months, and (e and f) after 15 years.

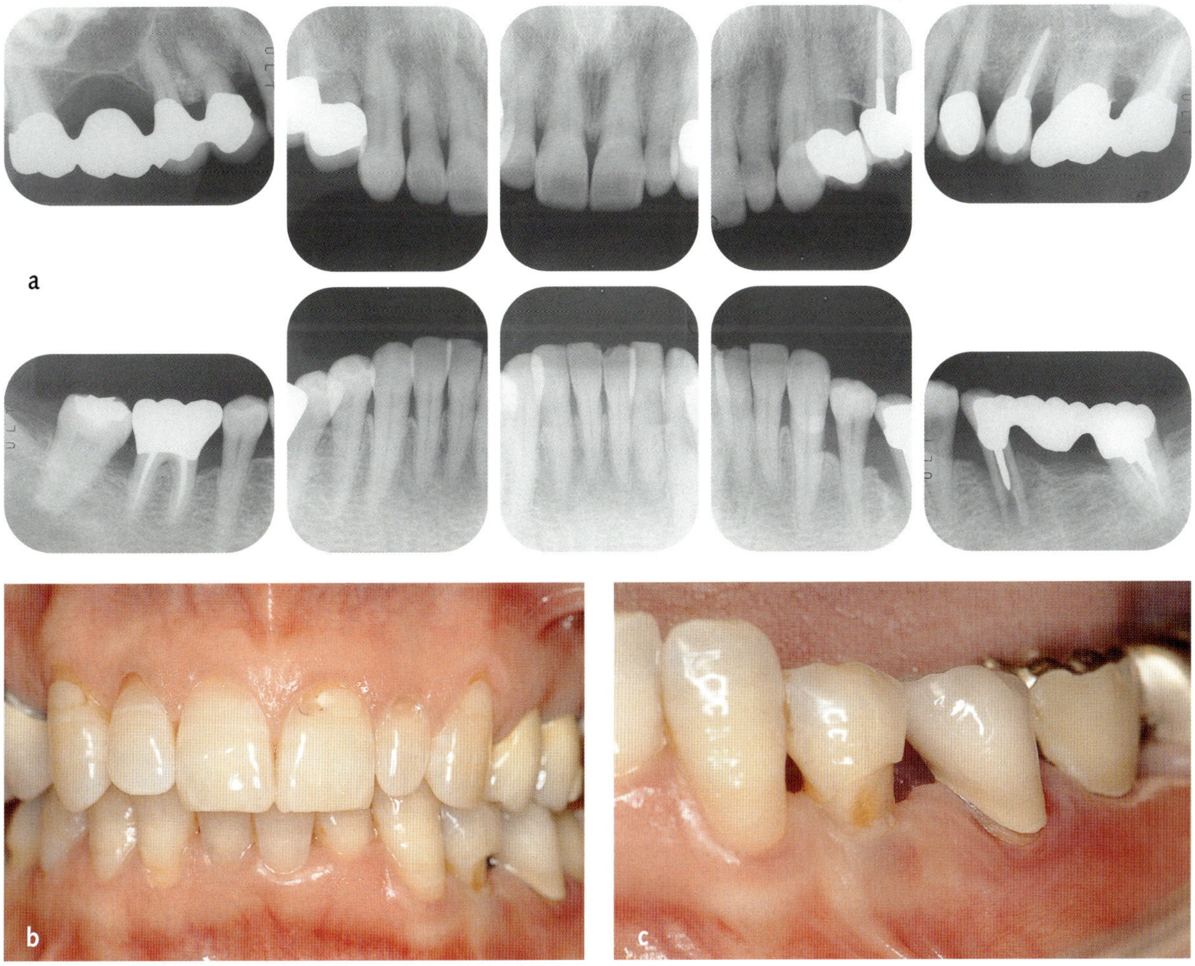

Fig 1-65 (a to c) There was a concern about the long-span design of the fixed partial denture connecting the mandibular left second premolar and molars (pontic: first molar) because clenching stress was concentrated in this area. Although crown morphology of the opposing teeth was corrected, she visited our clinic 15 years after the first visit (February 2001) with a root fracture. It is regrettable that her maintenance therapy was discontinued because if the situation had been monitored, this result could have been avoided.

Case 1-7 Restoration of biologic width and tooth-gingiva complex

Patient: *59-year-old woman at the time of first visit in 2000*

Chief complaint: *She started to have difficulty opening her mouth 2 months before the first visit. She had pain especially in the left TMJ area. Her left jaw felt somewhat heavy in the morning, and it was difficult to open her mouth. She had this symptom only in the morning at first, but had experienced difficulty opening her mouth at all times for a month by the time of her first visit. Her left temple and right shoulder felt stiff. She had a problem with her lower back.*

Diagnosis: *Chronic disc displacement without reduction of the left TMJ and anterior disc displacement with reduction of the right TMJ*

Although her chief complaint was the joint pain related to the disc displacement without reduction, advanced secondary caries was observed in all regions of her mouth (Fig 1-66). Crown lengthening was necessary to restore the biologic width of each tooth for occlusal reconstruction (Figs 1-67 to 1-75).

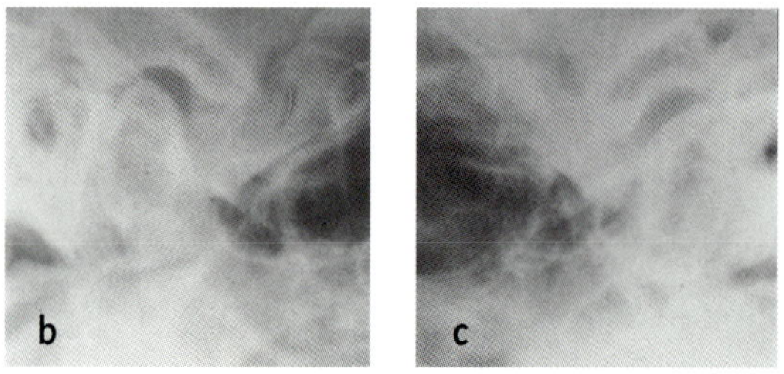

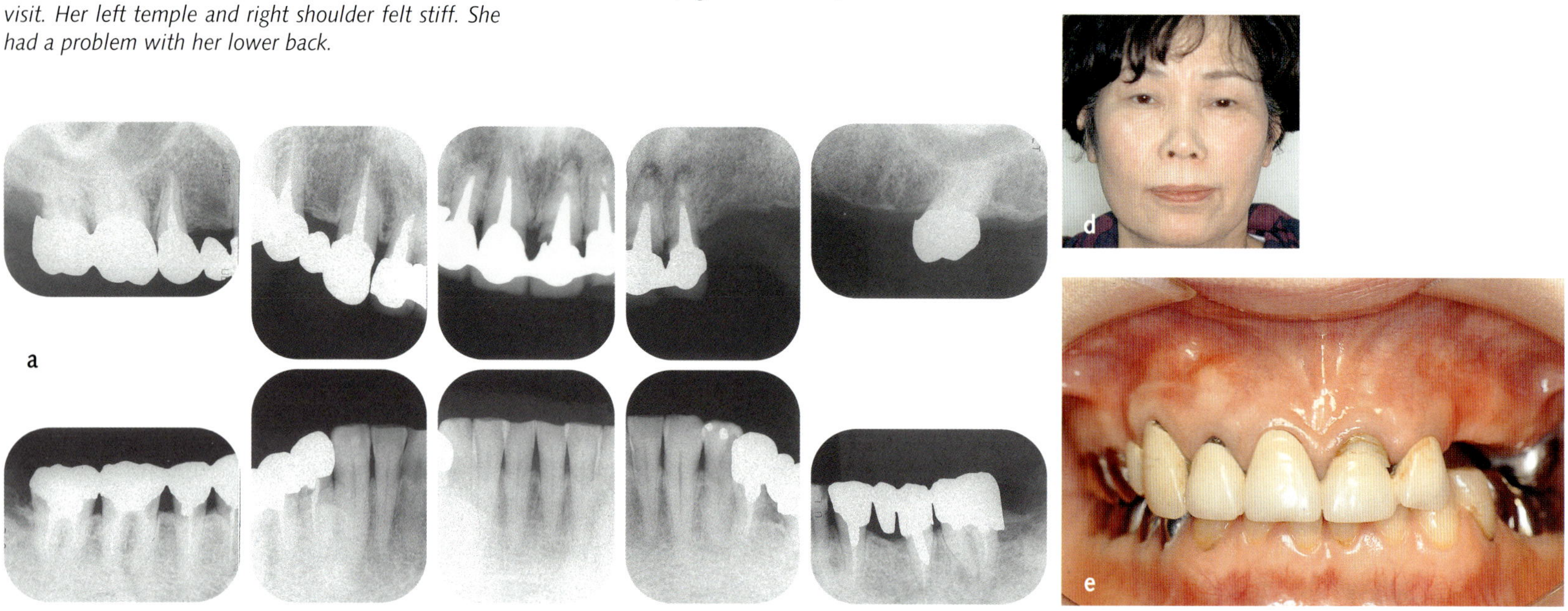

Fig 1-66 At the first visit. (a) The maxillary left canine, premolars, and first molar were missing. Disturbance of bone trabeculae was observed generally (occlusal trauma). Prostheses with poor fit, secondary caries, and inappropriate root canal treatments are seen in many teeth. Periodontal disease is generally mild, with periodontal pockets only at the maxillary right second molar and the four mandibular molars (7 to 8 mm). (b and c) ICP at the first visit. The left TMJ (c) seems to be pushed posteriorly. (d) Because of the disc displacement without reduction, the lip line is slanted, and the right and left eyes are different sizes. The maximum opening was 2.5 cm. The jaw was shifted to the left during opening. The right TMJ was diagnosed as anterior disc displacement with reduction based on the clinical symptoms. (e) The cervical line is lower on the right. All the restored teeth have deficiency in endodontic treatment and secondary caries.

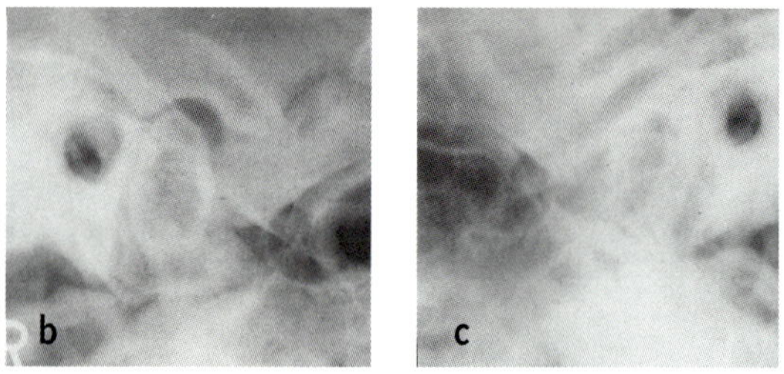

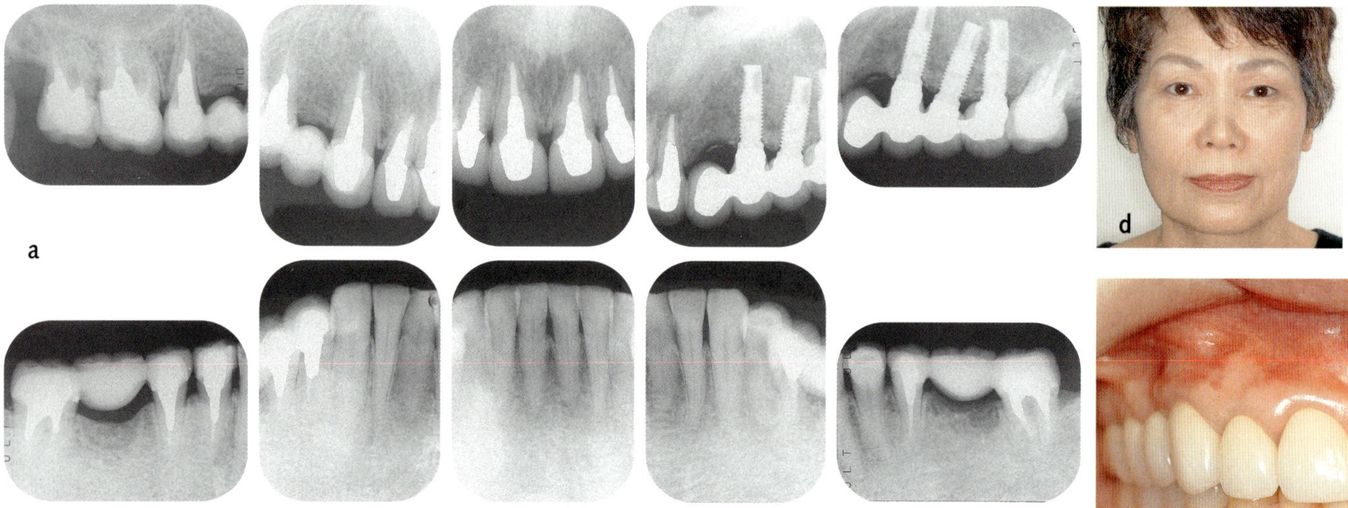

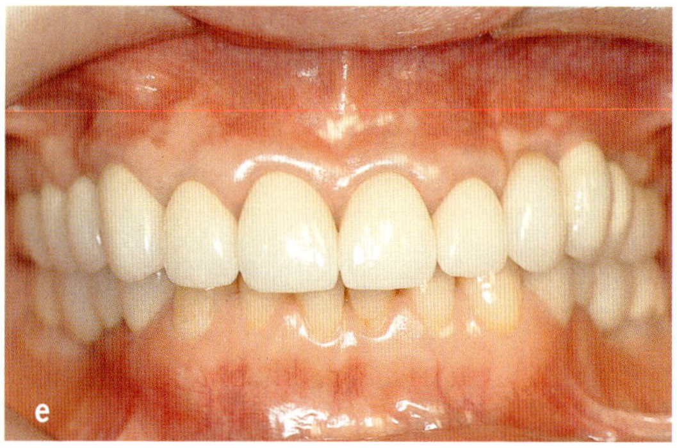

Fig 1-67 After the completion of treatment (approximately 2 years after the first visit). (a) The mandibular left first molar was extracted because of a perforation and the mandibular right first molar because of root fracture. In the maxillary left premolar–first molar area, vertical and buccal ridge augmentation was conducted with bone grafting and guided bone regeneration (GBR) with a resorbable membrane. Also, sinus lift procedure was conducted using an osteotome. (b and c) ICP 2 years and 3 months after the first visit. The left condyle (c) is located slightly more anteriorly than it was before treatment. (d) The imbalance between the right and left sides of the face has been corrected. The maximum opening was increased to 4.0 cm. Although the left condyle is not on the disc, joint symptoms disappeared. It is considered clinical healing. The right condyle is on the disc. (e) The occlusal plane has been improved.

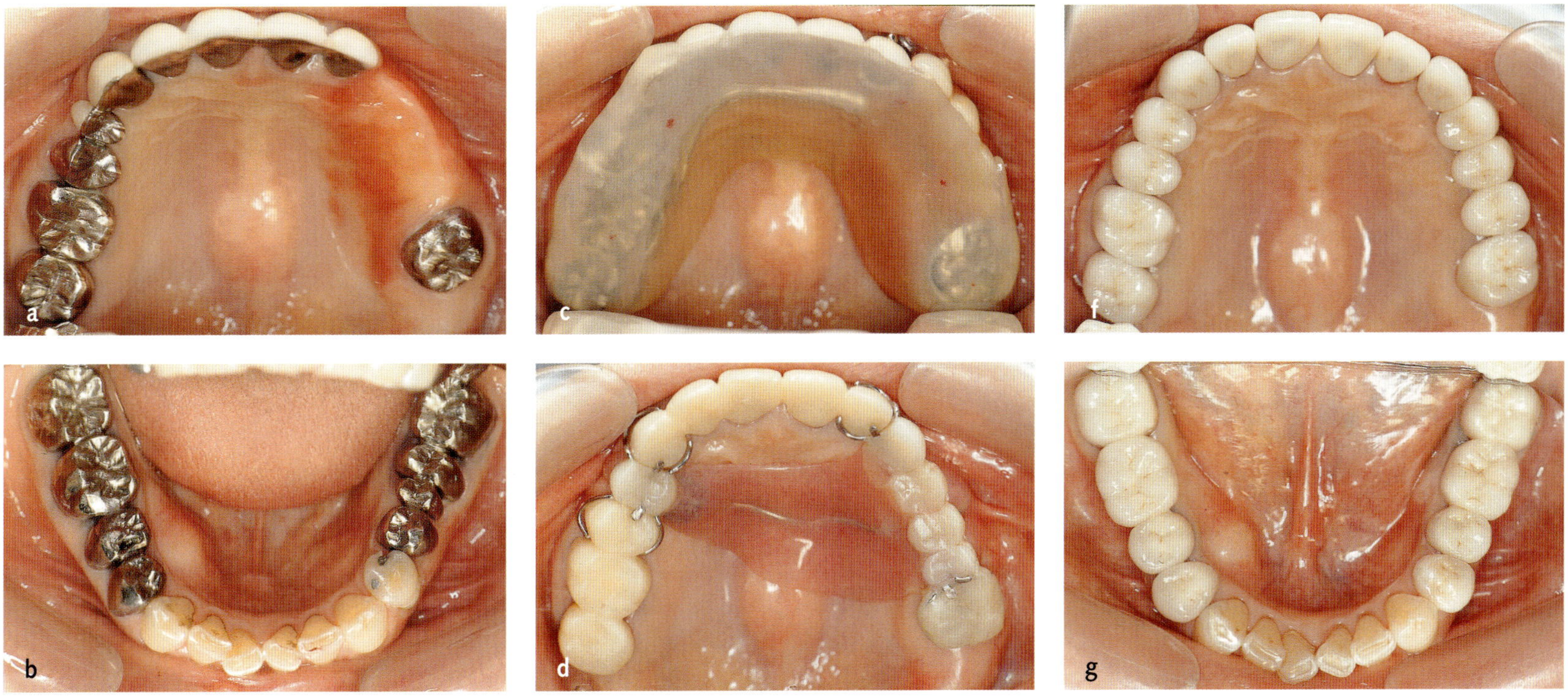

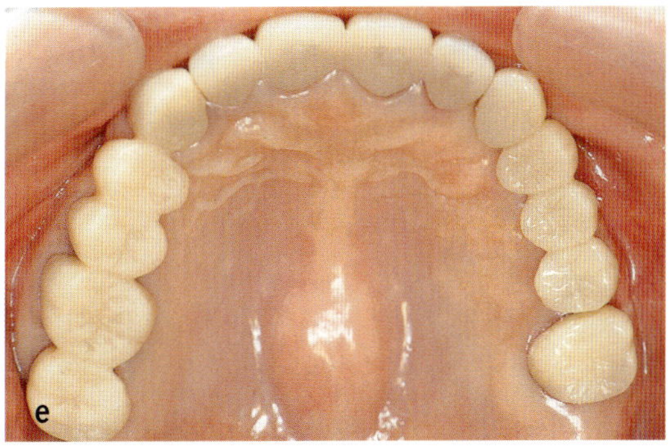

Fig 1-68 Occlusal views before and after treatment. (a and b) Occlusal views at the first visit. The maxillary left canine, premolars, and first molar were missing. The soft tissue indicates the pressure from a denture. In the maxilla, porcelain-fused-to-metal crowns connecting the incisors, crowns on the right molars and left second molar, and a fixed partial denture connecting the right canine and premolars (pontic: first premolar) are observed. In the mandible, the left arch is inclined lingually. Inappropriate root canal treatment, root fracture, and root caries are seen. (c) A bite plane is used to improve the mandibular position. (d) The mandibular position is corrected, and clinical crown lengthening is conducted. The oral environment is improved tooth by tooth, through endodontic treatment, dowel posts and cores, GBR for the maxillary left premolar and first molar area, and implant treatment. The fourth provisional restoration and a provisional denture are shown. (e) The final provisional restoration. (f and g) Completion of restoration after the delivery of all-ceramic crowns for all teeth, including in the maxilla Procera single crowns for the incisors, In-Ceram fixed partial denture connecting the right canine and premolars (pontic: first premolar), and In-Ceram single crowns for the right molars and left second molar. Note the symmetric arch shape. Those prostheses were copied from the provisional restoration as accurately as possible.

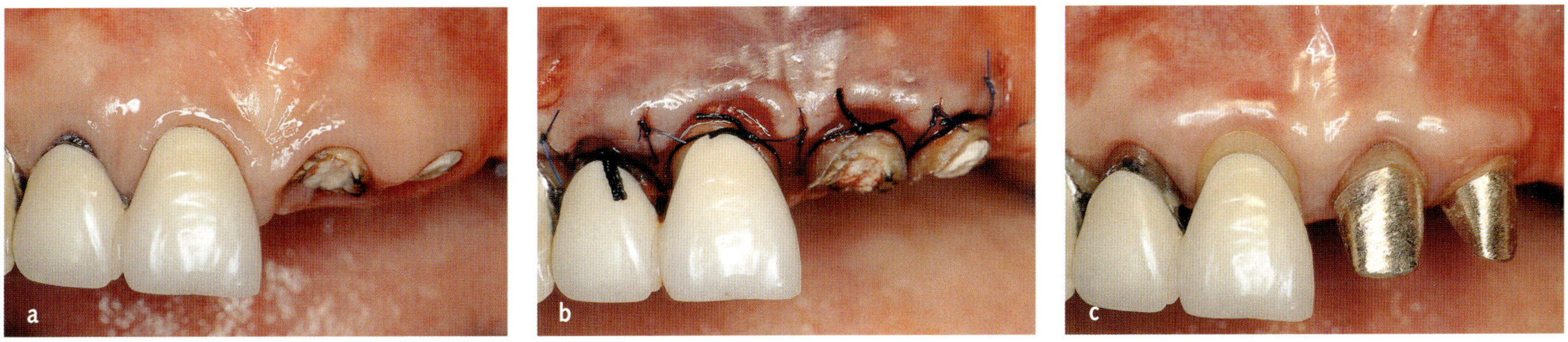

Fig 1-69 Clinical crown lengthening to obtain biologic width. The incision design, the flap design, and the method of bone correction used in the clinical crown lengthening procedure are chosen based on whether sufficient attached gingiva is available in the area, whether the gingiva is thick or thin, whether periodontal pockets are shallow or deep, and/or whether an esthetic problem is likely to occur. Particular attention should be paid to the position of the adjacent teeth on both sides and the degree of scalloping because they affect bone reduction volume. (a) The gingiva is thin, and the attached gingiva is very limited. (b) A partial-thickness flap was raised. A sulcular incision was made on the buccal side to raise a flap with scalloping. Horizontal and vertical bone reduction was conducted to achieve a scalloped shape and to secure biologic width. (c) One month after surgery. A healing period of at least 6 months is allowed while endodontic treatment and dowel posts and cores are provided.

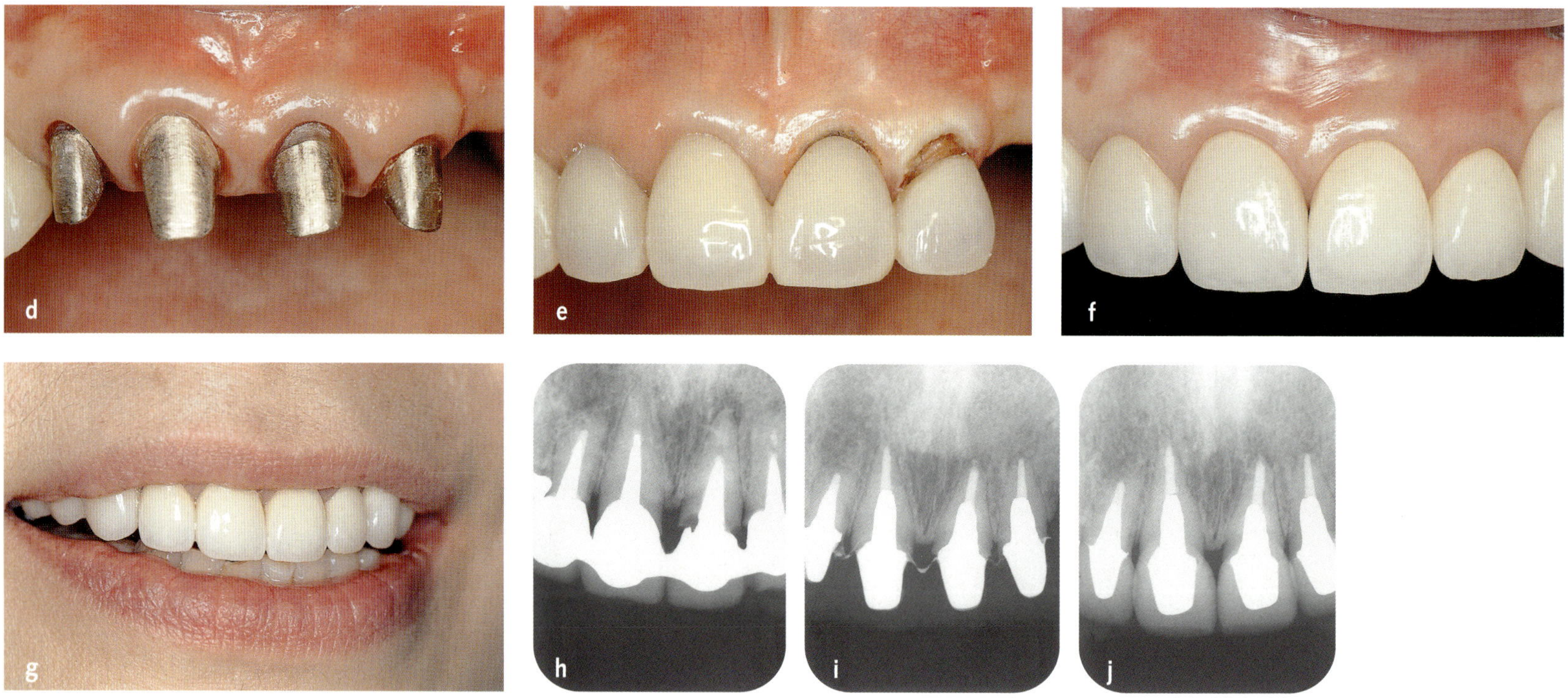

Fig 1-69 (cont) (d) Six months after surgery. Subgingival preparation is conducted gradually to complete subgingival contours. The thick gingiva at the maxillary left incisors (particularly the lateral incisor) led to creeping attachment coronally, making the cervical line higher on the left. (e) Gingivoplasty was conducted to adjust the cervical line. (f) Procera all-ceramic single crowns were delivered for the maxillary incisors. The cervical line is aligned. The interdental papillae are conserved. (g) The incisal edges are in harmony with the lower lip. (h) Periapical lesions, secondary caries, and disturbance of bone trabeculae (occlusal trauma) at the first visit. (i) At reevaluation. (j) At the delivery of prostheses. Disturbance of bone trabeculae and periapical lesions are improved.

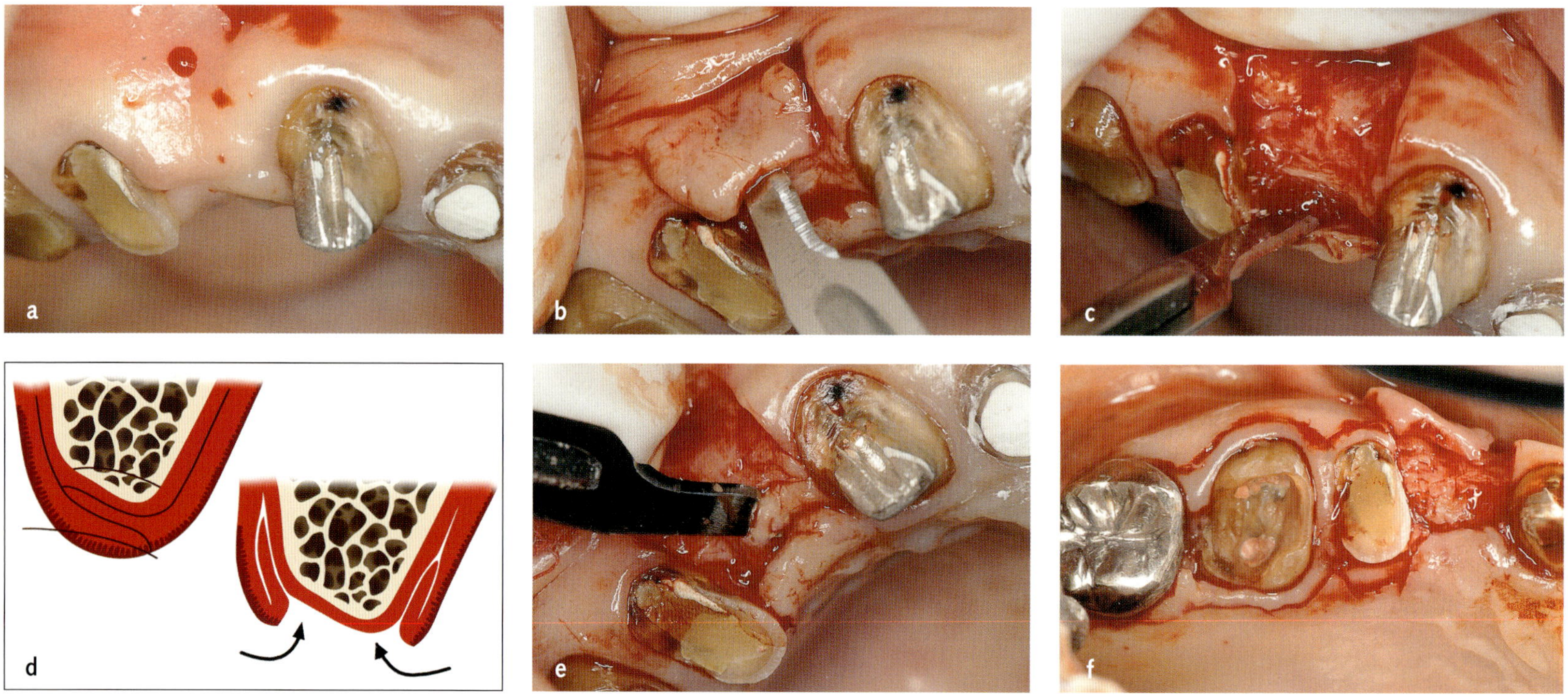

Fig 1-70 Ridge augmentation in the edentulous area and clinical crown lengthening. (a to d) Roll technique is used on the buccal and lingual sides in the missing area. Although sufficient gingival tissue is available at the crest of the maxillary right first premolar area (Seibert class I), attached gingiva on the buccal side will be lost if gingivoplasty is conducted. Accordingly, the buccal and lingual partial-thickness flaps were laterally repositioned. (e) Connective tissue on the crest is thinned. (f) Attached gingiva was sufficient, and the gingival thickness was moderate. Therefore, resective surgery with full-thickness flaps and bone reduction was performed. Clinical crown lengthening was conducted for subgingival caries. Scallop-shaped inverse bevel incisions were made to raise full-thickness flaps around the maxillary right second premolar and molars.

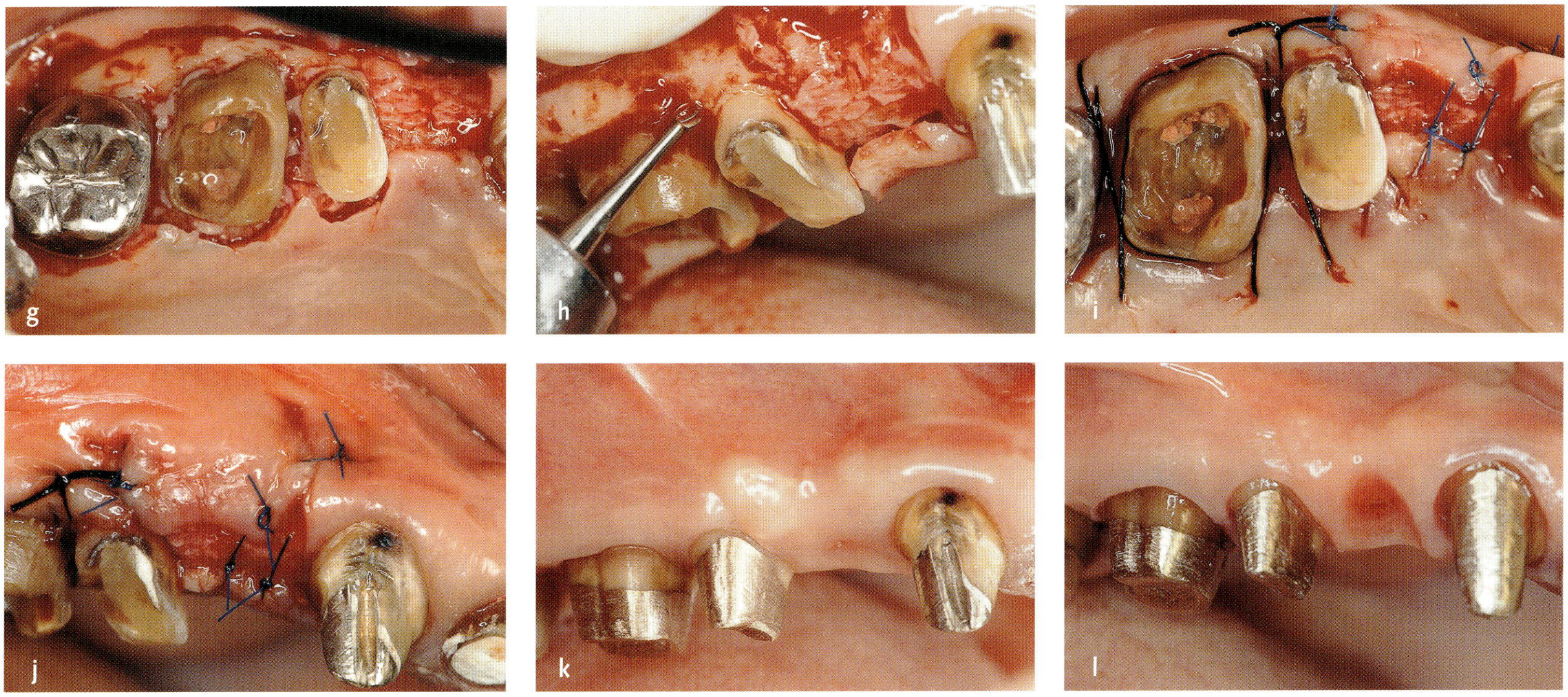

Fig 1-70 (cont) (g and h) After the gingival tissue was removed as one piece, bone reshaping was conducted with round burs and chisels to secure biologic width. (i and j) Suturing. (k) Clinical photograph taken 2 months after surgery. Sufficient attached gingiva is obtained. (l) Clinical photograph taken 7 months after surgery. Tooth by tooth, treatment progresses through endodontics, dowel posts and cores, and subgingival preparation. After gingivoplasty, the ovate pontic is to be refined.

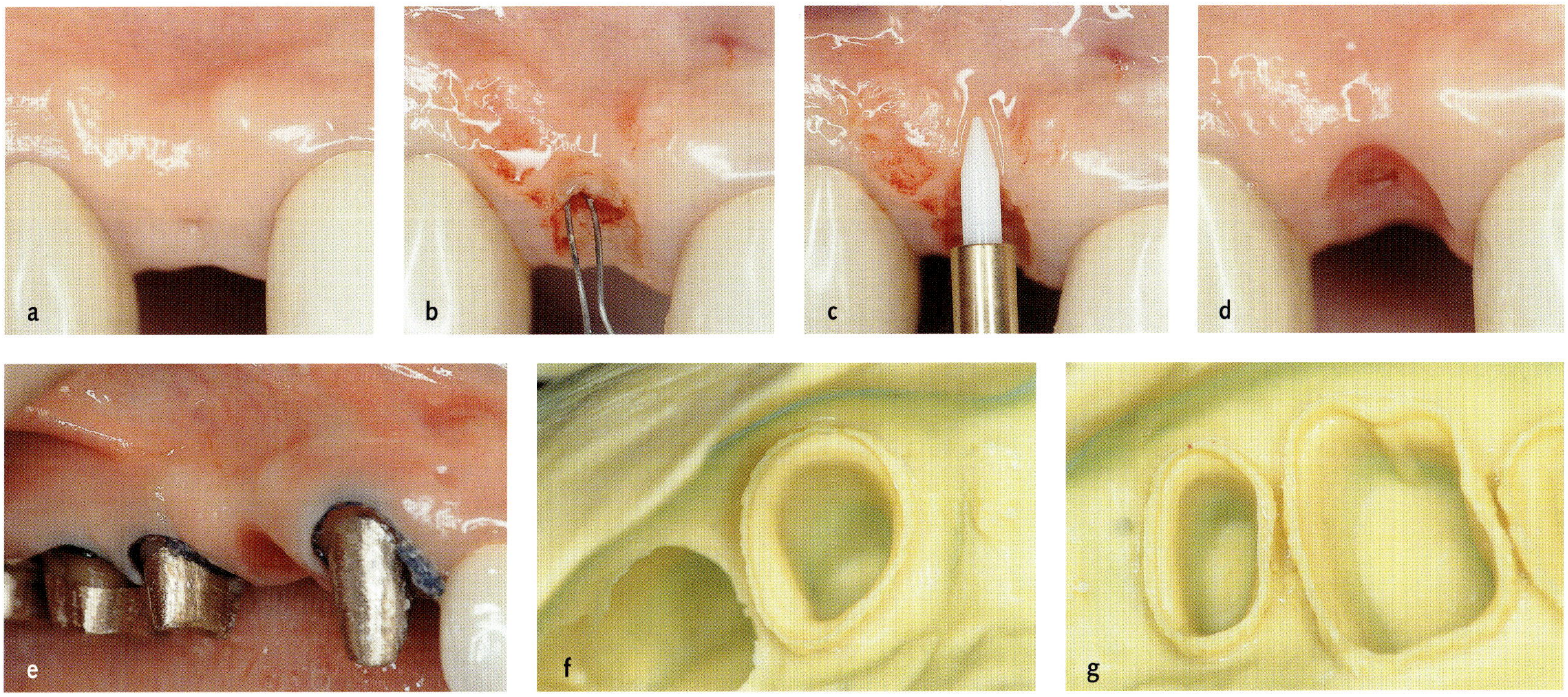

Fig 1-71 Ovate pontic. (a) Eight months after roll technique was applied buccally and lingually. Sufficient soft tissue is available in the pontic region. (b) Using electric cautery, the tissue is prepared to receive the base of the pontic. (c) A porcelain bur is used to further trim the gingiva. (d) Soft tissue 3 weeks after the trimming. Autopolymerizing resin is added to the pontic of the provisional restoration to complete an ovate shape. (e to g) After confirming keratinized gingiva, balance of interdental papillae with adjacent teeth, and conformity of the cervical line, HIT impression is taken with double retraction cord technique. The margins of the provisional restoration are frequently adjusted to ensure subgingival contour for the completion of the prostheses with good tissue support.

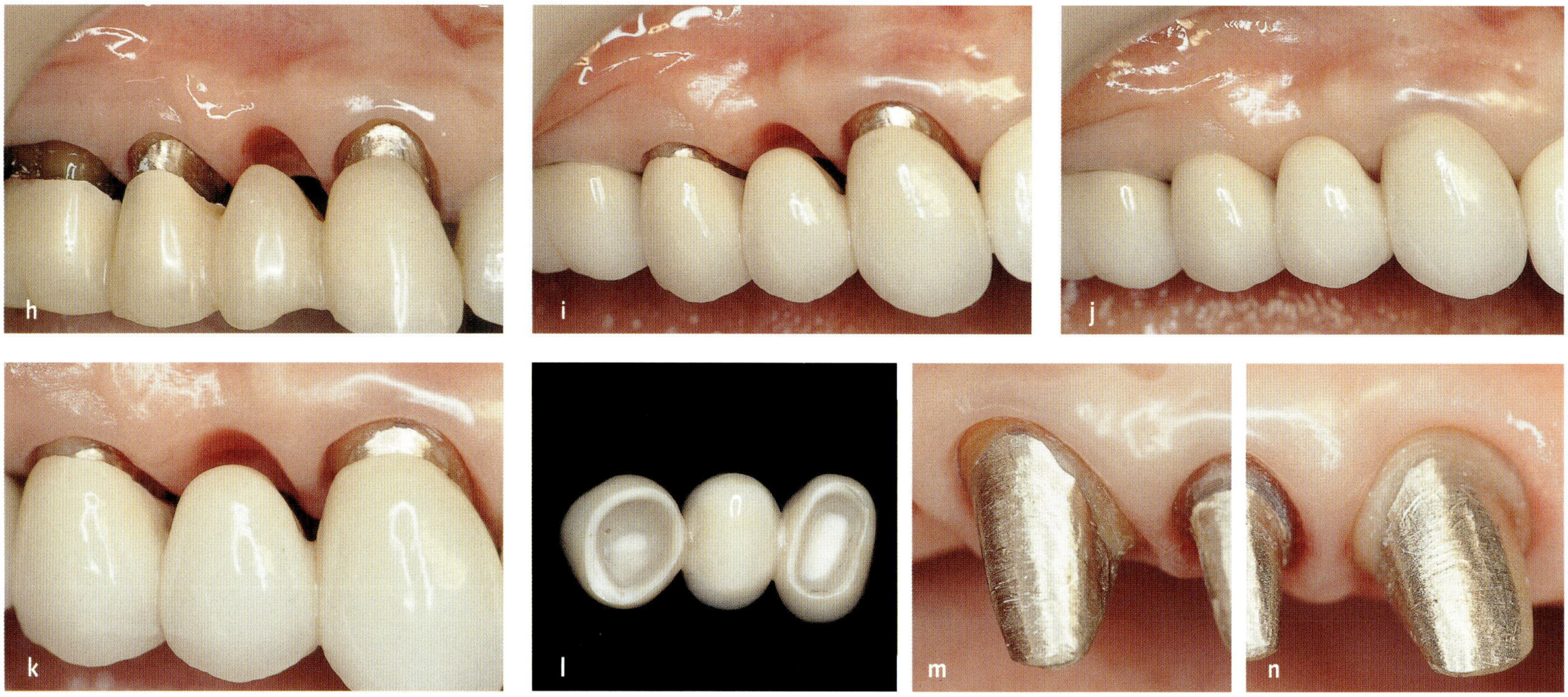

Fig 1-71 (cont) (h) The final provisional restoration. The final prosthesis should follow the final provisional restoration as closely as possible, which can present a challenge. (i and j) The final prostheses are delivered. Conditions are stable. Interdental papillae are restored and in good harmony with the prostheses. (k) Abutment teeth and the pontic region. Note interdental papillae (transitional forms between the buccal and lingual papillae and the gingival col). (l) In-Ceram all-porcelain fixed partial denture. (m and n) Clinical photographs taken 2 weeks after temporary cementation. Delicate and balanced gingival col are obtained. JRVT dowel posts and cores.

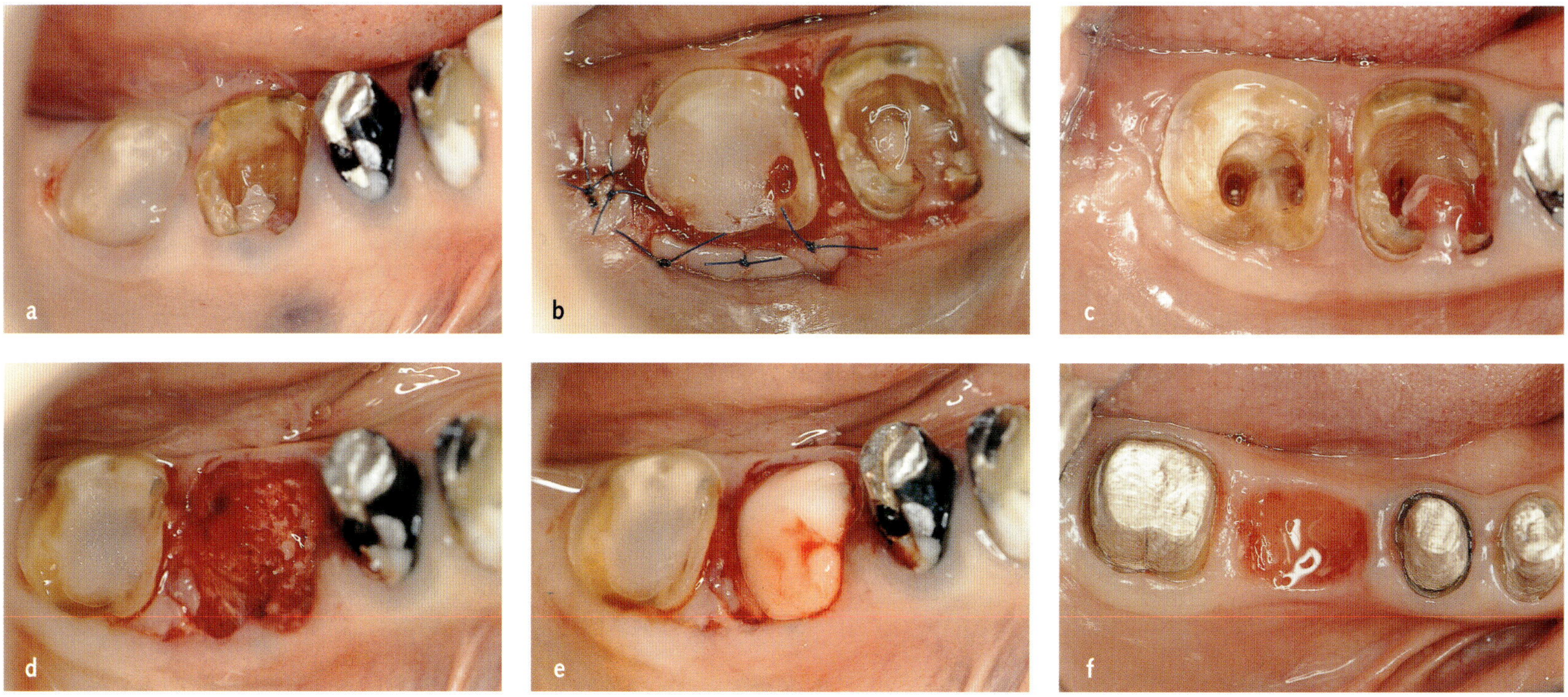

Fig 1-72 Healing of an extraction socket and formation of an ovate form. (a) Subgingival caries at the mandibular right premolars and molars. The second molar has only a residual root. There is a perforation at the septum of the first molar. The second premolar has noticeable black discoloration. (b) In order to confirm the possibility of saving the tooth, at first crown lengthening was conducted only for the second molar. Because there was no attached gingiva and the gingiva present was thin, partial-thickness flaps were raised and repositioned apically (with bone resection). (c) Crown lengthening resulted in healthy dentin and attached gingiva for the mandibular right second molar. A gingival polyp was observed at the floor of the pulp chamber of the adjacent first molar, and it was determined that the tooth could not be saved. (d and e) After extraction of the mandibular right first molar. CollaPlug was inserted in the extraction socket to enhance healing. (f) During the following 6-month healing period, root canal treatment was conducted for the mandibular right premolars and second molar. (The second molar has a separating dowel post and core.) Also, periodontal conditions were to be improved.

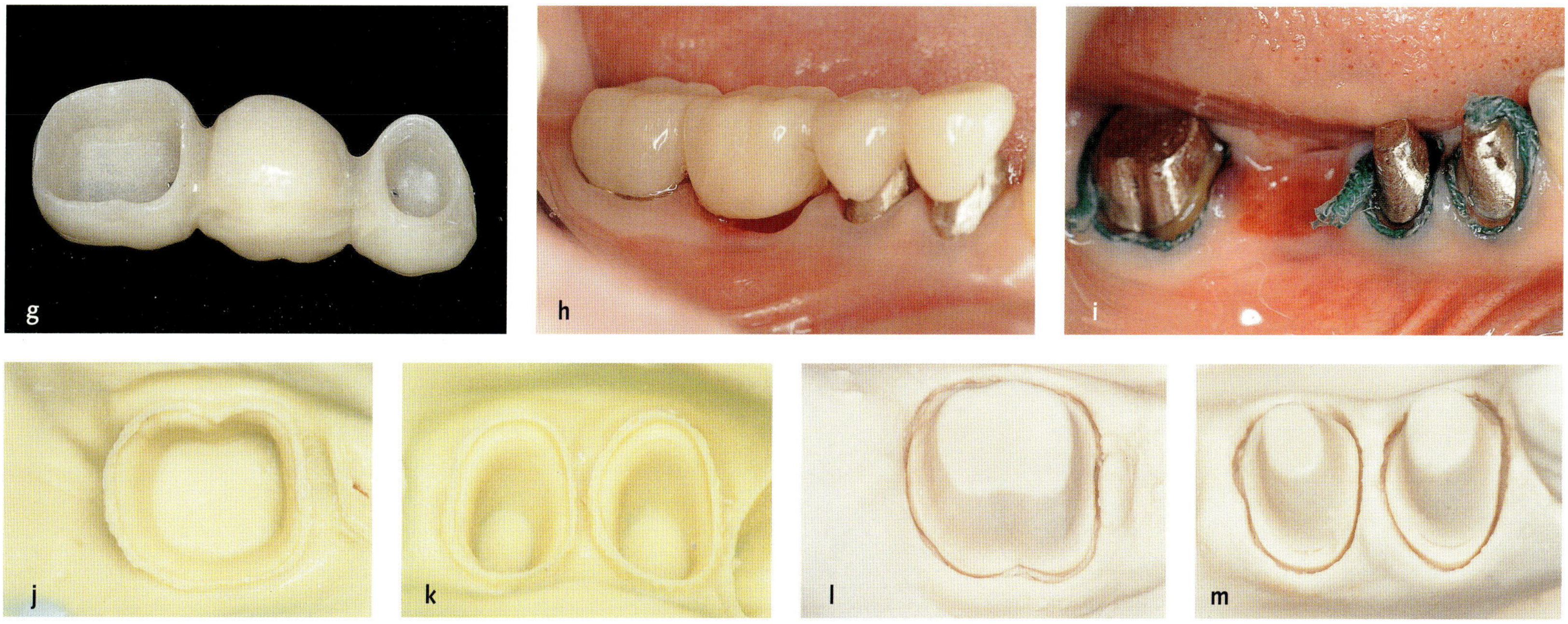

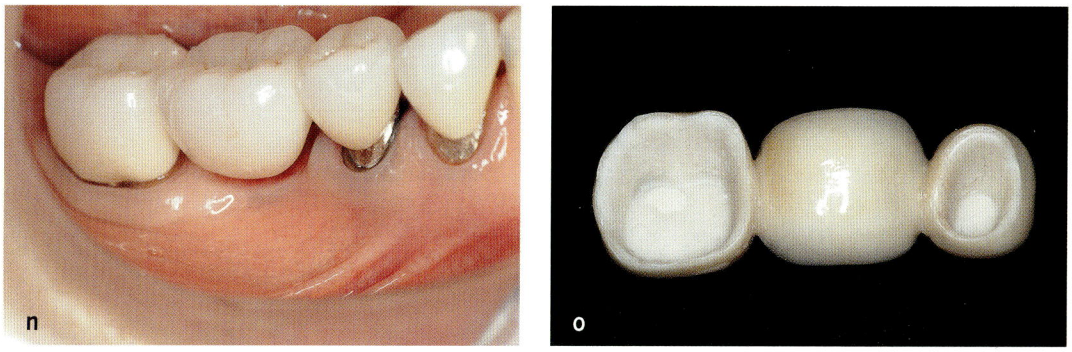

Fig 1-72 (cont) (g) Autopolymerizing resin is added to the base of the pontic to create an ovate shape. (h) Conformity between subgingival contours and interdental papillae was enhanced. (i) HIT impression was taken using the double-cord technique with PreCord and Ultrapak in accordance with the gingival sulci. (j to m) HIT impression. Clear preparation margins are shown. The double-cord technique allows this result without damage to the gingiva. (n) Trial of the final prosthesis, which follows the contour of the provisional restoration. Note the transition of natural gingival col form. (o) In-Ceram all-ceramic fixed partial denture connecting the mandibular right second premolar and molars (pontic: first molar).

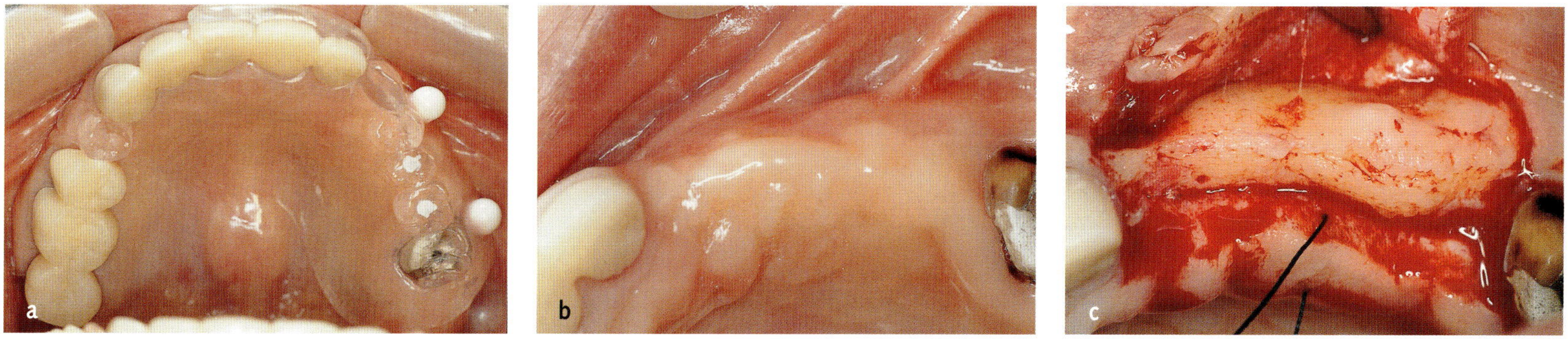

Fig 1-73 Implant placement in an edentulous area. (a) Planning for implants using a template. (CT scan was conducted with the template on.) (b) Before surgery. (c) Slip incision was made on the palate. Full-thickness flaps were raised. Palatal bone resorption was observed. There was almost no bone left in the area of the canine.

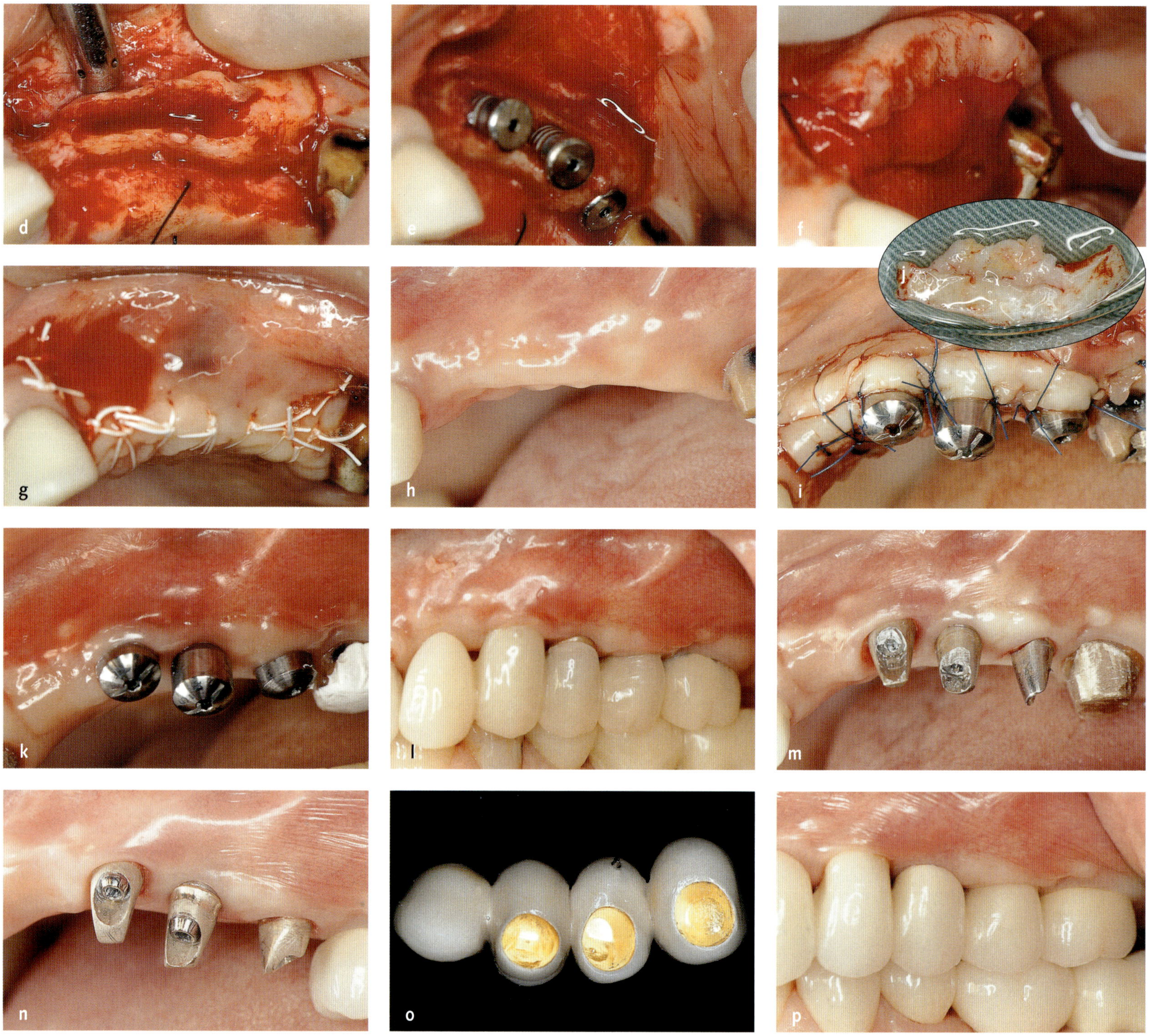

Fig 1-73 (cont) (d) The bone was split and inclined palatally. Three double-threaded implants were placed (3.75 × 13 mm). (e) To achieve conformity of the cervical line from the maxillary left lateral incisor to the second molar, implants were exposed over the bony crest. A releasing incision was used on the flap under the mucogingival junction. (f) The bone graft was covered with resorbable membrane (vertical bone augmentation). (g) Vertical mattress suture. (h) After 1 month. Conditions are stable without gingival dehiscence. (i and j) After 8 months. Because the cover screws were exposed as a result of pressure from the removable denture, soft tissue augmentation was conducted. Connective tissue graft with epithelium was obtained from the palate in the area from the maxillary left canine to the second molar and transplanted. (k) After 1 month. (l) After 2 months. Provisional restoration. (m) Provisional abutments. (n) Final abutments. (o) Porcelain fixed partial denture with cantilever. (p) Thirteen months after implant placement.

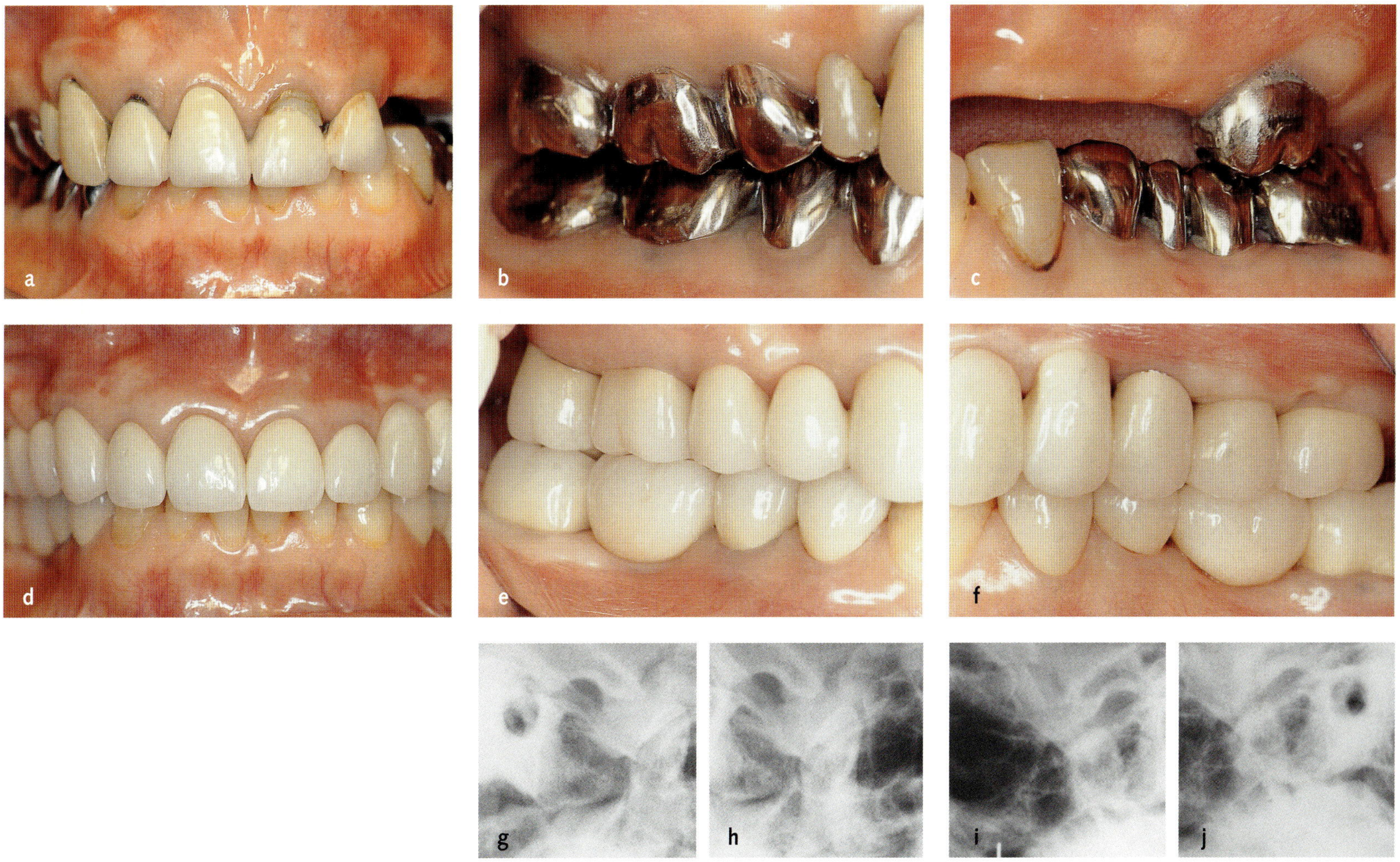

Fig 1-74 Homeostasis of the occlusal plane, the bone level, and the gingival level. (a to c) At the first visit. (d to f) Crown-lengthening procedures were completed at each region, and homeostasis of the occlusal plane, the bone level, and the gingival level was restored. (Prostheses by Chojiro Masuda, RDT.) (g and h) Before treatment, the condyles were pushed posteriorly and did not move much, even during maximum opening. The anterior part of the top of the condyles seems to be worn down. (i and j) After treatment, the condyles move significantly during maximum opening.

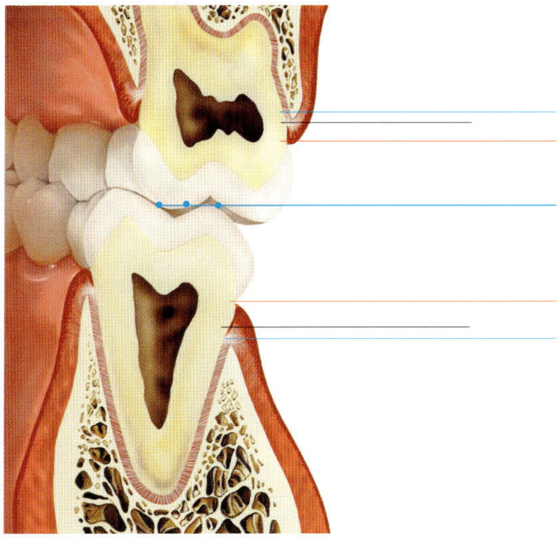

Homeostasis

Biologic width serves as an important guideline in the restoration of periodontally compromised teeth and teeth with subgingival caries. This hypothesis is based on the concept of homeostasis as mesenchymal tissue having a certain width of ectodermal tissue between it and the outermost layer of tissue. This homeostasis is, from a tooth-unit perspective, the width of healthy root surface required for connective tissue attachment and epithelial attachment. In a dentition-unit expression, it can be redefined as the attachment level and continuity of the cervical scallop line. The distance between the occlusal plane (the plane formed by cusp-to-fossa contact points at intercuspation) and the bony crest should fall within a certain range. In the posterior region, scalloping of the bone and gingiva and the overbite of the cusps become more shallow. Since they are constant in each tooth type, symmetric appearance results. This distance will not change if lost clinical crown is lengthened via extrusion. When a clinical crown is lengthened surgically, crown height is increased prosthetically.

This viewpoint of dentition-unit homeostasis is clinically important. Conditions without symmetry suggest abnormality. Homeostasis is lost when forces are not in balance (see chapter 2) or attachment is lost because of inflammation. In this case, priority should be given to restoration of homeostasis, which is restoration of the occlusal plane and bone leveling. Thus, in occlusal reconstruction, homeostasis of the distance between the occlusal plane and the bony crest is the first priority. In other words, when inflammation control and an appropriate jaw position are established, bone leveling is conducted, envisioning the adjustment of the occlusal plane. This is the comprehensive treatment plan.

Comprehensive Diagnosis of Occlusion-Unit Pathology and Treatment Goals

Harmony between tooth-unit morphology and occlusion-unit function

Examination of occlusion is divided broadly into two categories: examination of static (or morphologic) occlusion—such as the relative positional relationship and contact relationship between the maxilla and mandible and border movements of mandible—and examination of dynamic (or functional) occlusion—such as postural habits expressed in the dentition, sleep postures, the rhythm of masticatory movements, mandibular movement paths, contact balance, and the intensity of occlusal force.

The occlusion-unit approach (Case 1-8) aims at the central masticatory pattern, masticatory muscles, and temporomandibular joints, which are closely connected with dentition-unit static occlusion. In examination of dynamic occlusion, it is determined whether dentition-unit morphology and occlusion-unit functions are harmonized. For example, whether guidance is excessive or insufficient has to be evaluated not merely from a morphologic point of view but in harmony with the central masticatory pattern. Also, when there is hypertonia of circumoral muscles, a differential diagnosis needs to be made to determine whether it is merely a result of the central masticatory pattern or triggered by excessive guidance or occlusal interferences.

Case 1-8 Interdental spaces treated with an occlusion-unit approach

Although one must be cautious when changing a jaw position, there is even more risk involved in leaving a shifted mandible as it is and addressing only the resulting problems. When loss of occlusal support, malocclusion of a dentition, abnormality of a joint, and/or other conditions are associated with a problem in the mandibular position, inevitably the mandibular position itself will have to be addressed. When the intercuspal position is relatively stable, the clinician is forced to decide whether to cope with the patient's chief complaint only as an emergency measure or to conduct full-mouth reconstruction. Leaving the problem of the mandibular position as it is and treating the resulting problems often causes iatrogenic complications.

Patient: *49-year-old woman at the time of first visit in 1998*
Chief complaint: *Sensitivity to cold at the maxillary left incisors and protruding anterior teeth*

The etiology of this case is relatively uncomplicated, relating solely to a problem with the mandibular position. The occlusal plane is higher on the left and the diastema between the maxillary central incisors is apparent. Periodontal disease is not a significant problem. Although the maxillary left first molar has a Class II furcation involvement, periodontal pockets are about 3 mm in all the regions. The diagnosis is anterior disc displacement with reduction of the left TMJ. Treatment should be focused on the larger problem of the mandibular position, rather than closing the interdental spaces (Figs 1-76 to 1-80).

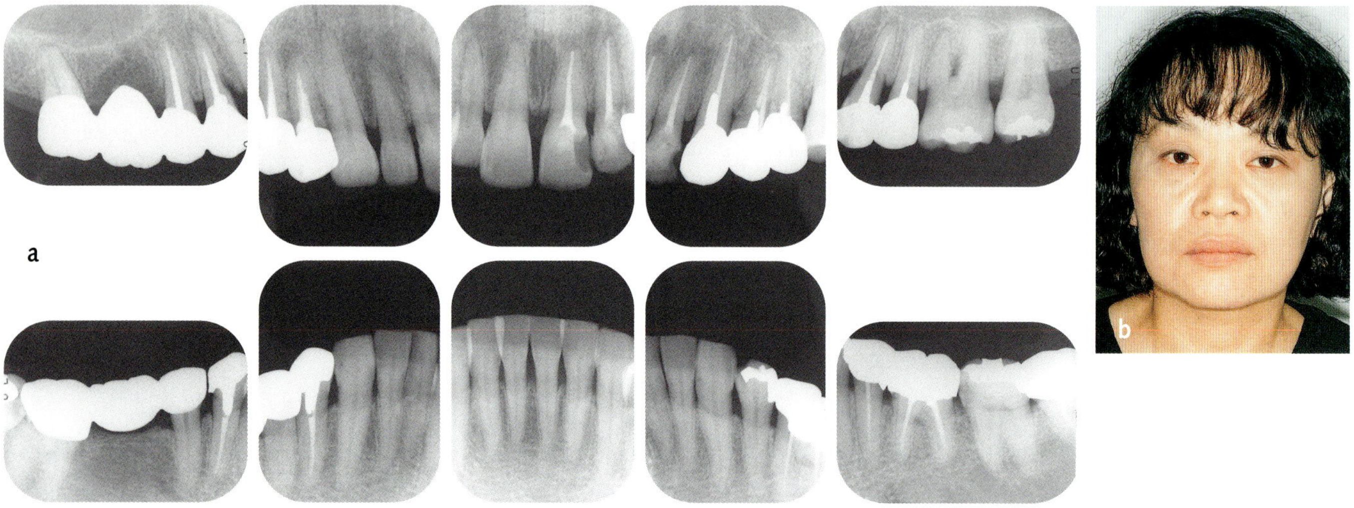

Fig 1-76 The patient complained of a feeling that the jaw receded, sensitivity to cold at the maxillary left incisors, a diastema between the maxillary central incisors, and protruding anterior teeth. She experienced painful headaches, stiff shoulders, and a stiff neck. One-time clicking sound was observed during opening the mouth on the left side. (a) There is a root fracture of the maxillary right second molar and Class II furcation involvement of the maxillary left first molar. Disturbance of bone trabeculae and condensing osteitis are observed, indicating traumatic pathology. (b) The left corner of the mouth is higher than the right, the left masseter is hypertrophic (left clenching), and the intermaxillary distance is shorter on the left side.

Ideal occlusion and pathologic occlusion

There is wide diversity in static occlusion. Even if an occlusion that is generally considered ideal is provided, not all patients adapt to it easily. Also, there is ethnic or racial difference observed in ideal occlusal relationships. This is easily understood if we adopt a hypothesis that masticatory movements are regulated by a central pattern generator in the brain stem. The authors consider that one of the major causes of pathologic occlusion is disharmony between this central masticatory pattern and peripheral movement paths.

The authors term typical pathologic occlusions caused by disharmony between central and peripheral occlusions *tight occlusion* and *loose occlusion* (see chapter 2). In loose occlusion, efficiency in biting off food is decreased because of excessive occlusal wear of posterior teeth, and masticatory movements are larger and wider in anteroposterior and lateral directions. With such an occlusal relationship, because of great masticatory forces and lateral forces applied to the teeth, periodontal supporting tissue is subject to severe stress. On the other hand, tight occlusion presents with high cusps and steep cusp angles in terms of tooth-unit pathology, which makes it difficult to slide smoothly from the intercuspal position in anteroposterior and lateral directions. There are also dentition-unit tight occlusions in which teeth are almost locked and cannot move, which seems to induce clenching. It also causes excessive tension in the temporomandibular joints, masticatory muscles, and circumoral muscles, generating external forces that jolt the teeth.

Tight occlusion often seems to be caused by the guidance provided to an individual with a grinding masticatory pattern through orthodontic treatment or full-mouth fixed partial dentures, which make masticatory movement paths artificially vertical.

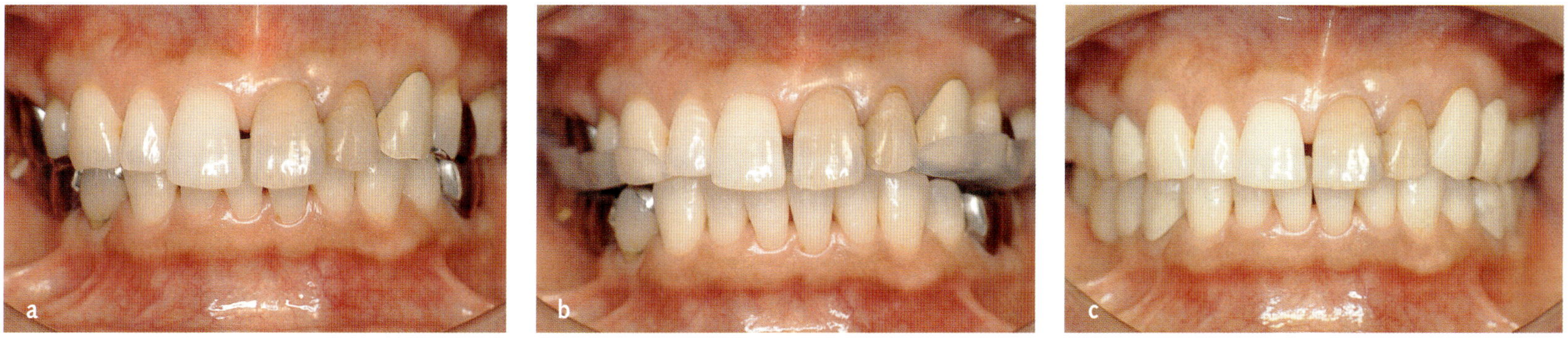

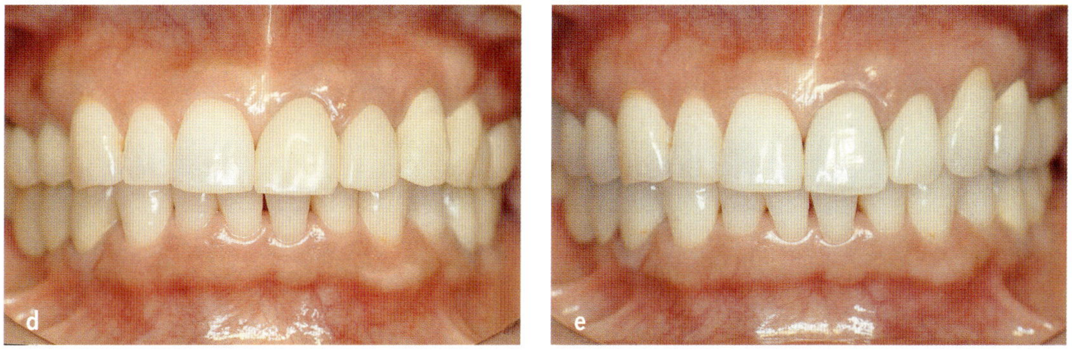

Fig 1-77 Intraoral frontal view of changes in mandibular position. (a) At the first visit. Remarkable loss of vertical height. The mandible is shifted in the left posterior direction. (b) A stabilization bite plane was delivered to guide the jaw to a relaxed position. (c) While conducting root canal treatment and post-and-core buildup, teeth are replaced with provisional restorations based on the relaxed jaw position. Implants were placed in the maxillary right molar region. (d) The final provisional restoration. The mandible's shift to the left is now improved, with the midline almost aligned. (e) Collarless porcelain restoration on the maxillary left incisors and canine and metal-ceramic restorations on the posterior teeth, 3 years and 5 months after the first visit.

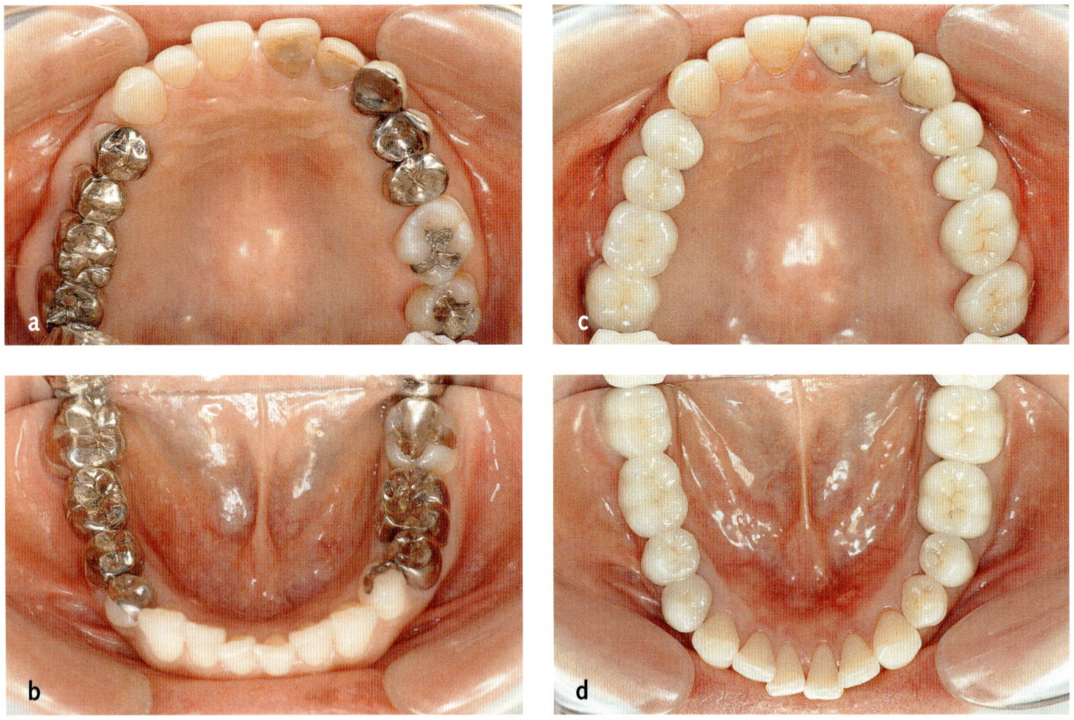

Fig 1-78 Occlusal views. (a and b) Arch form abnormality and malposition of teeth were observed. Curve of Spee was deep in the mandible. The left side had a reverse lateral curve. The buccal cusp of the maxillary left first premolar was high, holding the buccal surfaces of both opposing premolars. The occlusal surface of the mandibular left second molar was concave without a ridge, catching the lingual cusp of the opposing second molar. Because of these problems, the occlusal morphology of restorations on the left side was less than ideal. It was assumed that clenching developed as a result, with left TMD as a consequence. (c and d) After the occlusal reconstruction, integrity of the arches was obtained. The arch forms are symmetric. Implants were placed in the maxillary right molar region. (Prostheses by Kiyoharu Takada, RDT.)

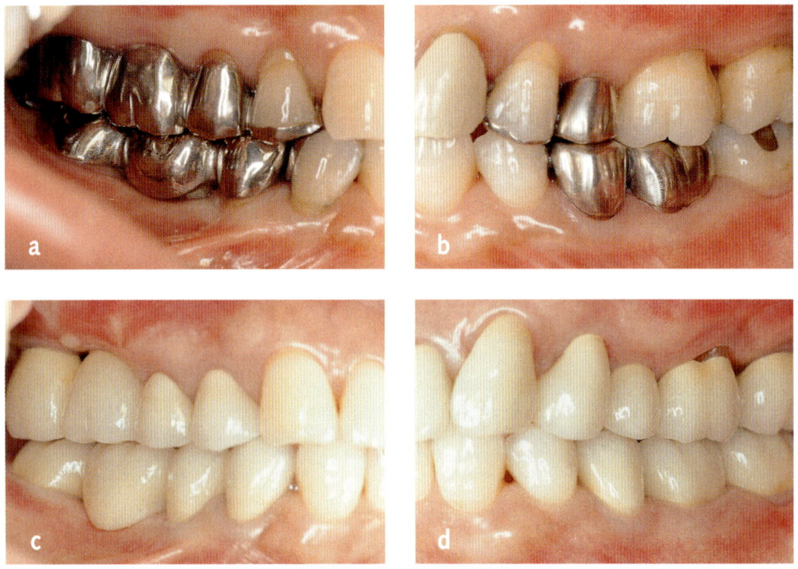

Fig 1-79 Lateral views. (a) Right side at the first visit. The dentition as a whole is depressed. (b) Left side at the first visit. The mandible is shifted to the left posterior, and the curve of Spee is deep. (c) Right side after treatment. Implants, which were placed immediately after the extraction of the maxillary right second molar and in a delayed manner after the extraction of the first molar, support the occlusion. (d) Left side after treatment. The left TMJ is on the disc. The mandible was advanced, increasing the vertical height of the posterior region.

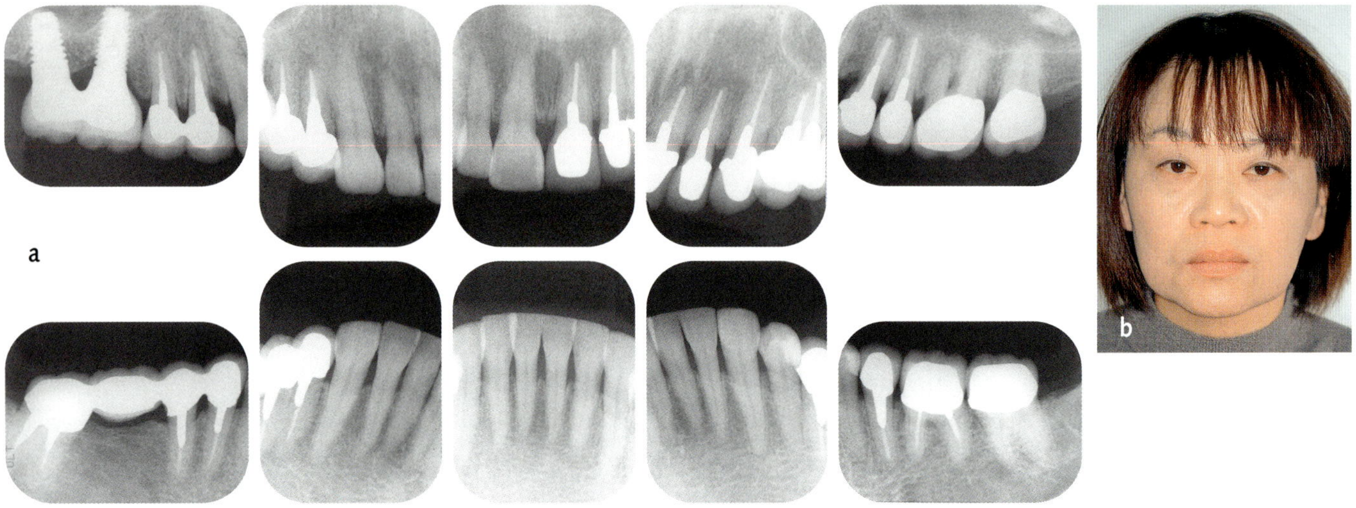

Fig 1-80 (a) Traumatic findings have disappeared. (b) The facial asymmetry is resolved, and the lower facial height is increased.

Treatment Goals and Maintenance in Cases with Occlusal Collapse

Examination

Occlusal collapse induces stomatognathic dysfunction via malposition, malformation, and loss of teeth with irreversible progressive attachment loss while also triggering systemic symptoms. When treating a patient with failed teeth, dentition, and/or occlusion, a diagnosis cannot be made without untying the intricately tangled threads of etiology, and in such cases collecting and analyzing information through examinations alone is not sufficient. These intricate factors must be explored through a process of examination of tissue responses to plaque control and force control, as well as reevaluation over a sufficient period of time.

Treatment objectives in occlusal collapse

Untreated loss of supporting tissue and tooth loss due to advanced periodontal disease, tooth malalignment, and deleterious habits and postures of the tongue or circumoral area cause pathologic migration of teeth, eventually leading to occlusal collapse with abnormal dentition or occlusion.

Although the progress of occlusal collapse may slow naturally, it will not stop altogether or resolve itself without therapeutic intervention. Because of this, the value of therapeutic intervention tends to be overestimated. Still, in treatment, the emphasis should be placed on bringing out the patient's natural healing ability to the maximum level.

The objective of treatment in occlusal collapse is restoration and maintenance of harmony in occlusal functions. Accordingly, reconstruction of occlusal collapse requires comprehensive treatments and therapies that skillfully combine control of inflammation and forces (Cases 1-9 to 1-11).

Constructing treatment objectives

Treatment objectives are constructed by evaluating the healing ability of the individual in a trial-and-error treatment process. An unlimited number of individual differences exist within a living body. Therefore, the clinician must determine to what extent the jaw function and morphology can be changed in each individual patient. It is futile to envision an ideal result independent of the healing ability of the individual.

The ultimate goal is to achieve maximal effect with minimal treatment within the possible limits. With that said, in constructing treatment objectives in occlusal collapse cases, priority should be given not to conservation of local tissue and/or restoration of ideal morphology but to restoration of occlusion as a whole and, eventually, recovery of systemic health. Consequently, treatment objectives and treatment methods are diverse, reflecting individual differences, such as age, expectation of esthetic recovery, and lifestyle. Treatment objectives and treatment methods should be decided based on sufficient informed consent. Even when a patient is highly dependent on specialists, the patient's perspective should be considered; a judgment should not be made only from a medicodental viewpoint.

Case 1-9 Considerations for functional rehabilitation and lifetime maintenance and stability

Patient: *53-year-old woman at the time of the first visit in 1990*

Chief complaint: *Her tongue was sore from abrasion, particularly in the regions of the tip and the right dorsum, and she could not chew hard food*

The oral examination at the first visit yielded the following observations: (1) indentations on the cheeks and tongue as well as anterior tongue thrusting; (2) instability of the ICP; (3) nonfunctional attrition in all molars and the mandibular anterior teeth, resulting in significant flaring in the maxillary and mandibular anterior regions, which was suspected to have caused the decrease in vertical height; (4) probing and radiographic examination indicated moderate to locally severe chronic periodontitis with furcation involvements in the maxilla and mandible; (5) degree 2 mobility for the maxillary incisors and mandibular right lateral incisor and second molar and degree 1 for the remaining teeth; (6) no jaw malfunction (clicking, trismus); (7) convex facial profile with hypertrophic masseter and relaxed lips, exposure of the maxillary central incisors between the lips, and suspected grinding; and (8) incorrect crown-root ratio (Figs 1-81 to 1-95).

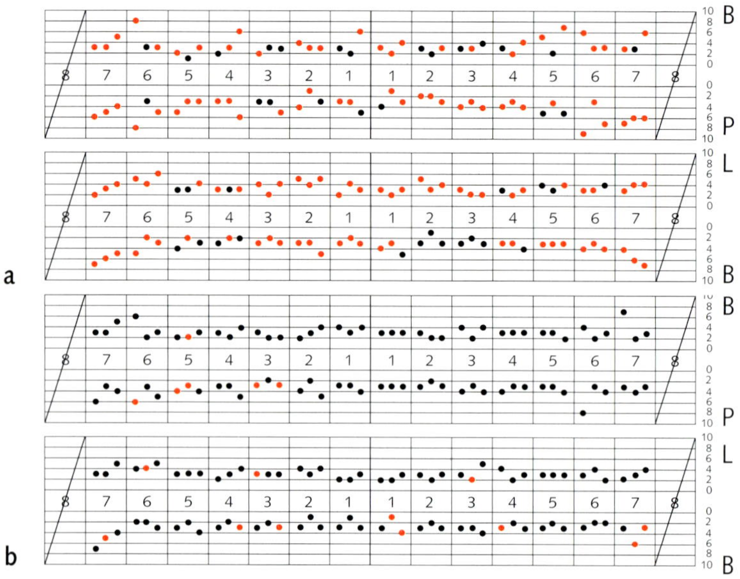

Fig 1-81 Probing charts. Red indicates bleeding. (a) At the first visit. (b) Six months after the first visit. Subsequently, periodontal surgery was conducted in all areas except the anterior mandible.

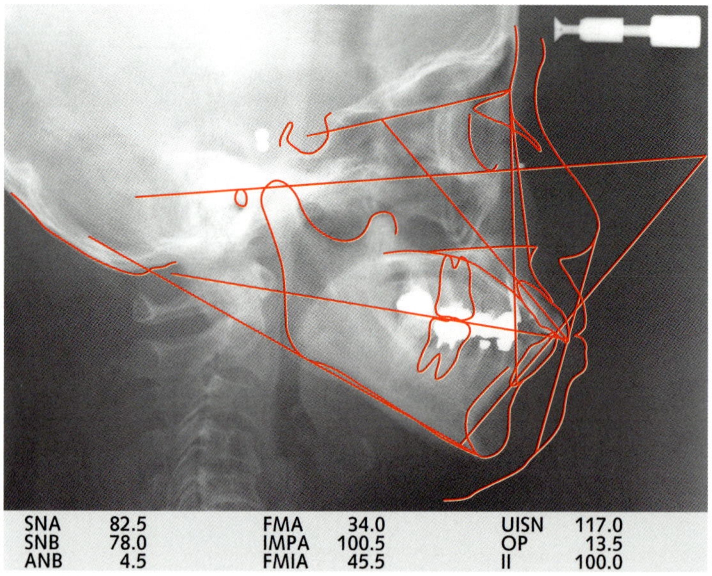

Fig 1-82 Lateral radiographic cephalogram at the first visit.

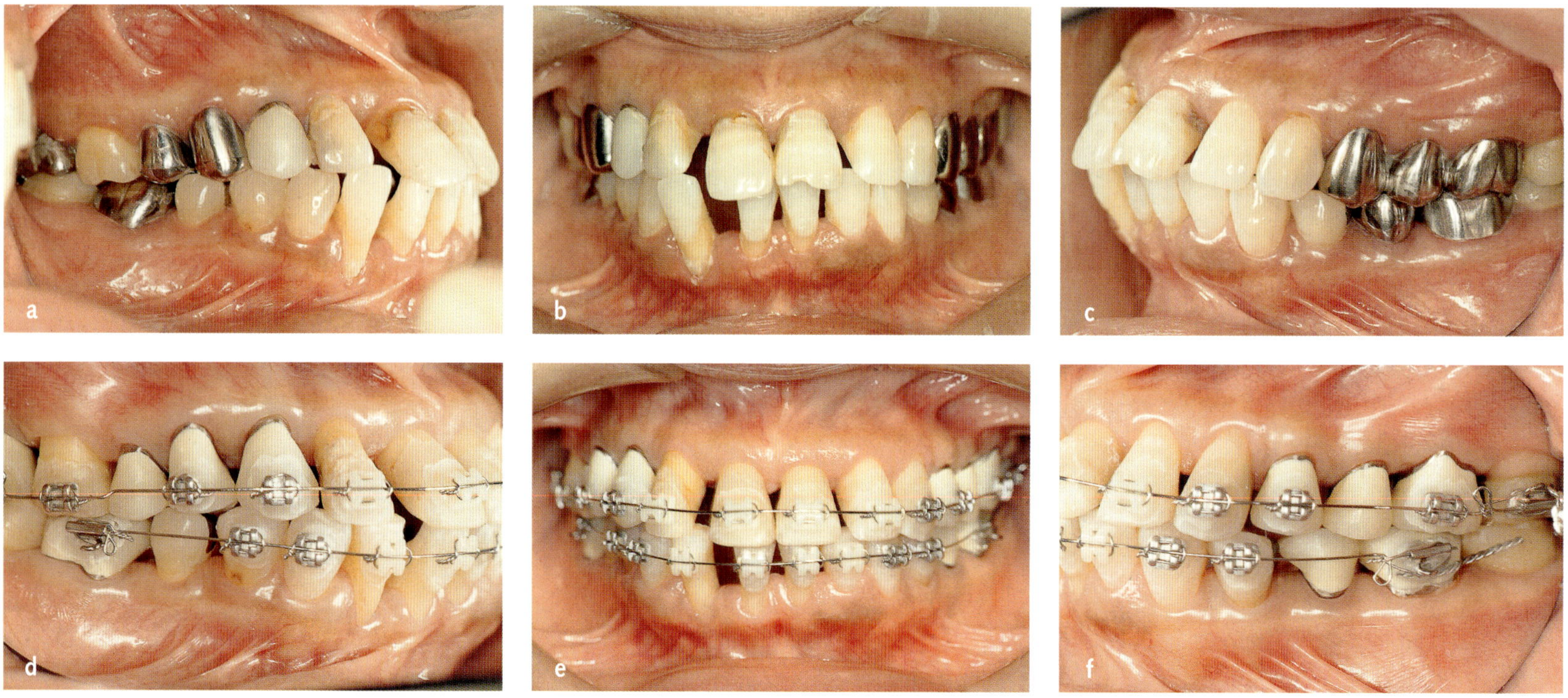

Fig 1-83 Occlusal reconstruction. (a to c) At the first visit. Due to periodontitis and bruxism, the anterior teeth are protruded, while the posterior teeth are intruded. (d to f) At 1 year and 8 months after the first visit. To improve furcation involvements and infrabony defects at the right molars, regenerative therapy using guided tissue regeneration (GTR) was conducted, followed by orthodontic tooth movement. Brackets were not attached to the left second premolars. The mandibular left molars were splinted with twisted wire.

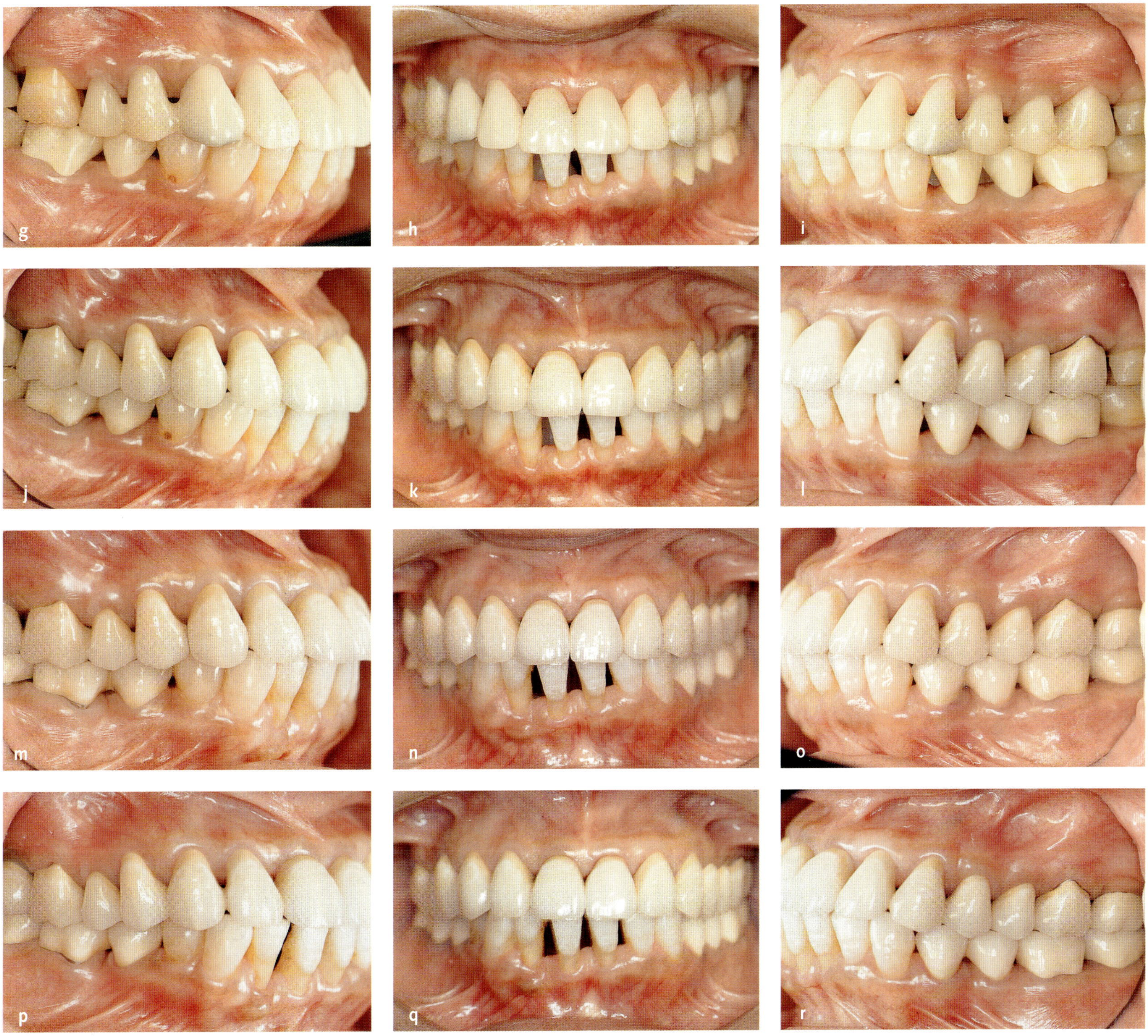

Fig 1-83 (cont) (g to i) Final provisional restoration. (j to l) Delivery of the final prosthesis (periodontal prosthesis), about 3 years after the first visit. The maxillary left and mandibular second molars have not received crown restorations. Relatively shallow canine guidance is provided. (m to o) At 8 years and 8 months after the first visit, 5 years and 8 months after delivery of the final prosthesis. The maxillary left and mandibular second molars received crown restorations. A new restoration was required for the mandibular right second molar. (p to r) At 12 years and 1 month after the first visit, 9 years and 1 month after delivery of final prosthesis. Note the shallow overbite of the anterior teeth to avoid overloading.

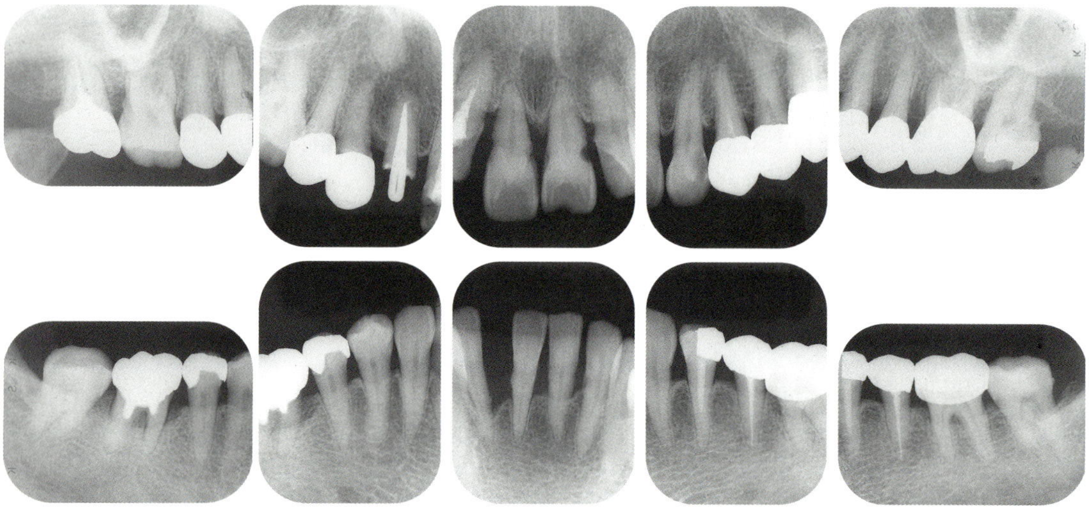

Fig 1-84 Full-mouth radiographs at the first visit. Moderate level of bone defects. The first molars exhibit class II furcation involvement. Secondary occlusal trauma is observed for all teeth.

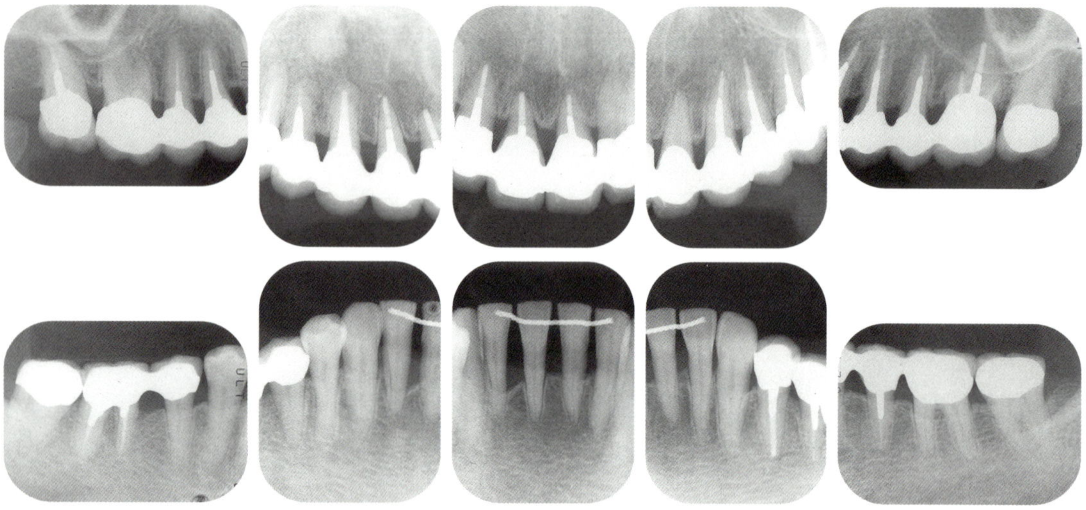

Fig 1-85 Full-mouth radiographs 5 years after the first visit, 2 years after the delivery of final prosthesis. As a result of periodontal therapy, tooth movement (harmony of morphology among adjacent and opposing teeth/dentition), and periodontal prosthesis (control of forces), there is improvement in periodontal tissue and secondary occlusal trauma, as well as bone regeneration. The maxillary central incisors and left canine underwent pulpectomy. Root canal treatment was conducted in the maxilla for the right lateral incisor, second premolar, and second molar and the left premolars and first molar and in the mandible for the left first premolar and the right first molar.

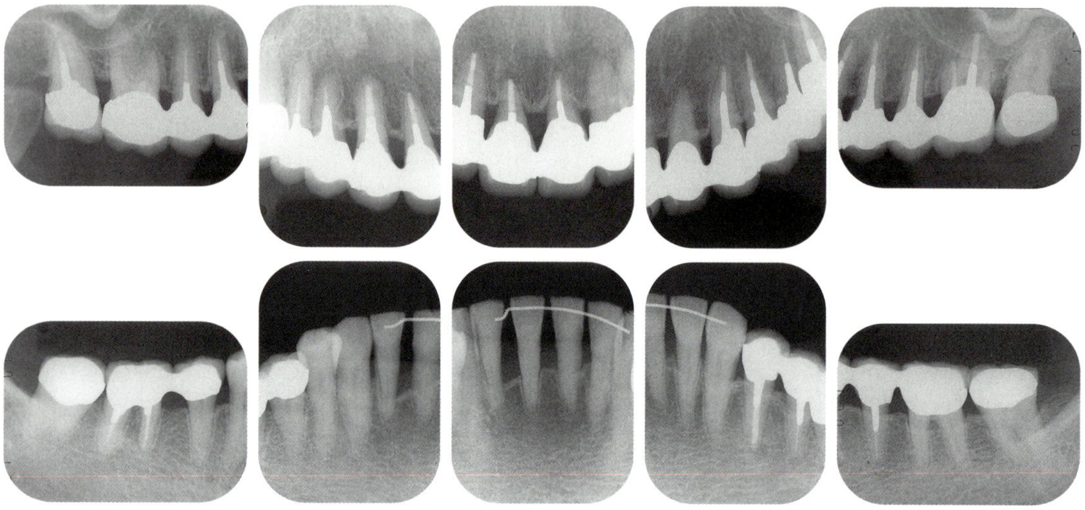

Fig 1-86 At 12 years and 3 months after the first visit. Additional treatment was provided for all second molars.

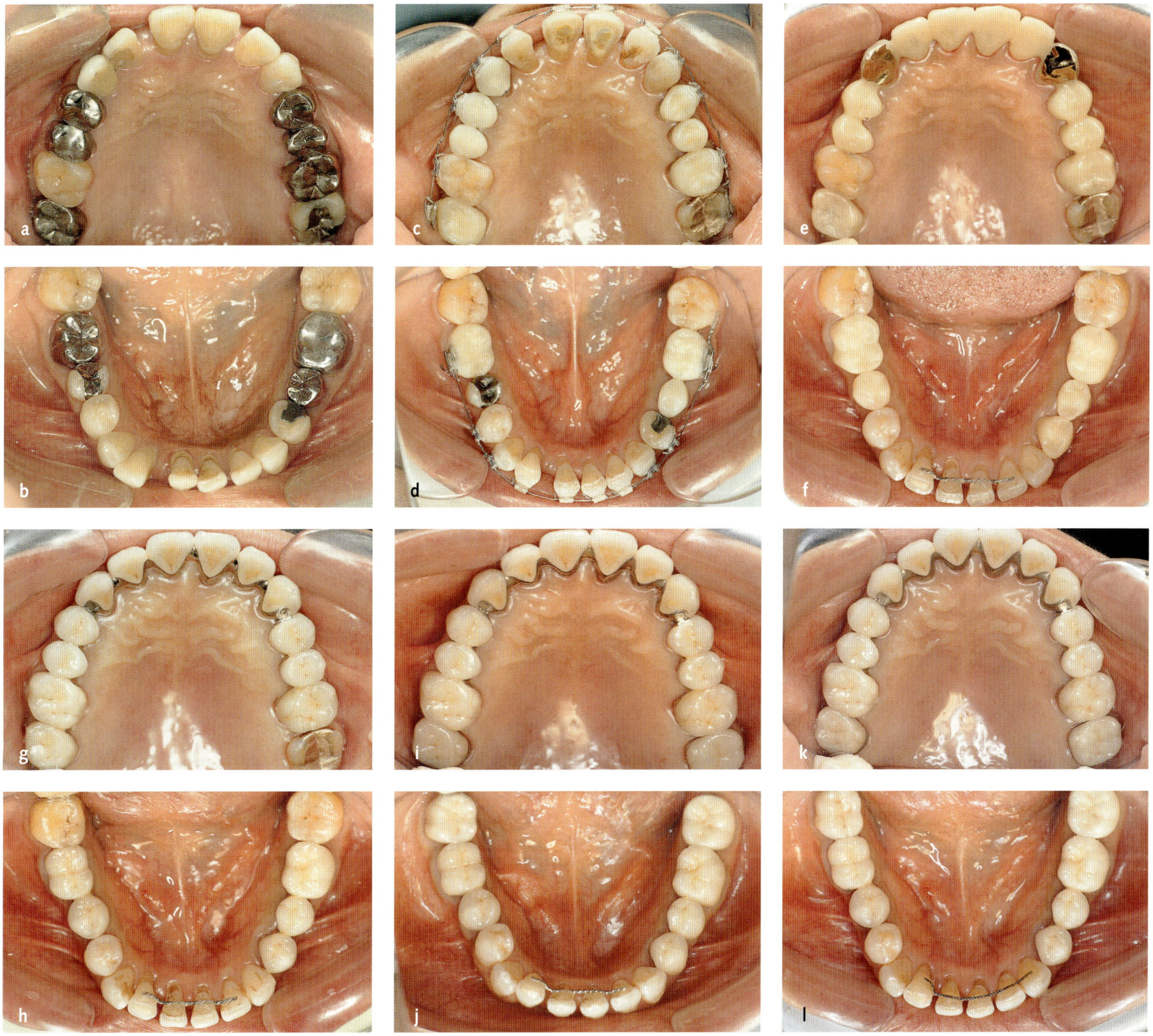

Fig 1-87 Reconstruction of both arches. (a and b) The causes of flaring are an unphysiologic mandibular position, advanced periodontal disease, inferior prostheses, a habitual wide path of masticatory movement, tongue thrusting, and/or grinding. Great care is taken in elucidating these complex collapse factors. In the mandible, the posterior teeth are flat and worn, and the anterior teeth are extremely worn. (c and d) Access flap for the maxillary anterior teeth, from canine to canine. After GTR with resorbable membrane for maxillary first molars, tooth movement was conducted to achieve harmony of morphology among adjacent and opposing teeth on the provisional restoration. Also for the mandibular right molars, tooth movement was conducted after regeneration therapy. After roughly restoring buccolingual positions of teeth by reshaping (in the area of the mandibular right lateral incisor) and myofunctional therapy, multiple brackets were applied. Intentional tooth movement is limited to the mesiodistal direction. (e and f) Final provisional restoration, 2 years and 5 months after the first visit. (g and h) Delivery of final prosthesis after remounting, 3 years after the first visit. All teeth in the maxilla from the right second molar to the left first molar are splinted (a collarless design is used from second premolar to second premolar). Keyways for splinting are located distal to the maxillary canines. The mandibular first molars have porcelain-fused-to-metal crowns, and the left premolars and right second premolar have collarless crowns, which are connected. Crown restorations are provided on the maxillary left and mandibular second molars because their extreme attrition was causing instability of the occlusion. (i and j) Occlusal view 8 years and 3 months after the first visit. The maxillary second molars, which had problems with fit, and severely worn teeth were restored again 1 year and 6 months after the delivery of final restoration. The mandibular right second molar also was restored again because of a fracture. (k and l) Occlusal view 12 years after the first visit, 9 years after delivery of final restoration. (Prostheses by Tsugumichi Kawasaki, RDT.)

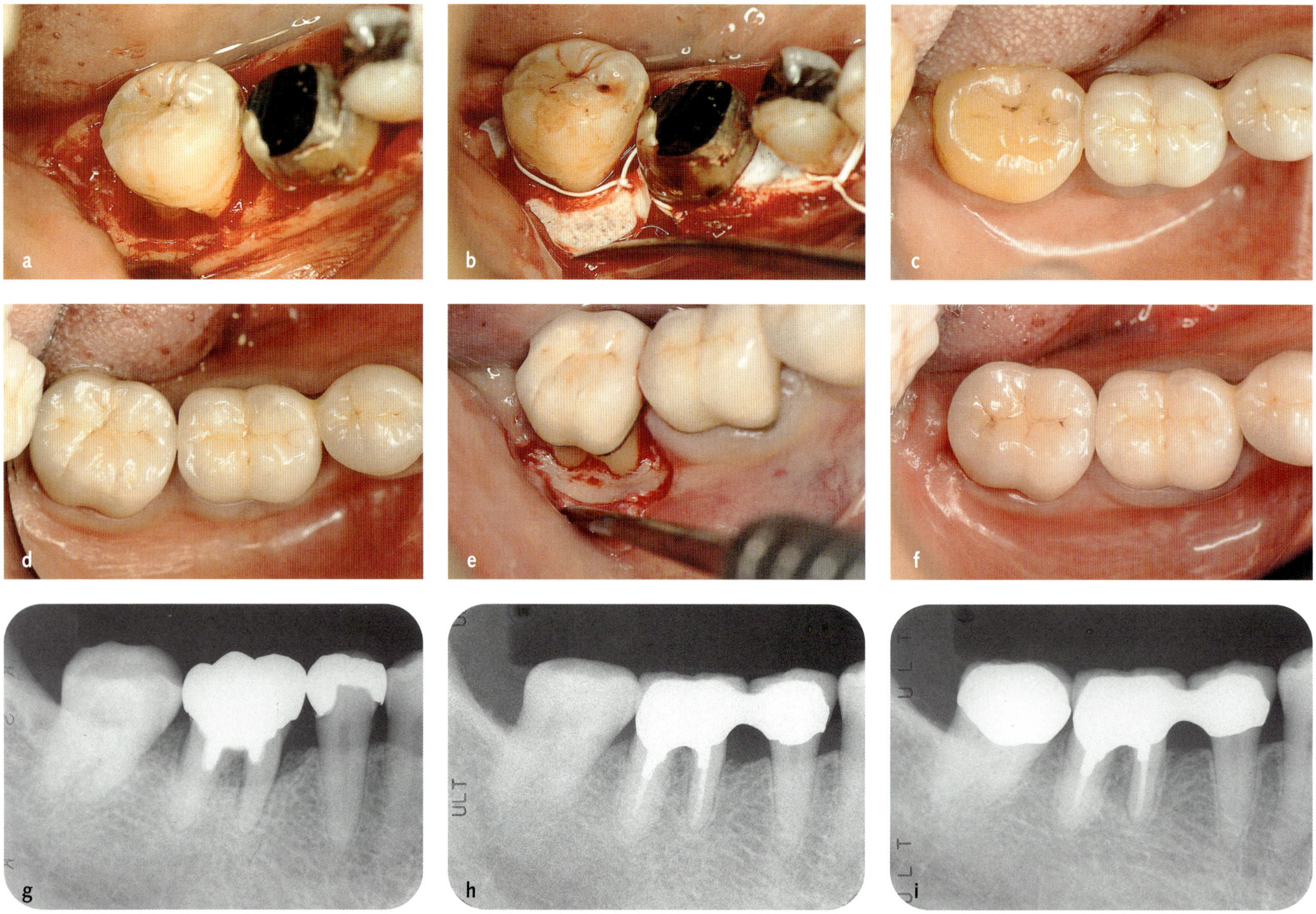

Fig 1-88 Treatment and follow-up for the mandibular right bone defect. (a) Seven months after the initial therapy. The mandibular right molars have class II furcation involvement, with the second molar presenting with a circumferential defect and a worn occlusal surface. (b) GTR membrane was applied to the buccal and distal sides of the second molar as well as the lingual and mesial sides of the first molar. (c) Two years and seven months after treatment. No restoration, only occlusal equilibration, was conducted for the second molar. (d) About 6 years after the first visit (January 1996). The second molar received crown restoration. (e) Bone regeneration at the second molar was confirmed at reentry. (f) Nine years and one month after the first visit. A new crown was delivered to the second molar. (g) Radiograph at the first visit. Class II furcation involvement and occlusal trauma at the mandibular right molars. (h) After treatment (3 years and 6 months after the first visit). (i) Conditions are stable 12 years after the first visit.

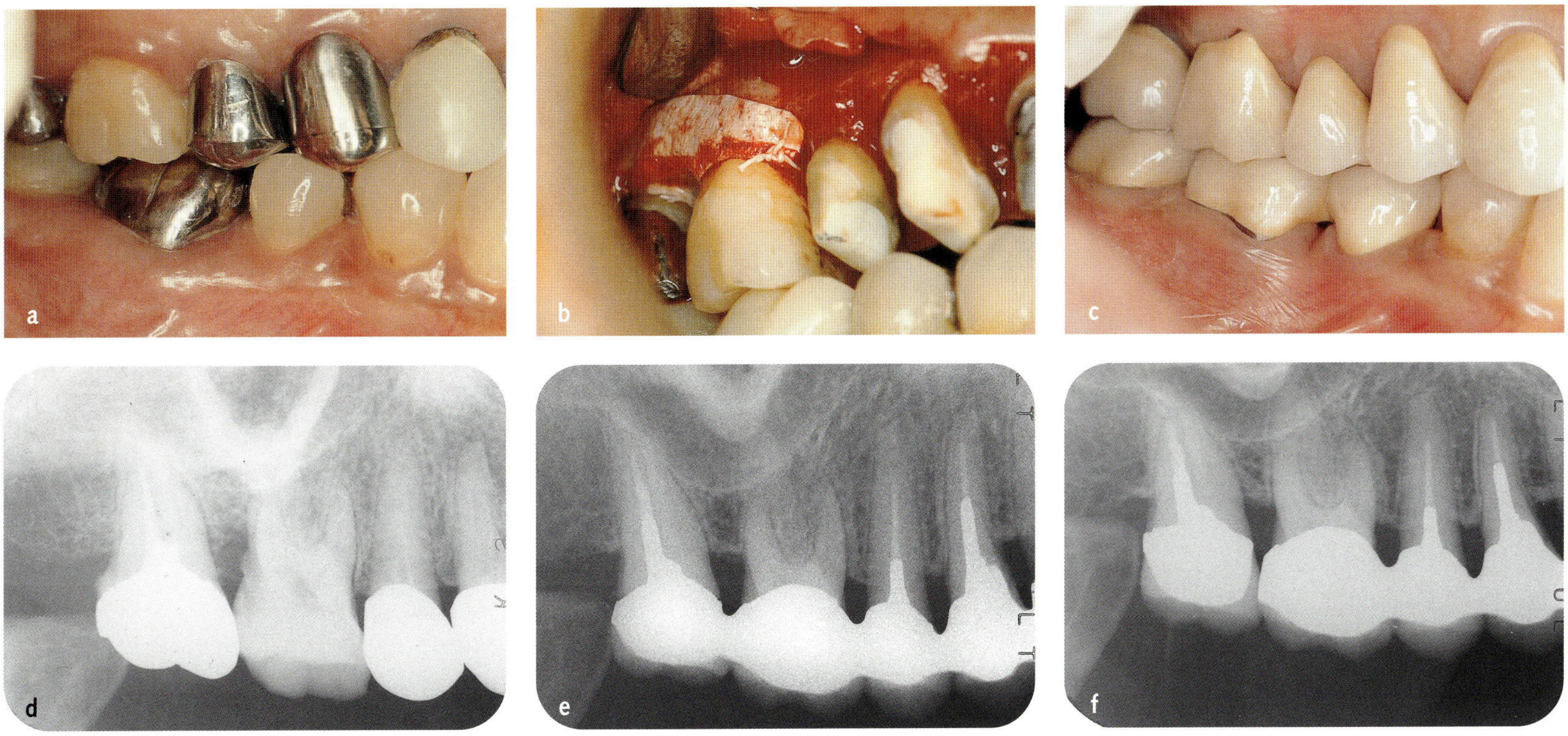

Fig 1-89 Treatment and follow-up in the maxillary right quadrant. (a) At the first visit. (b) Regeneration therapy (using Gore-Tex membrane) for the class II furcation involvement distal to the first molar. (c) Conditions are stable 11 years after treatment. (d) At the first visit. The first molar shows class II furcation involvement and occlusal trauma. (e) About 3 years and 6 months after the first visit. (f) About 11 years after the treatment (May 2002). Tissue regeneration is confirmed.

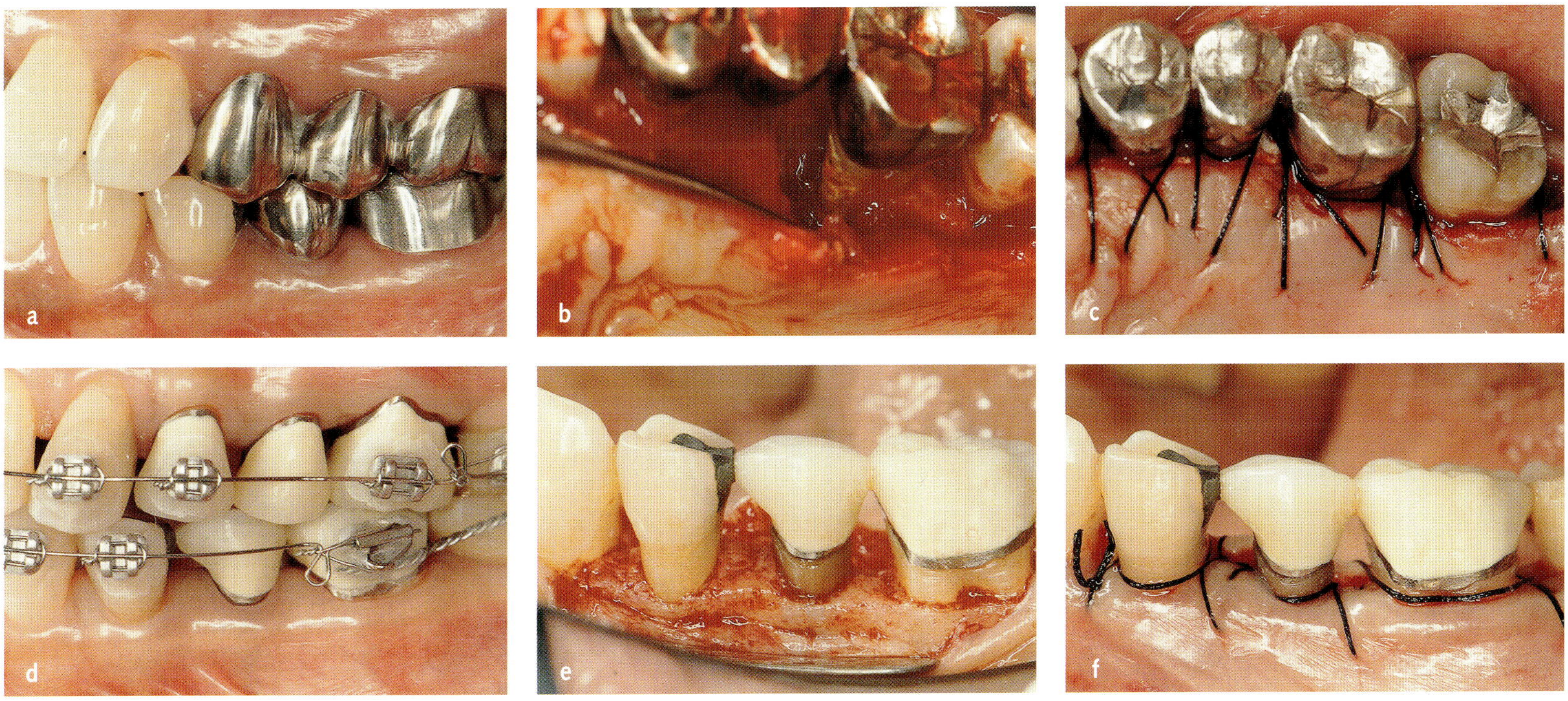

Fig 1-90 Improvement on the left side for easy maintenance. (a) At the first visit. (b and c) GTR for infrabony defects at the maxillary left second premolar and first molar (1 year after the first visit). (d) Tooth movement. (e and f) After tooth movement (2 years and 2 months after the first visit). To alter the surrounding thick gingiva, which is difficult to maintain, full-thickness flaps were elevated. The area was covered with shelf-like thick bone. Osseous surgery was conducted to achieve a maintainable environment.

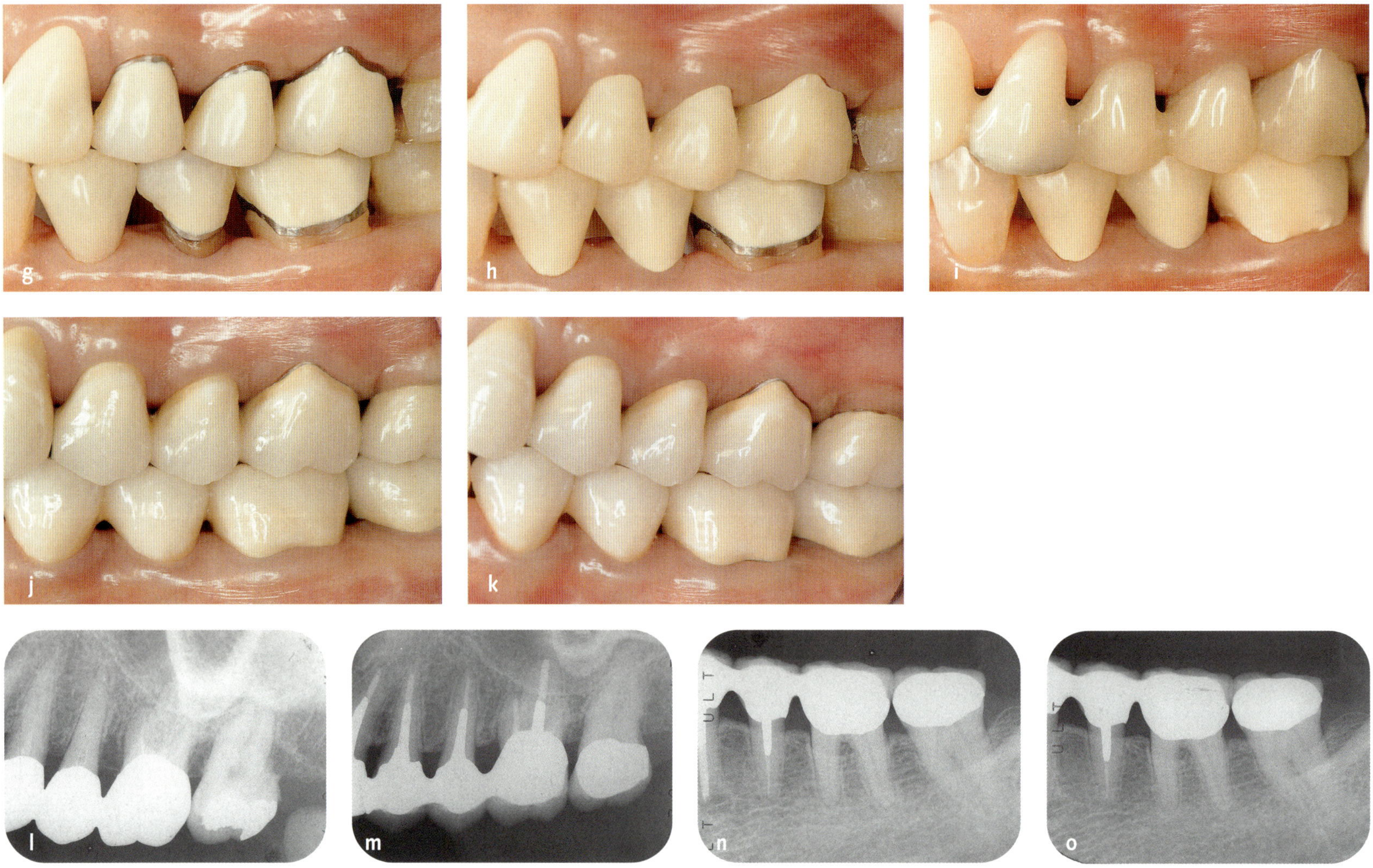

Fig 1-90 (cont) (g) Sufficient time is allowed for the healing of periodontal tissue. (h and i) Tooth by tooth, final provisional restoration was delivered, a process that took 3 months. (j) Delivery of final prostheses. (k) Nine years after the delivery of final prostheses. Conditions are stable. (l) Radiograph at the first visit, showing bony defects and occlusal trauma. (m) Conditions are stable 12 years and 3 months after the first visit. The maxillary left second molar was restored 9 years after the delivery of final prostheses. (n) Delivery of final prostheses. Traumatic findings at the mandibular left first molar. (o) Note improvement of the traumatic findings of the mandibular left first molar as a result of restoration of the adjacent second molar.

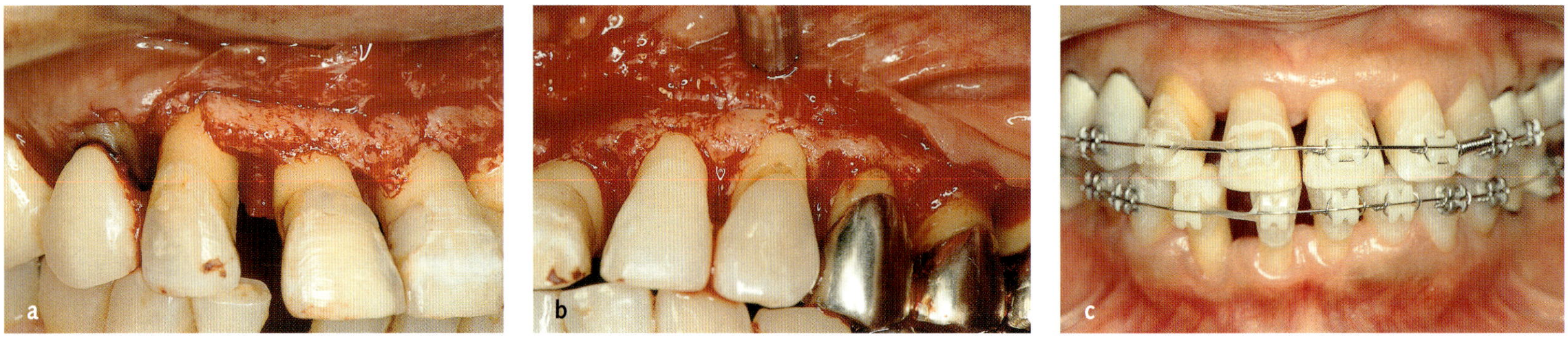

Fig 1-91 Severe bony defects and esthetic considerations. (a and b) A full-thickness access flap was raised for thorough debridement and prevention of gingival recession. (c) The height of the brackets was aligned to the attachment level to adjust the bone level, cervical line, and interdental papillae. The incisal edges of the maxillary incisors and the mandibular right lateral incisor were ground for adjustment (1 year after first visit).

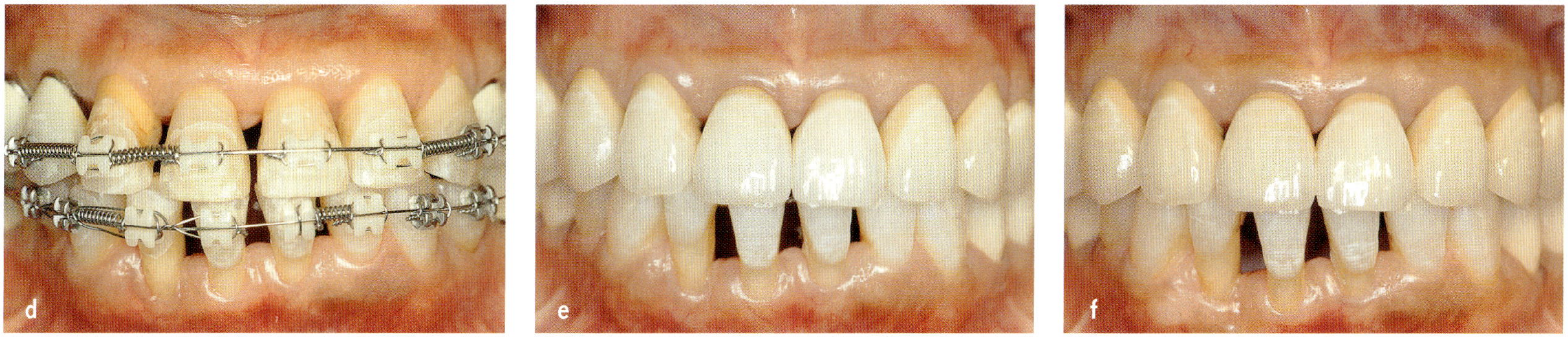

(d) Intentional tooth movement is limited to the mesiodistal direction. Buccolingual positions of teeth are restored as a result of myofunctional therapy (January 1992). (e) Delivery of cross-arch splint (February 1993). Conformity of the cervical line and the occlusal plane is achieved. (f) January 2002. A case of comprehensive treatment, harmonizing the whole body with the mandibular position, the mandibular position with the dentition, and the dentition with the position and morphology of each tooth.

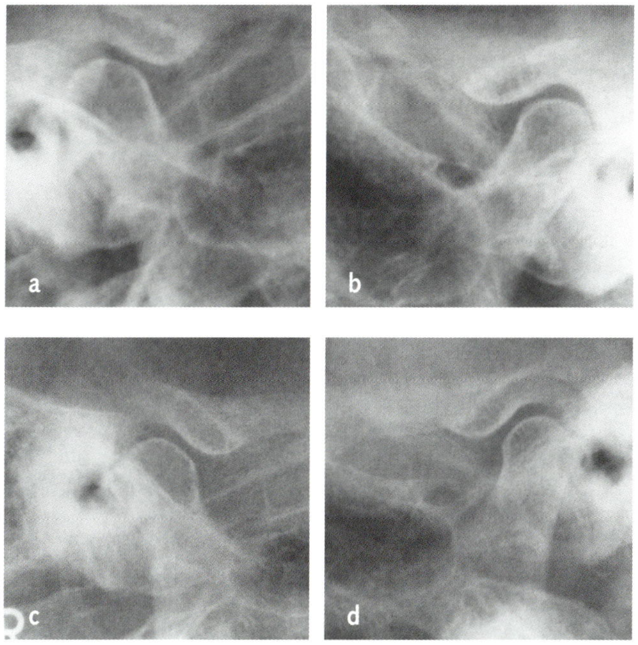

Fig 1-92 TMJ radiographs. (a and b) ICP at delivery of final prosthesis: (a) right TMJ; (b) left TMJ. (c and d) After about 9 years: (c) right TMJ; (d) left TMJ.

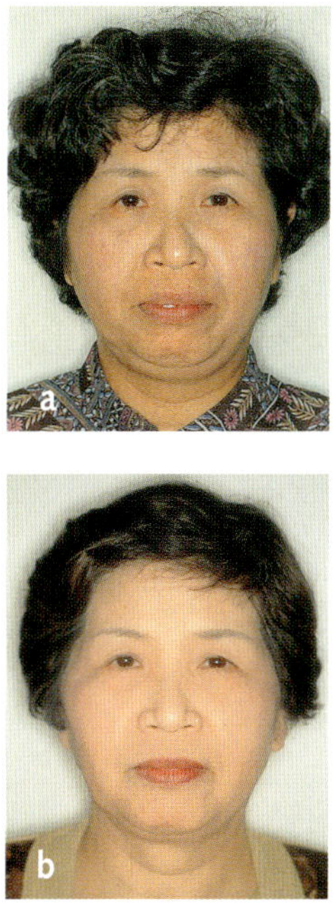

Fig 1-93 Facial photographs. (a) At the first visit. Masseter muscles are hypertrophic and tense. The lips are protruding, and she cannot close them completely. (b) Two years after delivery of final restoration.

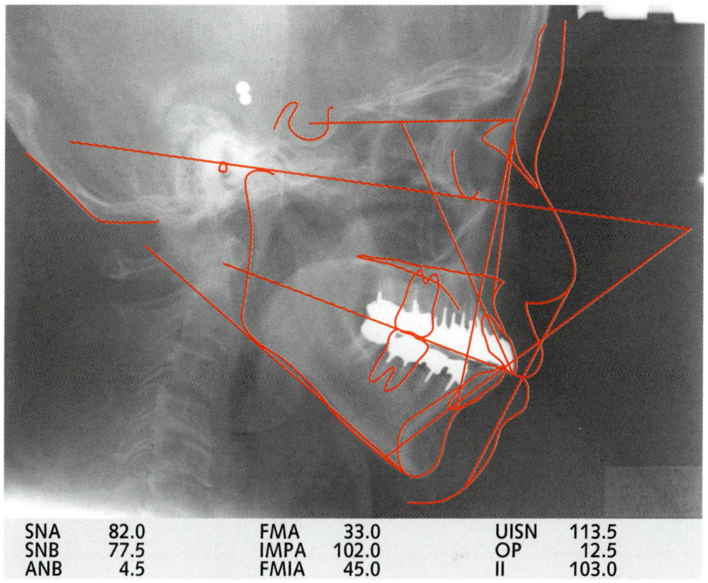

Fig 1-94 Lateral radiographic cephalogram at delivery of final prosthesis.

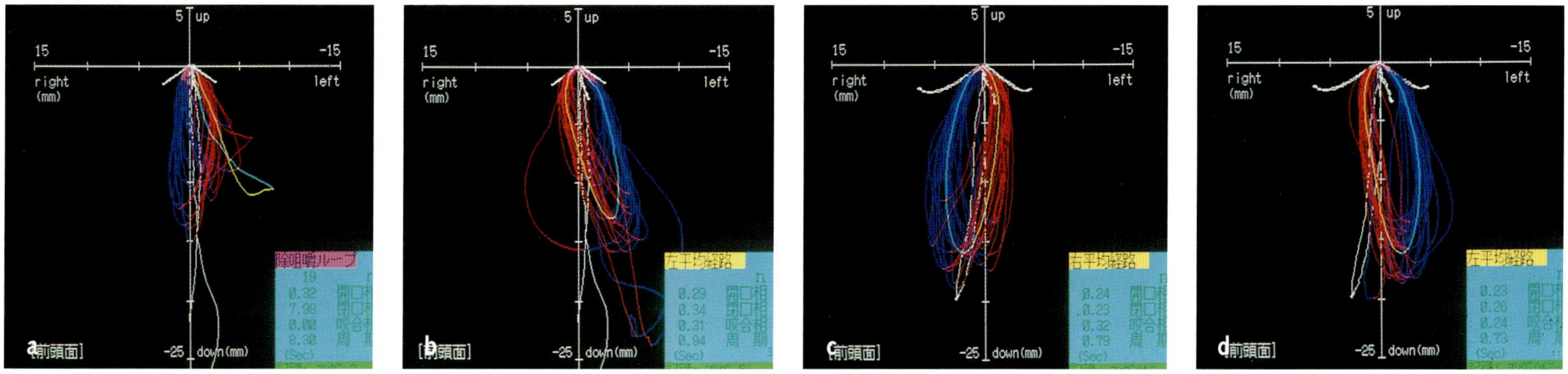

Fig 1-95 (a and b) Chewing paths 3 months after delivery of final prosthesis but before restoration of the second molars. Right (a) and left (b) chewing motions on the frontal plane are shown. Although it forms a cycle, rhythm is not stable, and both the opening phase and the closing phase have variability. ICP is stable. (c and d) Chewing paths after reshaping of the mandibular incisors (worn surfaces were adjusted to give sharpness), 2 years after delivery of final prosthesis. Chewing motions are of a grinding type, but functions have begun to stabilize. With less variability, the buccolingual width of the motion is narrowed. Wide opening and comfortable chewing are achieved. It was confirmed that masticatory movement became more vertical through crown restoration of the second molars and reshaping. There is some concern about the finding that left-side chewing (d) follows the tracing of the border movement. (c) Right-side chewing.

Case 1-10 Coping with difficulties during maintenance

Patient: *46-year-old woman at the time of first visit in October 1982*
Chief complaint: *Dislodgment of crowns on the maxillary left lateral incisor and canine and swelling of the gingiva at the mandibular left first molar*

The prognosis of a clinical case that requires full-mouth treatment is dependent on maintenance. During the long maintenance period, unexpected troubles almost always will occur. Any problems should be addressed while they are still easily manageable. This patient originally did not have a significant tendency toward periodontal disease. Dental caries and compromised restorations have brought occlusal collapse (Figs 1-96 to 1-106). Generally, when patients are compliant with regular maintenance, control of periodontal disease is relatively predictable. However, in patients with many restorations, often secondary caries and root fractures come to the clinician's attention only after problems arise. In a long-term follow-up, it is often found that when treatment has been performed to control forces, secondary caries is hidden in restorations. It is clear from follow-up observations that restored teeth are more likely to be subject to such troubles than natural teeth, nonvital teeth more than vital teeth, and abutment teeth of a fixed partial denture more than abutment teeth of crown restorations. Clinicians must consider how damaging it would be for a patient's quality of life to reduce healthy enamel, to extirpate dental pulp, or to extract a tooth unnecessarily.

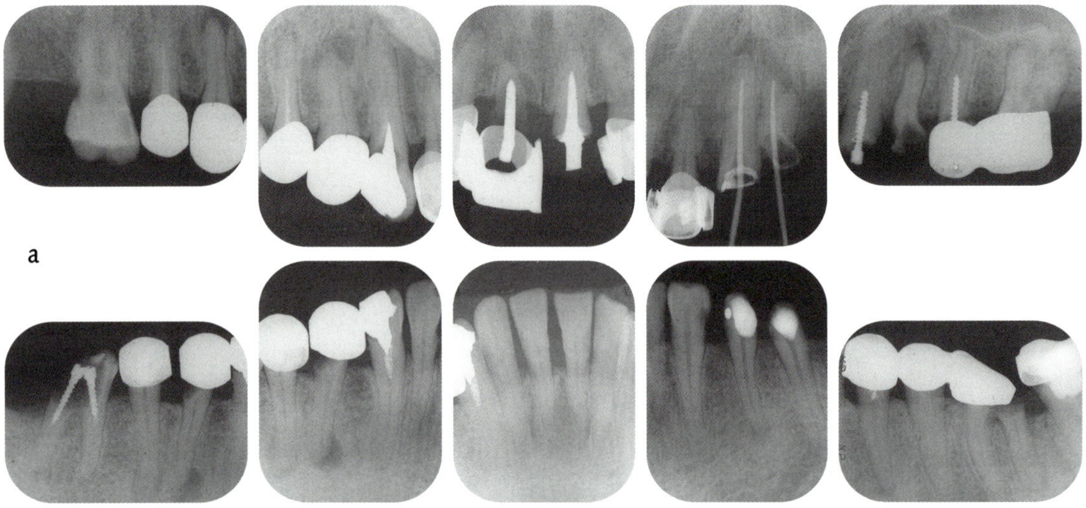
a
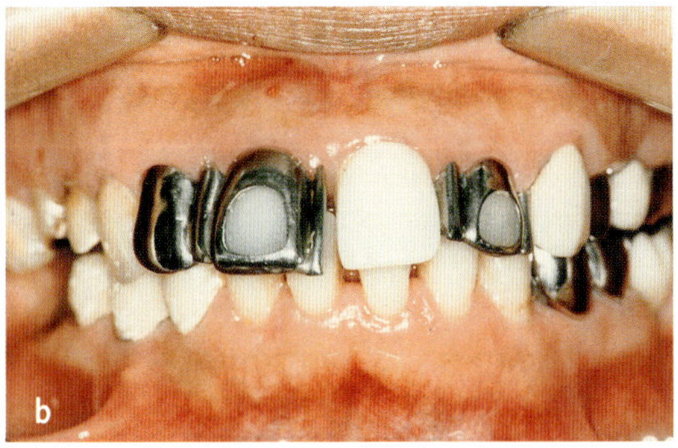
b
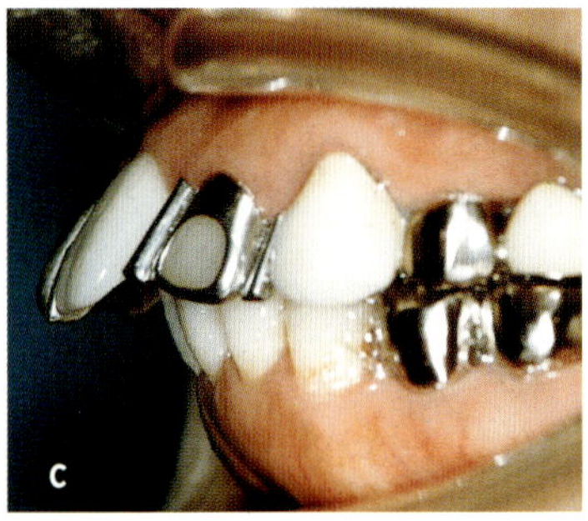
c

Fig 1-96 (a to c) At the first visit. She presented with dislodgment of crowns on the maxillary left canine and first premolar, among others. Because of the occlusal collapse of the posterior regions and the trauma to the anterior teeth associated with her profession as a diver, the anterior teeth are significantly flared. Secondary caries and periapical legions are observed in many teeth. At the time of the first visit, the type of prosthesis in place was not uncommon, although it is not often seen today. Although this restoration design inhibits oral hygiene, gingival inflammation is mild. Bony defects in the mandibular anterior region are considered to be derived mainly from trauma, judging from their shape. She frequently ingests sugar because of the intense physical labor associated with her profession. Also, because she has to keep a snorkel between her teeth, attrition and trauma of the teeth due to clenching were observed.

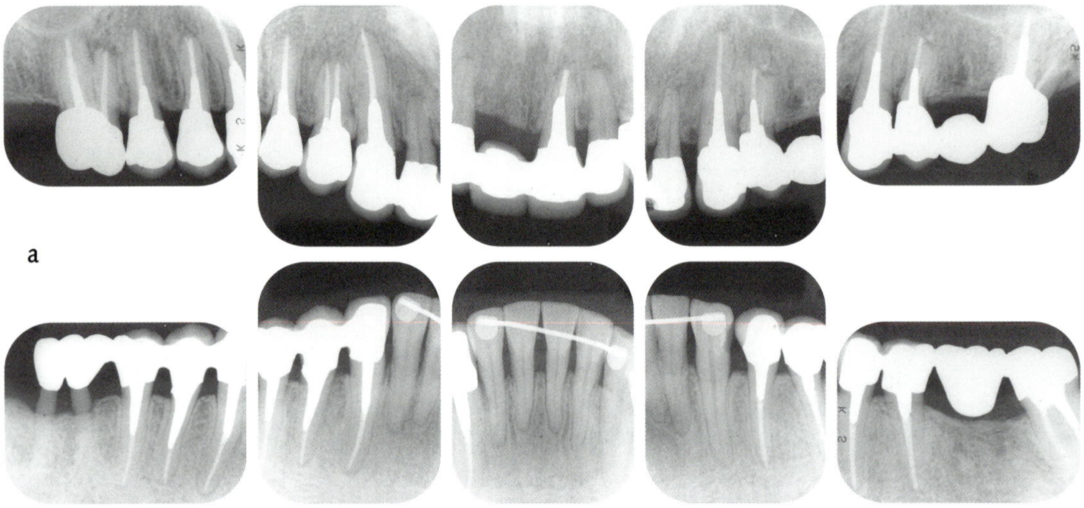
a
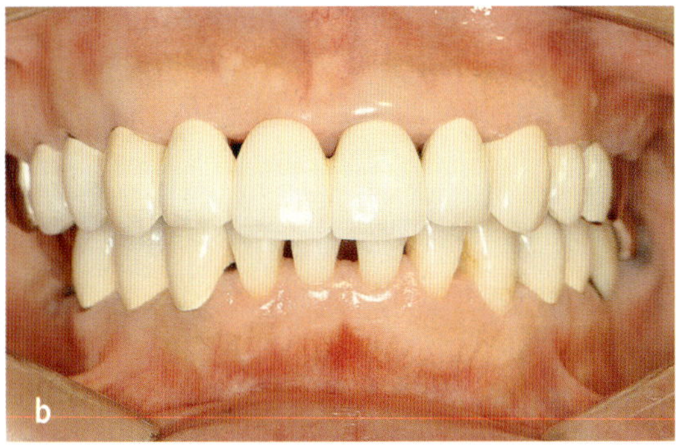
b
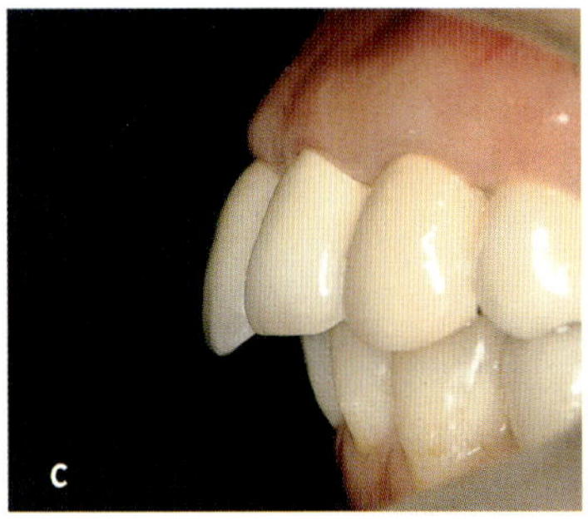
c

Fig 1-97 (a to c) About 1 year after delivery of final prostheses.

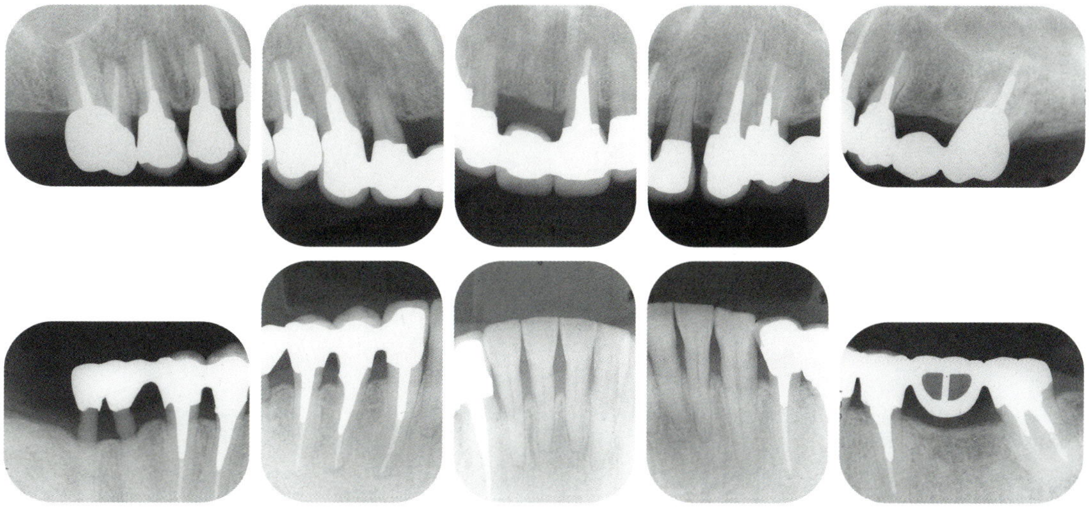

Fig 1-98 Radiographs 8 years and 7 months after the first visit, about 6 years after delivery of final prostheses. The patient was compliant with regular maintenance, and conditions have been maintained without significant problems.

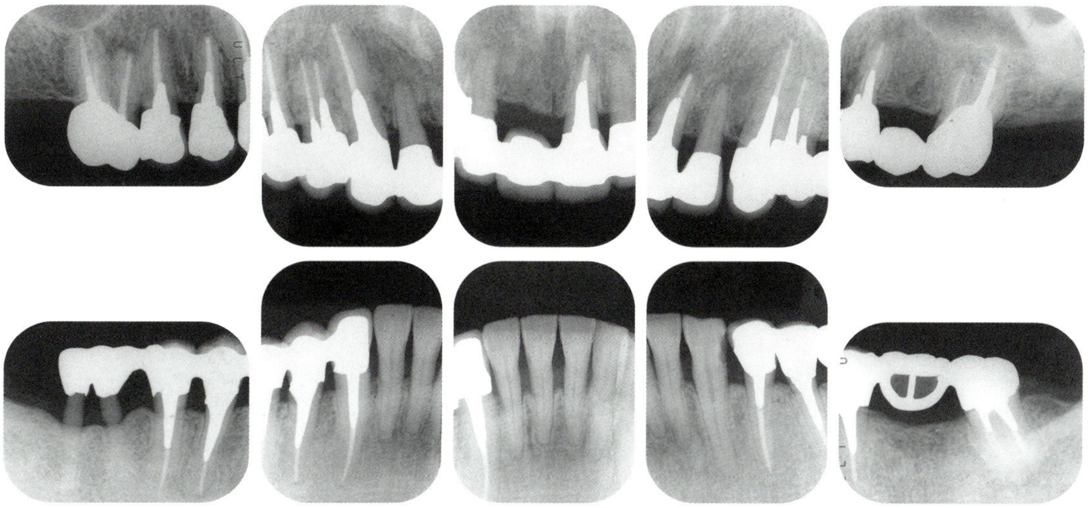

Fig 1-99 Radiographs 11 years and 2 months after the first visit.

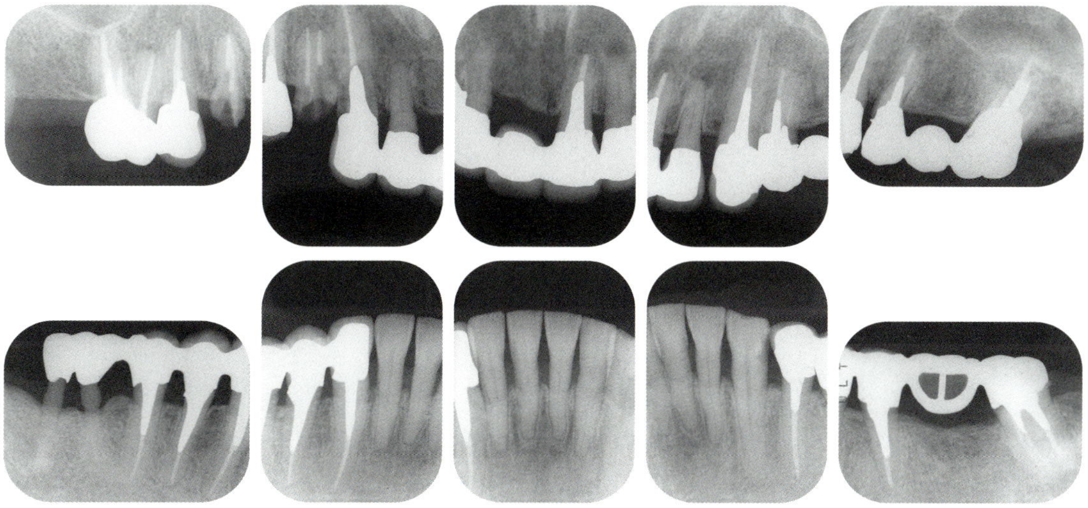

Fig 1-100 Dislodgment of crown on the maxillary right first premolar and secondary caries at the adjacent canine, 13 years and 3 months after the first visit.

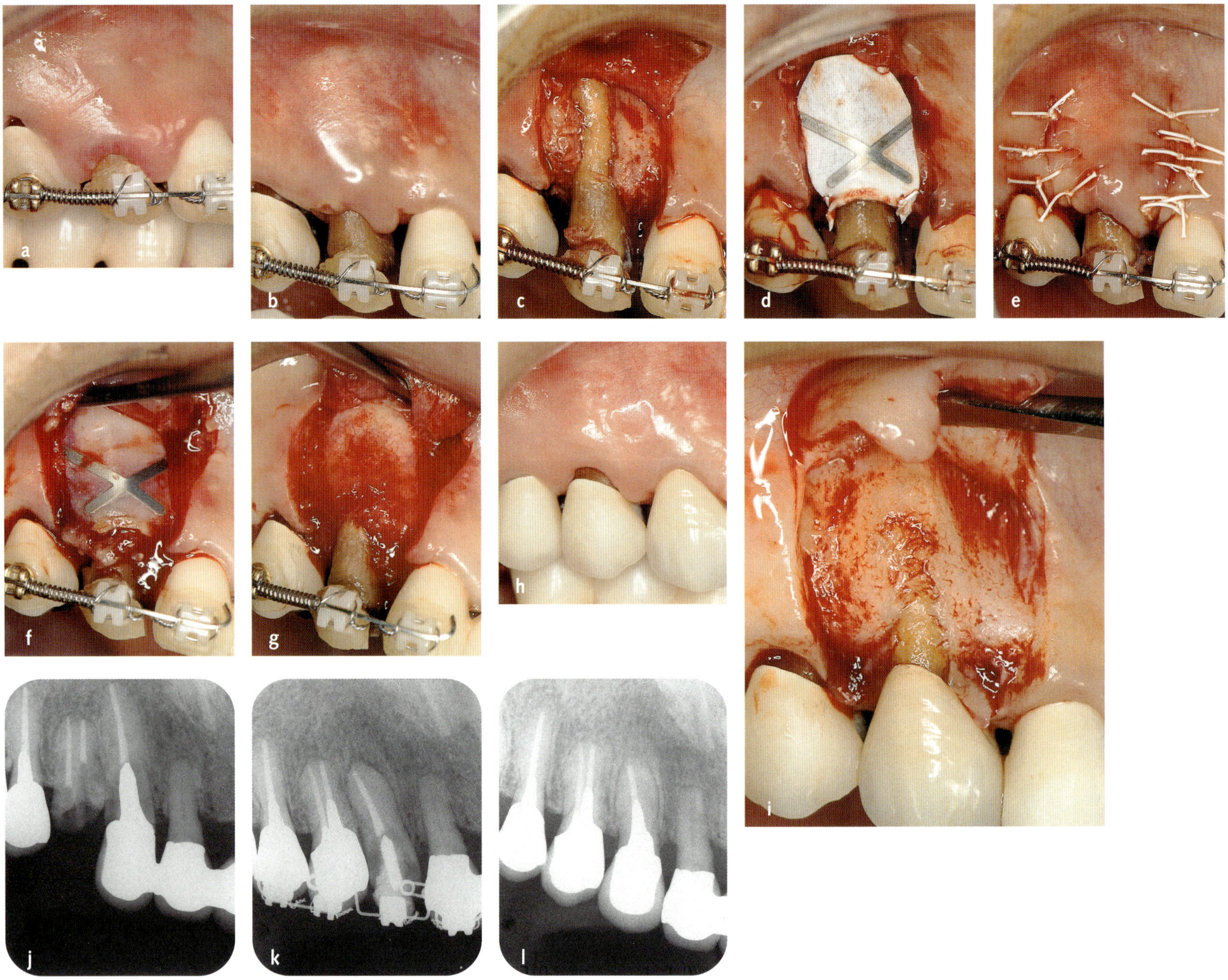

Fig 1-101 (a and b) Clinical situation 13 years and 3 months after the first visit. A fistula was formed on the buccal side of the maxillary right canine, and subgingival caries and a fracture line were observed. The tooth was orthodontically extruded, and a full-thickness flap was raised on the buccal side. (c to e) Titanium-reinforced nonresorbable membrane was used in GTR for bone regeneration. (f and g) The membrane was removed about 2 months after surgery. (h and i) Reentry was performed about 8 months after surgery. Bone was regenerated on the buccal side. (j) Dislodgment of the maxillary right first premolar crown and secondary caries of the adjacent canine. (k) Completion of orthodontic extrusion of the maxillary right canine. (l) Delivery of final restoration. Bone regeneration at the maxillary right canine is confirmed.

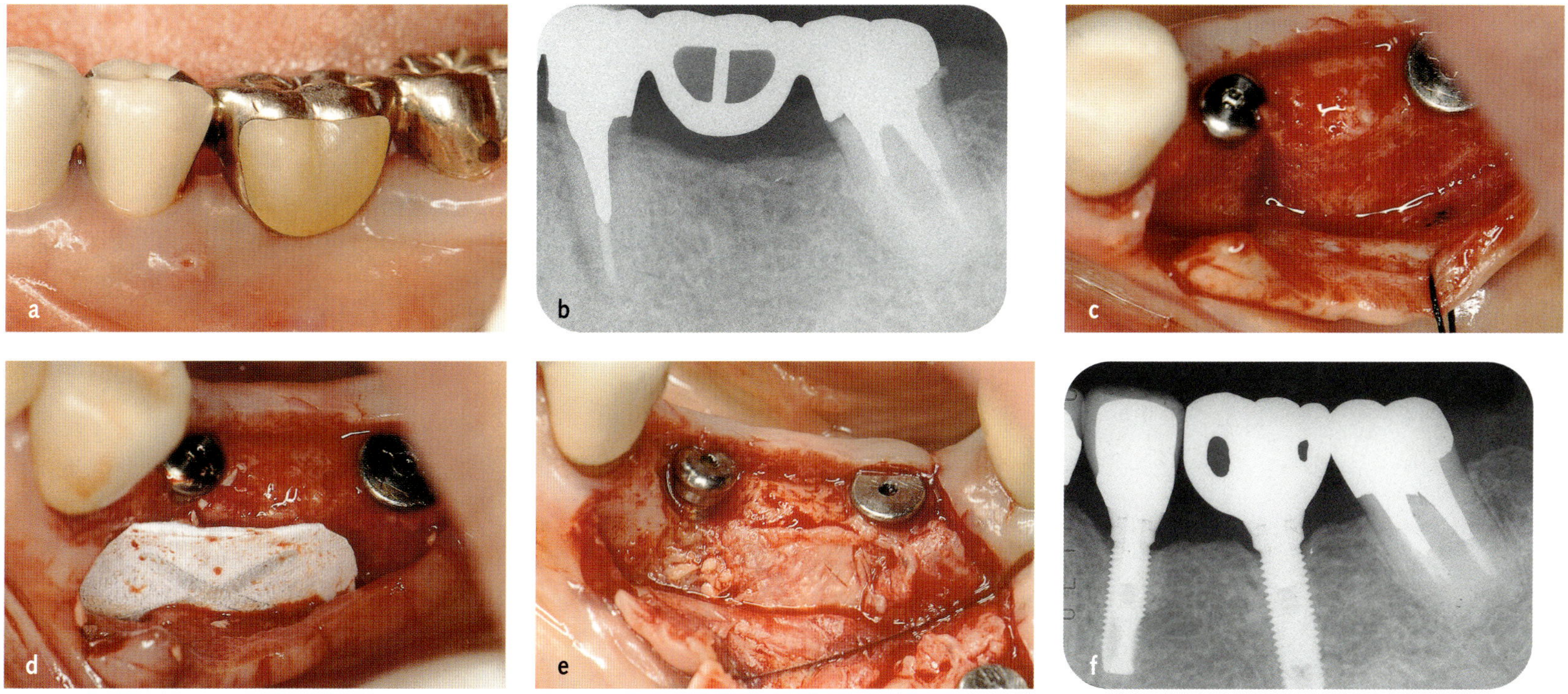

Fig 1-102 (a and b) Clinical situation 14 years and 6 months after the first visit. A fistula was formed on the buccal side as a result of the root fracture of the mandibular left second premolar. The tooth was considered hopeless and extracted. (c) Implant placement 7 months after the extraction. On the buccal side, the flap was started as full thickness, and then a partial-thickness flap was made at the apical portion, starting around the mucogingival junction. (d) Titanium-reinforced nonresorbable membrane was used on top of the autogenous bone graft. The mucoperiosteal flap was placed back and tightly sutured. (e) The membrane was removed about 5 months after surgery. Bone regeneration was confirmed. (f) Radiograph 16 years after the first visit.

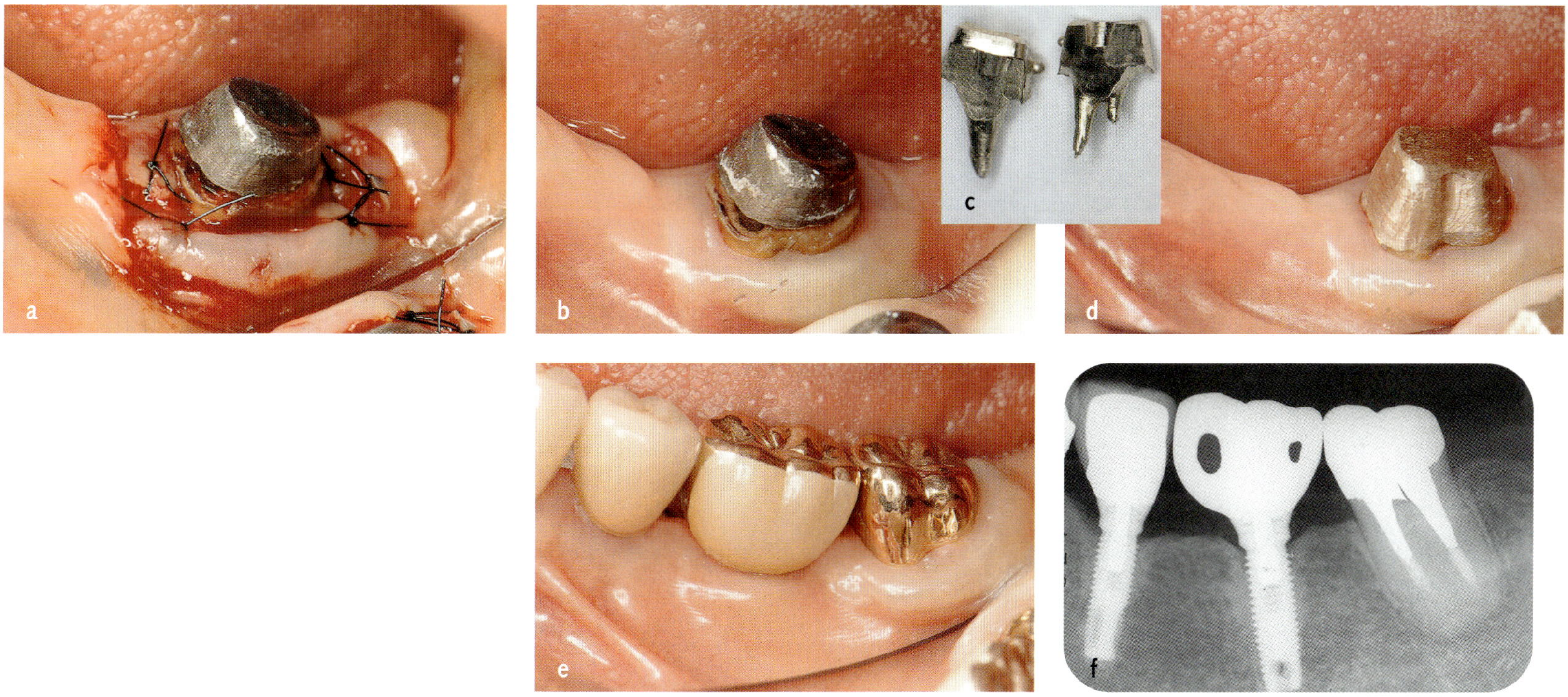

Fig 1-103 (a and b) After extracting the fractured mandibular left second premolar, crown lengthening and vestibular extension were conducted about 15 years after first visit to obtain biologic width for the mandibular left second molar, which had subgingival caries. (c and d) After crown lengthening, a separating post-and-core restoration (type IV gold) was delivered. The authors use type IV gold alloy for post-and-core restorations to avoid discoloration of abutment teeth and the metal color shadow in the gingiva caused by silver alloy posts and cores. (e) Implant restoration and the mandibular left second molar with a new restoration 16 years and 5 months after first visit. (f) Radiograph taken about 20 years after the first visit.

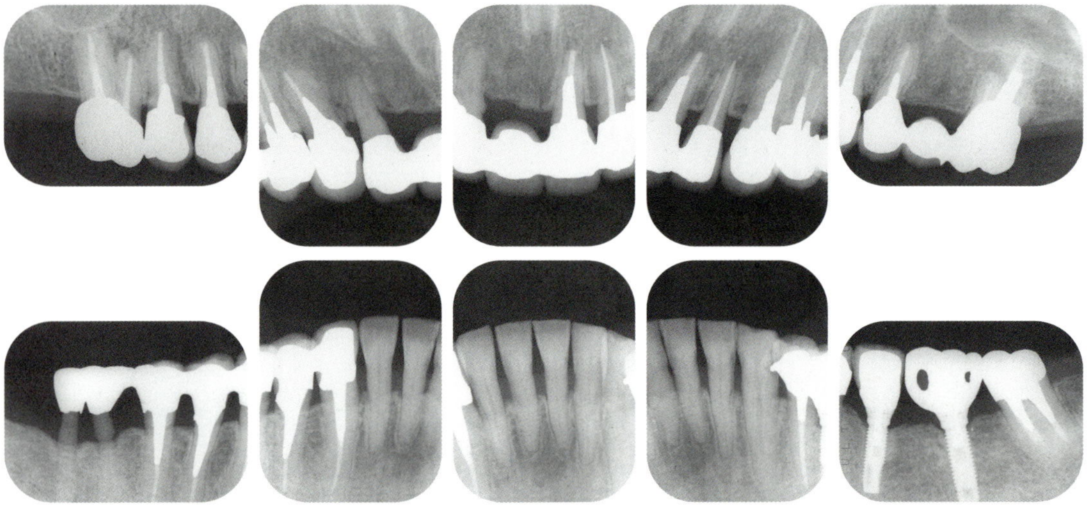

Fig 1-104 Radiographs 16 years after the first visit, about 14 years after delivery of final prostheses.

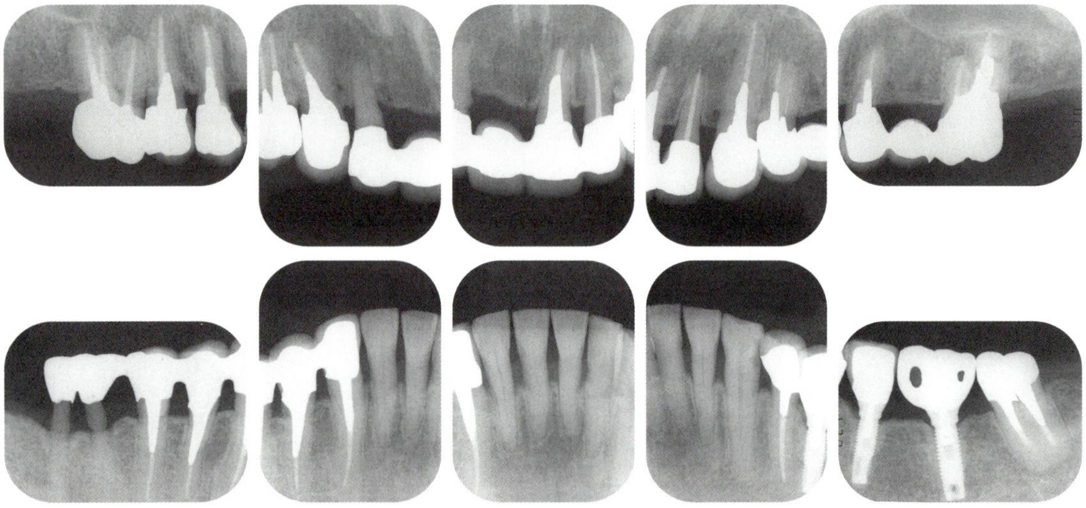

Fig 1-105 Radiographs 18 years after the first visit, about 16 years after delivery of final prostheses.

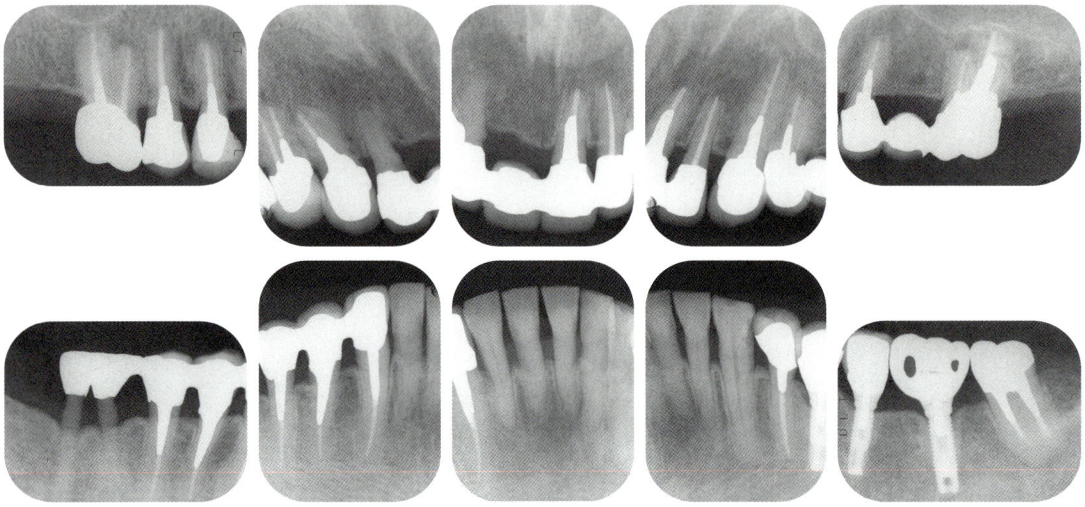

Fig 1-106 Radiographs about 20 years after the first visit.

Case 1-11 Challenges in caries control

Patient: *55-year-old woman at the time of first visit in October 1984*
Chief complaint: *Fracture and dislodgment of the maxillary anterior fixed partial denture*

Good confidence of the patient was obtained at an early stage, and active treatment was started relatively early. The patient stopped visiting us 6 years after treatment. During a 5-year absence, she suffered from hypertension, insomnia, angina pectoris, osteoarthritis of the knee, tension headache, and tinnitus, among other ailments. She was sensitive to her physical conditions because her elder brother died of a malignant tumor. When she visited us in 1996, secondary caries was observed in all abutment teeth. Her treatment should have taken into consideration that she had a strong tendency for dental caries. The mandibular posterior fixed partial dentures were remade in the following year, but re-treatment of the maxilla would have been too complex. Finally, 17 years after the first visit, the maxilla was re-treated to receive a Konus telescopic denture (Figs 1-107 to 1-113).
The patient was 55 years old at the first visit and is 72 years old now. Maintenance care is particularly difficult in middle-aged and elderly patients.

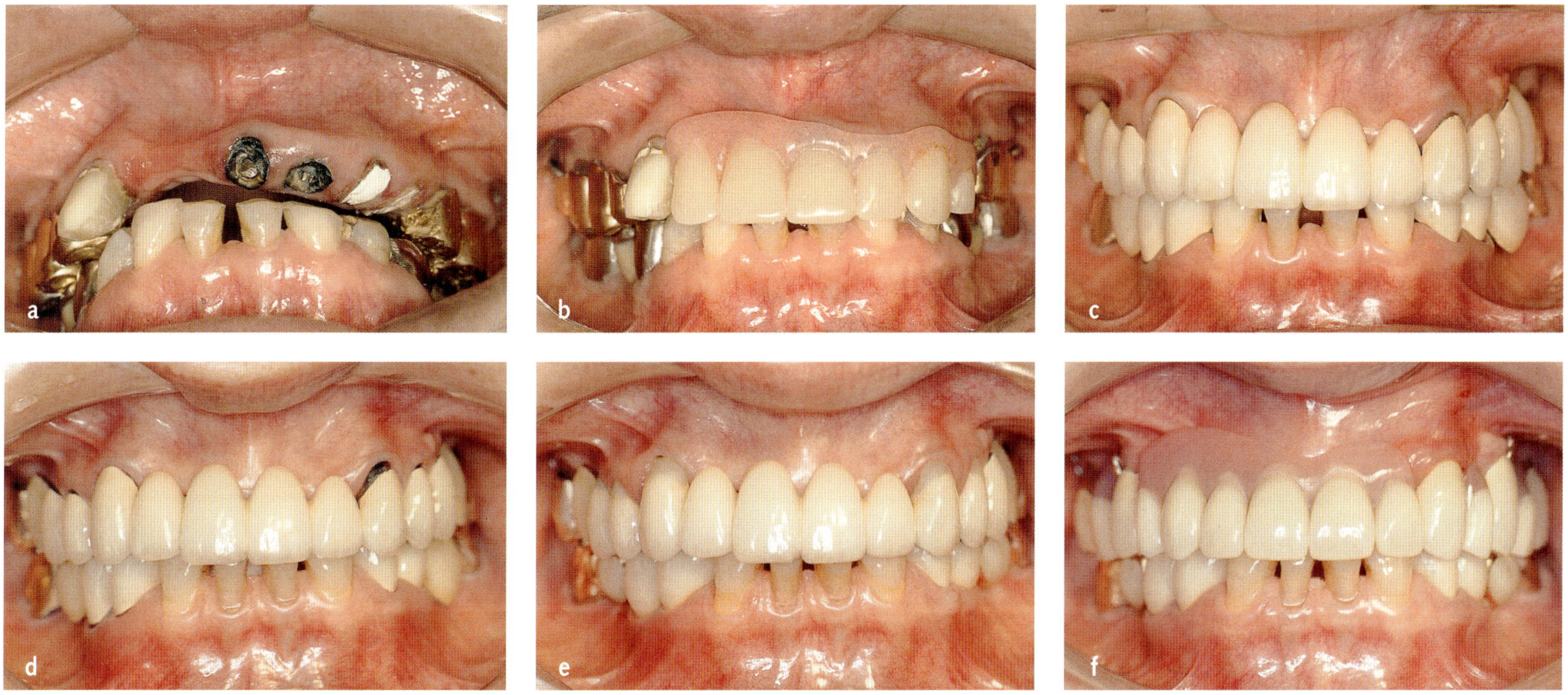

Fig 1-107 Frontal views from the first visit to about 17 years after treatment. (a) At the first visit. The patient visited us because of the fracture and dislodgment of a maxillary anterior fixed partial denture. (b) On the first day, an overdenture was fabricated with autopolymerizing resin and wire clasps as an emergency measure to restore esthetics to a certain degree. (c) Delivery of final prostheses, 1 year and 2 months after the first visit. The vertical dimension was increased in a reasonable manner by several provisional restorations. Disturbance in the occlusal plane was resolved as well. (d) Maintenance progressed smoothly until she stopped visiting the office. She returned after a 5-year absence, 12 years after the first visit. She said she was suffering from hypertension, insomnia, angina pectoris, osteoarthritis, and tension headache. Secondary caries was present in all abutment teeth. (e) New fixed partial dentures were made for the mandible, and resin composite was used in the maxilla to restore the areas affected by secondary caries. (f) Konus telescopic denture in the maxilla, 17 years after the first visit.

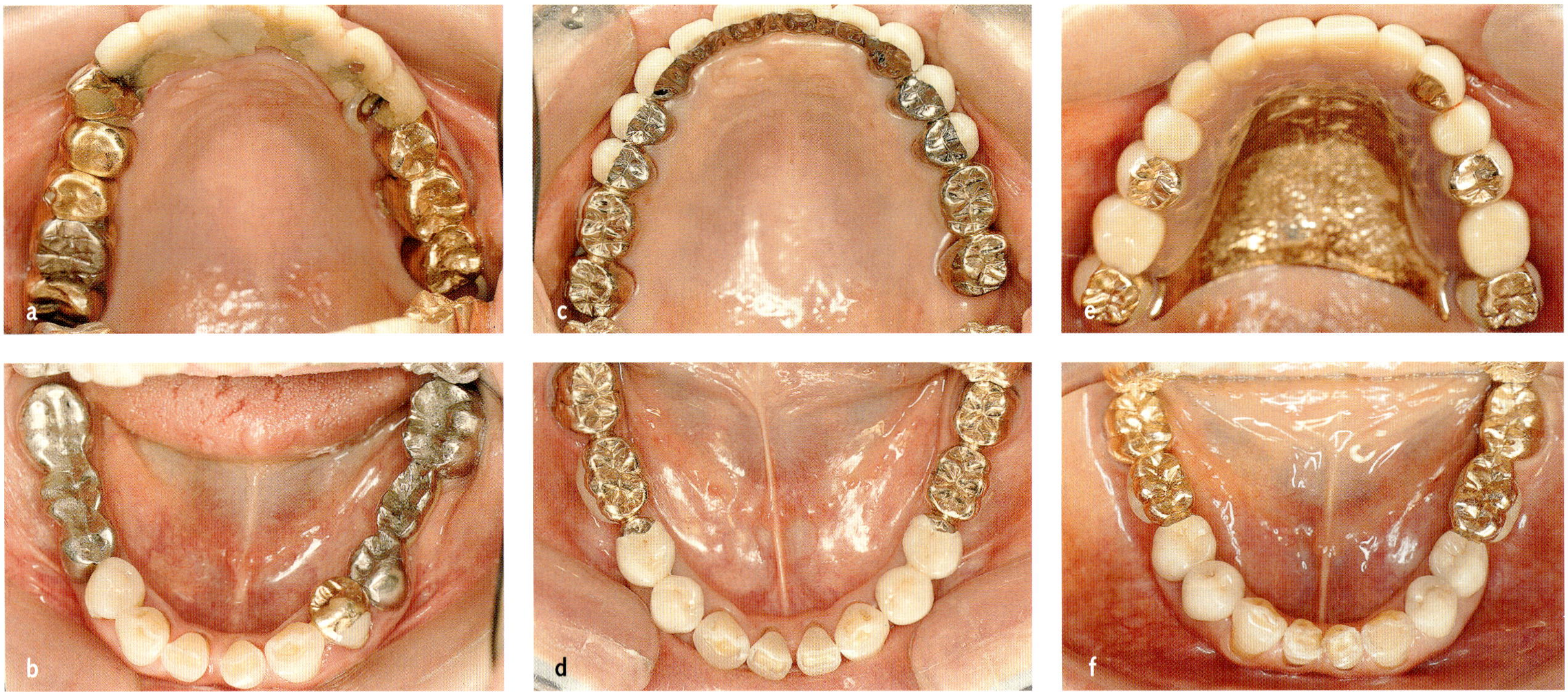

Fig 1-108 (a and b) At the first visit. Considerable problems in both dental arches due to poor prostheses, subgingival caries, and gingival inflammation. (c and d) One year after delivery of final prostheses, three years after the first visit. Restorations for all molars (pontics: first molars) are made of type IV gold. Porcelain-fused-to-metal fixed partial dentures have been provided for the maxillary incisors, canines, and premolars (pontics: incisors) and crowns have been placed on the mandibular premolars. (e and f) Konus telescopic denture in place, 17 years after the first visit.

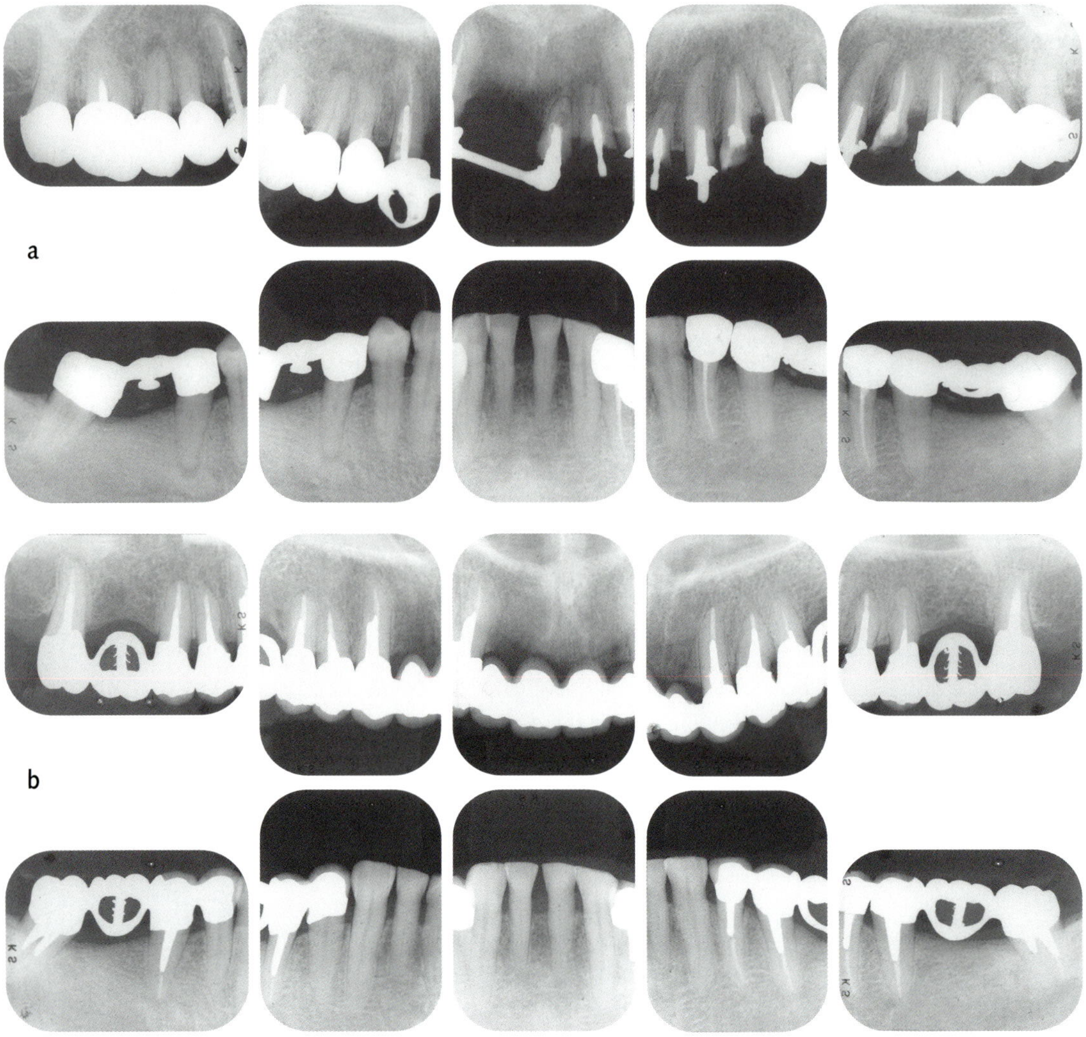

Fig 1-109 Full-mouth radiographs. (a) At the first visit. The maxillary left incisors exhibited subgingival caries. The teeth were extracted because of the unfavorable crown-root ratio due to trauma-related advanced root resorption. The maxillary first molars showed subgingival caries and furcation involvements and were strategically extracted. (b) Three years after the first visit. The maxillary first molars, premolars, and right canine had subgingival caries and received resective periodontal surgery, including bone recontouring.

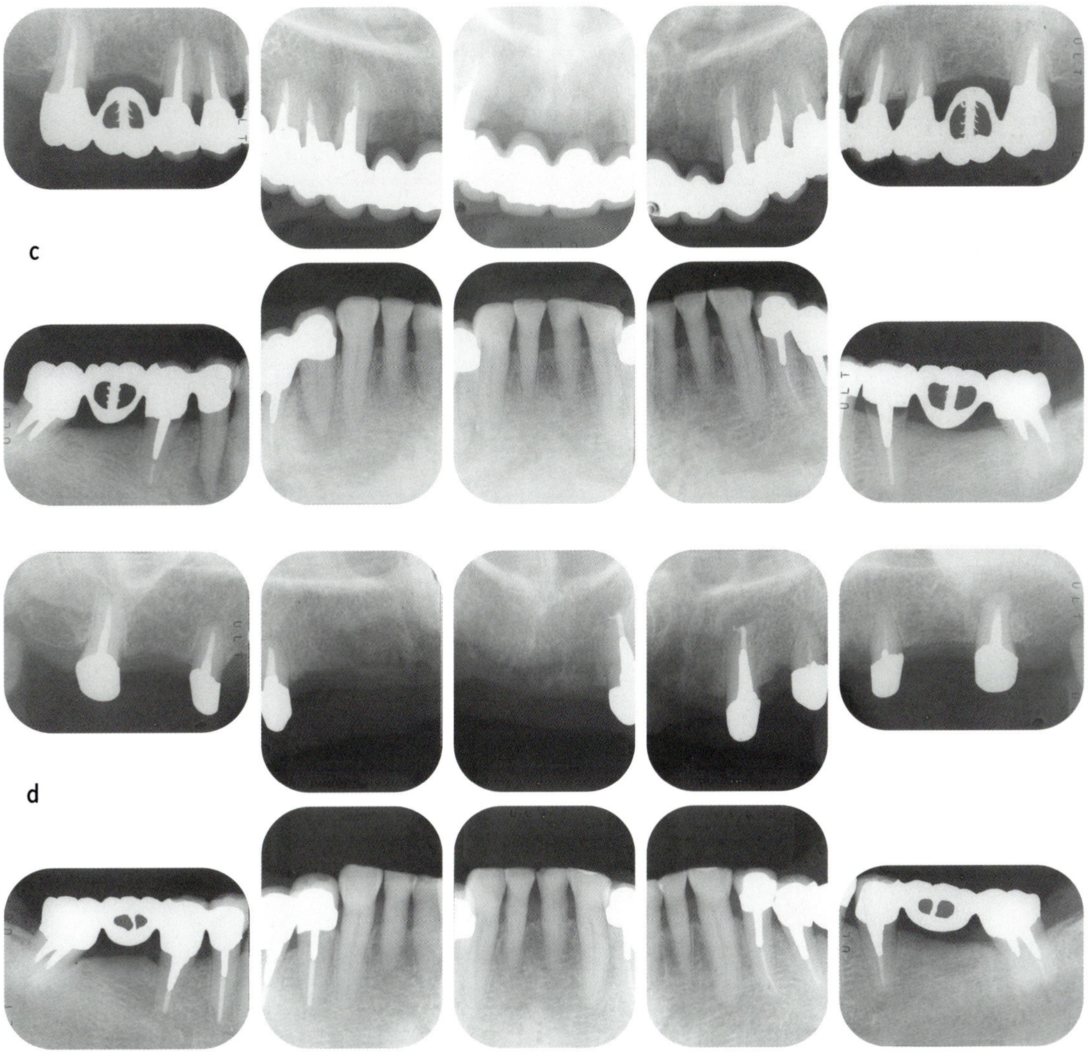

(c) About 12 years after the first visit. Secondary caries in all the abutment teeth. (d) Seventeen years after the first visit.

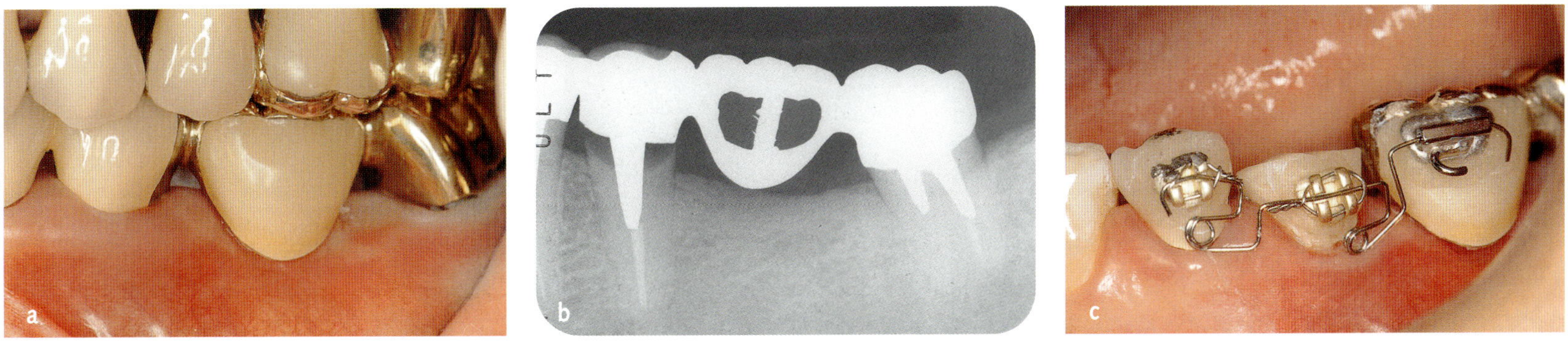

Fig 1-110 Treatment of deep secondary caries of abutment teeth. (a) Twelve years after delivery of final prostheses. The patient had almost no symptoms. (b) Dentin is lost almost to the bony crest level as a result of secondary caries. (c) Because there was no problem with the crown-root ratio, the mandibular left second premolar was orthodontically extruded. Twisted wire was used on the lingual sides of the mandibular teeth from the right canine to the left first premolar for splinting.

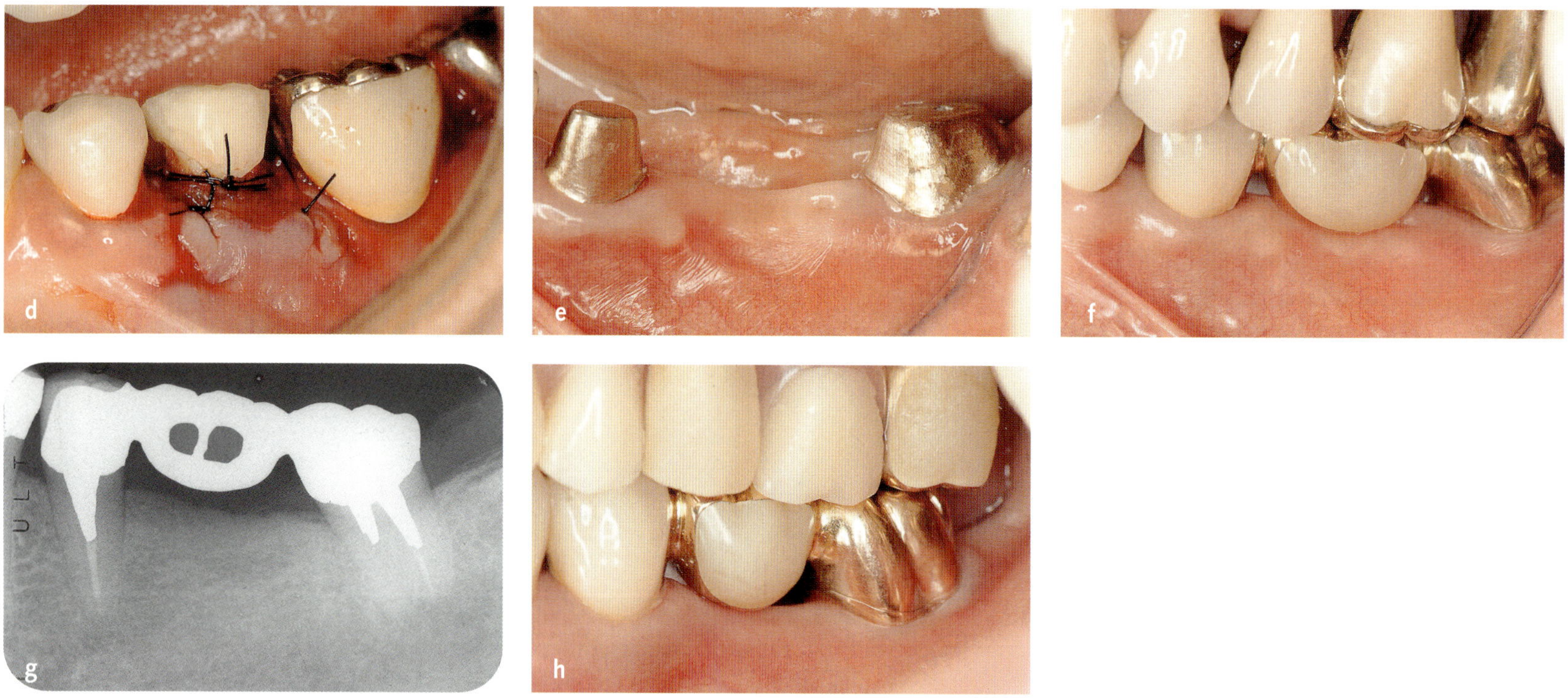

Fig 1-110 (cont) (d) Surgery including osseous recontouring to harmonize the cervical line and the bone level with the dentition. (e) Abutments were remade to ensure parallelism and to prevent root fractures. (f) Delivery of the new prosthesis, 13 years after the first visit. (g) Four years after delivery of the new prosthesis, seventeen years after the first visit.

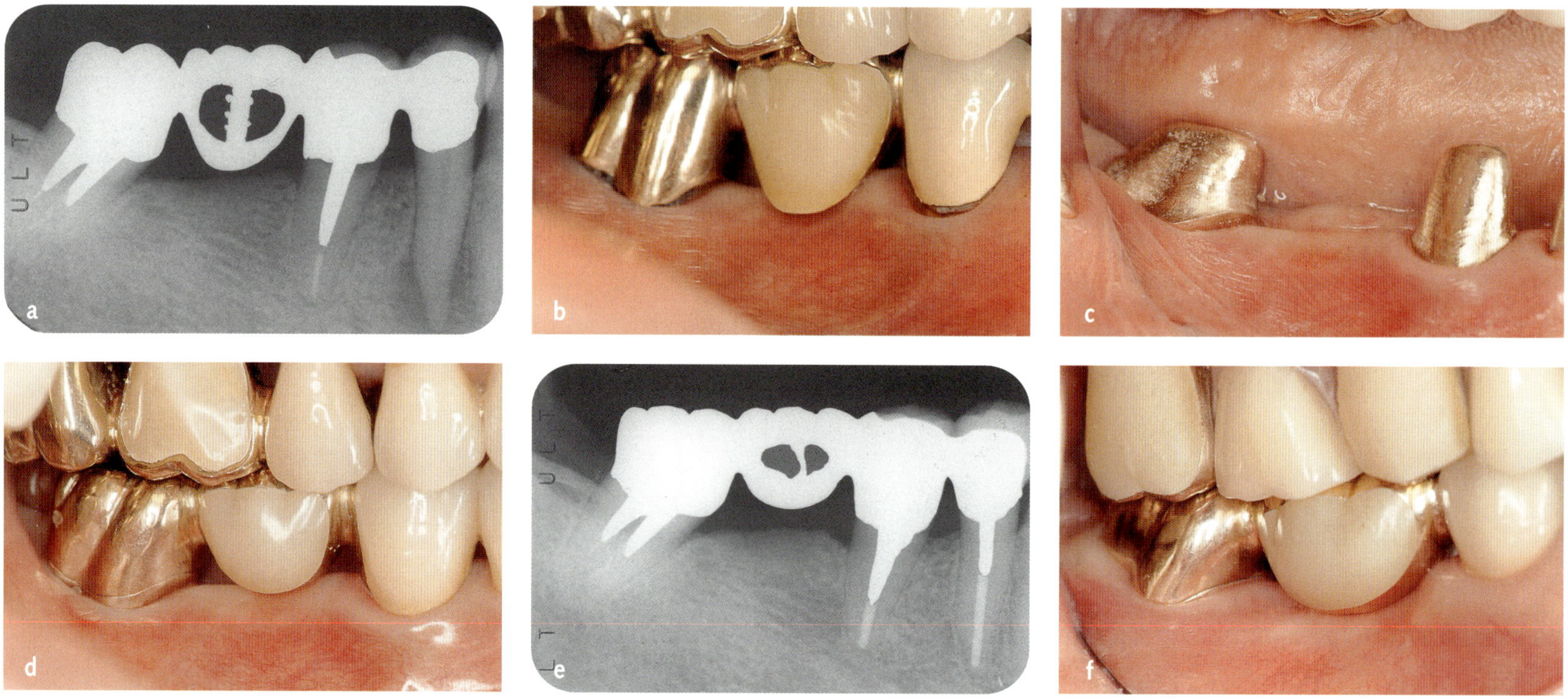

Fig 1-111 Fabrication of a new fixed partial denture. (a and b) 12 years after delivery of prostheses. Secondary caries in the mandibular right premolars and second molar. The first premolar has a periapical lesion. (c) Abutments were remade for the mandibular right second premolar and second molar. (d) Delivery of the new prosthesis, 13 years after the first visit. (e and f) Four years after delivery of the new prosthesis, seventeen years after the first visit.

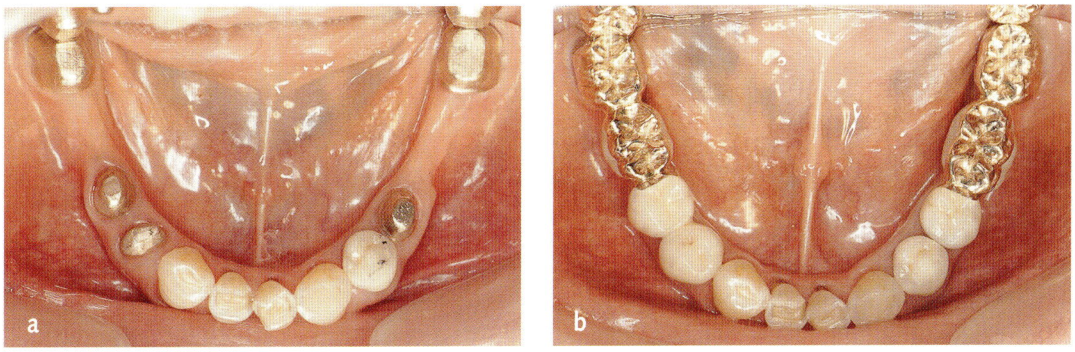

Fig 1-112 (a and b) Delivery of the new prosthesis, 13 years after the first visit. New abutments and fixed partial dentures for the mandibular premolars and molars (pontics: first premolars and first molars) were fabricated.

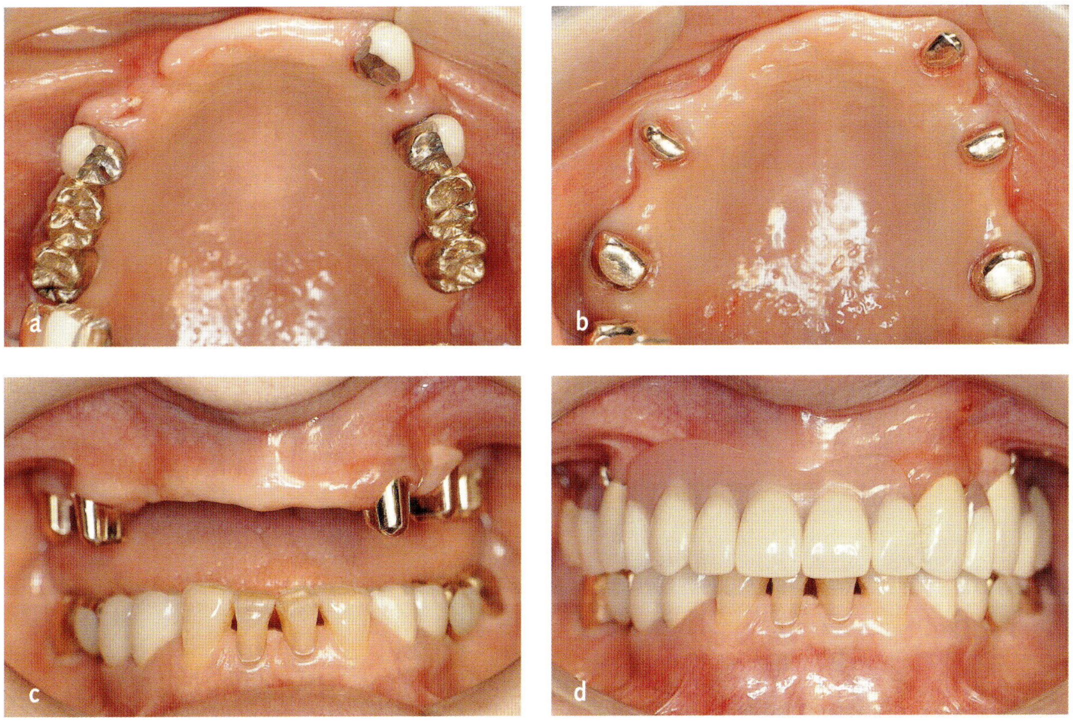

Fig 1-113 Recovery of the maxilla. (a) Sixteen years after the first visit. Secondary caries progressed further to jeopardize the maxillary right canine and left first premolar, abutment teeth of the fixed partial denture. A measure could have been adopted earlier to avoid tooth extraction; however, it was too much of a large-scale intervention to be feasible. (b) After 9 months. Root canal treatment and dowel posts and cores were provided, and Konus telescopic abutments were delivered. (c and d) The maxilla receives a telescopic denture 17 years after the first visit.

Chapter 2

Forces Affecting the Stomatognathic System and Their Control

Forces in the Stomatognathic System and Occlusal Therapy

Occlusal therapy

Occlusal therapy, or the control of forces in the stomatognathic system, is not merely a special therapy to treat jaw dysfunctions and is often misunderstood. Just as inflammation control (via plaque control) forms the most fundamental therapy for all oral diseases, occlusal therapy is a basic therapy that should never be neglected in dental health care. Occlusal therapy can be a piece of information regarding a patient's chewing habits or a morphologic modification of the occlusal surfaces of restoration. It may include some correction of a patient's posture and/or slight correction of a relationship between cusps and fossae that are too tightly interdigitated. With such slight intervention, patients may experience unexpected comfort. Consequently, this basic therapy may prevent future onset of anomalies in occlusion and jaw dysfunction.

Basic occlusal therapy is the elimination of the visible factors that are destructive to harmonious occlusion. We will be bold and say that it is not sufficient that a patient's casts be mounted on the articulator for examination of occlusion or that a patient's conditions be evaluated in view of occlusion theory. Rather, the assessment of occlusion in a patient should start with sufficient observation of the entie body (Box 2-1).

Box 2-1 What is occlusion?

In what is called *occlusion theory*, border movements are usually discussed. This may be understandable, considering that occlusion theory originated in the fabrication of complete dentures and was developed as a theory about the artificial construction of occlusal surfaces. However, because a living body is involved in functional movements, first we have to observe functional movements. Then we should start by identifying what factors maintain occlusion and what factors cause occlusion to collapse (Table 2-1).

Table 2-1 Factors in occlusal collapse

- Missing teeth; abnormality in occlusal surfaces
- Shift of mandibular position
- Abnormal activities of circumoral (eg, lip, tongue, and orbicular muscle of mouth) and masticatory muscles
- Habits (eg, resting the cheek on the hand during sleep)
- Posture
- Inflammation of tooth-supporting tissue

Dynamism of forces exerted in the stomatognathic system

It may be easily believed that the major forces exerted in the stomatognathic system are generated by masticatory muscles. However, attention also should be paid to the tongue, circumoral muscles such as the orbicular muscle of the mouth and the buccinator muscle, habits, and posture. Being weak forces, these factors play their major role through continuous exertion. The shape or position of bone or tooth can be altered by slight force (5 g/cm^2 or less). Therefore, these forces may cause slight deviation of teeth or a small facet in occlusal surfaces, and such changes may lead to changes in mandibular position and/or systemic posture. Such forces also may cause a change in the occlusal surface of a tooth. As function generates morphology and morphology affects function in biomechanical systems, there is dynamism, in which a cause becomes a result, a result once again becomes a cause, a microscopic change generates a macroscopic distortion, and a macroscopic distortion causes a microscopic deviation. Slight occlusal interference can affect a mandibular position, which may result in changes in posture and physical injury (see Case 2-4). Posture and habits also may affect dentition, which can trigger destruction of periodontal tissue (see Case 2-8). A significant level of individual difference is involved, and similar conditions may not necessarily invite the same problem. For this reason, it is difficult to define uniformly what is pathologic (Box 2-2).

Box 2-2 Good occlusion

Whether occlusion is "good" or "bad" is specific to each individual body. Clinicians cannot evaluate one patient's occlusion based on comparison with average or ideal standards. Having said that, it may be safe to say that conditions for "good occlusion" are as shown in Table 2-2. Having an image of good occlusion will help clinicians to rationally narrow perspectives in clinical practice and to facilitate detection of abnormality.

Essentials of occlusal therapy

Occlusal therapy starts with detection of signs of parafunction from a patient's motions or from findings in the face or oral cavity. Points that disturb occlusal harmony are detected, slight modifications are made, and responses are carefully interpreted (reevaluation); this last process should never be omitted. Even when a patient complains of jaw dysfunction, its solution will be found in an extension of adjustment of those small force imbalances. Claiming treatment of jaw dysfunction, some clinicians attempt to create ideal occlusion based on a certain theory. However, seemingly abnormal morphology is affected by systemic balance, and the balance may be kept with the morphology. On this account, it is highly risky to correct the occlusal plane, occlusal curvature, and occlusal vertical dimension in a uniform manner for all patients.

Morphology represents functions, and functions are an expression of morphology. Morphology and functions are like two sides of the same coin. Reading invisible functions from morphology is a key to solve a puzzle of occlusion.

Based on clinical experiences, almost all clinical cases with an abnormality in jaw function including temporomandibular disorders will take a favorable turn if "an appropriate mandibular position in the whole body" and "appropriate occlusal morphology including dentitions" are restored. However, an ideal mandibular position is not to be forced on a patient by a clinician. Also, occlusal morphology must be in harmony with a patient's masticatory pattern. It is not rare that some forces causing displacement or deformation of mandibular position, jaw bone, dentition, and/or tooth axes are overlooked and only the occlusion is treated. In addition, failures in clinical practice have resulted from the practice of capturing occlusion merely as a static relationship, forgetting that morphology and functions of occlusion constantly continue to remodel themselves according to their changes and neglecting such chronologic changes. Clinicians also must understand that symptoms and patients' complaints may be different, depending on individual differences in lifestyle or sensitivity. Some patients are not aware of a difference of 5 mm, while others are bothered by a difference of 10 mm. As long as a patient complains of some abnormality, clinicians have to adjust themselves to have the same level of filter as the patient.

Guichet (1970) defined occlusal disease as "a general term for pathological changes for which disharmony of occlusion serves as an onset factor or an aggravating factor." In other words, he considered that various symptoms, including excessive attrition for a patient's age, pulpitis, damage in periodontal tissue, TMD, stiffness and pain in the neck, chronic headache, excessive muscle spasm, and trismus, are all derived from disharmony of occlusion. Needless to say, it is not acceptable to consider occlusion alone as the causative factor of such symptoms. However, if factors other than occlusion, such as psychological stress, habits, and posture are carefully taken into consideration, concepts proposed by Guichet are still applicable today (Case 2-1).

Table 2-2 Signs of good occlusion

- No anteroposterior or lateral shift against the whole body
- Reasonable maxillomandibular distance
- Stable intercuspal position (ICP):
  Mandibular dentition inside the maxillary arch
  Appropriate curve of Spee and curve of Wilson
- Smooth, laterally symmetric and anterior border movement paths
- Functional movement paths of natural, regular cyclic motions in a stable range
- Harmony of border movement paths and functional movement paths
- Occlusal contacts in harmony with habitual, central mastication patterns

Case 2-1 Forces in the stomatognathic system and occlusal therapy

Patient: *40-year-old man at the time of first visit in 1998*
Chief complaint: *Occasional pain in right temporomandibular joint (TMJ) area*

Symptoms: *No joint noise, mobility disturbance, headache, facial myalgia, or fatigue was noted. The patient was conscious of clenching. No grinding was observed. He had a habit of chewing on the left side and stiff (right) neck and (right) shoulder. He slept on his right side. He often chewed gum.*

Facial findings: *The patient had a brachyfacial-type facial pattern. A raised right corner of the mouth, deep nasolabial groove, and tension of right facial muscles suggested that he was a right-side bruxer.*

Clinical findings: *Crowding and a crossbite were observed at the second premolars on the right side (Figs 2-1 to 2-4). The left side had a Class I relationship and the right side had a Class II relationship. On the right side, maxillary and mandibular tooth axes were lingually inclined, the occlusal plane was lowered, and the whole arch was lingually distorted. Severe abfraction was noted on the right side. The maxillary right first premolar was lingually inclined, holding the mandibular right first premolar. The lingual cusps of the maxillary right second molars were caught in the central fossae of crowns on the mandibular second molars. One lingual cusp of maxillary right second molar had degenerated, leaving the molar a single lingual cusp.*

Diagnosis: *Tight occlusion on the right side is considered to have caused clenching, which induced pain in the right TMJ and type I* or type II TMD.*
The right side had a Class II relationship because of the crowding, which was further affected by sleep posture, which invited lingual inclination of the right teeth, including the maxillary right first premolar. The large lingual cusp of the maxillary right second molar was caught by the opposing mandibular right second molar and could not move freely. The case was diagnosed as clenching caused by tight occlusion.

Treatments and progress: *The patient was instructed to correct sleep posture, and reshaping was conducted (Fig 2-5). The buccal cusp of the maxillary right first premolar was shortened, and the area around the fossa of the mandibular right second molar was ground to release the opposing tooth. Grooves were made on the B slope of the maxillary right first molar. For the maxillary right second molar, the B and C slopes were narrowed, and the distal side of the A slope was ground to eliminate posterior interference. Facets were narrowed on the A slope of the mandibular right first molar; the A slope of the maxillary left first premolar; the C slopes of the maxillary left second premolar, first molar, and second molar; the A and C slopes of the mandibular left first molar; and the A slope of the mandibular left first and second premolars. Grooving was conducted for the mandibular first molars. After reshaping (Figs 2-6 and 2-7), lateral sliding movement of the mandible was facilitated and clenching was stopped, which eliminated the pain at the right TMJ. The stiffness of the shoulder and neck also disappeared. The right corner of the mouth was no longer raised, and the facial asymmetry was diminished (Fig 2-8). Occlusal forces and chewing were more balanced (Figs 2-9 and 2-10).*

**The classification of TMD was made according to the recommendations of the TMJ Study Group (1986).*

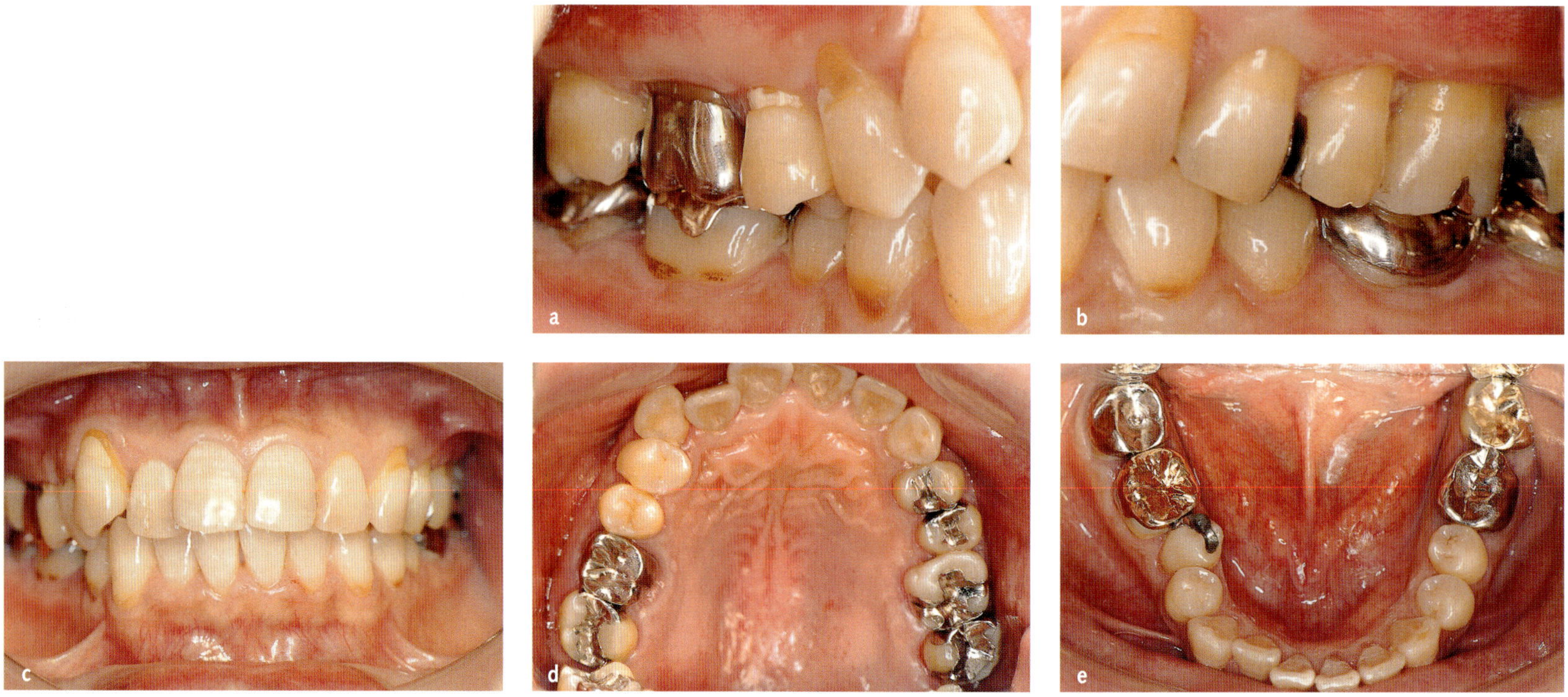

Fig 2-1 (a to e) At the first visit. On the right side, tooth axes are lingually inclined, the occlusal plane is lowered, and the whole arch is lingually distorted. Severe abfraction is noted on the right side. The maxillary right first premolar is lingually inclined, holding the mandibular right first premolar. The lingual cusps of the maxillary second molars are caught in the central fossae of crowns on the mandibular second molars.

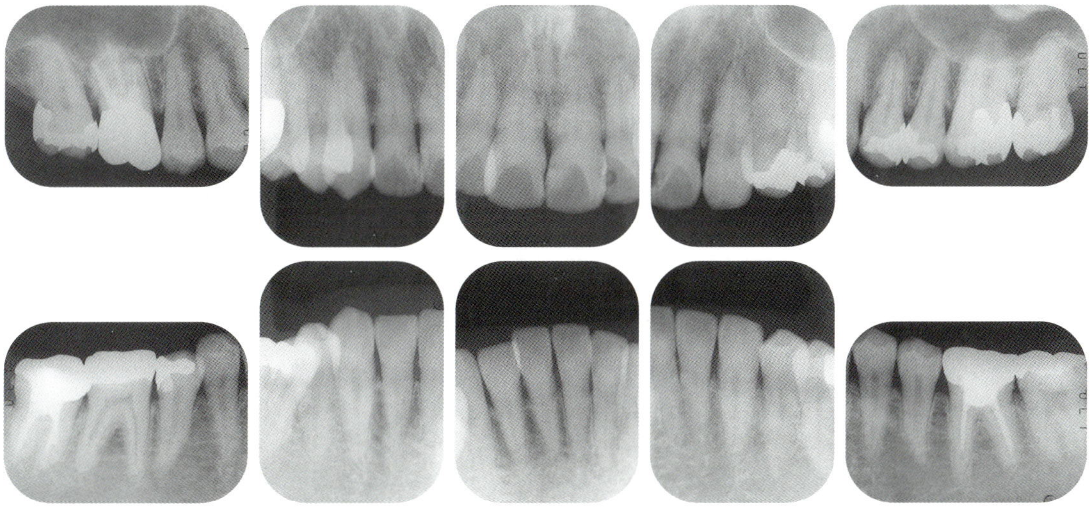

Fig 2-2 At the first visit.

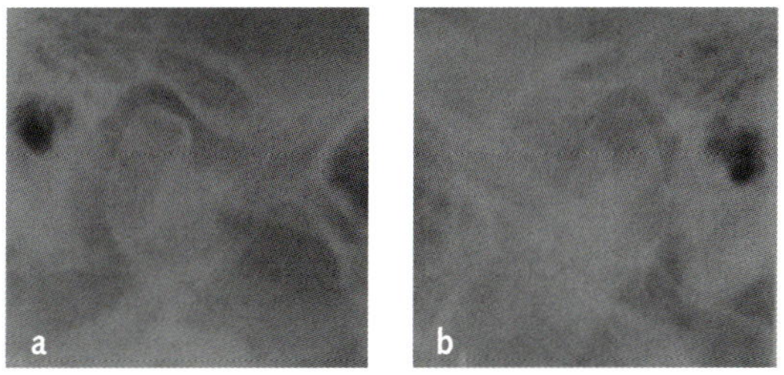

Fig 2-3 Transcranial plain radiographs at intercuspal position at the first visit. (a) Right TMJ. (b) Left TMJ. If the condyles are well developed, habits are less likely to lead them off the disc.

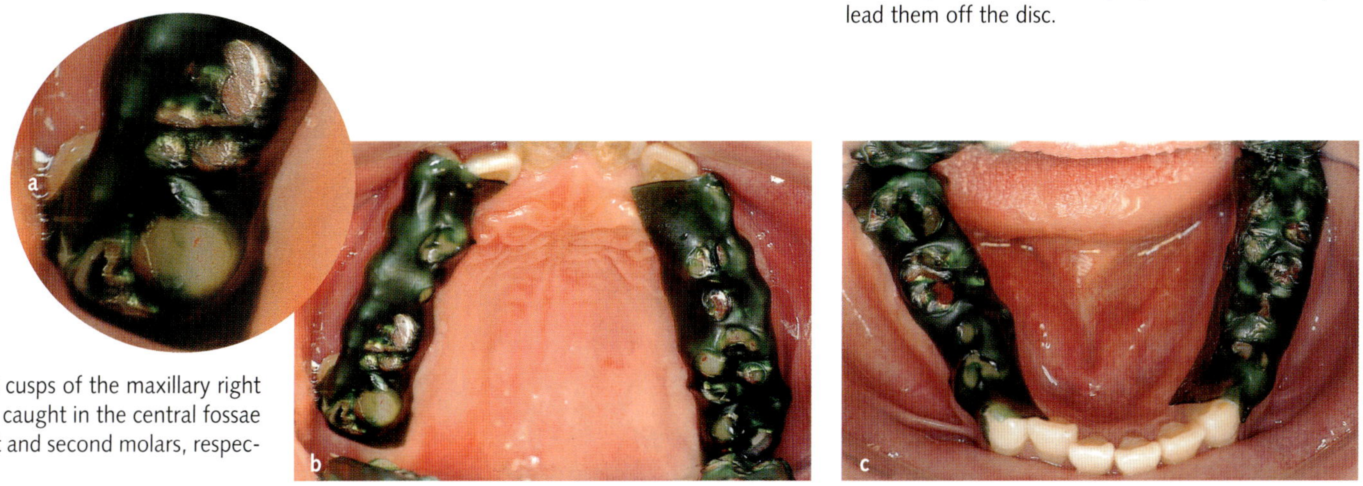

Fig 2-4 (a to c) The lingual cusps of the maxillary right first and second molars are caught in the central fossae of the mandibular right first and second molars, respectively.

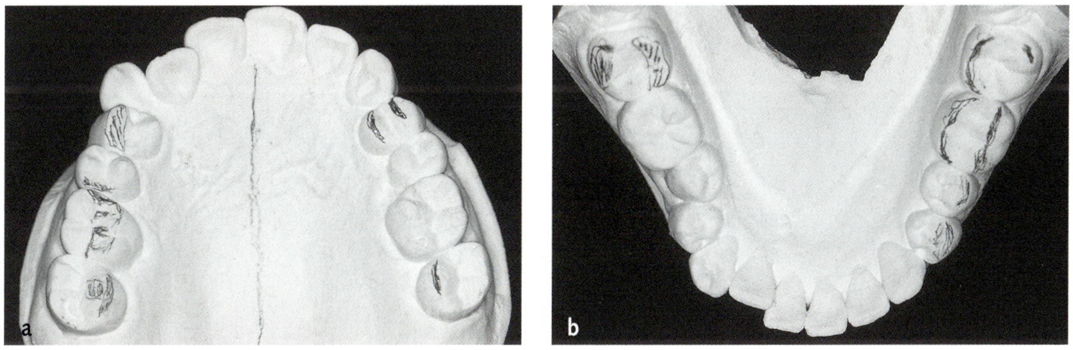

Fig 2-5 (a and b) Areas of reshaping are roughly shown.

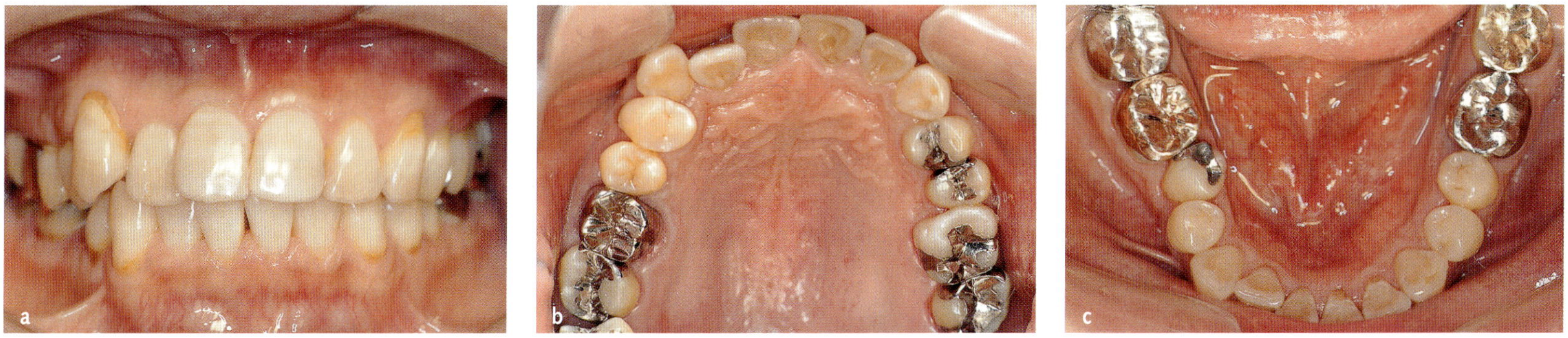

Fig 2-6 (a to c) Photographs taken after about 5 months.

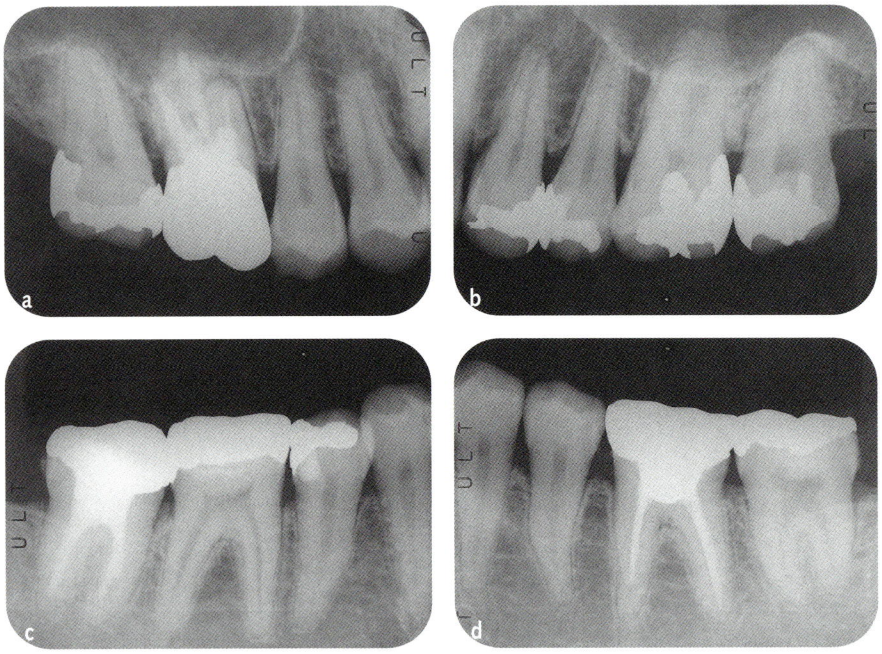

Fig 2-7 (a to d) Radiographs show that the lamina dura on the left side is more distinct.

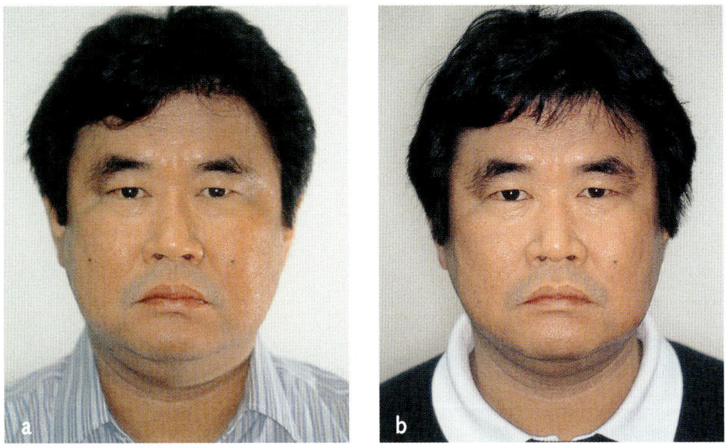

Fig 2-8 (a) Facial appearance before treatment. A clenching habit can be observed on the right side. He chews on the left side, where hypertrophy of masseter is noted. (b) Facial appearance after 5 months. Clenching as well as stiffness in the shoulders and neck have disappeared. The right corner of the mouth is no longer raised, and the facial symmetry has been improved.

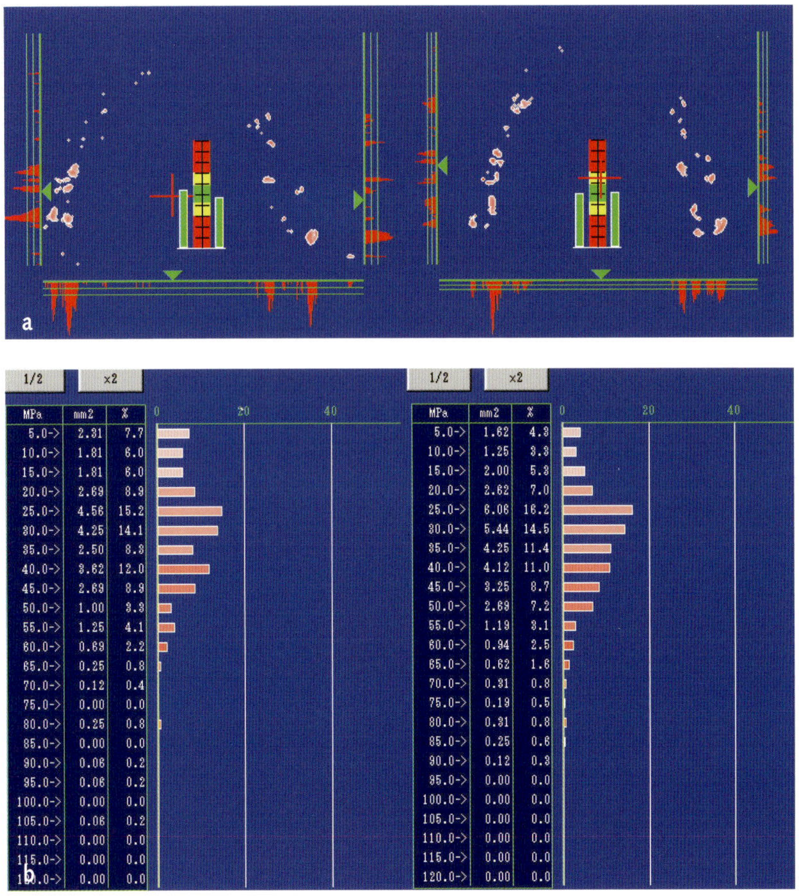

Fig 2-9 (a) The Occluzer reveals improvement in the balance of occlusal force from *(left)* the first visit to *(right)* 5 months later. The occlusal force has increased and the center of occlusion is more centralized. (b) The histogram indicates that, compared to *(left)* the first visit, *(right)* the distribution after 5 months is closer to a Gaussian distribution with a better balance in force.

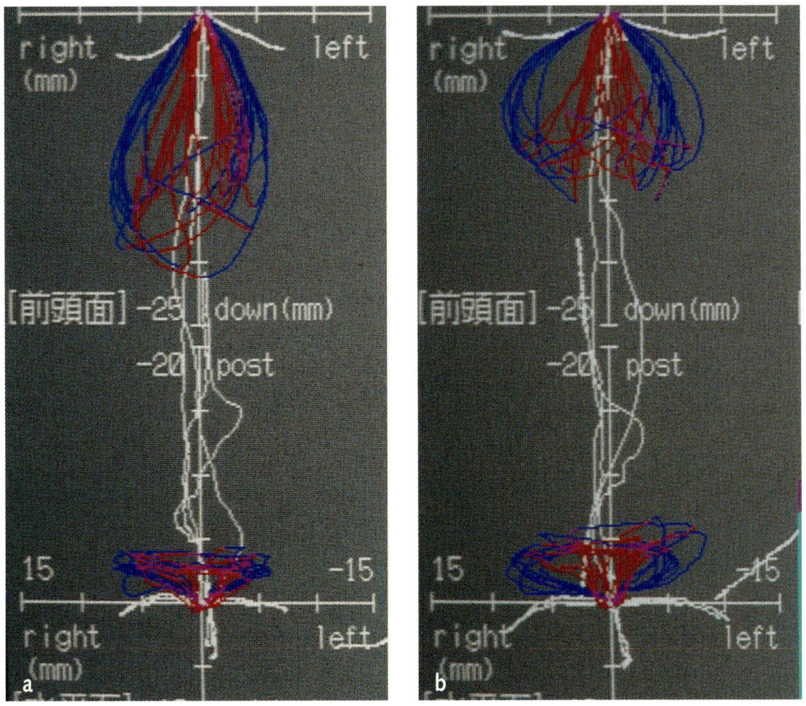

Fig 2-10 Sirognathograph of unconscious chewing (a) at the first visit and (b) after 5 months. *(top)* Frontal plane; *(bottom)* transverse plane. Before treatment, the right side border movement path was lower; this situation improved after treatment to facilitate lateral movement. Although this is a wide chewing cycle, this falls within a range of individual differences. Smooth mastication is achieved.

Examination and Diagnosis of Stomatognathic Functions

Reading signs of parafunction

The secret of occlusal therapy lies in examination, which is to read signs of parafunction. After history taking, visual inspection, palpation, and auscultation, the diagnosis can be established for most cases. Although equipment, including the mandibular movement analyzer, and radiographs are used as needed, they are intended for confirmation of diagnosis and objectification. Like cephalograms in orthodontic diagnosis, although very useful, they are "not something to totally rely on but to shed light on our route." For example, even when similar data are obtained by the mandibular movement analyzer, the clinical presentations of such cases are often different. Consequently, a diagnosis made based only on the mandibular movement analyzer is prone to be mistaken. Occlusion continues to change every day, or even every moment. If some intervention is made, the position of the mandible, for example, will change instantly. Slight differences (0.1 to 0.2 mm) will not be manifested on an articulator. It will be almost impossible to conduct an examination every time some change occurs. Even if an examination is performed, most changes are not shown. Therefore, data obtained by examination equipment should be regarded as supplementary to examinations with the five senses. Still, inexperienced clinicians should always train themselves, collecting as many materials as possible to find some agreement between the results of examinations based on their own five senses and the results based on equipment. We collect examination materials in the order shown in Table 2-3.

Narrowing the focus

The authors start from the face to the occlusion unit to the dentition unit to the tooth unit, narrowing the focus to examine the possible signs of parafunction (Fig 2-11). We imagine how those signs observed in four levels are related. We search for the root of parafunction, surmise how pathologic conditions have produced changes in the time course, and imagine what kind of problems they may invite in the future. In addition, we consider how the pathology is expressed in relation to inflammation, as if we are solving a puzzle.

Table 2-3 Collection of examination materials

- Photographs: clinical, facial, habits, posture of the whole body
- Radiographs: dental, TMJ, scanogram, orthopantogram, cephalogram
- Probing chart
- Study casts
- TMD chart
- Sirognathograph
- Gnathohexagraph
- Balancer
- Occluzer
- Confirmation of habits

Face*1

Occlusion-Unit
- Mandibular position (relaxed position)
- TMJ*2 (visual inspection, auscultation, palpation, and manipulation)
- Occlusion (maxillary and mandibular arches)

Dentition-unit*3

Toot-unit*3
- Teeth and periodontal tissue

***1 Face** In the facial examination, facial types (dolichofacial or brachyfacial) and profile types (straight, concave, or convex) are observed to predict possible pathologic conditions. For example, when there is a significant difference between the levels of right and left masseter hypertrophy, not only should chewing habits be noted, but also it should be conjectured whether the hypertrophy was caused by one-sided chewing or bruxism so that it can be linked to clinical and TMJ examinations. Also, facial observations should include possible shift and asymmetry of lower face, muscle tension, skin tone, skin texture, complexion, symmetry of eye size, eyelid line, distortion of the nose, nasolabial groove, lip line, dryness, and swelling.

***2 TMJ** First, with the clinician's fingers at the patient's right and left TMJ areas, the patient is allowed to open and close the mouth as the clinician palpates to assess rotation and translation of the condyles, the difference between right and left movements, and resistance. Simultaneously, auscultation is conducted for noise, and mouth opening is examined. When a clicking sound is heard, the patient is allowed to open and close in a different position to examine whether the noise disappears.

***3 Dentition, teeth, and periodontal tissue** Examination is conducted to assess maxillary and mandibular occlusion, to find if there is a narrow or distorted dental arch, and to assess teeth and periodontal tissue. We feel that there are some distinctive forms observed in the bodies and faces of current young adults (see Box 2-3) and pay attention to these characteristics at examination.

Fig 2-11 Examination for signs of parafunction.

Characteristics of occlusion and bruxism

Bruxism is the most well-known parafunction and is divided broadly into two categories: clenching and grinding. Bruxism is considered to have central and peripheral causes. Most clenching cases are related to tight occlusion (Fig 2-12) while most grinding cases are related to loose occlusion. Therefore, treatment for clenching is just the opposite of that for grinding, although both are regarded as bruxism. For clenching, areas of tight occlusion caused by excessive guidance are to be released, for which a stabilization-type splint is useful. On the other hand, for grinding, loose occlusion caused by lack of guidance is to be converged to a certain cycle. In this regard, a stabilization-type splint will not bring about dramatic results because it does not provide guidance.

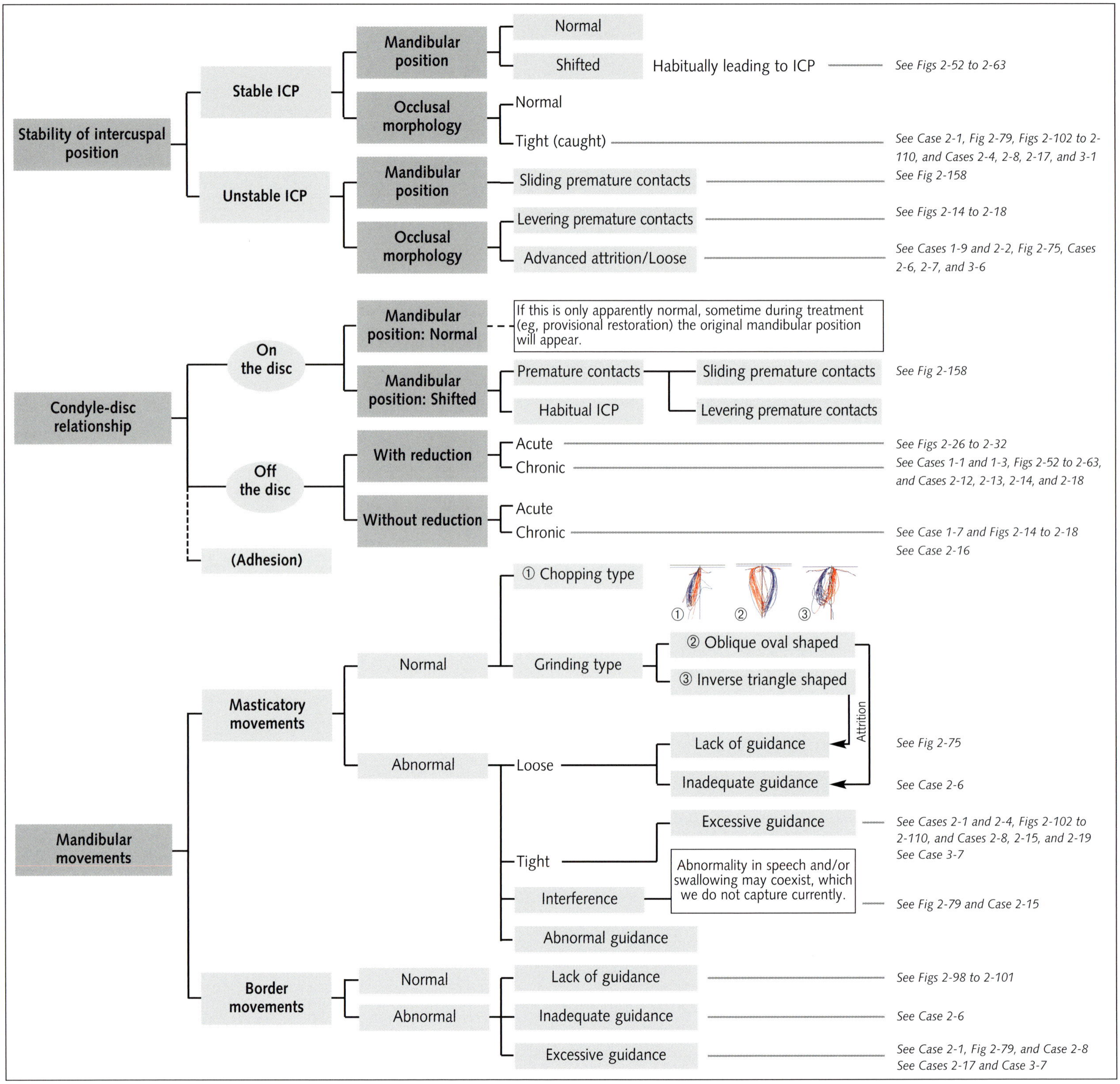

Fig 2-12 Concepts of occlusal analysis.

Unstable intercuspal position

In examination of stomatognathic functions, we focus on whether there is an abnormality in mandibular position, an abnormality in dental occlusion, or both. When there are no major problems in the TMJ area, the stability or instability of the intercuspal position will be the key. When ICP is unstable, whether or not the mandibular position has a problem has to be determined (Figs 2-12 and 2-13). A patient with unstable ICP has a problem in either the mandibular position or the occlusal morphology.

If relaxed position and ICP coincide and central and peripheral movement paths are harmonious, most occlusal problems will be solved.

Occlusal instability caused by premature contacts

Premature contacts that cause instability of occlusion are divided into sliding contacts and levering contacts. With a sliding premature contact, during closing, the mandible will shift anteriorly or laterally due to the sliding. With a levering premature contact, during closing, the mandible will rotate around a fulcrum point. It has been reported that such leverage affects the joints. In our experience, levering premature contacts are observed in patients with open bite and tongue habits where the relationship between the condyle and the fossa is loose and muscle strength is low. Obvious cases like that shown in Figs 2-14 to 2-18 are rare. Generally, it is a subtle movement that can be perceived with the senses.

In a dentition with a levering premature contact, if the patient bites heavily, a fulcrum point is escaped and intercuspation is achieved. Therefore, if occlusal morphology is corrected at that position, leverage will only worsen. In examination for premature contacts, contacts made at a feather-touch bite should be observed. These patients are less likely to develop serious joint problems, probably because muscle force is limited. Still, mere grinding of premature contact areas without elimination of the root cause may not necessarily stabilize the occlusion. When tongue habits cause an open bite, repeated occlusal adjustment will only reduce the vertical dimension without eliminating premature contacts.

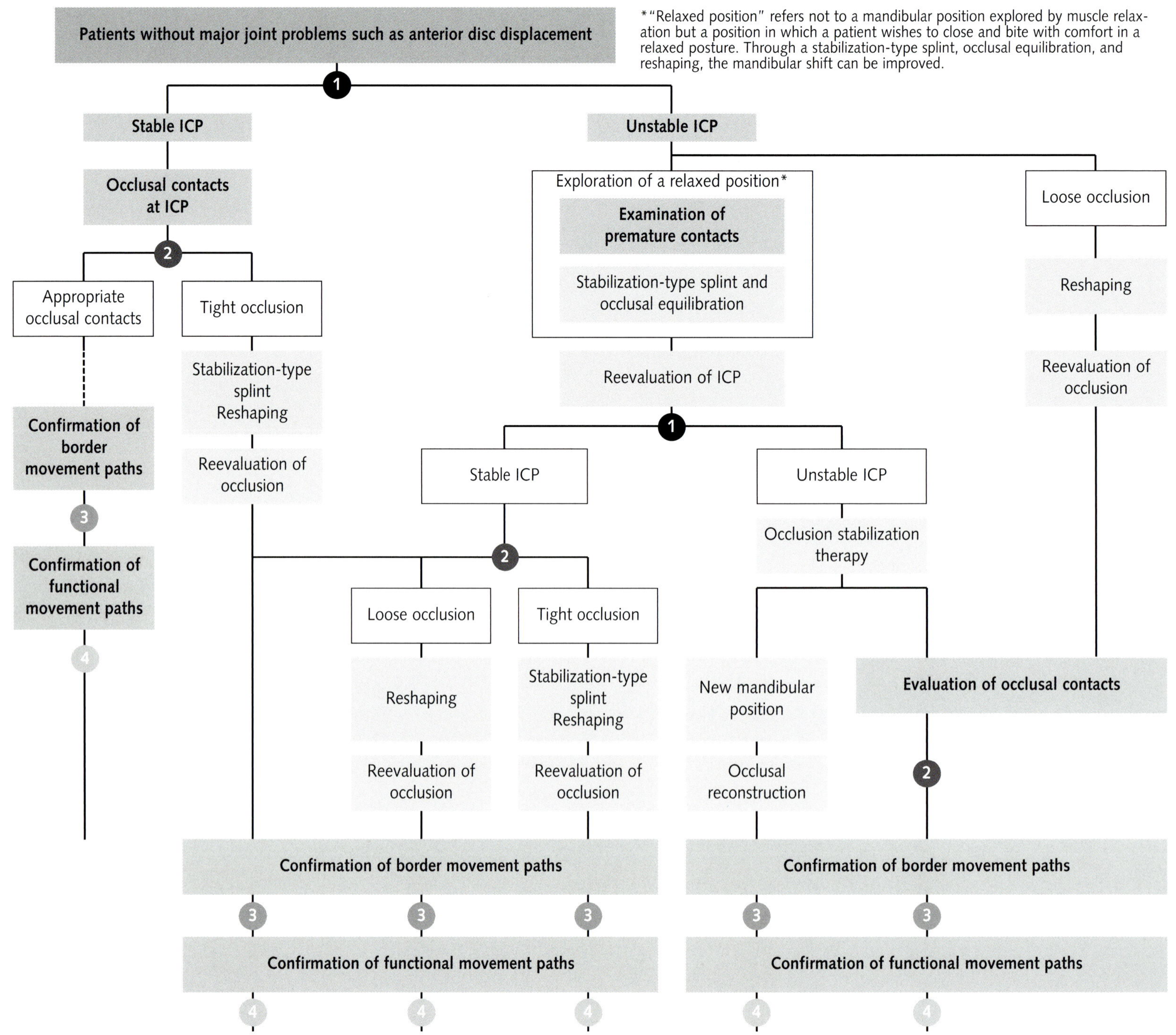

1 Examination of the stability of ICP
- Does it somewhat "click to" ICP? Can a patient tap at the same position in a stable manner?
- In a relaxed, reclined sitting position or a standing position, a patient is allowed to bite in a position they wish.
- Slight movement in a range of about 0.5 mm immediately before reaching ICP should not be overlooked.

2 Evaluation of occlusal contacts
- When a mandible starts to move from ICP, it can move quickly and smoothly.
- With loose occlusion, greater force is required to bite off food, which leads to muscle fatigue as well as damage to teeth, periodontal tissue, and joints.
- Tight occlusion, in which cusps catch on each other, causes clenching.

3 Confirmation of border movement paths
- Guidance and cuspal interference are examined.

4 Examination of functional movement paths
- Functional movement paths are inferred from occlusion and occlusal morphology.
- Evaluation with a mandibular movement analyzer is performed.

Fig 2-13 Procedures in occlusal therapy.

Conspicuous levering premature contacts

The patient in Figs 2-14 to 2-18, a 25-year-old woman, said that she had pain and clicking in the left TMJ several years before her first visit. However, no pain or noise was noted at the first visit. She said the jaw felt heavy when she chewed on the left side, and she had symptoms including left shoulder stiffness and headache. Anterior disc displacement without reduction was observed. She had a Class II, division 1 malocclusion with crowding. Her facial type was dolichofacial. The point A–nasion–point B (ANB) angle was 7.5 degrees. After extraction of all four maxillary premolars, myofunctional therapy (MFT) and active orthodontic treatment with full brackets (2 years 3 months) were conducted. However, the occlusion was not stabilized.

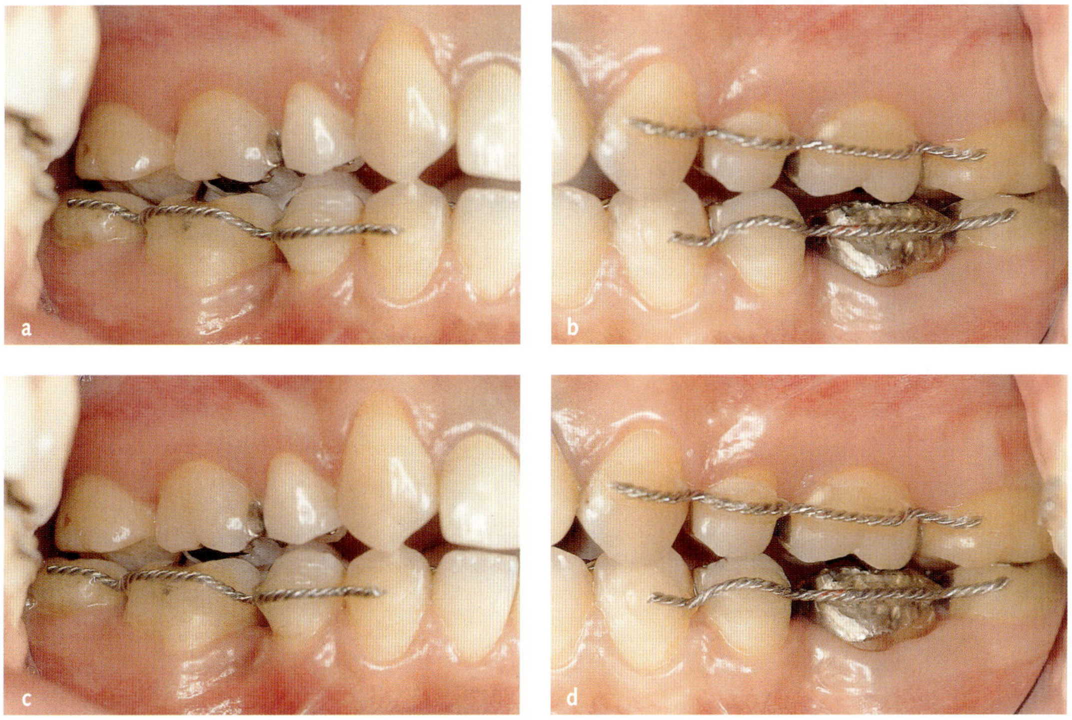

Fig 2-14 Premature contacts. (a and b) When lightly tapped, the maxillary left second molar and mandibular left second molar contact with 2 mm remaining overjet. Twisted wire is used for fixation. A relaxed position and ICP are not consistent (with about a 2-mm gap). Symptoms such as left shoulder stiffness and headache are resolved. (c and d) When the patient occludes strongly, the right-side bite is lowered with a fulcrum point at the maxillary and mandibular left second molars, and the left joint is stretched. At right-side chewing, the mandible is shifted to the right lateroposterior direction. At left-side chewing, the mandible is shifted to the left.

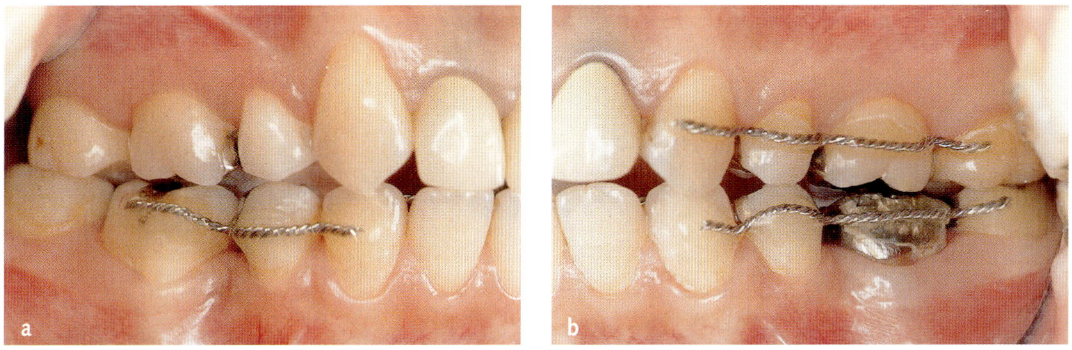

Fig 2-15 (a and b) Occlusal equilibration was conducted for the B slopes of the maxillary and mandibular left second molars, which acted as a fulcrum. Myofunctional therapy and splint therapy were also conducted. However, the patient's habit of putting her tongue between maxillary and mandibular teeth was not corrected, nor was the open bite improved. At 4 years 3 months after the first visit, another intense approach was made to correct the tongue habit. In a similar manner to previous treatments, occlusal equilibration was conducted for the B slopes of both left second molars, gradually and slightly in two sessions, so that the two molars occlude in such a way that an articulating paper lightly slips off. The discrepancy between the relaxed position and ICP falls in a range of about 1 mm.

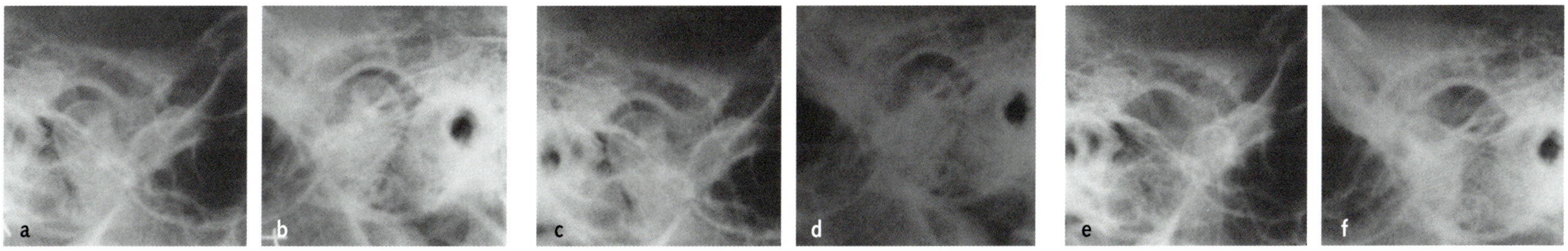

Fig 2-16 Articular space. (a) Right and (b) left TMJs when the teeth are lightly tapped together. The left TMJ remains in an anterior displaced position. (c) Right and (d) left TMJs when the teeth are strongly occluded. The right articular space is narrower, and the left articular space is stretched. The right and left condyles rotate like a seesaw, or with the action of a lever. (e) Right and (f) left TMJ at maximal opening (38 mm). The left condyle does not get over the anterior process.

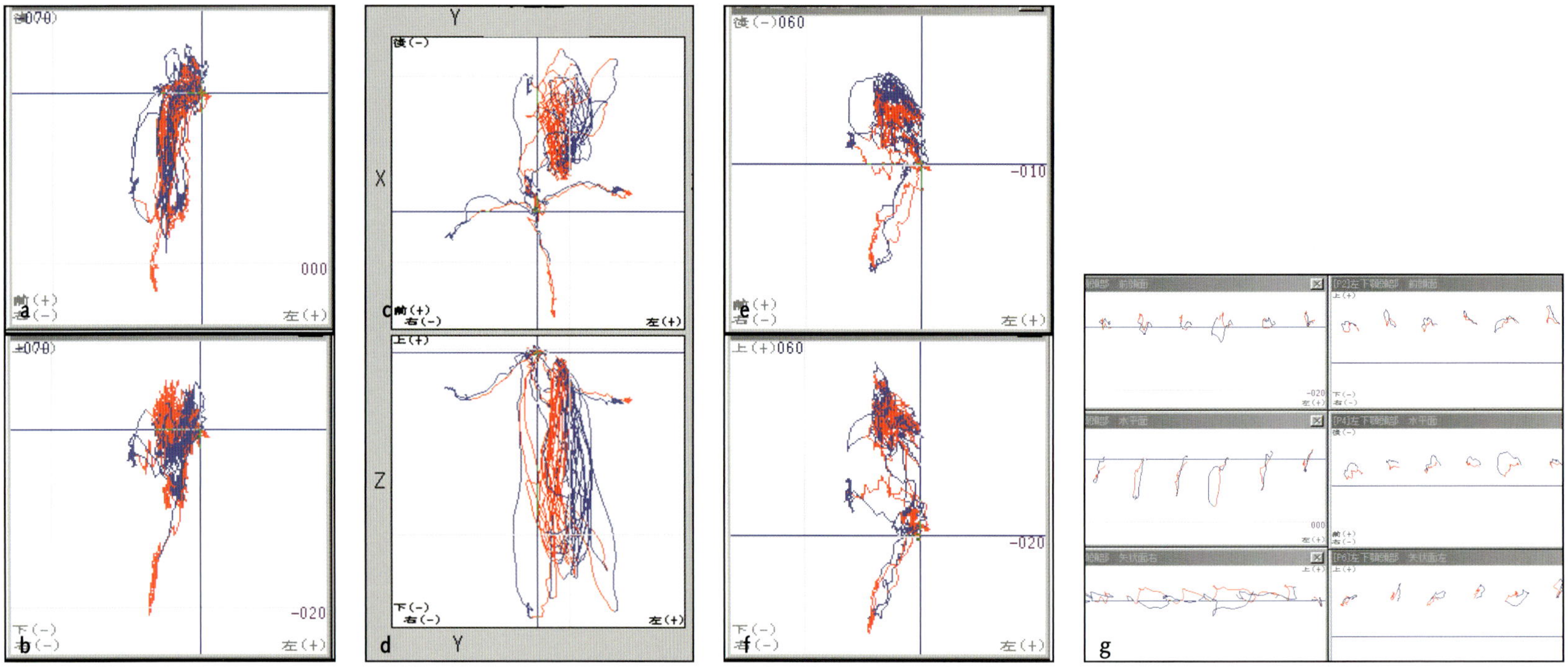

Fig 2-17 Functional movements of incisal areas and condyles observed with the Gnathohexagraph. Tracing of border movements is started from a light tapping position. At both right-side and left-side chewing, starting points and terminal points are laterally, posteriorly, and inferiorly located. Especially, they are located extremely posteriorly at left-side chewing. Movements of right and left condyles at left-side chewing (left condyle at working side and right condyle at nonworking side) takes place in a posterior, superior position by about 5 mm, which is totally different from the ending of the border movement. Similar results are obtained with the Sirognathograph, which enhances reliability. (a) Right condyle on a transverse plane during left-side chewing. (b) Right condyle on a frontal plane. (c) Incisal point on a transverse plane during left-side chewing. (d) Incisal point on a frontal plane. (e) Left condyle on a transverse plane during left-side chewing. (f) Left condyle on a frontal plane. (g) Cycles of condylar movements are individually observed. Condylar movements at left-side chewing are shown. *(left)* Right condyle (nonworking side); *(right)* left condyle (working side). Movement of the left condyle (working side) is located posteriorly and superiorly by as much as 5 mm. The right condyle (nonworking side) generates disordered cycles in an anterior, inferior direction.

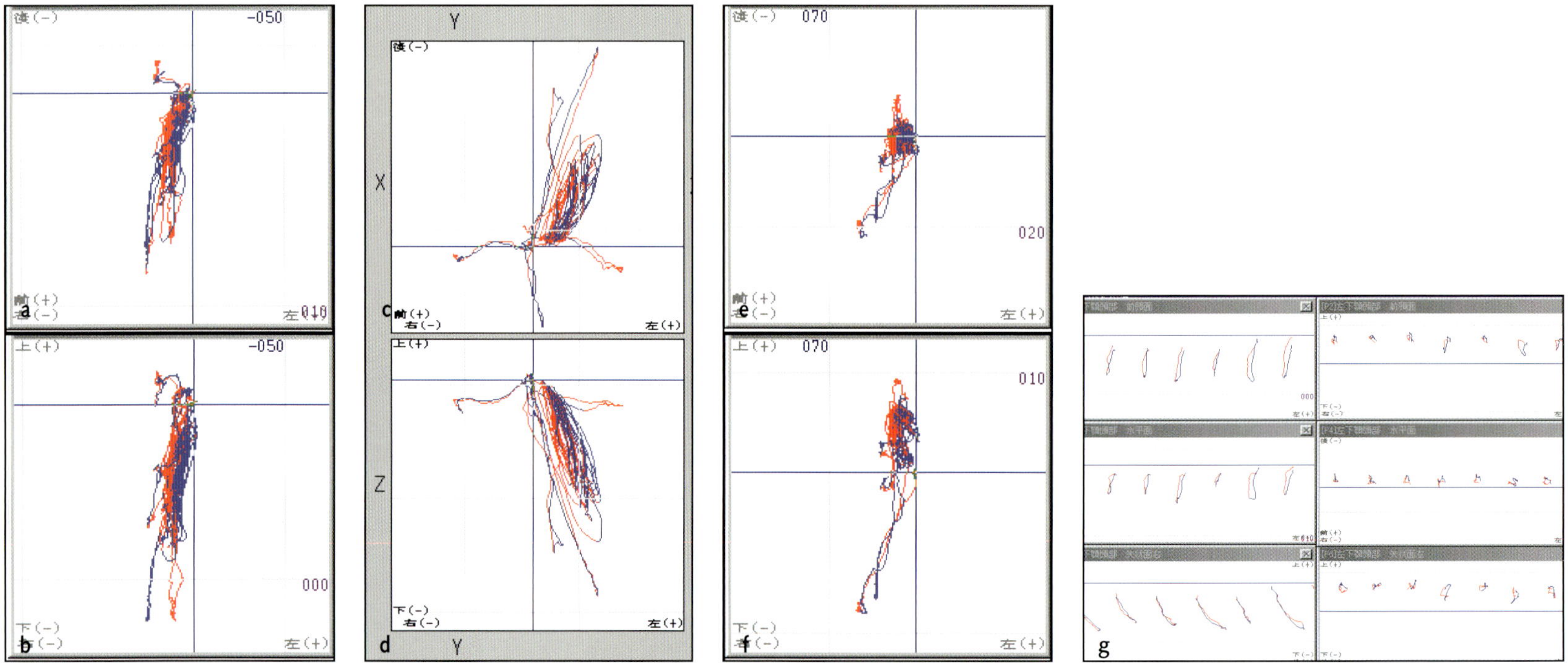

Fig 2-18 Functional movements of incisal areas and condyles after a second round of MFT. At both right and left sides, ending of movements is still posterior to ICP. Still, the discrepancy becomes smaller, and the endings of movements are converging. (a) Right condyle on a transverse plane during left-side chewing. (b) Right condyle on a frontal plane. (c) Incisal point on a transverse plane during left-side chewing. (d) Incisal point on a frontal plane. (e) Left condyle on a transverse plane during left-side chewing. (f) Left condyle on a frontal plane. (g) Cycles of condylar movements after a second regimen of MFT are individually observed. Condylar movements at left-side chewing are shown. Condylar movements are more organized.

Individual Differences and Jaw Functions

Occlusion

Naturally, each individual is different. Neither diet nor plaque accumulation is the same. Even with the same level of plaque accumulation, the development of inflammation is different. Furthermore, individual differences in occlusion are more diverse and complicated, because there is dynamism involved in which function shapes morphology and morphology enables function. Microscopically, a slight accessory ridge, the shape of a fissure, attrition on an occlusal surface, and slight tooth mobility will affect functions. Macroscopically, the posture of the whole body, the patient's lifestyle, and the patient's personality will have an influence. These are entangled in a complex manner to establish pathologic conditions. In determining the pathologic condition of the stomatognathic system, clinicians have to capture such dynamic relationships, which are typically represented in a facial pattern.

Facial patterns

Ricketts divided facial growth patterns into brachyfacial, dolichofacial, and mesiofacial patterns. The most common types of facial pattern are brachyfacial (Fig 2-19) and dolichofacial (Fig 2-20). Their morphologic characteristics are shown in Table 2-4, and characteristics of the pathologic conditions that are likely to result are described in Box 2-3. Although there are no statistics available, it seems that brachyfacial patterns have decreased and dolichofacial patterns have increased among current adolescents. In patients with a brachyfacial pattern, special attention should be paid to the periodontal tissue around molars. Reshaping of molar occlusal surfaces with advanced attrition is effective. Also, although a factor of skeletal overbite is involved, raising the bite often encounters resistance. Patients with a dolichofacial pattern are likely to have a discrepancy between the condyle and the disc, and they skeletally have a tendency to open bite. The mandible of a brachyfacial patient is L-shaped, while that of a dolichofacial patient is obtuse. According to Baba, the face of the Japanese is changing from a brachyfacial type to a dolichofacial type, and the angle of the mandible is changing from a right angle (L shape) to an obtuse angle. Such a change in the mandible has a potent influence on the stomatognathic system in the onset of, progression of, and recovery from diseases. Cases 2-2 and 2-3 present the treatment of typical brachyfacial and dolichofacial patients, respectively.

Disease patterns and facial patterns

With regard to jaw function disorders for which individual differences are significant, it facilitates understanding to consider the onset, type, and progress of diseases as well as occlusal collapse in roughly two categories according to facial patterns. Most dolichofacial patients have insufficiently developed condyles, which as a result are smaller compared to the fossae. Because of this, the articular space is wide, and condylar movement has more play. Consequently, when factors that cause condylar shift are present, including one-sided chewing, interference, and habits, condyles are likely to shift off the disc. Often occlusion is unstable, and mandibular shift is likely to occur.

On the contrary, most brachyfacial individuals have well-developed muscles, and, unlike dolichofacial patients, even if the same forces are applied, their condyles are less likely to shift off the disc. Rather, because of the strong force of their mastication, they are prone to the onset of TMD symptoms as a result of tooth attrition, compression of the jawbone, and a decrease of vertical dimension.

Because most Japanese subjects have a grinding-type chewing pattern, insufficiency of guidance is likely to progress, and, coupled with rolling movement (see Fig 2-75), cusps will become M shaped through attrition. This change often causes locking of maxillary and mandibular molars. When this is combined with inflammation of periodontal tissues and trauma, rapid loss of supporting tissue is expected.

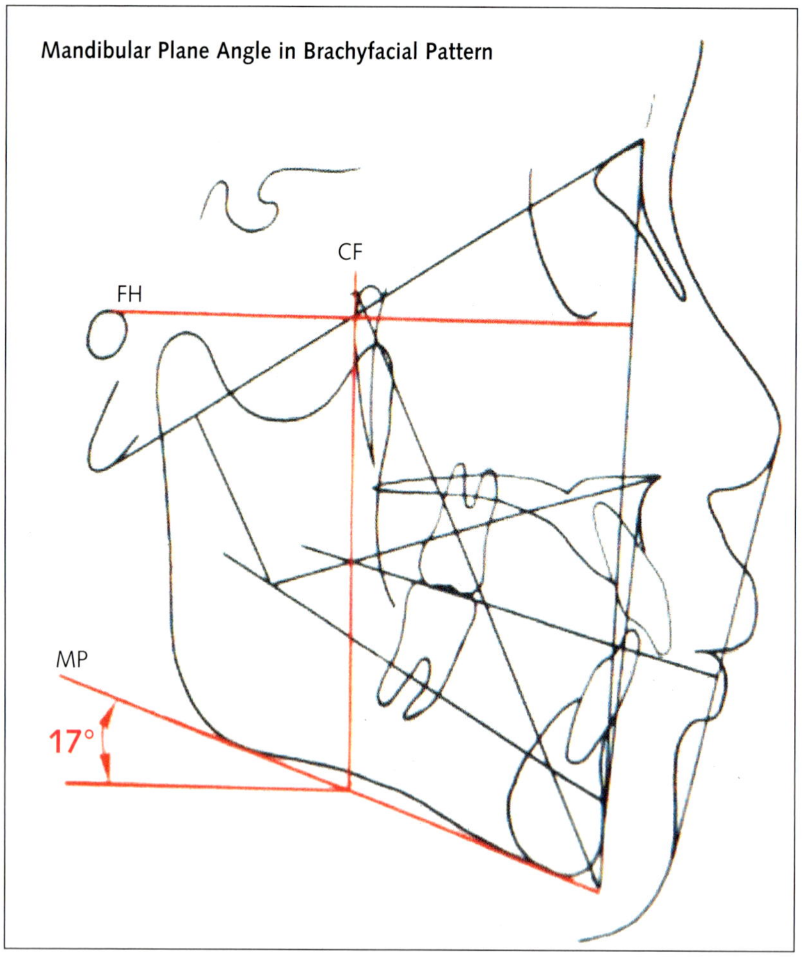

Fig 2-19 Cephalogram of the patient in Case 2-2 (brachyfacial pattern).

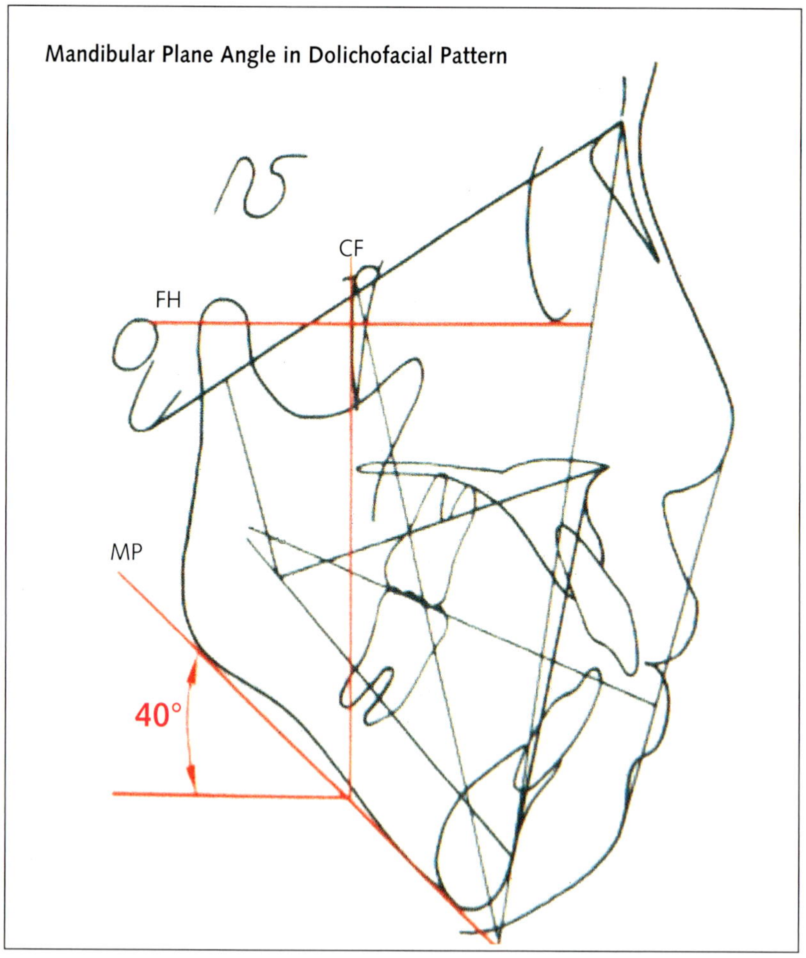

Fig 2-20 Cephalogram of the patient in Case 2-3 (dolichofacial pattern).

Table 2-4 Facial patterns and their characteristics

Characteristics of the brachyfacial pattern	Characteristics of the dolichofacial pattern
• Masseter action is strong. • The mandibular angle and vertical component of the face are small (small Frankfort horizontal–mandibular plane angle [FMA]): L-shaped face. • The vertical maxillomandibular distance tends to be shortened because of attrition. • The mastication pattern is more horizontal, which tends to cause lateral forces on teeth. • Secondary occlusal trauma tends to develop because of attrition and inflammation, which may cause loss of molars. • Molar loss invites deep bite and flaring of the anterior teeth in many cases. • Condyles are large, and disc displacement is less likely to occur. • Joint noise may be noted as a result of disc perforation caused by a decreased vertical dimension, for example.	• Masseter action is weak. • The lower face is narrow and long (large FMA), and the mandibular angle is large: open L-shaped face. • There tends to be a low tongue and crossbite at molars. • Open bite tends to develop because of the lateral thrust of the tongue. • Often the airway is narrow, causing mouth breathing. • The lip seal is weak. • Condyles are small, and disc displacement is more likely to occur. • Mandibular shift is like to occur.

Box 2-3 Impressions of the physical characteristics of adolescents

The following are the subjective impressions that the authors have of the physical characteristics of today's adolescents:

Body type
- Short torso and small face
- Poorly muscled
- Poor carriage; rest their chins on their hands due to weak back muscles (Figs 2-21 and 2-22).

Face
- Retruded maxilla and/or mandible; prominent midnose and chin
- Inverse triangle–shaped lower face
- Thin and weak mastication muscles
- Small and narrow maxilla and mandible
- Open L–shaped mandible
- Large gonial (Go) angle and FMA
- Large occlusal plane (OP) angle
- Asymmetric lower face
- Dolichofacial type increased

Dentition
- Increased crowding, mandibular retrusion, and open bite

Teeth
- Increased number of congenitally missing teeth (second molars, third molars, maxillary lateral incisors, maxillary second premolars, mandibular second premolars, and mandibular central incisors)
- Macrodontia of the maxillary central incisors
- Microdontia of the maxillary lateral incisors
- Giant mesiolingual cusps and small or no distal cusps of the maxillary second molars
- Tendency to impaction of the second premolars
- Short and thin tooth roots
- Narrow roots of multirooted teeth
- Tendency to single root

TMJ
- Shallow articular fossae
- Small, underdeveloped condyles
- Wide articular space, giving much play in movement of the condyle, likely to cause displacement between condyle and disc

Periodontal tissue
- Thin gingiva
- Narrow attached gingiva
- Less dense bone

Tongue
- Narrow tongue and tongue space; not stable in palatal space
- Weak tongue muscle
- Inability of the tongue to adhere to the palate
- Increase of low tongue and tongue thrust

Lips
- Increase of lip-biting habits
- Loose lips as a result of mouth breathing

Habits (Mostly, resting the cheek on the hands and postural habits during sleep)

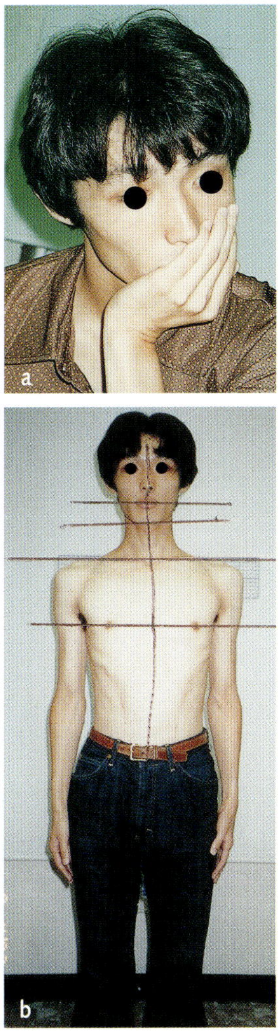

Fig 2-21 (a and b) Case 2-20.

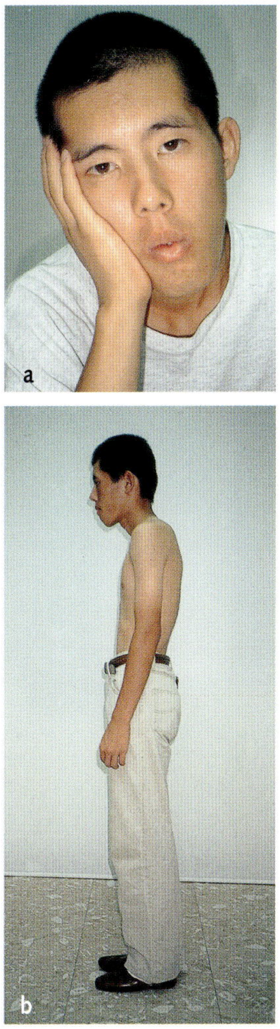

Fig 2-22 (a and b) Case 2-9.

Case 2-2 Posterior occlusal collapse in a typical brachyfacial-type patient

Patient: *61-year-old woman (a traditional flower arrangement instructor) at the time of first visit in 1991*
Chief complaint: *Masticatory dysfunction accompanied by mobility of a fixed partial denture extending from the maxillary right central incisor to the maxillary left lateral incisor (pontic: maxillary left central incisor), as well as mobility of the mandibular left premolars*
Medical history: *Diabetes mellitus and hypertension*
Diagnosis: *Moderate to severe periodontitis, missing molars because of severe bite force and inflammation, and flared-out anterior teeth*
Treatment plan: *Bite raising, uprighting of anterior teeth, and recovery of molar occlusal support*

This was a typical patient with a brachyfacial pattern who had severe periodontal disease and a risk factor of diabetes. When molar occlusal collapse occurs in this facial type, the decrease of vertical dimension is advanced even further by the strong force of masseters, horizontal masticatory movements, and other forces. In this patient, at the first visit, molar occlusal support had been already lost, with extrusion of the opposing teeth (Fig 2-23). Accordingly, the occlusal surfaces of the mandibular denture teeth were replaced by metal, the stability of the denture was enhanced, the load bearing for the ridge was reduced, and preservation of the mandibular position was expected (Figs 2-24 and 2-25). Also, the vertical dimension was recovered, and attention was paid to occlusal morphology to reduce the burden on periodontal tissue. During provisional restoration, constriction screws were used in the maxilla to narrow the arch width, and elastics were used to incline anterior teeth lingually (2-month active orthodontic treatment). After natural extrusion, a fixed partial denture was delivered to mandibular left second premolar, which was eventually extracted in 1999. The patient was instructed to be aware of clenching. We advised her to wear the splint when she had to cut a hard branch for her flower arrangements. After treatment, masseter hypertrophy as well as the mandibular shift to the left were alleviated.

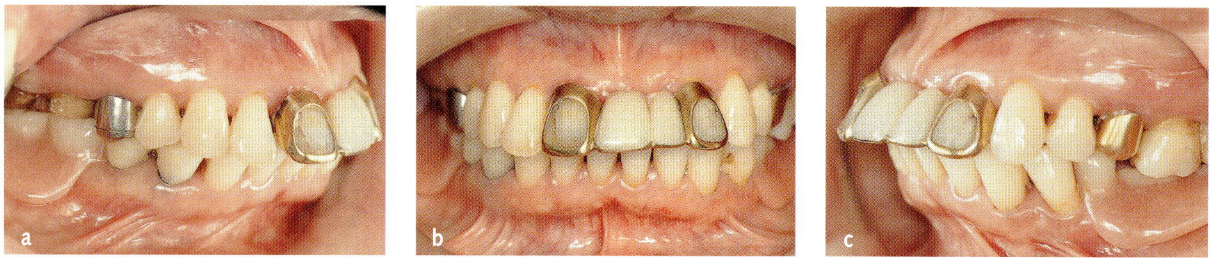

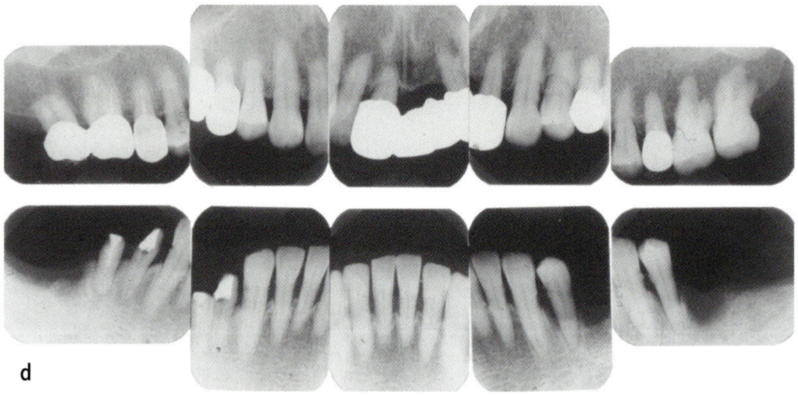

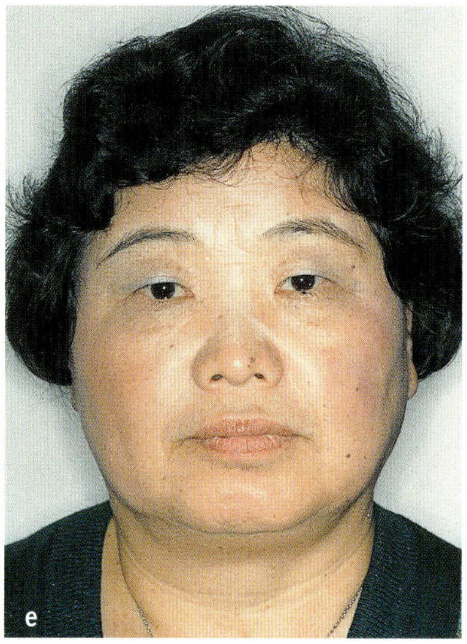

Fig 2-23 (a to e) At the first visit, molar occlusal support was lost, and the vertical dimension was conspicuously decreased. The mobility of the fixed partial denture extending from the maxillary right central incisor to the maxillary left lateral incisor (pontic: maxillary left central incisor) and the mobility of the mandibular left premolars were significant. Although the lower face was shifted to the left, the condyle was not off the disc.

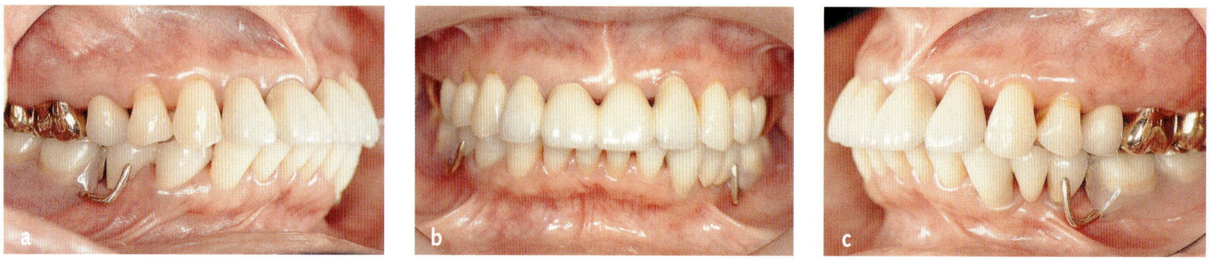

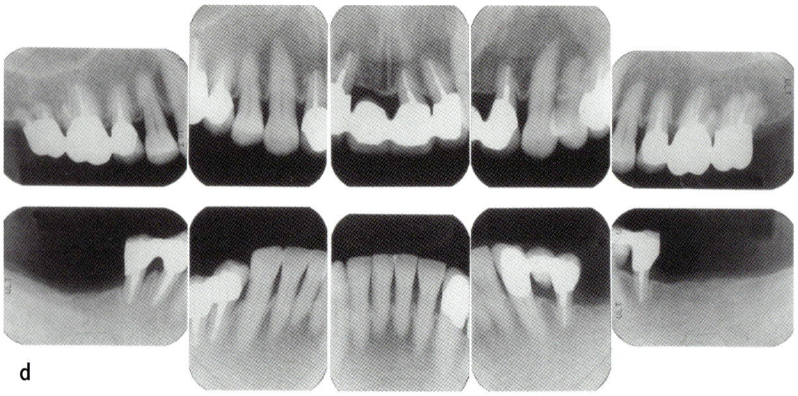

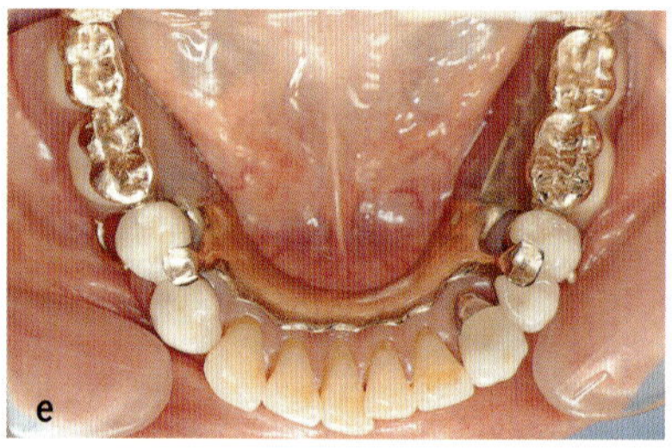

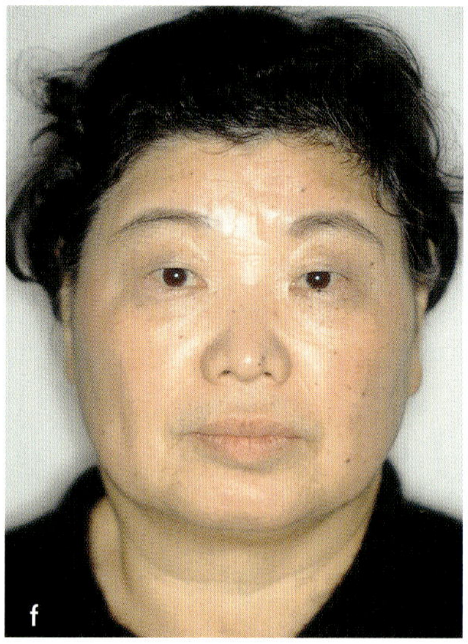

Fig 2-24 (a to f) The occlusal surfaces of the mandibular denture teeth were replaced by metal, and the patient was instructed to be aware of clenching. The mandibular shift to the left was reduced.

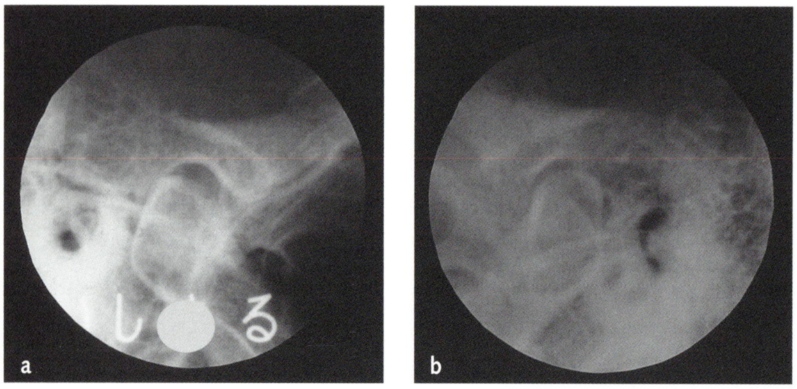

Fig 2-25 Transcranial plain radiographs at the first visit. (a) Right and (b) left TMJs at closing. The morphology of condyles is well developed. Although the right condyle seems to be posteriorly displaced, this is not abnormal clinically. With this morphology of the condyle, there is no space for disc displacement even if some force is applied as a result of the patient's oral habits.

Case 2-3 Disc displacement in a typical dolichofacial-type patient

Patient: *17-year-old boy at the time of first visit in 1992*
Chief complaint: *Pain in the right TMJ area, trismus, and restriction of mandibular movement*
Diagnosis: *Labial inclination of the maxillary anterior teeth caused by a lower lip–biting habit. Right-side chewing, caused by a habit of resting the left cheek on his left hand and interference at the second molar, as well as other reasons invited right disc displacement with reduction. Figures 2-26 to 2-32 detail his treatment.*

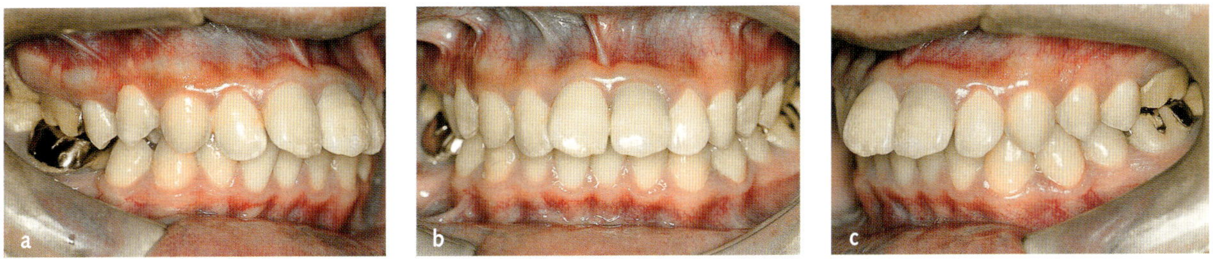

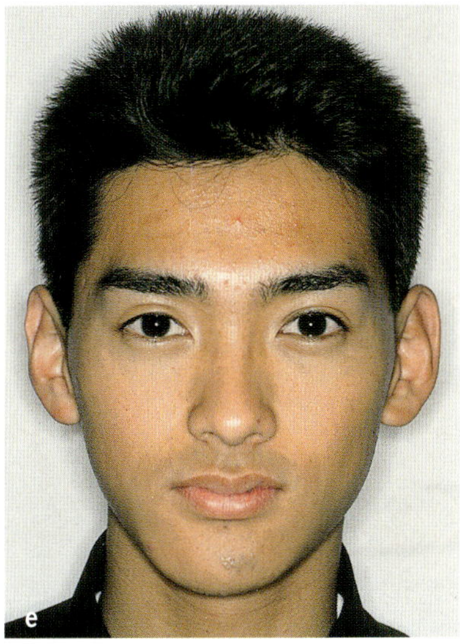

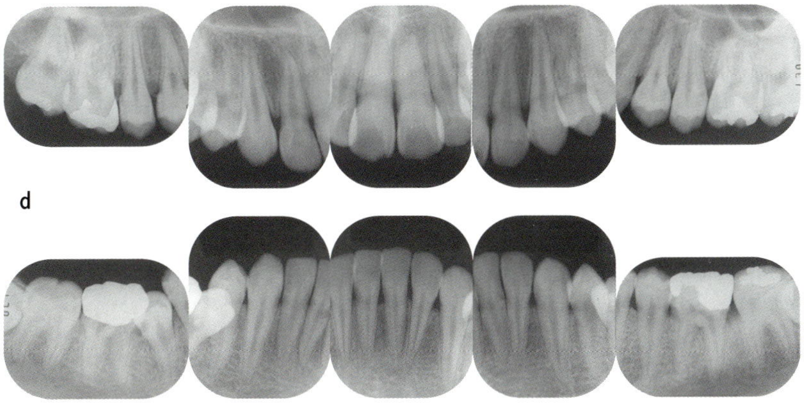

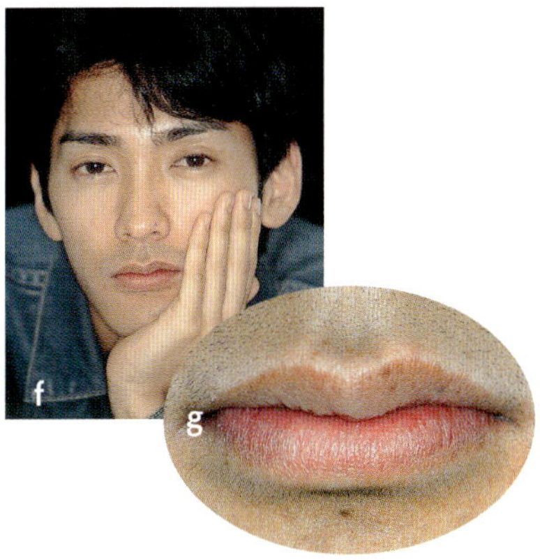

Fig 2-26 (a to d) At the first visit, typical anterior disc displacement with reduction (right condyle off the disc) is observed. Cuspal interference is noted for the left second molars. The occlusal force is weak. (e) The lower face is shifted to the right. He has the habits of (f) resting his left cheek on his left hand (photograph shows reenactment 5 years later) and (g) biting his lower lip.

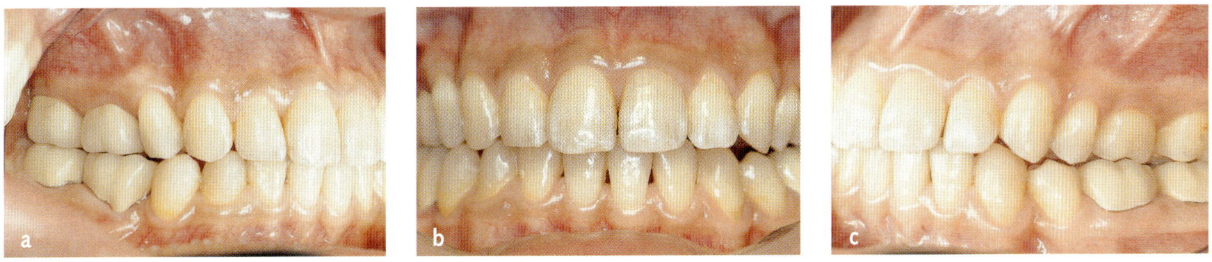

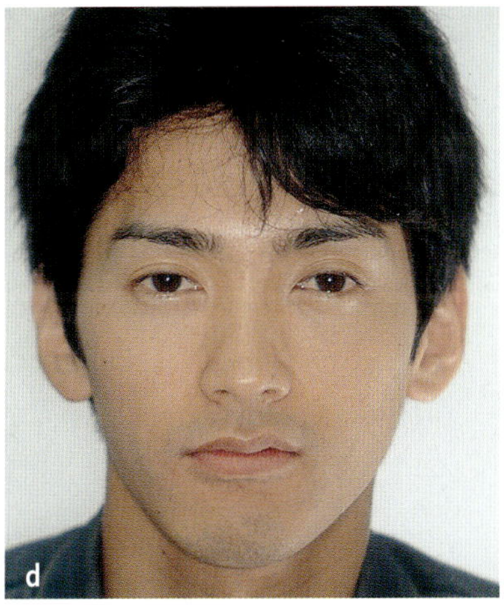

Fig 2-27 (a to d) Photographs taken after about 8 years. Because the right condyle is still off the disc and is not stabilized even after orthodontic treatment, the occlusal surface of the right molar was raised by a crown restoration to bring the condyle "on the disc."

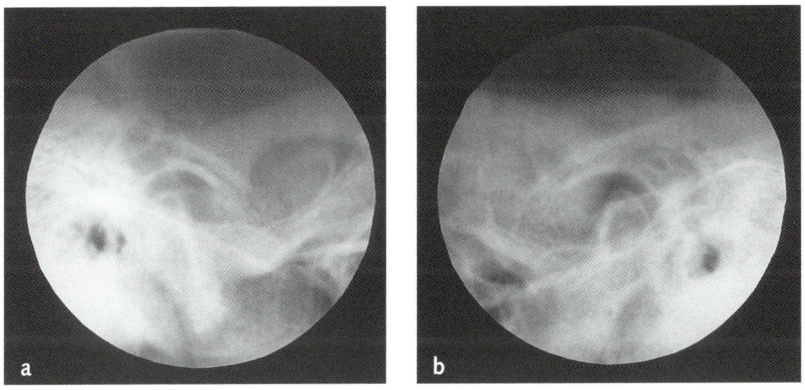

Fig 2-28 Transcranial plain radiographs show the inadequate morphology of the condyle, which is a common feature of a dolichofacial pattern. (a) The right condyle is especially poorly developed. The right condyle is off the disc. Because of a wide articular space, such a condyle comes off the disc when forces are applied, for example, from a habit. (b) Left condyle.

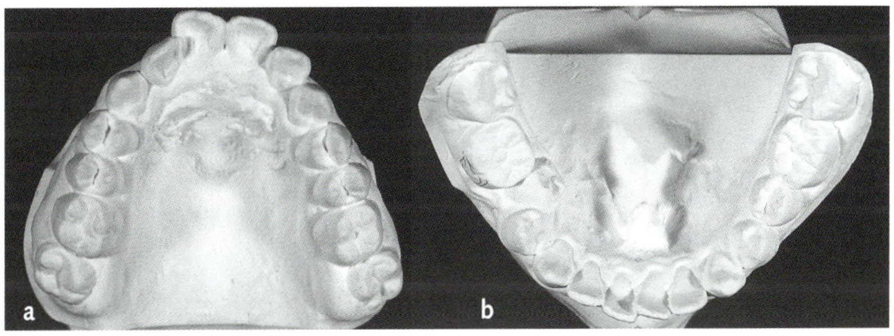

Fig 2-29 At the first visit. Because the maxillary second molars erupted with buccal inclination and the mandibular second molars are lingually inclined, there is interference, especially at the B slopes of the maxillary and mandibular left second molars. Also, because the mesiolingual cusps of the maxillary second molars are large and pointed, this seems to have intensified the interference at the B slopes.

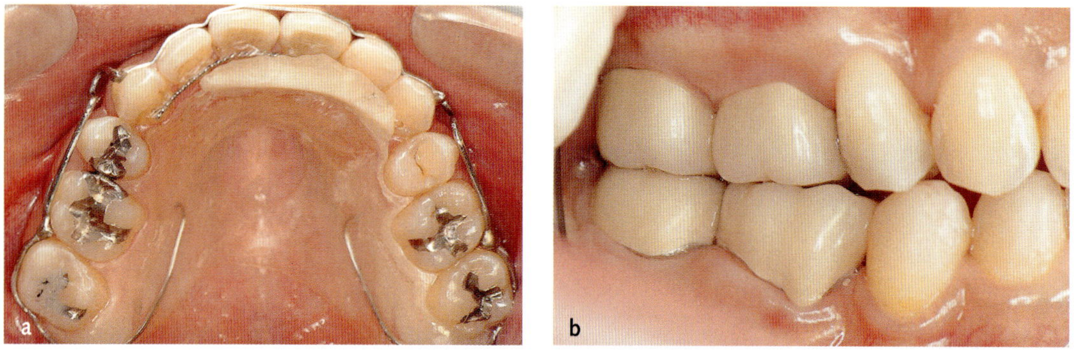

Fig 2-30 A guiding slope is added to the retainer of the maxillary anterior teeth to prevent the right condyle from coming down during sleep. Eventually a hybrid, superhard resin crown restoration was provided for the right molars.

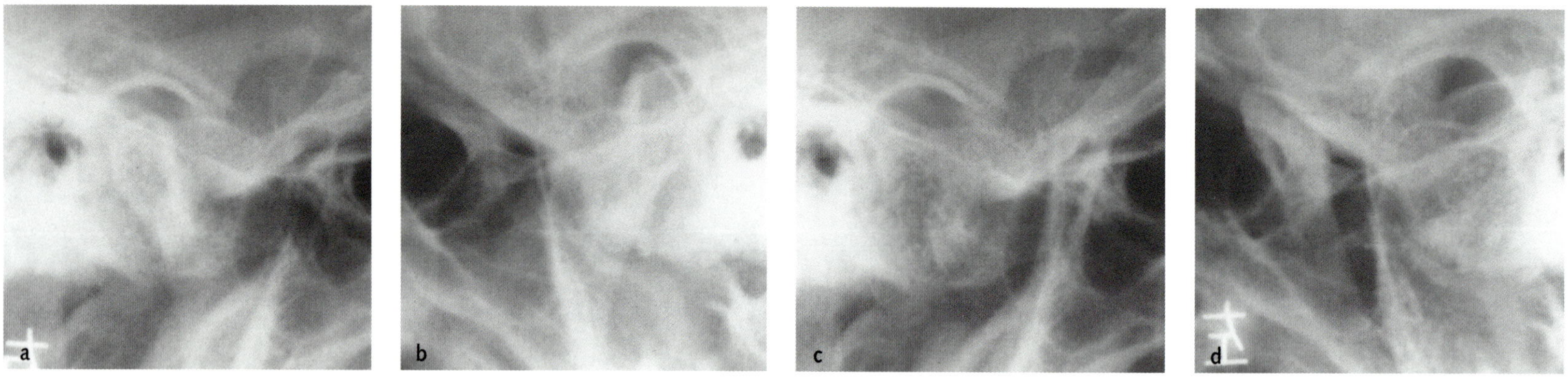

Fig 2-31 Transcranial plain radiographs taken 6 years after the first visit, showing the (a) right and (b) left condyles on the disc. (c) Right and (d) left TMJs at maximal opening.

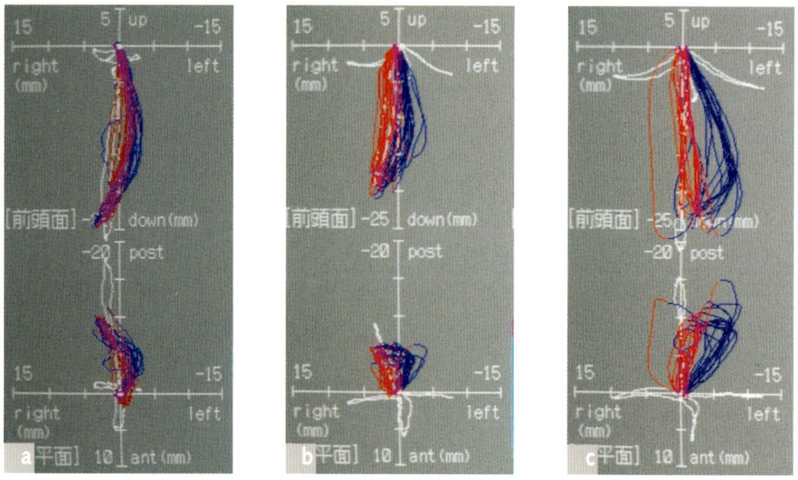

Fig 2-32 Sirognathographs, all completed during left-side chewing. *(top)* Frontal plane; *(bottom)* transverse plane. (a) At the first visit. Because the right condyle is off the disc, the turning point in the left cycle is pulled to the right while the right cycle is normal. The small deviation between opening and closing suggests that this is an acute disc displacement without deformity or displacement of the posterior band. (b) After orthodontic treatment. Although the condyle remains off the disc, the width of the masticatory movement path has been expanded. The range of motion posterior to the disc is increased, suggesting that the condition is getting old. (c) After crown restoration. The turning point has been shifted to the left, suggesting that mastication is conducted at an on-the-disc position.

History of present illness: *At the onset of the disease, which was 1 month prior to his visit, the patient had significant pain on mouth opening. However, he was prescribed a stabilization-type splint by a dentist who referred the patient to us, and the pain had been relieved when we examined him. This was a typical acute anterior disc displacement with reduction in a typical dolichofacial-type patient. The open L–shaped mandibular angle, narrow lower face, FMA of 33.5 degrees, prominent nose, and large Go angle are typical characteristics observed in dolichofacial types.*

Right anterior disc displacement with reduction: *Because of buccoversion of the maxillary second molars and lingual inclination of the mandibular second molars, interferences of the B slopes, especially the left-side B slopes, were severe, causing right-side chewing. Buccoversion of the maxillary second molars and lingual inclination of the mandibular second molars may be caused by discrepancy, which is often observed in dolichofacial types. Because of their tendency to attrition, the maxillary second molars had large, conical mesiolingual cusps, which intensified the interferences of the B slopes. The condyles were poorly developed, especially on the right, which was also affected by dysfunction. Because of this, the condyle had more play in the articular fossa, which was likely to invite deviation. It was surmised that the posterior shift of the mandible was caused by his habits of resting the cheek on the left hand and biting the lower lip in addition to his right-side chewing. The large overjet may also have been associated with the lower lip–biting habit.*

Treatment progress: *A repositioning splint was used to put the condyle on the disc. As anterior displacement resulted as the splint was removed, orthodontic treatment was started. The active treatment was conducted from August 1992 to April 1995 with a full-bracket system. A Class I relationship was achieved on the left side but not on the right side. The midline was still shifted to the right. The right disc was easily dislocated anteriorly. Eventually, crown restorations were provided to provide occlusal support on the right side, and the condyle was given an on-the-disc relationship.*

Like this patient, the number of dolichofacial-type individuals with weak occlusal force is increasing among young generations, and therefore the number of patients who are likely to have trouble with their TMJs is also increasing.

Concepts of Biomechanics and Remodeling

System to maintain optimal morphology for function

A living body always experiences secondary morphologic changes in response to changes in functions or remodeling and functional changes in response to changes in morphology. It is said that organisms have a system to maintain optimal morphology for their functions. Based on this hypothesis, it is believed that pathologic functions will lead to pathologic morphology and that pathologic morphology will invite pathologic functions. While healthy organisms maintain homeostasis while repeating metabolism, links of pathologic functions and pathologic morphology, if left alone, will develop into a vicious circle, resulting in malfunctions and occlusal collapse in stomatognathic systems.

Recovery of appropriate occlusal morphology

The principal measures we take in dentistry are modification of morphology. For masticatory dysfunctions, recovery of appropriate occlusal morphology, including maxillary and mandibular dental relationships, is often the most effective therapy (Box 2-4).

When proper occlusal morphology is given, muscle spasms will be eliminated. Also, muscles, bone, joints, and periodontal ligaments will be released from compressed conditions. In most cases, the occlusal vertical dimension will increase naturally, and the mandible moves forward. A living body gradually remodels itself, allowing a more natural and reasonable position for the mandible against the cranium. Needless to say, an articulator does not remodel itself. It cannot express a subtle change in the mandibular position or premature contacts associated with that change. Consequently, optimal occlusal morphology has to be recovered according to the changing mandibular position. Although it is easy to say, it is sometimes extremely difficult to accomplish clinically.

Sensitive patients may complain of discomfort with 0.1 to 0.2 mm of occlusal contact change. Clinicians must use their senses to perceive slight changes, based not on theory or examination data but according to a patient's sensitivity. With placement of a subtle groove (0.1 to 0.2 mm deep, about 1.0 mm long) to divide the B slope and C slope, clenching is resolved for some patients, and they are relieved from headache. Slight improvement in morphology will greatly change functions, including mastication and speech, and the morphology of the muscles and dentition will change in accordance to such functional changes, as is shown by Case 2-4, the first clinical case that clearly taught the authors the relationship between reshaping and remodeling in the living body.

Improvements that follow occlusal therapy

We have experienced that, by recovering relaxed occlusion, symptoms such as orofacial pain, head and neck pain, tinnitus, and obstructed feelings of the ears are relieved. However, we do not believe that occlusal therapy should be conducted with the goal of improving of such symptoms or assuring a patient of improvement. It is merely that improvement may be obtained in some cases as a result of recovery of a natural, relaxed occlusion. This is because the causes of pain and discomfort of these kinds are diverse and are deeply associated with a patient's sensitivity, with which we can agree based on a number of experiences. Having said that, when various occlusal anomalies do exist, clinicians should not disregard the patient's complaint by simply determining that the main cause is psychologic and solely relying on counseling for resolution. A dentist must make maximal efforts to restore a comfortable oral environment with minimal invasion, listening to the patient's complaints and looking for the causes.

Box 2-4 Reshaping (reestablishment of occlusal morphology)

We define reshaping as the conversion of large-surface occlusal contacts to small ones to enable smooth, buccolingual and anteroposterior gliding from a position of interdigitation. Conventionally, grinding of the inclined planes of cusps was advocated within the scope of selective grinding, based on the mesial upper-distal lower or buccal upper-lingual lower methods. Adjustment of natural enamel in accordance with such principles, however, is not only meaningless but also dangerous, possibly inviting occlusal collapse.

Reshaping is designed to provide an occlusal relationship close to the ideal to the existing teeth and/or restorations with minimal invasion. Relationships between ridges and fossae are corrected, developing three-dimensional contact relationships against opposing teeth that are reflected in articulating papers and occlusal indicator wax. Not only grinding but also the use of resin may be conducted. Special attention should be paid to grinding. Areas that must be removed are prudently confirmed and ground little by little with a carbide bur. Functional occlusal examination equipment may be used for evaluation during the procedure.

Case 2-4 Improvement of tight occlusion and remodeling

Patient: *28-year-old woman at the time of first visit in 1993*
Chief complaint: *For a week, somewhat dull, heavy pain was felt from the left TMJ area to the left mandibular base. Pain was felt whether the mouth was open or closed. Dizziness and nausea continued. Due to severe palpitations, pain in the chest was felt during work.*
The patient reported left-sided migraine and a heavy feeling in the jaw beginning when she was 20 years old. When she visited us, she complained of a facial pain felt under the ear and a tight, dull feeling in the mid- and lower face on the left side. Her treatment is shown in Figs 2-33 to 2-50.

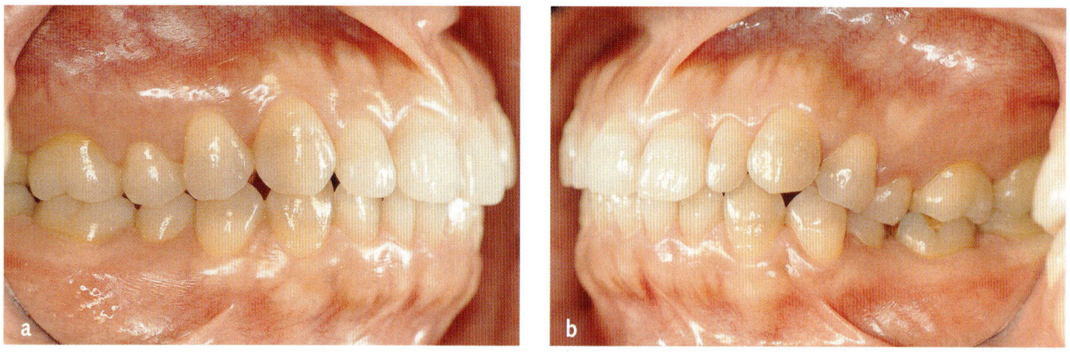

Fig 2-33 (a and b) At the first visit, the dentition is distorted on the left side as if pushed lingually. Especially, the maxillary left second premolar, first molar, and second molar and the mandibular left second premolar, first molar, and second molar are deeply engaged anteroposteriorly, and free gliding is not possible.

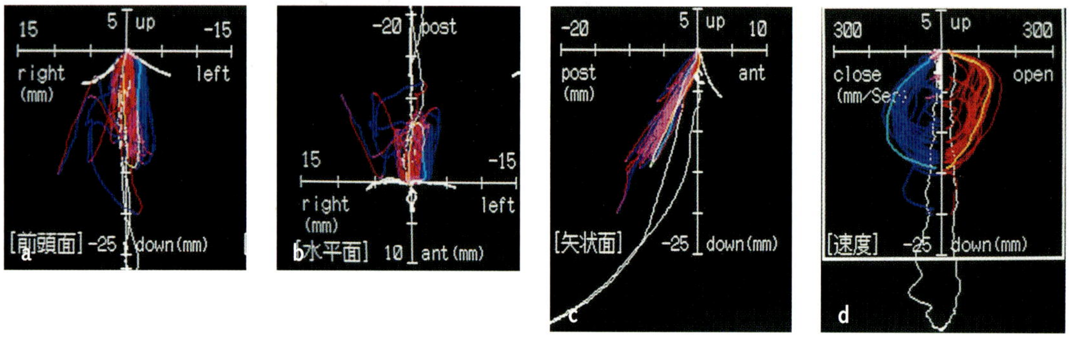

Fig 2-34 Sirognathographs taken during left-side chewing at the first visit. (a) Frontal plane. (b) Transverse plane. (c) Sagittal plane. (d) Velocity. This patient's habitual mastication is conducted on the left side. At the first visit, the occlusal phase is longer than the closing phase, which is consistent with the patient's complaint that her left occlusion felt locked. On the frontal and transverse planes, the opening paths are not stable when getting around excessive guidances, and closing paths have limited freedom because of lateral guidances. On the sagittal plane, opening is possible only after initial opening in the anterior and inferior direction. The closing path reaches ICP from downward.

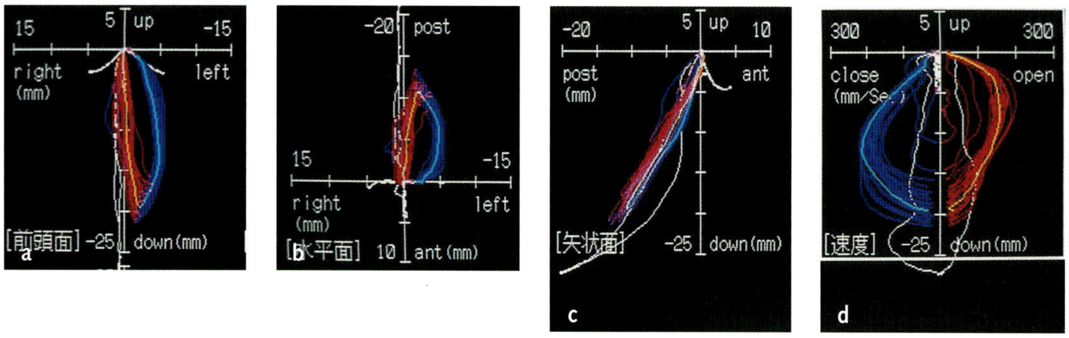

Fig 2-35 (a to d) Sirognathographs taken during left-side chewing after 1 year 5 months. (a) Frontal plane. (b) Transverse plane. (c) Sagittal plane. (d) Velocity. Discrepancies between opening and closing paths have decreased, forming stable large cycles. Anterior and inferior movement at opening still remain.

It was surmised that lingual inclination of the left molars and crowding invited occlusal interferences at the left molars and excessive guidance. Also, it was believed that clenching was not connected with deep engagement of the fossae and cusps.

The main treatment plan included correction of the lower lip–biting habit, muscle relaxation using a stabilization-type splint, and elimination of interferences and excessive guidances via reshaping to provide freedom in occlusion.

The buccal cusps of the lingually inclined mandibular left first and second molars were firmly engaged in central fossae of maxillary left first and second molars. With the mesial inclination of molars and crowding of the premolars, this disturbed free gliding. Through the improvement in occlusion, an improvement of function materialized gradually, which, as a result, improved the morphology.

Since crowding remains in this patient, there is the possibility that symptoms may recur, in which case orthodontic tooth movement will be required. If there is no recurrence, we believe it is appropriate to complete the case with basic therapies alone. This patient originally had a convex profile. Resolution of crowding may result in a further convex situation or may require tooth extraction. As such, the authors believe orthodontic treatment should be avoided if conditions are improved.

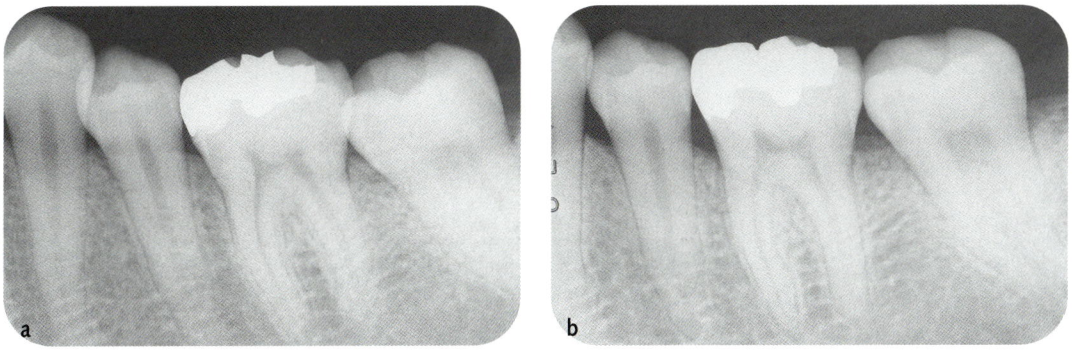

Fig 2-36 Left molars (a) at the first visit and (b) after 1 year. The mandibular left second premolar, first molar, and second molar are being uprighted naturally.

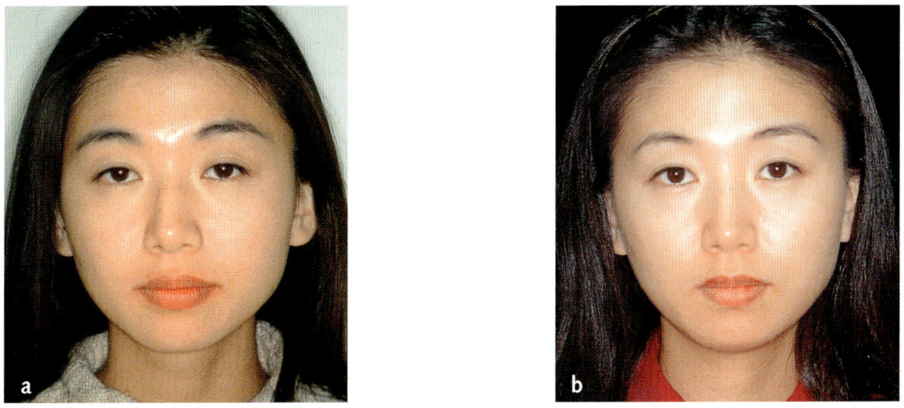

Fig 2-37 (a) Frontal view of the face at the first visit. The left and the right sides of the face are asymmetric. The left masseter is hypertrophic. The mandible is slightly shifted to the left. She has a convex profile with an ANB angle of 6.0 degrees. Tenderness is observed in the temporalis, masseter, lateral pterygoid, and sternocleidomastoid muscles as well as the TMJ and around the ear on the left side. Stiffness is observed in left shoulder, occipital region, neck, and back. She is slightly built. (b) Photograph taken 9 months after the first visit. Facial symmetry is improved. Her eyes are better defined, and her skin tone is improved. On the whole, the facial appearance is healthier.

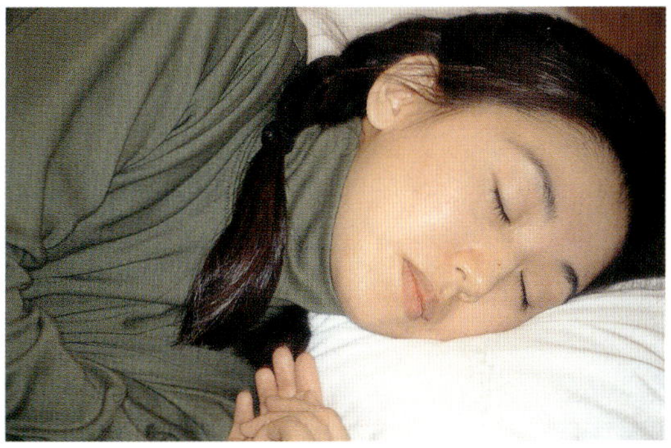

Fig 2-38 Sleep posture. She often slept on her left side with the pillow applied to the lower face. She said she felt tired when she awoke in the morning. Because she was a slender woman, this level of sleep posture probably caused deformity of the dentition. We were still somewhat doubtful at this time, because we had only started to pay attention to habits and posture. Later, as we experienced results in a number of patients, we were convinced of the significance of the effects of posture.

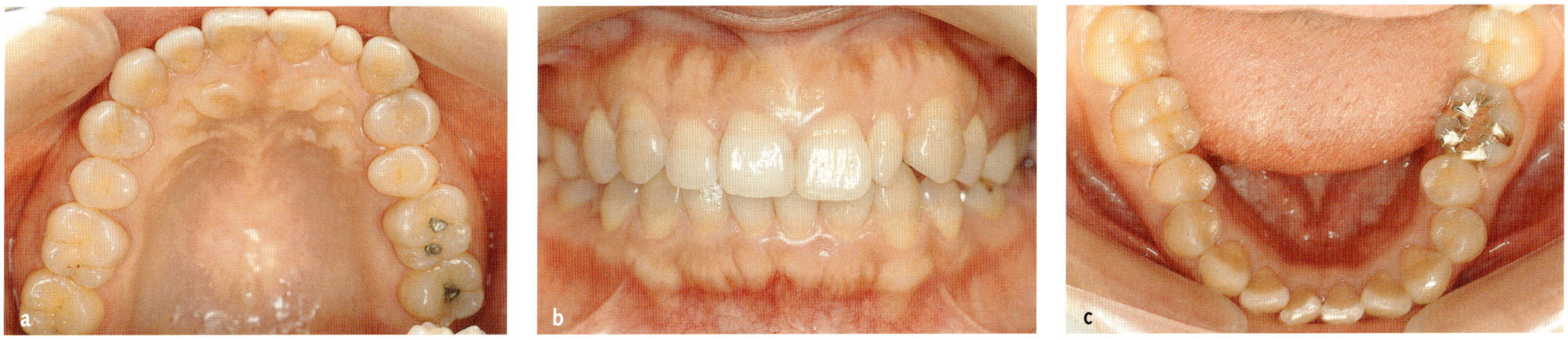

Fig 2-39 (a and b) At the first visit, the left and right sides of the maxillary arch are asymmetric. Although the right side is slightly shifted lingually, the left molars are conspicuously shifted to the lingual side. (c) In the mandible, the molars are lingually inclined. This type of collapse of the arches suggests that some unphysiologic, external force, such as a habit of resting the cheek in the hand, is being applied.

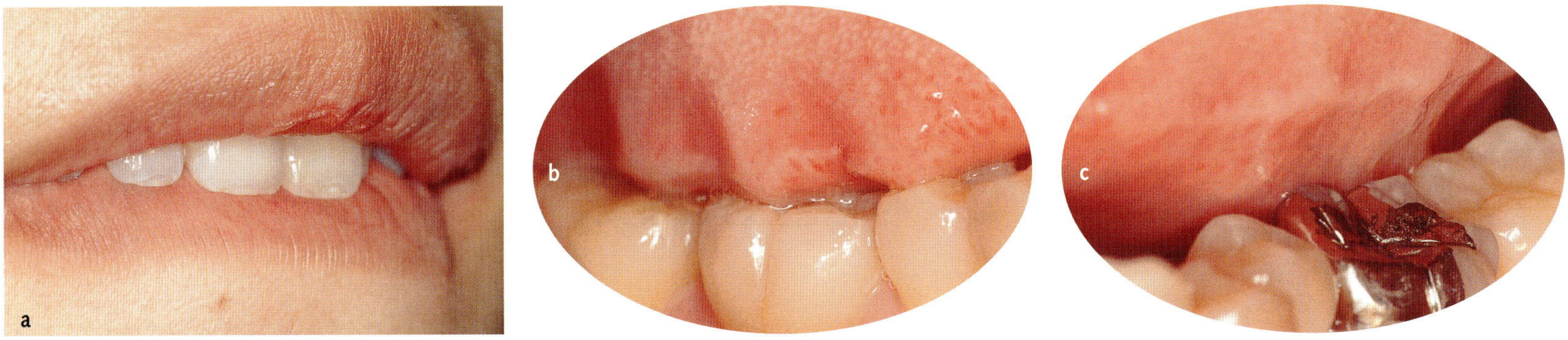

Fig 2-40 (a) Because of the patient's habit of biting and licking her lower lip, the border of the lower lip has become brownish. (b and c) Distinctive impressions of molars are noted on the sides of the tongue. The tongue is in a low position, and the patient has a severe habit of pressing the tongue against teeth. During swallowing, the tongue is not thrust forward, but the apex of the tongue is located anteriorly.

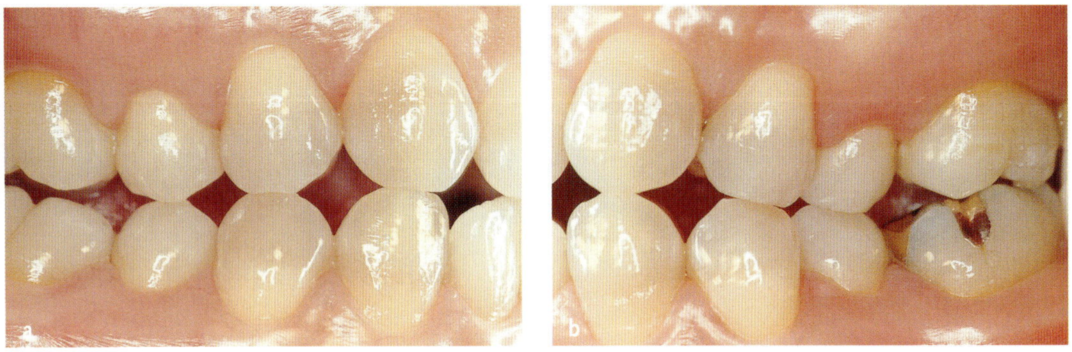

Fig 2-41 (a) Right and (b) left lateral movements at the first visit. Group function guidance is noted for the maxillary right canine, first premolar, and second premolar and for the maxillary left canine, first premolar, second premolar, and first molar.

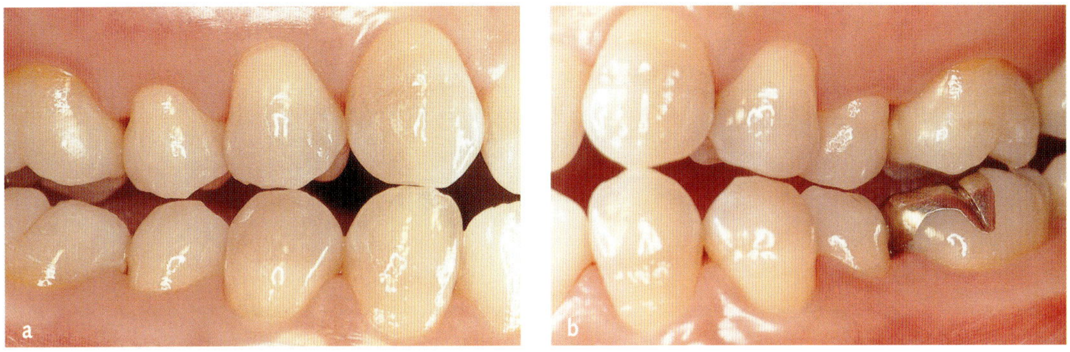

Fig 2-42 (a) Right and (b) left lateral movements after 1 year. Mostly canine guidance is achieved.

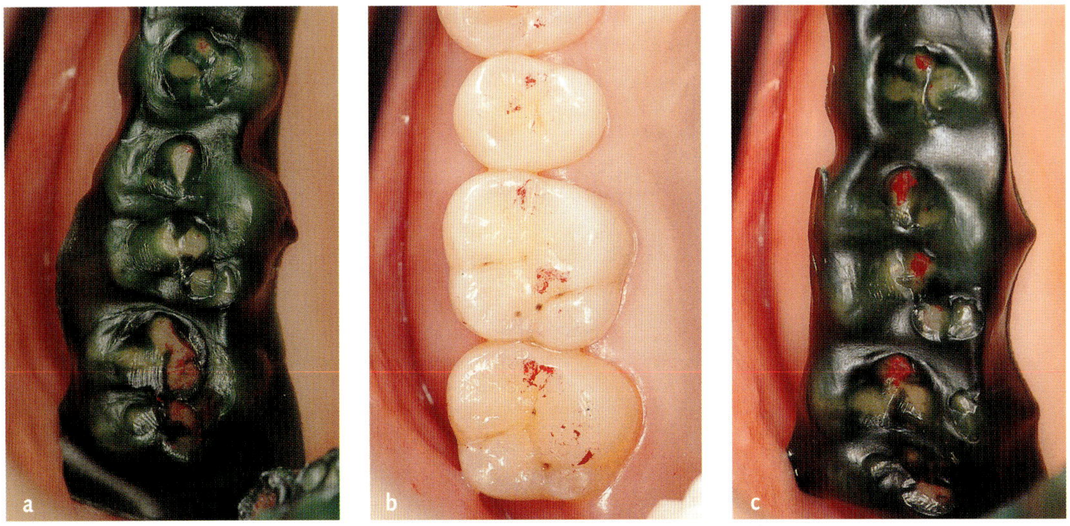

Fig 2-43 Right maxilla. (a) After red articulating paper is used, occlusal indicator wax is applied. The surfaces are reduced while the points marked with the articulating paper are maintained. Adjustment of the B slope is most difficult. Care is taken not to reduce functional cusps. (b) The same region about 6 months after the reshaping. (c) The same region about 11 months after the reshaping. The contact areas have become smaller.

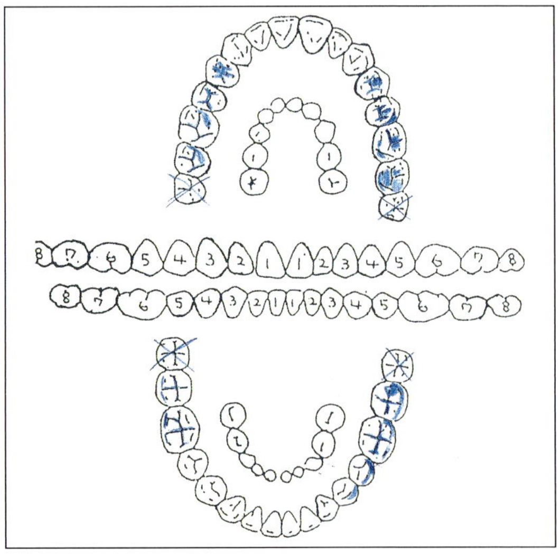

Fig 2-44 The record shows areas that were reshaped over many sessions. Blue indicates grinding, and red indicates addition. This chart is attached to the patient's medical record every time.

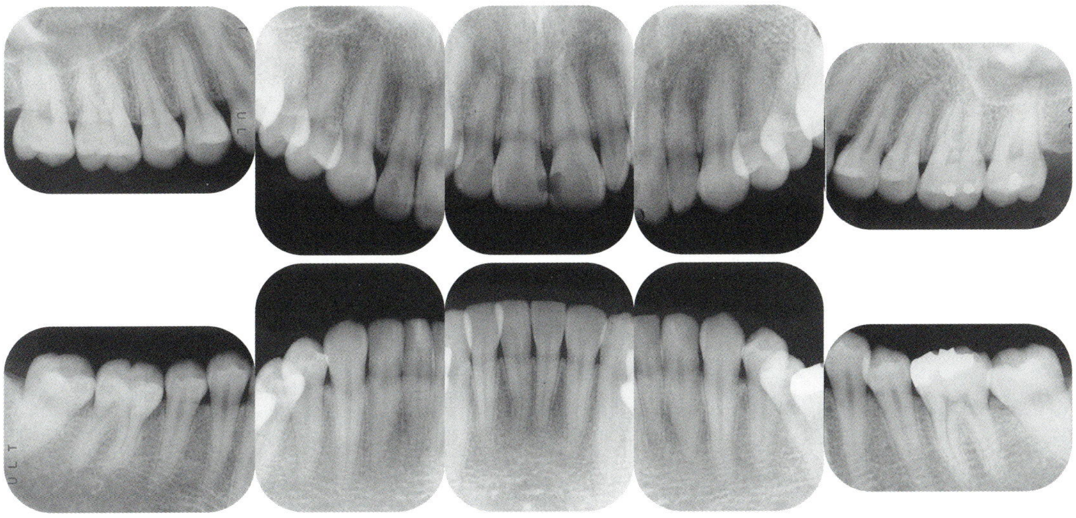

Fig 2-45 Full-mouth dental radiographs taken at the first visit. Right and left molars in the mandible are inclined mesially. Although the condition of alveolar bone is mostly normal, some bone resorption is noted, including the disappearance of the lamina dura at mesially inclined areas. Widening of the periodontal space is noted at the maxillary left second molar, suggesting that a rolling force is applied.

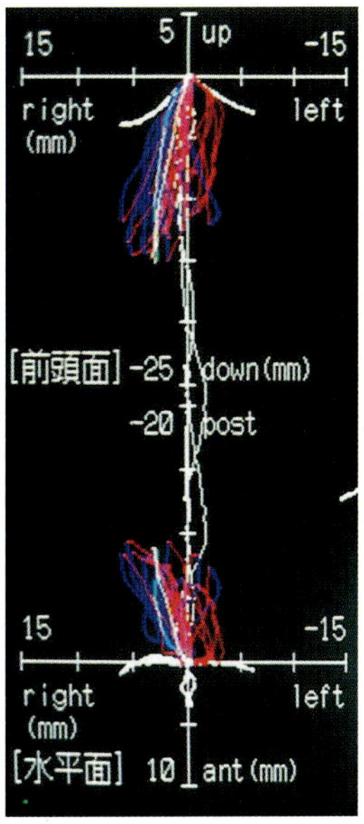

Fig 2-46 Sirognathographs of right-side chewing at the first visit.

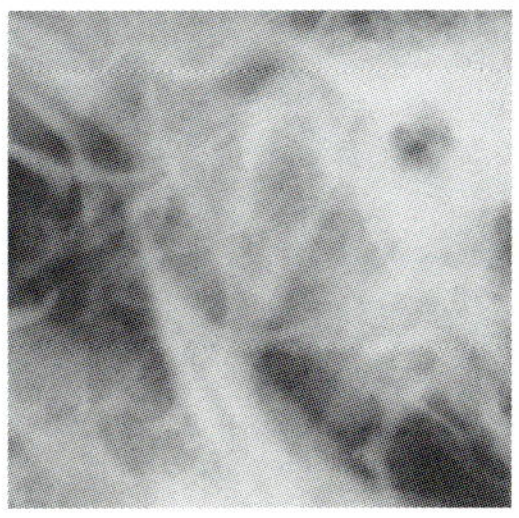

Fig 2-47 Transcranial radiograph of the left TMJ area at the first visit. The articular space is narrowed, suggesting that the vertical dimension is decreased for some reason.

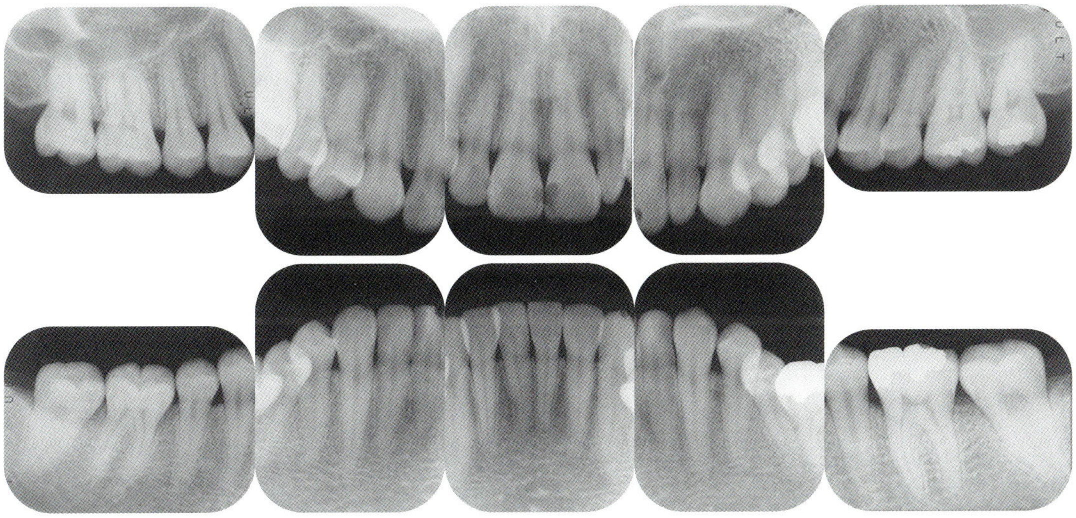

Fig 2-48 Radiographs taken after 1 year. Right and left molars in the mandible are uprighted naturally.

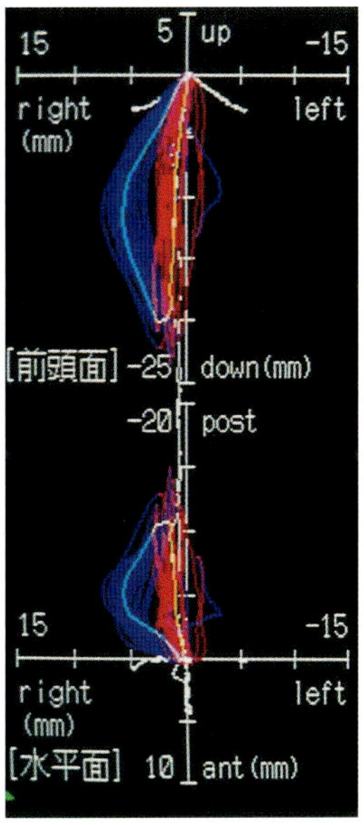

Fig 2-49 Sirognathographs of right-side chewing after 1 year 5 months. Vertically, more than a 2-cm opening is achieved with a steady cycle. Excessive guidance at opening is not completely eliminated.

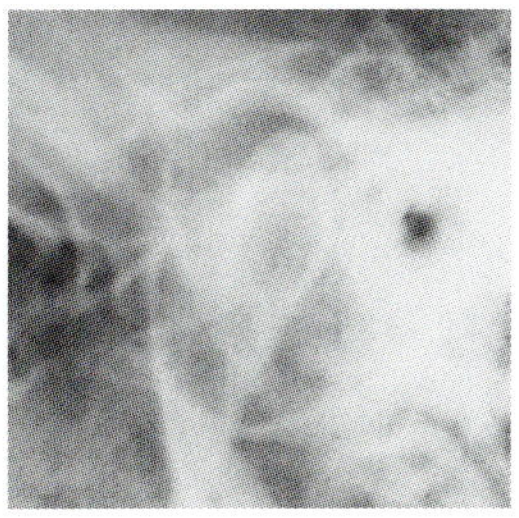

Fig 2-50 Transcranial radiograph of the left TMJ area after 1 year. Although the change is not definite, the compressed articular space seems improved.

Optimal Mandibular Position

Changeable nature of the optimal mandibular position

Discussion about mandibular positions originated in the search for the optimal mandibular position with regard to the cranium, based on the structure of the joints and muscles. It is a concept that disregards the workings of nature to advocate a separate ideal mandibular position when the intercuspal position is stable. Protocols that give the highest priority to condylar position come from articulators. Although it may be going too far to say this, condylar positions in the living body may change from day to day. Bone tissue goes through successive cycles of addition and resorption, the balance of which changes according to the slight changes of forces applied as well as morphologic changes. Therefore, there is no fixed, unchangeable position in the living body. Changes are especially considerable in the cranium, which is made up of a number of bones. It is possible that the morphology and position of the articular fossa in the temporal bone may change (see Cases 2-18 and 2-20). Consequently, we do not find significant meaning in the search for the condylar position in the articular fossa. Rather, the highest priority for obtaining the optimal mandibular position should be placed on a relaxed muscular position and a stable intercuspal position. In particular, the idea that a clinician should guide a patient's mandible to the ideal position, regardless of the method used, is dangerous. An appropriate mandibular position is not something that a clinician should decide but rather that the living body will tell us.

Clinicians should skillfully read the position where a patient is relaxed and wishes to chew. When good occlusion is attained, a living body will manifest good functions and remodel itself to better morphology, changing its mandibular position to more relaxed one. We read the mandibular position and provide a more appropriate occlusion for it. We believe that clinical practice is repetition of such processes until occlusion is stabilized.

Finding a relaxed mandibular position

As shown in Box 2-5, first, at a standing position, a patient is instructed to relax the entire body to eliminate muscle tension. The patient is allowed to relax the jaw and tap the teeth together, and an approximate mandibular position is determined. While the patient is relaxed, only light stimuli for tapping are given from the base of the mandible. After a relaxed position is found, premature contacts, restrictive cusp interferences, overlap, and occlusal contacts that are pushing the mandible posteriorly and superiorly are eliminated to recover a stable intercuspal position and await changes in the living body. At every visit of the patient, the relaxed position is determined, and the tapping process is repeated. This is a basic examination, like plaque elimination and probing in periodontal pockets.

Stability of occlusal positions

Such morphologic improvement allows smooth functions, and when functions become natural and reasonable, morphologic remodeling will occur. By repeating this process, tense muscles, compressed or excessively stretched articular spaces, ligaments, and periodontal ligaments will slowly remodel themselves like compressed floss silk regains its shape. An appropriate mandibular position will emerge as obstacles to natural healing are gradually detected and eliminated.

A mandible that has been in a shifted position for a long time will not immediately return to its original position if interferences are removed. It may take several years in some cases. It seems natural that such a process will take so long, considering that distortions in the cranium and other parts of the body have to be resolved and balance of the whole body has to be improved. The fact that a condylar position itself does change constantly should be fully recognized.

Elimination of interferences and rough reshaping of occlusal surfaces will allow the natural shift of the mandible to a relaxed position. It is necessary that we do not overlook this position but rather capture it. The living body will cure itself. We just remove stumbling blocks to help the process. Even if the condyle is located slightly anteriorly in the articular fossa, it should be regarded as a correct condylar position as long as an occlusal position is relaxed and stable at that position. Also, although it is preferable that the disc be reduced, it is a kind of clinical healing to secure the articular space with the condyle off the disc, if reduction of the disc would cause disharmony with occlusal contacts. Having said that, in our clinical experiences, very few cases were completed in which the condyles remained off the disc.

Habitual mandibular position versus optimal mandibular position

The process to find the optimal mandibular position in the whole body may take a long time in some cases. The control of forces in the stomatognathic system cannot be started without a critical mind asking, "Where is the mandibular position?" With this question, we emphasize the importance of always challenging the truth of a patient's mandibular position as it appears. Just because the intercuspal position is stable when the patient is allowed to bite, we cannot conclude that there is no discrepancy between ICP and centric relation (CR). Finding the optimal mandibular position is not that simple. As discussed earlier in this chapter, the position and the relationship of the condyle to the articular fossae are not reliable. After reshaping of restricted, tight occlusion areas, a mandibular position may change even when the habitual intercuspal position is stable.

During occlusal therapy, at every visit, a patient is allowed to tap the teeth together in a relaxed manner, and the mandibular position is confirmed. Even with so much effort, we still sometimes find a sudden change of the mandibular position during orthodontic tooth movement. For example, habitual bite position may be affected by crowding, or a mandibular position may shift as cusps are engaged more deeply because of a different speed of movement for the maxillary and mandibular arches. Also, in some cases, the mandibular position will emerge clearly only after final restorations are delivered to allow a bite with light force, or the mandible is shifted to a stable position after maintenance phase is started.

Box 2-5 Finding a relaxed mandibular position

The thumb and the index finger of the clinician are placed lightly at the right and the left sides of the mandible and the middle finger is placed at the base of the mandible to apply light stimuli in an upward direction (Fig 2-51). At a standing position, the patient is allowed to close slowly and gently himself or herself with the clinician's hand placed at the mandible, and the position is recorded. Attention is paid not to cause sliding or rotation. Generally, compressed areas will start to open. As the patient becomes relaxed, compression of masseter and temporalis muscles and joints will be released, allowing disocclusion of the molars and contacts at the anterior teeth. If the results of this relaxed tapping are not stable during the treatment process, grinding of interferences and addition of light-curing resin are repeated. As relaxed tapping is stabilized, the mandible will further relax to manifest the optimal mandibular position. The final mandibular position is perceived by visual, auditory, and tactile sensations.

- Visual sensation: Slight movement of the mandible, a gap, or a distortion when teeth are touched together should not be overlooked.
- Auditory sensation: High-pitched, clear occlusal sound should be noted.
- Tactile sensation: The strength of vibration of the teeth at occlusal contacts should be felt by fingers.

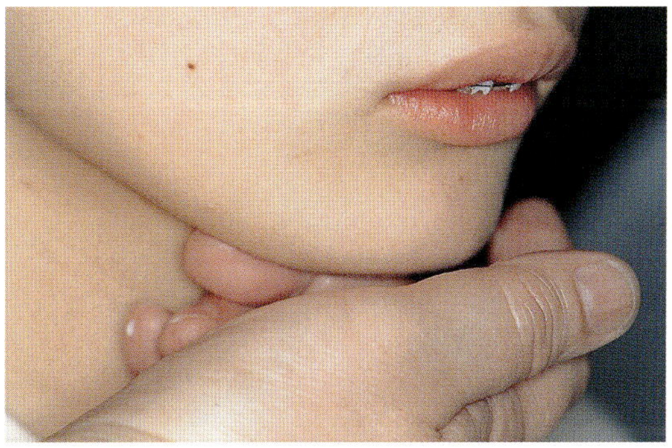

Fig 2-51 The clinician provides only light stimuli in an upward direction.

Starting from the optimal mandibular position

The 29-year-old woman in Figs 2-52 to 2-63 had experienced pain in the jaw when she awakened in the morning for about 4 years. Every morning, after one click of the jaw, the pain of the left TMJ area disappeared and movement became easy. Her four first premolars had been extracted because of crowding when she was about 10 years old, but no orthodontic treatment was conducted. With this level of information, a rough diagnosis could be made. Nevertheless, at facial examination, the tilt of the face and asymmetry of each part of the face were noted as significant. Here, we asked ourselves: "Why the shift to the left? Why the left clicking? Where was the original position of the mandible?"

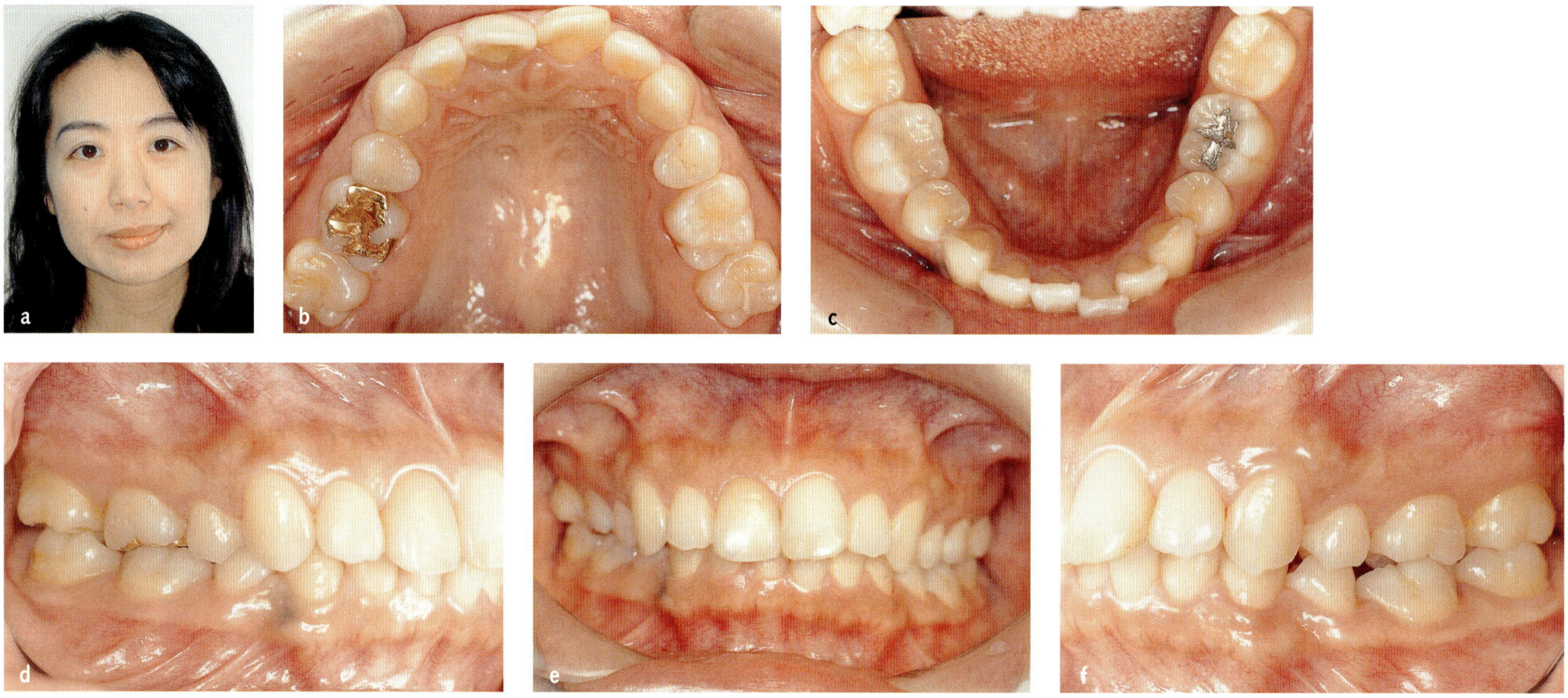

Fig 2-52 (a) The head tilt to the right, muscle tenderness in the left TMJ area and left shoulder and neck, tension in the left masseter, and the lip line tilt to the right are noted. (b to f) The occlusal plane is lower on the left, the mandibular dentition is shifted to the left (about 2 mm), and there is deep overlap. The lingual inclination of maxillary canines, the lingual inclination of the premolars (especially on the right), and the labial inclination of maxillary left central incisor and mandibular left central incisor are observed. The mandibular arch is V shaped with an intense curve of Spee. The arch is flat on the right side, suggesting an external force from the right. The axes of the molars are mesially inclined. The molar relationship is Class I on the right side and Class II on the left.

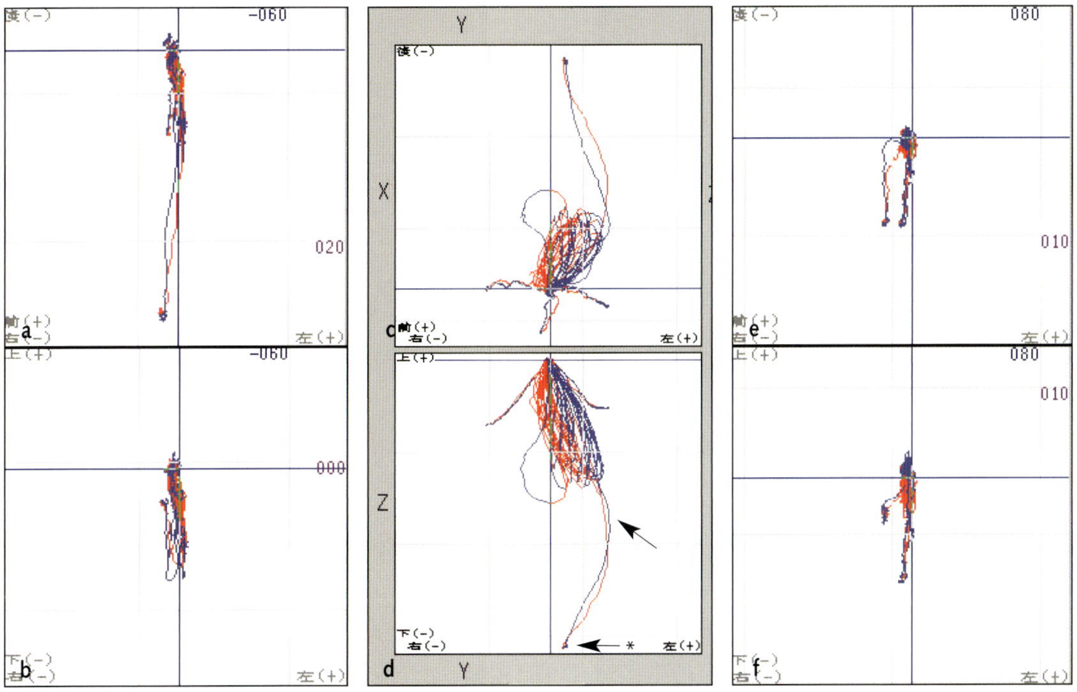

Fig 2-53 Examination of functional movements with a Gnathohexagraph shows that the opening path is shifted to the left *(arrow)* before reaching the maximal opening but there is no shift at the maximal opening *(arrow with asterisk)*. Also, there is no step suggesting that the condyle comes off the disc. Because movements of the left TMJ are limited during masticatory movements, the turning point is on the left side even with right-side chewing. ICP is stable. Although guidance is abnormal (maxillary left canine and mandibular left canine) during opening, the cycle is mostly normal. Observation of the movements of the condyles during right-side chewing indicates that the right condyle moves more anteriorly than the left. The working-side condyle may be moving forward for compensation because the nonworking-side *(left)* condyle does not move. (a) Right condyle on a transverse plane during right-side chewing. (b) Right condyle on a frontal plane. (c) Incisal point on a transverse plane during right-side chewing. (d) Incisal point on a frontal plane. (e) Left condyle on a transverse plane during right-side chewing. (f) Left condyle on a frontal plane.

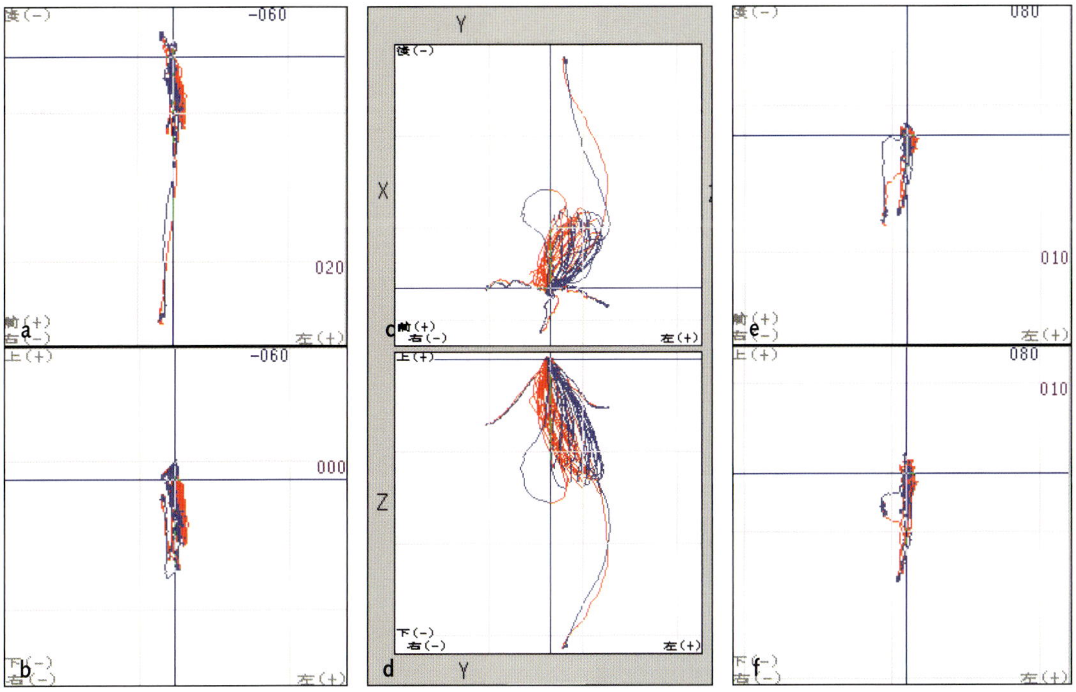

Fig 2-54 During left-side chewing, inadequate movement of the left condyle is not an issue. (a) Right condyle on a transverse plane during left-side chewing. (b) Right condyle on a frontal plane. (c) Incisal point on a transverse plane during left-side chewing. (d) Incisal point on a frontal plane. (e) Left condyle on a transverse plane during left-side chewing. (f) Left condyle on a frontal plane.

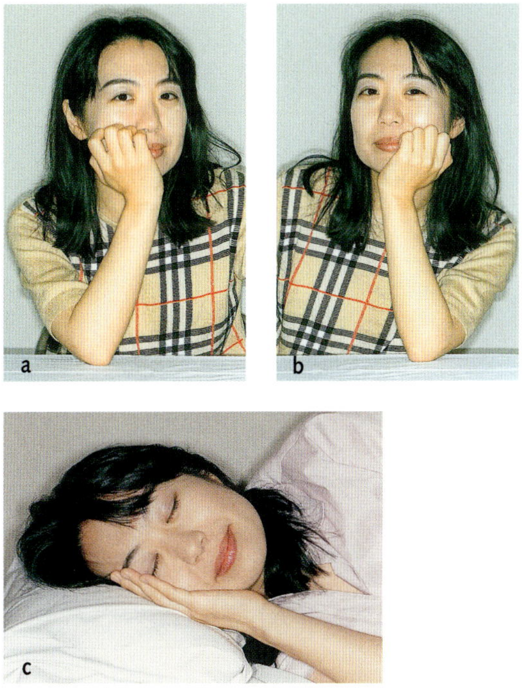

Fig 2-55 (a and b) The patient has a habit of resting her right and left cheeks in the hands, which seems to have triggered lingual inclination of molars. (c) She sleeps on her right side with her right hand under the right cheek. It is surmised that this sleep posture caused a flat arch on the left and pushed out the left central incisors labially. This posture puts the left condyle off the disc during sleep.

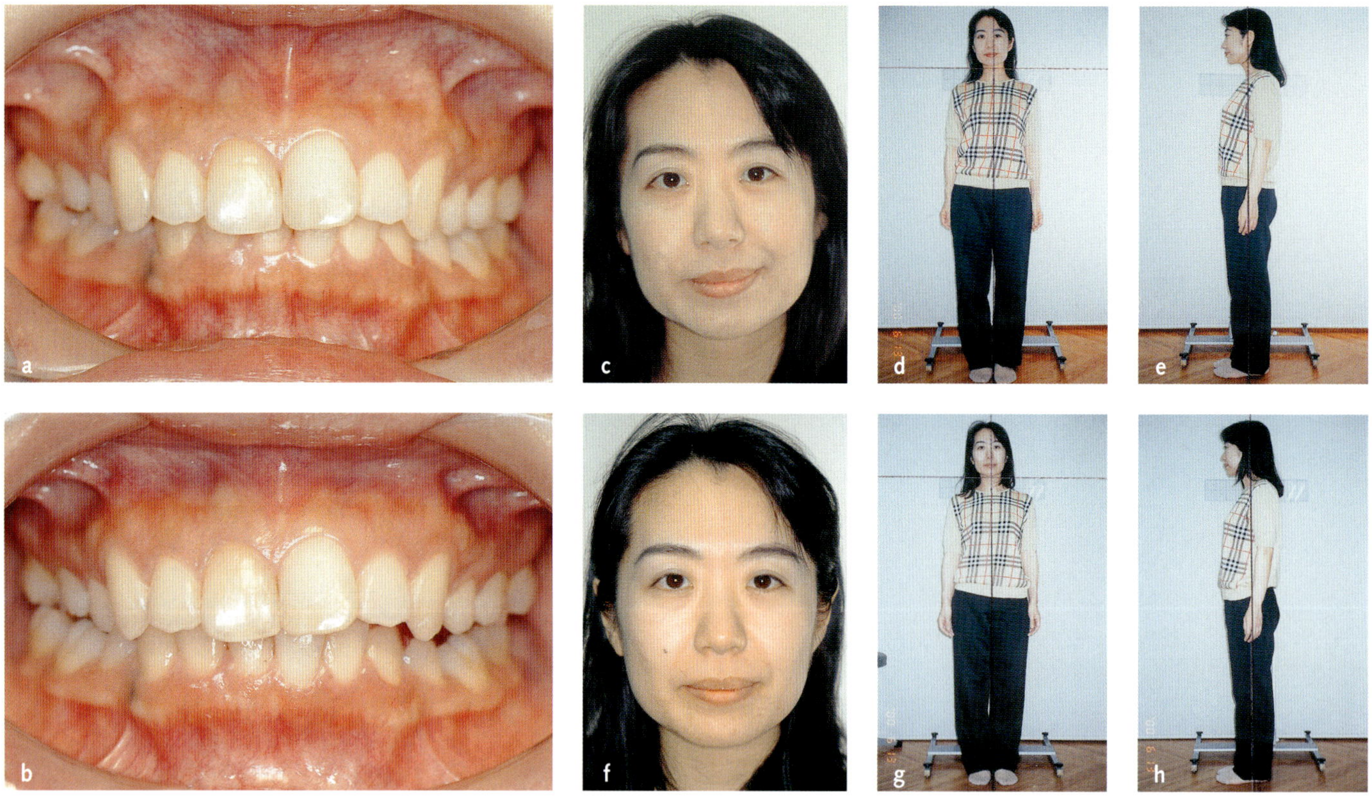

Fig 2-56 (a) Intercuspal position at the first visit. (b) Relaxed position at the first visit. When the patient is allowed to tap lightly in the relaxed position, the midline is shifted to the right by about 2 mm. All the treatments start from here. Preferably the tooth axis of the maxillary right canine should be changed by orthodontic treatment. (c to e) ICP at the first visit. When the mandible is retruded, the head comes forward. Some clinicians used to advocate adapting the most posterior position as CR for bite registration. If the mandible is pushed backward, however, the head and the neck are thrust forward for more comfort, which results in a stoop. (f to h) Relaxed position at the first visit. When the mandible is at the relaxed position, the tilt of the head and the distortion of the whole body disappear instantly.

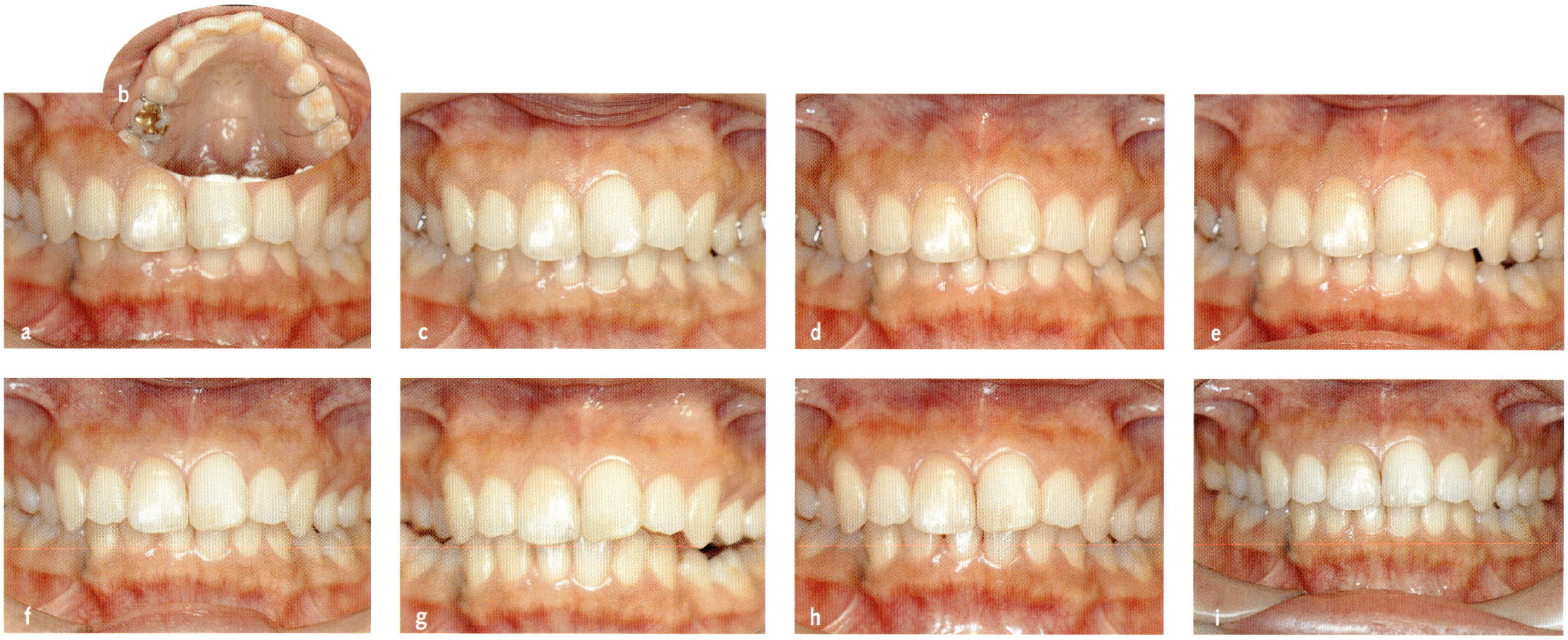

Fig 2-57 Clinical changes induced by a relaxed positioning splint. (a) ICP at the first visit. (b) Relaxed positioning splint. (c) Because a weaker curve of Spee is favorable, the maxillary arch is not in active treatment. (d) After 1 month of use of the splint, intermittent symptoms of being off the disc have disappeared. (e) At the same time, the guiding slope is adjusted. (f) Photograph taken after another month. The procedure has been repeated. (g) After another month, the relaxed position starts to appear on the right. (h) Photograph taken 4 months after delivery of the splint. The vertical dimension is increased and the mandible moves forward. (i) Photograph taken 1 year 8 months after the first visit. Throughout the period, the splint has been used at night only. The vertical dimension is increased, crowding of the maxillary and mandibular arches is resolved, cervical lines are aligned, and the imbalance of the occlusal plane is reduced to a certain degree. Resin composite has been added to the area of attrition on the mandibular left canine.

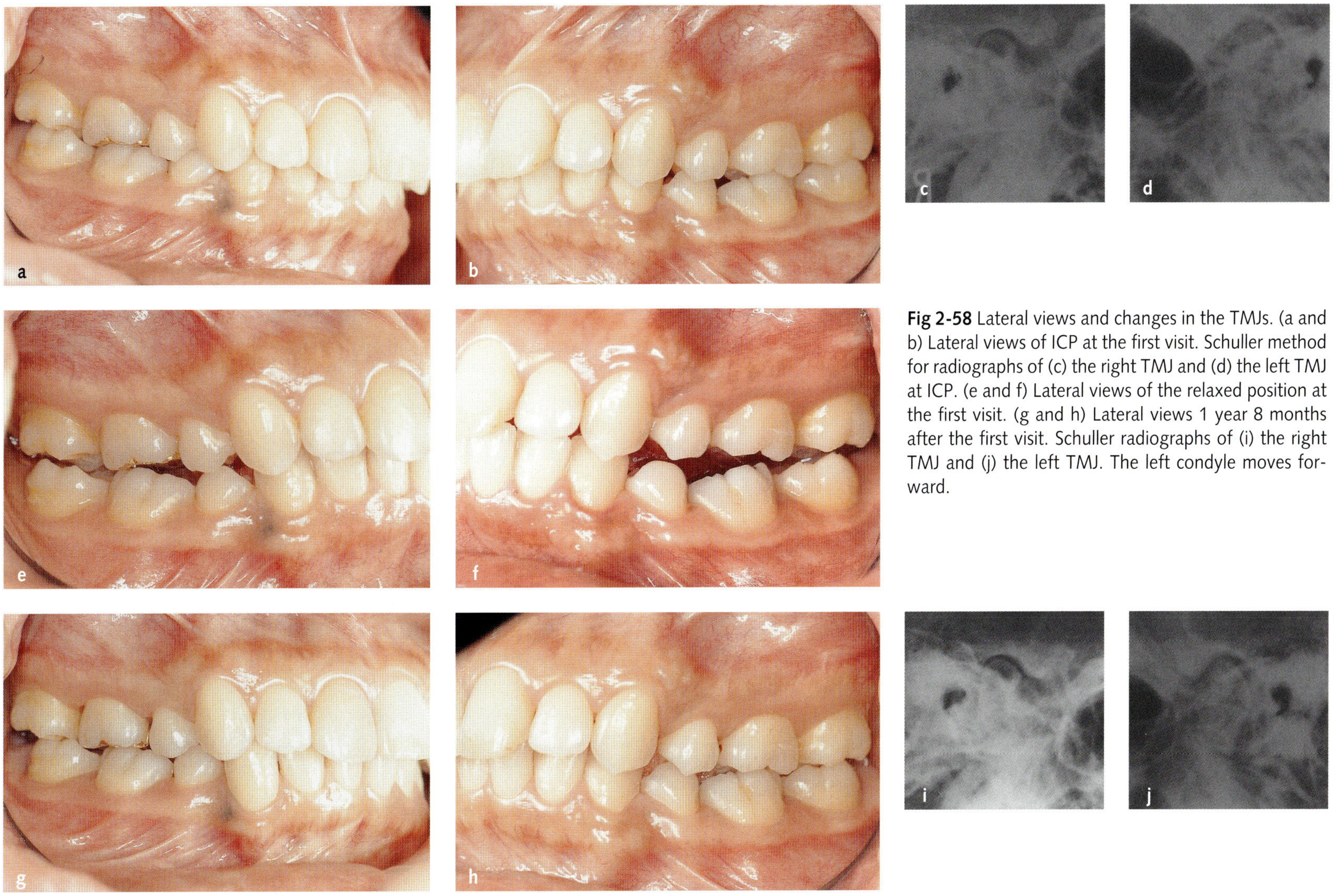

Fig 2-58 Lateral views and changes in the TMJs. (a and b) Lateral views of ICP at the first visit. Schuller method for radiographs of (c) the right TMJ and (d) the left TMJ at ICP. (e and f) Lateral views of the relaxed position at the first visit. (g and h) Lateral views 1 year 8 months after the first visit. Schuller radiographs of (i) the right TMJ and (j) the left TMJ. The left condyle moves forward.

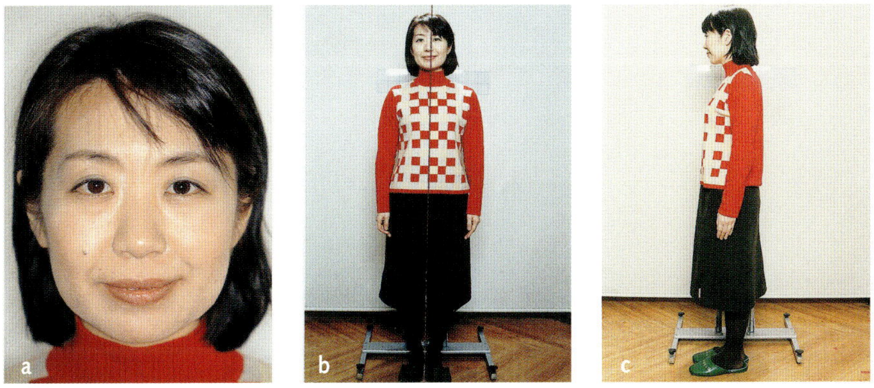

Fig 2-59 The patient's posture 1 year 8 months after first visit. Although the left corner of the mouth is still slightly higher, improvement is noted. Symptoms around the left TMJ have resolved.

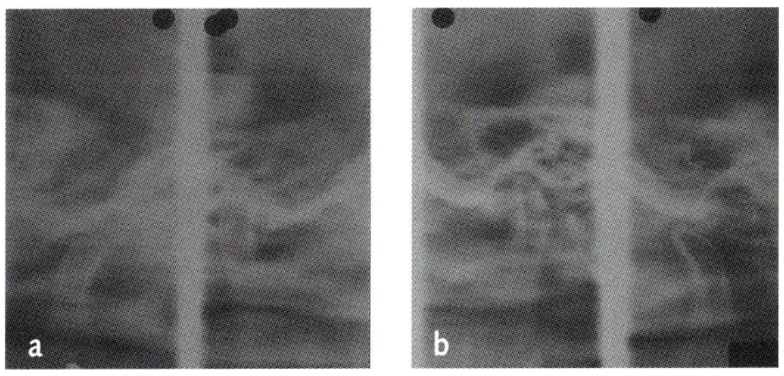

Fig 2-60 Scanograms (tomograms) of the (a) right and (b) left TMJs at the first visit. The morphology of the left condyle suggests retrograde degeneration.

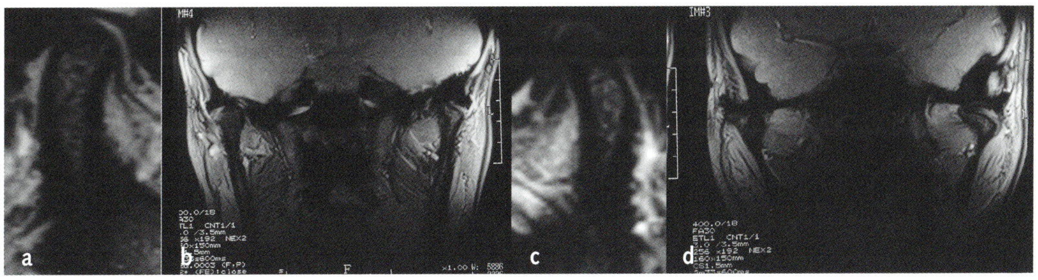

Fig 2-61 Magnetic resonance images of the TMJs. (a to c) Coronal and sagittal sections at ICP. (d) Coronal section at maximal opening.

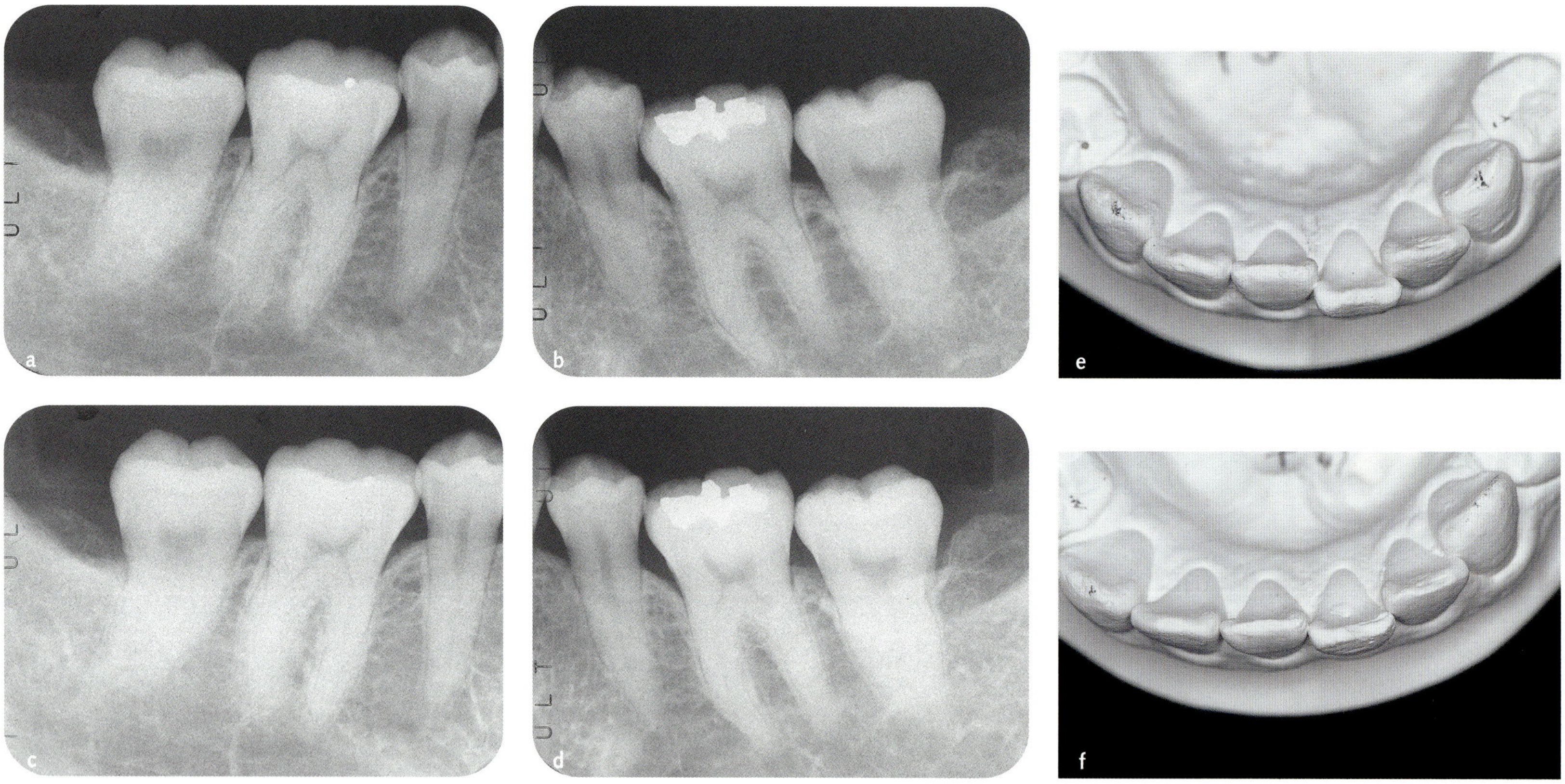

Fig 2-62 Uprighting of the mandibular molars. (a and b) Right and left molars are inclined mesially to a significant degree at the first visit. (c and d) After 1 year 8 months, the mandibular position has moved forward and the vertical dimension of occlusion has increased, uprighting the molars naturally. Compared to the condition (e) at the first visit, (f) at 1 year 8 months, labioversion of the mandibular left central incisor is improved and the tooth is incorporated in the dental arch.

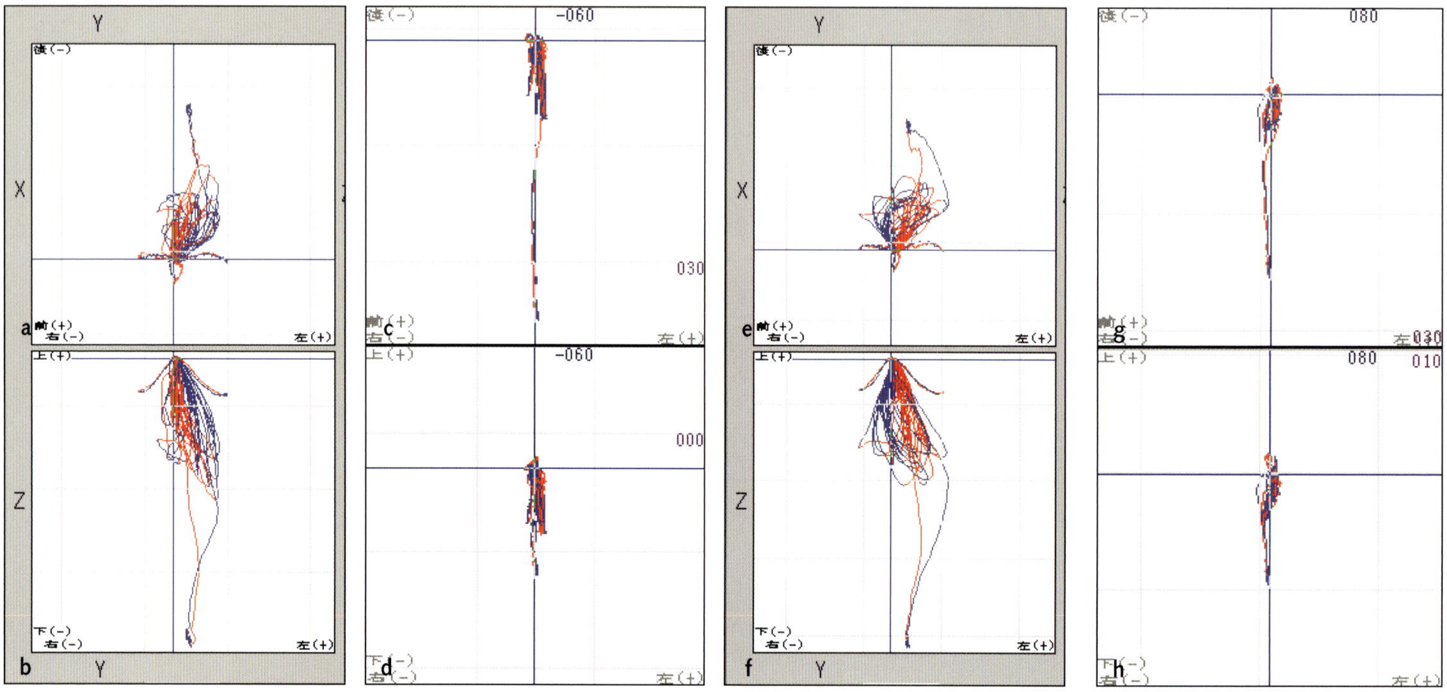

Fig 2-63 Examinations of functional movements posttreatment. (a and b) At left-side chewing, the change in the mandibular position is not detected on a Gnathohexagraph. The delay on the left side at opening is diminished, reducing the pull to the left. (a) Incisal point on a transverse plane. (b) Incisal point on a frontal plane. (c to h) At right-side chewing, movements of the left condyle are improved compared to movements at the first visit. (c) Right condyle on a transverse plane. (d) Right condyle on a frontal plane. (e) Incisal point on a transverse plane. (f) Incisal point on a frontal plane. (g) Left condyle on a transverse plane. (h) Left condyle on a frontal plane.

Functional Movements of the Mandible: Condylar Movements

Misperceptions in occlusion theory based on border movements

Through the use of mandibular movement–analyzing equipment, clinicians can observe real-time functional movement paths of each patient. Clinical application of such equipment has greatly revised occlusion theory, which used to be based on the analysis of border movements.

Because it was established on the model of articulators and based on border movements, occlusion theory has given various false impressions to clinicians. By definition, an articulator is a substitution of relationships of maxillary and mandibular arches using a simple model. Unlike the jawbone, an articulator neither remodels nor bends. Teeth supported by periodontal ligaments show complicated movements, while teeth made of plaster or dental stone show no mobility. Moreover, for such a mechanical model to be established, there has to be an ideal condylar position (CR), and it has to be the rotation center of the mandible. Analysis of mandibular movements has proven that such a hypothesis does not hold true in most patients.

Review of clinical procedures

An understanding of functional movements of the mandible and the concept of an appropriate mandibular position (discussed in the previous section) has significant implications, and fundamental review of many clinical procedures is required, including centric bite registration method, concepts about occlusal interference, proper overlap for molars, and appropriate occlusal morphology (see the section entitled, "Occlusal Morphology From the Viewpoint of Masticatory Movements").

Individual differences in the working-side condyle during function

What kind of behaviors does a condyle show during functional movements? Because condylar movements cannot be directly observed and are very delicate, they had to be created by imagination so that the occlusion theory could be developed. Routine use of mandibular movement–analyzing equipment reveals that functional movements of condyles have many variations. Often condyles show totally different movements even when the movements of the occlusal surfaces look exactly the same. An understanding of condylar movement paths has a high diagnostic value for determining an appropriate method of bite registration and making a diagnosis of occlusal interference.

Posterior movement of the working-side condyle

In movements of the working-side condyle during functional movements, individual differences are significant. Posterior movement from ICP is not rare (Fig 2-64). There are not necessarily many cases showing stable cyclic movements of the condyle centering around the stable condylar position during function. As more and more individuals have poorly developed condyles with significant play, an increasing number of patients do not exhibit stable cycles.

Observation of condylar movements in many patients indicates that posterior movement of the working-side condyle is observed in more patients than expected. Since observed by a measuring instrument designed by Lundeen and Gibbs (Box 2-6), condylar movements have been believed to have a general behavior as reported. It seems, however, some specific cases were observed with a flawed measuring method in a distorted manner. One of the major problems is posterior movement of the working-side condyle. Observation of condylar movements by Gibbs' replicator was conducted in a limited number of patients. Even if examination had been conducted in many patients, however, posterior movement of the working-side condyle could not have been observed because of a major mistake in the method: the reference plane was set so that it was higher posteriorly.

In the past, movement paths of incisal points and condylar points measured with Gibbs' mandibular movement measurement device have been introduced as typical masticatory movement patterns. Measurement by Gibbs, however, did not accurately reproduce physiologic movements because of inappropriate determination of the reference plane and restrictions of natural movement by the heavy, bulky facebow and clutch used in the mouth.

Also, although pictures showing stable cyclic movements of the working-side condyle and wide anterior reciprocation of the nonworking-side condyle were introduced as typical examples of normal movements, this type of movement path is merely one example among various variations in condylar movements. It is surmised that posterior movements on the transverse plane were difficult to identify with Gibbs' measurement device because of its inappropriate reference plane.

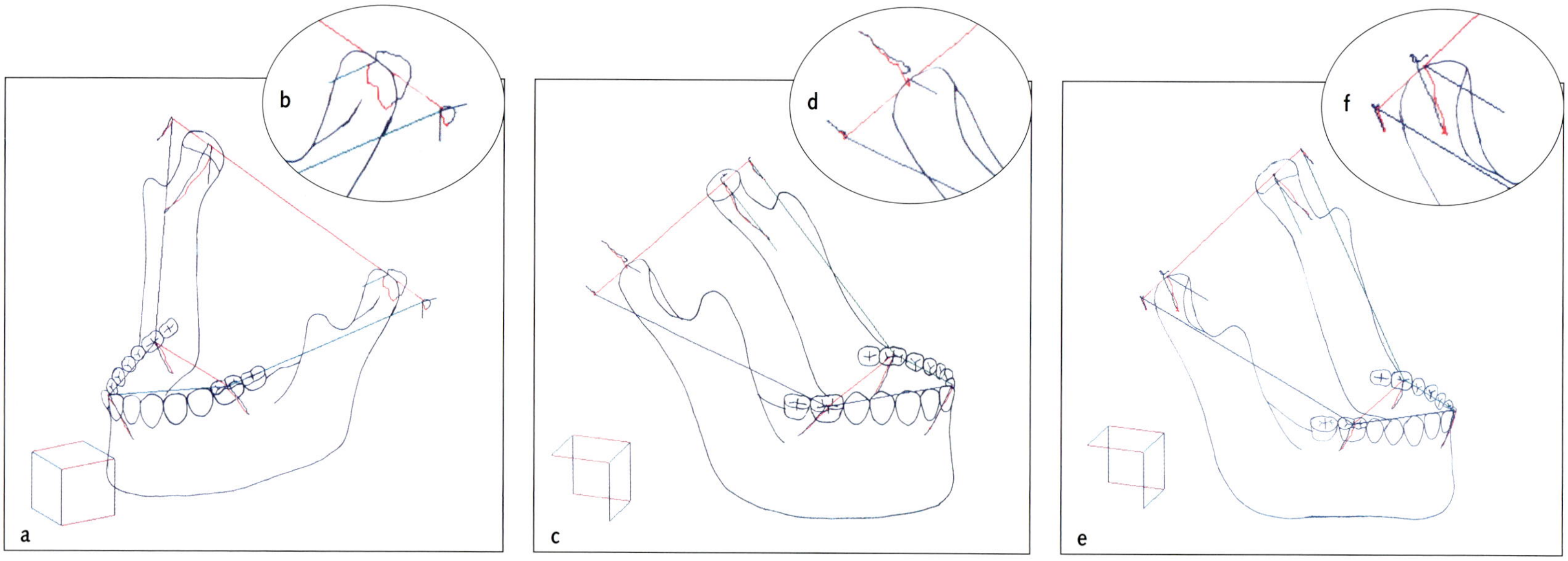

Fig 2-64 Individual differences in condylar movements. (a) Posthealing of a patient with previous symptoms of TMD (left-side chewing). (b) Working-side condyle. (c) Patient with mandibular protrusion and without symptoms of TMD (right-side chewing). (d) Working-side condyle. (e) Patient with Type I TMD (right-side chewing). (f) Working-side condyle. The angle shown in a three-dimensional display *(bottom left)* is the same for these three cases. These examples show that the working-side condyle exhibits various movements. The condylar positions are located on skin in these figures but in reality are actually about 10 mm deeper. On the condyles, enlargement of a single cycle movement is shown.

Box 2-6 Problems with typical masticatory movement patterns described by Lundeen and Gibbs

Study of mandibular functional movements was a matter of great concern for occlusion researchers, because they have a conclusive influence on the occlusal morphology of restorations. Among other subjects, research to record the three-dimensional position and relationships of the mandible to the maxilla along the time axis (record of movements with six degrees of freedom) attracted attention in the 1960s to the 1980s. What was introduced in *Advances in Occlusion* (Lundeen and Gibbs) is well known in Japan as "typical masticatory movement patterns." Gibbs (1966) developed a device to optically record mandibular movements (Fig 2-65) and later published several studies on detailed functional movements of the mandible using the equipment. In the 1980s, Lewin (1981) developed a measuring device, which was later succeeded by the current Sirognathograph. Although various other devices have been developed for precise measurement of functional movements, the method that Gibbs and Lundeen introduced has been understood as a typical one with regard to condylar movements during function.

However, their device was incapable of capturing posterior movements because of its inappropriately designed reference plane. Also, the heavy, bulky clutch had to be used in the mouth, which restricted natural movements. As a result, the equipment did not allow detailed expression of physiologic conditions. In addition, because of their small sample size, they seem to have made mistakes in determining what is an individual difference, or natural variability, and what is typical.

Figure 2-66 is an example of a movement path shown as a "typical masticatory movement pattern." Gibbs' record of mandibular movements seems to have had different shapes on the transverse plane and the sagittal plane because the head frame was too highly positioned posteriorly. When the reference plane is too high at the posterior end, the angle between the reference plane and the occlusal plane will be smaller. This will give a wider projection on the transverse plane. The sagittal plane will be closer to the vertical, and opening will appear larger on the frontal plane.

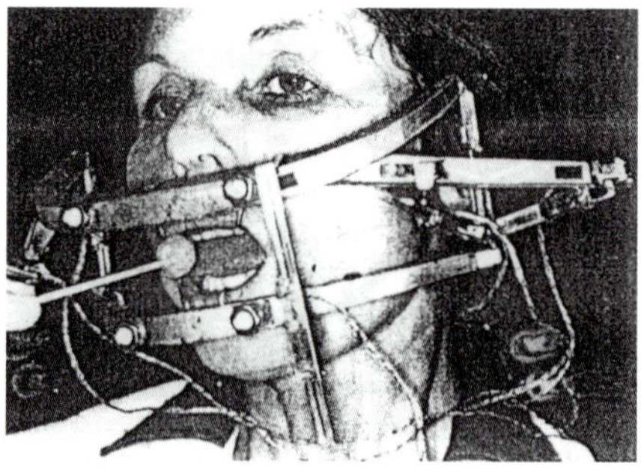

Fig 2-65 Measuring instrument for determining mandibular movement paths. From Lundeen and Gibbs.

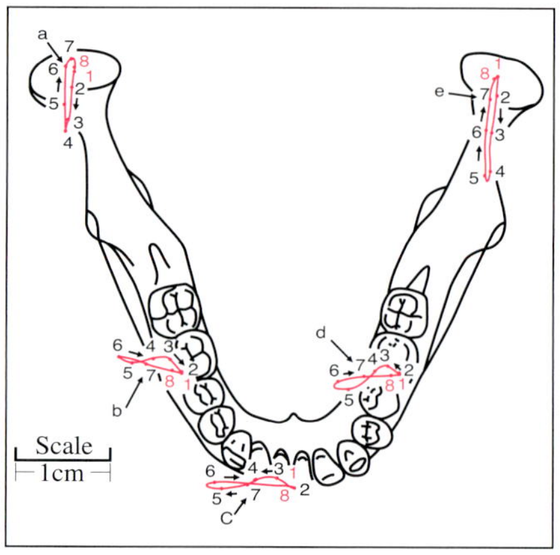

Fig 2-66 "Typical masticatory movement pattern." Cheese, right-side chewing. From Lundeen and Gibbs.

Changes in the working-side condyles before and after orthognathic surgery

The woman in Fig 2-67 had a Class III malocclusion and a typical chopping-type chewing pattern; the working-side condyles clearly moved posteriorly before treatment. After orthognathic surgery, however, the working-side condyles of this patient started to move anteriorly in masticatory movements, as shown in Gnathohexagraphs. As shown in this case, condylar movements may change by 180 degrees as a result of changes in occlusion.

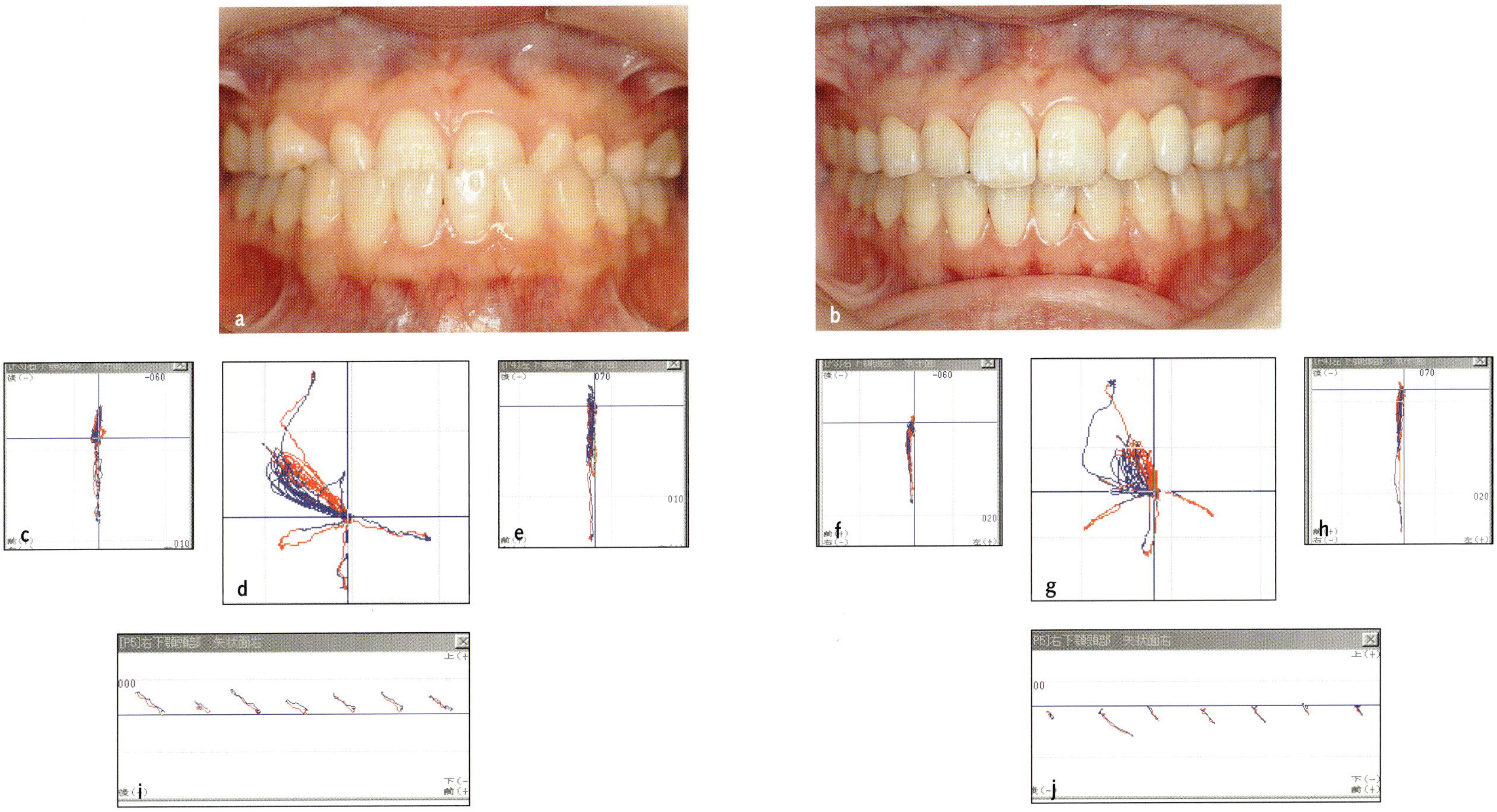

Fig 2-67 (a) Frontal view before orthognathic surgery. (b) Frontal view after orthognathic surgery (after 4 years 3 months). (c) Transverse projection of the right condylar movement path (working side). (d) Transverse projection of movement paths of the incisal point during right-side chewing before orthognathic surgery. (e) Transverse projection of the left condylar movement path. (f) Transverse projection of the right condylar movement path (working side). (g) Transverse projection of movement paths of the incisal point during right-side chewing after orthognathic surgery. (h) Transverse projection of the left condylar movement path. (i) Transverse projection of individual cycles of the right condylar movement path during right-side chewing before orthognathic surgery. (j) Individual cycles of the right condylar movement path after orthognathic surgery.

Problems caused by posterior movements of the condyles

In our clinical experience, when a patient with a one-sided chewing habit and mild anterior disc displacement on the habitual chewing side is instructed to chew on the other (healthy) side, sometimes clicking will disappear and the immobility will be alleviated. If working-side condyles merely move anteriorly and inferiorly, such movement alone is unlikely to cause reduction of the disc. When a patient with posterior movements of the working-side condyle chews on the healthy side, the nonworking side, or the affected side, will always be pulled anteriorly and inferiorly, which seems to cause disc reduction. This was our hypothesis, which could be confirmed by Gnathohexagraphs. We learned that working-side condyles do move in various ways even when movements of the occlusal surfaces look very similar. The movements may include reciprocation or cyclic motion in a posterior and superior direction. By definition, in a patient with condyles moving posteriorly and superiorly, posterior displacement is highly likely to occur, and asymmetry of the lower face tends to be enhanced by one-sided chewing. Also, habits such as one-sided chewing can be a factor for occlusal collapse in some patients, which seems to be related to posterior movements of the condyles (Box 2-7).

Box 2-7 Posterior movements of working-side condyles

In commonly accepted theories, it was not considered that working-side condyles move posteriorly during functional movements (see Figs 2-64 and 2-67). Clinically, however, we have observed some patients with a one-sided chewing habit in whom the condyle is posteriorly off the disc and whose condyles come on the disc only when they chew on the healthy side. The concept of posterior movements of working-side condyles explains this phenomenon.

Box 2-8 Centric bite registration

In many individuals, sliding movement of the condyles starts from the initial phase of opening. Consequently, when bite registration is conducted at 6 to 7 mm opening with no force applied to the mandible by a clinician, the registered position will be anterior to ICP (Fig 2-68). Conventional registration of "centric relation," with the mandible pushed backward, was intented to force rotational movement. When a subject is allowed to open experimentally with a chin cap, the anterior sliding component of condyles decreases and a rotational locus is obtained. In theory, in subjects with limited play in the TMJs and well-developed condyles, bite registration with a certain degree of posterior force seems to provide centric bite records with a relatively high reproducibility. Still, an artificial load should not be applied to the mandible to manipulate a mandibular position in order to obtain an appropriate position, because we do not use chin caps when we eat.

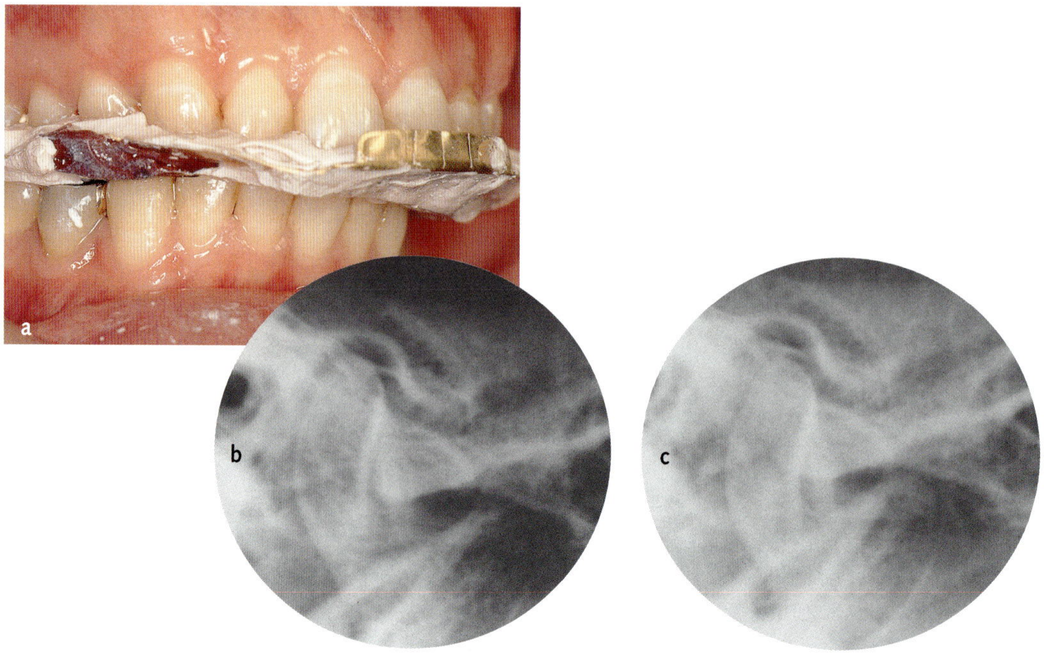

Fig 2-68 (a) Centric bite registration. The opening in the anterior region is 6 to 7 mm. Experimental transcranial radiographs of (b) the right condyle at ICP and (c) the right condyle at centric bite registration are compared. In this case, the incisal opening was 5 to 8 mm during registration. The condyle clearly slides anteriorly and inferiorly. Therefore, if this registration is transferred to an articulator as it is, the mandible will be positioned more anteriorly than it actually is.

Anterior sliding of condyles and reproducibility of mandibular positions

As the mandibular behaviors during function came to be understood distinctly, the issue of mandibular positions (condylar positions), which used to be a matter of debate, can be clearly explained (Box 2-8).

When full-mouth restorations were fabricated as one piece based on a centric bite record, we often found that the occlusion was incorrect at try-in. We started to fabricate the prosthesis for one third of the arch at a time while preserving the provisional restoration for the remaining areas to maintain the vertical dimension. With this approach, the discrepancy in the mandibular position was mostly resolved. This discrepancy seems to be an error caused by registration of the occlusal record at a centric bite with 6 to 7 mm opening. When the centric bite record is obtained, often the mandible has already started translating (Fig 2-69). Although it has been advocated that the mandible shows hinge movement at an early phase of opening (about 10-mm incisal opening), mandibular movement–analyzing equipment shows that such hinge movement is rather rarely observed and that many subjects present a translating component from the initial phase of opening (see Fig 2-69).

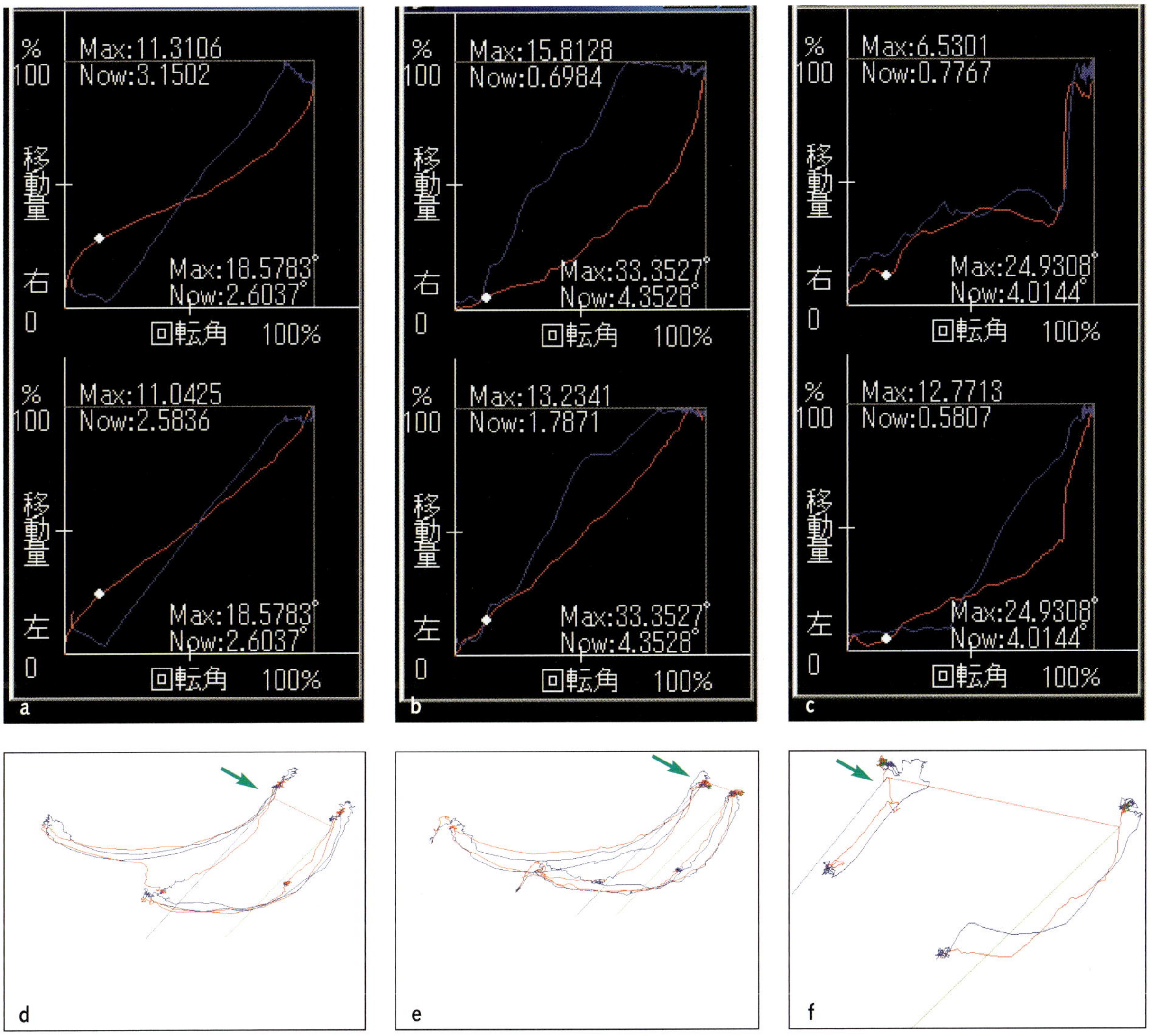

Fig 2-69 Movements and rotation angles of condyles, as shown on a Gnathohexagraph. Incisal opening is 4 mm (vertical axis: movement; horizontal axis: rotation angle). Neither of these two subjects has abnormality in their TMJs. (a) At about 4 mm opening from ICP with no force applied, the right and left condyles are at 3.1 mm and 2.5 mm, respectively. The rotation angle is at 2.6 degrees, while the maximum is 18.6 degrees. Translation started in an early phase of opening. It does not show hinge movement as conventionally advocated. (b) Three-dimensional display of condylar movements at 5-mm opening with 0 g of force. The end point of the green line indicates the condylar position at 5-mm opening. (c) For the same subject, 800 g of force was applied to the mandible. At about 4-mm opening, the right and left condyles are at 0.7 mm and 1.8 mm, respectively. The rotation angle is at 4.3 degrees, while the maximum is 33.4 degrees. When force is applied to the mandible, motion in an early phase of opening is closer to hinge movement. (d) At 5-mm opening while 800 g of force is applied. (e) At about 4-mm opening in another subject. The right and left condyles are at 0.8 mm and 0.6 mm, respectively. The rotation angle is at 4.0 degrees, while the maximum is 24.9 degrees. This subject shows small translation or movement with rotation. This type is rare. (f) At 5 mm-opening with no force applied.

However, if one wishes to obtain a mandibular position that is reproducible, relatively fine hinge movement can be obtained by registering a centric bite record while applying some force to the mandible (Box 2-9). With this approach, the anterior translating component of the mandible is reduced. When a patient is allowed to open while attempting to pull the mandible posteriorly, relatively fine hinge movement is shown. Although this practice is acceptable in patients with well-developed condyles, slight force applied to the mandible will change the condylar positions in patients with a wide articular space. This is considered to be an extremely important issue, because the numbers of individuals with a wide articular space are increasing.

Box 2-9 Hinge axis and manipulation to centric relation

Measurement of condylar movements with a chin cap applied reveals hinge-like movements (Table 2-5). Because anterior translation starts in an early phase of opening, it is necessary to apply posterior force to obtain a reproducible mandibular position (Fig 2-70).

I had the opportunity to have my mandibular position recorded by a distinguished American clinician. Using the Dawson technique, this clinician explained that no force was applied. However, I clearly felt that too much posterior force to endure was applied. Later, I wore a chin cap and found that the feeling was similar to that of application of about 600 g force.

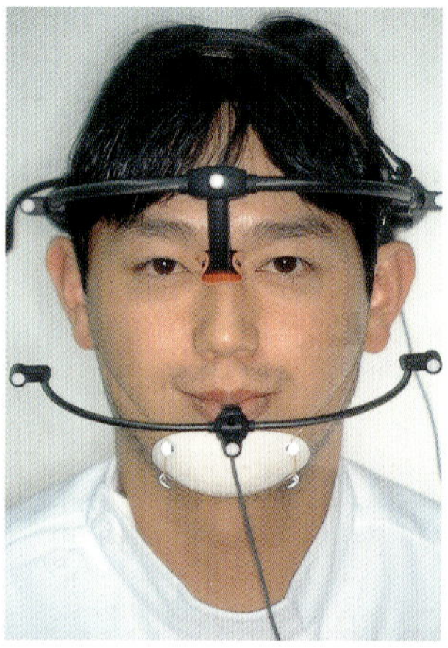

Fig 2-70 Experimentally, the chin was pushed posteriorly to record opening and closing movements.

Anterior and inferior movement of condyles when 0 g, 300 g, or 1000 of g force is applied to the chin (data from one subject)

Opening at incisal point	0 g	300 g	1000 g
ICP	0.0 mm	0.0 mm	0.0 mm
2.0 mm	2.5 mm	0.7 mm	1.0 mm
5.0 mm	3.0 mm	1.1 mm	1.0 mm
10.0 mm	4.2 mm	2.3 mm	2.0 mm

Functional Movements of the Mandible: Occlusal Movements

Which morphology for which functions?

From occlusal equilibration to occlusal reconstruction, procedures for correction of tooth morphology and maxillomandibular relationships are conducted to improve and recover function. How do we define recovery of function? Without a clear answer to that question, we cannot attempt treatment. In conventional occlusion theory, however, changes in morphology are discussed with a goal of achieving morphology that is, or is considered to be, "better." In other words, measures have been discussed without an objective or a target image of function in mind. In this book, we discuss occlusal morphology in relation to function.

Individual differences in chewing patterns

Functional movement paths are divided into the grinding type, in which the horizontal component is relatively large and the mandible moves toward the nonworking side initially at opening, and the chopping type, in which cyclic movements are conducted only on the working side (Figs 2-71 and 2-72). In addition to the large horizontal component, movement paths of the grinding type are characterized by initial opening toward the nonworking side, entering the working side, and then reaching ICP from the posterior and lateral direction. When chewing cycles (frontal surface) are examined separately, oblique egg–shaped tracings and inverse triangle–shaped tracings, which include horizontal grinding and cutting at ICP, are noted. Conventionally, it was considered that, as attrition progressed, or guidance became insufficient, oblique egg–shaped movement paths change into the inverse triangle–shaped movement, or lack of guidance. However, these are originally two different chewing patterns. It is probable that each human has his or her own chewing pattern by nature, and functional movements are conducted by both this central pattern and peripheral guidances. The appearance of oblique egg–shaped and inverse triangle–shaped tracings seems to be derived from the central mastication pattern. We believe that central mastication patterns include the chopping type and the grinding type and that grinding-type subjects have diminished guidance or lack guidance due to attrition.

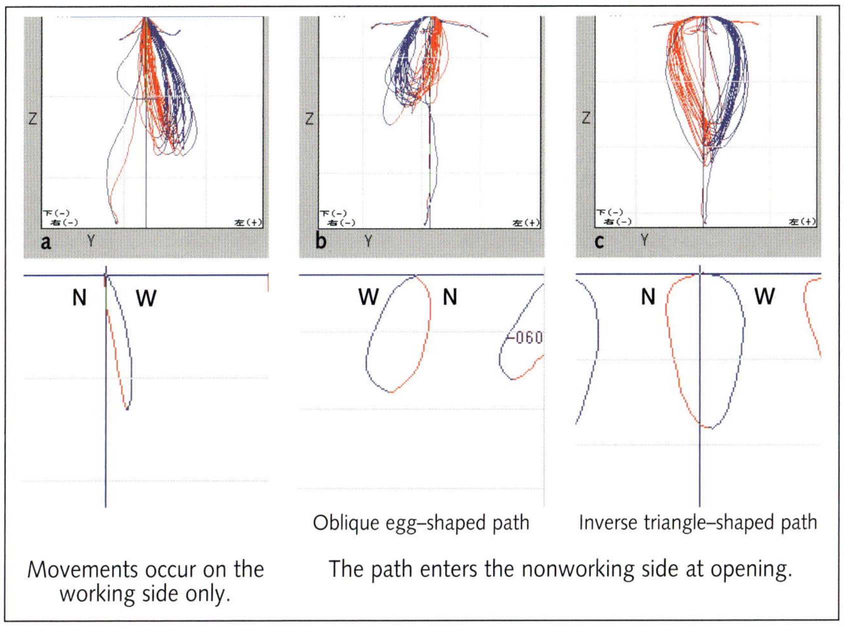

Fig 2-71 Individual differences in chewing patterns. (a) Chopping type. (b and c) Grinding type. N = Nonworking side, W = Working side.

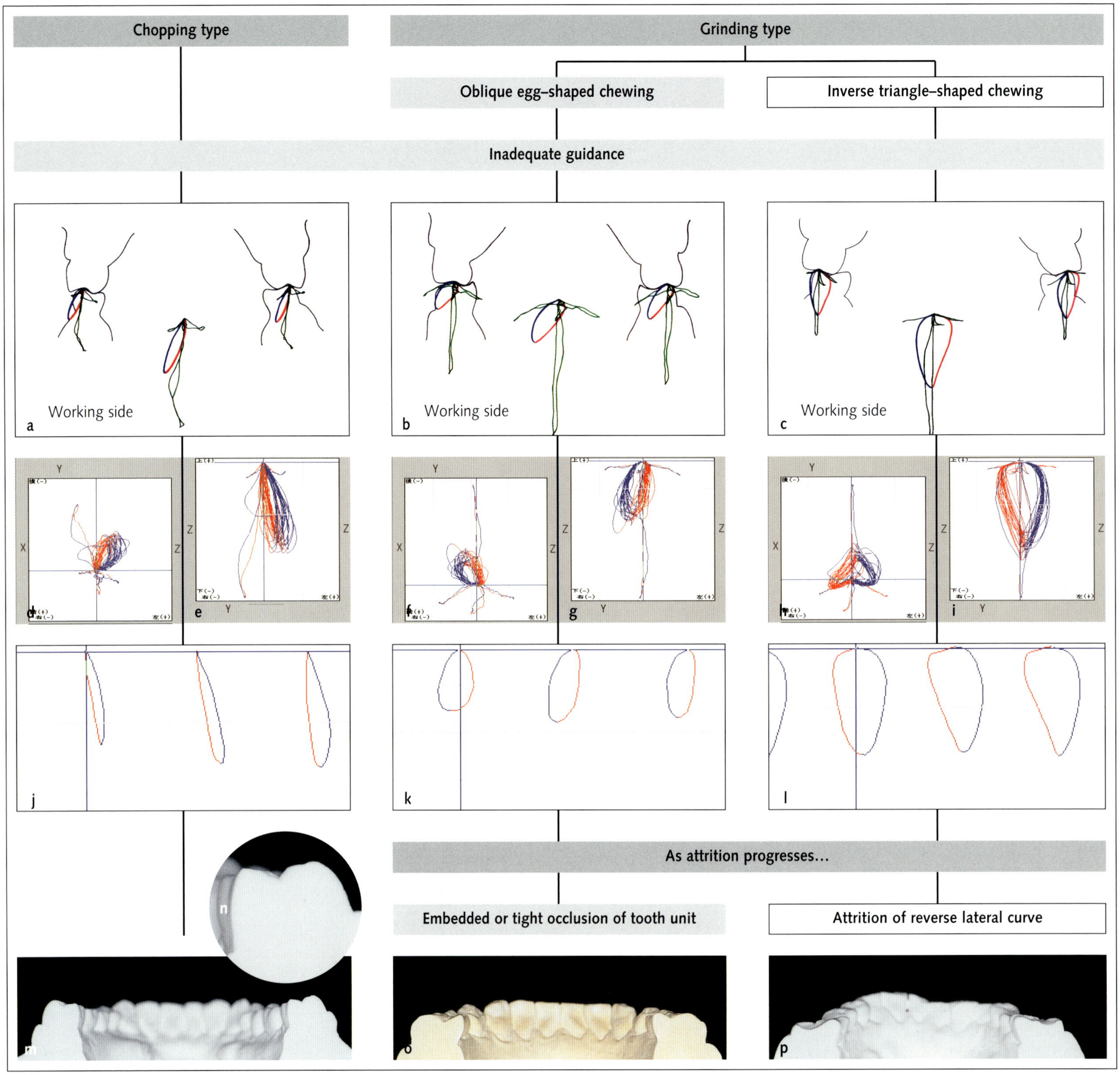

Fig 2-72 Individual differences in chewing pattern and progress of attrition. (a) Masticatory movements occur as a cyclical movement only on the working side. The width of the cycle is narrow, and tooth wear is limited. (b) The mandible initially opens to the nonworking side and enters ICP from the working side. Compared to the chopping type, the grinding type is more likely to cause attrition and be affected by interferences. (c) This type grinds food with almost horizontal movements like herbivorous animals. The movement is highly likely to cause attrition. At opening and closing, the working-side path and the nonworking-side path are largely different in their shape. As opening takes place on the nonworking side in a horizontal manner, the maxillary teeth tend to be flared buccally. (d and e) Movements of the mandibular anterior teeth during left-side chewing on the (d) transverse plane and (e) frontal plane. (f and g) Movements of the mandibular anterior teeth during right-side chewing on the (f) transverse plane and (g) frontal plane. (h and i) Movements of the mandibular anterior teeth during left-side chewing on the (h) transverse plane and (i) frontal plane. (j) Incisal movement cycles (left-side chewing) on the frontal plane of a chopping-type subject are shown separately. (k) Incisal movement cycles (right-side chewing) on the frontal plane of a grinding-type subject are shown separately. (l) Incisal movement cycles of a grinding-type subject with lack of guidance are shown. (m and n) The morphology and height of cusps are less likely to cause interference. This type is rare among Japanese patients. (o) The external slopes of the buccal cusps (A slopes) are worn horizontally, while the internal slopes of the lingual cusps (C slopes) are worn obliquely. This is believed to have been caused by rolling-type chewing and the time lag between the working side and the nonworking side. (p) Reverse lateral curved attrition seems to have been caused by horizontal grinding-type chewing and the time lag between the working side and the nonworking side.

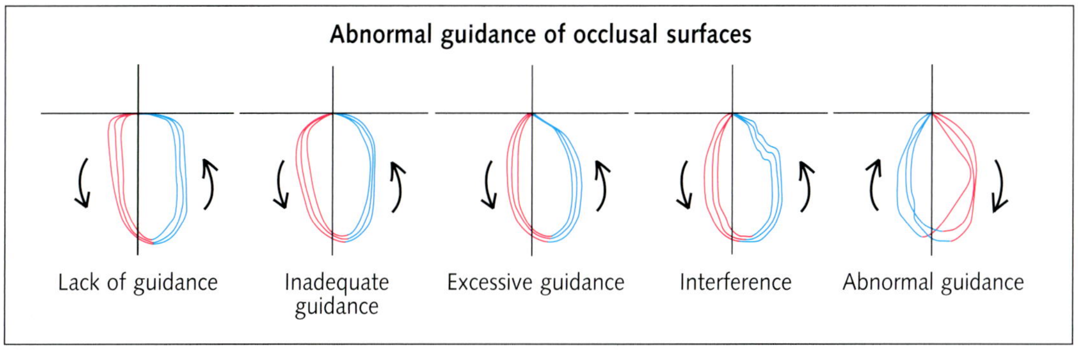

Fig 2-73 Excess, inadequate, or lack of guidance. Maruyama classified chewing patterns accompanied by abnormal guidance (the frontal plane of functional movements).

Oblique egg–shaped pattern and inverse triangle–shaped pattern

In patients with the inverse triangle–shaped chewing pattern, as attrition progresses, there will be a lack of guidance and gradual wear of mandibular buccal cusps that form the reverse lateral curve. Attrition in this type of patient does not often cause problems in periodontal tissues. On the other hand, in patients with the oblique egg–shaped chewing pattern, as will be discussed later, when attrition progresses, the maxillary and mandibular teeth catch on each other and form a typical tight occlusion of tooth unit (see the section entitled, "Tight Occlusion Versus Loose Occlusion"). This is likely to invite clenching and occlusal trauma.

Harmony between the central pattern and peripheral morphology

When occlusal tables are wide and flat, the subject will have a wide chewing pattern. However, no matter how wide the occlusal table, a subject who originally had a chopping-type pattern will never develop a grinding-type pattern with lack of guidance. On the contrary, if occlusal tables are narrowed too much, it will be manifested as excessive guidance or reverse. For example, if occlusal tables with high cusps are created in a grinding-type subject with lack of guidance, either trauma to the teeth or clenching will result.

Each living body has its own central chewing pattern. If peripheral occlusal surface morphology deviates largely from the pattern, mastication will not work. In such a case, it will be manifested as a pathologic condition in a weak part of the system, such as trauma to the teeth, disturbance of chewing, or loading of the joints or muscles.

Time lag between the working side and the nonworking side and occlusal morphology

Functional movement measurements obtained by early analytical equipment did not contribute to an accurate understanding of mandibular movements. Current mandibular movement analyzers allow simple measurement of six degrees of freedom at any point on the mandible. In addition, the time lag between the working side and the nonworking side as well as posterior movement of the working side during opening now can be captured (Fig 2-74). Also, because functional movements in a number of cases can be easily recorded in detail, significant information with regard to appropriate occlusal morphology is obtained.

Relationships between masticatory movements and occlusal morphology in a typical grinding-type (oblique egg–shaped) subject are shown in Fig 2-75.

In masticatory movements, the velocity of movements of the working side and the nonworking side is not the same. Movements of occlusal surfaces and condyles are not parallel either. According to observations using a Gnathohexagraph, the working side, the nonworking side, the condyles, and the occlusal surfaces of the mandible generally shift with a slight time lag in the following order: the working-side condyle, the working-side occlusal surfaces, the nonworking-side occlusal surfaces, and the nonworking-side condyle. Then they reach ICP in the same order. This order is common to chopping-type and grinding-type movements. In the oblique egg–shaped grinding pattern, which is observed in many Japanese subjects, rolling-type movement paths with multiple centers of rotation are observed.

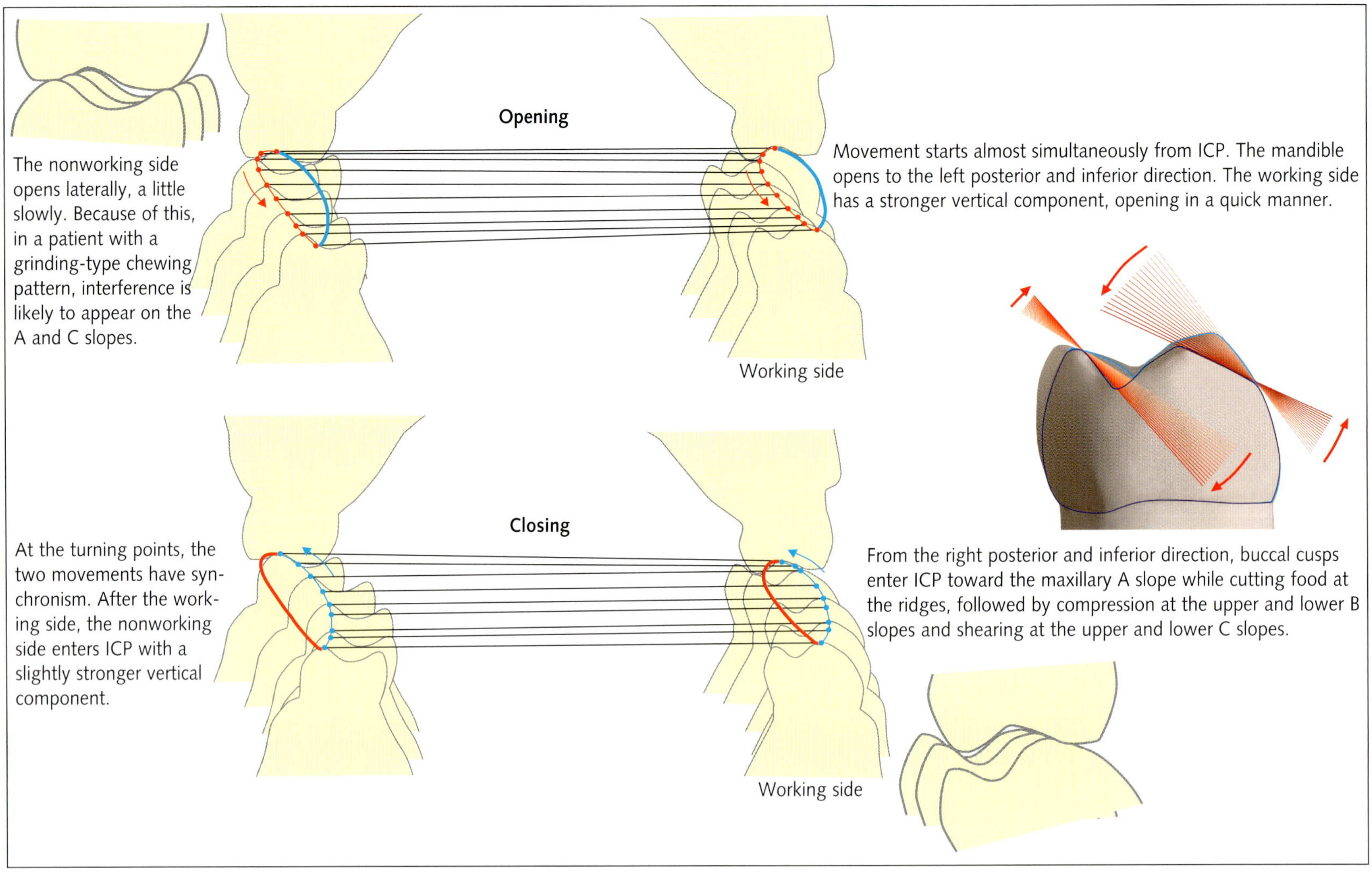

Fig 2-74 Time lag between the working side and the nonworking side. The time lag between the working side and the nonworking side produces a steep C slope. On mandibular molars, abruptly increasing attrition is found more often on C slopes than on A slopes. In conventional occlusion theory, it was believed that the working side and the nonworking side enter ICP simultaneously. If this were the case, there should be no difference in the angles of the A slope and C slope resulting from attrition. This discrepancy of angles can be explained by the time lag in movements of the working side and the nonworking side: First, the working side interdigitates from a somewhat lateral direction, and then, with some delay, the nonworking side interdigitates somewhat vertically. The time lag between the right and the left, or the working side and the nonworking side, corresponds to the difference in the angles between A slope and C slope. Therefore, the process should be understood not as if interdigitation takes place simultaneously in a shearing manner at the A slope and C slope but as if food is cut like scissors between the A slope cusp and ridge, pressed and chopped on the B slope, and lastly, sheared off at the C slope like a shearing machine.

On the working side, food is present, receiving occlusal pressure first and depressing the teeth. Without a small time lag, the nonworking side would have contact first, and it would be difficult to grind food. The existence of a small time lag is reasonable in this sense.

Anterior and lateral guidances and masticatory movement paths

Based on the argument that tooth contacts observed on an articulator have some diagnostic meaning for jaw function, the discussion of mandibular movements often has focused on the anterior and lateral guidances of maxillary and mandibular tooth contacts. In activities of daily living, most mandibular movements should be functional movements, including swallowing, speech, and mastication, and border movements should be limited. In the frontal plane, masticatory movements seem to exist within border movements that can be reproduced on an articulator. In the transverse plane, however, the masticatory movement path is located laterally and posteriorly. Moreover, even in the vicinity of ICP, the border movement path and the masticatory movement path do not necessarily overlap each other (Table 2-6).

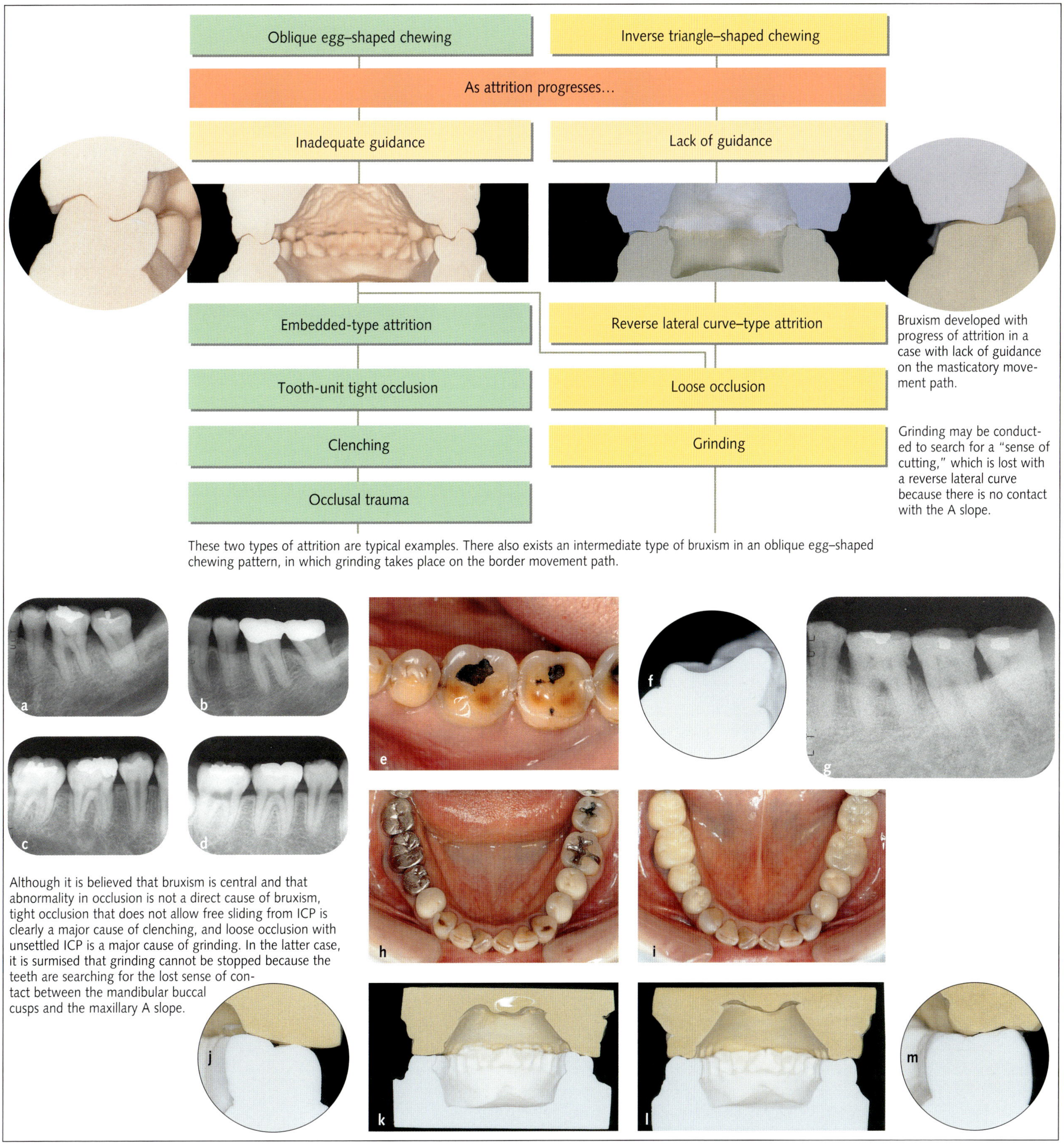

Fig 2-75 Relationship between progress of attrition and parafunction. (a and b) Traumatic findings, including loss of attachment, and their improvement. (c and d) Reversible traumatic findings (widening of periodontal space, turbulence of bone trabeculae, and disappearance of lamina dura) without loss of attachment and their improvement as well as recontouring. (e to g) Lack of anterior guidance caused excessive attrition and bruxism caused TMD. After the restorative treatment, grinding ceased. (h and i) Attrition has progressed because of lack of guidance. Also, the crown morphology has further accelerated a reverse lateral curve at mandibular right first and second molars. (j to m) With just the removal of the crowns on these molars, the 10-year-old grinding habit of this 61-year-old woman has been stopped. Bruxism occurs because there are teeth with a reverse lateral curve. It will not occur without poorly shaped teeth.

Lundeen and Gibbs showed movement paths in the frontal plane, trying to differentiate normal and abnormal through the relationship between masticatory movements and border movements. In their presentation, however, what is regarded as "normal" clearly has excessive guidance at opening, what is regarded as "occlusion with attrition" of a bruxer is a grinding-type pattern, and what is regarded as "malocclusion" should be judged within the scope of individual differences in masticatory movements.

Although anterior and lateral guidances are often the focus of attention in discussions of movements guided by occlusal contacts, masticatory movements generally head toward a lateroposterior and inferior direction. For mandibular movements to be considered normal, certainly it is necessary that the mandible move smoothly toward the anterior direction in a symmetric manner, with the focus on border movements. However, if there is interference in a posterior and inferior direction, smooth masticatory movements will be hindered. Also, even if movements are mostly symmetric based on observation at the incisal point, the path comes down significantly on the lingual side of molars on both sides. Because of this, the B slope is actually less likely to have interference than was conventionally believed. In the transverse plane, most movements head toward a lateroposterior direction (see Fig 2-72).

Movements guided by the occlusal surfaces of teeth and functional movements seem to go through the same area on the coronal projection but are totally different on the horizontal and sagittal projections, the former being anterior and the latter posterior. Among these movements, only the border movements of condyles and mandibular incisors are expressed on articulators. Therefore, clinicians should recognize that occlusal diagnosis with articulators examines only a part of mandibular movements.

Table 2-6 Inadequacies of the mandibular movement analyzer

1. Depending on how the reference plane is determined, a projected movement path will change significantly.
2. Because masticatory movement paths are projected on the Frankfort horizontal plane, expressed loci will be different because of different occlusal plane angles.
3. It is not possible an appropriate mandibular position in the whole body is to be expressed. If there is a habitual ICP it will be shown as a stable ICP.
4. The opening movement is different at the right and the left sides, for example, when condyles are large or there is clenching, in which case observation of movement paths alone will give the impression that the condyles are off the disc.

Box 2-10 Inadequacies of the mandibular movement analyzer: 1

Because a mandibular movement analyzer projects three-dimensional movements on a plane, projected movement paths will differ greatly, depending on how the reference plane is determined. Movement paths projected on the transverse and the sagittal planes include significant error. Even if the measurement device is accurately positioned in relation to the Frankfort horizontal plane, the projection of the same amount of rotation will be greatly different in the transverse plane and in the sagittal plane, depending on the angle formed by the Frankfort horizontal plane and the occlusal plane. Consequently, in the projection in the transverse plane, the same amount of rotation will be presented as a posterior cycle in an individual with a dolichofacial pattern and as a transverse cycle in an individual with a brachyfacial pattern. Also, although this is not realistic because of intricate measurement, if the occlusal plane is regarded as the reference plane, the transverse projection on the Frankfort horizontal plane that we observe has emphasized posterior movement of occlusal surfaces. Note that the anteroposterior movements of condyles are disregarded.

Fig 2-76 (a to c) Projected movement paths differ greatly, depending on how the reference plane is determined.

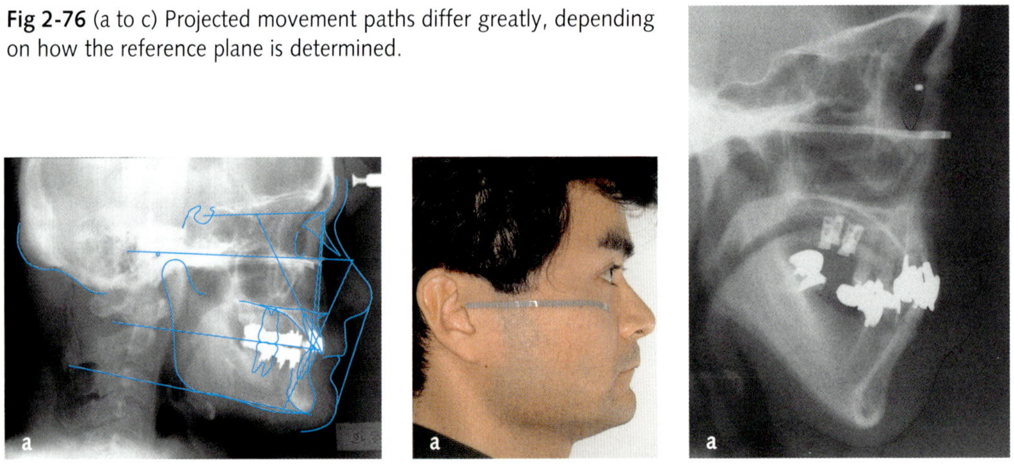

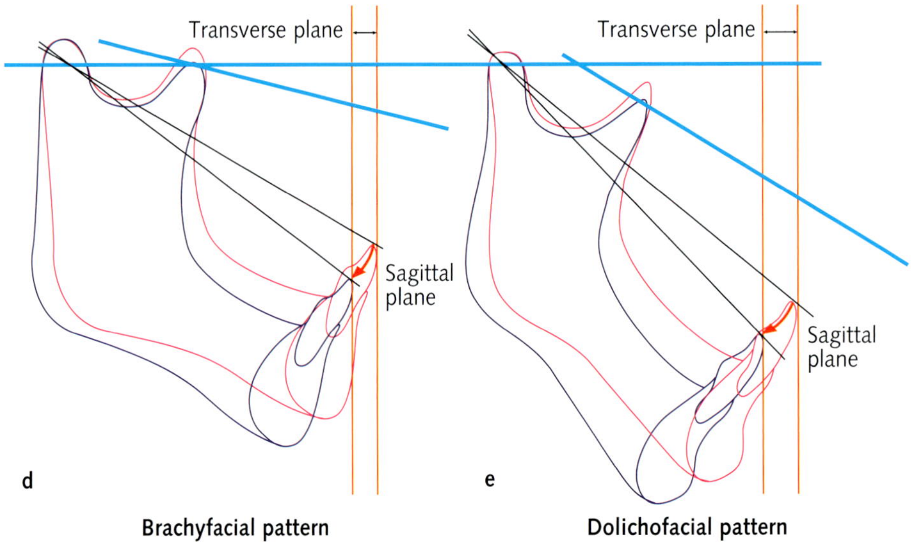

Texture of food, muscle force, and occlusal morphology

Movement paths during mastication are different during the chewing of soft, hard, or fibrous (hard and elastic) food. When tough, fibrous food is chewed, wide mastication is conducted using muscles. Here, mastication is widely affected by the position, height, and width of buccal and lingual cusps. With soft food, the role of cusps is limited, because only narrow movements are conducted within the occlusal tables. If a patient cannot bite off soft, thin food, the morphology of small accessory ridges should be examined. When a patient has a small mastication cycle and weak masticatory force, accessory ridges are likely to interfere with movements. Thus, when a patient complains of "some contact," "slipping," or "discomfort," the cause of which a clinician cannot detect, interference by small accessory ridges should be suspected.

On the contrary, when a patient does not have problems with muscle force but has difficulty eating fibrous food, disharmony between the centrally controlled mastication pattern and occlusal surfaces, including cusps, is suspected. Also, there must be some play, or a wedge-shaped space, between buccal interior and exterior slopes (Figs 2-79 and 2-80), so that different widths of movement paths can be accepted, depending on food texture. In other words, appropriate overbite and overjet are necessary for molars also.

Box 2-11 Inadequacies of the mandibular movement analyzer: 2

Is the transverse plane (or Frankfort horizontal plane) or the occlusal plane the basis for a diagnosis? The Frankfort horizontal plane is the basis of a diagnosis. When the diagnosis is based on the occlusal plane, a horizontal component appears strong. There is not much difference between the two projections in the case of a brachyfacial subject, but a posterior component will be smaller in a dolichofacial subject, which will make it difficult to detect interferences immediately posterior to ICP.

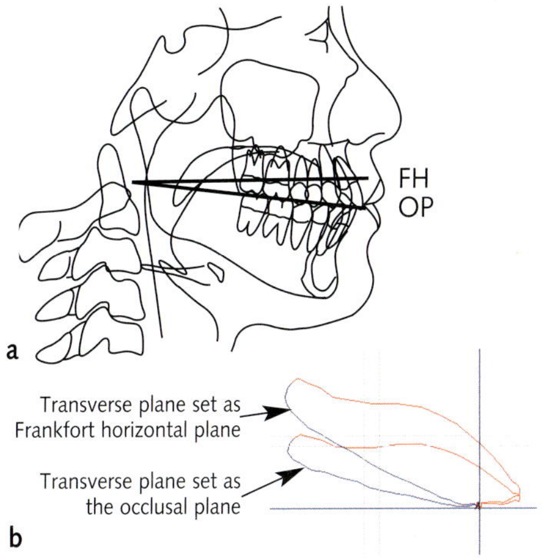

Fig 2-77 (a) Frankfort horizontal (FH) should be the basis for a diagnosis rather than the occlusal plane (OP). (b) Patient with an occlusal plane angle of 9 degrees.

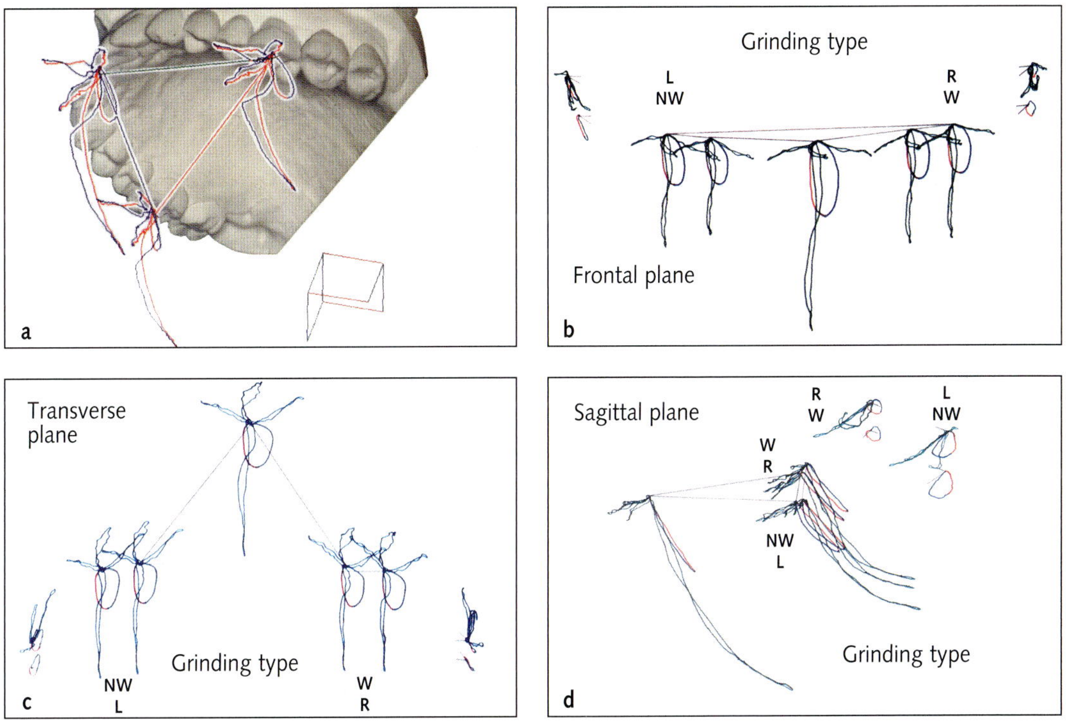

Fig 2-78 Anterior and lateral movement paths and masticatory movement paths (oblique egg–shaped). (a) A Gnathohexagraph is used to superimpose masticatory movement paths and anterior and lateral guidances at the mandibular incisal point and occlusal surfaces of the first molars on the maxillary occlusal surfaces; this reveals that the masticatory movement path exhibits a cycle in a posterior and inferior direction. (b to d) Frontal, transverse, and sagittal projections of masticatory movements and anterior and lateral guidances of a grinding type indicate that (b) in the frontal plane, incisal points are symmetric and at molars on the both sides the paths come down, because interferences are less likely to occur on the nonworking side during closing. (c) In the transverse plane, at the posterior cycle, the lingual side of the lateral border movement comes forward. (d) The sagittal plane projection shows that the anterior component during closing is large.

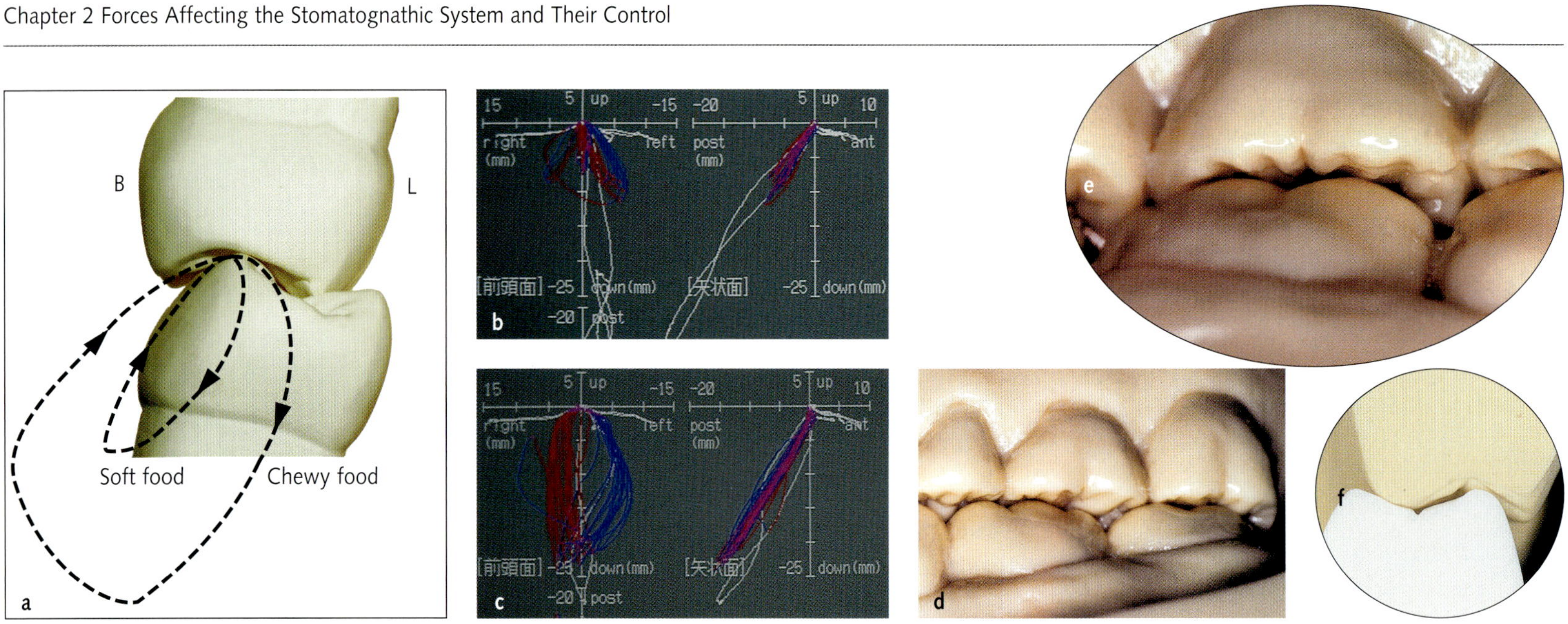

Fig 2-79 (a) Difference in the movement path due to different textures of food. (b) Coronal and sagittal projections during chewing of soft food. (c) Coronal and sagittal projections during chewing of chewy food. (d to e) Lateral overjet.

Correct masticatory movements

As for factors needed for correct masticatory movements, an appropriate mandibular position should be obtained in the whole body; joints and muscles should have no problems; border movements guided by occlusal surfaces should be symmetric and glide lightly and smoothly; and molars should show some disocclusion. Also, masticatory movement paths should naturally become vertical without following border movement paths, and lateral overjet and overbite should be present to allow comfortable chewing of food with different textures details the masticatory movements that fulfill these requirements. This is an example of right-side chewing in a patient who exhibits bruxism.

Unless ideal masticatory movements are understood in detail, it is impossible to determine the best occlusal morphology. When occlusal surfaces are observed in still images and when masticatory movements are observed in slow-motion video images, morphology itself appears different.

Box 2-12 Correct masticatory movements.

1. When food enters the mouth, the mandible opens to the left in a posterior and inferior direction. The tongue is used to place the food on the occlusal tables of the right molars. The right working side opens with a strong vertical component, and with some delay, the left nonworking side then opens with a strong vertical component. Because of this pattern, interference during opening is more likely to appear on the A and C slopes of the nonworking side than on the B slope of the working side.
2. At the turning point, the nonworking side catches up when both sides come to the same position in the cycle.
3. From the right posterior, the mandible closes in an inferior direction. Maxillary right buccal cusps aim at the A slopes in the maxillary arch, grinding food at the ridges and entering ICP. Food falls buccally toward the vestibule.
4. Food is pressed and ground at the upper and lower B slopes.
5. Shortly after that, the upper and lower C slopes enter ICP with a strong vertical component to grind and cut food to the tongue space.
6. The nonworking side enters ICP with a strong vertical component.

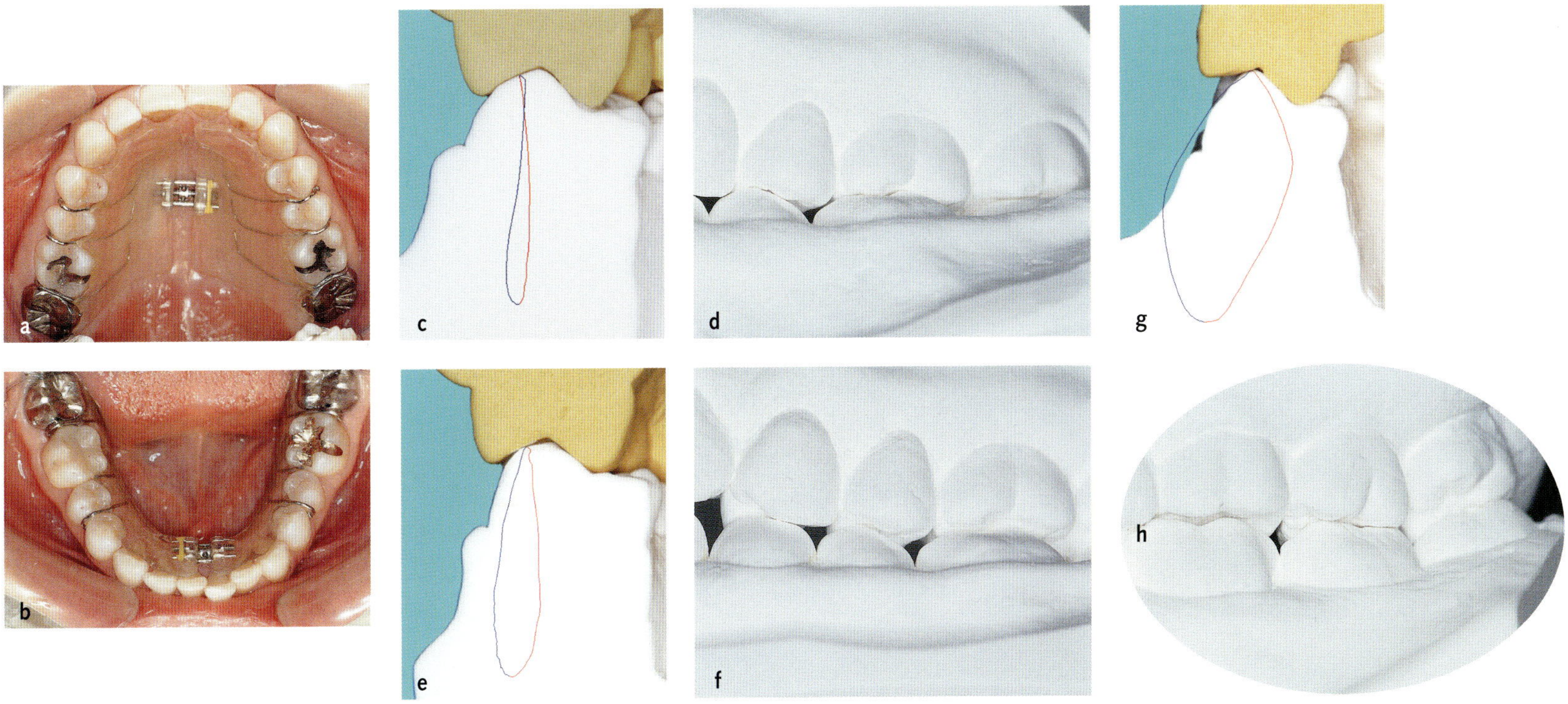

Fig 2-80 Play in lateral overjet and tight occlusion. (a and b) The dental arches are laterally expanded with screws, uprighting the lingually inclined molars. (c and d) Before treatment. This is a type I TMD patient who has a conspicuous deep bite. As diagnosed, the arches are narrowed because of habits, causing clenching, a deep bite, and lingual inclination of molars and resulting in tight occlusion. Under this vicious circle, the patient complains of stiff shoulders, headache, and pain in the neck and jaw. (e and f) After lateral expansion. The dental arches have been laterally expanded with screws, uprighting the lingually inclined molars. Because the unpleasant symptoms were clearly decreased by this lateral expansion, the patient looked forward to tightening the screws once a week. As the teeth uprighted, the mandibular buccal cusps, which used to be caught in the maxillary central fissures, started to rise, creating triangular spaces of play and channels for food spillage on the A slopes. (g and h) In contrast, the lateral overjet is too shallow. The movement path shown on the casts is in the coronal section of the same area.

Interferences of molars and condylar movements

Routine use of a mandibular movement analyzer in clinical practice has clarified the influences of molar interferences on condylar movements. With examination of border movements, it was not possible to understand what kind of molar morphology would cause interference during functional movements. Currently, it is understood that molar interference causes more significant condylar movements than earlier imagined. Here, relationships between cuspal interference and TMJ symptoms are once again brought into perspective. Occlusion and TMD are deeply related to each other.

One representative type of cuspal interference is interference of nonworking side molars, in which the B slopes of the nonworking side molars have contact before the working side. The interference of the nonworking side molars was generally considered to inhibit normal movements of the mandible. However, when an onlay is delivered to experimentally cause lateral interference of the B slope on an articulator, it does not cause interference during functional movements if the lateral interference is minor. This is because, except in extreme grinding that closes along the border movement path, the nonworking side molars enter ICP with a strong vertical component and the working side opens with a strong vertical component during opening. Consequently, this is less likely to cause interference for functional movements (coronal projection). In other words, as observed on the articulator, no interference will occur at the B slopes.

Then, posterior interference was intentionally added to the B slope. As a result, it entered ICP from an anterior direction to avoid the posterior interference and opened anteriorly for both the working and the nonworking sides, although the degree was different.

During mastication, opening occurs with a slide in a somewhat posterior, lateral, and inferior direction. In a grinding-type pattern, it initially opens toward the nonworking side. In right-side chewing, occlusal surfaces on the right side open somewhat vertically to left posteroinferior direction, and, with some delay, occlusal surfaces on the left side open slightly laterally. Because of this, interference during opening is more likely to appear on the A and C slopes of the nonworking side than on the B slopes of the working side. When border movements are reproduced on an articulator, it appears as if interference is likely to occur on the slopes of the working side. Even if border movements seem to have interferences, as for masticatory movements, the A and C slopes on the nonworking side should be observed in a patient's mouth. The C slopes of the nonworking side often have a morphology that will hold the C slopes of the maxillary arch because of attrition. This is likely to cause interference on the nonworking side as well as excessive guidance on the working side (see Fig 2-74).

Significance of interference on functional movement paths: Experiment 1. Nonworking side and posterior interferences during closing.

To observe cuspal interference during functional movement, an onlay was experimentally delivered to a subject who exhibited mostly an average grinding-type pattern (Fig 2-81). The onlay was delivered to the inner slope (B slope) of the lingual cusp of the maxillary left first molar so that nonworking-side and posterior interference could be generated at closing of right-side chewing (Fig 2-82). As a result, the subject started chewing on the right side and, from the day of the delivery of the onlay, complained of a heat sensation in the right TMJ area, pain and heaviness of the shoulder, and pain and weakness of the temporal muscle area (Box 2-13). On day 3, symptoms included tension of the left neck, which subsided in about a week. Later, the subject had pain on percussion of the maxillary left first molar, which subsided in about 10 days. At this time, mandibular movements (Figs 2-83 to 2-85) changed in the movement paths on the noninterference side, as the border movements on the interference side changed. When there is an interference on either the opening path or the closing path, both masticatory movement paths will change their shape.

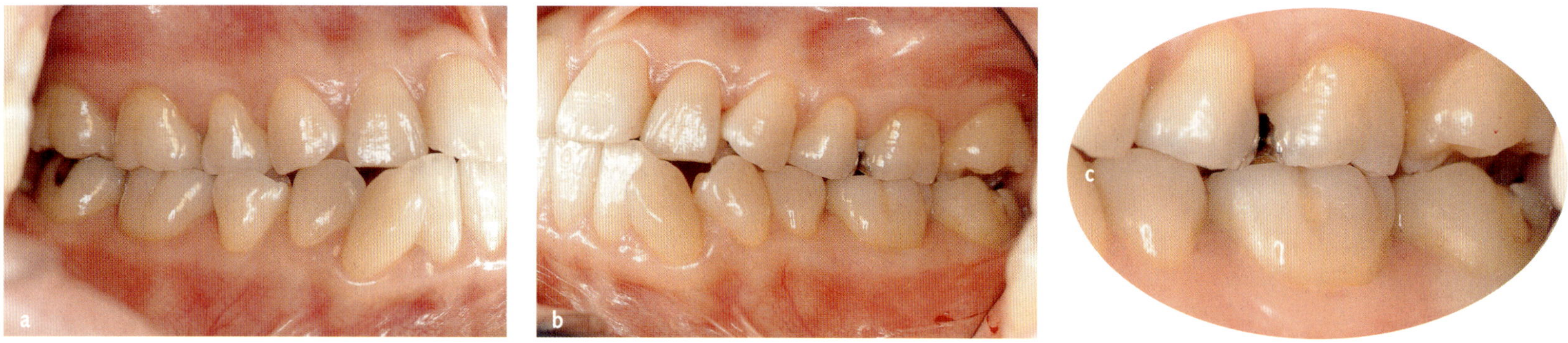

Fig 2-81 (a and b) The subject mostly exhibits an average grinding-type chewing pattern. The maxillary right and left canines are missing. (c) An onlay is delivered to the B slope of maxillary left first molar to create nonworking-side and posterior interference. ICP is not changed.

Box 2-13 Experimental interference: Diary of the subject

Wednesday, October 6
An onlay was delivered on the maxillary left first molar. Immediately after the delivery, a tight feeling and difficulty in biting was felt. Especially when I bite on the left side, I feel like it is hitting against a stone. I notice that I am trying to chew on the right side. After a while, I felt hot in the right TMJ area and heavy in the right shoulder.

Thursday, October 7
It is still difficult to chew on the left side. During right-side chewing, I can clearly feel that I am trying to avoid the B slope of the maxillary left first molar at closing. In the afternoon, I dismissed the heat sensation at the right TMJ from my mind, but the right temporal muscle was tense and the shoulder hurt.

Friday, October 8
In the morning, I found the right-side symptoms were improved. But now, the left side of the neck felt very tense. Also, the left temporal muscle hurts and feels heavy.

Saturday, October 9
I am getting used to this interference. The pain of the left temporal muscle does not bother me, but tension of the neck still continues. It is more like myalgia rather than stiffness. When I chew on the left side, I feel it does not cut well. It is mostly grinding. I cannot chew a sheet of dried seaweed.

Sunday, October 10
Tension of the left neck is awful. I can turn my head to the left but not to the right, as it hurts terribly.

Tuesday, October 12
Now I do not feel tension of the neck much. During left-side chewing, it feels like biting dry rice.

Wednesday, October 13
During left-side chewing, discomfort is felt at the maxillary left first molar. Mild percussion pain was felt at the palatal root of the maxillary left first molar.

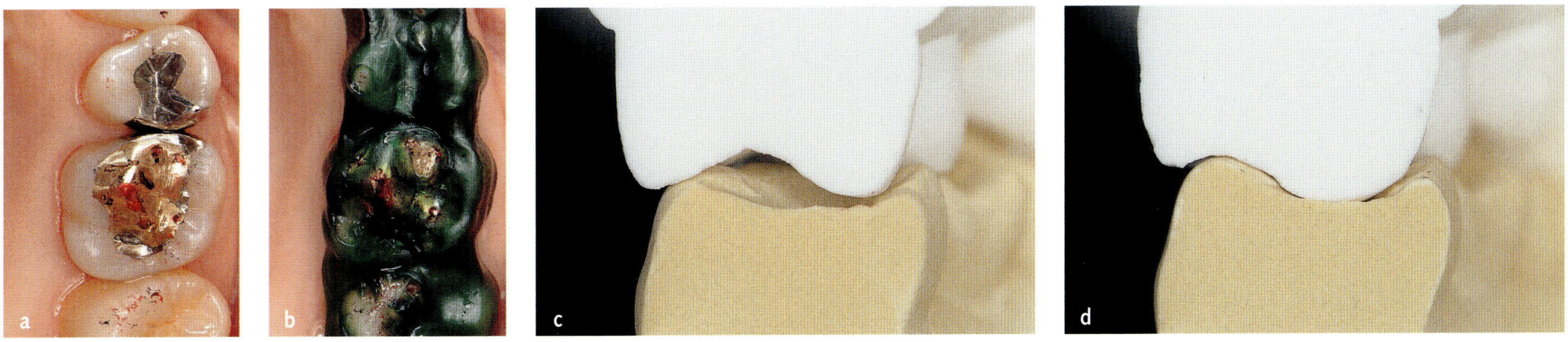

Fig 2-82 (a and b) An onlay is placed on the B slope of maxillary left first molar to create nonworking-side and posterior interference. ICP is not changed. Cross sections from the posterior direction are shown (c) before delivery and (d) after delivery of the onlay.

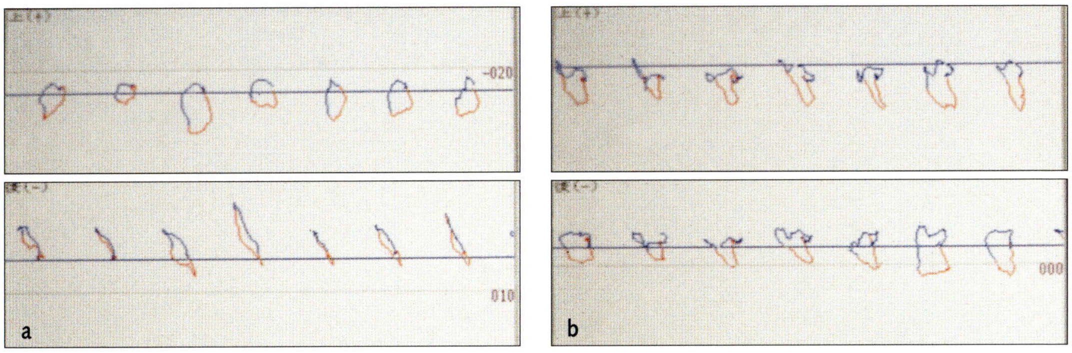

Fig 2-83 Disturbance in the condylar movements of the working side, shown from the *(top)* frontal plane and the *(bottom)* transverse plane.(a) Individual cycles of condylar movement paths during right-side chewing are shown before interference was created. (b) Significant disruption has been caused in the working-side condylar movements.

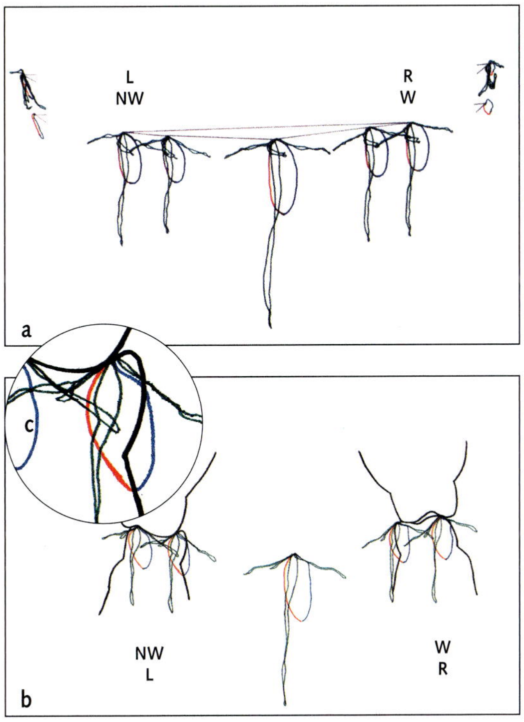

Fig 2-84 Interference of the B slope on the frontal plane. (a) Before delivery of the onlay, mostly standard grinding-type paths are observed although a relatively large portion goes along ICP. (b and c) After the delivery of the onlay, because of the lateral interference of the B slope of the maxillary left first molar, a larger area overlaps with the border movement path. The border movement path of the inside of the maxillary left first molar, where no treatment was performed, has a stronger angle.

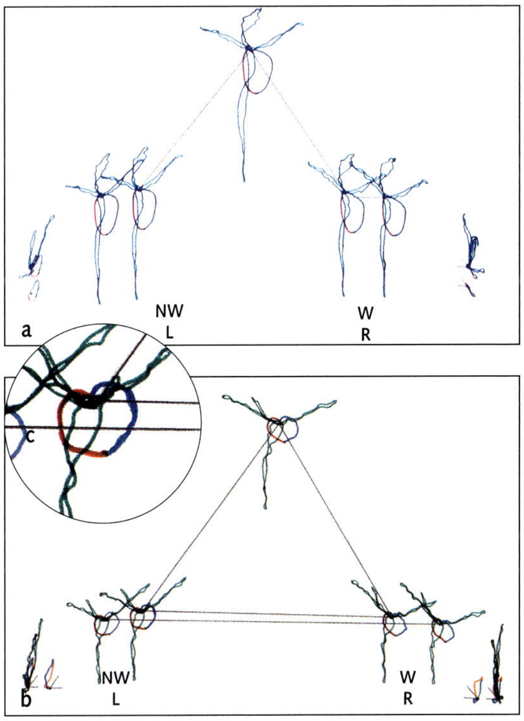

Fig 2-85 Posterior interference on the transverse plane. (a) Before delivery of the onlay, mostly standard paths are observed, although a relatively large portion goes along ICP. (b and c) After the delivery of the onlay, the path moves anteriorly first and then enters ICP at closing, avoiding the posterior interference. At opening, the path also moves anteriorly first.

Significance of interference on functional movement paths: Experiment 2. Tight holding of the C slope.

Figures 2-86 to 2-88 show the response after experimental placement of a tightly holding onlay on the C slope of the mandibular left first molar. The onlay was intended to raise the C slope and hold the outer slope of the maxillary lingual cusp. Immediately after delivery, it was difficult for the subject to move the jaw horizontally, which caused some anxiety (Box 2-14). The subject originally chewed on the right side, but the right-side chewing was not smooth after delivery of the onlay, and it became difficult to open smoothly. During left-side chewing, which was more comfortable for the subject, slow biting movements were needed. At closing, as teeth came into contact, it was very tiring for the subject, because contact at the onlay was avoided. When the subject awakened in the dental chair, some tension was felt on the left lower back. Gradually, a tense feeling was developed in the neck. After meals, a heat sensation was felt at the left TMJ. Although the subject became accustomed to the B slope interference in about a week (see Figs 2-81 to 2-85), it was not easy to get accustomed to this tightly holding interference on the C slope.

Box 2-14 Experimental interference: Effects on the subject

An onlay was delivered to raise the C slope and hold the outer slope of the maxillary lingual cusp (see Fig 2-86). Some symptoms were noted at the TMJ area on the interfering side. Comparison of the movement paths before and after delivery of the onlay (see Fig 2-87) reveals significant disruption of the closing path; the opening path was also affected. Opening on the nonworking side indicated reverse chewing, and closing on the nonworking side showed movement specific to excessive guidance.

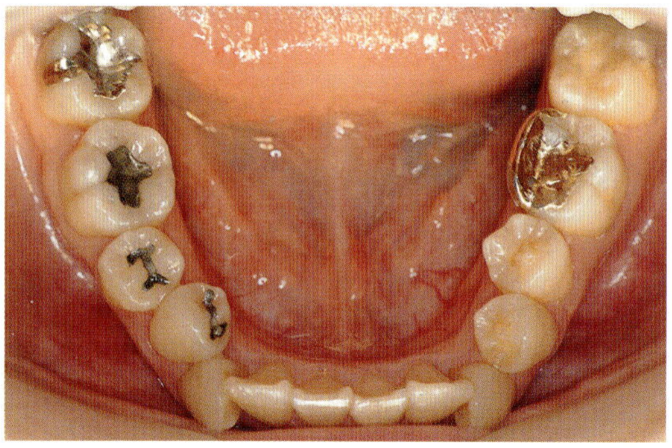

Fig 2-86 An onlay is delivered to raise the C slope and hold the outer slope of the maxillary lingual cusp.

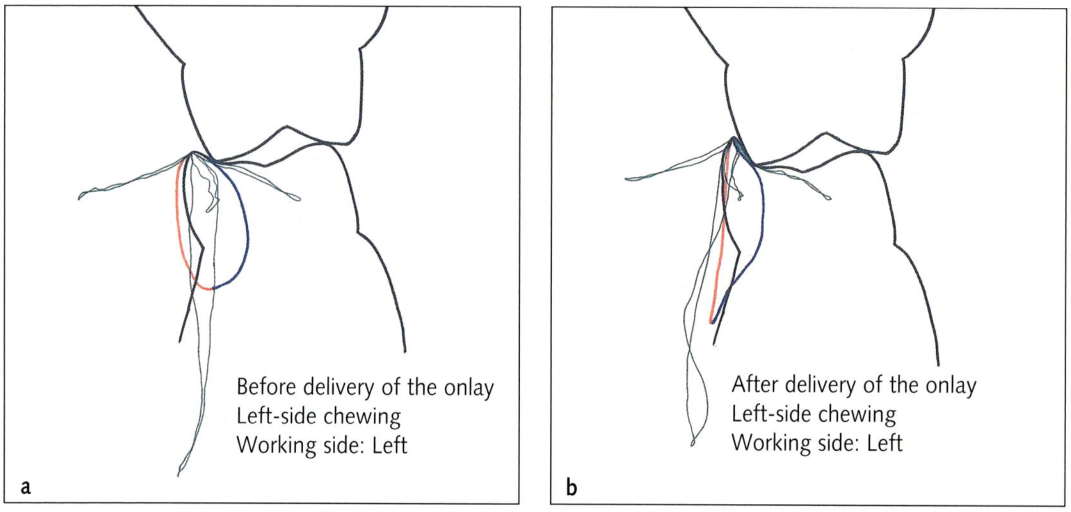

Fig 2-87 Clear evidence of how relations between border movements and masticatory movements will change if the C slope in the mandibular arch is raised. (a) Before interference. (b) The C slope has been raised to give create guidance on the working side at closing and interference on the nonworking side at opening.

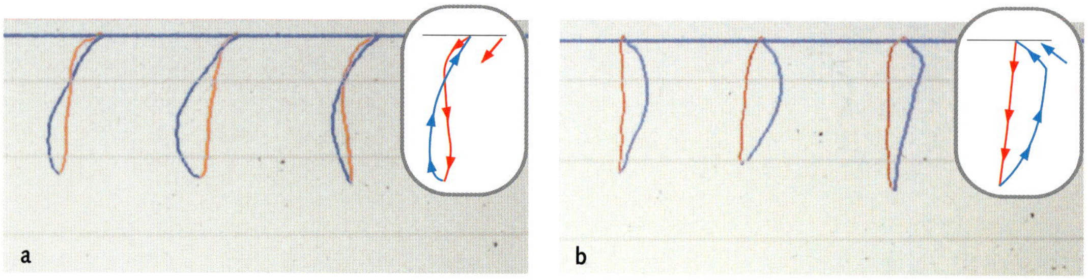

Fig 2-88 (a) Reverse actions are generated by the nonworking side interference during right-side chewing at opening. As the onlay of the mandibular left first molar hits against the C slope of the maxillary left first molar, it cannot open to the nonworking side, and shows this reverse movement on the way. The frontal projection of the incisal area is shown. (b) Left-side chewing at closing. Movements are disrupted at closing (excessive guidance). Opening shows a straight path. The frontal projection of the incisal area is shown.

Posterior interferences at opening and closing

At the initial stage of opening and closing, often the mandible slides slightly posteriorly. Therefore, attention should be paid to posterior interference, which tends to be overlooked because it is not reproduced in simulation on an articulator. Still, posterior interference is likely to cause difficulty in chewing and symptoms of TMD. On an articulator, only anterior and lateral border movement paths are observable. The mandible moves in an inferior and posterior direction in the initial phase of actual opening and closing.

Also, when an occlusal interference is noted on an articulator, clinicians tend to think that teeth contact each other at that point. In functional movements, however, the living body shows movement to avoid the interference, which results in trauma in another area that cannot be predicted on the articulator. This is the reason why occlusal interference and trauma are not consistent. In short, functional movement paths do not necessarily converge with border movement paths.

For example, in a patient with stable ICP and no premature contacts on border movement paths, signs of trauma are sometimes observed in the periodontal tissues of the maxillary anterior teeth. For this situation, posterior interference is suspected. Namely, the mandible first moves inferiorly and anteriorly and then moves down posteriorly, when the interference occurs. When either the opening path or the closing path has interference, the shape of the whole mastication cycle will be changed. Therefore, distortion of masticatory movement paths should be regarded not as disorder of the movement paths but as a suggestion of interference in the vicinity of interdigitation (Box 2-15). Also, when there is an obstacle on the masticatory movement path, the subject tends to learn it and avoid it. When flaring out of teeth or porcelain chipping is noted in a maxillary anterior area, possible posterior interference may be suspected.

Significance of interference on functional movement paths: Experiment 3. Crossbite.

The buccal tables of the mandibular left second premolar and first molar were extended to cause crossbite (Fig 2-89).

With no guidance of the A slope, there is no guidepost when the subject enters ICP. As a result, the cycle becomes unstable, showing reverse or crossover trajectories (Figs 2-90 and 2-91). Because masticatory movement always starts with a cutting action, the A slope is needed. Consequently, in a patient with crossbite, the C slope is used for cutting.

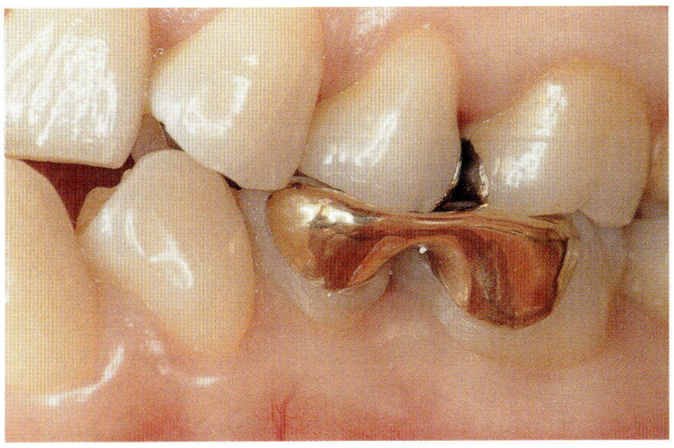

Fig 2-89 The buccal tables of the mandibular left second premolar and first molar and mandibular left second premolar were extended to cause crossbite.

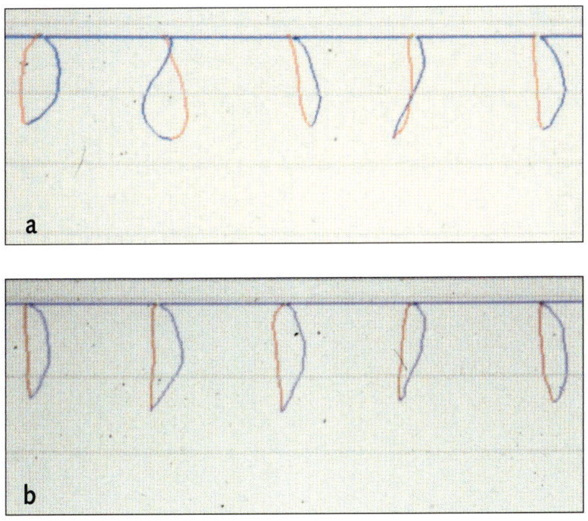

Fig 2-90 (a) Observation of individual cycles of left-side chewing at the mandibular incisors in the frontal plane immediately after the crossbite was created reveals an irregular shape of the opening path and a reversal on the closing path. (b) Observation after 1 week shows no irregularity of the cycles, which seems to indicate learning by the patient.

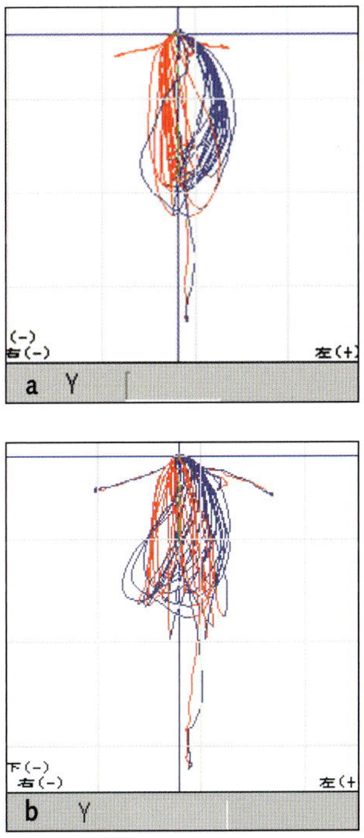

Fig 2-91 When crossbite is created, the variability of ICP and chewing is increased. (a) Before and (b) after delivery of the restoration.

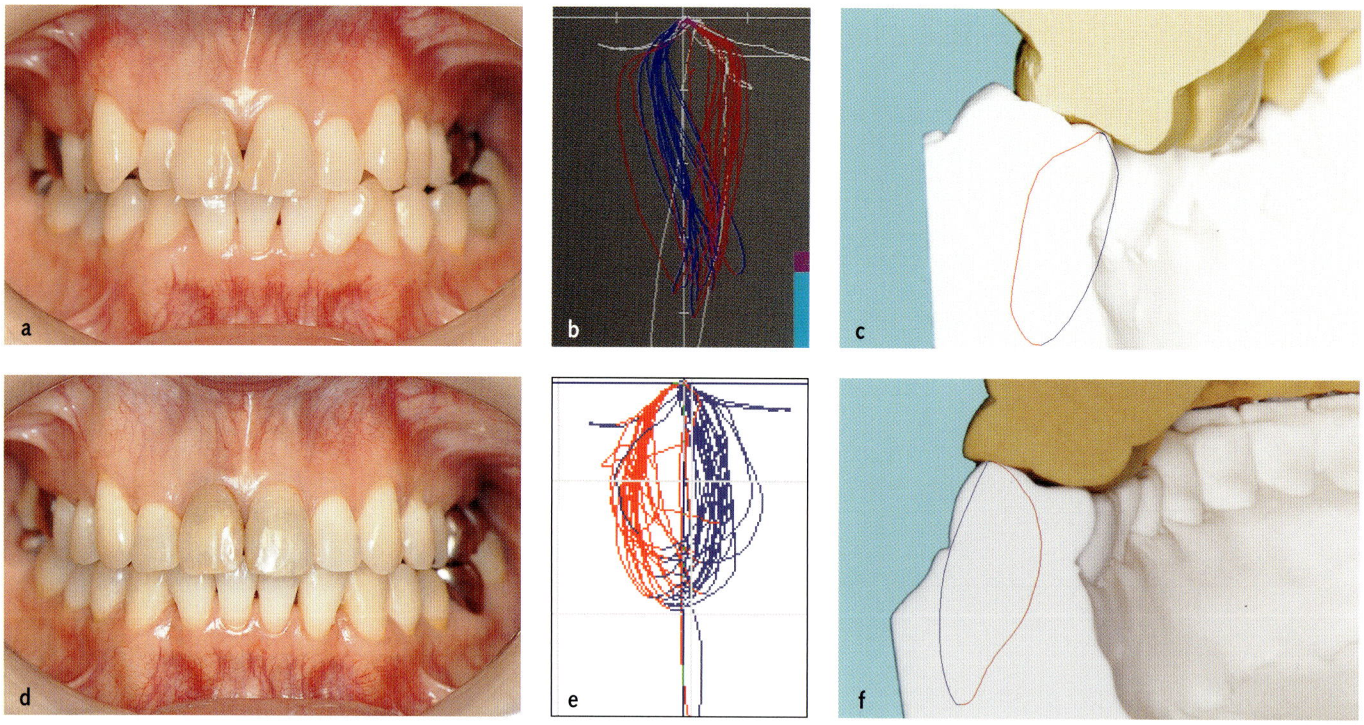

Fig 2-92 Improvement of crossbite and convergence of chewing. Chewing cycles are compared in the frontal plane (a to c) before and (d to f) after crossbite was created. In a case with posterior crossbite, because there is no A slope to bite into, a reverse cycle is drawn to bite at the C slope. For implant-supported prostheses, some clinicians narrow the occlusal surfaces to reduce occlusal load, resulting in no contact at the A slope. From the viewpoint of biting and cutting food, this has an adverse effect.

Box 2-15 Conclusions derived from experimental abnormal chewing (see Figs 2-81 to 2-92)

- TMD symptoms may be caused by abnormal morphology of occlusal surfaces.
- Even when TMD symptoms are derived from posterior interference, the interference cannot be detected on an articulator.
- Posterior interference on the closing path cannot be found in a border movement examination but may become an obstacle in functional movement.
- When there is mobility and flaring out of anterior teeth, posterior interference should be suspected.
- Interference will also change the border movement of the noninterfering side.
- When there is disruption of the opening path, the existence of interference not only on the opening path but also on the closing path should be suspected.
- Because masticatory movement always starts with a cutting action, the A slope is needed.
- When the A slope, or the target at closing, is lost, ICP becomes unstable and a reverse cycle may be generated.

Occlusal Morphology From the Viewpoint of Masticatory Movements

Masticatory movements and occlusal morphology

What kind of occlusal morphology is appropriate for the living body? In what case can occlusal morphology be considered interference? What kind of morphology is needed for comfortable chewing? What kind of morphology will unnaturally inhibit sliding movement of the mandible? What should we use as a reference for appropriate occlusal morphology? Clearly, appropriate occlusal morphology should allow efficient functional movements.

When one or two teeth are missing but adjacent teeth are present on both sides, there is a direct method available to reproduce occlusal morphology from functional movements. Clinically, occlusal morphology has been discussed via border movements reproduced on an articulator. However, thanks to the development of the mandibular movement analyzer, now clinicians can easily observe functional movements, which provides an understanding of occlusal morphology.

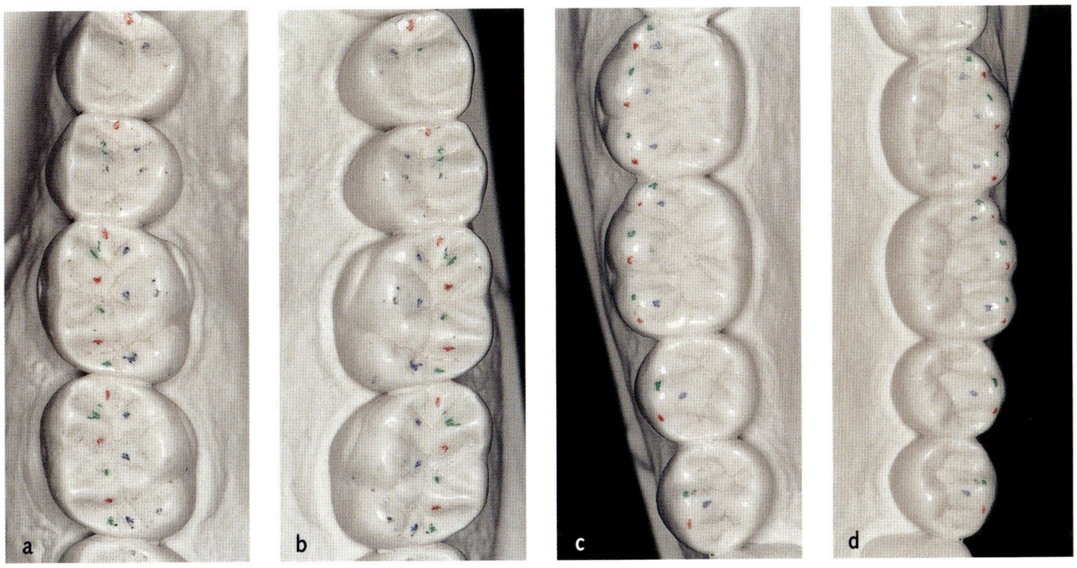

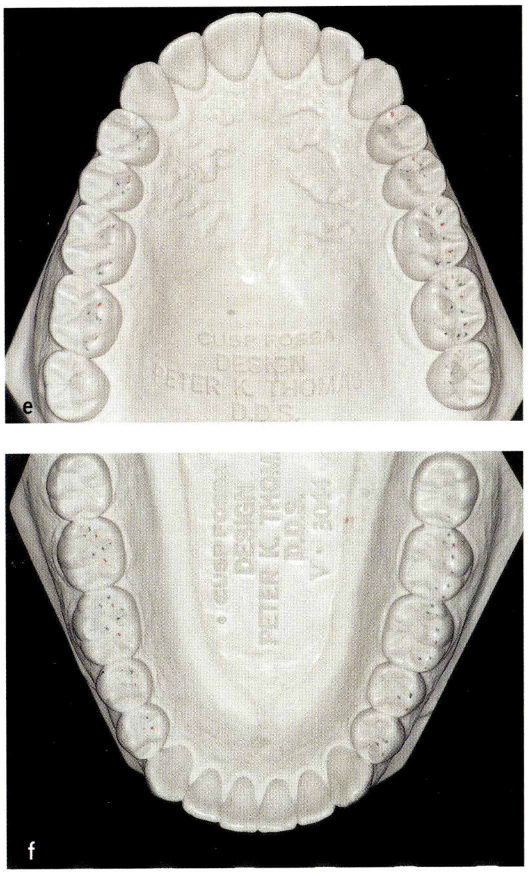

Fig 2-93 (a to f) Models designed by P. K. Thomas are considered a typical example of ideal occlusal morphology. However, the cusps are too steep and fossae are too deep to serve as an average occlusal morphology for Japanese individuals, most of whom exhibit grinding-type chewing patterns. The authors used this model as a reference after shallowing the upper A, lower B, and C slopes and removing the posterior interference of maxillary molars.

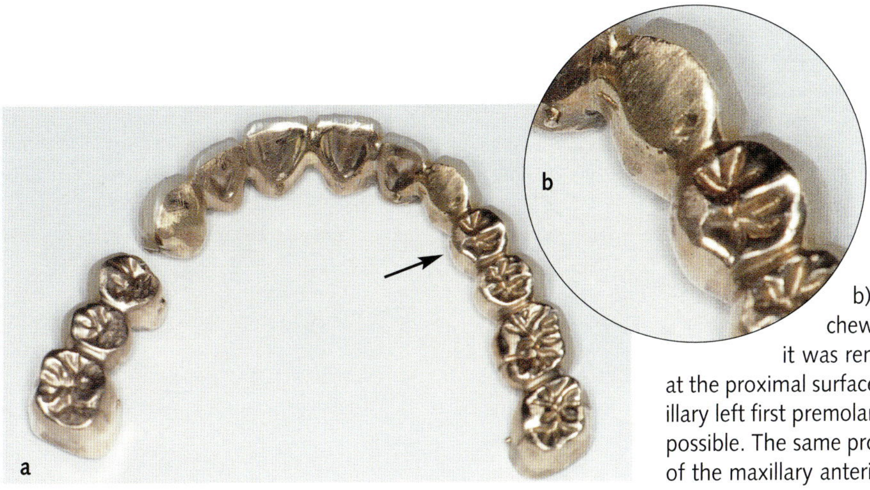

Fig 2-94 Seemingly ideal occlusal morphology that has a serious problem. (a and b) The patient brought this prosthesis for examination, claiming to be unable to chew. Because the cost of treatment was so high, the patient kept the prosthesis after it was removed. At first glance, it looks like an ideal splint. However, the marginal ridges at the proximal surfaces are generally high. Especially because the buccal and lingual ridges of the maxillary left first premolar are connected *(arrow)*, sliding from ICP to a lateral and posterior direction is not possible. The same problem applies to the maxillary left second premolar. The shovel-like palatal shape of the maxillary anterior teeth is deep.

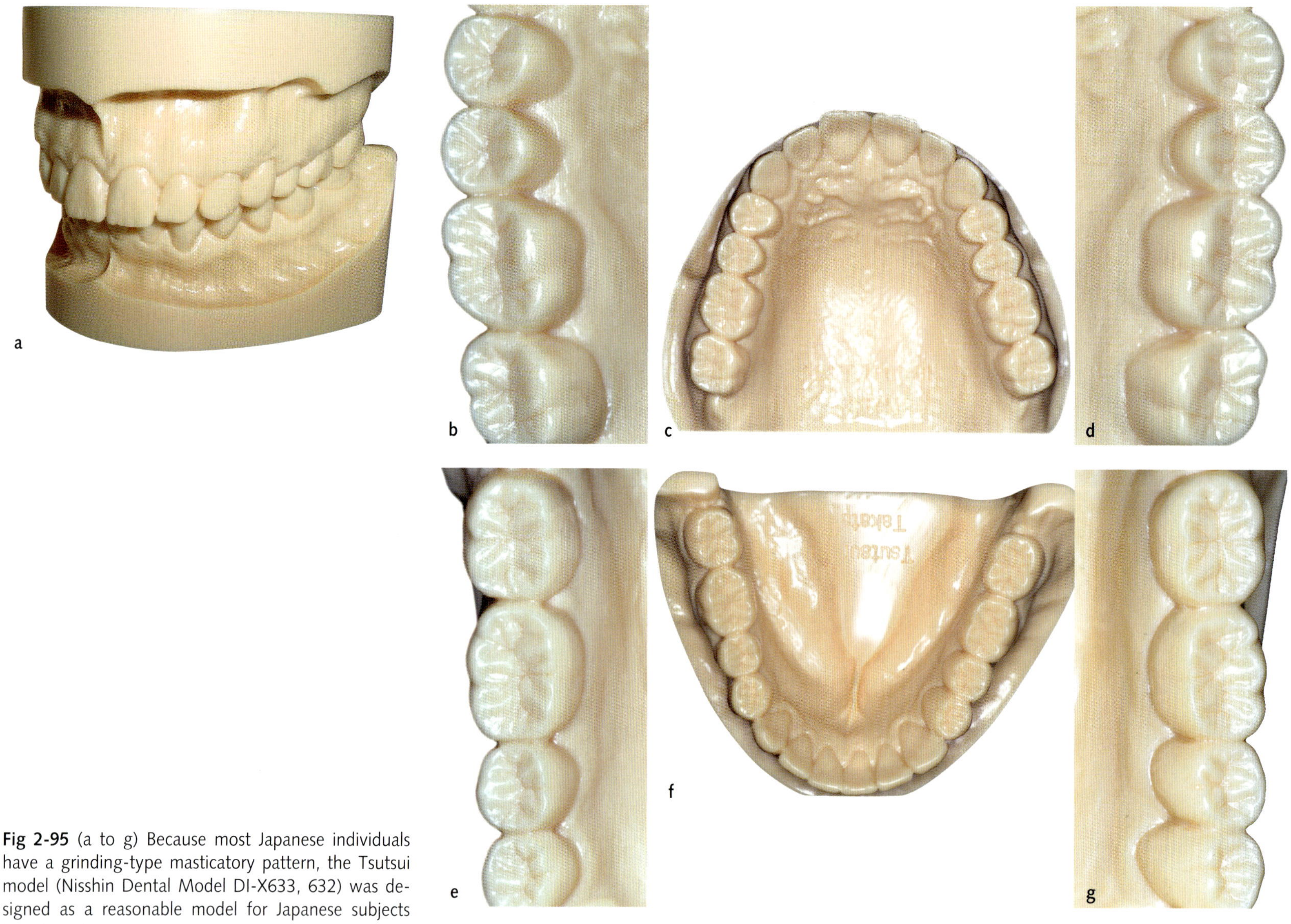

Fig 2-95 (a to g) Because most Japanese individuals have a grinding-type masticatory pattern, the Tsutsui model (Nisshin Dental Model DI-X633, 632) was designed as a reasonable model for Japanese subjects based on their masticatory movements.

Model for ideal occlusal surfaces

What kind of occlusal surfaces should a dentition have as an ideal model? It is not only needed as a reference for wax-up of full-mouth rehabilitation. When provisional restoration is fabricated at chairside and to have the skill to perceive a subtle abnormality in occlusion, clinicians require a clear and solid image of an ideal model. Conventional dentition models were constructed to recreate a chopping-type masticatory pattern with high cusps and steep occlusal surfaces, which are common in many Western patients (Fig 2-93). For this reason, in an extensive crown restoration case, it is often observed that tight occlusion is given, which restricts the functional movements of a patient (Fig 2-94). The authors designed the Tsutsui model with the intention of creating a model of occlusal surfaces that would accept the average masticatory movements of Japanese subjects (Fig 2-95).

This model has occlusal surfaces in harmony with oblique egg-shaped, grinding-type masticatory movements, which are observed in many Japanese subjects (Fig 2-96). In comparison with the models of P. K. Thomas and H. C. Lundeen that have been prevalent as an ideal model, the occlusal morphology from the viewpoint of masticatory movements must fulfill the requirements outlined in Box 2-17. Also, if occlusal surfaces are examined or new occlusion is provided for a therapeutic purpose, the principles noted in Box 2-18 should be considered. If a therapeutically created occlusion is incorrect, it is not only dysfunctional but also may cause iatrogenic pathologic conditions.

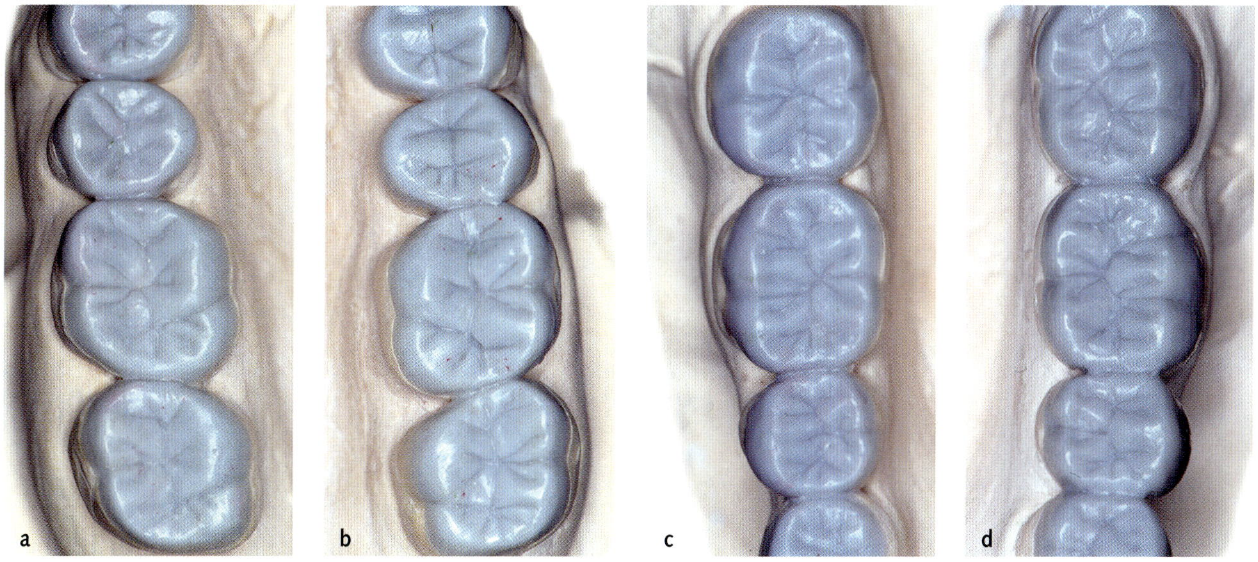

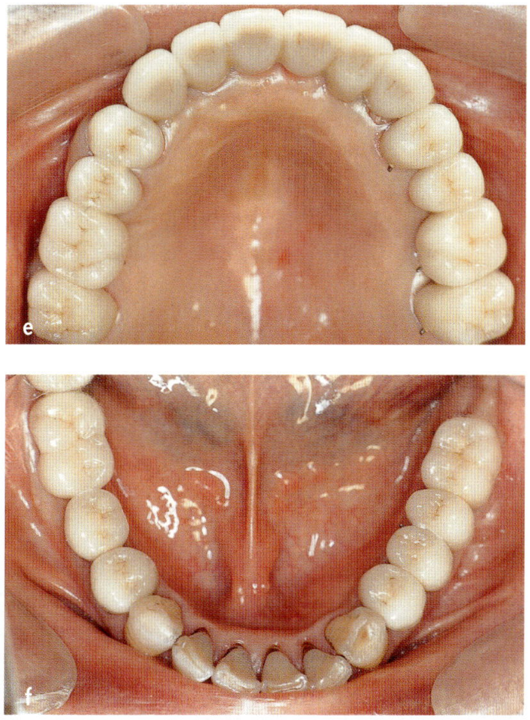

Fig 2-96 (a to f) Examples of wax-up and crown restorations based on the Tsutsui model.

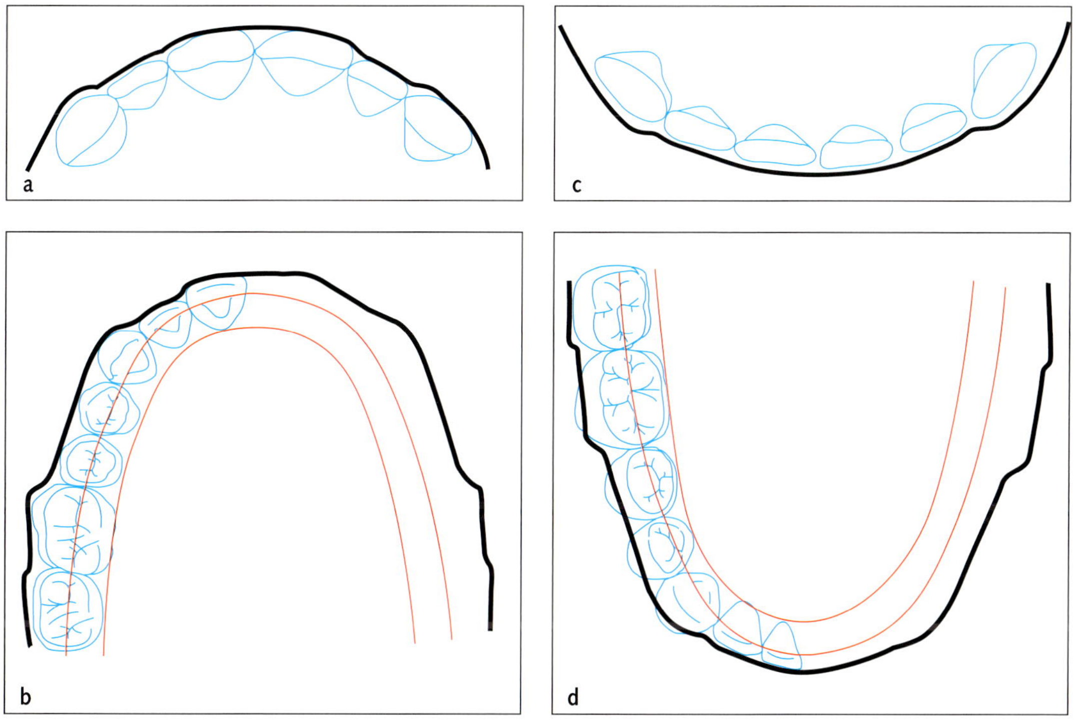

Fig 2-97 (a to d) An ideal arch in orthodontics includes an ideal arch form of the buccal surfaces of the dental arch.

Morphology of the dentition

The morphology of the dentition includes a three-dimensional curve of occlusion (curve of Spee and lateral curve), a symmetric occlusal plane with a certain inclination to the cranium, tooth axis with regularity in accordance with each tooth type, and a certain arch form.

The buccal surfaces of the maxillary and mandibular anterior teeth draw a somewhat continuous arc (Fig 2-97), standing in alignment with the central fissures of the molars. The contours of the labial surfaces reflect the difference in labiolingual thickness (highly variable among individuals), which has a slight concavity at the lateral incisors, emphasizing the projection at canines. The labial contours of the mandibular anterior teeth are continuous for the four incisors and slightly projected at the canines. This form of labial contour is distinctively shown in an ideal arch in orthodontics. An ideal arch for the maxillary arch has an inset between the central incisor and the lateral incisor in the maxillary arch and offset between a lateral incisor and a canine (see Fig 2-97).

Box 2-16 Requirements for occlusal morphology from the viewpoint of masticatory movements

- The morphology allows expression of individual differences in chewing cycles (see Fig 2-71).
- The occlusal table (of the mandibular arch against the maxillary arch) does not cause interference in chewing with individual differences.
- The occlusal table has an appropriate width: If the occlusal table is too narrow, it will be very uncomfortable for a patient. If it is too wide, the chewing cycle will be wide and unstable (likely to cause loose table and to generate lateral forces).
- Some space (play) at the A slope is necessary to accept different consistencies (hardness and softness) of food (see Fig 2-79). For hard food, an occlusal table suitable for a wide chewing cycle is needed. For soft food, effective accessory ridges are needed.
- Because oblique egg–shaped grinding (exhibited by most Japanese subjects) results in a time lag in condylar movements (between the working side and the nonworking side), food is cut like scissors from the posterior and lateral direction of the A slope, pressed and chopped on the B slope, and sheared off at the C slope like a shearing machine.
- Cusp-to-fossa contact should involve convexity against convexity.
- Cusp-to-fossa contact should be neither too shallow nor too deep (should be stable at three points and allow resistance-free movement).
- The occlusal surfaces should have grooves or spillways for food.

Box 2-17 Principles of examination of occlusal surfaces and treatment of malocclusion

- Border movement paths and masticatory movement paths are different. The clinician must have a good understanding as to the benefits and limitations of conventional occlusal analysis.
- Does the A slope have sufficient space (play)?
- Do the fossae of the maxillary arch consist of convex surfaces?
- Areas where interference is likely to appear should be well understood:
  - Interference posterior to ICP: At the initial opening of masticatory movements, often the path starts in a lateral posteroinferior direction. If there is a posterior interference and occlusion is shallow, the path initially goes forward, which is likely to cause porcelain chipping, flaring out, and mobility of anterior teeth.
  - Interference of lingual C slope: If the C slope of the maxillary arch is closely held at closing on the working side, it will invite tight occlusion, causing interference at opening on the nonworking side and a reverse cycle.
  - Projection at the upper and lower A slope: Guidance will be excessive at closing on the working side, causing crossover release.
  - Projection at the upper and lower B slope: This is likely to cause interference at closing on the working side.
- Lack of guidance will cause loose occlusion, leading to grinding.
- Excessive guidance will cause tight occlusion, leading to clenching.
- For patients who exhibit grinding, the occlusal table should be narrowed with guidance.
- For patients who exhibit clenching, guidance should be made shallower to facilitate movements.
- A stabilization-type splint is an effective means for reducing clenching in patients with a tight occlusion.
- For patients with loose occlusion and grinding, a stabilization-type splint will eliminate guidance, worsening grinding.

Tight Occlusion Versus Loose Occlusion

Differences between tight occlusion and loose occlusion

During occlusal examinations, the clinician first must confirm that a patient's ICP is stable in a relaxed condition and then must determine if the mandible can move from ICP in a reasonable manner (see Fig 2-13). In earlier sections, this chapter introduced viewpoints of occlusion, namely, tight occlusion and loose occlusion, and we discussed how tight or loose occlusion is constructed in a tooth unit.

Generally, involuntary parafunction of the mandible is called *bruxism*. Clenching, observed mostly in patients with tight occlusion, and grinding, observed mostly in patients with loose occlusion, should be handled with totally opposite approaches. For patients who exhibit clenching, tight conditions should be released. A stabilization-type splint will improve situations dramatically. On the other hand, a stabilization-type splint is not very effective for treatment of grinding, because loose movements should be converged to eliminate grinding.

Management of loose occlusion

Patients with unstable ICP have a problem with either their mandibular position or their occlusal morphology. Therefore, finding an optimal mandibular position should have the highest priority compared to anything else in treatment related to occlusion. To correct loose occlusion, either guidance should be given or reshaping is conducted to narrow the occlusal table slightly if the occlusal surfaces have attrition. Grooving is performed for the occlusal surfaces. With this treatment, masticatory movements with a strong horizontal component will change to those with a strong vertical component.

Management of tight occlusion

Because tight occlusion is caused by occlusal surfaces that hold each other too closely, excessive guidance, or close holding of the maxillary and mandibular dentitions, the causes should be determined and tightly holding areas should be released. More specifically, for tooth-unit tight occlusion, areas of excessive guidance and interferences should be reshaped. For dentition-unit tight occlusion, the dental arch should be expanded. Consequently, the chewing cycle that is too narrow should be widened to a moderate degree.

The occlusion associated with clenching and the occlusion associated with grinding are totally opposite. How to cope with them is also quite different. Bruxism, which clinically includes these two parafunctions with opposite meanings, must not be discussed as a single entity.

Temporary measures for management of loose occlusion

A 50-year-old woman first visited us with a chief complaint of dislodgment of a prosthesis (Figs 2-98 to 2-101). With infraversion and labioversion of the maxillary left canine and linguoversion of the maxillary left lateral incisor, the left canine guidance was lost. Chewing occurred on the right side and the left side, making occlusion unstable. This is a typical loose occlusion case accompanied by symptoms such as neck pain and fatigue of both eyes. Compared to tight occlusion, loose occlusion is less likely to cause major problems. Because of a hesitation to undertake extensive invasive procedures, temporary canine guidance was given. The patient became comfortable with this treatment and reported no stiffness of the neck, even during driving. She has used these provisional crowns for a long time only at night.

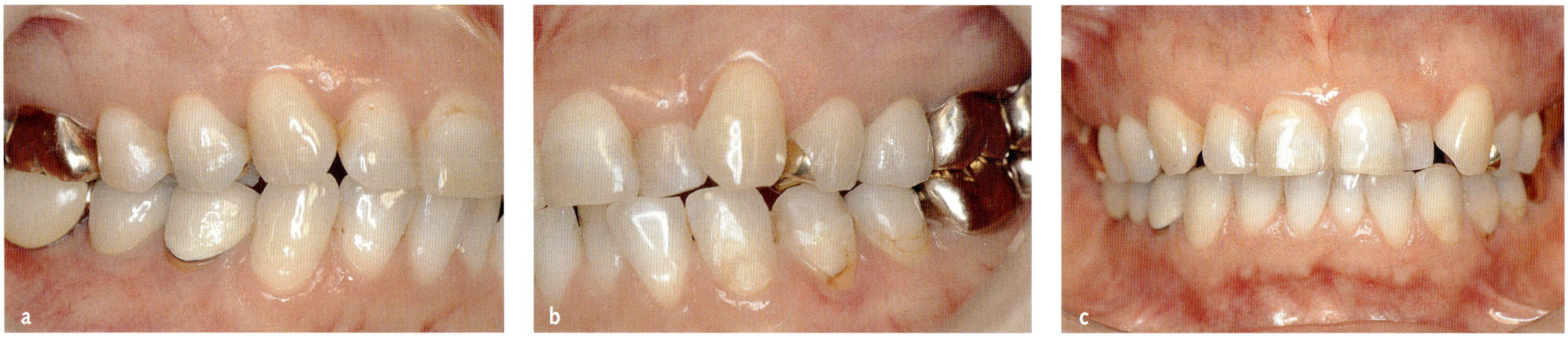

Fig 2-98 (a to c) The occlusion is unstable because of infraversion and labioversion of the maxillary left canine and linguoversion of the maxillary left lateral incisor. Although she was instructed to chew on the right side, the mandible quickly moves to the left.

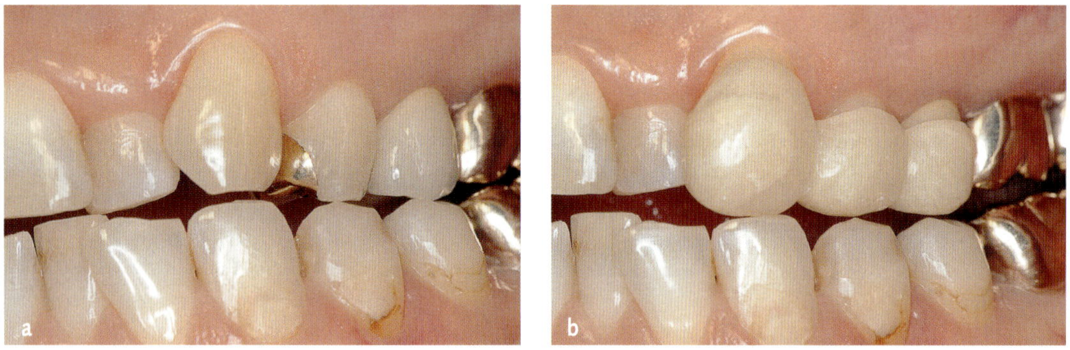

Fig 2-99 Because (a) the left canine guidance has been lost, (b) provisional crowns are fabricated to add thickness to the lingual side. These crowns are used only at night, without causing any changes in ICP. This temporary measure helps to resolve the patient's neck pain and has been used for 2 years.

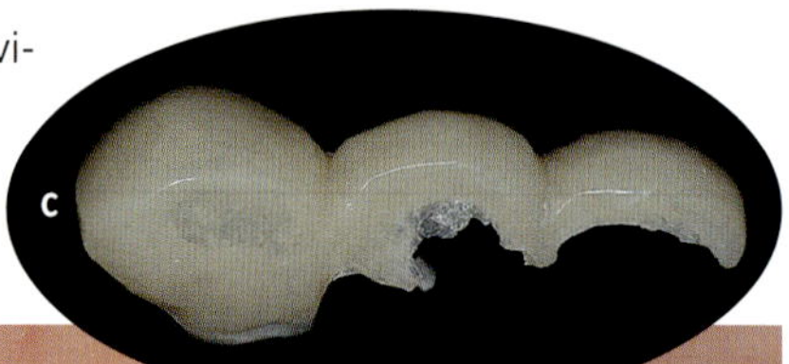

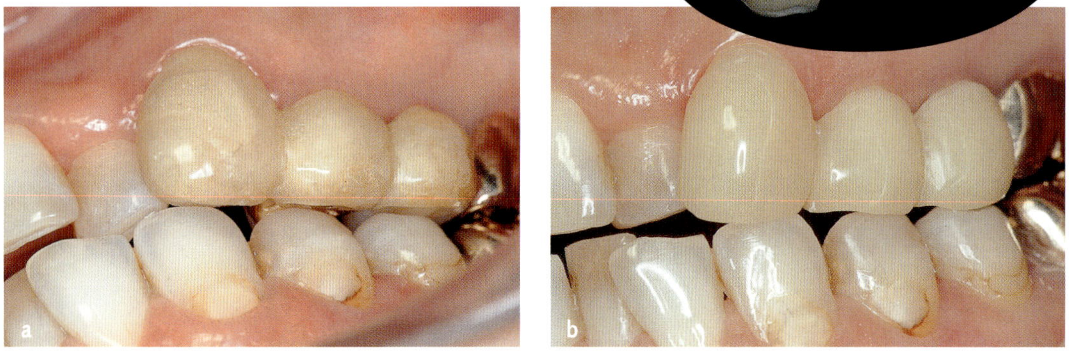

Fig 2-100 Photographs taken after 2 years 10 months. Because of (a) wear on the occlusal surface, (b and c) new crowns are fabricated to provide similar lateral guidance for the right and left sides without a change in ICP.

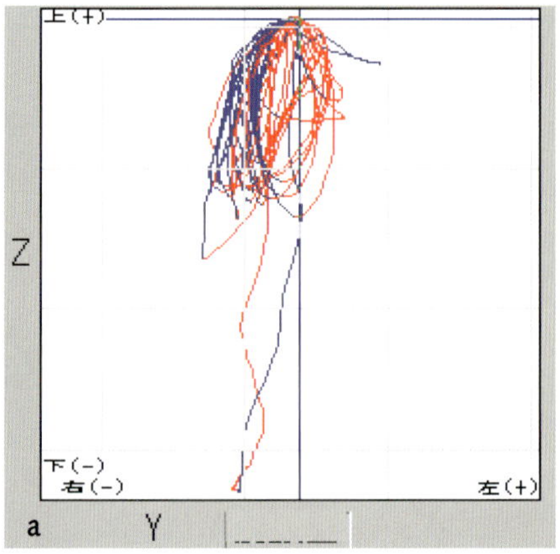

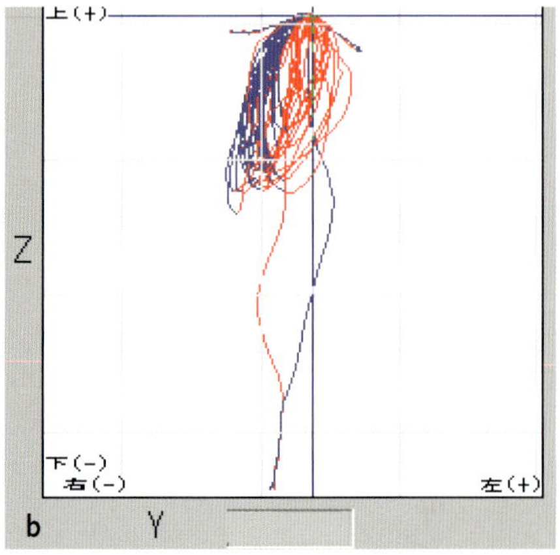

Fig 2-101 Coronal projection of incisal points using a Gnathohexagraph. (a) When the crowns are not used, wide, horizontal chewing cycles are observed; some reverse cycles suggest some interference. (b) When the crowns are used, both right-side chewing and left-side chewing show acceptable cycles.

Clenching derived from tooth-unit tight occlusion

The 55-year-old woman in Figs 2-102 to 2-110 presented with acute symptoms of a periodontal abscess. She had almost abnormal tension in the circumoral muscles. Although she was instructed not to clench her teeth, she clenched frequently. Because of dislodgment of inlays, the molars became intercuspated with each other too tightly, causing clenching and occlusal trauma. Case 2-5 presents the treatment of another patient whose deep curve of Spee and tight occlusion resulted in tooth clenching.

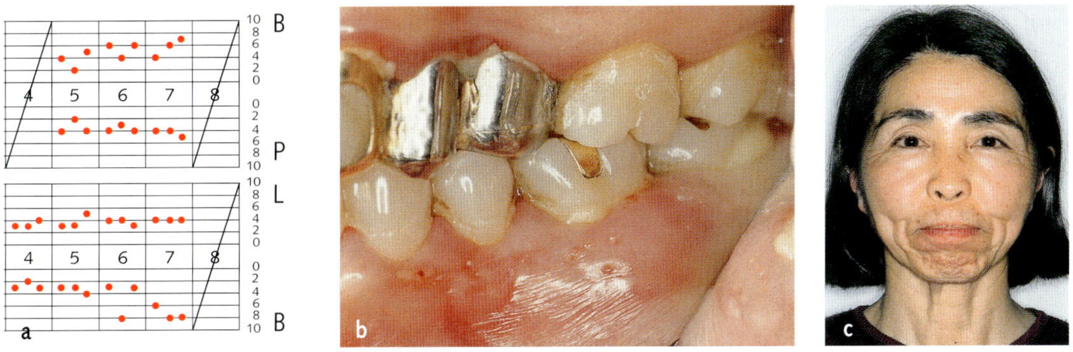

Fig 2-102 (a) Probing chart of the left molars at the first visit. Red indicates bleeding points. (b) There is a periodontal abscess at the mandibular left first molar. (c) The patient's face at the first visit is shown. She often clenches with full force.

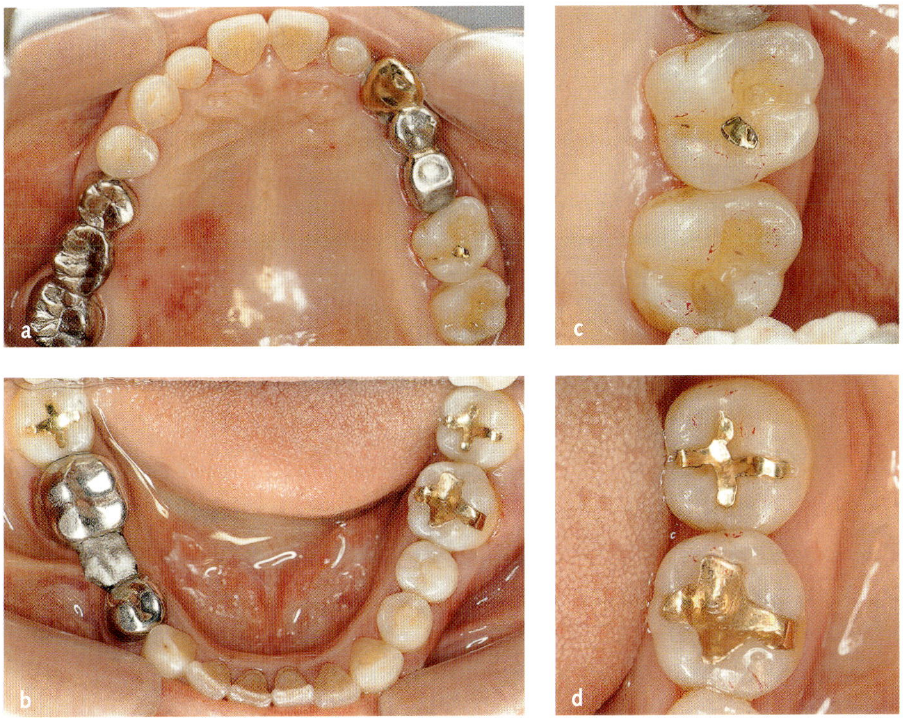

Fig 2-103 (a and b) Occlusal views at the first visit. The periodontal probing depths are 3 to 8 mm with moderate to severe periodontitis. The buccal probing depth at the mandibular left first and second molars is 8 mm. (c and d) Inlays on the maxillary left first and second molars have been dislodged.

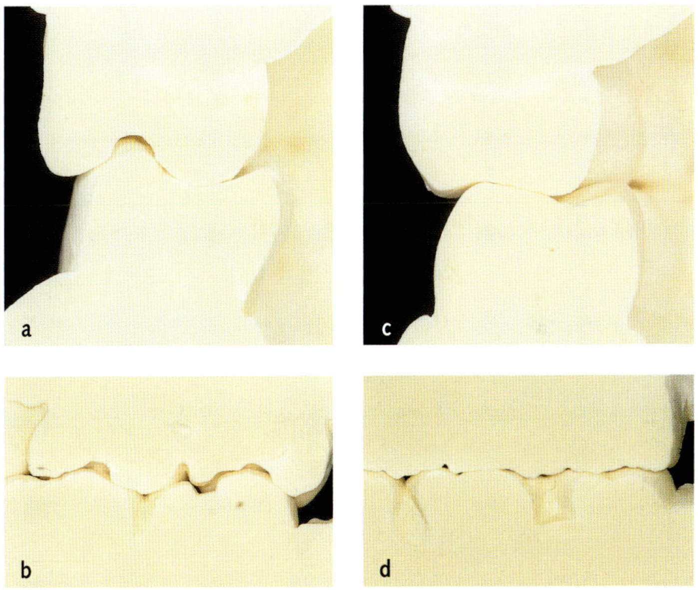

Fig 2-104 Cross sections of study casts at the first visit and after crown restorations. (a and b) At the first visit, the buccal cusps of the mandibular left first and second molars are deeply intercuspated to the maxillary left first and second molars, from which inlays have dislodged in a buccolingual and mesiodistal manner. Because no movements are allowed in the anteroposterior and lateral directions, clenching results, sending jiggling forces to the teeth. (c and d) After crown restoration, the occlusal tables become slightly narrower. Both occlusal surfaces are convex.

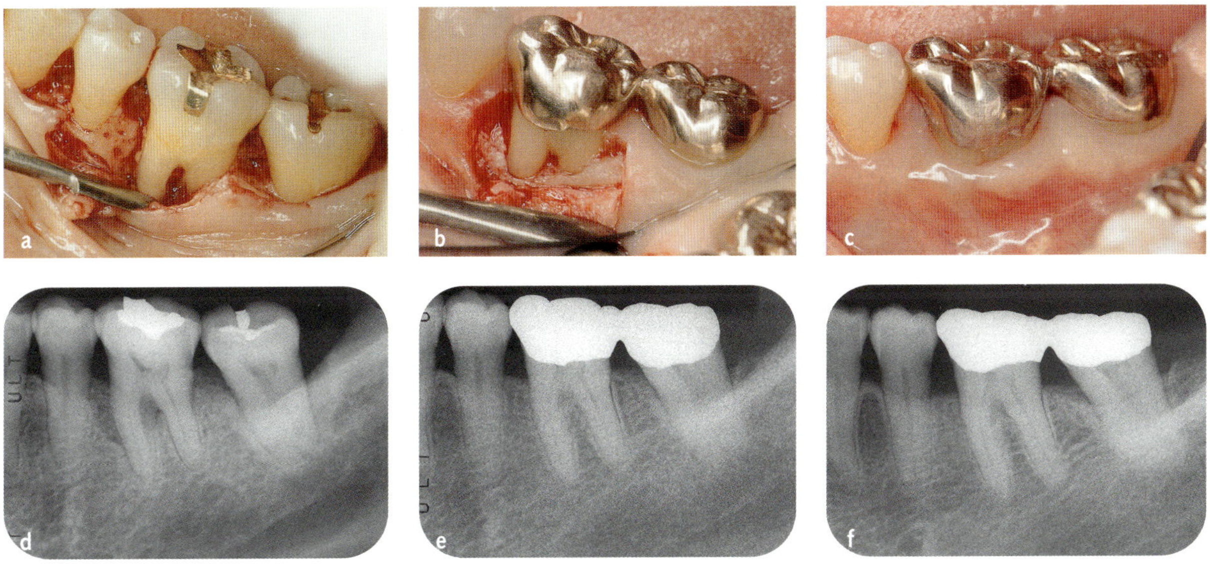

Fig 2-105 Improvements in the mandibular left first molar. (a) Six months after the first visit. Furcation involvement at the mandibular left first molar is noted as well as a traumatic, vertical infrabony defect. (b) Photograph taken 6 years 7 months after the first visit. (c) Photograph taken 7 years 4 months after the first visit. (d) Radiograph taken at the first visit. (e) Radiograph taken 3 years 8 months after the first visit. (f) Radiograph taken 7 years 4 months after the first visit.

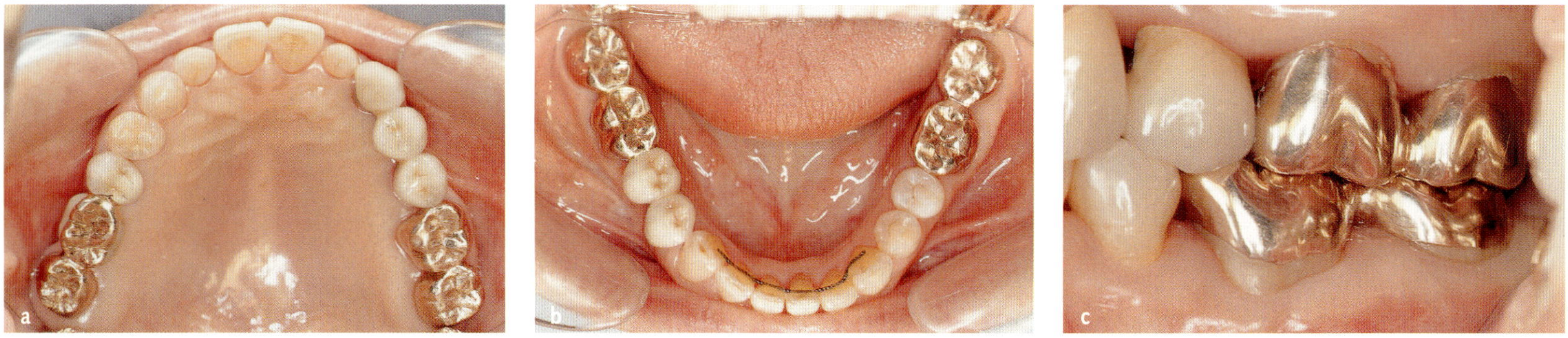

Fig 2-106 (a to c) Photographs taken 5 years 6 months after the first visit.

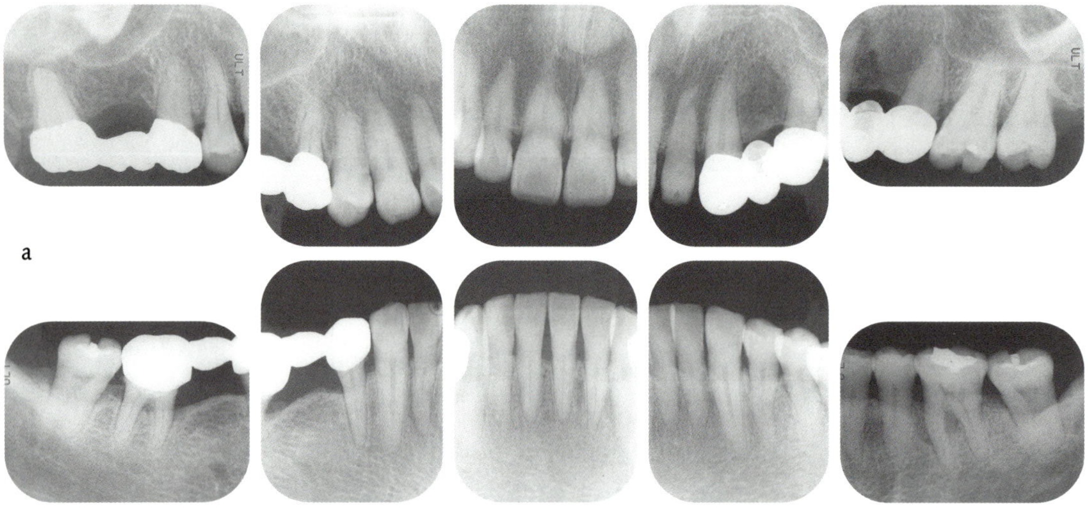

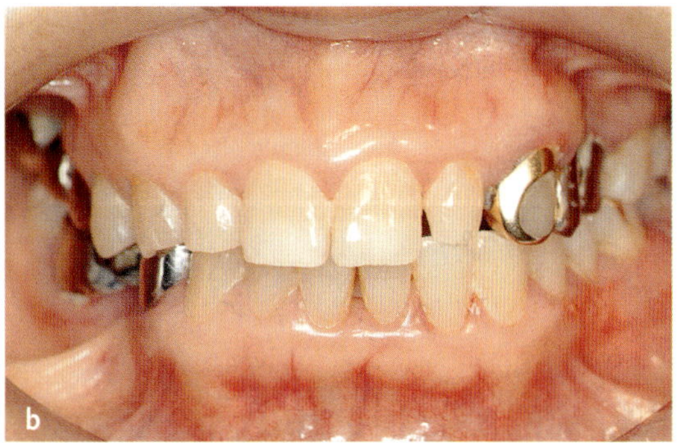

Fig 2-107 (a) Radiographs and (b) photograph taken at the first visit.

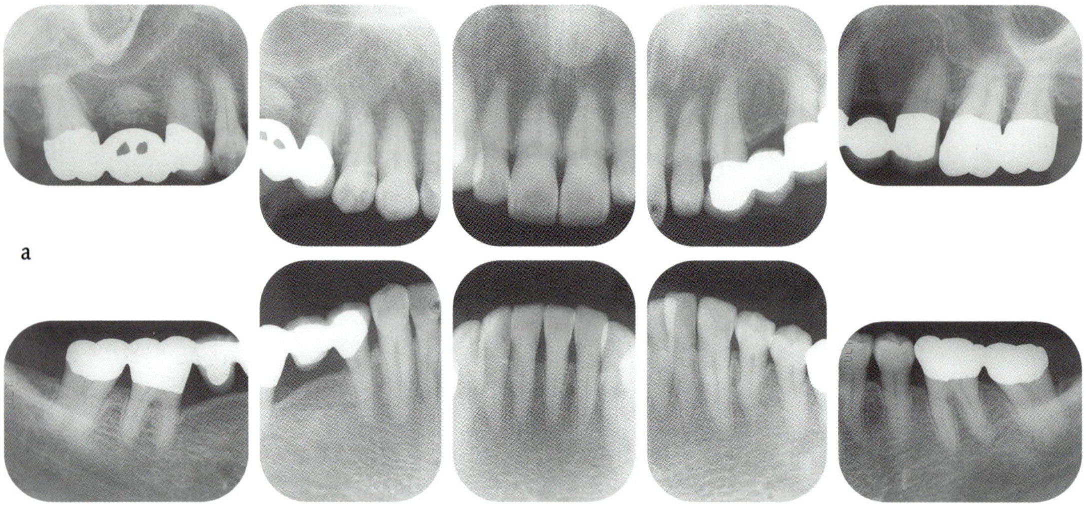

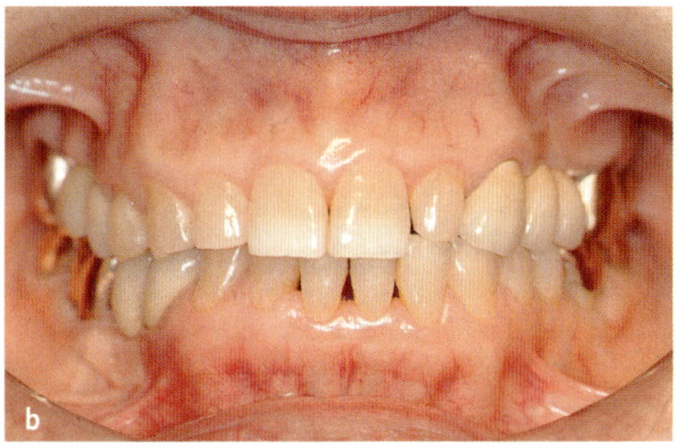

Fig 2-108 (a) Radiographs taken 3 years 1 month after the first visit. (b) Photograph taken 5 years 6 months after the first visit.

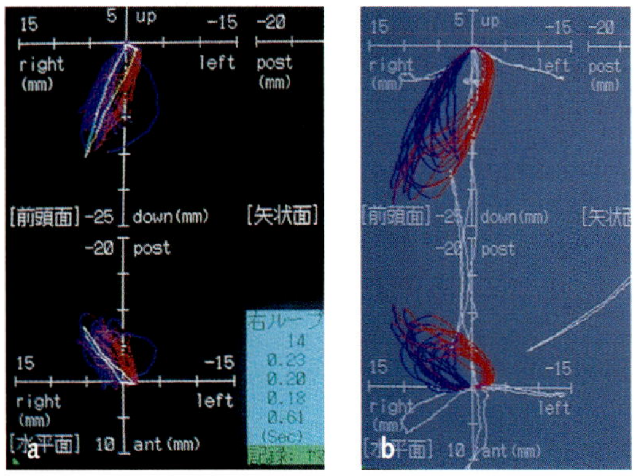

Fig 2-109 Coronal projections of right-side chewing (gum). (a) Projection 3 months after the first visit. Movement paths are very thin, like a needle. (b) Projection 4 years 11 months after the first visit. Movement paths are mostly standard.

Fig 2-110 Facial appearance 3 years 1 month after the first visit. The extreme tension of circumoral muscles has disappeared.

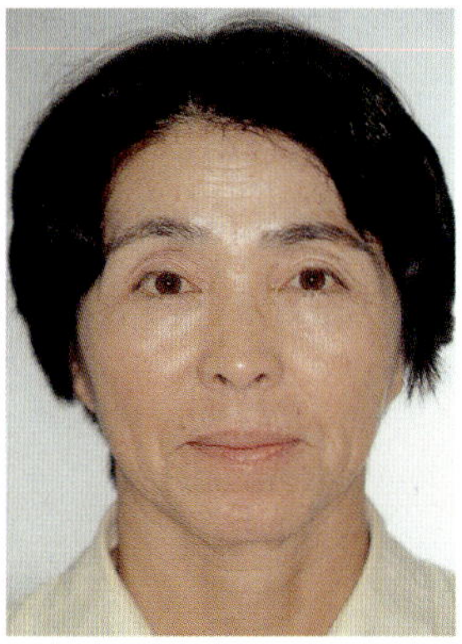

Case 2-5 Deep curve of Spee and malfunctions of the jaw (tooth-unit tight occlusion)

Patient: *59-year-old woman at the time of first visit in 1996*

Chief complaint: *The feeling that something is wrong with her occlusion, including stiff shoulders and tinnitus*

The deep curve of Spee tended to invite tight occlusion with too-close interdigitation of the maxillary and mandibular dentition in an anteroposterior direction, causing clenching. This patient had tension in the masseter at the first visit; her lower face was shifted to the left, and the lip line was higher at the left end. She had surgery in her left meniscus 1 year previously. She also had severe periodontitis, and there were limits to what could be done in our treatment. Still, correction of curve of Spee alone resolved TMD symptoms, such as severe shoulder stiffness, tinnitus, and headache, from which she had been suffering for 2 to 3 years, 6 months, and 4 to 5 years, respectively (Figs 2-111 to 2-114).

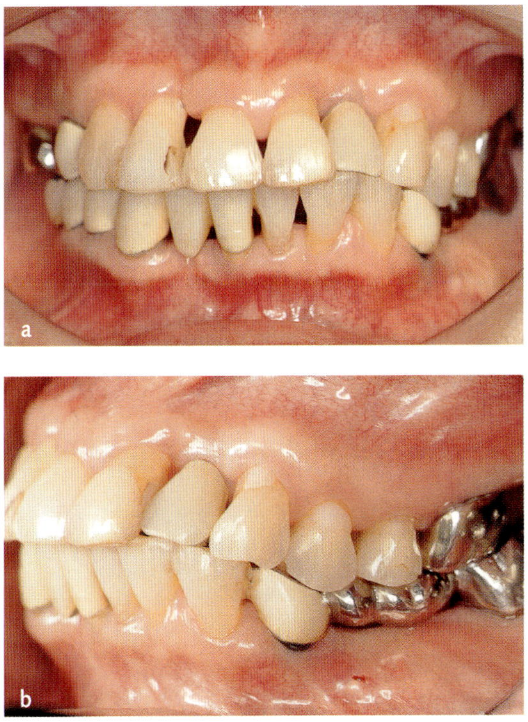

Fig 2-111 (a and b) At the first visit, the curve of Spee on the left side is extremely deep.

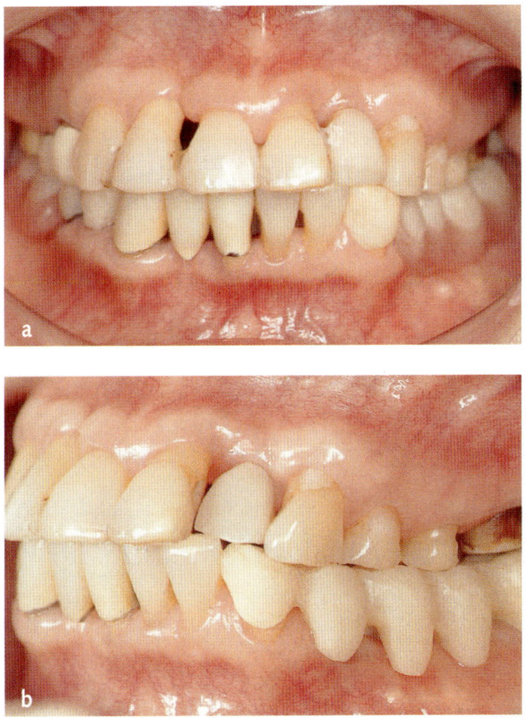

Fig 2-112 (a and b) Provisional restorations have been provided to correct the occlusal plane. Crown lengthening is not possible because of the seriously compromised periodontal support in the maxillary left posterior region. The symptoms of TMD have been relieved at this time point.

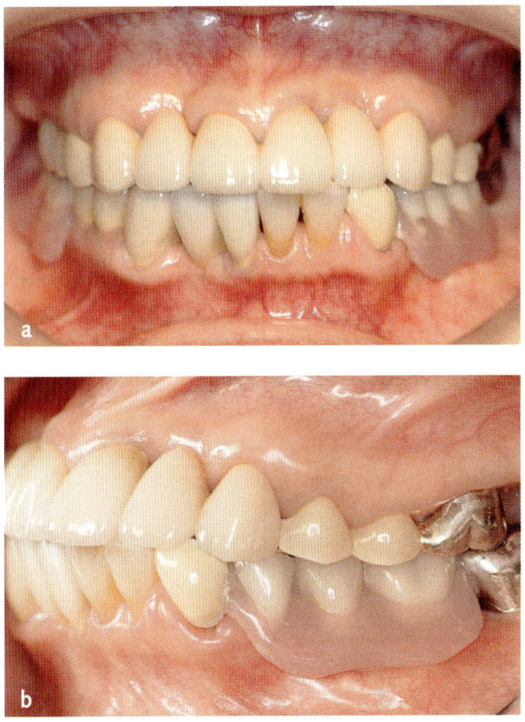

Fig 2-113 (a and b) After orthodontic tooth movement, final prostheses are delivered.

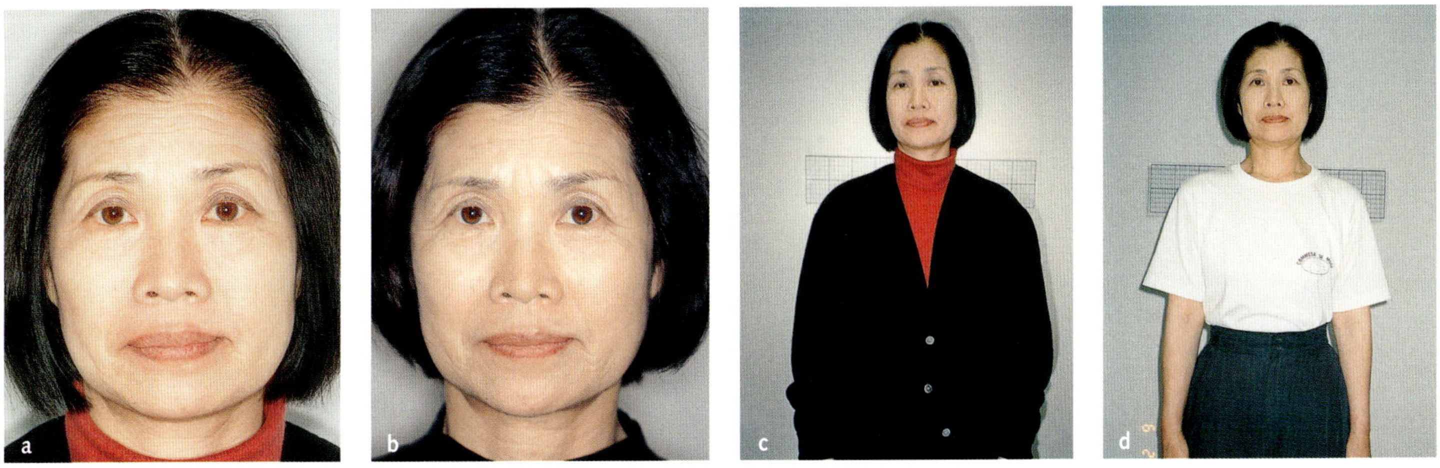

Fig 2-114 Frontal views (a and c) at the first visit and (b and d) after 4 years 5 months. The left masseter still has some tension, but the lip line is no longer slanted, and the balance has been improved.

Diagnosis and Management of Abfraction

Abfraction

Pathologic loss of hard tissue resulting from biomechanical loading, or abfraction, is observed most commonly in cervical areas (Figs 2-115 to 2-117 and Box 2-18). This is considered to have been caused by repeated stress concentrations on the cervical areas during clenching, which invites loss of tooth hard tissue substance through fatigue, similar to metal fatigue. McCoy has called clenching-related symptoms characterized by abfraction *dental compression syndrome* (DCS).

Figs 2-115 to 2-117 Typical abfraction case.

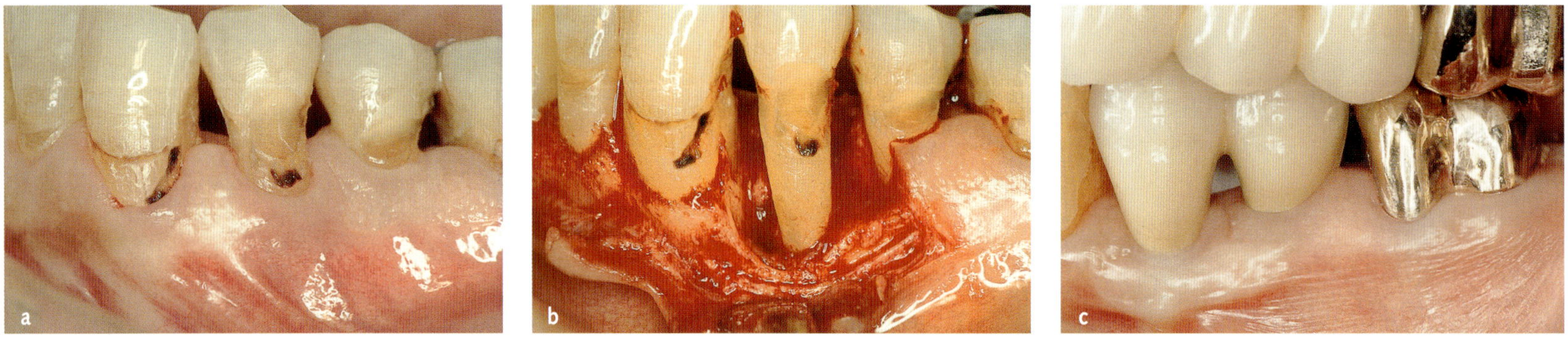

Fig 2-115 Abfraction is the manifestation of parafunctional occlusal forces in teeth and periodontal tissue. It is often manifested in wedge-shaped defects in a cervical area and a bony defect with a similar shape. In this patient, it is manifested as destruction of teeth and supporting bone. (a) Initial therapy is completed 4 months after the first visit (September 1990). Periodontal pockets at the mandibular left first premolar were 10 mm buccally and 6 mm lingually several days after the first visit. Although probing depths have decreased to 9 mm and 4 mm, respectively, at completion of initial therapy, there is no significant improvement. (b) Photograph taken 9 months after the first visit. At the time of guided tissue regeneration, bone is lost almost to the level of the apex. (c) After guided tissue regeneration, free gingival grafting was conducted. Photograph taken 2 years 1 month after grafting.

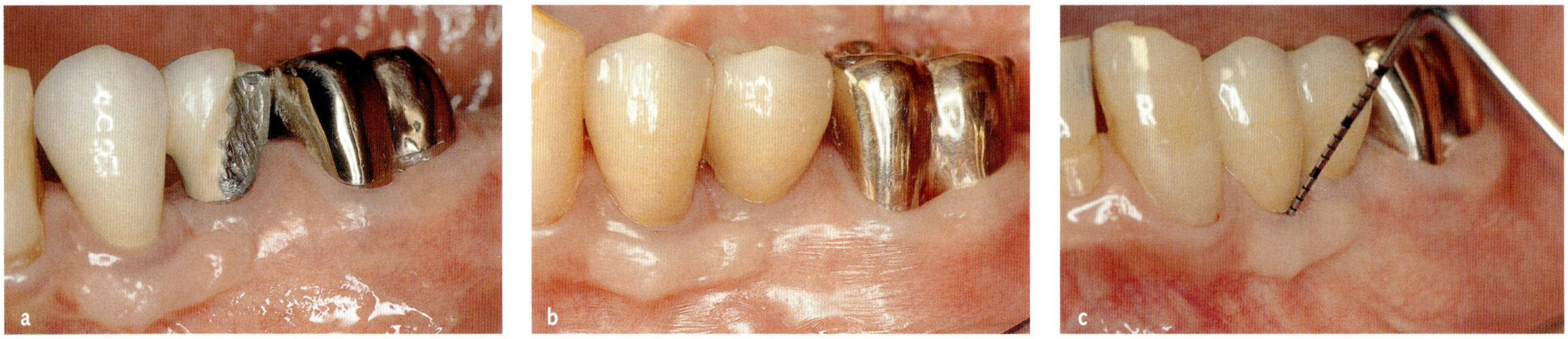

Fig 2-116 Recurrence of the powerful destructive force. (a) Photograph taken about 11 years after the first visit, or about 9 years after completion of prosthetic treatment. Probably because of another shift of the mandibular position, the facing material of the mandibular left second premolar has fractured. (b) A new prosthesis is delivered 6 months after the fracture (September 2001). (c) Periodontal probing depths are maintained as mostly healthy (November 2001).

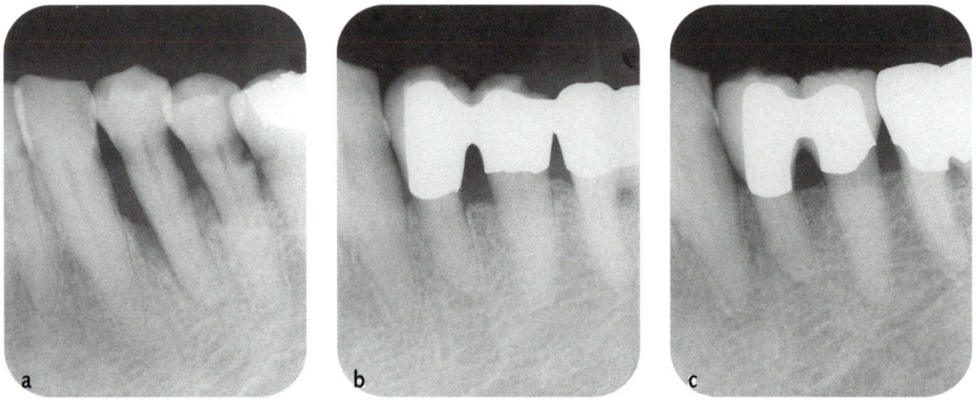

Fig 2-117 Radiographs showing natural tooth extrusion and regeneration of supporting bone. (a) Radiograph taken at the first visit. (b) After 5 years, due to natural extrusion and guided tissue regeneration, the bone level is improved. At that time, autogenous bone grafting was not conducted in combination with guided tissue regeneration. (c) Radiograph taken about 12 years after the first visit.

In patients with loose occlusion and without stable ICP, grinding is likely to occur. These subjects tend to exert stronger forces to bite because their occlusal morphology is not suitable for biting. On the contrary, in dentitions with very tight occlusion where anteroposterior or lateral (right or left) sliding from ICP is not easy, clenching is likely to occur. This is also one of the dental compression forces.

Reshaping

McCoy advocates coronoplasty or correction of crown morphology to control forces when abfraction is observed. Coronoplasty is reduction of an occlusal contact surface that has been widened too extensively by attrition. By sharpening the morphology of functional cusps, burden of forces for the oral system. We have applied these concepts in our regimen of reshaping, which includes not only partial reduction of teeth with attrition but also the addition of material to restore the original anatomy and morphology of the teeth.

Indications for reshaping are not limited to those cases mentioned by McCoy as characterized by DCS. Cases involving morphologic changes in teeth, periodontal tissue, and TMJs may also be included in the indication. Similarly, morphologic correction of a restoration or crown restoration with poor morphology in occlusal surfaces can be conducted. Reshaping is a minimally invasive procedure to restore dentitions to a fine arch form as well as a stable mandibular position, functional movements without obstacles, and a good balance between the maxillary and mandibular arches. In reshaping, occlusal morphology is considered from the viewpoint of masticatory movements. Reduction and addition should be recognized as procedures to restore and maintain the relationships of cusps, fissures, and fossae between a pair of teeth in a series of reconstructive processes.

Box 2-18 Abfraction (dental compression syndrome)

Abfraction causes not only attrition or wedge-shaped defects but also microdestruction of enamel, wavy destruction of cementum, and increased risk of root caries, inviting destruction of teeth (Fig 2-118). Also, in supporting tissue, occlusal trauma as well as periodontal tissue destruction are typical. In a preceding stage, widening of the periodontal space, disappearance or thickening of the lamina dura, compact osteitis, and trabecular turbulence are observed radiographically. Abfraction also seems to be deeply related to bony defects in furcation involvement and exostoses.

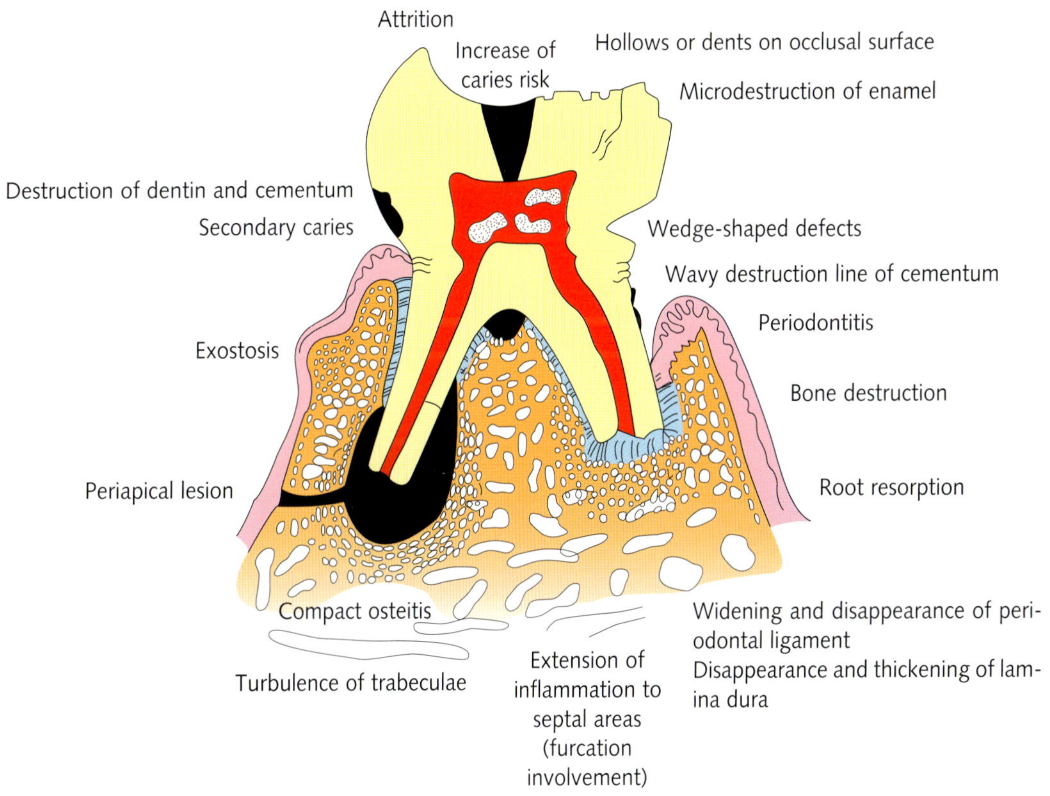

Fig 2-118 Characteristics of DCS (Courtesy of Dr K. Shimokawa.)

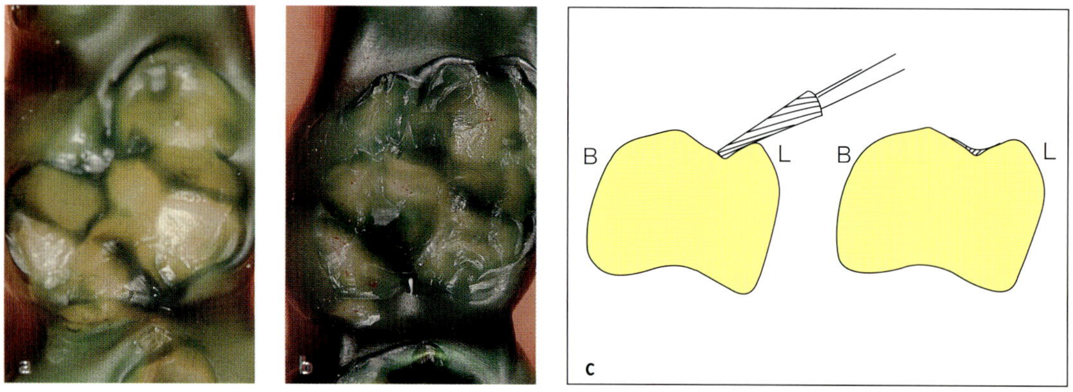

Fig 2-119 Buccolingual reshaping and grooving. (a) After marking with articulating paper at ICP, the patient is instructed to bite on indicator wax to find contact surface locations. (b) Grooving is conducted in fissure areas. The buccal slope of the maxillary teeth and the lingual slope of the mandibular teeth are slightly reduced to narrow the occlusal table. Also, the A slope of the mandibular buccal cusps and the C slope of the maxillary lingual cusps are adjusted, maintaining points on the articulating paper, to change wide surface contacts to narrow surface contacts. (c) Grooving or preparation of fissures is conducted. The tips of well-cutting carbide burs (F1 or F3) are used to make fissures slightly deeper.

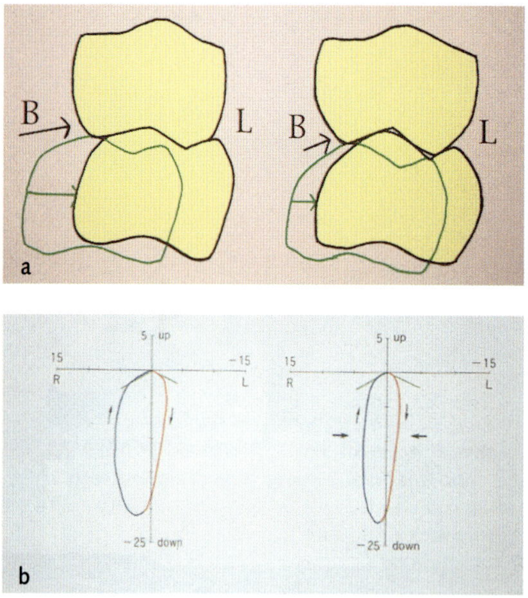

Fig 2-120 Reshaping and associated changes in chewing patterns. (a) Buccolingual reshaping. (b) Changes in the chewing pattern (frontal plane).

Indications and contraindications for reshaping

A dentition without an established mandibular position is contraindicated for reshaping. Although some anteroposterior discrepancy between ICP and CR is allowed, lateral or vertical shift is not an indication. A patient with short crowns resulting from to severe attrition or a patient with severe TMD symptoms would instead require an increase of vertical dimension, through crown restorations, for example. Partial reshaping may be conducted to alleviate muscle spasms.

Force control forms basic therapy together with plaque control. Unlike inflammation in gingiva, however, the normality or abnormality of function is difficult to judge. It is not possible to determine whether attrition is physiologic or nonphysiologic all at once. It is preferable to conduct three-dimensional analysis of the mandible during functional movements as a means of diagnosis and to reevaluate with a similar method. In the case of prostheses, active reshaping should be conducted if a flat surface or an occlusal surface tightly holds its opposing tooth.

Verticalization

Reshaping produces the same results as "verticalization (naturalization)," advocated by Lee. Reshaping makes an occlusal surface convex, dividing a large surface into several small ones in practice (Fig 2-119). With this change alone, compressive force is reduced, and the patient feels much more comfortable. This will facilitate shearing of food, create grooves for food spillage, reduce excessive loading of teeth, and direct occlusal forces toward the long axis of the tooth.

Through reshaping, widened occlusal tables are narrowed, and chewing patterns are verticalized by the appropriate interdigitation of cusps and guidance (Fig 2-120).

As a result of reshaping, mastication should be facilitated, chewing or biting habits should be resolved, and stabilization of ICP and the dentition should be obtained (Case 2-6). Morphologically, such changes can be observed through verticalization of teeth and restoration of the vertical dimension of occlusion.

Case 2-6 Correction of widened chewing

Patient: *56-year-old man at the time of first visit in 1997*
Chief complaint: *Sensitivity to cold water in a maxillary left molar*
Gingival recession was noted during the examination. A first glance revealed that this patient had the typical face of a grinding-type occlusion. His symptoms were diagnosed as being the result of hypersensitivity caused by the excessive lateral force applied to the molars. The excessive force was the result of a widened chewing cycle, which was developed by the progression of left-side attrition originating from left-side chewing.
Treatments: *As a basic therapy, reshaping was conducted after a resin restoration was placed in the fractured area. Also, the patient was instructed to chew on both the right and left sides in a well-balanced manner. Hypersensitivity was resolved at this stage. As a definitive therapy, crown restoration was conducted for the molars to adjust the crown morphology. This treatment was restricted to a minimal level of invasion (Figs 2-121 to 2-125).*

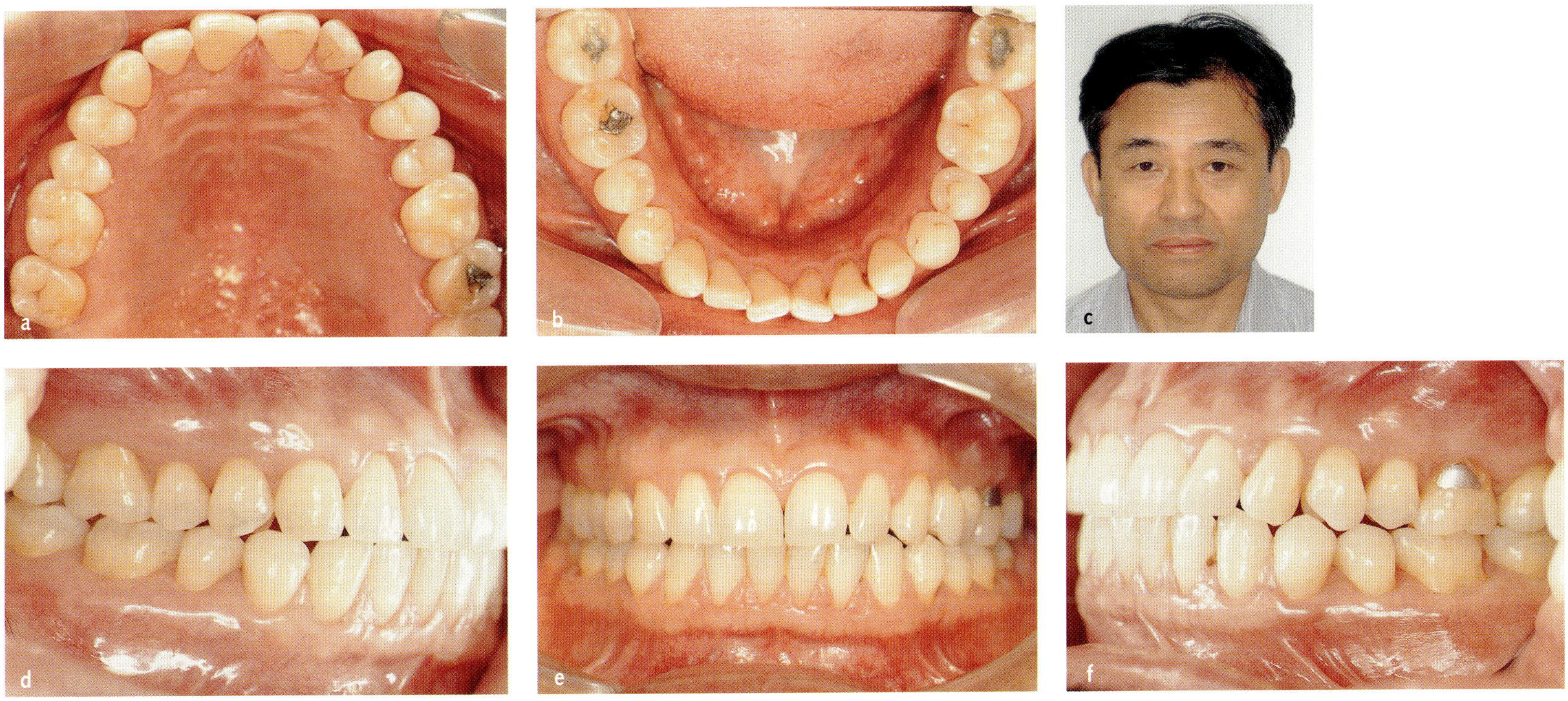

Fig 2-121 (a to f) The patient visited us with chief complaint of sensitivity to cold water. This is an almost completely Class I occlusion. Being a brachyfacial type, he has generalized attrition. Attrition on the left side is relatively noticeable. The left arch has been laterally expanded. This cone-shaped attrition suggests attrition of the oblique egg–shaped occlusion, which caused inadequate guidance.

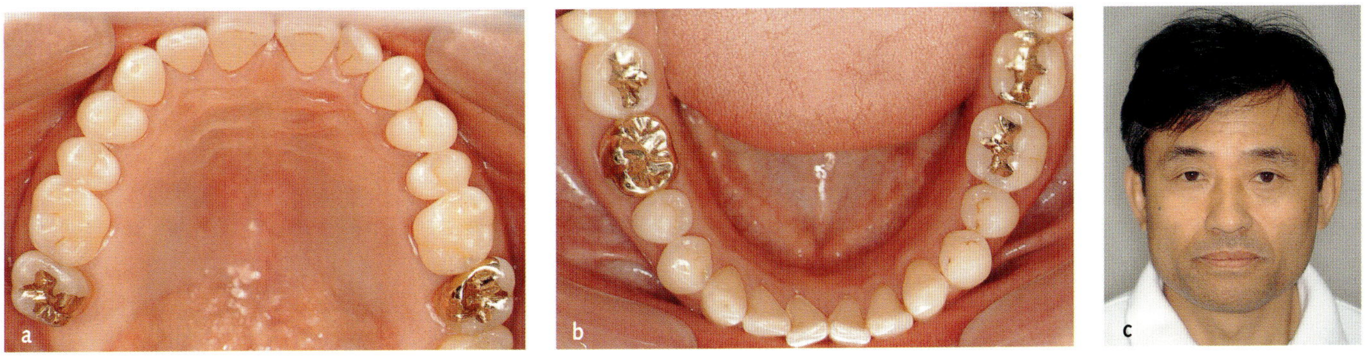

Fig 2-122 After treatment. (a and b) As a definitive therapy for occlusion, inlays or crown restorations were delivered to all four second molars and both of the mandibular first molars to adjust crown morphology. (c) The right and left masseter muscles are in a better balance.

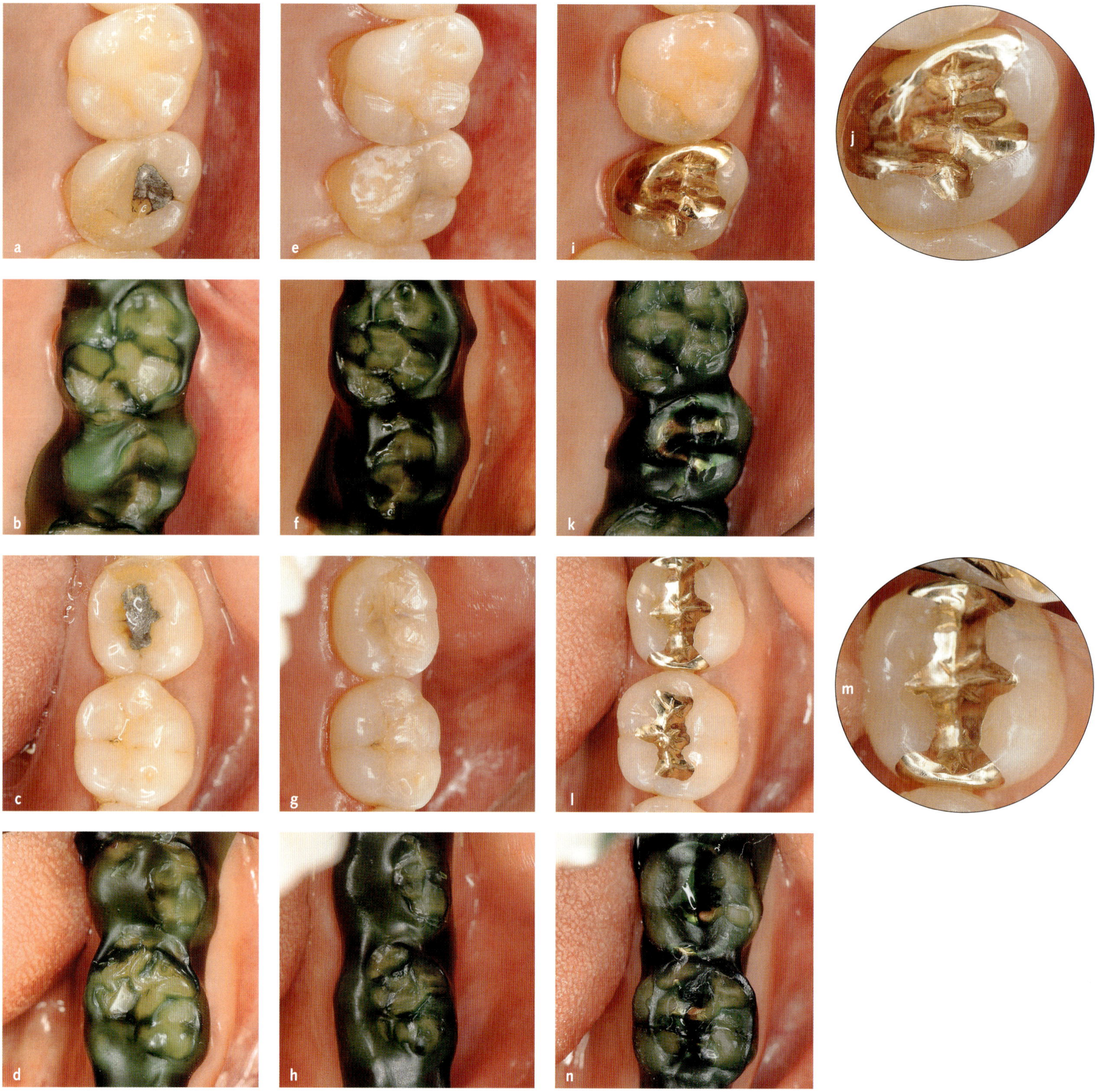

Fig 2-123 Progress of reshaping. (a to d) Before treatment, all of the A, B, and C slopes are interdigitated with surfaces. In particular, the lingual side of the maxillary left first molar is tightly held by the C slope of the mandibular tooth. Because the maxillary and mandibular teeth are almost locked, the mandible cannot move in a relaxed manner. In order to unlock near ICP, a strong force will be required, which also involves lateral movement of teeth. Extremely thin indicator wax in the area of central fissures indicates that the cusp tip of the opposing tooth is deeply interdigitated. (e to h) Reshaping has been conducted, narrowing the occlusal table and grooving. In particular, the emerging or rising area of the C slope in the mandibular arch has been reduced to decrease holding of the maxillary C slopes. The use of grooving to divide connected slopes into two slopes can reduce both the tightly interdigitated areas and force. (i to n) After crown restoration. Attention is paid to developing occlusal morphology with which food can be bitten off with light force. The teeth are grooved for food spillage, and the size of the occlusal table is selected carefully. The occlusal morphology is developed to ensure the stability of ICP, smooth onset of movement, and lack of interference. Articulating paper will not reveal the three-dimensional occlusal relationships. Kerr occlusal indicator wax (Kerr/Sybron) will provide a good idea about three-dimensional space, including surfaces, points, grooves, and holding of maxillary and mandibular teeth.

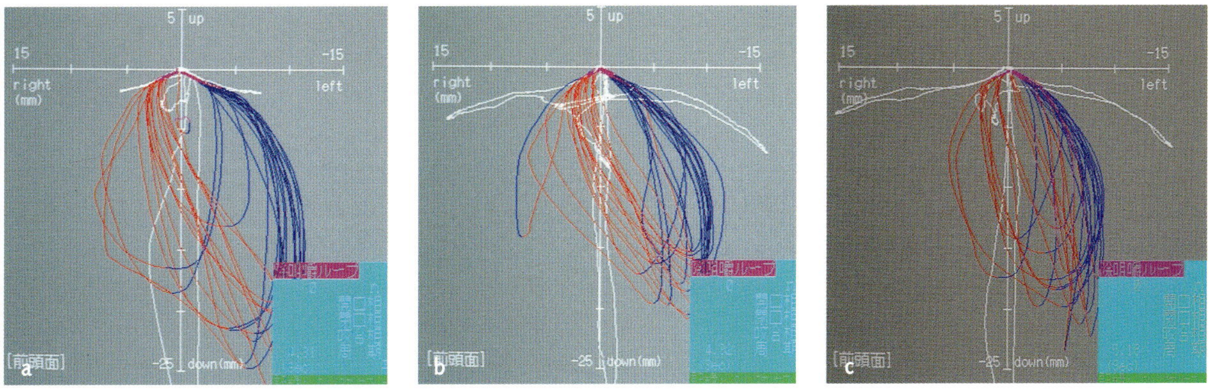

Fig 2-124 Chewing on the frontal plane (left-side chewing). (a) Before treatment record of left-side chewing. (b) Record after reshaping. (c) Sirognathograph after placement of crown restorations. This is a grinding-type pattern, opening first to the nonworking side. Through the processes of reshaping and crown restoration, the wide grinding observed at the first visit has gradually converged, so that there is a decrease of areas of travel following border movement paths.

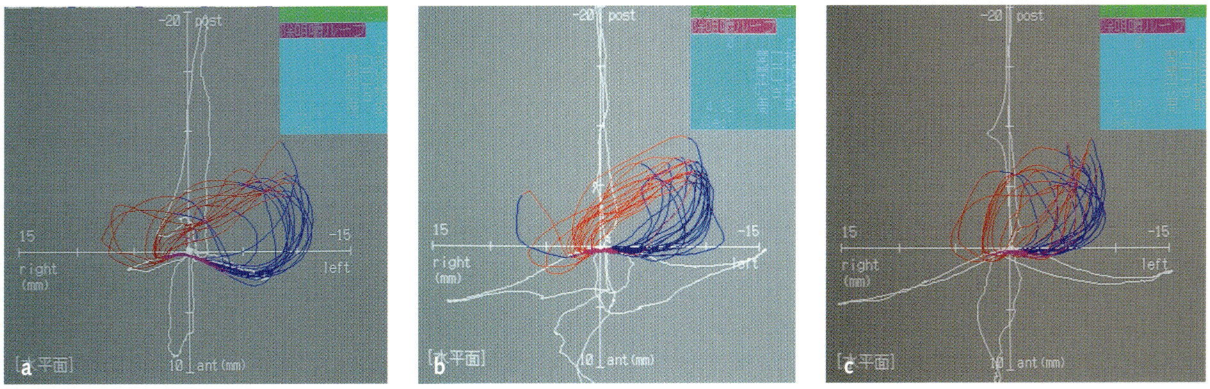

Fig 2-125 Chewing on the transverse plane (left-side chewing). (a) Record before treatment. (b) Record after reshaping. (c) Record after placement of crown restorations. Although both opening and closing paths previously followed border movement paths in their large portion, after treatment the paths have developed a posterior cycle with very little travel through border movement paths to enter ICP. In other words, horizontal chewing has been verticalized. Forces causing lateral movement of the teeth and attrition have been reduced.

Box 2-19 Typical presentation of dental compression syndrome

Typical examples of DCS are clinically observed as abfraction. Abfraction is a defect of hard tissue caused by a type of fracture of tooth structure in which stress is concentrated due to flexion of teeth when they are compressed and loaded. Abfraction may occur not only in enamel but also in dentin and cementum.

Signs of DCS are not limited to abfraction. Dental compression syndrome may be manifested as hypertrophy of the masseter muscles, symptoms in the TMJ area, myalgia in maxillofacial areas, headache, wavy lines in enamel or dimples on the occlusal surfaces of molars, wavy lines or deformity of restorations, resorption of supporting bone and exostosis, change in taste (metallic taste, acidity), and recession of marginal gingiva. It also may be related to tooth mobility, dehiscence of bone, decrease of the vertical dimension, morphologic changes in the TMJ, and a mandibular shift.

Habits of Circumoral Muscles and Myofunctional Therapy

Myofunctional therapy for circumoral muscles

Myofunctional therapy (MFT) was designed for improvement of imbalance of circumoral muscles or abnormal swallowing behaviors. Originally MFT was developed in orthodontics as training to eliminate tongue habits in children with an open bite. However, just as plaque control is needed for control of inflammation, normal functioning of circumoral muscles is needed for control of functions. Control of muscular forces of the oral area as well as correction of morphology constitute the most basic treatment in all dental therapies. MFT is a therapy for muscles in oral area. Not only the tongue, lips, cheeks, and masticatory muscles, but also habits and postures should be covered in instructions. Chewing habits, mandibular shift, habitual behaviors, and postures are closely related each other, and they cannot be considered separately. Abnormal muscle morphology, strength, and movement patterns are deeply related to a number of dental diseases, including periodontal disease, malocclusion, and occlusal problems.

Potential for change: The roles of the clinician and the patient

Although sometimes functions are improved by the adjustment of morphology alone, in most cases, simultaneous approaches are taken to improve function while morphology is adjusted. One of the most important approaches to improving functions is MFT. Some clinicians do not wish to take this approach, claiming that it is difficult to obtain the patient's cooperation and predictability is low. However, it is not logical to leave the causes of the current problems untreated and try to adjust morphology. In rehabilitation, medical professionals have to define patients' roles, so that these individuals also can have their share of responsibility. Furthermore, leaving the situation unchanged will not provide a cure.

In treatment processes, it is necessary to define "what can be changed," "what cannot be changed," and "what is difficult to be changed" one by one with a patient. Mutual understanding between the clinician and the patient is essential. For example, the patient may have the attitude, "I will make greater effort because I want to be more comfortable," or the clinician may have to say, "If lip habits cannot be corrected, we have to accept the situation at this level." In that sense, MFT is a very basic therapy that cannot be avoided in dental practice.

Tongue position and habits

Normal tongues at rest stay in the palate space. Most of the force or pressure from the tongue during function (such as speech or swallowing) should be received by the palate, not by the teeth. In pronunciation of plosives, force from the tip of the tongue is received by the area near the incisal papilla of the palate. However, in a patient with a low tongue or tongue thrusting habits, during functions, force from the tip or the lateral part of the tongue is received by teeth (Figs 2-126 to 2-130). In addition, tongue force at rest may affect the morphology of the dentition and jawbone. A tongue in an incorrect position or with poor morphology will cause a morphologic anomaly of the dentition or the jawbone. Dysfunctions of the tongue may apply jiggling forces to teeth.

When the tongue is stable in the palate and normal swallowing is conducted, a mandibular position will be stable. For this reason, it is said that "the tongue decides a mandibular position." A low tongue or a tongue thrusting habit will be a factor to push the mandible forward. If the tongue is inserted between the maxillary and mandibular teeth, it will cause open bite and ICP will not be stabilized. When the tongue position is not stable, a hole can be prepared in an incisal papilla area of a plate-type appliance or removable denture so that the patient can learn the appropriate position for the tongue.

An anterior tongue thrusting habit can be corrected if the patient is conscious of the habit. However, the cure rate for lateral tongue thrusting and low tongue is low. It is sufficiently meaningful if a patient understands that it is inappropriate to push teeth with the tongue.

Figs 2-126 to 2-130 Improvement of a tongue habit and treatment of open bite treatment with myofunctional therapy.

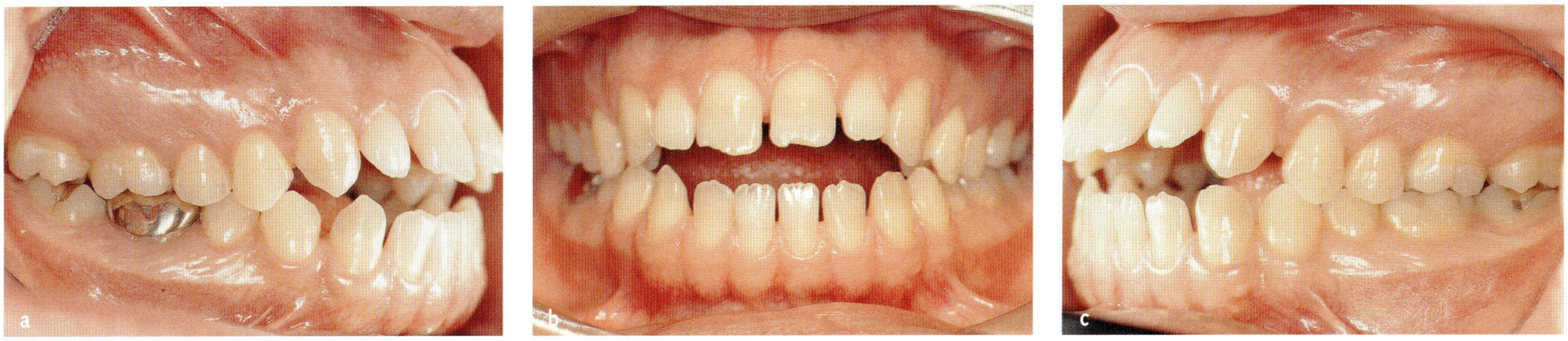

Fig 2-126 An 18-year-old man at the first visit (1997). (a to c) He has an open L–shaped mandible with an ANB angle of 3.5 degrees. Instructions for tongue training are provided.

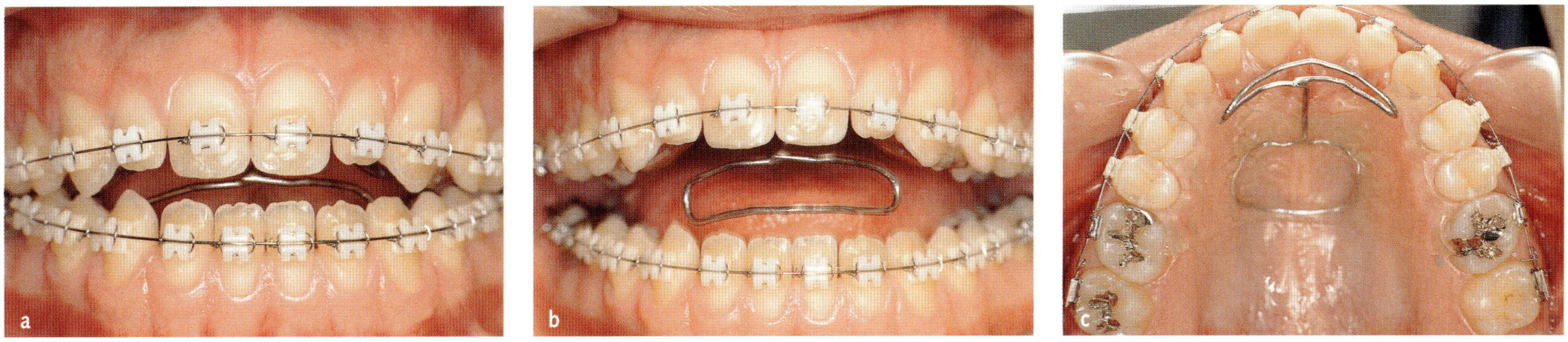

Fig 2-127 A tongue guard with ball clasps may be delivered simultaneously with full brackets. (a to c) In this case, however, the device is delivered when active treatment of molars is mostly completed (5 months after the first visit). In the treatment of protrusion in children with tongue habits, because anterior teeth require anchorage, the patients are trained not to push the teeth with the tongue or increase tongue strength. In this case, no retention is provided to the plate. The plate is designed not to stay in place without tongue support. It also serves as motivation to push up the tongue against the palate.

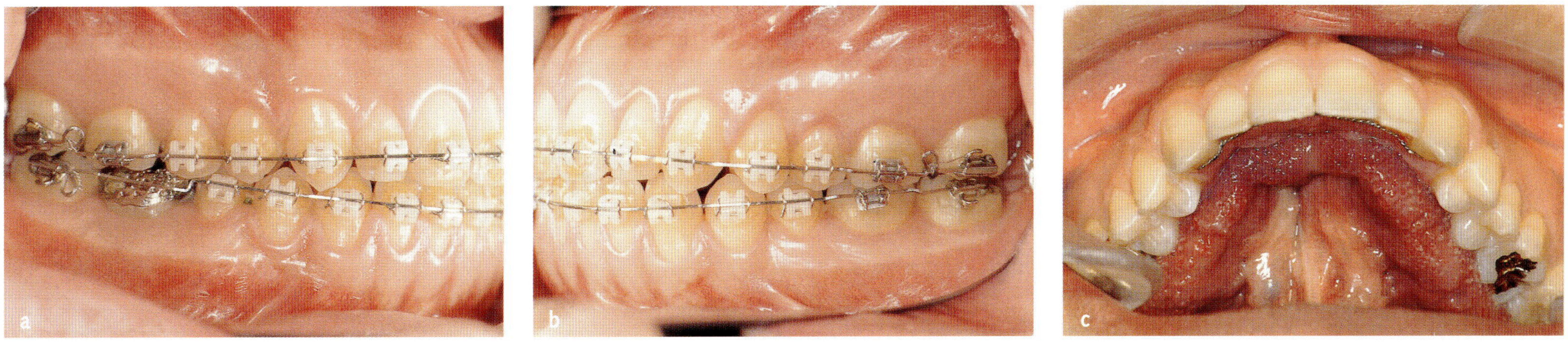

Fig 2-128 (a and b) Active orthodontic treatment was conducted for 1 year 8 months. (c) Through training, the patient has learned to stick the tongue to the palate.

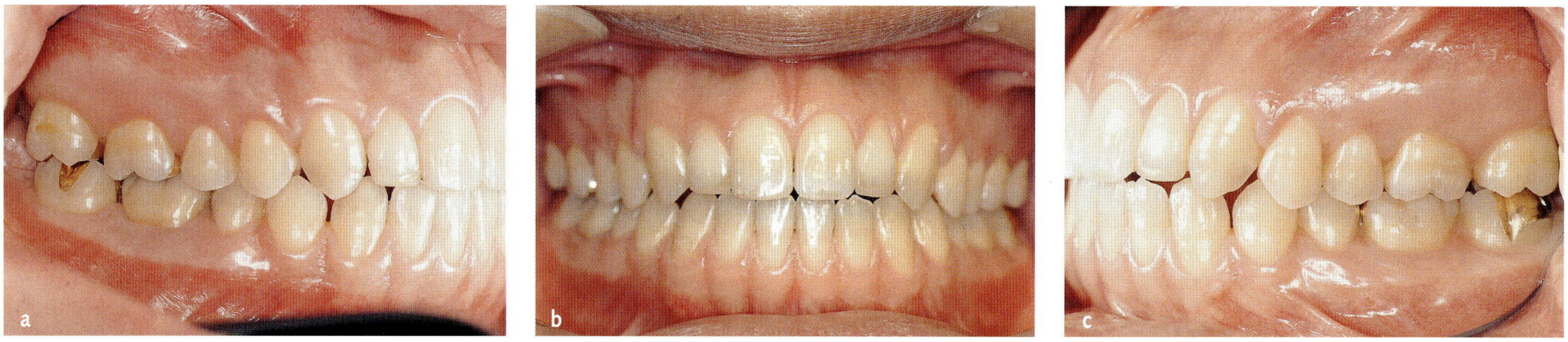

Fig 2-129 (a to c) Photographs taken 2 years 3 months after the first visit. This condition cannot be maintained without improvement in muscle functions, especially the elimination of tongue habits.

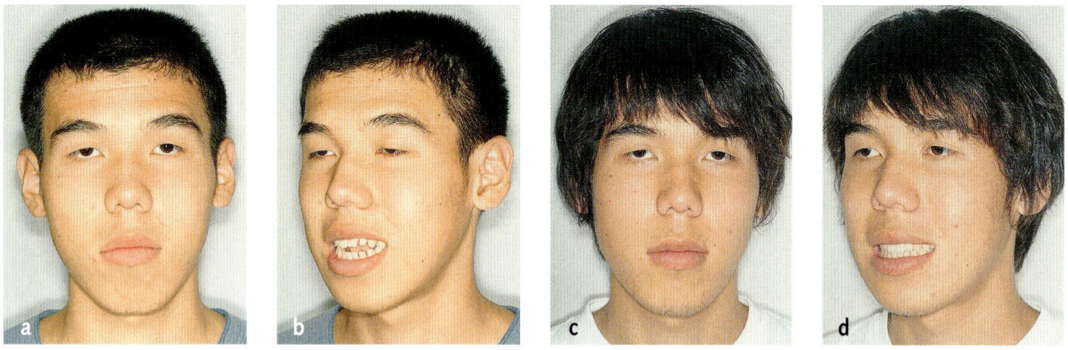

Fig 2-130 Changes in the face. (a and b) Before treatment, at 18 years old, the patient has an open L–shaped face. (c and d) Appearance after treatment, at 20 years old.

Lips and cheeks

Lips are supposed to relax when at rest and seal anterior teeth. Abnormality in lip morphology and functions may cause anterior malocclusion and invite esthetic and/or functional problems. Also, relaxation of lips and mouth breathing will dry the anterior gingiva and accelerate gingival inflammation.

Abnormalities of the lips are divided into the categories of malformation and malfunction. With regard to malformation of lips, when the upper lip is short, a patient may extend the lower lip to close the mouth, because lip seal is not possible under a relaxed condition. This situation may be improved by training to extend the upper lip. Although thick lips are generally relaxed and weak, sometimes the muscle itself is thick. Myofunctional therapy will be helpful for the former situation but not for the latter. In patients with maxillary protrusion, the lower lip may unavoidably come underneath the maxillary anterior teeth. Even after correction of malformation, a habit of biting the lower lip may remain. Various lip habits may not be corrected even when no morphologic abnormality is involved. Lip habits are more difficult to correct than tongue habits and are also awkward in terms of the stability of the anterior dentition.

Cheek abnormalities include tensing or puckering up the mouth, which is not as common as lip habits. In a patient with tight occlusion who clenches, crown-shaped indentations are often observed on the insides of the cheeks.

Relationship of Chewing Habits and Postural Habits to Occlusal Collapse

Chewing habits and occlusal collapse

Although congenital imbalance in morphology and aging are not negligible as factors to destroy harmony in the stomatognathic system, acquired factors such as inflammation, occlusal trauma, imbalance in the circumoral muscles, habits, and postures play more important roles and can be controlled.

A habit of one-sided chewing can cause occlusal collapse (Case 2-7). The maxillary arch of the biting side tends to flare out buccally and the vertical dimension tends to decrease from attrition and compression. One-sided chewing naturally invites a shift of the mandibular position to the side of habitual mastication. This shift is more significant for a subject with posterior shift of the working-side condyle. Turning to either direction while eating will cause the mandibular shift to that direction. In a patient with one-sided chewing, the masseter will develop clear hypertrophy in a month, causing imbalance between the right and left muscles. When hypertrophy of the masseter on either side is present, it is difficult to judge whether the patient still exhibits one-sided chewing on the hypertrophic side or whether the hypertrophy is the remains of a previous chewing habit. The current chewing side is determined by the tone, fresh-looking nature, and complexion of the skin, because the functional side has better complexion and freshness.

One-sided chewing causes mandibular shift and arch expansion. The shift of mandibular position will lead to a twist or distortion of the whole body. Therefore, when one-sided chewing is likely to be related to occlusal collapse, a patient is instructed to chew on the side opposite to habitual mastication until the right and left sides achieve some balance. When good balance is attained, the patient is informed of the signs of one-sided chewing and instructed to touch the masseter and view himself or herself in a mirror.

Postural habits: A forgotten influence on stomatognathic balance

Although often an important factor in the destruction of stomatognathic balance, postural habits do not usually attract attention. Proffit attached much importance to the "influences of functions on development of teeth and face," and pointed out that a prone position, one kind of sleeping habit, used to be regarded as the main cause of Class II occlusion and that leaning habits, such as resting the chin on the hands, were considered to be the cause of facial asymmetry. Still, he denied the direct influences of those habits.

In orthodontic treatment, however, as we accumulate clinical experience that teeth do not move in the same manner in different patients even though the same type of appliance is used, we are once again reminded of the importance of postural habits. Indeed, we have had repeated clinical experiences that correction of habits improved morphology and promoted improvement.

Case 2-7 Chewing habits in a patient with strong occlusal forces

Patient: *52-year-old man at the time of first visit in 1991*

Chief complaint: *A concern about the progress of periodontal disease*

Periodontal probing depths were 10 mm in some areas, and degree of tooth mobility was 1 to 2. Periodontitis was moderate to severe. The patient's occlusion was Class II on the right side and Class I on the left side. The maxillary left canine was slightly labially inclined with some extrusion and mobility (degree 2), while the maxillary right canine was lingually inclined. Compared to the right, the left teeth exhibited more wedge-shaped defects at the cervical areas of maxillary and mandibular teeth, suggesting habitual left-side chewing.

Although the morphology of the maxillary left canine was corrected to reduce occlusal load, after some time, the tooth became somewhat mobile because of overloading. This process was repeated several times. The reasons seemed to be that the patient was more likely to chew on the left side because of the right side Class II and left side Class I occlusion, the habitual left-side chewing promoted left-side attrition, and the mandibular left first premolar exhibited buccoversion.

Treatments: *(Figs 2-131 to 2-139):*

1. *Instruction in right-side chewing*
2. *Inflammation control and establishment of periodontal tissue with morphology that was less likely to attract plaque and, even with some plaque accumulation, was less likely to break down*
3. *Reshaping to narrow the widened occlusal table, form cusp-to-fossa relationships, and establish occlusal morphology to facilitate biting off food*
4. *Arrangement of the dentition: Tooth movement of the mandibular left first premolar and reshaping to adjust the morphology so that cusps and fissures had a smooth flow in the arch.*

Healing process. *The following changes seemed to appear:*

1. *Horizontal chewing with a high variability was converted to vertical chewing with less variability.*
2. *Compressive forces subsided.*
3. *The vertical dimension was restored.*
4. *The left-side chewing was converted to right-side chewing. To a certain degree, natural recovery was achieved in the dentition, tooth positions, and tooth axes.*

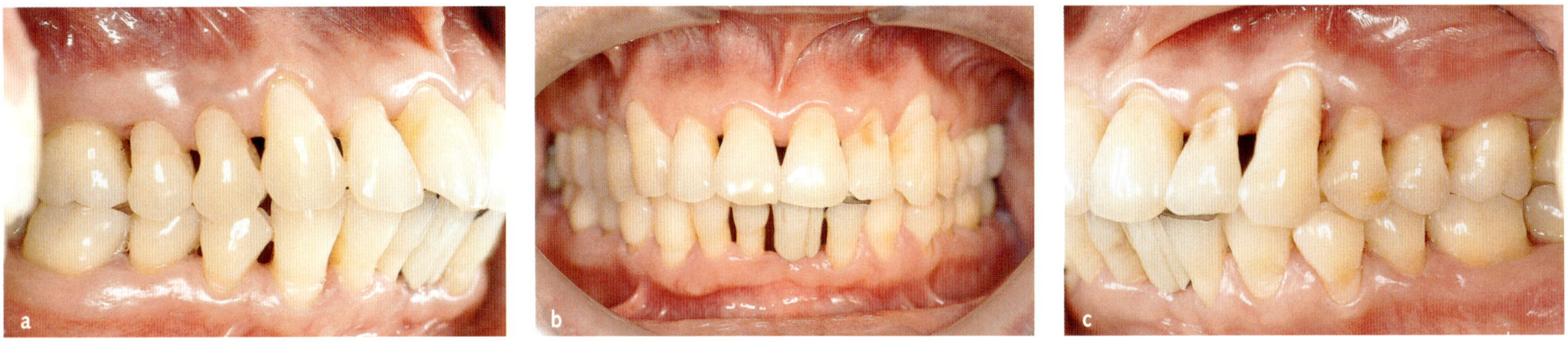

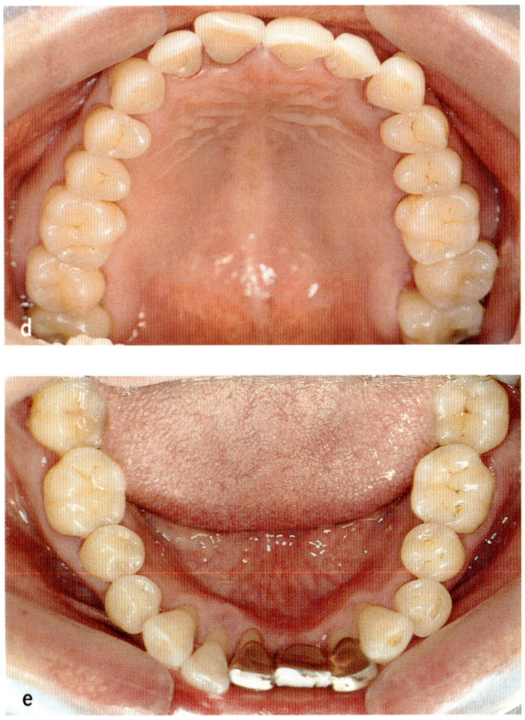

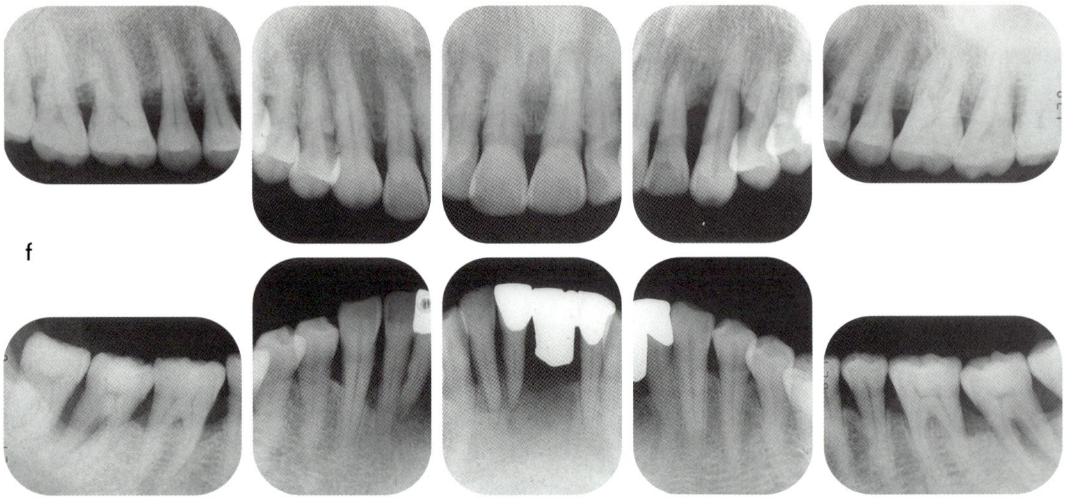

Fig 2-131 At the first visit, the patient was concerned about the progress of periodontal disease. (a to c) Wedge-shaped defects are observed at cervical areas of the maxillary left lateral incisor, canine, first premolar, and second premolar and the mandibular left canine, first premolar, second premolar, and first molar. The maxillary right third molar, maxillary left third molar, mandibular left second and third molars, and mandibular right second and third molars were extracted. Periodontal therapies, including regeneration therapy, were conducted. The extruded maxillary left canine was reshaped and a resin composite restoration was placed. A new fixed partial denture was fabricated, extending from the mandibular left lateral incisor to the mandibular right lateral incisor (pontic: mandibular left central incisor). (d and e) Although both the mandibular left second molar and mandibular right second molar are lingually inclined, the buccolingual inclination of molars is different: the right molars are lingually inclined while the left molars are uprighted. The left teeth have more severe attrition with dimples on the occlusal surface. Because of attrition, the relationships between cusps and fissures or between ridges and fossae are not sharp, resulting in poor cutting quality. Buccoversion of the mandibular left first premolar is problematic. (f) Radiographs reveal horizontal bone loss at the mandibular anterior teeth and severe vertical bone loss at the mandibular molars, especially at the mandibular second molars, which are mesially inclined and hopeless. The maxillary left canine also has severe bone loss. The maxillary right and left molars have moderate vertical bone loss.

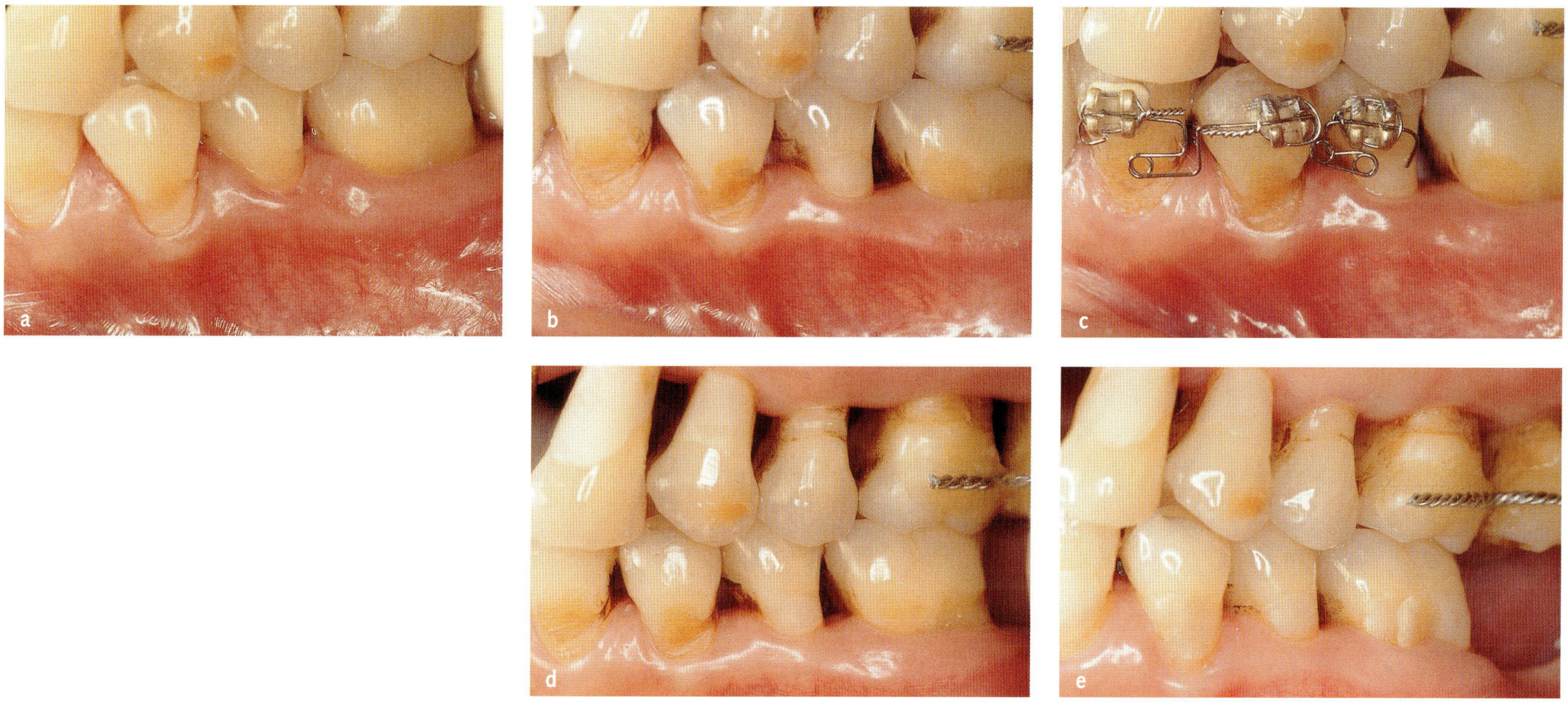

Fig 2-132 Progression of DCS. About 1 year after the first visit, maintenance therapy was started. About 3 years later, worsening of DCS signs was noted on the left side compared to the right side, including wedge-shaped cervical defects and attrition. The patient seemed to exert excessive force to chew because of worn, flat occlusal anatomy. (a) Photograph taken at the first visit. (b) Photograph taken after 3 years 6 months, before orthodontic tooth movements. Wedge-shaped defects at the mandibular left first premolar and molar have advanced. Toothbrushing may be involved. (c) During tooth movements. Disking has been conducted for the mandibular left canine, first premolar, and second premolar, and brackets have applied to correct the position of mandibular left first premolar with buccoversion so that the tooth will be incorporated in the dental arch. Twisted wire is used on the lingual side to anchor the mandibular left lateral incisor, canine, second premolar, and first molar, to move mandibular left first premolar alone. The duration of active orthodontic treatment was 4 months. After resin composite was used to restore dimples on occlusal surfaces, general reshaping was conducted. Occlusal tables were slightly narrowed and grooving was conducted to restore occlusal morphology to facilitate chewing. Disking was conducted for the mandibular left canine, first premolar, and second premolar; the amount of disking corresponded to a space obtained by one session of orthodontic movement. When the space was not sufficient, disking was repeated as necessary. (d) Photograph taken after 4 years 9 months, after completion of orthodontic movements. Wedge-shaped defects have not advanced much in the prior 1 year 3 months. (e) Photograph taken 8 years 10 months after the first visit.

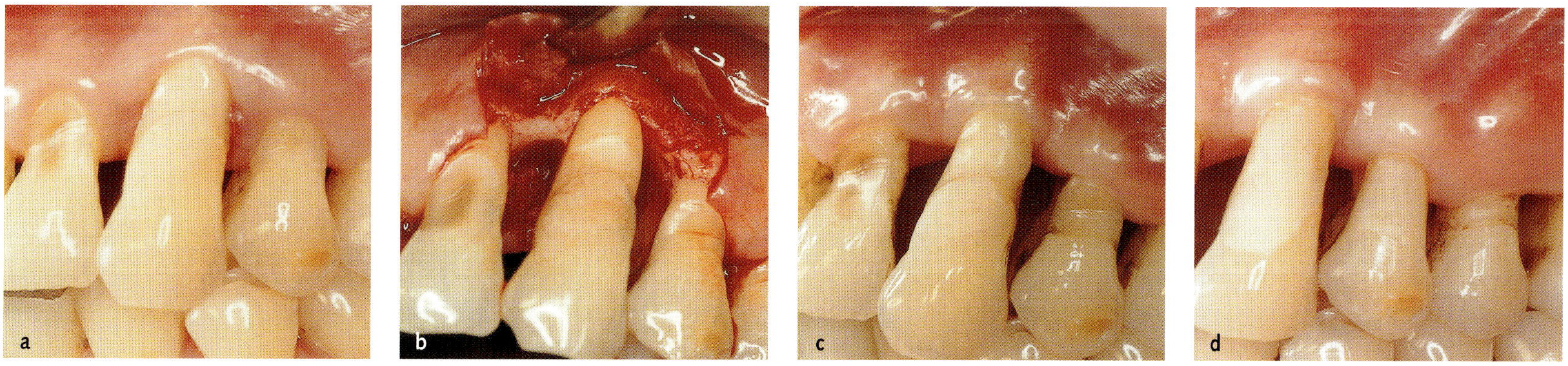

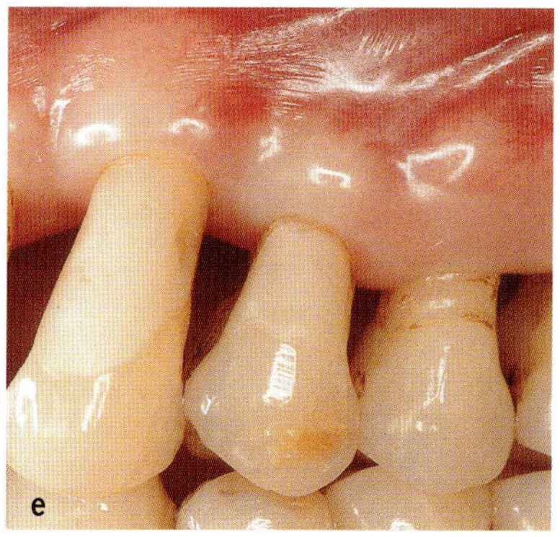

Fig 2-133 Vertical bone loss resulting from trauma. (a) Because of attrition, a chewing pattern is established so that the mandible slides from the lateral direction to enter ICP during function, which has invited concavity of the bone and gingiva. (b) Alveolar bone at the maxillary left canine exhibits vertical bone loss. The left-side arch is flared out because of left-side chewing, which has forced the tooth root out of the bone housing and invited dehiscence and concavity of the labial bone. Tooth mobility cannot be controlled, probably because of lateral occlusal forces applied to extruded teeth. (c) About 10 months after treatment, the maxillary left canine has been extruded. The incisal edge has not been ground yet. The labial gingiva is thin. (d) After 3 years 6 months, the gingival margin at the maxillary left canine is more aligned. The tip of the cusp has been reshaped several times to adjust the morphology in accordance with extrusion. (e) After 5 years 7 months, the gingiva at the maxillary left canine is thickening, becoming equalized with gingiva at the maxillary left lateral incisor and maxillary left first premolar.

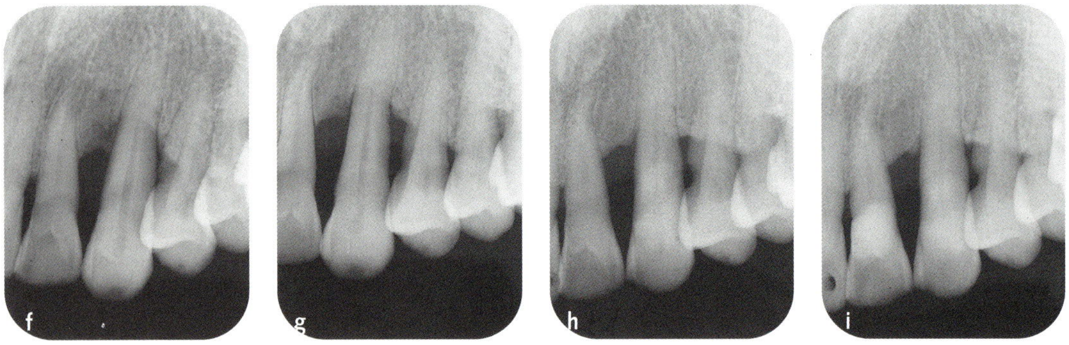

Fig 2-133 (cont) (f) Radiograph taken at a similar time point as (a). (g) Radiograph taken 2 months after treatment. (h) Radiograph taken 4 years 9 months after the first visit. (i) Radiograph taken 10 years 9 months after the first visit.

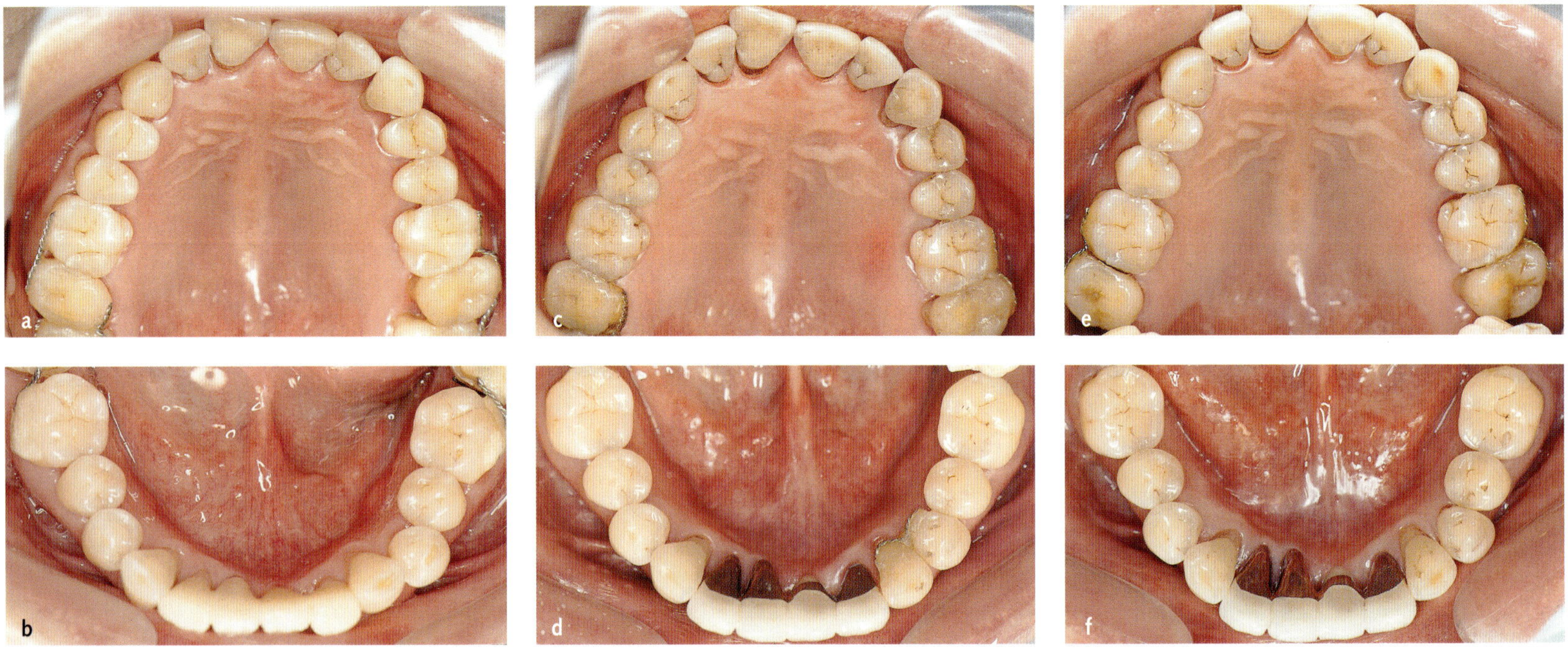

Fig 2-134 Improvement of one-sided chewing. (a and b) Twisted wire is used to splint the maxillary molars to prevent extrusion of the maxillary second molars and to splint the mandibular left canine and first premolar to prevent relapse after orthodontic movements. The maxillary right third molar, maxillary left third molar, mandibular left second and third molars, and mandibular right second and third molars were extracted later. (c and d) After 4 years 9 months, the maxillary arch shows a change of the left arch form from a box shape to a U shape as well as symmetry between the maxillary canines. The labioversion of maxillary right central incisor been advanced. Although the unbalanced buccolingual inclinations of the tooth axes of the maxillary canines have been somewhat improved, the patient still feels more comfortable chewing on the left side and does so easily. Toothbrushing is well done, and inflammation is mostly under control. (e and f) Photographs taken after 11 years. A resin composite restoration was placed and reshaping was conducted after the mandibular left first premolar was moved back in the dental arch and the arch form was put in order. The symmetric flow of the left and right cusp tips and the alignment of the central fossae of individual teeth will create symmetric, fine chewing cycles with little variability. The difference in angulation between the right and left molars is slightly ameliorated.

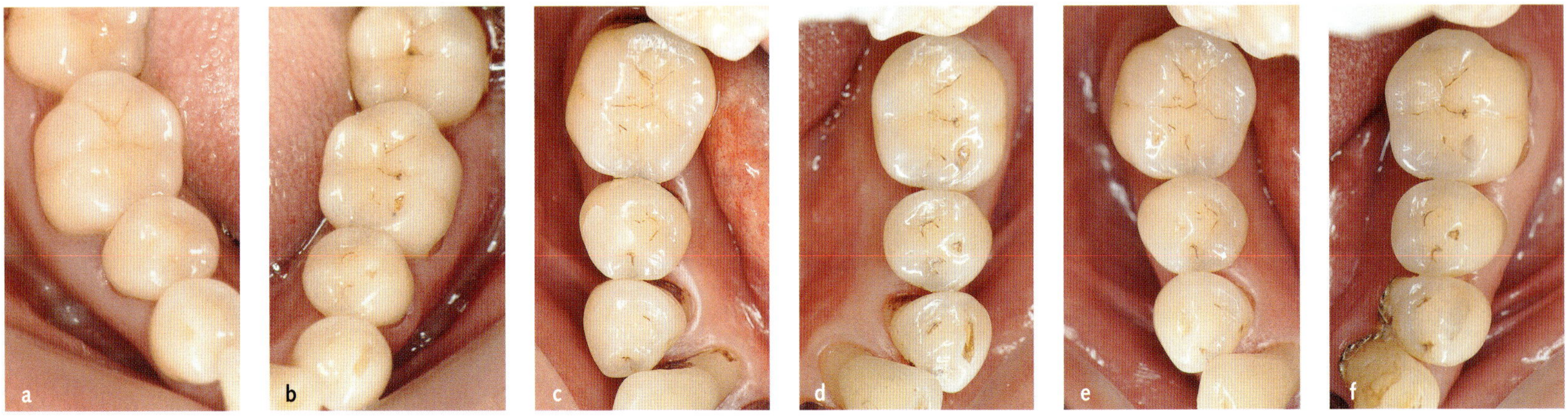

Fig 2-135 Occlusal surfaces. (a and b) At the first visit, the mandibular left occlusal surfaces show area contacts, indicating no spillway for food. The right molars also show attrition, but to a lesser degree than the left side. (c and d) After 3 years 6 months, the buccoversion of the mandibular left first premolar has advanced. The attrition of left teeth has diminished, increasing the size of dimples. (e and f) Photographs taken after 4 years 9 months. The buccolingual width has been slightly reduced to narrow the occlusal table. Grooving has been added to fossae. The buccal cusp tip lines and central fossa lines are being organized.

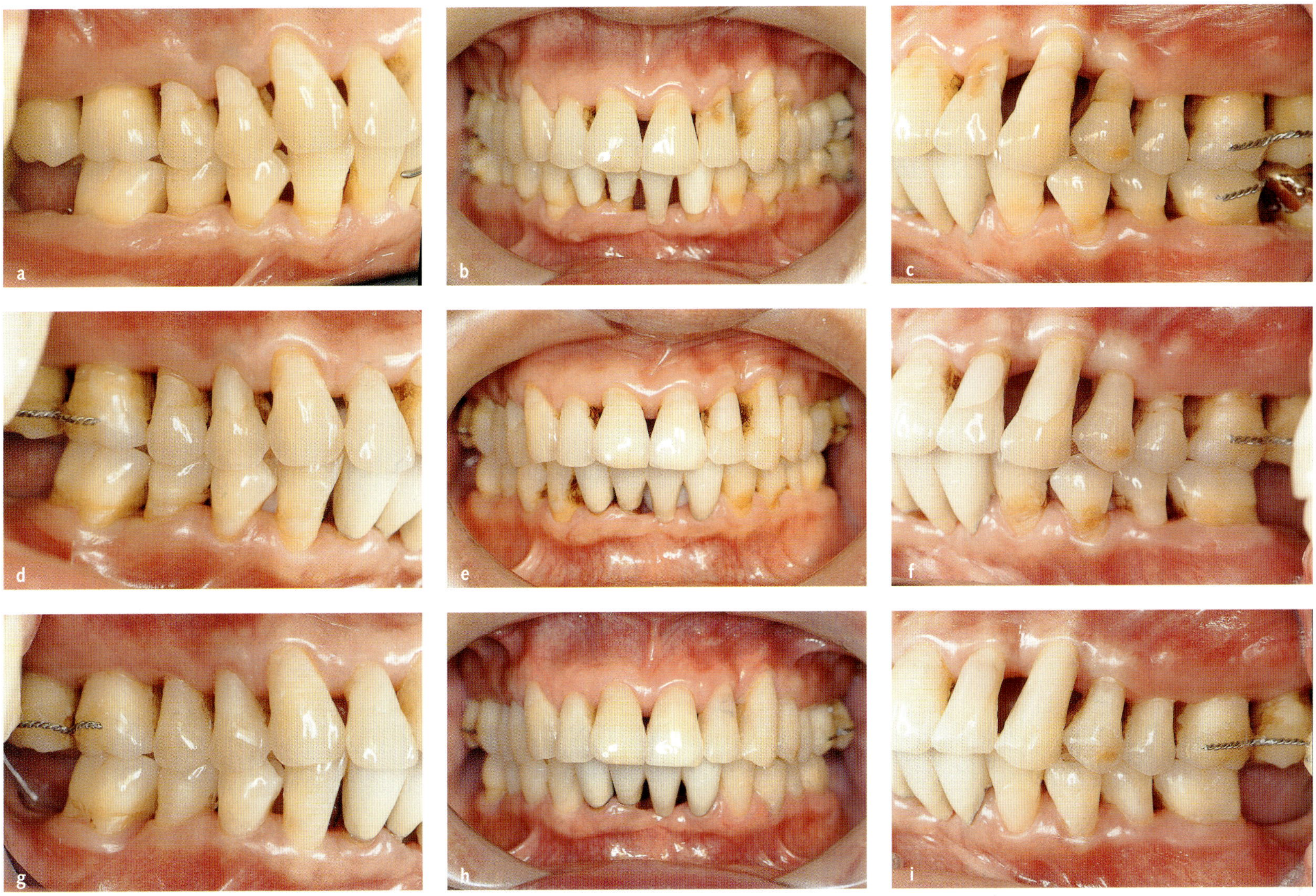

Fig 2-136 Treatment progress. (a to c) Photographs taken 10 months after the first visit. (d to f) Photographs taken 4 years 1 month after the first visit. Although gingival recession at the mandibular right first molar has progressed, the probing depth is decreasing. The gingiva shows a healthy, pink color on the right side, but it is still reddish at the mandibular left first premolar. (g to i) Photographs taken 11 years after the first visit.

Fig 2-137 Evaluation of functional movements. (a) A Sirognathograph of left-side chewing after 3 years 5 months (before force control) shows cycles with too-wide lateral movement and high variability. When a dental arch is not in good alignment, the chewing cycle has severe variability, depending on the position where food enters. The opening path to the nonworking side includes an appropriate cycle to move to the working side from the vicinity of the maxillary right canine and a cycle showing wide lateral grinding movement. The closing path also goes round laterally to enter ICP. The flat occlusal surfaces of the molars or a lack of continuity among teeth, including buccoversion of the mandibular left first premolar, seem to have formed this closing path. (b) Reduced variability and better-organized cycles are observed after 4 years 5 months (after force control). There are two closing paths showing mastication at the premolars and molars. Although the cycle at the premolars is acceptable, the one at the molars still exhibits a wide occlusal table and variability.

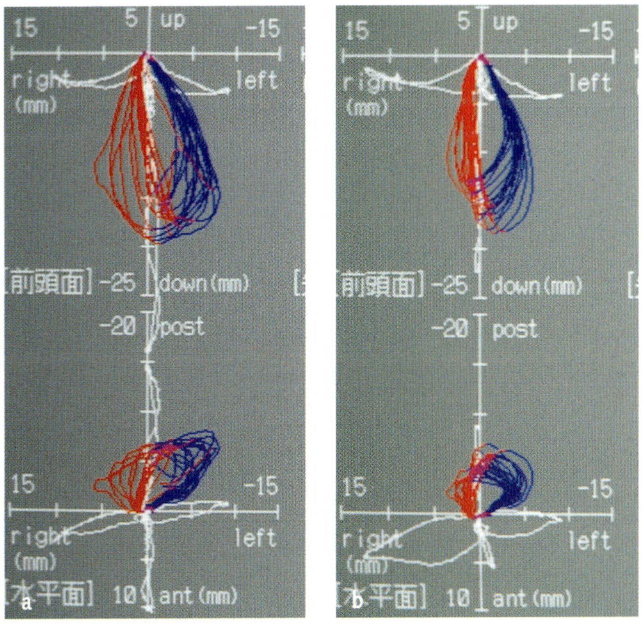

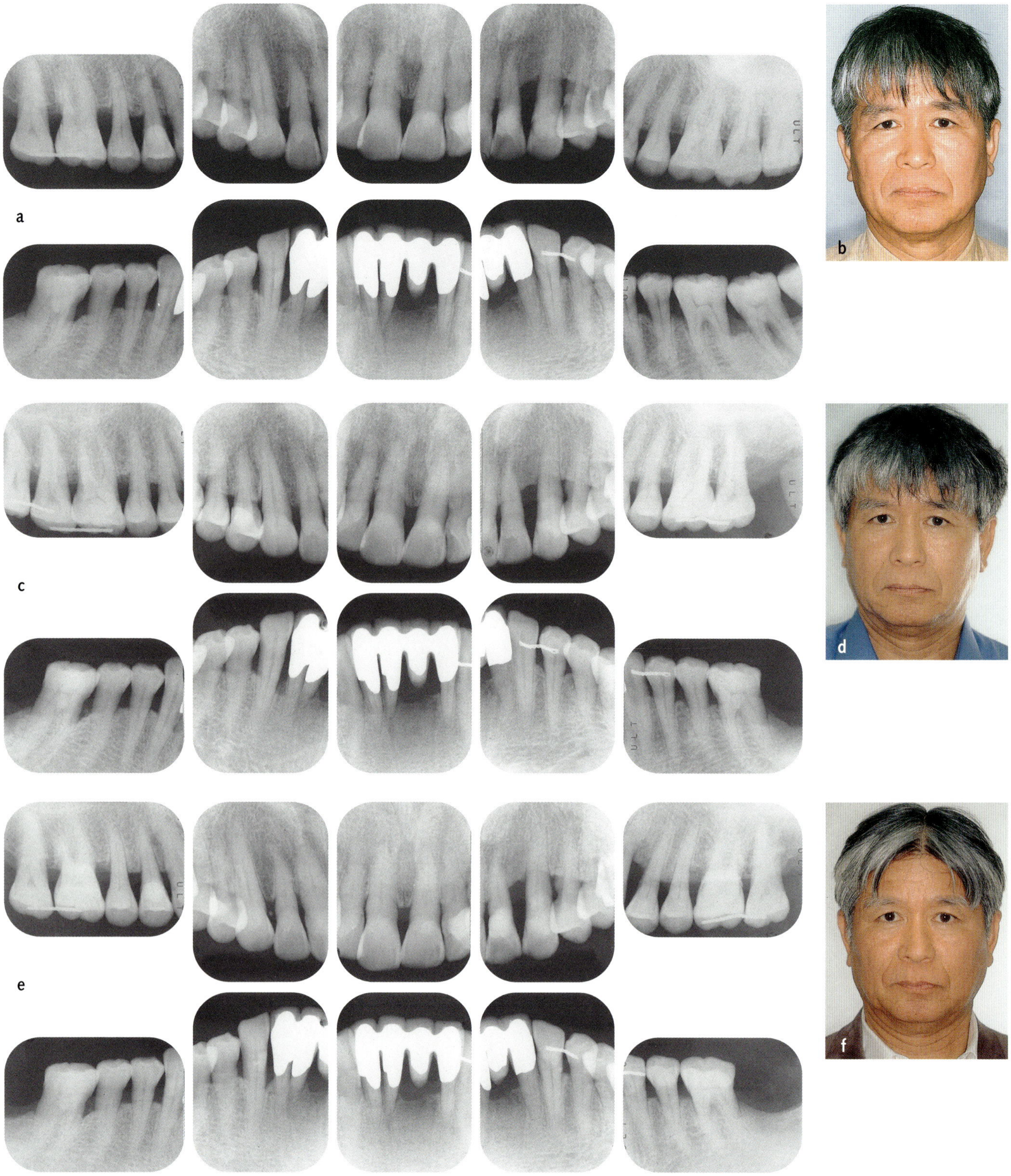

Fig 2-138 (a) Radiographic follow-up 5 years after the first visit. Signs of DCS have become conspicuous. (b) A photograph of the face (taken 3 years 6 months after the first visit) reveals that the lip line is higher on the right side and the nasolabial sulcus is deeper on the right side, which suggests clenching on the right side. The left masseter is tense, indicating left-side chewing. (c) Radiographs taken about 8 years after the first visit. After 4 years 9 months. The alveolar hard line at the crest is mostly established, showing overall improvement. The vertical bone loss at maxillary left canine has been flattened and ameliorated. (d) The face is gaining balance. (e) Full-mouth radiographs taken 10 years 9 months after the first visit. (f) A photograph of the face (taken 6 years 10 months after the first visit) reveals that the left masseter is thicker. On palpation, the left masseter feels larger in strain. The patient seems to be chewing on the left side.

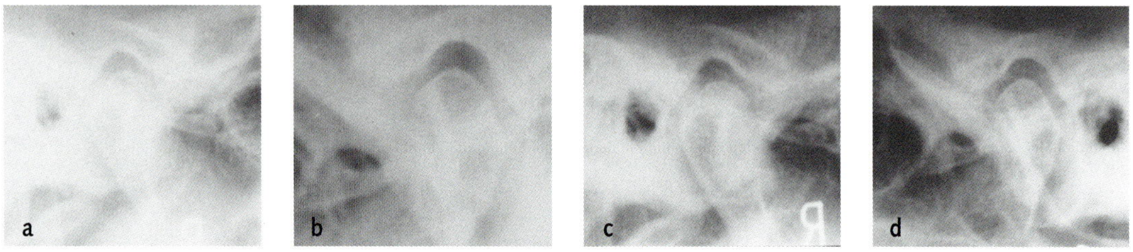

Fig 2-139 Radiographs of the TMJs. (a) Right and (b) left TMJs at ICP after 3 years 7 months. The right TMJ shows deep concavity at the articular fossa and the large, solidly built condyle. These muscles and joints may well cause attrition even with some interference of the teeth. (c) Right and (d) left TMJs at ICP after 4 years 1 month.

Connection of postural habits to occlusal collapse and TMD symptoms

Shift of the lower face including displacement of the maxilla (see Cases 2-18 and 2-20), arch deformity and asymmetry (Case 2-8), lingual inclination of tooth axes (see Case 3-1), and asymmetry in the occlusal plane (see Figs 2-52 to 2-63) are among other pathologic conditions that we have often treated. All of these will be a significant factor in occlusal collapse. Shift of the lower face may invite distortion of the trunk or TMD symptoms. Most patients complaining of TMD symptoms may experience amelioration of their symptoms after only a change in their daily lives, such as postural and chewing habits.

Postural habits may not be detected immediately (Fig 2-140). Often patients will not admit their habit, even if one is found. When there is some trouble in treatment, patients will not admit that one of the reasons for the trouble is their habit. As a clinician dealing with the lower face, a dentist should pay more attention to the fact that the oral cavity is affected by habits such as sleep posture (Case 2-8) and resting the cheek in the hand (Case 2-9).

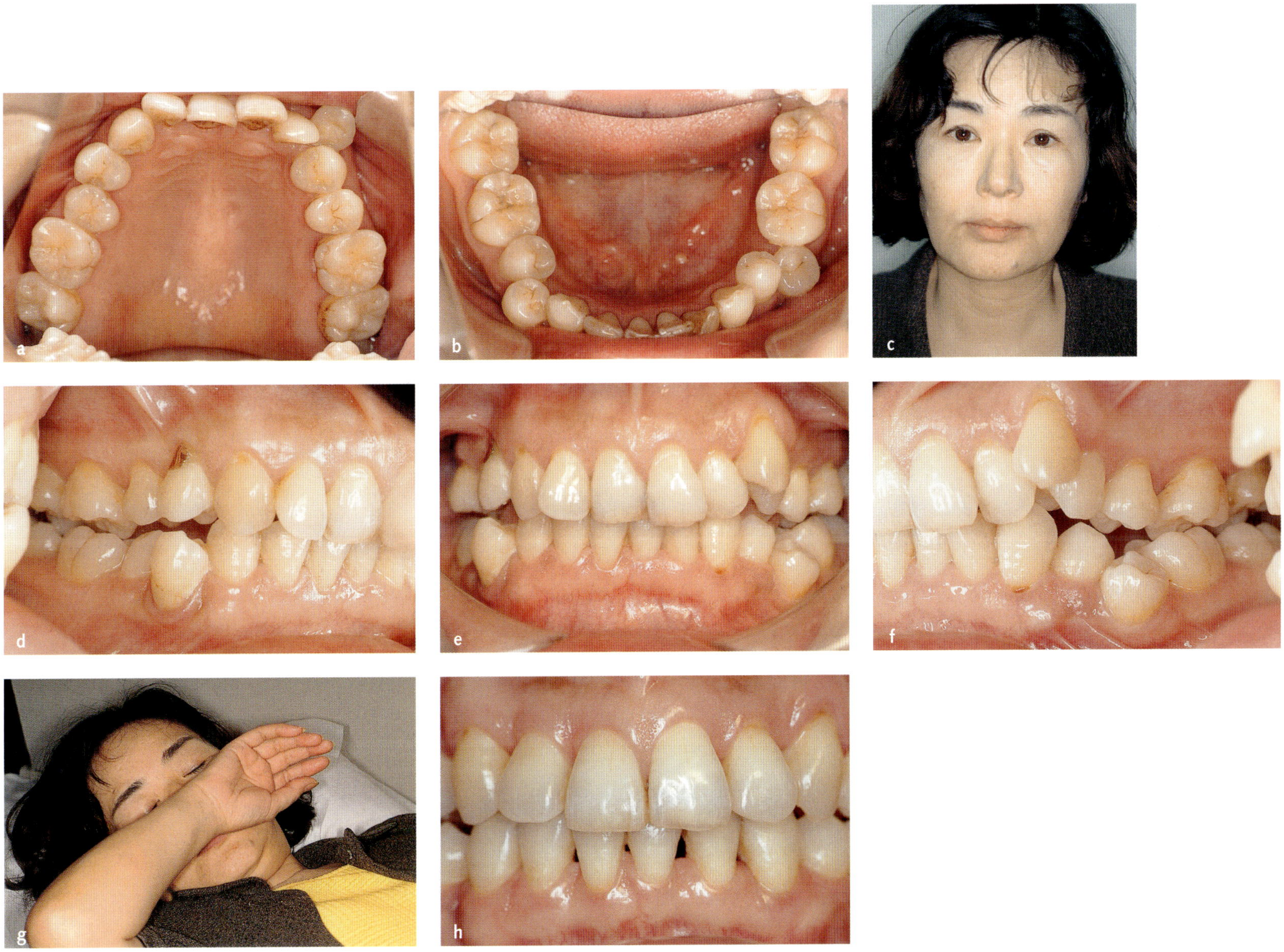

Fig 2-140 Postural habits may not be detected immediately. (a to c) A 52-year-old woman complained that she started to have some space between molars about 1 year previously and it became difficult to chew. She also felt some discomfort in the anterior teeth and suffered from headache, stiff shoulders, and pain in the back. (d to f) Buccal views at the first visit. She complained that she felt as if maxillary anterior teeth had moved lingually, which bothered her because the tongue felt it. Crowding is conspicuous with labioversion of the maxillary left canine, mandibular left second premolar, and mandibular right first premolar. There is no occlusion distal to the premolars. Although lateral thrust of the tongue is noted, this seems secondary because attrition is also present. This seems to have resulted from bite opening caused by lingual inclination of maxillary and mandibular anterior teeth. Still, there is no sign of a lip biting habit, and she said she did not have a habit of sleeping in a prone position. (g) Although we did not identify the cause, we had a discussion with the patient at every visit, suspecting that there must be some habit. Eventually we learned that she was sleeping with her hand on the face. (h) Photograph taken after treatment.

Case 2-8 Significant role of habits in occlusal collapse

Patient: *47-year-old woman at the time of first visit in 1978*

Chief complaint: *Required restoration of missing teeth*

In 1978, restoration was conducted with a Konus telescopic denture for the mandibular arch, which was supported by abutments (mandibular left first and second molars and mandibular right lateral incisor to mandibular right second molar). Fixed partial dentures were also fabricated, one extending from the maxillary right first premolar to the second molar (pontic: maxillary right first molar) and one with abutments on the maxillary left second premolar and first molar (pontic: maxillary left second molar). Over the following 17 years until 1995, the mandibular left second premolar and mandibular right central incisor were extracted, and the mandibular denture was remade four times. This was because a denture ulcer frequently formed on the lingual gingiva of the mandibular left side and the patient complained of pain even after denture adjustment. The telescopic denture was broken many times. At each occasion, the denture had to be adjusted, repaired, and remade.

The right arch of maxilla showed a lingual inclination. The protrusion of the anterior teeth increased, especially at the maxillary right central incisor, which had extrusion and significant labial inclination. Gingival recession occurred at the maxillary right second molar, resulting in severe root exposure.

The denture ulcer was always found on the lingual side of the left mandible, the denture was broken frequent-

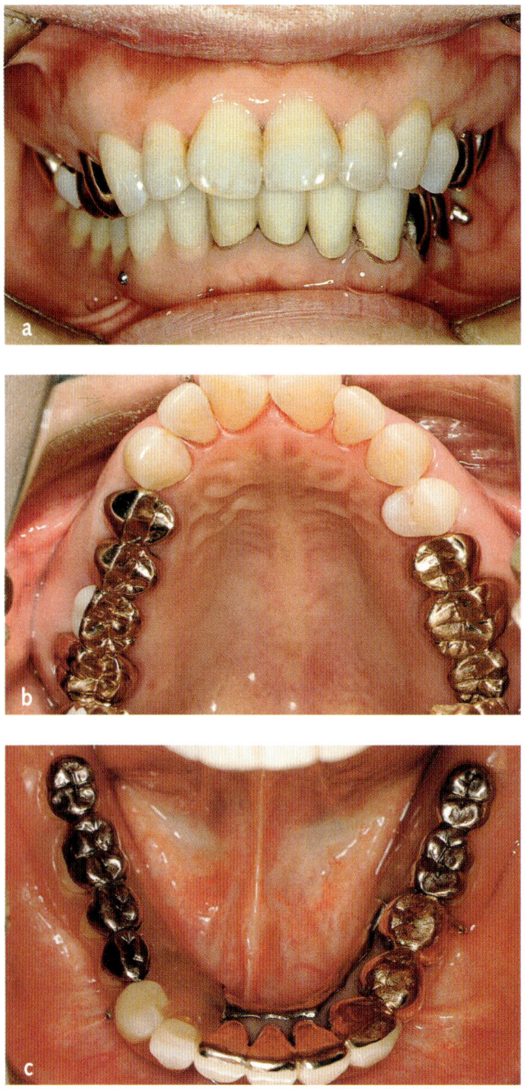

Fig 2-141 At completion of treatment in September 1978. (a) The maxillary right arch is lingually inclined. The roots of the maxillary right second molar are exposed. The maxillary central incisors, especially the right central incisor, are rotated. (b) A fixed partial denture extends from the maxillary right first premolar to the second molar (pontic: maxillary right first molar). A fixed partial denture with abutments on the maxillary left second premolar and first molar replaces the maxillary left second molar. (c) A telescopic denture is supported by abutments on the mandibular left first and second molars and from the mandibular right lateral incisor to the right second molar.

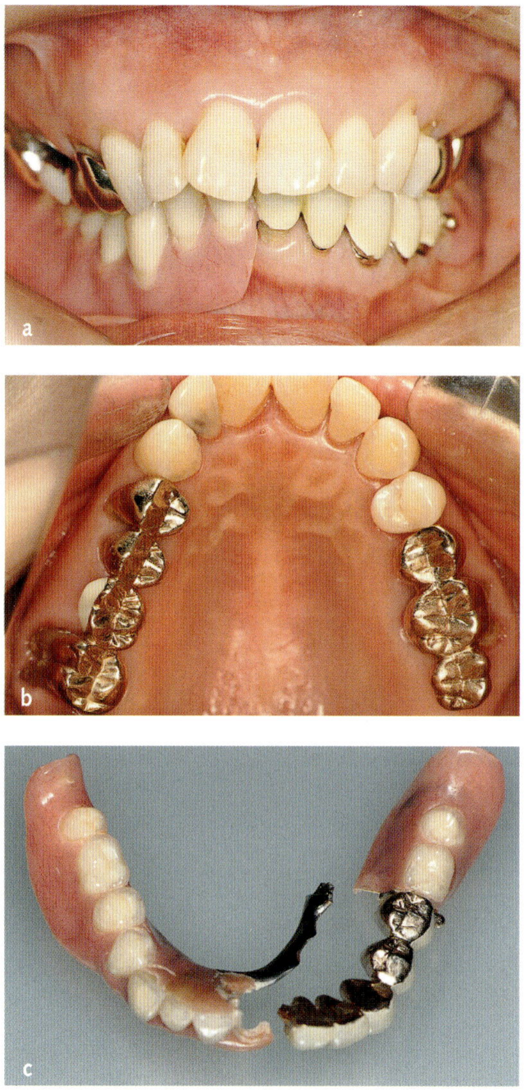

Fig 2-142 Ten years after the first visit. (a) As a whole, the bite has become deeper and protrusion has advanced. (b) The lingual inclination and extrusion of the maxillary right arch have progressed. (c) February 1989. The mandibular right central incisor has been extracted. The denture has been remade three times in 10 years. The denture has fractured frequently.

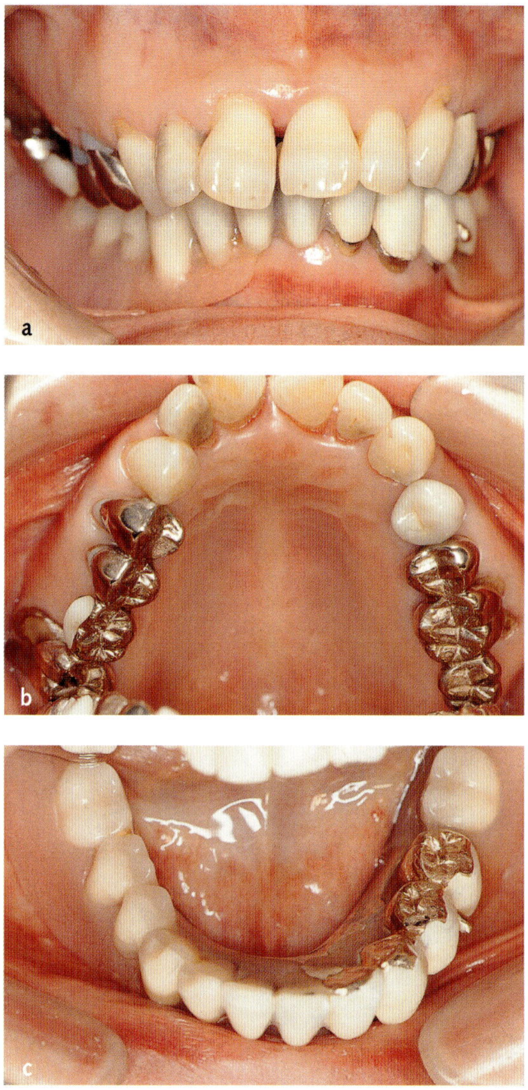

Fig 2-143 July 1995, 17 years after the first visit. (a) For 10 years she has suffered from symptoms including headache, shoulder stiffness, fatigue, and inability to raise the right shoulder. Because she felt relieved when she removed the denture from the mouth, she did not wear the denture when she was at home except at mealtime, which is a sign that indicates a problem with the occlusion of the denture. (b) Lingual inclination and extrusion of the maxillary right arch have further progressed. (c) The mandibular left second premolar has been extracted, and the fourth telescopic denture has been fabricated. The mandibular right denture teeth are lingually inclined in accordance with the opposing maxillary arch.

ly, and the maxillary anterior and maxillary right segments of the arch were deformed. In addition, there was root exposure of the maxillary right second molar. About 17 years passed while we were wondering what was wrong. Inspired by Nishihara, we questioned the patient and found that her sleeping habit was to place her right hand under her cheek.

Treatment: *We first instructed the patient to stop the habit and then adjusted the occlusion through orthodontic treatment and provided new prostheses. It is now 24 years since the first visit of the patient. She is free from all the previous symptoms, including headache and shoulder stiffness, and lives in good health. Her treatment is detailed in Figs 2-144 to 2-150.*

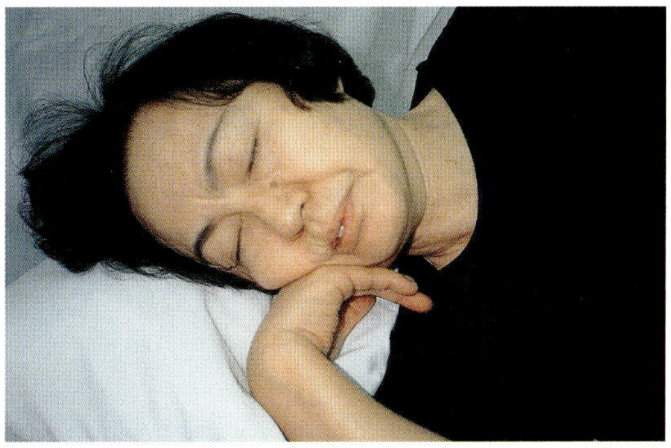

Fig 2-144 September 1995. It was found that her habit of putting her hand on the cheek played an important role. A report by Nishihara prompted us to this discovery.

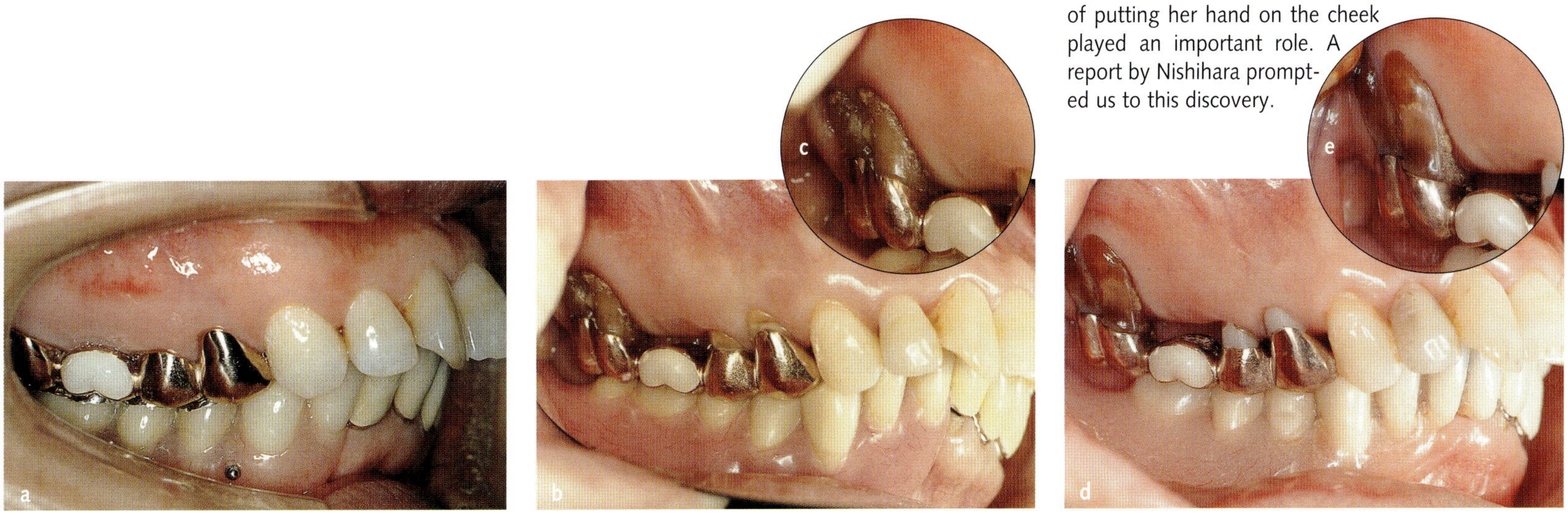

Fig 2-145 Change in curve of Spee and buccal root exposure of the maxillary right second molar. (a) In 1981, the change in curve of Spee and buccal root exposure of the maxillary right second molar are not yet observed. (b and c) In 1988, the buccal roots of the maxillary right second molar have started to be exposed. No specific inflammation is visible. (d and e) Over 14 years, by July 1995, the curve of Spee has become more severe. The maxillary anterior teeth are labially inclined, showing deep bite. Bone resorption on the buccal side of the maxillary right second molar has progressed. A surprising degree of change is observed in the living body.

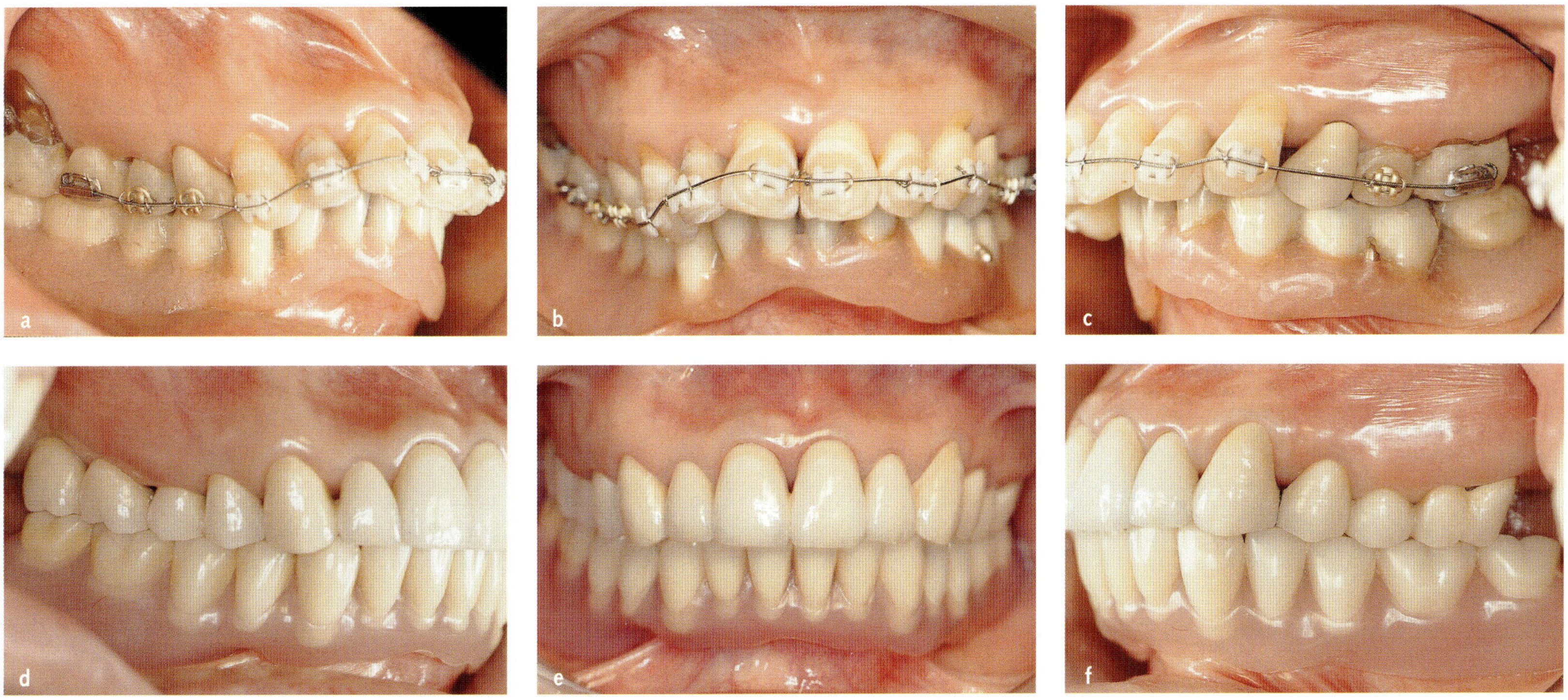

Fig 2-146 Reconstruction of occlusion. (a to c) In September 1995, the patient is instructed to correct the postural habit, and reconstruction of occlusion is started. The buccal roots of the maxillary right second molar have been amputated. After provisional restoration, the multibracket method is used for leveling. (d to f) Photographs taken in September 1997, after full-mouth rehabilitation, 19 years after the first visit. A full overdenture has been delivered for the mandible, with crowns of the abutment teeth located lingually. With buccal roots removed, the maxillary right second molar has only the palatal root, serving as an abutment tooth for a fixed partial denture extending from the maxillary right first premolar to the second molar (pontic: maxillary right first molar).

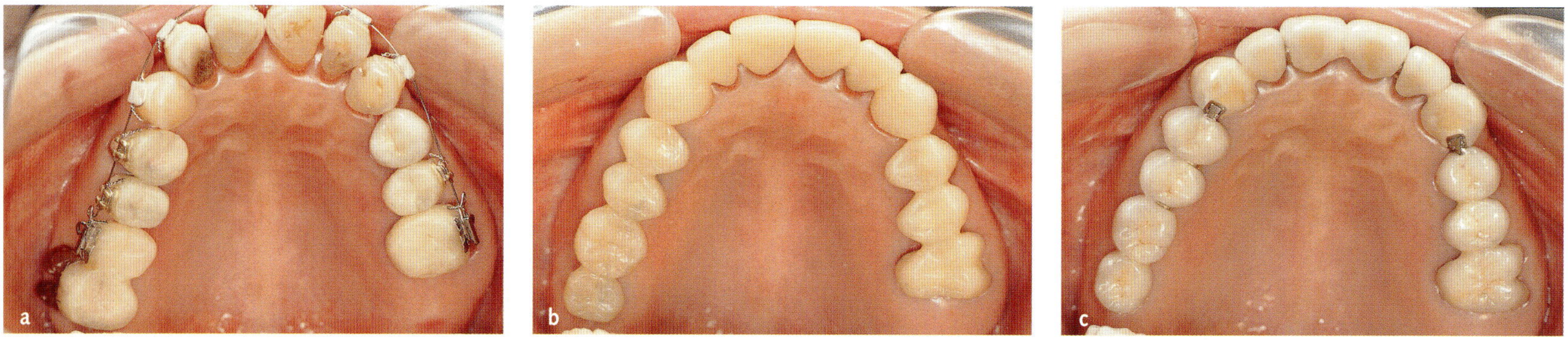

Fig 2-147 Improvement of the maxillary arch. (a) Photograph taken in October 1995. The multibracket method is used for leveling. (b) Photograph taken in December 1996. After tooth movement, a provisional restoration has been delivered. (c) Photograph taken in June 1997. A full splint has been fabricated with keyway joints between the maxillary right first premolar and right canine and between the left canine and left first premolar. Because the maxillary right central incisor was dislocated due to trauma in the course of orthodontic treatment, the appliance was removed and the maxillary right central incisor was splinted. Areas where orthodontic treatment was not completed satisfactorily have been treated prosthodontically.

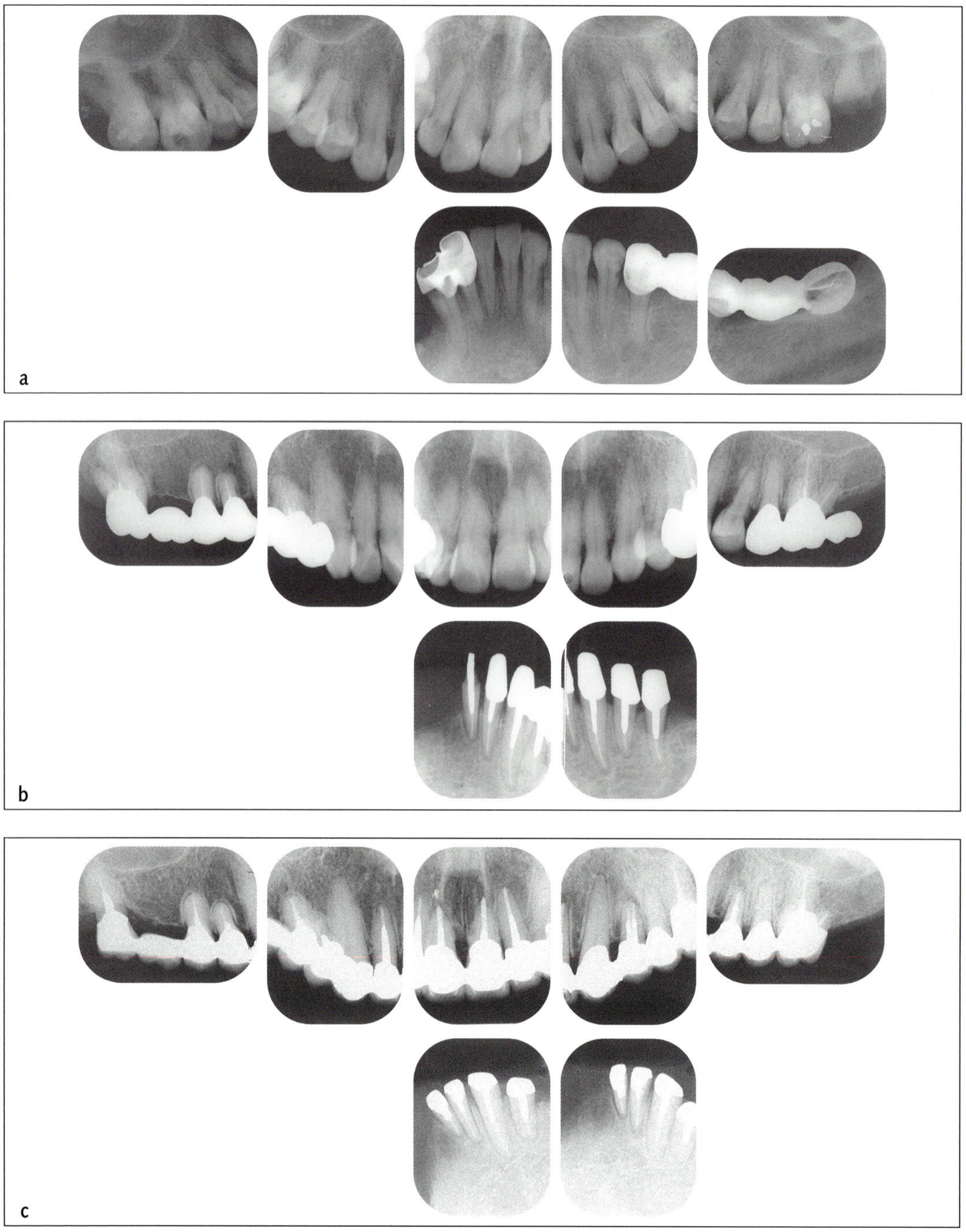

Fig 2-148 Full-mouth radiographs. (a) January 1978. (b) July 1988. (c) September 1997.

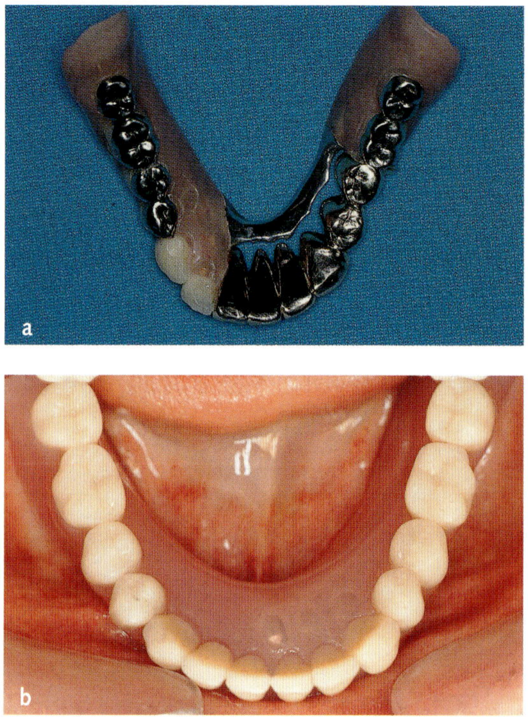

Fig 2-149 Mandibular denture. (a) 1978. (b) 1997.

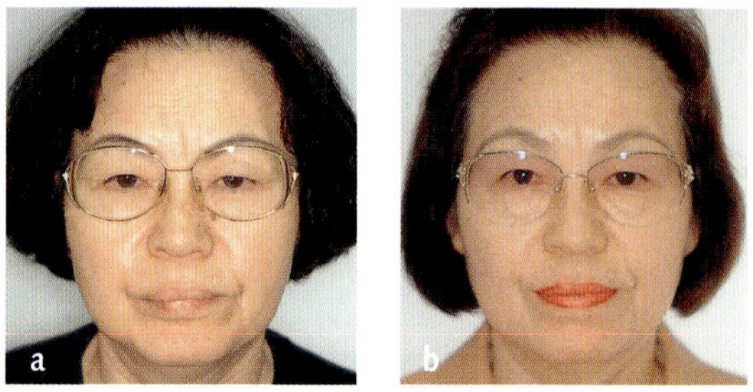

Fig 2-150 Facial change. (a) In September 1995, because of symptoms including headache, shoulder stiffness, fatigue, and inability to raise the right arm, the patient underwent repeated examinations at internal medicine, neurosurgery, and orthopedic surgery departments unsuccessfully to detect any abnormality. The circumoral muscles and sternocleidomastoid muscles are tense. Her face lacks animation. (b) In August 1997, the muscle tension is relieved, and she has a good complexion. Her face is full of life.

Case 2-9 Deformity of the lower face and distortion of the trunk caused by a habit of resting the cheek on the hand

Patient: *16-year-old boy at the time of first visit in 1995*
Chief complaint: *Crowding, open bite, and masticatory dysfunction*
Compared to his parents, the patient had a narrower head and neck with a long lower face, convexity, and a longer chin shifted to the left (Fig 2-151). These characteristics seem to have been mostly caused by acquired, environmental factors. Because of an open bite, the mandible rotated posteriorly and inferiorly, which led to a low tongue (Figs 2-152). As a result, the mandibular arch became wider, while the maxilla did not grow laterally; this pattern is likely to cause a posterior crossbite. In the maxilla, the palate became narrower and deeper and the maxillary arch became V shaped, which further hindered the tongue from entering the palatal space and maintained the tongue in a low position. Such morphology prevented the airway from widening, promoting a vicious circle of mouth breathing and rhinitis. In such cases, slight thickening of the nasal mucosa alone will cause nasal obstruction. The cephalogram at the first visit is shown in Fig 2-153. Figure 2-154 shows the maxillary expansion appliance and its results. Nearly 4 years after the first visit, when the patient was almost 20 years old, his low tongue was not cured yet, the vertical overlap was still shallow, and it continued to be difficult to close the lips without any improvement in the conditions (Figs 2-155 and 2-156).

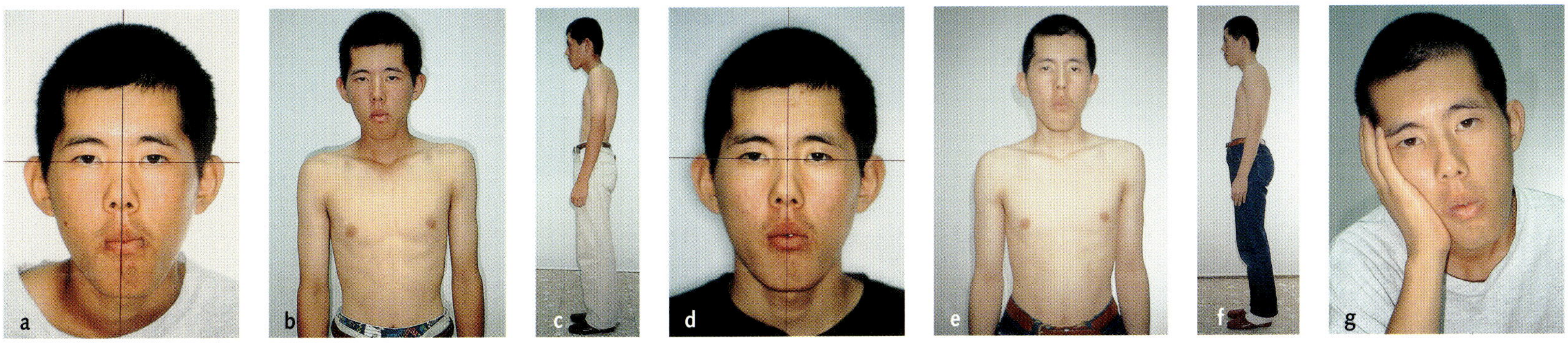

Fig 2-151 Distortion of the face and the body. (a to c) The face is narrow, and the lower face is especially long. Because of an imbalance between the length of the lower lip and the mandible, it is impossible for the patient to close the lower lip naturally. The chin is not well developed. The mandible is shifted to the left. Because of allergic rhinitis, he has been breathing through the mouth since his childhood. The face and the head are shifted to the right compared to the center of the body. The left shoulder and left nipple are higher. He is stooped and the head is positioned anteriorly. He played baseball as a child and has been suffering lower back pain for a year. (d to f) Photographs taken 5 months after the first visit. There is molar crossbite due to a laterally hypoplastic maxilla caused by mouth breathing and a low tongue. A removable plate appliance with an expansion screw is used for lateral expansion of the maxilla. By merely curing the patient's habit of resting the cheek on the hand and alleviating the crossbite, the facial asymmetry has almost been resolved and the facial complexion has improved. At this time, the habit has been cured, the maxillary dentition has been expanded, and the posterior crossbite has been decreased. The midline of the face and the head agrees with the midline of the body. Asymmetry of the shoulder and the nipple line has been slightly improved. His lower back pain naturally disappeared in about 1 month, after he stopped the habit of resting his cheek in his hand. (g) His habit of resting the cheek in the hand is revealed at the first visit. It is surmised that the mandibular shift to the left has been caused partially by this habit.

Fig 2-152 (a to e) Clinical conditions at the first visit. There is an open bite because of mouth breathing. The mandible is rotated posteriorly and inferiorly. The maxilla is narrowed due to a low tongue, which has caused a posterior crossbite. Because of the patient's habit of resting his cheek in his hand, external force was applied from the right, which moved the right teeth lingually and caused a more severe crossbite on the right side. Maxillary hypoplasia has caused crowding. It is surmised that the open bite has been caused by a tongue thrusting habit.

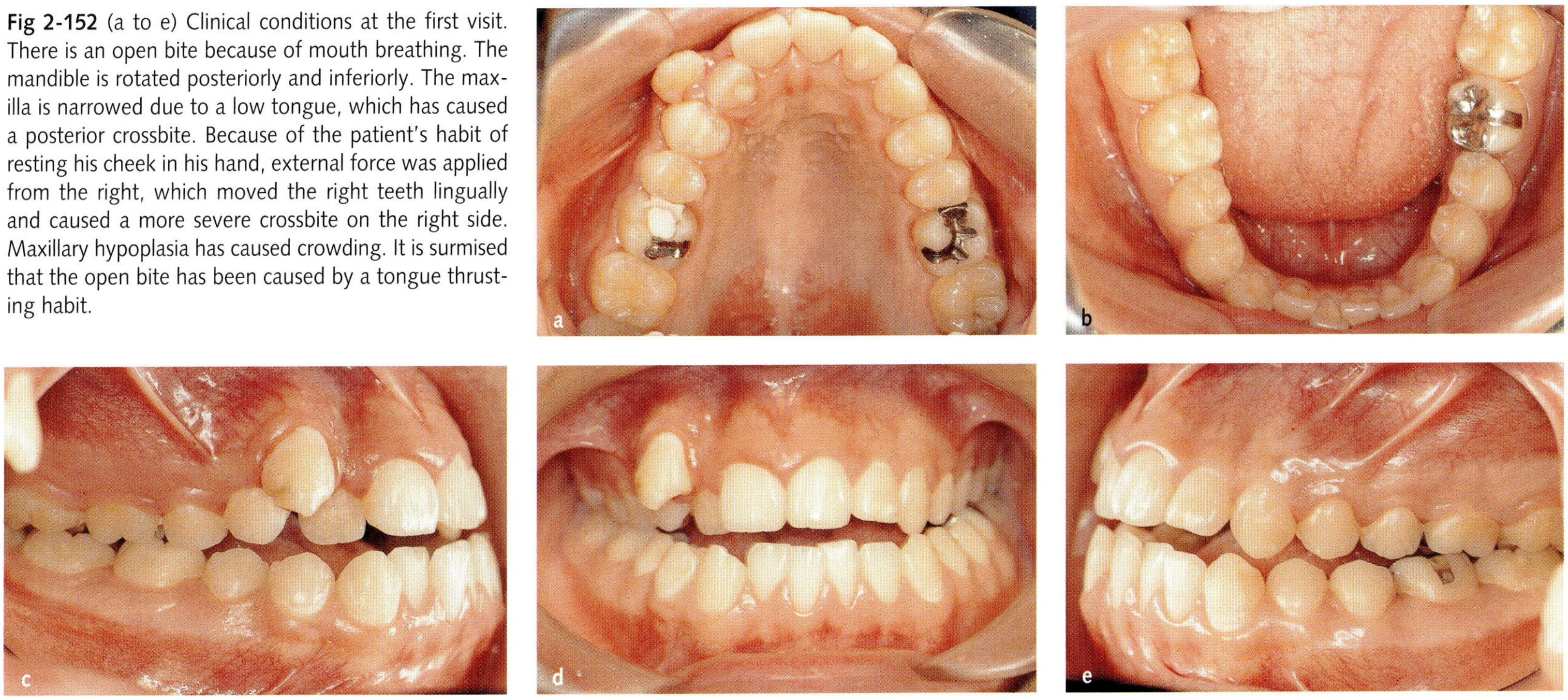

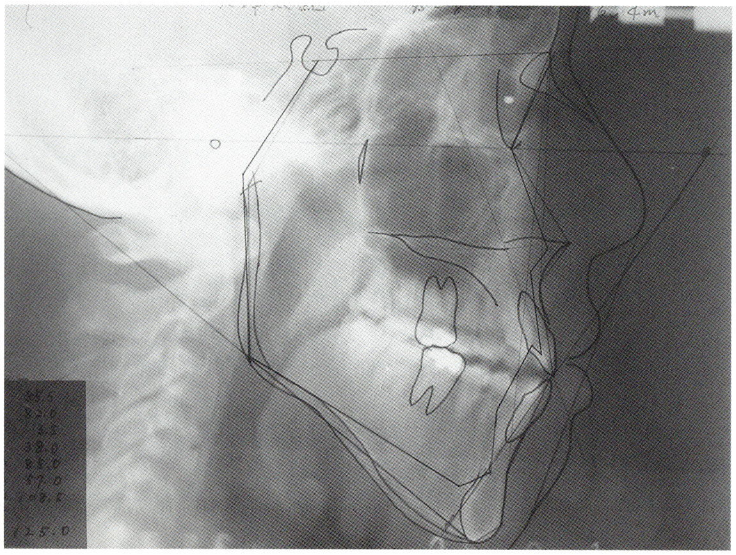

Fig 2-153 Analysis of the cephalogram at the first visit. Superimposition with profilogram. The mandible has a large Go angle with an open L shape. Sella-nasion–point A: 85.5 degrees; sella-nasion–point B: 82.0 degrees; ANB: 3.5 degrees; FMA: 38.0 degrees; mandibular incisor–mandibular plane: 85.0 degrees; Frankfort horizontal–mandibular incisor: 57.0 degrees; maxillary incisor–sella-nasion: 108.5 degrees; OP: 13.5 degrees; maxillary incisor–mandibular incisor: 125.0 degrees.

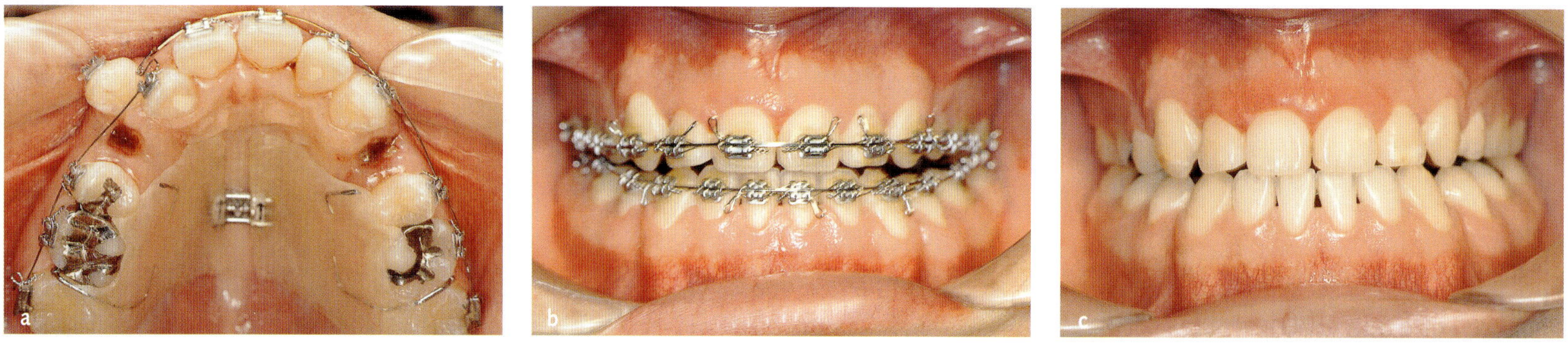

Fig 2-154 Arch expansion. (a) After extraction of the four first premolars, a removable plate appliance with an expansion screw is used for 3 months to laterally expand the maxilla (1 year 2 months after the first visit). (b) Photograph taken 1 year 9 months after the removable plate appliance was delivered. Multibrackets are used to adjust the dentition. Myofunctional therapy has been conducted from the first visit. However, because mouth breathing has not been eliminated, complete cure of the tongue habit is difficult. The mouth breathing and tongue habit have not been corrected, and the open bite is not completely eliminated. The posture has improved. (c) Photograph taken about 3 years after delivery of the appliance.

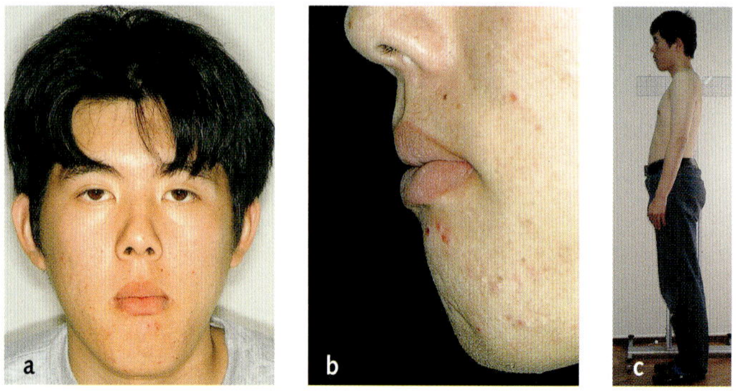

Fig 2-155 Changes in the face and the posture. (a and b) Photographs taken about 3 years 1 month after delivery of the appliance. (c) Photograph taken about 3 years 8 months after the first visit. The posture has improved considerably.

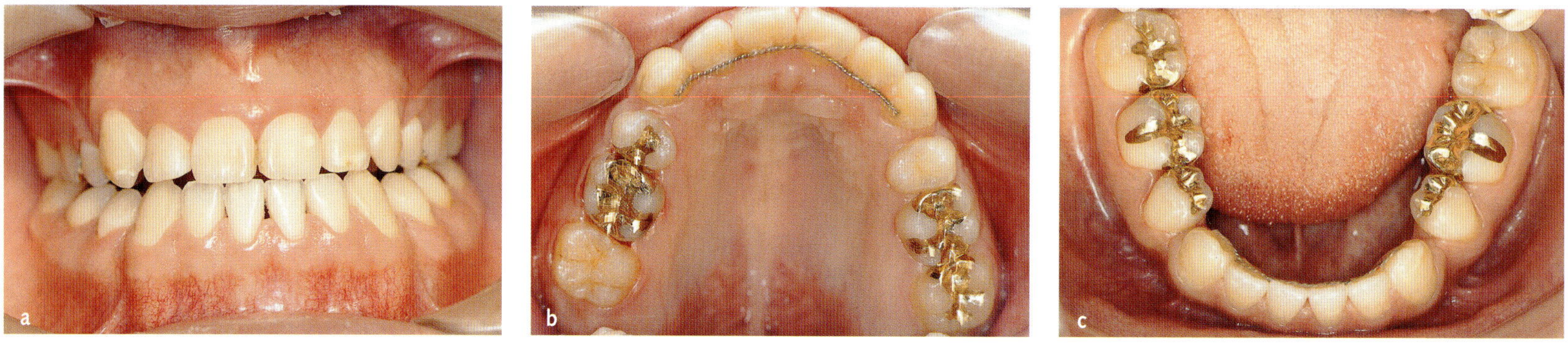

Fig 2-156 (a to c) Photographs taken 4 years 2 months after the first visit.

Pathologic Conditions Derived From Occlusion

Classification based on site of onset

A variety of causes lead to an anomaly of occlusion, including chewing habits, habits of circumoral muscles, malalignment of teeth, missing teeth, attrition, and poor restoration. Malocclusion will be manifested not only as a mandibular shift or an abnormality in occlusal surfaces but also as a wide range of unpleasant symptoms in teeth, periodontal tissues, TMJs, and distortion of the trunk.

We have classified the anomaly of occlusion according to the site of onset of pathology (Tsutsui's classification). Often the causes are interrelated, and it is not rare that an anomaly of occlusion will cause another habit. Also, the pathologic conditions show extremely wide variations, depending on the site of sympathetic onset.

In cases where an anomaly of occlusion is manifested in teeth and periodontal tissues, good results cannot be obtained even if high-quality inflammation control is possible.

Occlusion: The main cause of TMD symptoms

Some clinicians have negative opinions about relating TMD symptoms to occlusion, which seems to be because it is based on an incorrect perception about occlusion. Our theories about occlusion that we have discussed so far, combined with the patience to accept a patient's complaint and the careful application of delicate clinical techniques, will allow clinical confirmation that many TMD symptoms are derived from occlusion. When a patient complains of discomfort of occlusion, almost without exception, signs such as mandibular shift, abnormal guidance, and/or interference can be observed (Figs 2-157 and 2-158). If sufficient time is spent adjusting ICP to a position in which the patient can relax, significant amelioration of symptoms can result (Cases 2-10 and 2-11).

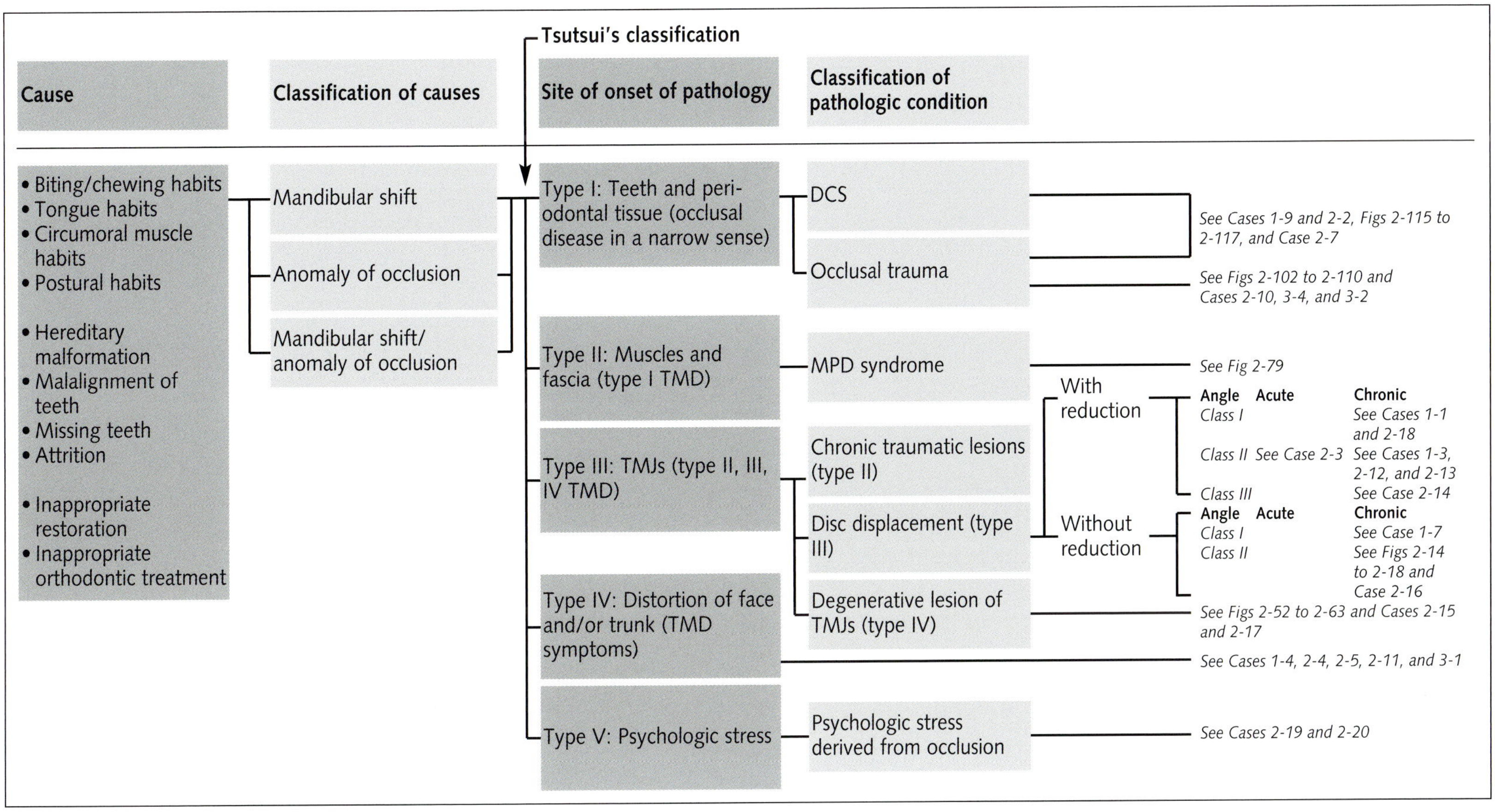

2-157 Pathologic conditions derived from occlusion.

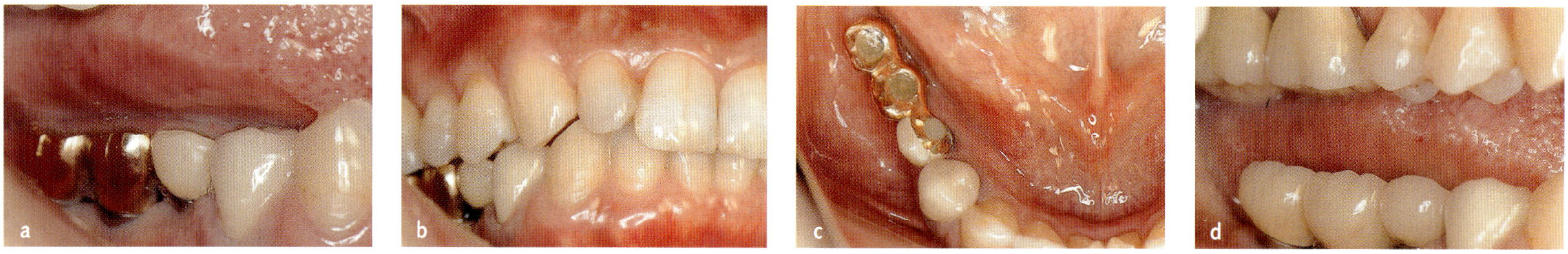

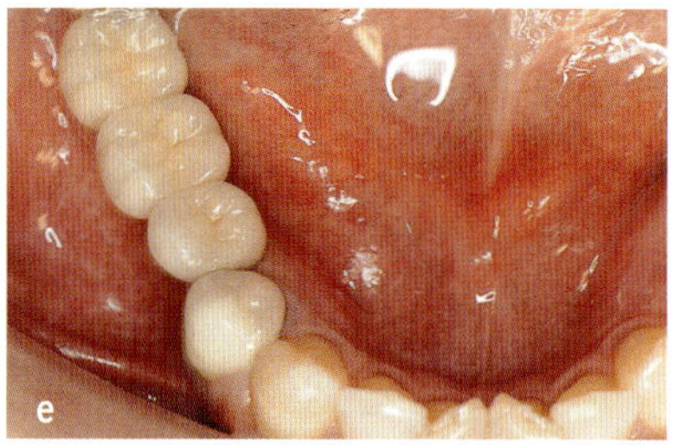

Fig 2-158 Glossodynia is a manifestation of an occlusal disorder in the tongue. Although glossodynia is said to appear suddenly, the mandible is shifted to the painful side or the vertical dimension is short on the painful side in most patients. (a) This patient visited us with a chief complaint of pain in the right side of the tongue, claiming that the pain started after a previous clinician placed implants in the right side of the mandible. Although the clinician ground the lingual side of the implant superstructure considerably, the pain was not resolved. This pain was caused by the fact that the mandible was shifted to the right as the A slope of porcelain restorations on the maxillary left first and second premolars formed premature contacts and the fact that the vertical dimension of the right side was short. (b and c) As the patient is allowed to tap in a relaxed manner at the first visit, the diagnosis is established immediately. ICP shows interdigitation on the right side. The patient originally had a shallow floor of the mouth and a large tongue, which invited the pain in the tongue when the mandibular shift occurred. (d and e) A superstructure has been newly fabricated and the mandibular position is improved. The pain has disappeared in spite of the bulge on the lingual side.

Also, although it is not appropriate to look for the cause in occlusion alone, because multiple factors are involved in accompanying unpleasant symptoms, they may be causes mutual to each other, forming a vicious circle in which an inappropriate mandibular position causes distortion of the trunk or promotes deleterious habits.

Suitability of occlusion

Seeking the main cause of unpleasant systemic symptoms in psychologic factors such as stress is not of help in the resolution of symptoms in many cases. Rather, an anomaly of occlusion may cause psychologic stress. Patients often feel strong psychologic stress because even their family members cannot understand the unpleasant symptoms that accompany an anomaly of occlusion. In conclusion, if it is possible to have reasonable agreement between a relaxed position and ICP and to have harmony between the central system and peripheral movement paths, symptoms of TMD will be ameliorated. When it is not possible to create such harmony, the possibility that another factor is involved should be considered. It is not rare that some unconscious behavior of the patient intended to correct the mandibular position actually is worsening symptoms.

Case 2-10 Anomaly of occlusion manifested in the periodontal tissues

Patient: *52-year-old woman at the time of first visit in September 1997*
Chief complaint: *Inability to chew because of severe mobility of the mandibular central incisors*
In this clinical case, while a bite plane was used to improve the mandibular position and occlusal plane, the occlusal surfaces of the provisional restoration were corrected and the existing prostheses were refabricated in a trial-and-error manner to ameliorate the mandibular shift to the right, decrease the vertical dimension on the right side, and restore physiologically harmonized morphology to the occlusal surfaces (Figs 2-159 to 2-168). The vertical dimension of the left side was slightly decreased.

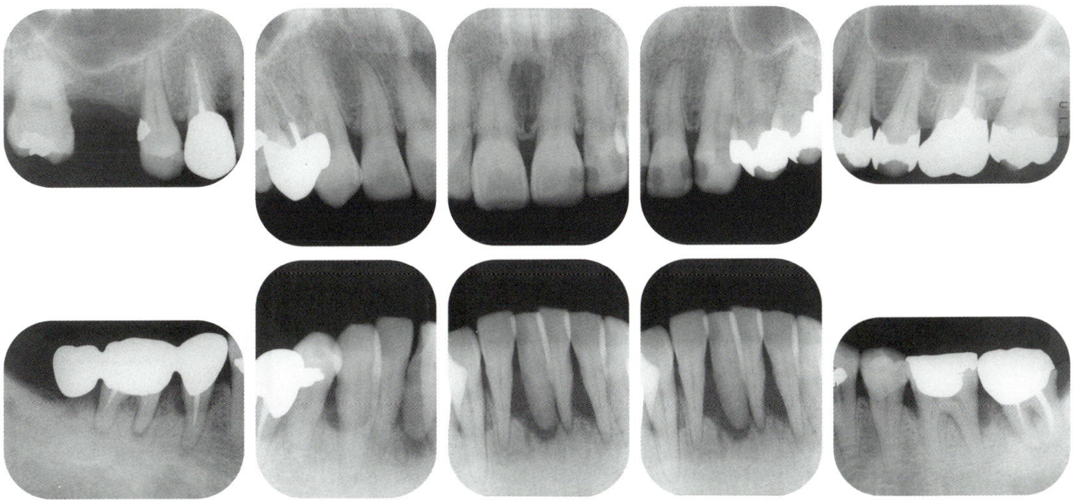

Fig 2-159 At the first visit (September 1997), findings of secondary occlusal trauma are noted. Class II furcation involvements at the mandibular left first molar and mandibular right first molar as well as Class III furcation involvement at the mandibular left second molar are observed.

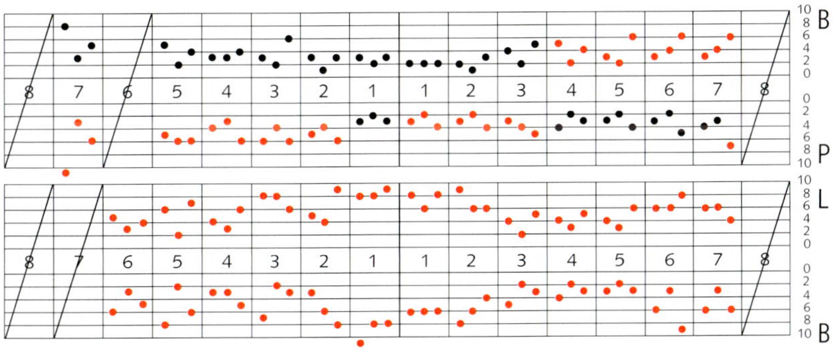

Fig 2-160 A little while after the first visit, probing depths at the mandibular anterior teeth and left molars are 6 to 9 mm (12 mm at the distal surface of the maxillary left central incisor). Red indicates bleeding points.

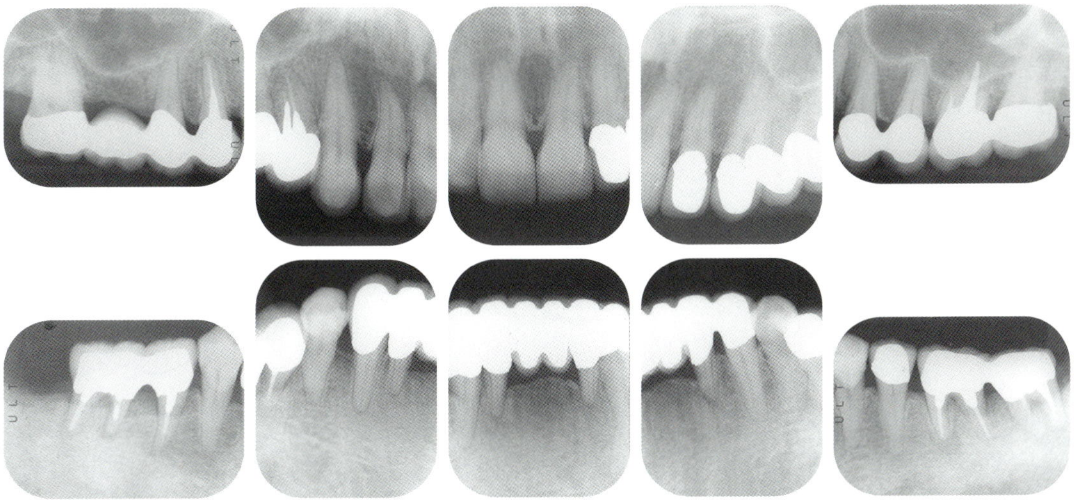

Fig 2-161 Radiographs taken 4 years 6 months after the first visit. The bone level has flattened. Bone regeneration and disappearance of traumatic findings are noted.

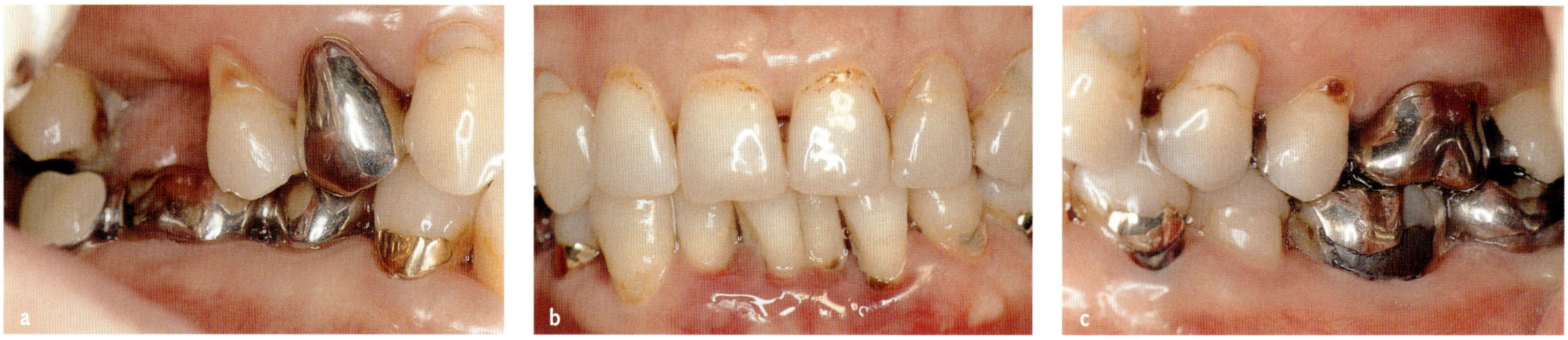

Fig 2-162 (a to c) Labial and buccal views at the first visit (September 1997). There was involvement of the sleep posture habit from the left side.

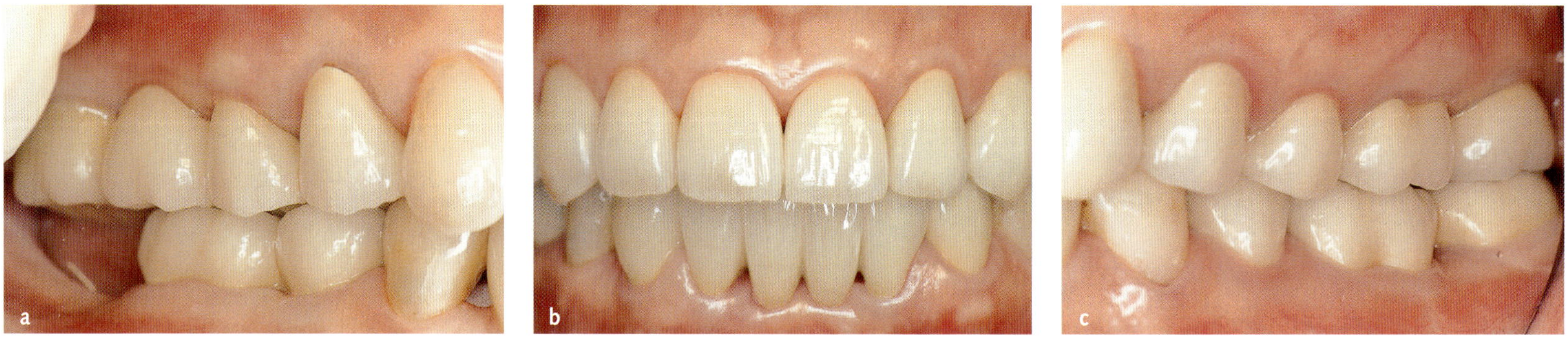

Fig 2-163 (a to c) Views at delivery of the final prostheses (January 2001).

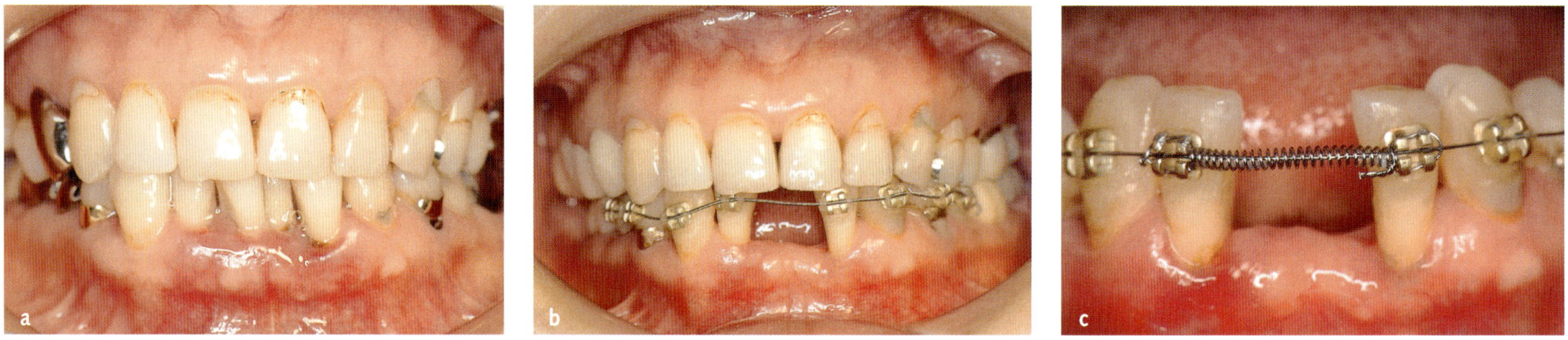

Fig 2-164 Orthodontic treatment of the mandibular anterior teeth. (a) After extraction of the hopeless maxillary right lateral incisor, right central incisor, and left central incisor and initial therapy, crowding of mandibular anterior area is corrected (June 1998). (b and c) Leveling of the bone is being conducted (August 1998).

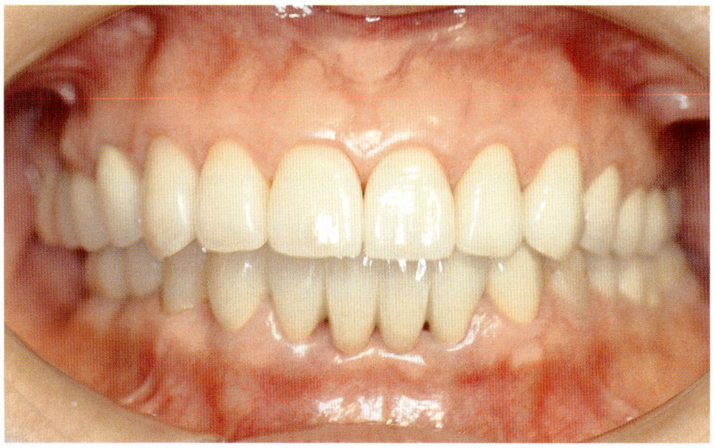

Fig 2-165 Change in the mandibular position. As a result of trial-and-error correction of the mandibular shift by provisional restoration and remodeling of the TMJ areas, the occlusal plane has improved. There is a slight decrease of the vertical dimension on the left side and a slight increase on the right side. The mandibular position has shifted to the left. Pontics at the maxillary right central incisor and maxillary left central incisor have an ovate design.

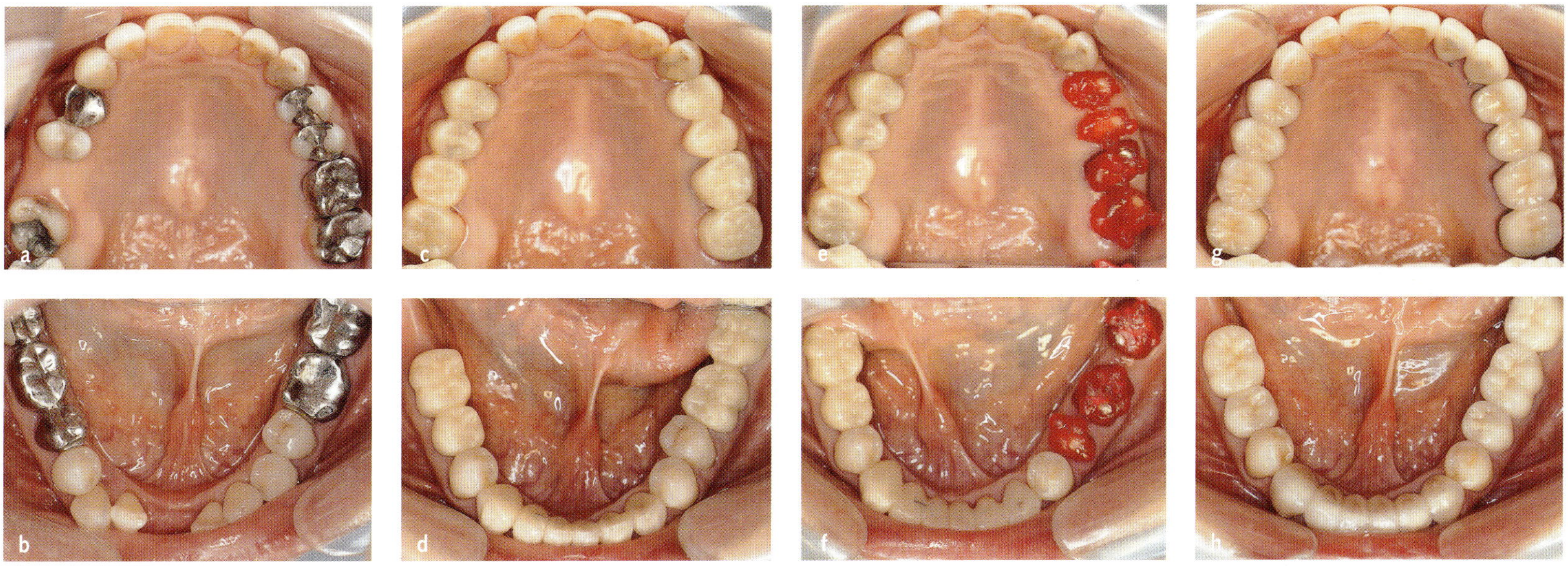

Fig 2-166 Improvement of the arch form. (a and b) Appearance at the first visit (January 1998). (c and d) Two years after the first visit, the arch form is improved by provisional restoration (January 2001). (e and f) After the left maxillary and mandibular segments are replaced by final prostheses, prostheses for the right maxillary and mandibular segments are cemented. (g and h) At delivery of final prostheses (January 2001), the arch integrity has been recovered. A clinical crown-lengthening procedure has been conducted for the maxillary right second molar. Connected crowns are placed on the maxillary right first and second premolars, maxillary left first and second premolars, and maxillary left first and second molars. Metal-ceramic connected crowns with a metal margin are delivered to the mandibular right second premolar and first molar. Splinted crowns are delivered to the mandibular left first and second molars.

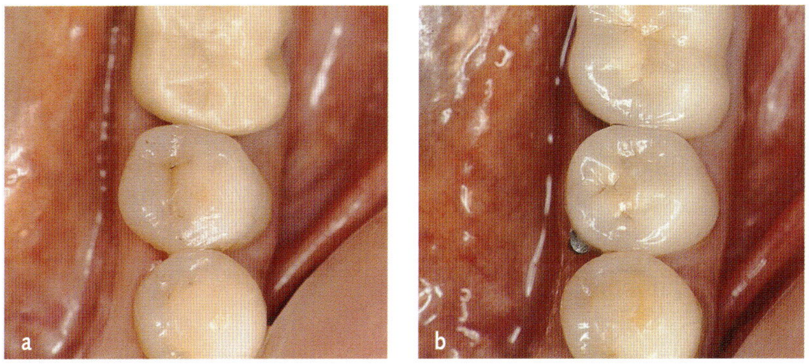

Fig 2-167 Prosthetic improvement of the occlusal morphology. (a) Photograph taken 2 years after the first visit. Although the enamel of the mandibular left second premolar is intact, lingual inclination is noted. (b) To prevent relapse of the mandibular position, the morphology of mandibular left second premolar has been prosthetically corrected. In advanced cases of occlusal collapse, aggressive therapeutic intervention is considered to be rational.

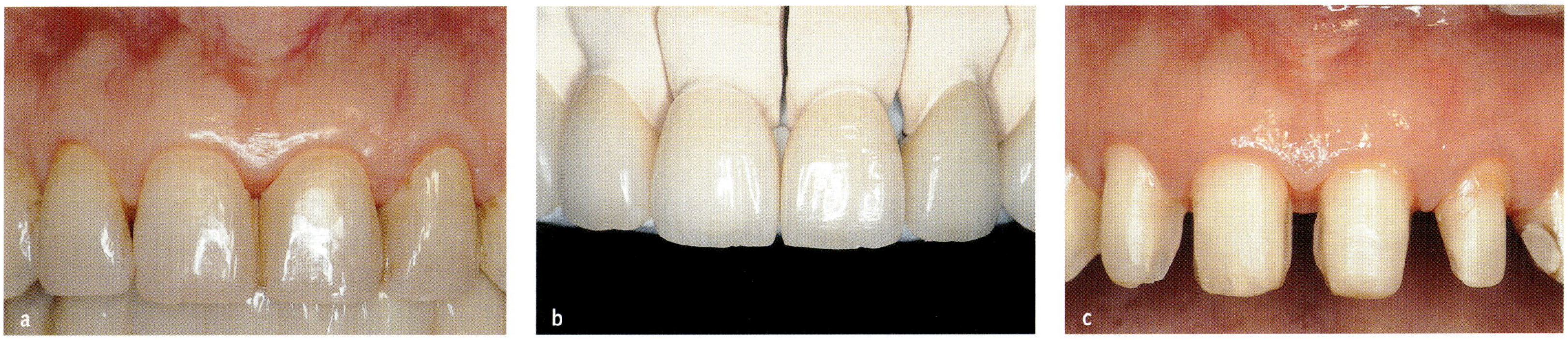

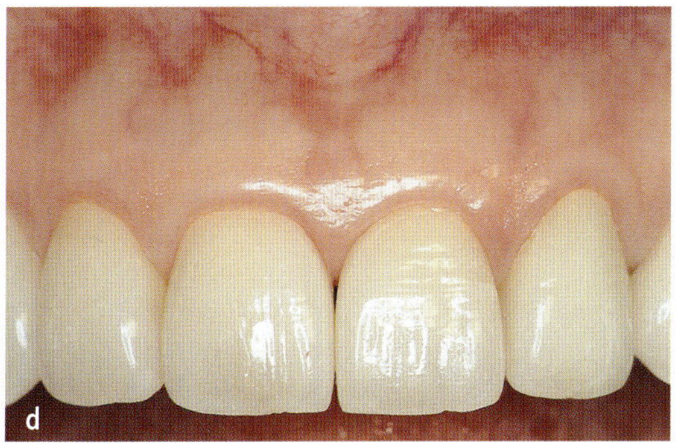

Fig 2-168 (a to d) Improvement of the crown morphology and esthetics of the anterior teeth. Laminate veneer restorations are fabricated to improve the tooth color of the maxillary right canine, lateral incisor, and central incisor and the maxillary left central incisor. Collarless porcelain prostheses are delivered to the maxillary left lateral incisor and canine to improve anterior guidance.

Case 2-11 Management of TMD symptoms accompanying a left posterior shift of the mandible

Patient: *37-year-old woman at the time of first visit in 1996*
Chief complaint: *Uncomfortable bite*
Case history: *The history is long. Table 2-7 is an excerpt from her own record. Treatment is detailed in Figs 2-169 to 2-184.*
Why did the patient feel that the left bite was high? The patient felt that the bite on the left side was too high and complained of abnormality in occlusion to the degree that she ground the left mandibular crown by herself (Box 2-20). Although she felt better immediately after grinding, after a while she began to feel again that "the left bite was high."

Thick metal-ceramic crown on the maxillary right central incisor. *A thick metal-ceramic crown had been applied to the maxillary right central incisor (see Fig 2-170). When the patient was allowed to tap in a relaxed manner, only the maxillary right central incisor has occlusal contact. It was surmised that, because the mandibular anterior teeth contacted the palatal side of the maxillary right central incisor, the mandible rotated to a left and posterior direction and was confined. As the left side received strong force, she felt it was relatively high. It was considered that, during orthodontic treatment, because an appliance was used and she could not bite strongly, the condition was similar to that of when splints were applied, without the mandible confined to the left.*

Individual differences. *If a similar, buccolingually thick restoration were delivered, the maxillary right central incisor would incline labially and the mandibular shift would not occur when periodontal support was inferior or lip pressure was weak. Or, if a condyle were poorly developed and small, it would come off the disc, which would be diagnosed much earlier.*
Systemic symptoms were located on the left side of the body alone, suggesting a mandibular shift to a left and posterior direction or a decrease of vertical dimension in general. However, her face, which should be shifted to the left, actually exhibited development of the right masseter and a shift to the right. This troubled us. The patient said she intentionally inclined her head to the right and chewed on the right side, because the mandibular shift to the left caused worsening of various symptoms (see Fig 2-171). We also learned that she slept on her left side, placing her hand, so that the mandible would be shifted to the right (see Fig 2-169). She was coping with the mandibular shift with postural habits.

Examination of the mandibular position. *The clinician's fingers were lightly applied to the dentition and the patient was instructed to tap so that teeth had light contacts. Fremitus was felt. A discrepancy between the teeth and occlusal contacts was confirmed. In this clinical case, when the patient was allowed to relax and tap while palpation was conducted at the first visit, fremitus was felt on the maxillary right central incisor when the mandible was in a position slightly right of ICP, and disocclusion at the left molars was noted. When the patient was instructed to "bite" tightly, the mandible entered habitual ICP, and the original mandibular position was no longer detected.*

Detailed treatment processes
1. At a second visit, a stabilization splint that was fabricated in a relaxed position was delivered.
2. By the third visit (2 weeks after the first visit), all the unpleasant symptoms had disappeared in an almost unbelievable manner, and an increase in body weight was noted. The maxillary right central incisor showed mobility. Occlusal contacts on the left molars were lost.
3. The lingual side of the maxillary right central incisor was ground for adjustment. Crowns on the left molars were removed and replaced by provisional crowns.
4. The patient was allowed to relax and tap, and areas with strong contact were ground for adjustment. Resin material was added to the occlusal surfaces of the provisional crowns.
5. Just 2 months after the first visit, her body weight had increased by 2.5 kg. She said unpleasant symptoms, such as nasal congestion of the left nostril, had been ameliorated.
6. Five months after the first visit, her fatigue disappeared. She said she was no longer sensitive to cold, even in a cold season.
7. Seven months after the first visit, periodontal therapy was conducted. Resin composite restorations were placed on the mandibular left canine and first premolar to provide provisional occlusion. Provisional restorations were delivered prior to fabrication of crown restorations for the maxillary right first and second molars; maxillary left first and second molars; mandibular left canine, first and second premolars, and first and second molars; and mandibular right second premolar, first molar, and second molar. It was surmised that food-cutting efficiency would be improved by metal occlusal surfaces, allowing resolution of the compacted conditions of muscles, jawbone and TMJs and leading to expansion of the vertical interarch distance as well as gradual disocclusion in the molars. Eventually, the final crowns for the mandibular left first and second molars were remade three times and that for the maxillary right central incisor was remade twice (see Fig 2-175).
8. Even after delivery of the final prostheses, this tendency continued and there was a stress on the maxillary right central incisor (see Fig 2-175), which was restored with Estenia hybrid ceramic. Her systemic conditions significantly improved. It may seem as if we intentionally raised the bite on the left side, which was not the case. Rather, material was added several times to stabilize the occlusion in accordance with remodeling of the body. At the end of treatment, the maxillary and mandibular midlines agreed with each other, and the overlap was shallower (see Fig 2-177). The left condyle was located slightly anteriorly. The body trunk had also become straight (see Fig 2-181).
Later it was found that her habit of exerting force in the right lips caused lingual inclination of the anterior teeth.

Table 2-7 Case history*

12 years old	Had a traffic accident; the left face was strongly hit and swollen.
14, 18 years old	Became slightly sick (related to current conditions) and visited an ophthalmologist with ocular pain (believing it was an eye disease).
22 years old	Found employment.
1 to 2 years after starting to work	Due to ocular pain, migraine, nasal congestion, tightness of the throat, shoulder stiffness, back pain, numbness of hands, nausea, and sense of severe fatigue, she visited internal medicine, ophthalmology, ear, nose, and throat, orthopedics, neurology, chiropractic, Chinese acupuncture and moxibustion, and neuropsychiatry departments. She also visited several dental clinics and was told that there was no abnormality of the occlusion.
28 years old	A metal-ceramic crown was placed on the maxillary right central incisor.
29 years old	Her body weight suddenly decreased, and she left her job. She happened to receive crowns on her teeth at a dental clinic and 3 days later experienced an improvement of physical conditions, including a disappearance of numbness of the hands.
30 years old	The maxillary right first premolar and maxillary left first premolar were extracted for orthodontic treatment (expecting improvement of protrusion and TMD symptoms).
About after 3 years	Orthodontic treatment was completed. During treatment, symptoms were ameliorated, and there was a relapse after the appliance was removed. Although new crown restorations were completed for the left molars, the symptoms were not resolved.
37 years old	At the first visit to our clinic, she was suffering from symptoms including a sense of fatigue, a dull pain in the left eye, left shoulder stiffness, and migraine of the left side.

*The patient received a resin composite restoration in the maxillary right central incisor in her teens, after which various symptoms appeared. It is mere conjecture to determine to what extent it is related to current disease. Because there are many suggestive episodes, an excerpt from the patient's record is presented.

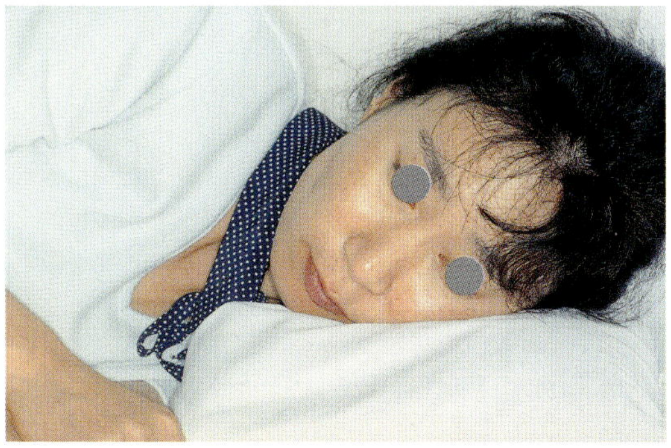

Fig 2-169 The patient was sleeping on her left, placing her hand under her pillow, intentionally shifting the mandible to the right.

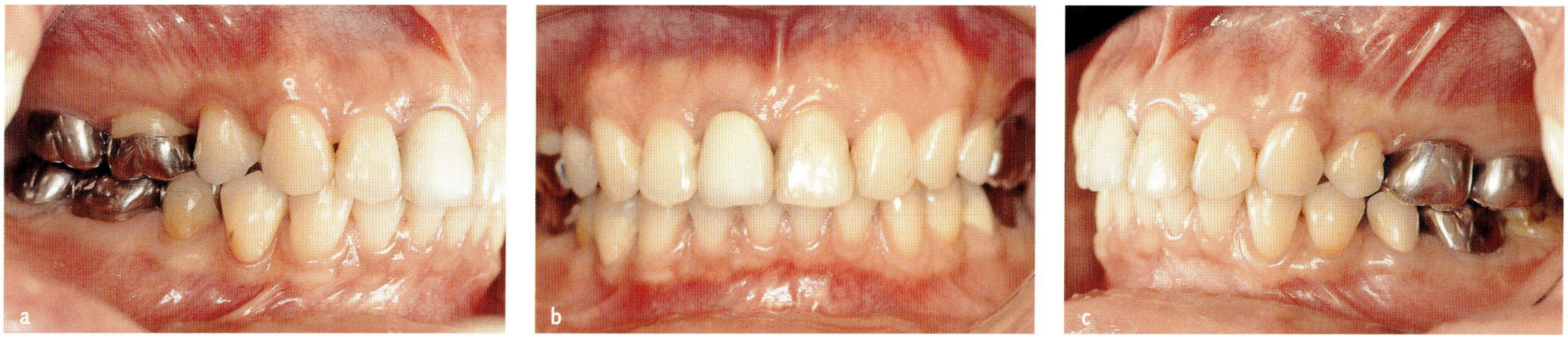

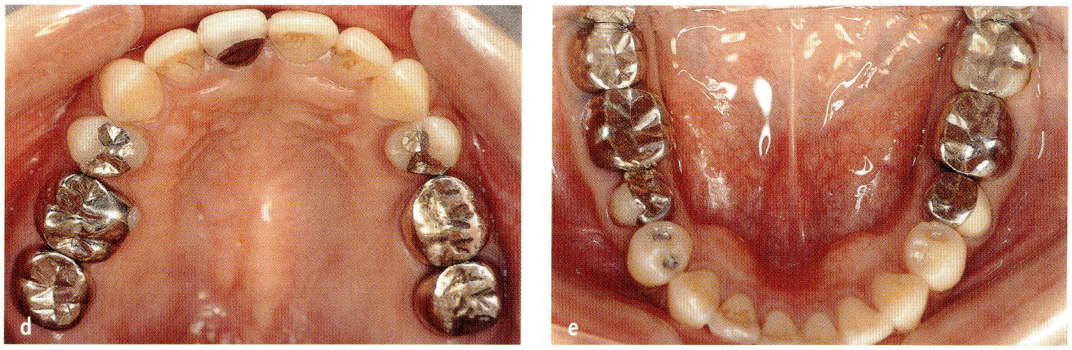

Fig 2-170 (a to e) Clinical conditions at the first visit. A thick metal-ceramic crown at maxillary right central incisor is noted at first glance.

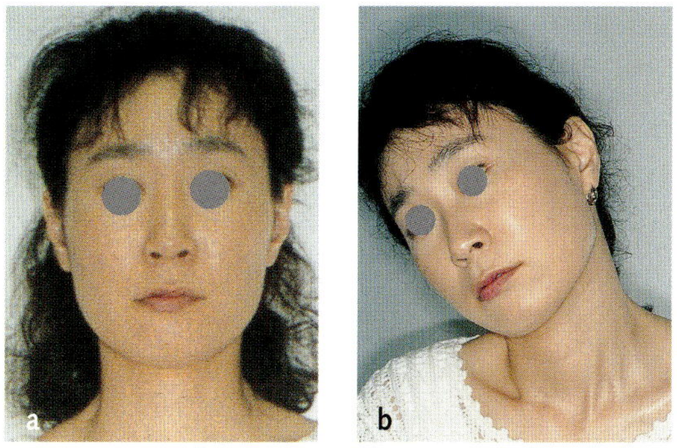

Fig 2-171 Generally, the mandible is often shifted to the side with symptoms, and the vertical dimension is lower on the same side. (a and b) This patient intentionally inclines her head to the right and chews on the right side, because the mandibular shift to the left causes worsening of various symptoms. If the metal-ceramic crown on the maxillary right central incisor contacts the mandibular anterior teeth, it is concluded that the mandible is rotated to the left and posterior direction and confined. Although systemic symptoms are located on the left side of the body alone, the frontal view of the face seems to exhibit development of the right masseter and a shift to the right.

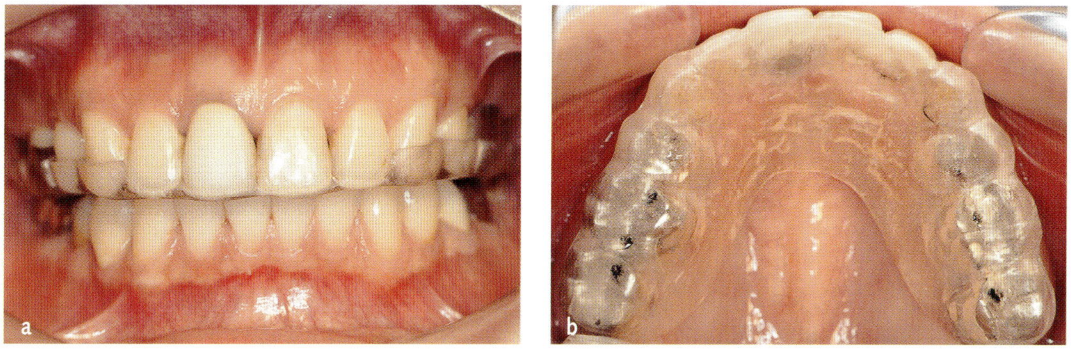

Fig 2-172 (a and b) Photographs taken 2 months after the first visit. A stabilization-type splint had been delivered at the second visit. By the third visit (2 weeks after the first visit), the unpleasant symptoms had disappeared and an increase in body weight was noted. The maxillary right central incisor showed mobility. Occlusal contacts on the left molars were lost.

Box 2-20 Patient complaint of "high bite"

When a patient claims "the bite is high," this means that he or she has a strong perception of sensitivity of the periodontal ligament. When one of the condyles is poorly developed or has a large articular space, a patient is likely to claim a high bite because burden of the periodontal ligament becomes stronger on the same side. If an area is ground for adjustment, as the patient often requests in such a case, naturally symptoms will be aggravated.

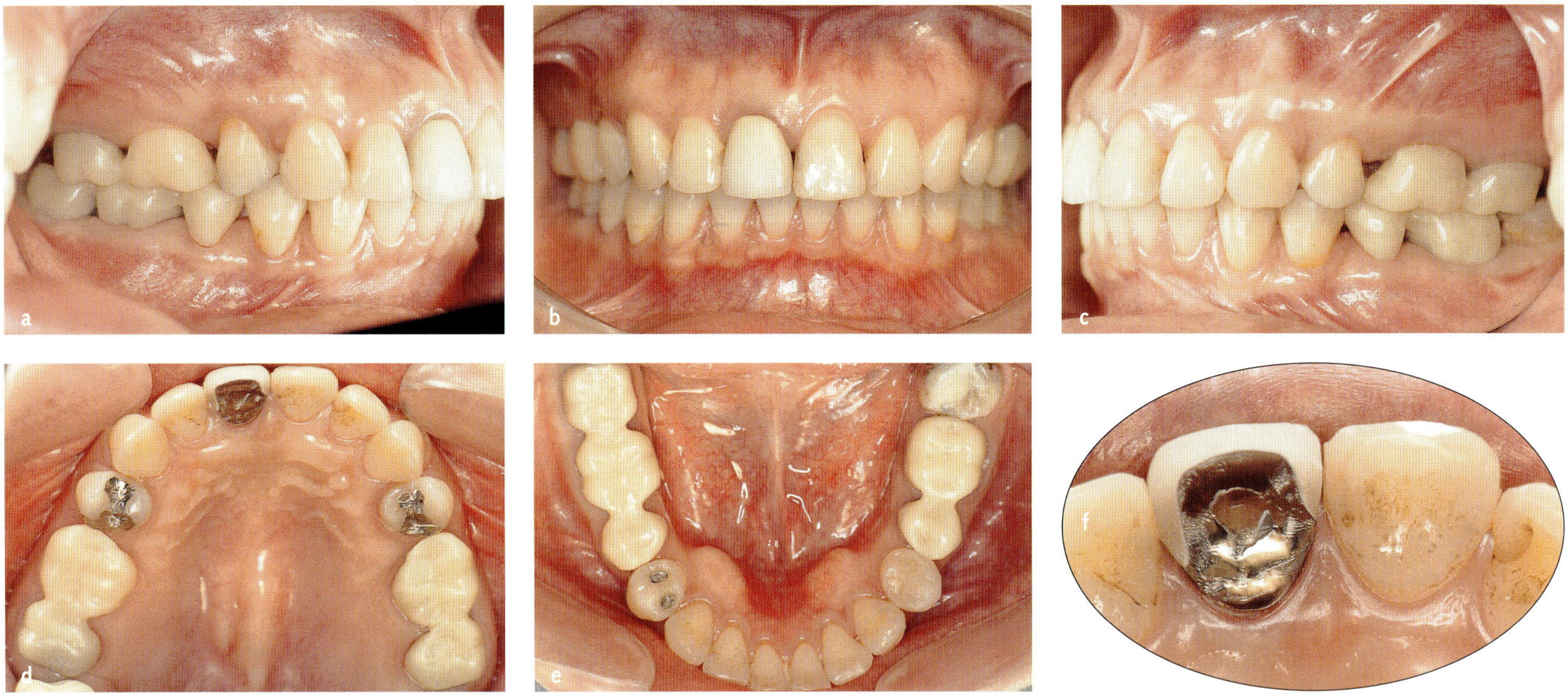

Fig 2-173 (a to f) Photographs taken 1 year 1 month after the first visit. The provisional restoration has been delivered. The patient is allowed to relax and tap, and for the areas where occlusal contacts have been lost, resin is added. With this treatment, the mandible returns to the right and the left vertical dimension increases. Generally, when a resin provisional restoration is replaced by metal, occlusal contacts at the molars become less tight. This is presumed to occur because muscles, the jawbone, and the TMJs are released from previously compacted conditions as food-cutting efficiency is improved and vertical interarch distance is increased.

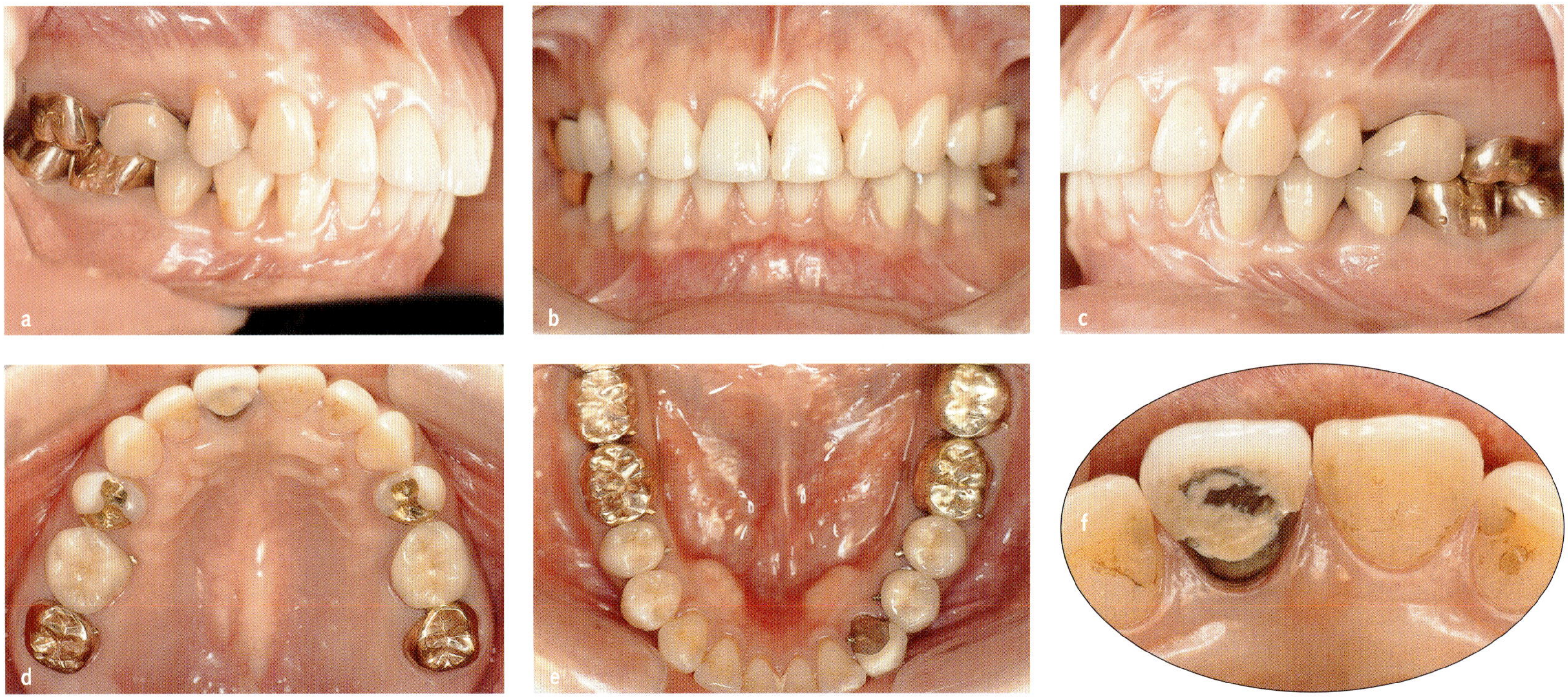

Fig 2-174 (a to e) Photographs taken 1 year 8 months after the first visit. Because the occlusal surface has been replaced by metal in the final prostheses, the vertical interarch dimension is further increased and molar occlusal contacts become less tight, adding stress on the maxillary right central incisor. Although these were intended to be final prostheses, eventually the final crowns for the mandibular left first and second molars were remade three times and the crown for the maxillary right central incisor was remade twice. (f) Photograph taken 1 year 11 months after the first visit. As we repeated adjustments, we ended up grinding the lingual surface.

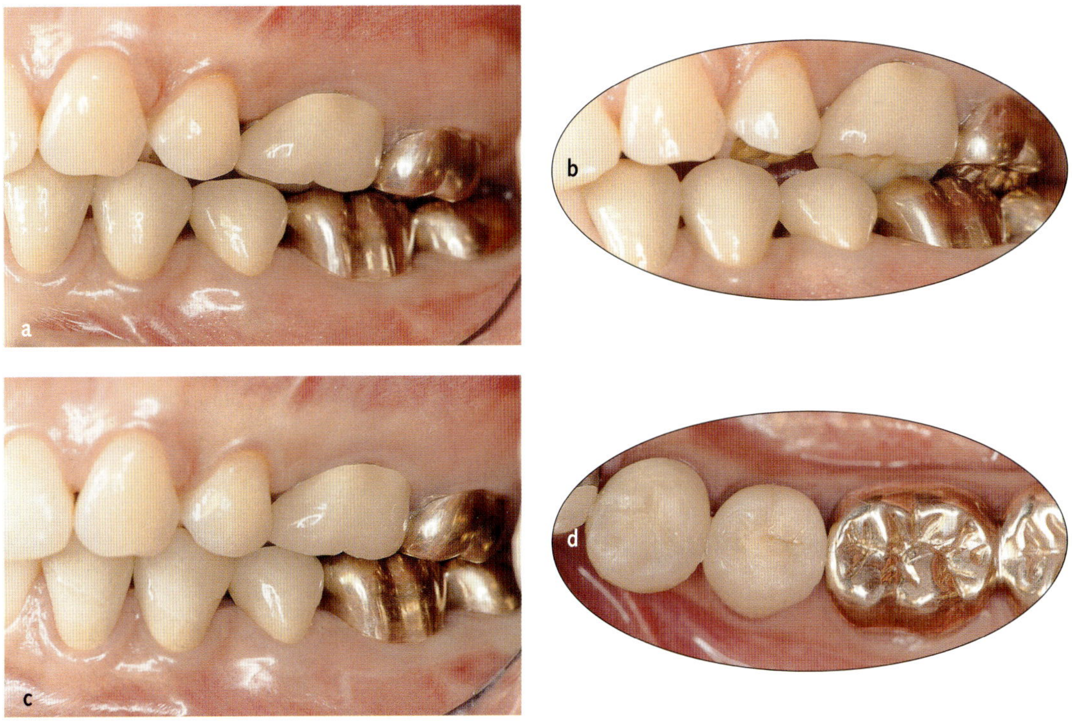

Fig 2-175 (a) Photograph taken about 3 years 1 month after the first visit. (b) The molar occlusal contacts became lost naturally. (c and d) Photographs taken about 3 years 3 months after the first visit. Resin composite has been added to the metal-ceramic crowns. It may seem as if we intentionally raised the bite on the left side, but rather material has been added several times to stabilize occlusion in accordance with remodeling of the body. The maxillary and mandibular midlines agree with each other, and the overlap is shallower.

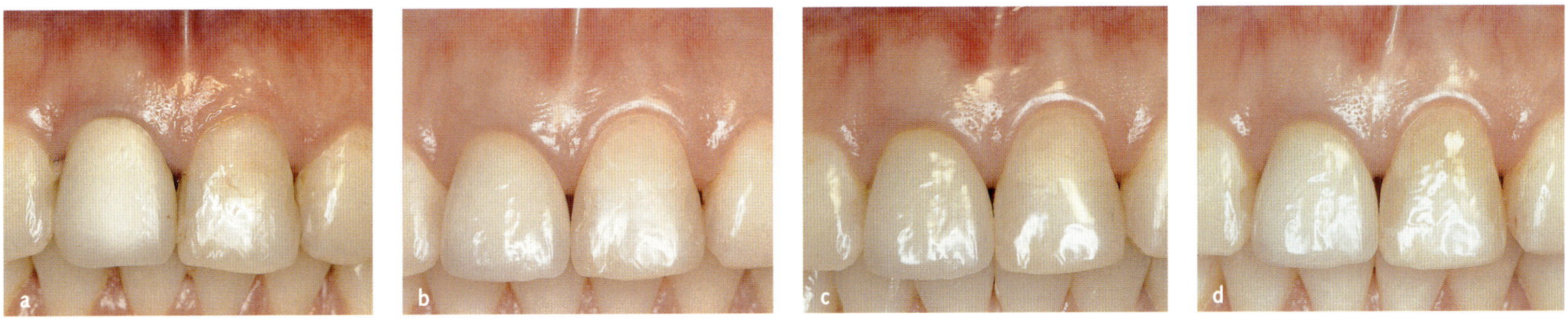

Fig 2-176 (a) Photograph taken at the first visit (1996). (b) Photograph taken 1 year 8 months after the first visit. (c) Photograph taken 3 years 6 months after the first visit. The maxillary and mandibular midlines are meeting with each other, and the overlap is shallower. Although the midlines agree, the gingival margin of the maxillary right central incisor is positioned slightly coronally. (d) Photograph taken 5 years 11 months after the first visit. Regarding the lingual inclination of the maxillary right central incisor, lateral incisor, and canine, it was found that the patient had a habit of exerting force in the right corner of the mouth (Box 2-21). This habit caused the lingual inclination.

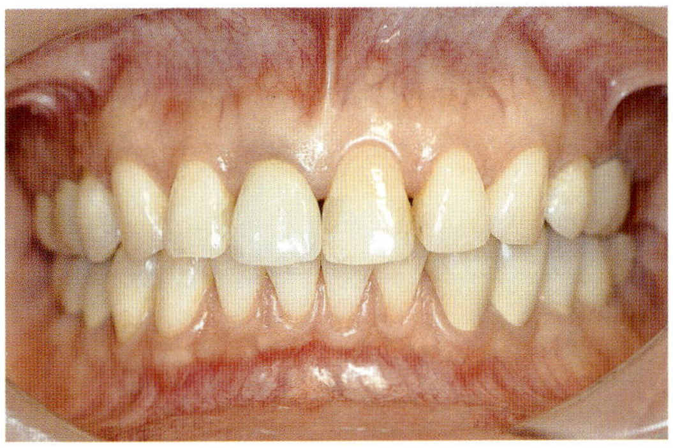

Fig 2-177 Photograph taken 5 years 11 months after the first visit. At 4 years 2 months, restorations for the maxillary right first and second molars, mandibular right first and second molars, and mandibular left canine, first premolar, second premolar, first molar, and second molar were newly fabricated. Compared to the condition at the first visit, the maxillary right canine is linguoverted, showing a discrepancy of the gingival margins of the maxillary central incisors. This has been caused by the patient's habit of exerting force in the right corner of the mouth.

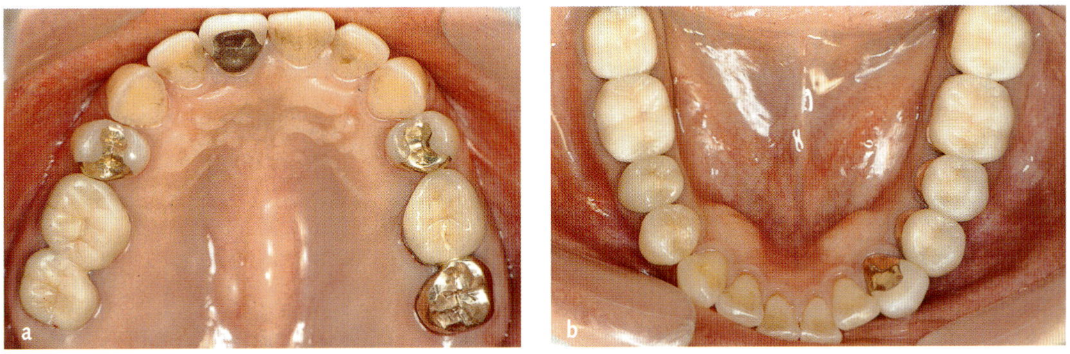

Fig 2-178 (a and b) Photographs taken about 5 years 5 months after the first visit.

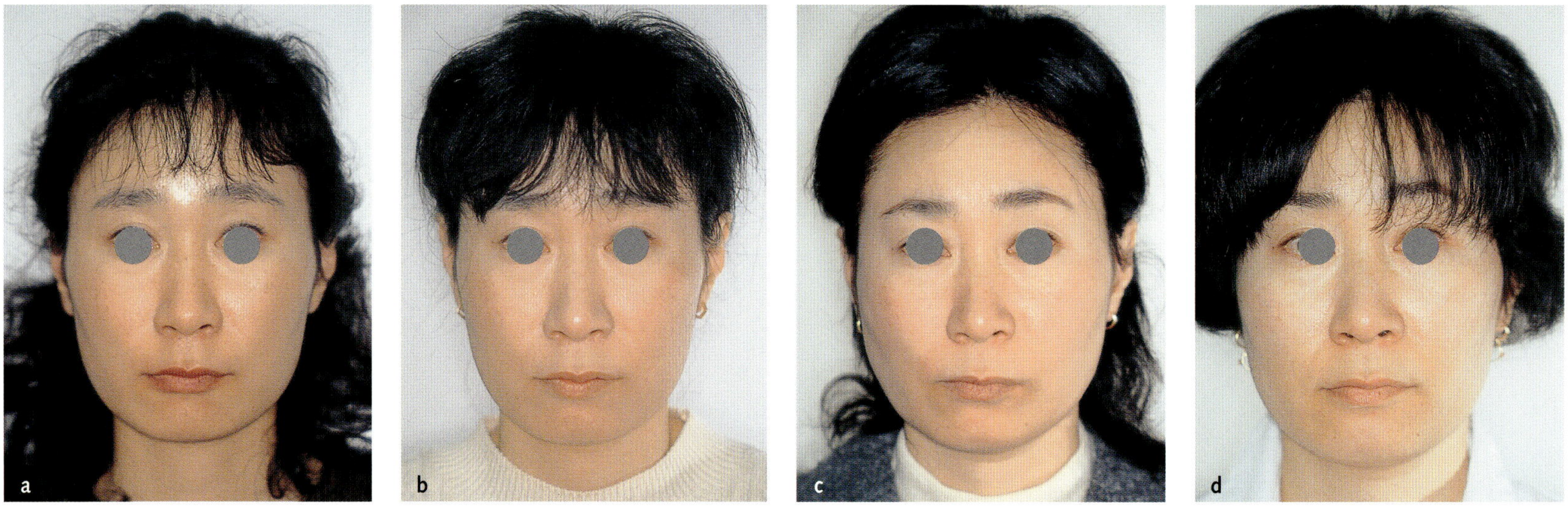

Fig 2-179 Facial appearance (a) 4 months after the first visit, (b) 2 years 7 months after the first visit, and (c) 5 years 5 months after the first visit. Her habit of exerting force in the right corner of the mouth has caused a deformity of the maxillary arch, including linguoversion of the maxillary right canine and an imbalance of the gingival margins of the maxillary central incisors. (d) Appearance after about 6 years. She has regained a calm face.

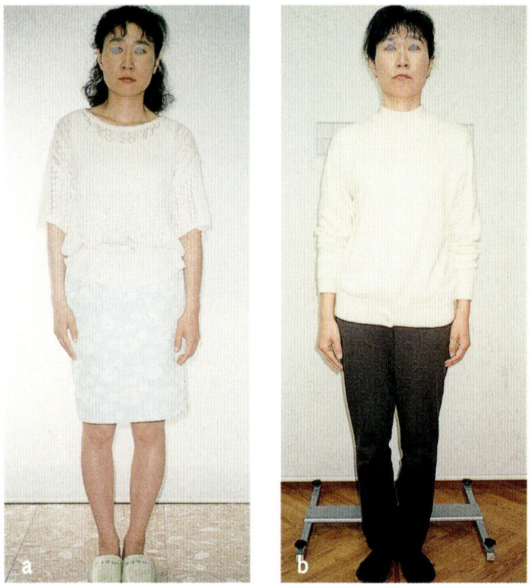

Fig 2-180 Posture (a) at the first visit, and (b) after 2 years 5 months. The body trunk has become straight.

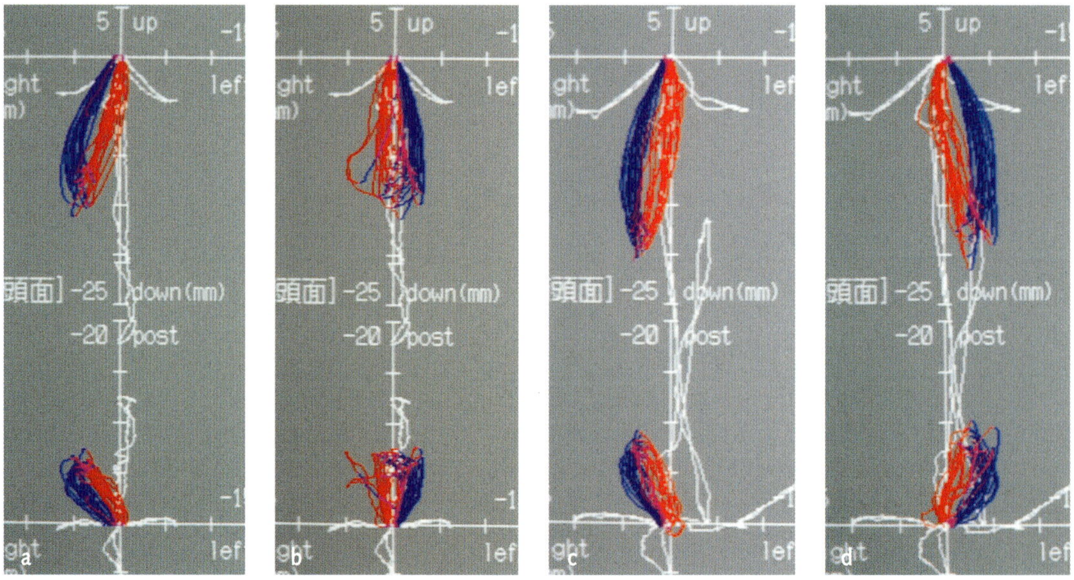

Right-side chewing 1 month after the first visit.

Left-side chewing 1 month after the first visit.

Right-side chewing about 2 years 5 months after the first visit.

Left-side chewing about 2 years 5 months after the first visit.

Fig 2-181 Change in masticatory movements as shown by Sirognathograph. (a and b) Frontal plane *(top)* and transverse plane *(bottom)* shortly after the first visit. ICP is mostly stable, and the mandibular movement analyzer does not show a problem in the mandibular position. When a patient bites into a habitual position, ICP appears to be stable. (c and d) Frontal plane *(top)* and transverse plane *(bottom)* after treatment. Compared to the situation at the first visit, chewing has become dynamic. The mandible has returned to the right, and the vertical dimension is increased.

Box 2-21 Change in the mandibular position

A long-term change in occlusion should be taken for granted as a part of systemic remodeling. However, careful attention should be paid to these changes, because sometimes a new detrimental habit may be detected.

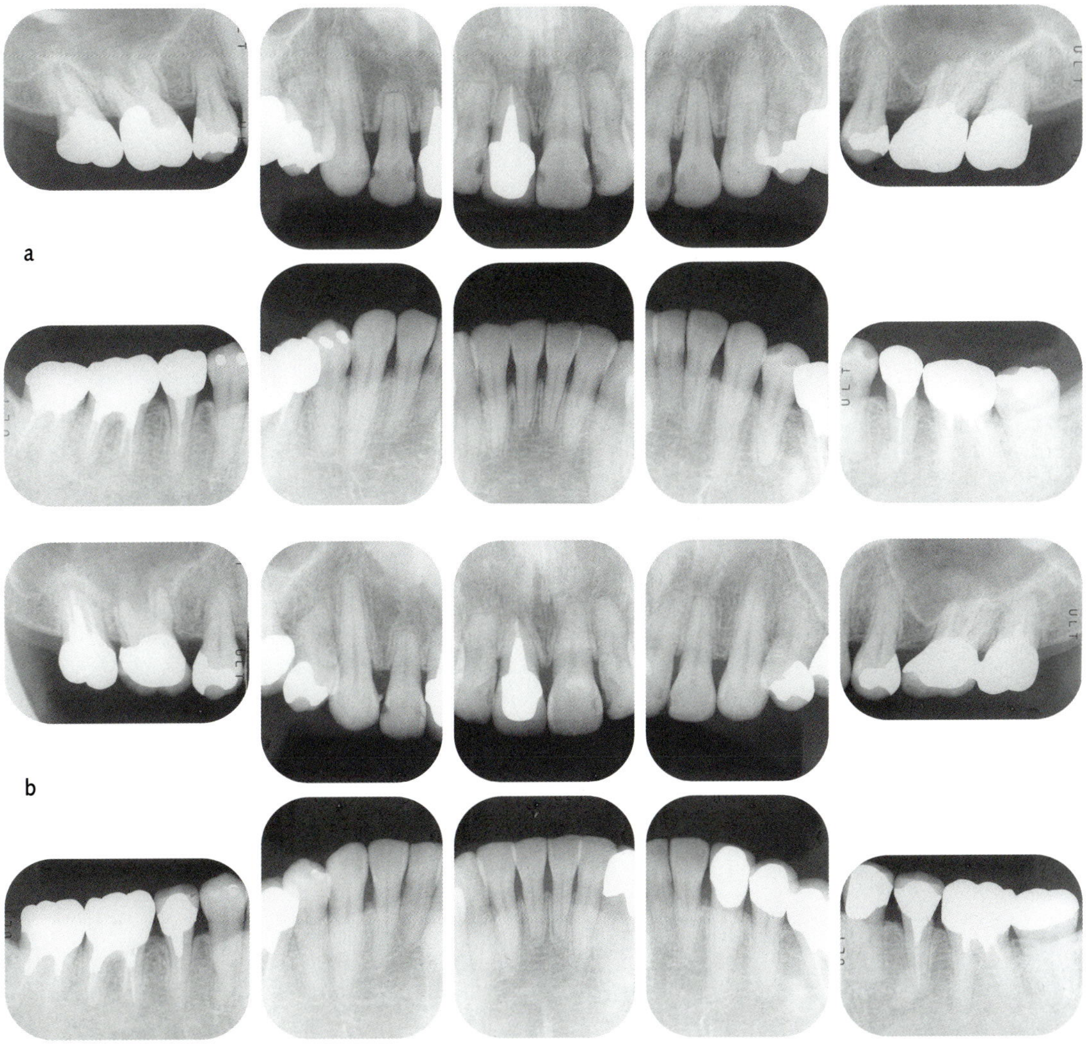

Fig 2-182 (a) Radiographs taken at the first visit. (b) Radiographs taken 2 years 1 month after the first visit.

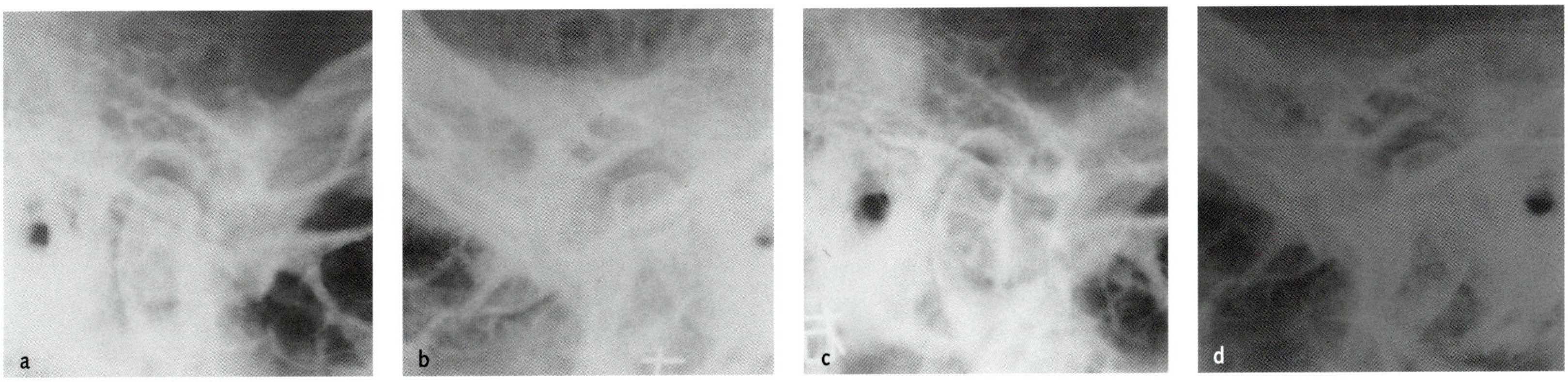

Fig 2-183 Transcranial plain radiographs (at ICP). (a) Right and (b) left TMJs at the first visit. (c) Right and (d) left TMJs about 1 year 11 months after the first visit.

Disc Displacement, Arthralgia, and Myalgia

Figure 2-185 is a schematic representation of the types of disc displacement. Cases 2-12 to 2-17 show the treatment of patients with various conditions affecting the TMJ.

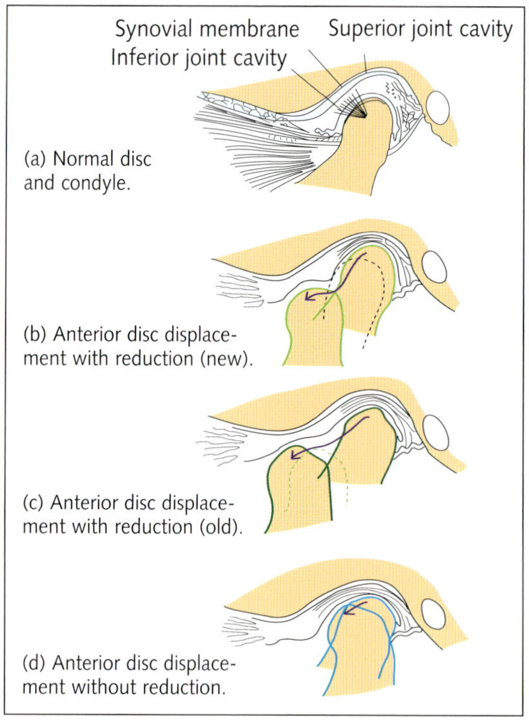

Fig 2-184 Displacement of disc and condyle and process of changes.

Case 2-12 Angle Class II malocclusion with anterior disc displacement with reduction

Patient: *21-year-old woman at the time of first visit in 1993*

Chief complaint: *Gingivitis and malalignment of the teeth, as well as clicking of the left TMJ at opening and closing*

She reported that she had experienced a disturbance of mouth opening for 2 or 3 years, but conditions were left untreated because there was no pain. It was surmised that the cause was the mandibular shift to the left, which compensated for linguoversion of the maxillary right lateral incisor (Fig 2-186). Still, the patient had the habits of sleeping in a prone position on her right and resting her cheeks on her hands, and it was concluded that these habits caused an off-the-disc condition of the left TMJ (Fig 2-187). She had a Class II, division 1 malocclusion (ANB = 6.0 degrees; IM = 96.5 degrees; maxillary incisor–sella-nasion angle = 113.0 degrees).

Discontinuation of the habits was a priority. After linguoversion of maxillary right lateral incisor was reduced, a splint was used to put the condyle on the disc. Although it was known that the mandible came forward after the condyle was on the disc, the final mandibular position was not yet known. Therefore, when the mandibular position was almost determined, a judgment had to be made whether the anterior teeth should be moved distally to fill extraction spaces or the molars should be moved mesially.

After extraction of the four first premolars, full brackets were applied for leveling (Fig 2-188). Later, a repositioning splint was delivered to put the left condyle on the disc. As gradual setback was observed, the final mandibular position for occlusal reconstruction was determined (Figs 2-189 to 2-193).

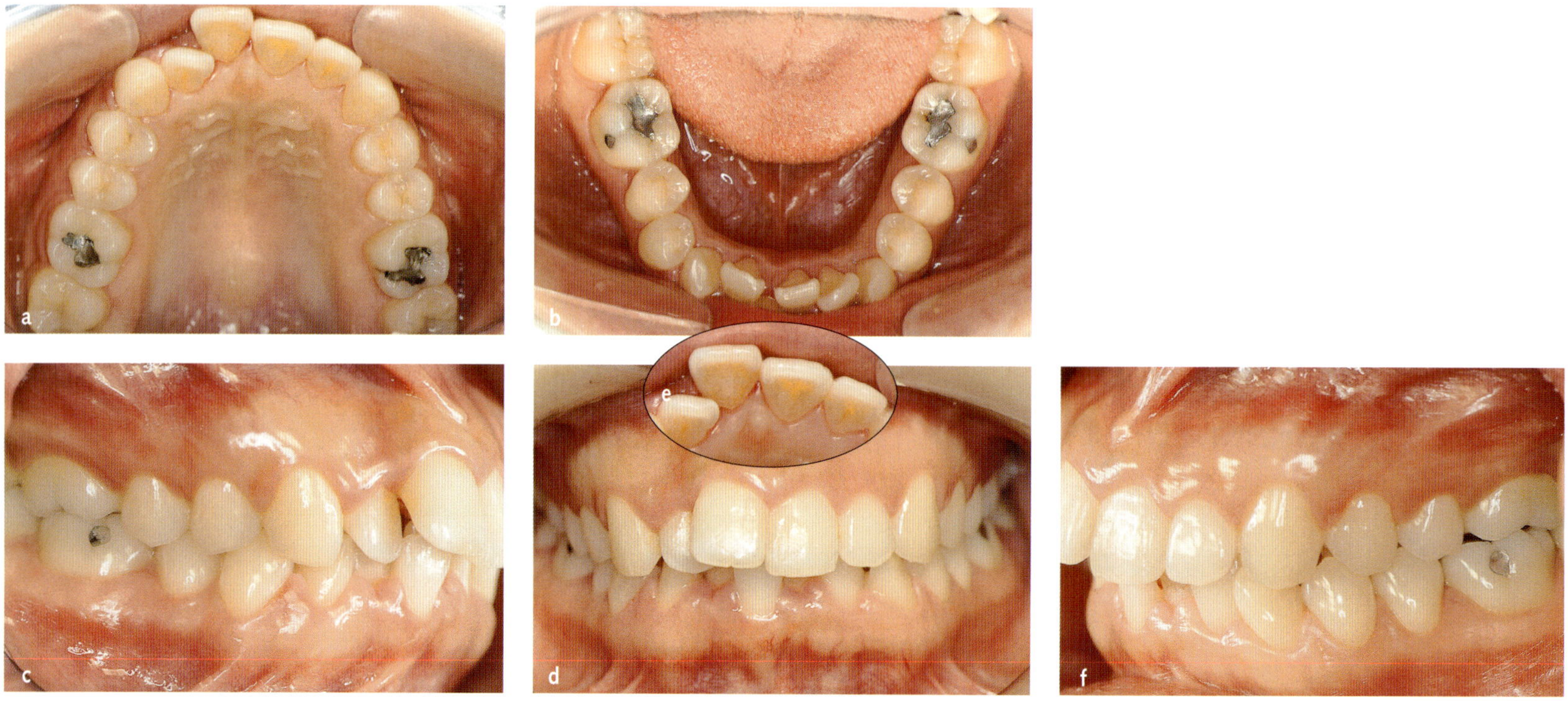

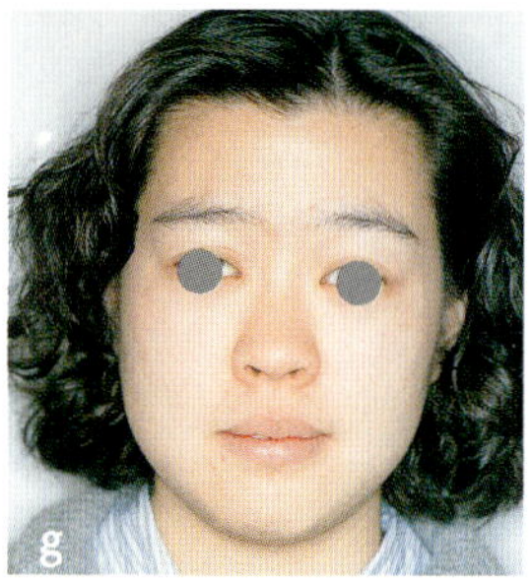

Fig 2-185 At the first visit. (a to f) Linguoversion of the maxillary right lateral incisor, labial inclination of the maxillary right central incisor, crowding of the mandibular anterior teeth, and different tooth axes of the maxillary canines are noted. It is suspected that lateral forces are being applied from both the right and the left. Linguoversion of the right side is especially notable, suggesting that some habit applies force from the right side. Tooth extraction is inevitable in this Class II, division 1 case. (g) The face shows the mandibular shift to the left. The left eye is in a lower position, the left corner of the mouth is in a higher position, and there is a decrease of vertical dimension on the left side.

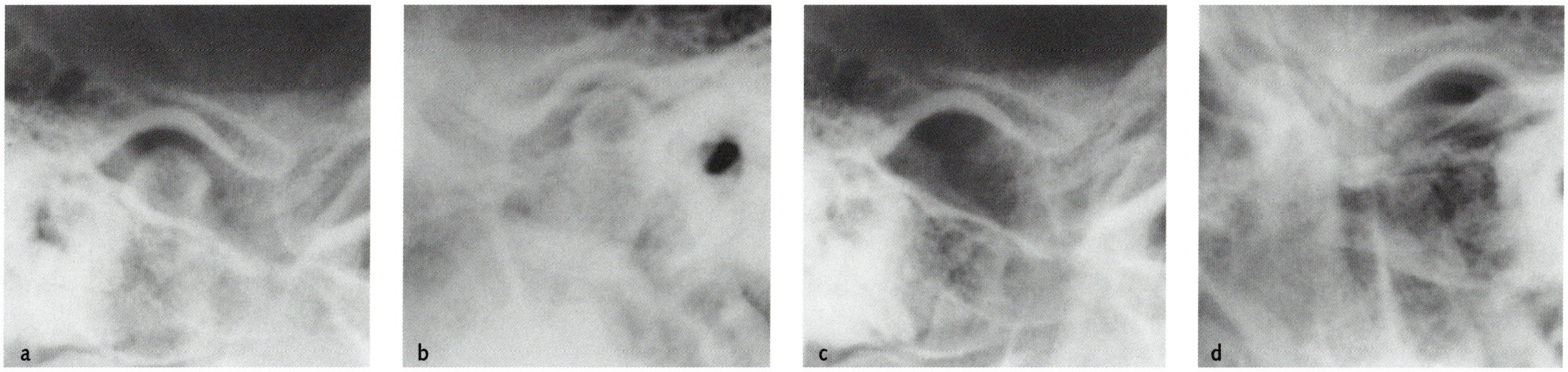

Fig 2-186 Radiographs of TMJs at the first visit. The posterior joint space of the left TMJ is narrow, and the condyle is pushed backward. (a) Right TMJ at ICP. (b) Left TMJ at ICP. (c) Right TMJ at maximal opening. (d) Left TMJ at maximal opening.

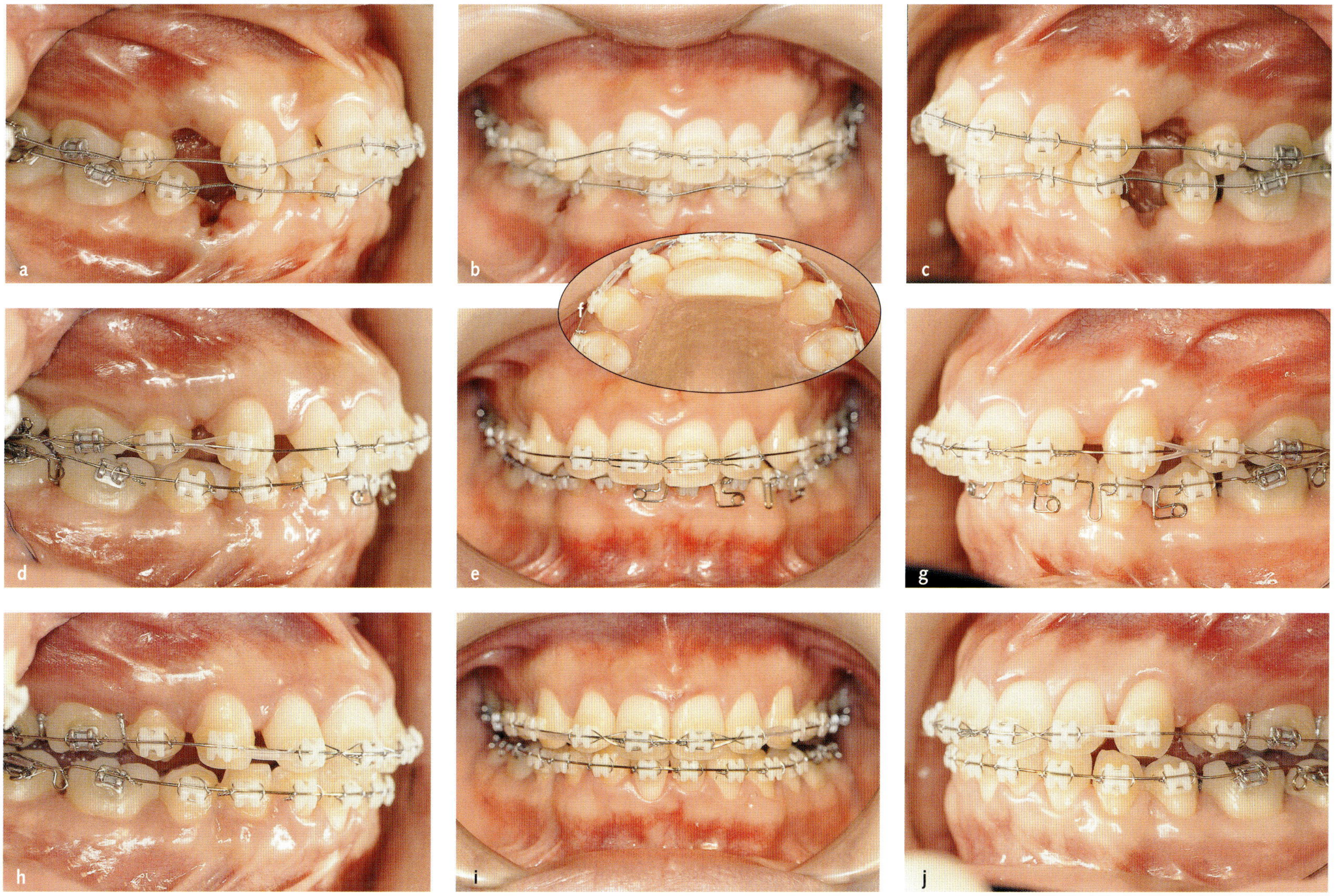

Fig 2-187 Multibrackets are delivered for the maxillary and mandibular arches. (a to c) Leveling. (d to g) To resolve crowding, the maxillary right and left canines are distalized. A repositioning splint is used to put the left condyle on the disc. (h to j) After the mandibular position has been mostly determined (1 year 2 months after the first visit), the buccal teeth are moved mesially, because they have been distalized too much.

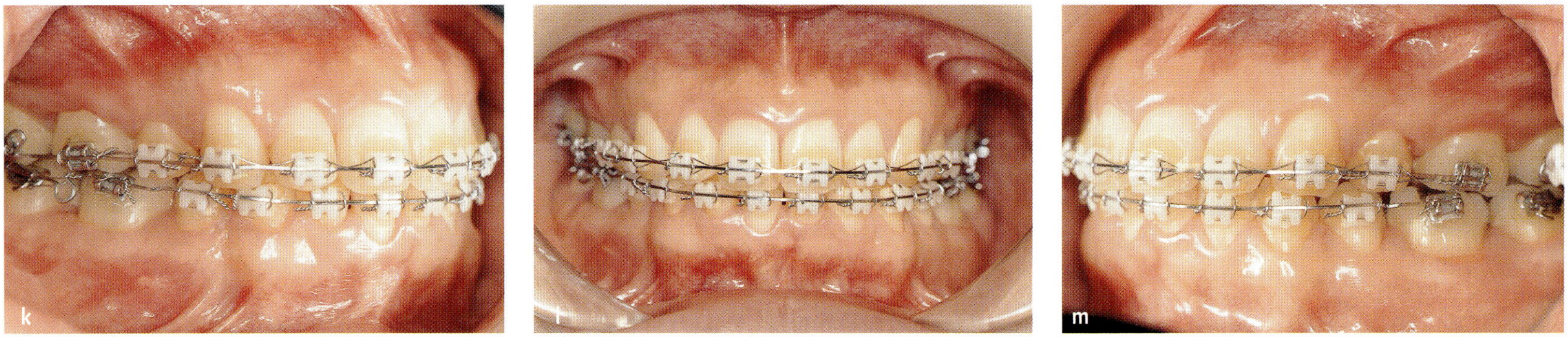

Fig 2-187 (cont) (k to m) Rectangular wire is used for finishing. The multibrackets were debonded after 2 years 9 months.

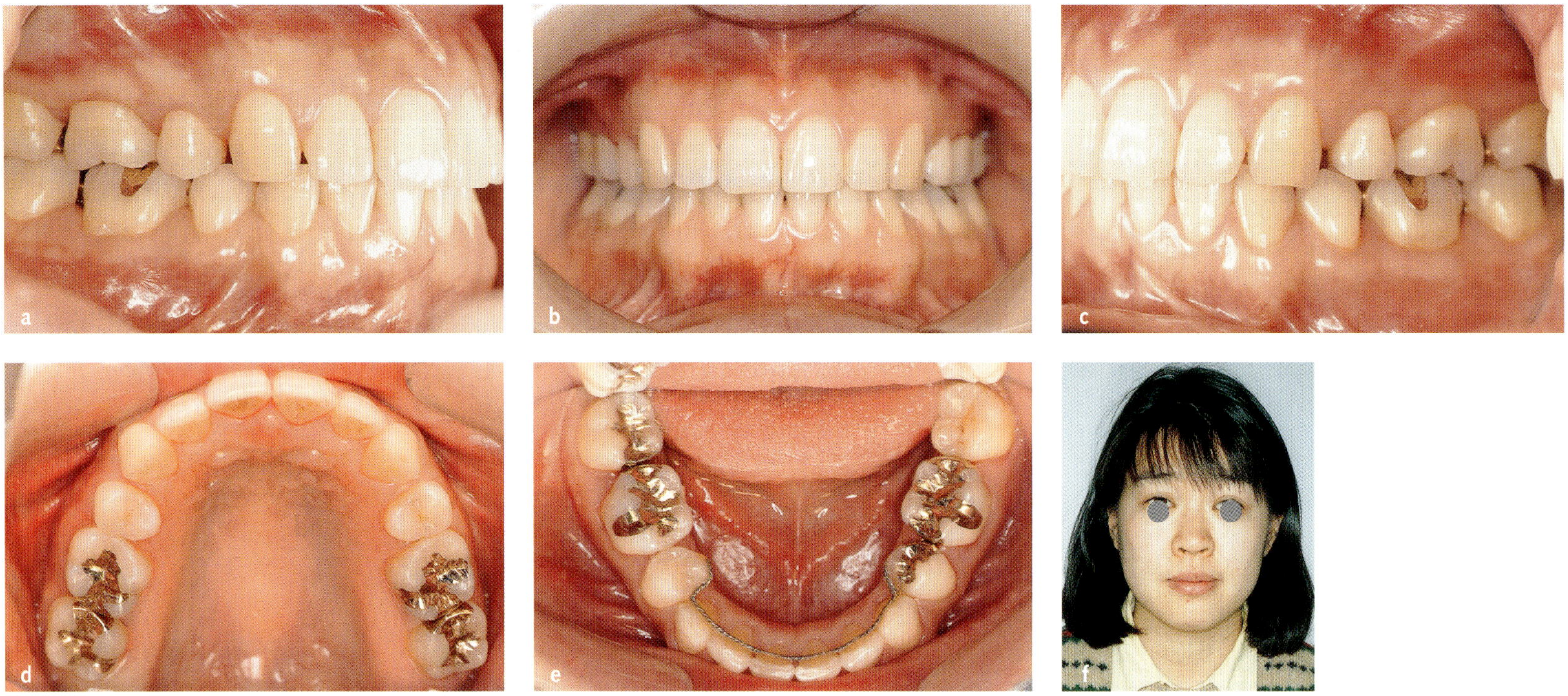

Fig 2-188 Posttreatment follow-up, 2 years 2 months after completion of active movement. (a to e) A retainer with a flap is used at night. Although the mandibular gingival margin and the width of attached gingiva had not been aligned when tooth malalignment was corrected, they have become well arranged after 3 years. (f) The face shows improvement of the previously shortened vertical dimension of occlusion on the left side.

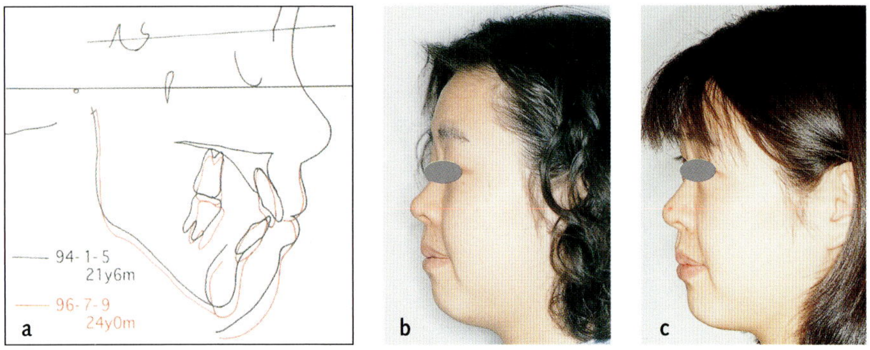

Fig 2-189 Profile views. (a) Tracings of the cephalograms before *(black)* and after *(red)* treatment show advancement of the mandible by 1.5 mm (ANB = 4.5 degrees). This is almost a Class I occlusion. (b) Profile before treatment. (c) Because this was originally an Angle Class II occlusion, improvement of the profile is significant.

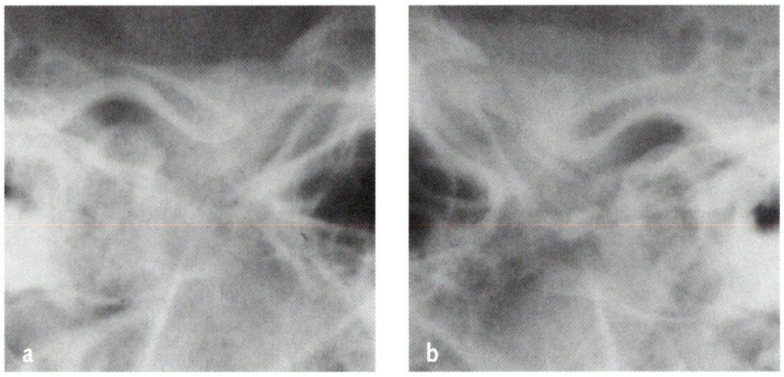

Fig 2-190 TMJ radiographs. Radiographs show that the TMJs are still unstable during orthodontic treatment (May 1996), 2 years 9 months after the first visit. (a) Right TMJ at ICP. (b) Left TMJ at ICP.

Fig 2-191 Comparison between functional movements around the time of the first visit and after 5 years. (a and b) About 1 month after the first visit. (a) During left-side chewing, the condyle is off the disc at maximal opening. (b) During right-side masticatory movements, on and off conditions are mixed. During opening from ICP, the left condyle comes off the disc and comes on the disc at about half opening, leading to the maximal opening. The patient says she intentionally speaks on the right side so that the condyle will not come off the disc. She knows this works for prevention. (c and d) After 5 years. Speed has not been developed yet, and the mastication is still somewhat unstable. Depending on how chewing is done, the condyle may come off the disc. Maximal opening path on the frontal plane, which used to be pulled to the left, shows improvement. However, opening and closing paths do not follow the same route, still being unstable. (c) Left-side chewing. (d) Right-side chewing.

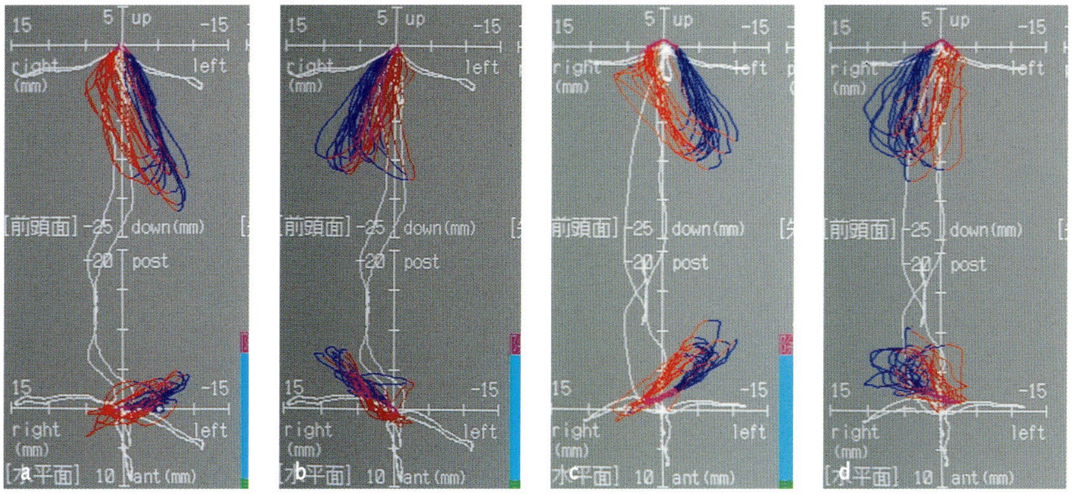

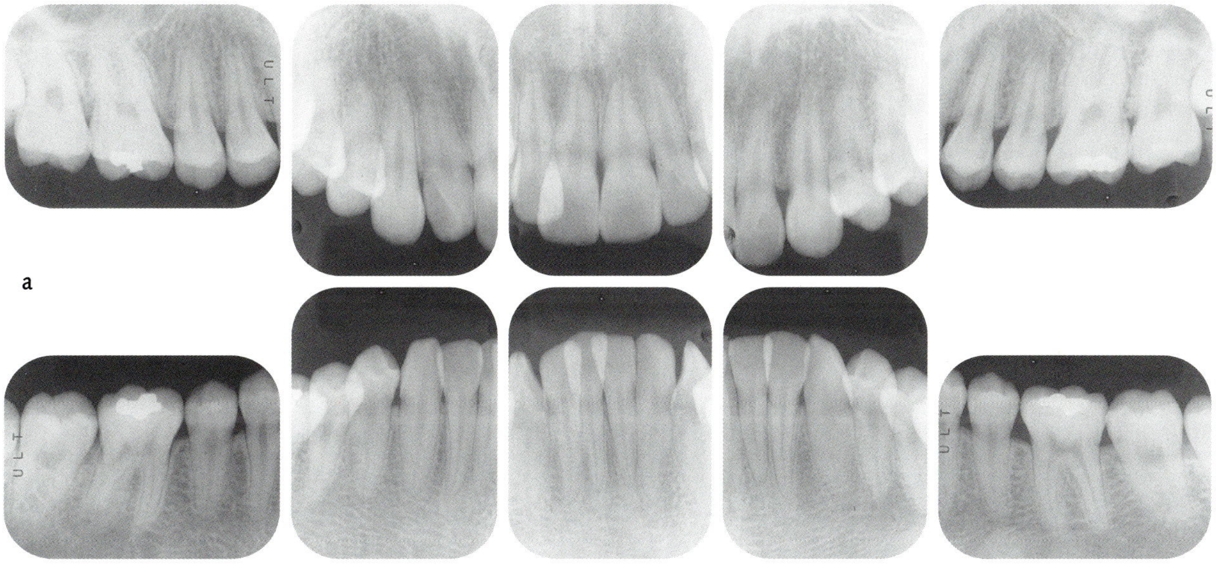

a

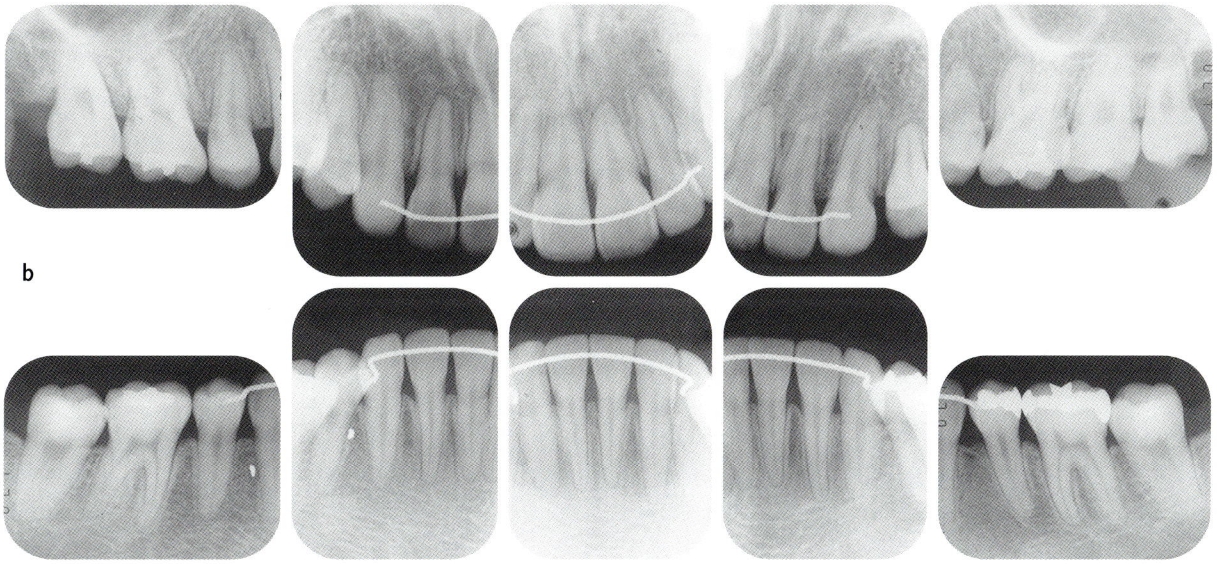

b

Fig 2-192 Full-mouth radiographs (a) at the first visit and (b) after 3 years 2 months. After the maintenance period started, the patient was instructed to chew more on the right side with a ratio of 7:3 between the right and the left. She was also advised to chew hard food on the right side, reconsider the position of her work desk, stop postural habits, and quit biting her lips. Often habits of posture and routine activities may relapse in the long-term. It is important that the patient understand the harmfulness of habits.

Case 2-13 Angle Class II malocclusion with anterior disc displacement with reduction

In an Angle Class II case with anterior disc displacement with reduction, if it is possible to place the condyle back on the disc, the abnormality in TMJ areas will diminish, occlusion will be improved more easily, and the profile will be improved without extraction. All of the joints, the occlusion, and the profile will be improved.

Patient: *56-year-old woman at the time of first visit in 1992*

Chief complaint: *Dislodgment of prostheses at the maxillary left lateral incisor and mandibular right first premolar*

The patient was aware of clicking of the right TMJ about 6 months before the first visit. She had neither pain nor other TMD symptoms. The right condyle was off the disc, which seemed to be because the condyle could not move to the left. Movement was prevented by the mesial inclination of the maxillary left second molar, which had resulted from a missing maxillary left first molar. Both the maxillary and mandibular arches were V shaped. Postural habits were not known. The mandibular left third molar also showed a mesial inclination because of a missing mandibular left second molar. She had a skeletal Class II malocclusion, ANB = 6.0 degrees, and she had a convex facial type. Her treatment is shown in Figs 2-194 to 2-200.

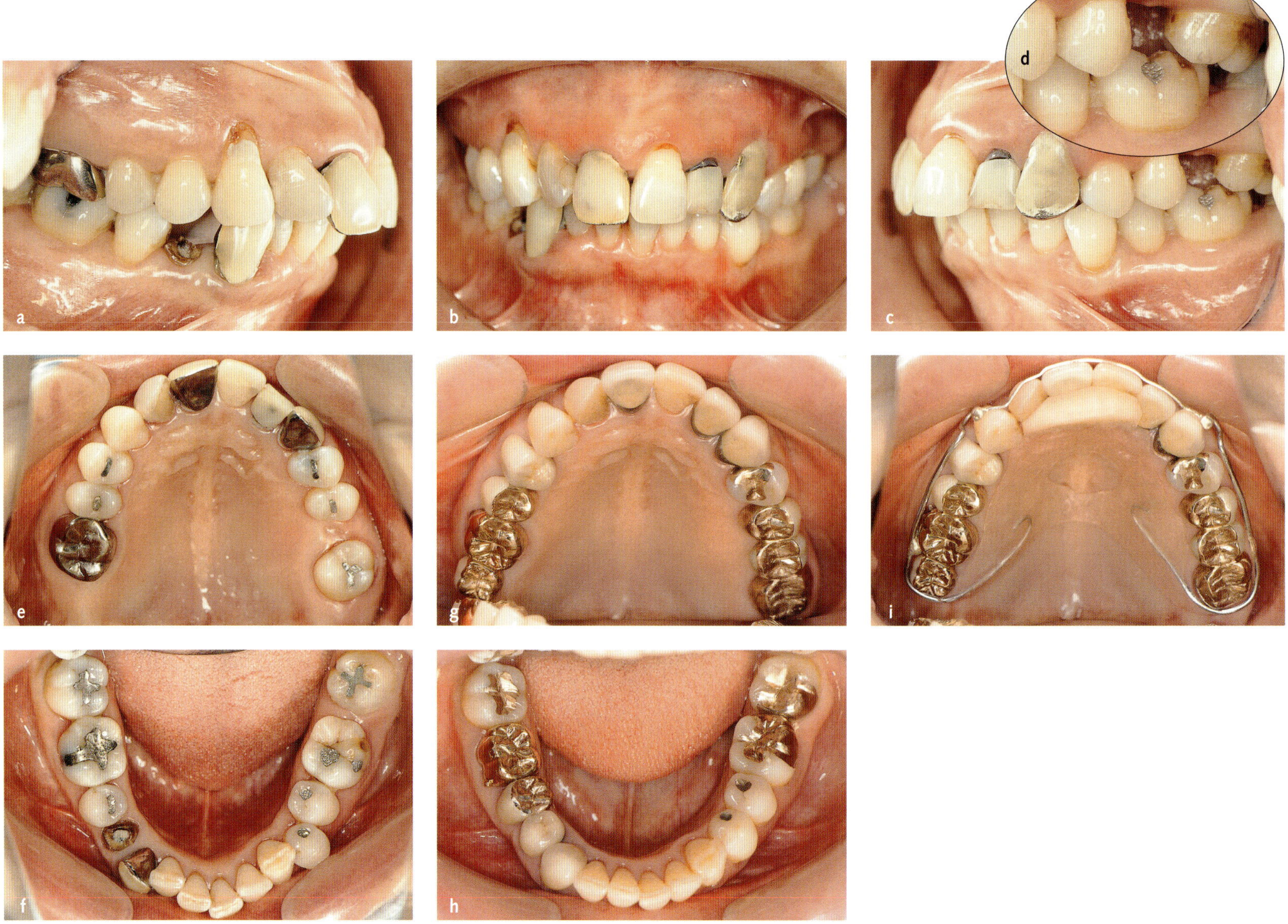

Fig 2-193 Improvement of the mandibular position and improvement of occlusion. (a to c) Clinical conditions at the first visit. (d) The distal cusp of the maxillary left second molar is deeply caught between the mandibular left first molar and the mandibular left third molar. (e and f) At the first visit, both the maxillary and mandibular arches are V shaped and constricted. (g to i) Photographs taken 7 years 2 months after the first visit, and 3 years 5 months after delivery of prostheses. Eleven months after the first visit, multibrackets were applied to the maxillary left first premolar, second premolar, and second molar and from the mandibular left second molar through the mandibular right second molar. The maxillary left second molar was uprighted, and a fixed partial denture was delivered extending from the maxillary left second premolar to the maxillary left second molar (pontic: maxillary left first molar). The mandibular left third molar was uprighted and the roots were advanced mesially so that the molar could participate in occlusion as a second molar. The arch was changed to a U shape. Orthodontic tooth movement was conducted for 1 year 6 months.

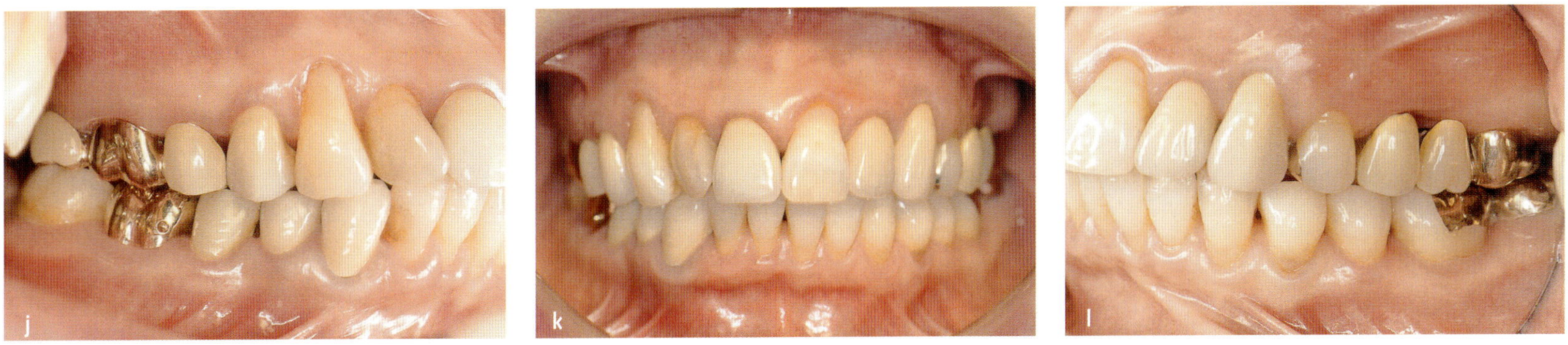

Fig 2-193 (cont) (j to l) Photographs taken 7 years 2 months after treatment. Crowding was resolved by disking of the mandibular left and right lateral incisors. The ANB angle has been reduced from 6.0 to 4.0 degrees.

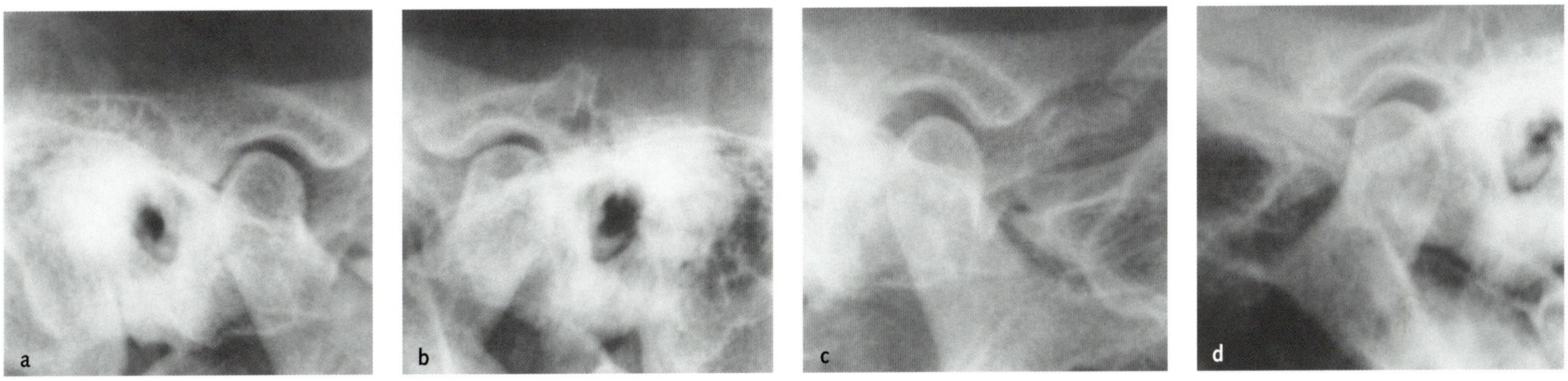

Fig 2-194 Radiographs of the (a) right and (b) left TMJs at the first visit. Radiographs of the (c) right and (d) left TMJs after orthodontic treatment; 3 months after delivery of the prostheses. The right condyle has moved anteriorly.

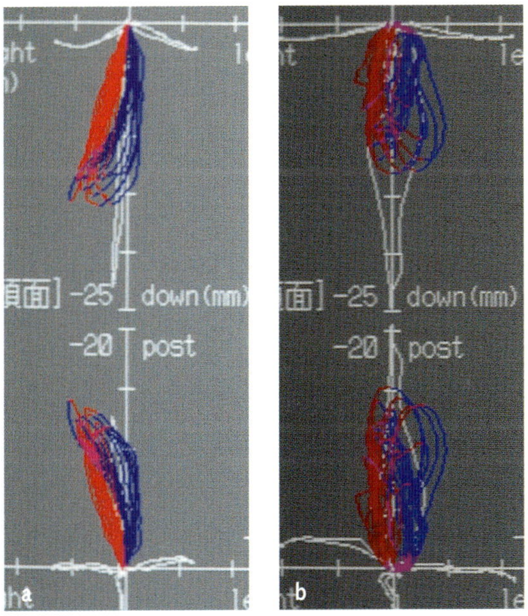

Fig 2-195 Masticatory movements. (a) Sirognathograph of left-side chewing 4 years after the first visit (March 1996). Although the condyle is on the disc at maximal opening, during function, all the turning points are on the right side, and mastication always takes place with condyles off the disc. (b) Sirognathograph made about 9 years after the first visit (February 2001). Although there is variability, turning points are on the left side, and during most of the mastication cycles the condyles are on the disc.

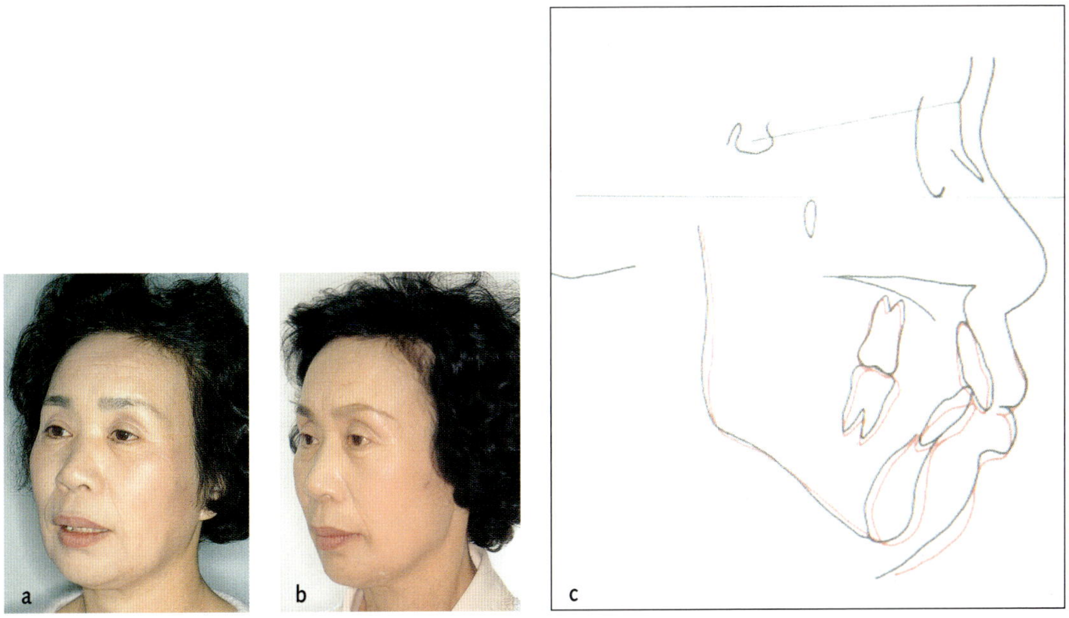

Fig 2-196 Changes in the face. (a) Appearance before treatment. (b) Appearance 6 years 5 months after the first visit. The ANB angle is 4.0 degrees, and the profile is improved. (c) Superimposition of preoperative *(black)* and postoperative *(red)* cephalogram tracings reveals advancement of the mandible and improvement of the profile.

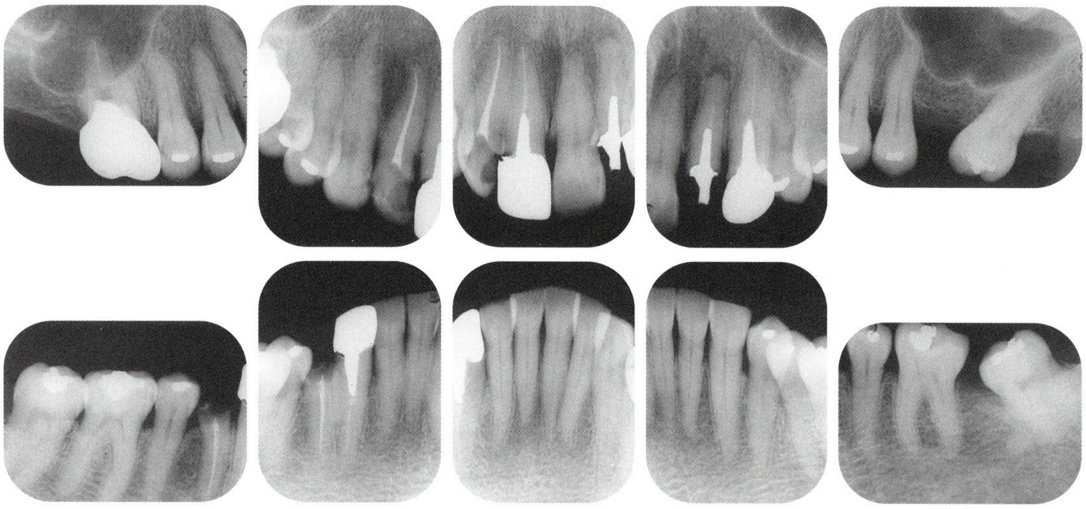

Fig 2-197 Radiographs taken at the first visit (January 1992).

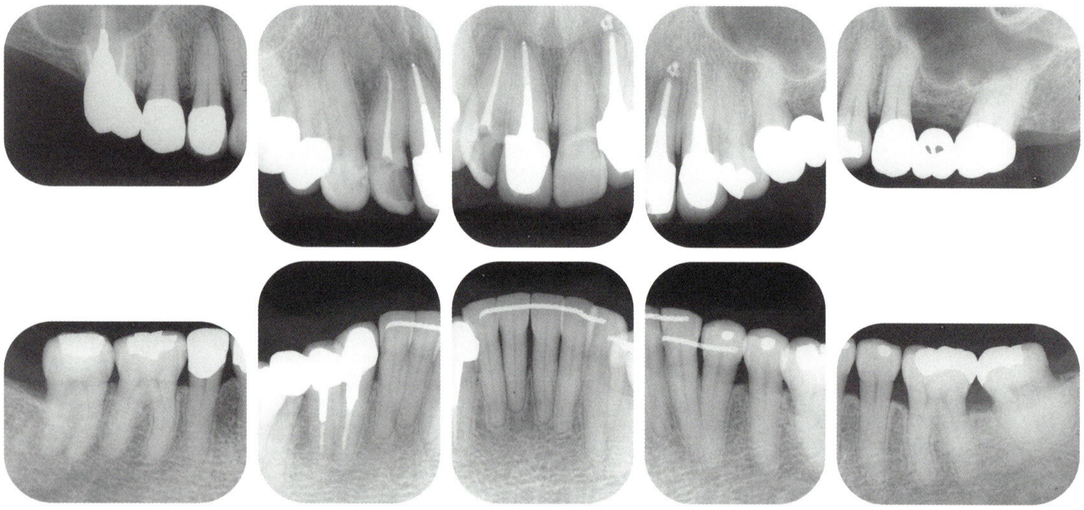

Fig 2-198 Radiographs taken after orthodontic treatment and completion of restoration (February 1996).

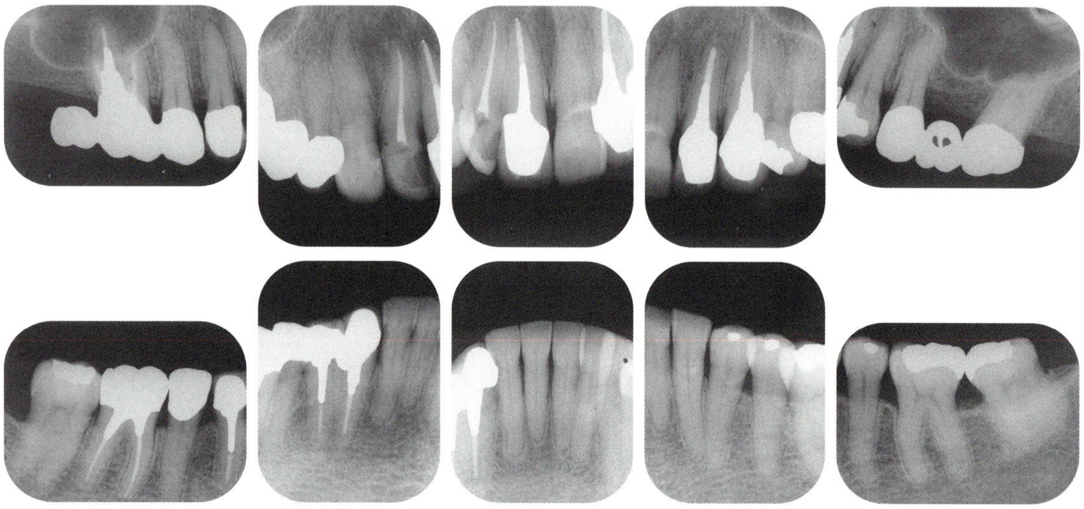

Fig 2-199 Radiographs taken 7 years 3 months after the first visit (April 1994).

Case 2-14 Angle Class III malocclusion with anterior disc displacement with reduction

Patient: *22-year-old woman at the time of first visit in 1998*
Chief complaint: *Trismus, pain of the right side during opening, and clicking of the right TMJ*
The patient had hypersensitivity at the cervical area of the maxillary right teeth. She had clicking and pain of the right TMJ during opening when she was 17 years old. At 17 and 18 years of age, she visited an oral surgeon. Although she received splint therapy, the symptoms were not alleviated.

A crossroads for occlusal reconstruction in an off-the-disc case is a degree of deformity and displacement of the disc. First, the posteriorly located condyle is brought back on the disc, and reconstruction of occlusion is considered on that position. In this particular case, the right molars indicated crossbite, which was misleading. However, treatment should be started with the search for a mandibular position with condyles on the disc. In this patient, the right condyle was off the disc. To bring the condyle back on the disc, the mandible was brought left and forward (Figs 2-201 to 2-215). Treatment of an Angle Class III case like this is difficult. The mandibular teeth have to be retruded while the condyles have to be pulled forward. Consequently, it is highly likely that the mandibular arch will require tooth extraction. The disc, which was pushed forward, and the condyle moved posterior and became stabilized after they acquired the on-the-disc condition.

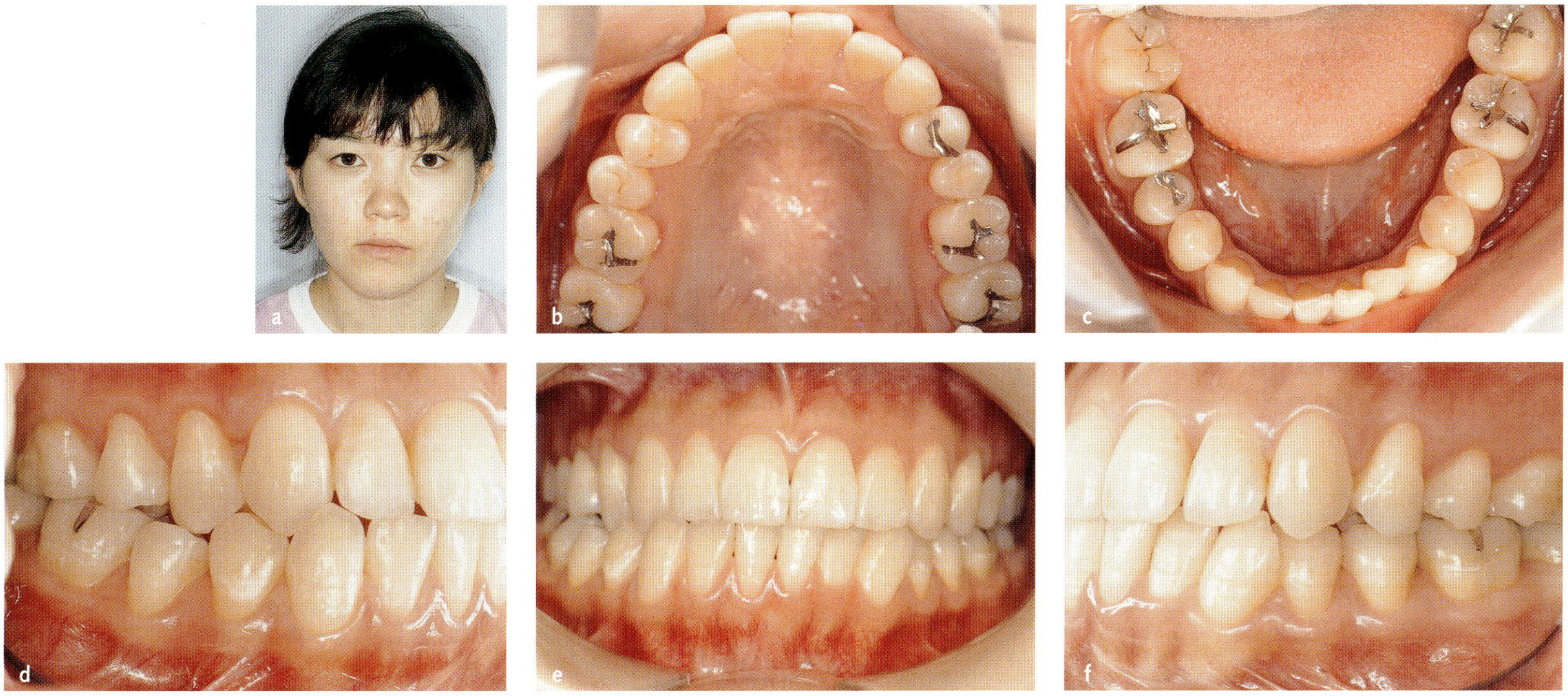

Fig 2-200 Photographs taken at the first visit. (a) This patient has a skeletal Class III malocclusion. The mandible is shifted to the right, and the vertical dimension is smaller on the right. The right masseter is tense, and the patient chews on the right side. The angle of the mouth is tilted and higher on the right side. The right and left eye lines and morphology are different. (b to f) At the first visit, the mandible is shifted to the right by 1.5 mm. Crossbite is observed for the maxillary right second premolar through the maxillary right lateral incisor and the mandibular right lateral incisor through the mandibular right second premolar. The overlap on the left side is normal but shallow, while the right side shows crossbite. Possibly because of some habit, the mandibular left canine through the mandibular right second molar are inclined to the left. Because of the low tongue, the maxillary arch width is narrow and the mandibular arch is large.

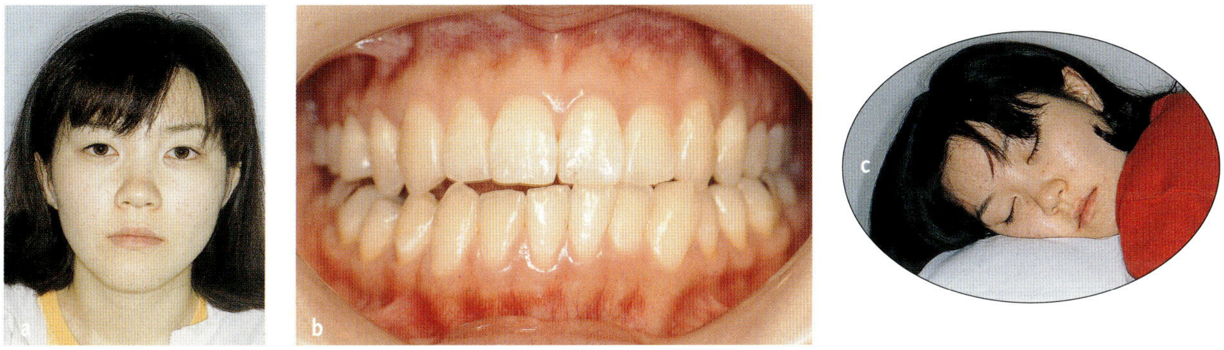

Fig 2-201 On the disc at the first visit. (a) Appearance of the face when the right condyle is brought on the disc at the first visit. The face as well as the shape and the lines of the eyes show symmetry. (b) The condyle is on the disc when the mandible is shifted to the left by 3.5 mm. Supposedly, the right side did not originally have crossbite, but the mandible was shifted to the right because the left side was unstable as a result of edge-to-edge occlusion of the left buccal teeth. (c) The patient has a habit of sleeping in a prone position on her right and a habit of resting the cheek on the right hand, causing the inclination of the mandibular teeth to the left.

It was surmised that the occlusion was not stable in this Class III patient because the mandibular arch was large compared to the maxillary arch (the low tongue and maxillary undergrowth), causing the mandible to shift in search of maximal occlusal contact and leading to unilateral crossbite. The mandibular arch was asymmetric with different occlusal planes for the right and the left sides, and the right side had a stronger curve of Spee because of habits. The mandibular arch had mild crowding. The patient had a habit of sleeping in a prone position on her right and a habit of resting the cheek on the right hand, which caused the inclination of mandibular teeth to the left.

When the mandible was shifted to the left by about 3.5 mm, after some clicking, smooth opening and closing were possible and pain was resolved. Hence, this case was diagnosed as disc displacement with reduction.

Treatment plans and procedures. *The mandible was shifted to the left to find a position that does not cause clicking, and the right condyle was brought on the disc so that reconstruction of occlusion could be considered in this position. With this movement, the width of the maxillary left buccal area became insufficient, and edge-to-edge occlusion of buccal teeth would result. Therefore, the left side of the maxillary arch was expanded while the mandibular position was maintained on the disc (basic treatment). It was hoped that this would stabilize occlusion. If not, one mandibular incisor would be extracted, the mandibular anterior teeth would be inclined lingually so that the mandibular arch would become smaller and to create an overlap and stabilize occlusion (definitive treatment).*

All of this was explained to the patient, and the treatment was started from the least invasive procedure.

Basic treatment of occlusion. *The patient was informed of the conditions of on and off the disc and instructed to routinely and intentionally bring the mandible to the on-the-disc position and intentionally chew on the left side in that position (tapping-like chewing).*

- *The patient was encouraged to discontinue her detrimental habits.*
- *The patient was given instructions about low tongue (and told to perform the intentional exercise of adhering the tongue in the palatal space every day).*
- *An appliance that served as both a repositioning splint and an appliance to expand the left side of the maxillary arch was delivered.*

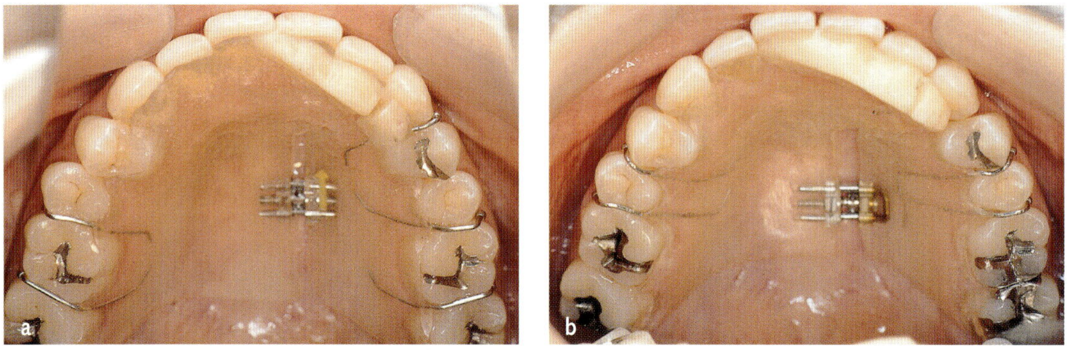

Fig 2-202 Repositioning splint and arch expansion appliance for the left part of the maxillary arch. After the appliance had been used for 10 months, clicking of the right TMJ diminished significantly. Disturbance of mouth opening as well as pain also decreased to the degree that they were no longer a concern for the patient. The right condyle was still off the disc at this time. (a) About 1 month after the first visit, a plate appliance with screws is applied to expand the area from the maxillary left canine to the maxillary left second molar. The appliance also serves as a repositioning splint. Because the patient wears this only at night due to her occupation, a one-quarter revolution is applied to the screws once a week. The appliance was used for 10 months and refabricated once during the period. (b) Photograph taken after the appliance for screw expansion and repositioning has been used for 10 months. About 2.5 mm of expansion has been achieved.

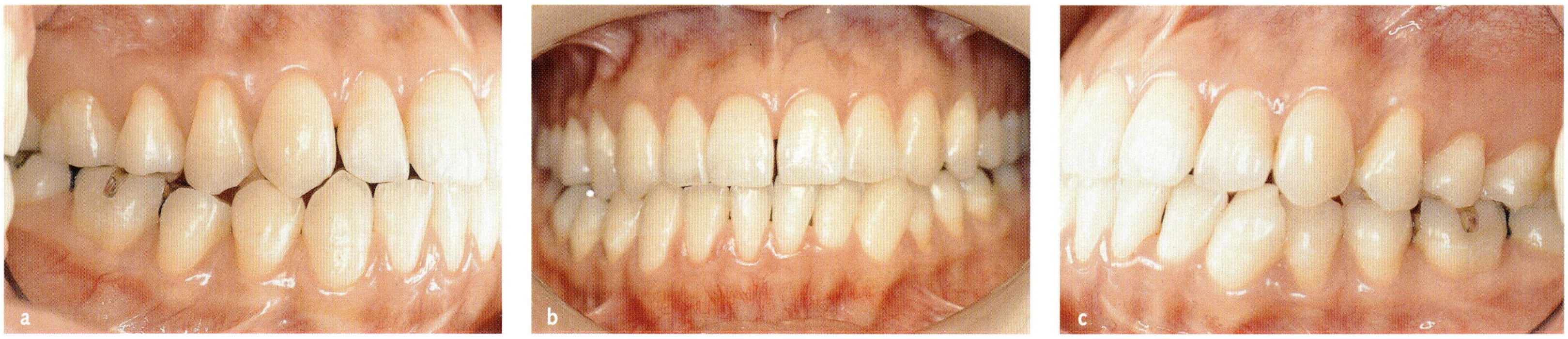

Fig 2-203 Decision-making for definitive treatment. If further stabilization of occlusion is desired, it is necessary to reduce the size of the mandibular arch so that mandibular anterior teeth will be aligned inside of the maxillary dentition, which can be achieved by extraction of the maxillary right second premolar, maxillary left second premolar, mandibular left first premolar, and mandibular right first premolar or by extraction of one mandibular incisor. Although the former approach will stabilize occlusion, it will require extraction of multiple teeth and a longer duration of treatment. The latter plan requires fewer teeth to be extracted, but occlusion is less likely to be stabilized. (a to c) Because the patient wanted further stabilization of occlusion, orthodontic treatment was conducted after tooth extraction. When the mandibular arch was made smaller and the anterior overlap was improved, clicking of the right TMJ disappeared and the condyle naturally came on the disc. Because of this irregular extraction, occlusion is Class III and not completely stabilized. Still, the condyle is mostly on the disc. As the root form of maxillary left first premolar became visible through the gingiva and gingival recession was started, it was judged as a limitation of expansion and the treatment was discontinued. The maxillary and mandibular midlines mostly agree, and the mandible has moved to the left by 1.5 mm. Because of this, clicking of the right TMJ has been reduced to a weak level. Although the condyle is still off the disc, discomfort disappeared. The facial shift to the right has also been reduced.

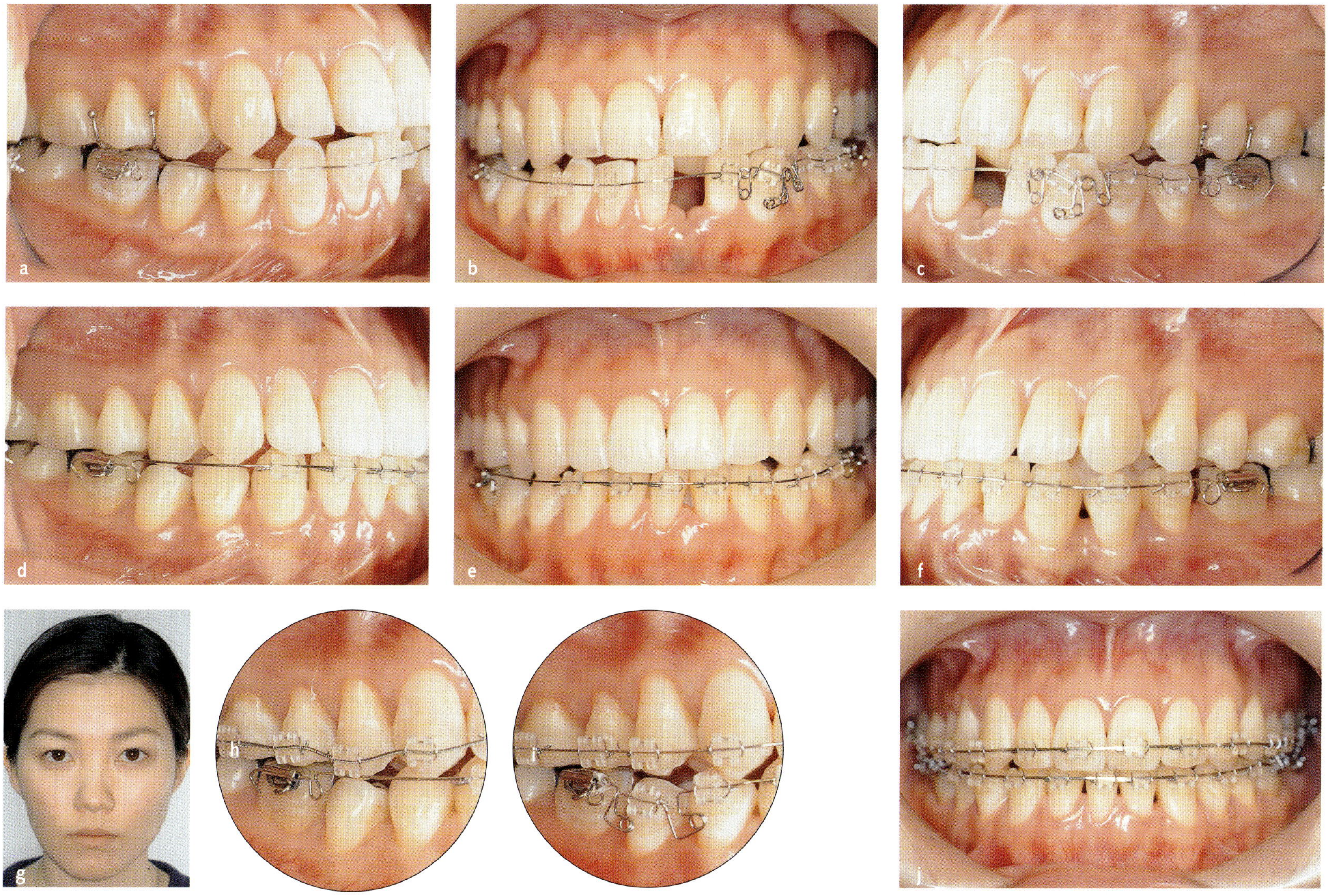

Fig 2-204 Definitive treatment after tooth extraction. (a to c) Basic therapy was reevaluated and counseling was conducted when the patient desired further stabilization of occlusion. After extraction of the mandibular left central incisor, multibrackets are applied to the mandibular arch. (d to f) Photographs taken 5 months after application of multibrackets to the mandibular arch. After 3 months, the mandibular anterior teeth moved lingually, clicking disappeared, and the condyles came on the disc naturally. (g) The mandibular shift to the right, tension of the right masseter, and the tilted lip line that was higher at the right end have mostly resolved. (h) The following month, multibrackets are applied to the maxillary arch as well. (i) Because the maxillary right first premolar and maxillary right canine have been extruded, bonding is conducted for the mandibular right first premolar and mandibular right second premolar to provide leveling after intrusion of the maxillary arch has progressed. Some time lag should be allowed, because extrusion takes place faster than intrusion. (j) Rectangular wire is used for adjustment of occlusion.

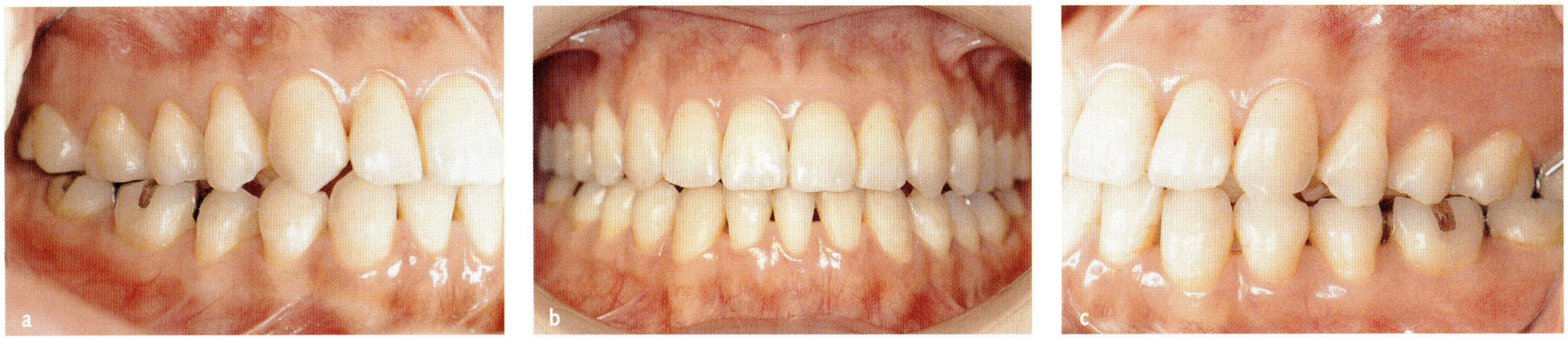

Fig 2-205 (a to c) At completion of active treatment, 1 month after removal of multibrackets. The duration of active treatment with multibrackets was 1 year 1 month. Because of the irregular extraction, tooth-to-tooth occlusion has been established. The right condyle is reduced nonfunctionally but sometimes comes off the disc during masticatory movements. Because the condyle comes off the disc when the patient is in the supine position, a flap is added to a retainer. For stabilization of occlusion and esthetics, an inlay for the mandibular left first molar has been newly fabricated with Estenia extrahard resin.

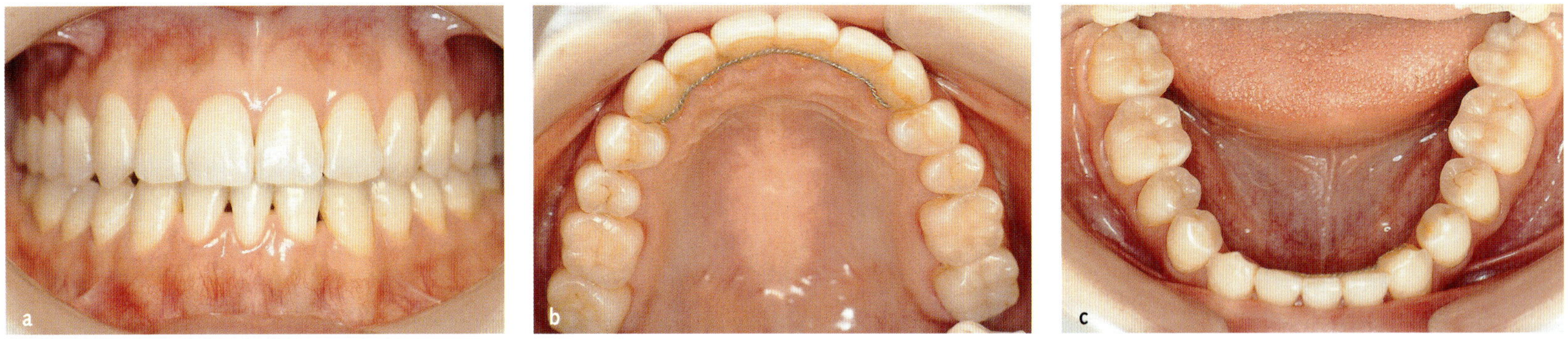

Fig 2-206 (a to c) Photographs taken 7 months after completion of active treatment, 1 year after fabrication of the new inlay. Currently, the retainer is used only at night and maintenance therapy is conducted. Postural habits and chewing habits are reassessed at each examination. The patient is instructed to masticate more on the left side with a 3:7 ratio between the right and the left sides and to chew hard food on the left side. Depending on how food is masticated and how food enters the chewing site, the condyle is still sometimes caught in an off-the-disc position.

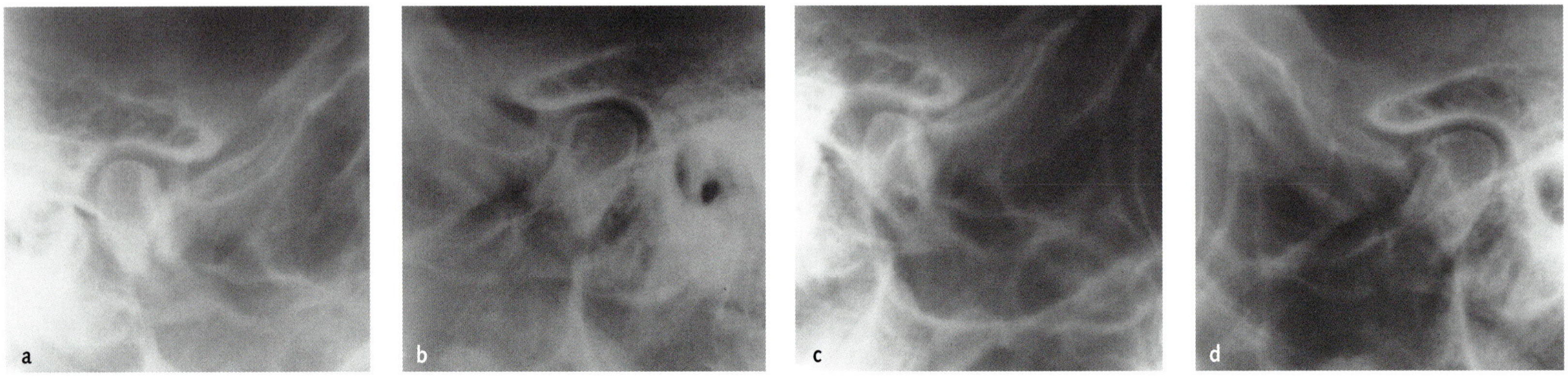

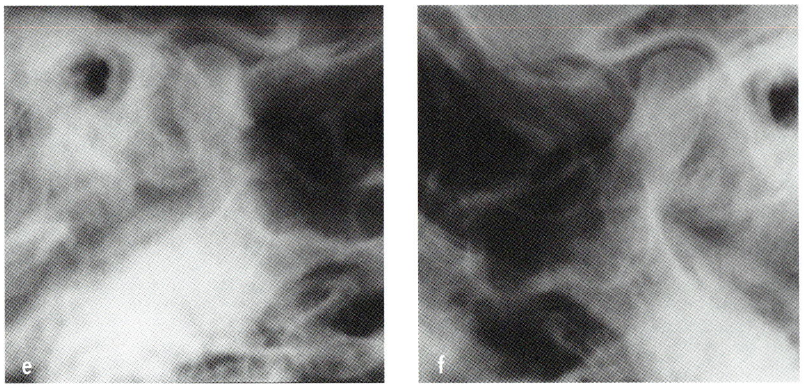

Fig 2-207 Changes in TMJ areas (Schuller radiographs). (a) Right and (b) left condyles at ICP at the first visit. The right condyle is off the disc. The left condyle is on the disc. (c) Right and (d) left condyles while the occlusion is at a position that allows the right condyle to be on the disc at the first visit. (e) Right and (f) left condyles after tooth movement. Although the both condyles are on the disc, the right condyle is more posteriorly located compared to its position at the first visit. Also, the disc is set back.

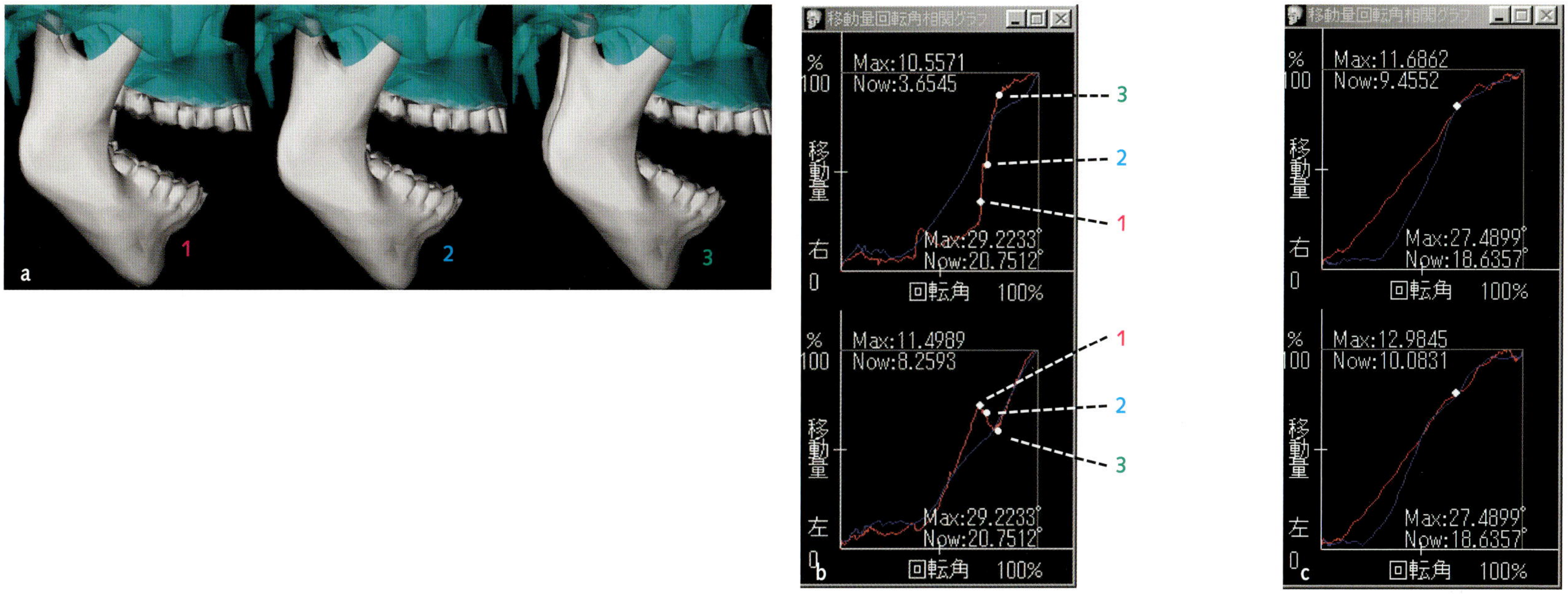

Fig 2-208 The Gnathohexagraph visualizes sliding and rotation components of condylar movements on the sagittal plane. The horizontal axis shows the rotation angle of the condyle (or the whole mandible), while the vertical axis indicates the amount of movement. Opening paths are shown in red and closing paths in blue. (a) At the first visit (September 1998). At 22-mm opening, the mandible is opening while being shifted to the right. The right condyle rotates first, followed quickly by translation. First, the condyle is not on the disc (1) and then it moves quickly on the disc at position (2). At position (3), the condyle is stabilized on the disc. During closing, the condyle stays on the disc while returning and then comes off the disc near ICP. (b) There is a time gap between clicking during opening and closing. This is because the longer the dysfunction exists, the more anteriorly the disc is pushed during opening; as a result, the condyle gets on the disc near maximal opening, moves backward and remains on the disc during closing, and slips off the disc near ICP. This means that, in reconstruction of the occlusion, the occlusion may well be stabilized in a condition before the condyle slips off the disc during closing. The left condyle translates while rotating, reduces its movement as the right condyle gets on the disc, and catches up with the right condyle to reach the maximal opening. (c) After treatment, the difference between the right and left condyles at maximal opening has become smaller, and the both condyles move while being on the disc. White points indicate the positions of condyles at 22 mm of opening. Functional movement paths include the trajectory of the right condyle with smaller movement and they sometimes indicate mastication with the condyle on the disc.

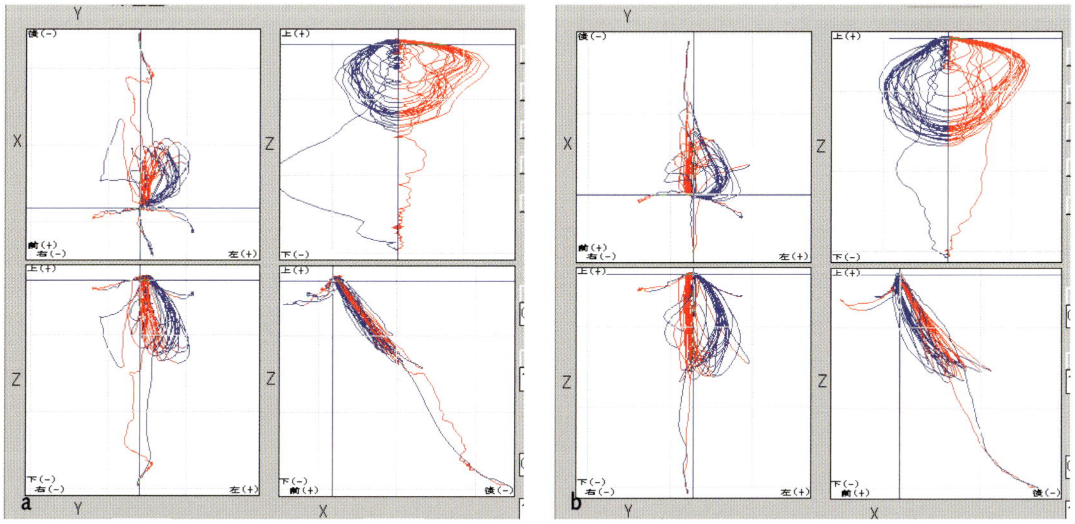

Fig 2-209 The Gnathohexagraph visualizes functional movements of incisal points. Left-side chewing in the transverse *(top left)*, frontal *(bottom left)*, and sagittal planes *(bottom right)*. Velocity *(top right)*. (a) At the first visit, the opening path is pulled to the right to reach the maximal opening. The condyle gets on the disc at about 2.5 cm and closes remaining on the disc until it gets off the disc near ICP. Functional movement paths have opening at about 1.0 cm with limited speed to conduct gentle chewing. However, depending on how the patient eats, condyles may repeat on-the-disc and off-the-disc conditions during mastication rather than staying off the disc all the time. (b) After removal of the appliance, the opening and closing paths at maximal opening are becoming consistent with each other mostly at the midline and the condyles are on the disc. Functional movement paths show reasonable speed and mastication with about 1.5 cm of opening. Still, depending on how the patient eats, condyles are sometimes off the disc.

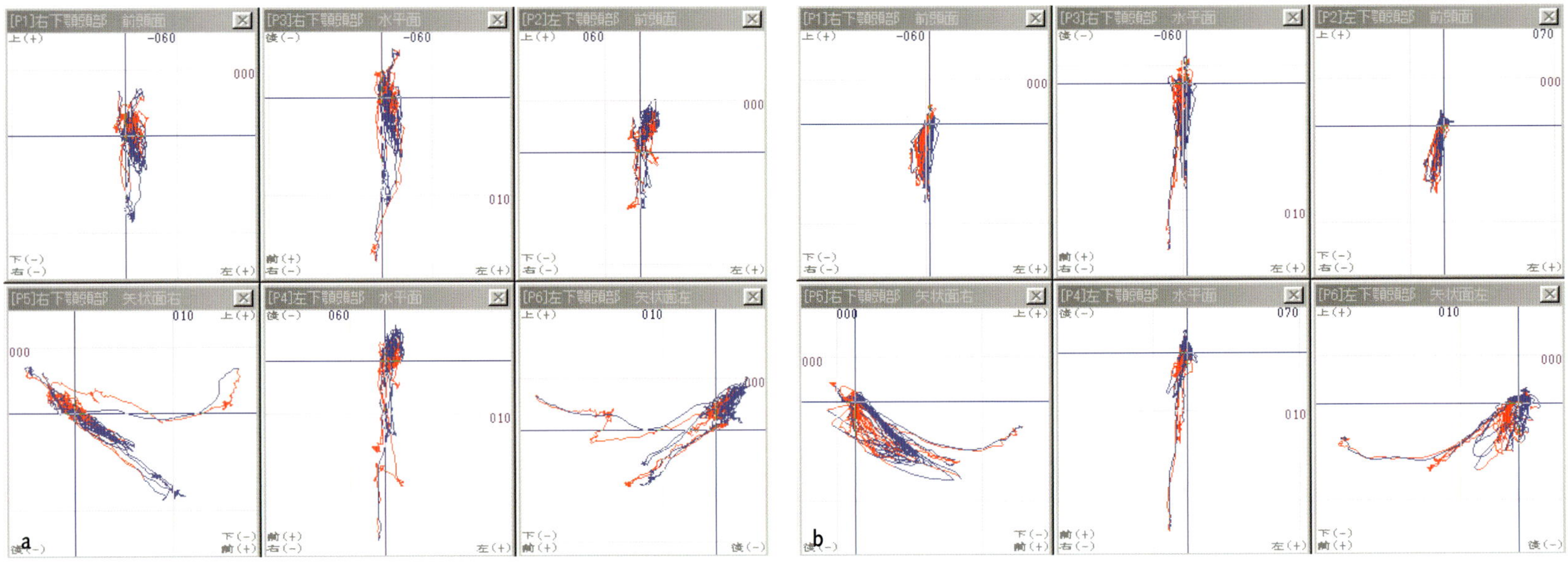

Fig 2-210 Gnathohexagraph presentation of condylar movements. (a) Left-side chewing at the first visit. (b) Left-side chewing after treatment. Movement of the working-side (left) condyle during function has changed from posterior and superior direction to an anterior and inferior direction. It is obvious that it changes depending on changes in occlusion.

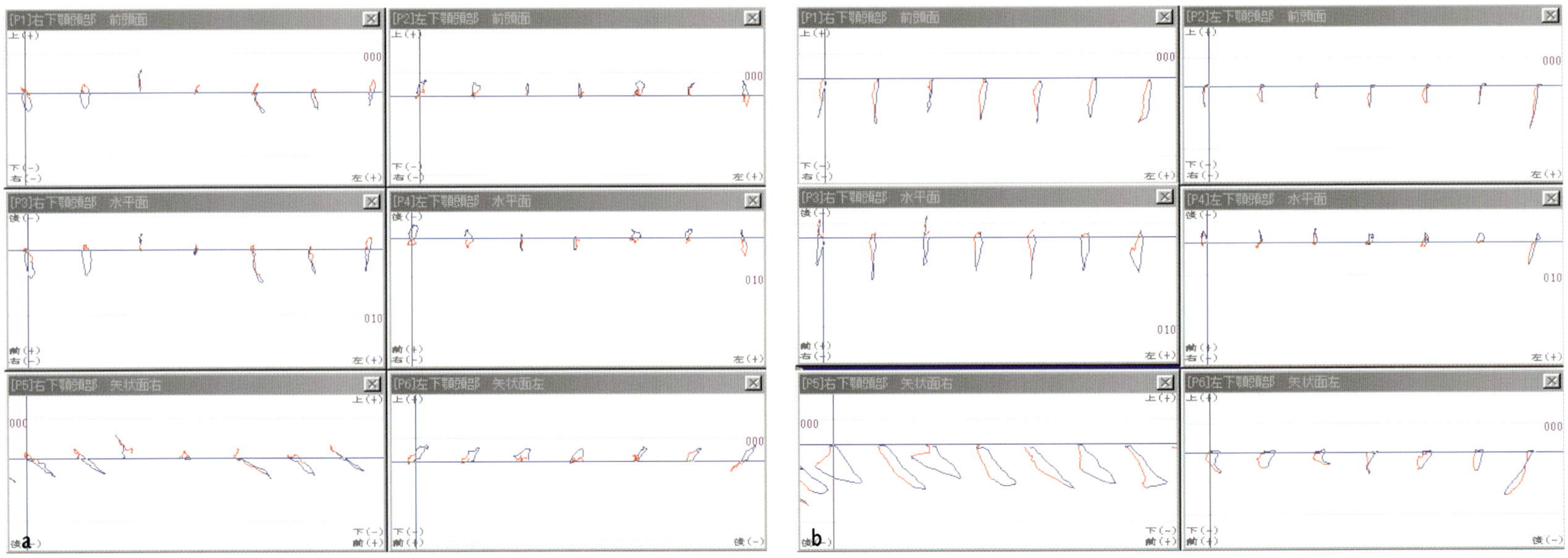

Fig 2-211 Individual presentation of cycles of the right *(left)* and left *(right)* condyles with the Gnathohexagraph in the frontal *(top)*, transverse *(center)*, and sagittal planes *(bottom)*. (a) Left-side chewing at the first visit. Movement of the nonworking-side (right) condyle is not stable in the anteroposterior and superoinferior directions from the stable condylar position or the condylar position at ICP. Also, the form of the cycles is irregular, repeating on and off the disc. The cycle of the working-side (left) condyle is also irregular. (b) Left-side chewing after treatment. Both the right and left condyles have the stable condylar position as a reference, and the right condyle conducts reciprocation in an anterior and inferior direction on the nonworking side. The left condyle shows smaller forms with more uniform shape on the working side than at the first visit.

Examination of TMJs with medical electronics equipment tells us whether a condyle is on or off the disc at each chewing point. The authors believed that the condyles should be off the disc if they are off the disc at maximal opening. However, analysis revealed that the condyles may be off the disc at maximal opening but on the disc during mastication as in this clinical case (see Fig 2-213), or they may be on the disc at maximal opening but off the disc during mastication. Equipment for examination of mandibular functional movements clarifies the relationship between the disc and the condyle during function that could not be examined with magnetic resonance imaging or radiographs, becoming effective means for examination and diagnosis of TMJs as well as reconstruction of occlusion. Also, such equipment enables actual proof of the connection between the whole body and occlusion.

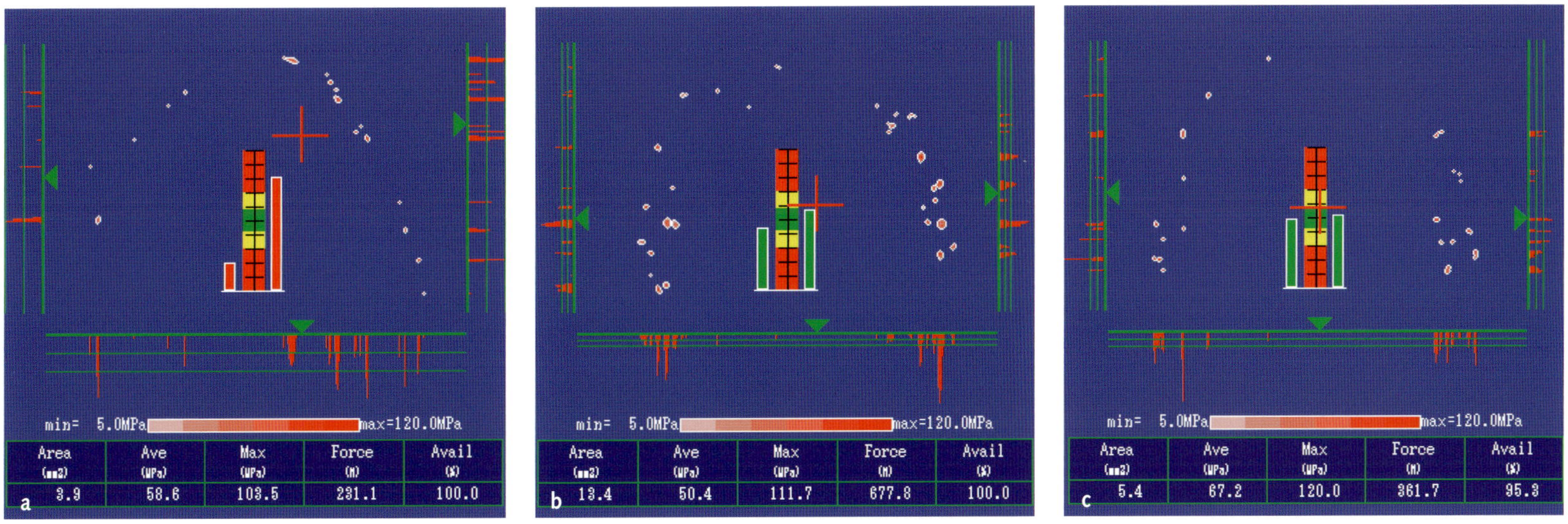

Fig 2-212 GC Occluzer presentation of the balance of occlusal forces. (a) At the first visit. Where occlusal force is applied is exhibited as white islands, which are hardly observed in the molar areas. The center of the occlusal forces, shown at the bottom, is the right anterior area. (b) Analysis 11 months after the first visit, after completion of basic treatment and expansion of the left maxilla. (c) Analysis 2 years 2 months after the first visit, after completion of definitive treatment and tooth movements. The center of occlusion is centralized, indicating that the occlusion is being stabilized.

Fig 2-213 Changes in the posture of the whole body. (a) At the first visit, ICP (the right condyle is off the disc; the left condyle is on the disc). (b) At the first visit, when the right condyle is put on the disc, facial inclination to the right is eliminated and the head is straightened. (c) Posture after completion of basic treatment and expansion of the left maxillary jaw (11 months after the first visit). Although the right condyle is still off the disc, the symptoms are ameliorated and the body posture has become straighter. (d) Profile at the first visit. The patient stands with her chest and buttocks pushed out. (e) Profile at the completion of basic treatment.

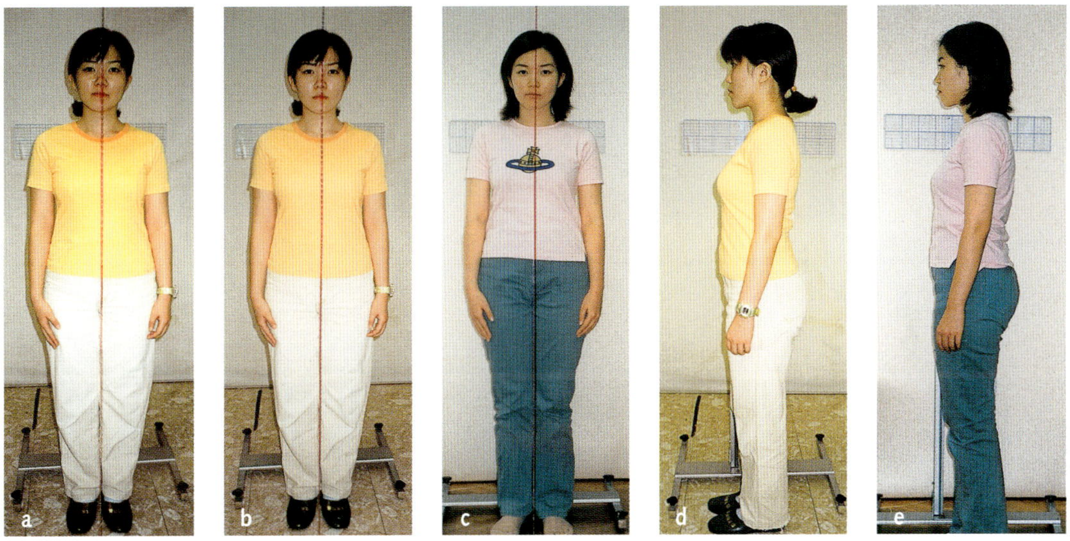

Fig 2-214 Observation of stability in the body's center of gravity using the Gravicoder. Measurement of the body's center of gravity is important for objectification of examinations. *(left)* Instability of the body while the patient stands for 30 seconds with eyes open; *(right)* instability while the patient stands for 30 seconds with eyes closed. (a) Results at the first visit in ICP. (b) Results at the first visit, at a position allowing the right condyle to be on the disc. Compared to the results found when the patient is in ICP, rolling of the body is smaller with the patient's eyes open or closed.

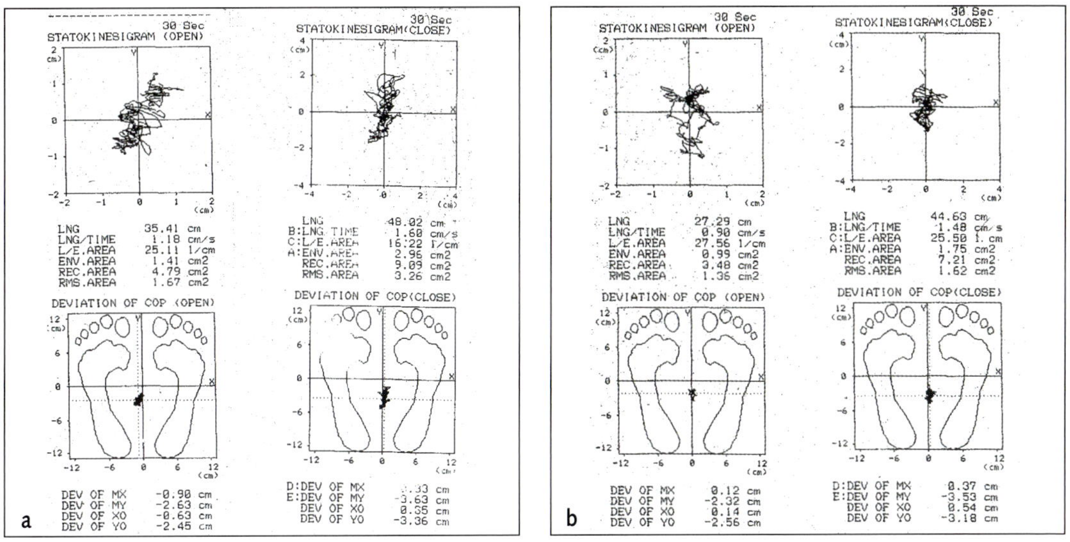

Case 2-15 TMJ pain caused by a trivial anomaly of occlusion

Patient: *42-year-old man at the time of first visit in 1999*

Figures 2-216 to 2-225 present the case. The patient first felt pain in the left TMJ 10 years ago and tried to chew on the right side, later developing pain in both TMJs. He received occlusal therapy, wearing removable splints (20K gold). He lost the mandibular arch splint, but continued to wear the maxillary arch splint. He exhibited nocturnal clenching.

The lip line was tilted so that the left corner of the mouth was higher than the right. The left nasolabial fold was deeper and the left cheek was more hypertrophic. Considering that he was originally a right-side chewer, left-side clenching was suspected (see Fig 2-224).

The axes of the maxillary right canine and maxillary left canine were different, with the former labially inclined the latter lingually inclined. This should naturally have caused right-side chewing and made left-side chewing difficult. The lingual inclination of the axes of the maxillary left canine, maxillary left first premolar, and mandibular left first premolar was unnatural, suggesting the existence of some postural habit involvement. The patient confirmed that he had a habit of resting his left cheek on the left hand (see Fig 2-222).

Diagnosis. *Because of his habit of resting his left cheek on his hand, the maxillary left canine was inclined lingually and rotated distally, causing excessive guidance on the left side, which invited clenching, a decrease of the vertical dimension, and an excessive burden for the TMJs. He represented type IV TMD. It was believed that the splints he wore diminished the burden for the TMJs, which relieved pain.*

Treatment and progress. *The splints were removed and the patient was instructed to stop the habit. The lingual morphology of the maxillary left canine was corrected so that similar guidance could be provided for both right and left sides. The other four sites that seemed to cause interference in masticatory movement paths were slightly reshaped (see Fig 2-223).*

By 5 or 6 hours after reshaping, clenching had disappeared. The molars (especially on the left) lost occlusal contacts. Because only anterior teeth had contacts, the patient was instructed not to insert his tongue or cheek between maxillary and mandibular molars so that we could wait for natural extrusion.

Extrusion of molars started to be felt after about 2 months, and the patient could eat a normal diet. Molars occluded with each other in about 4 months. He could eat hard food, and TMJ symptoms were almost completely gone. Except for instructing him to stop the habit of resting his cheek on his hand, the only intervention we made for improvement of symptoms in this case was grinding of the lingual surface of maxillary left canine.

Symptoms can be eliminated if splints are delivered as a temporary measure. However, delivering a splint without considering the cause of the complaint is merely sweeping a troublesome problem under the rug.

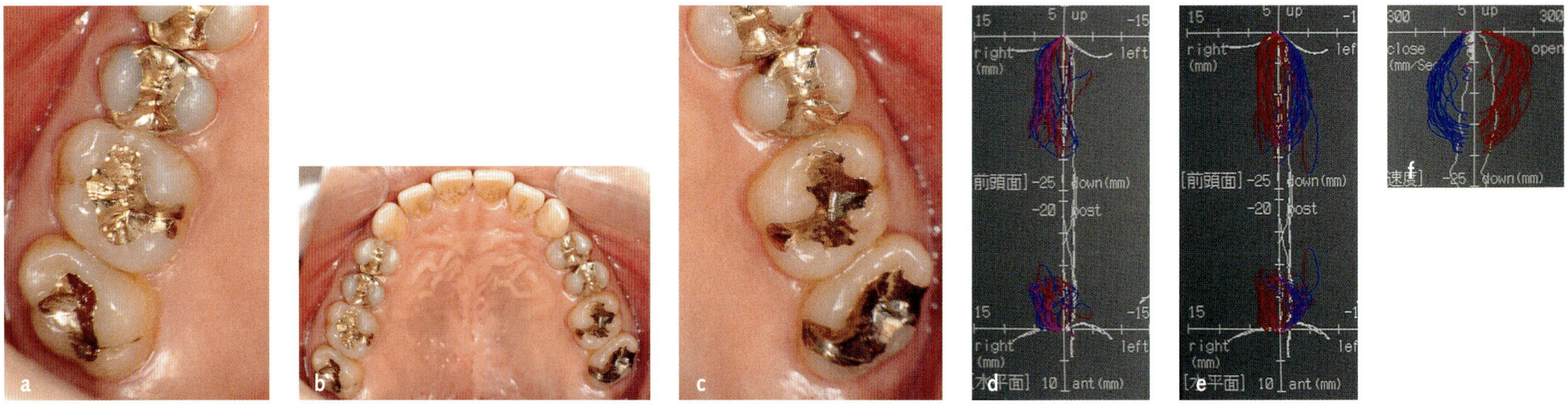

Fig 2-215 At the first visit. (a to c) The patient chews on the right side unconsciously. He may gently chew on the left side when he has pain in the right TMJ but chews on the right side when there is no pain. Without splints, the maxillary left canine causes interference during opening and prevents opening to the left, which leads to opening to the right side in a reverse manner. Sirognathographs of (d) unconscious chewing and (e) left-side chewing in the frontal plane *(top)* and the transverse plane *(bottom)*. (f) Velocity of unconscious chewing.

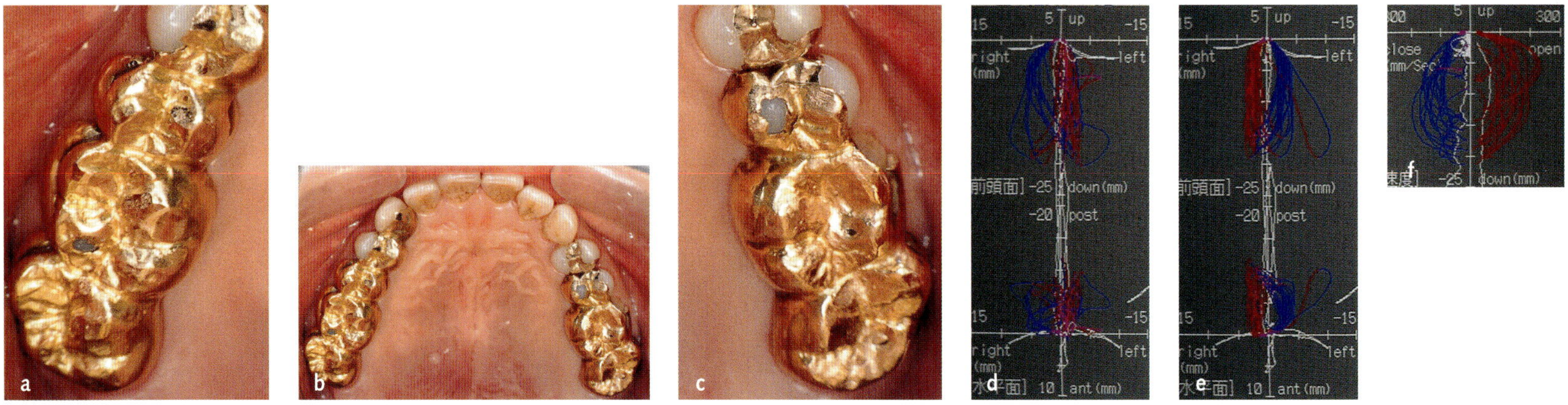

Fig 2-216 (a to c) When the splints fabricated 6 years ago are worn, interference of the maxillary left canine disappears, generating opening to the left and mastication with acceptable chewing cycles with good velocity. Sirognathographs of (d) unconscious chewing and (e) left-side chewing in the frontal plane *(top)* and the transverse plane *(bottom)*. (f) Velocity of unconscious chewing. The splints merely veil the cause of the problem.

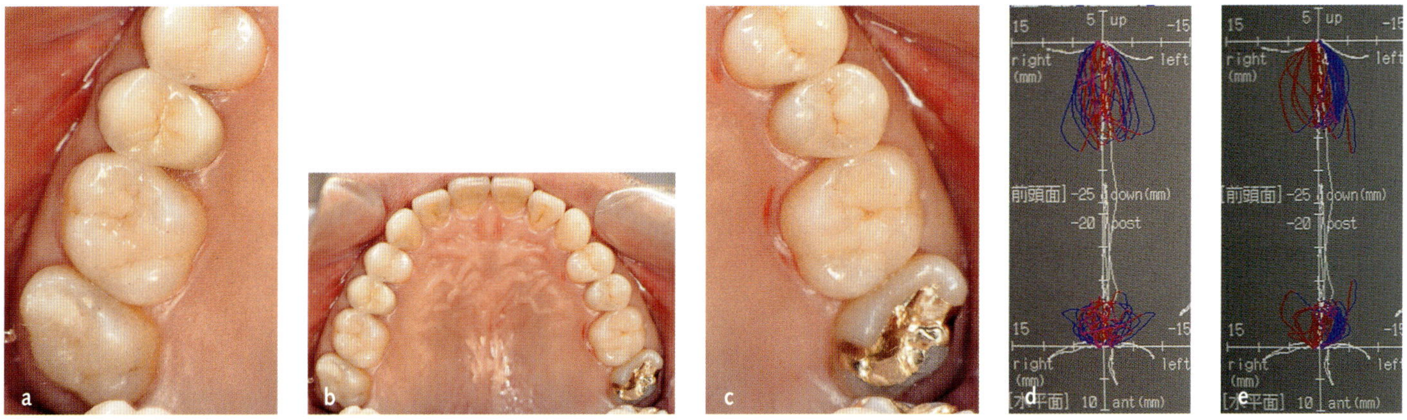

Fig 2-217 (a to c) After reshaping, he can chew with similar cycles for the right and the left. Sirognathographs of (d) unconscious chewing and (e) left-side chewing in the frontal plane *(top)* and the transverse plane *(bottom)*.

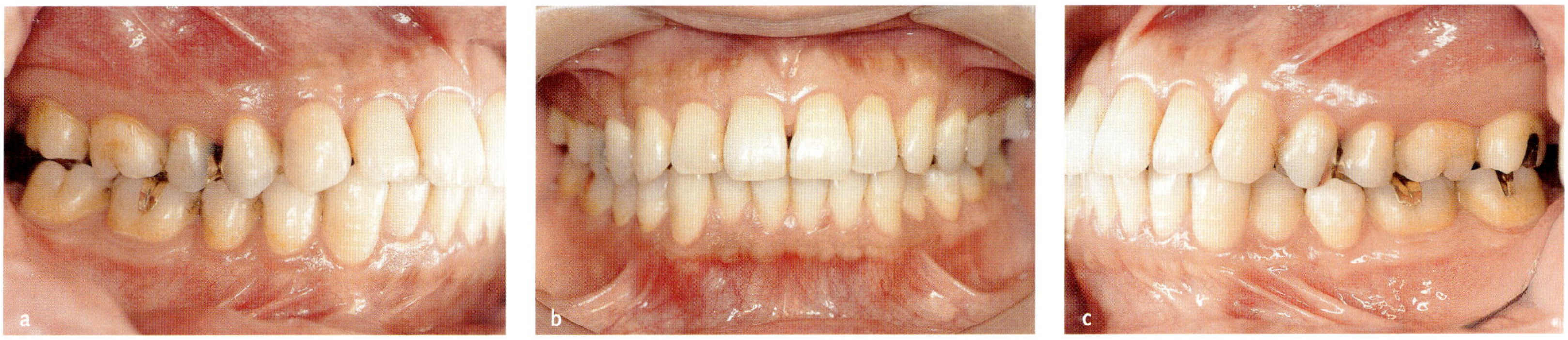

Fig 2-218 (a to c) At the first visit. This is mostly an acceptable Class I occlusion. The different inclination of the axes of the maxillary right canine and maxillary left canine are a concern. Different guidances of the maxillary right canine and maxillary left canine naturally cause right-side chewing.

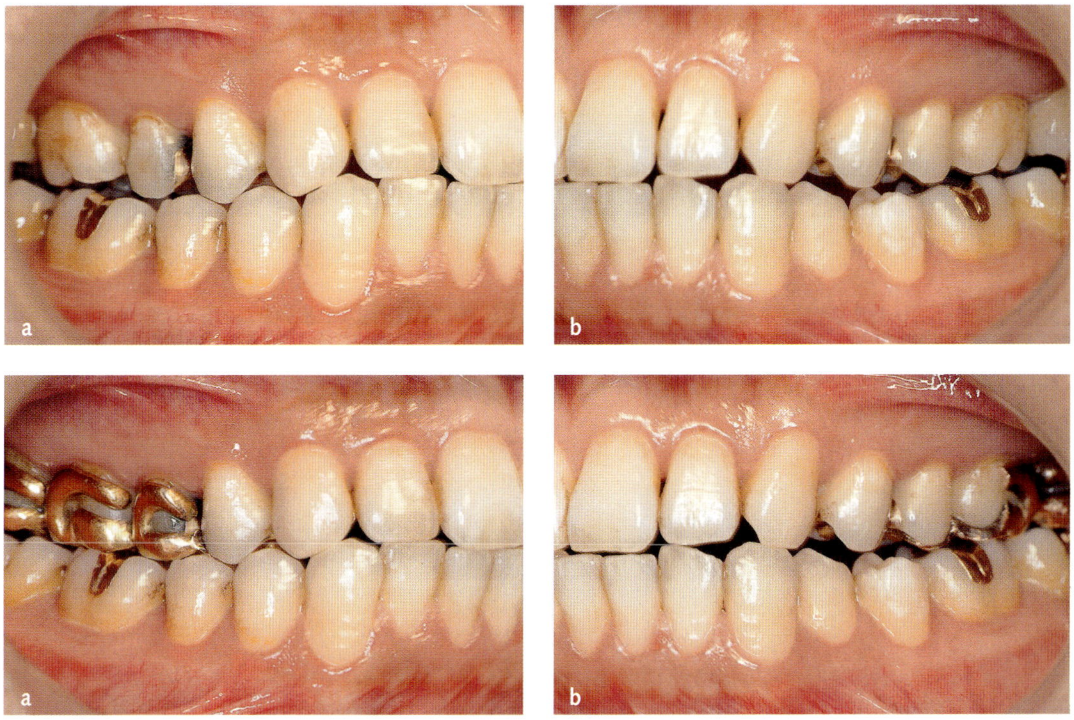

Fig 2-219 (a and b) Lateral guidance. The right side has group function of the maxillary right canine, maxillary right first premolar, mandibular right canine, and mandibular right first premolar, while the left side has canine guidance of the maxillary left canine and mandibular left canine. The left side has a larger amount of disocclusion. At lateral excursion, lingual inclination and rotation of maxillary left canine prevents excursion to the left, resulting in exertion of force and clenching. (c and d) The patient has worn these splints for the maxillary right canine to second molar and the maxillary left second premolar to second molar for 6 years. Lateral excursion with these splints generates guidance at the maxillary left canine, second premolar, first molar, and second molar, and the mandibular left canine, first molar, and second molar and allows smooth movement, while the right side has group function guidance.

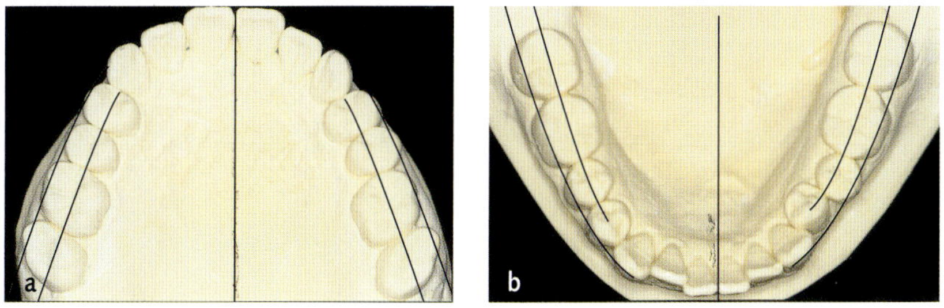

Fig 2-220 (a and b) Arch asymmetry. Curvature of the left side is distorted. It would be unlikely to have such asymmetry unless some external force had been applied to the maxillary left canine area. The left side of the mandibular arch is also distorted laterally.

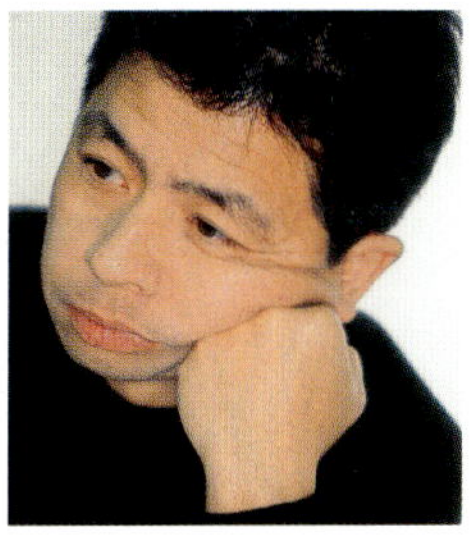

Fig 2-221 The patient had a habit of resting his left cheek on his left fist (reenactment).

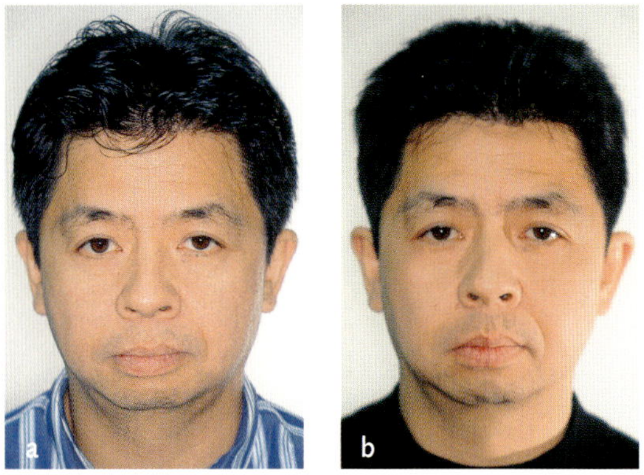

Fig 2-222 (a) The lip line is tilted and the left corner of the mouth is higher. The left nasolabial fold is deep, and the left masseter is hypertrophic. It is considered to be left-side clenching. (b) Facial photograph taken after 5 months shows a slight improvement of the tilted lip line. The left nasolabial fold is still deeper. The level of tension in the right and the left cheeks is similar.

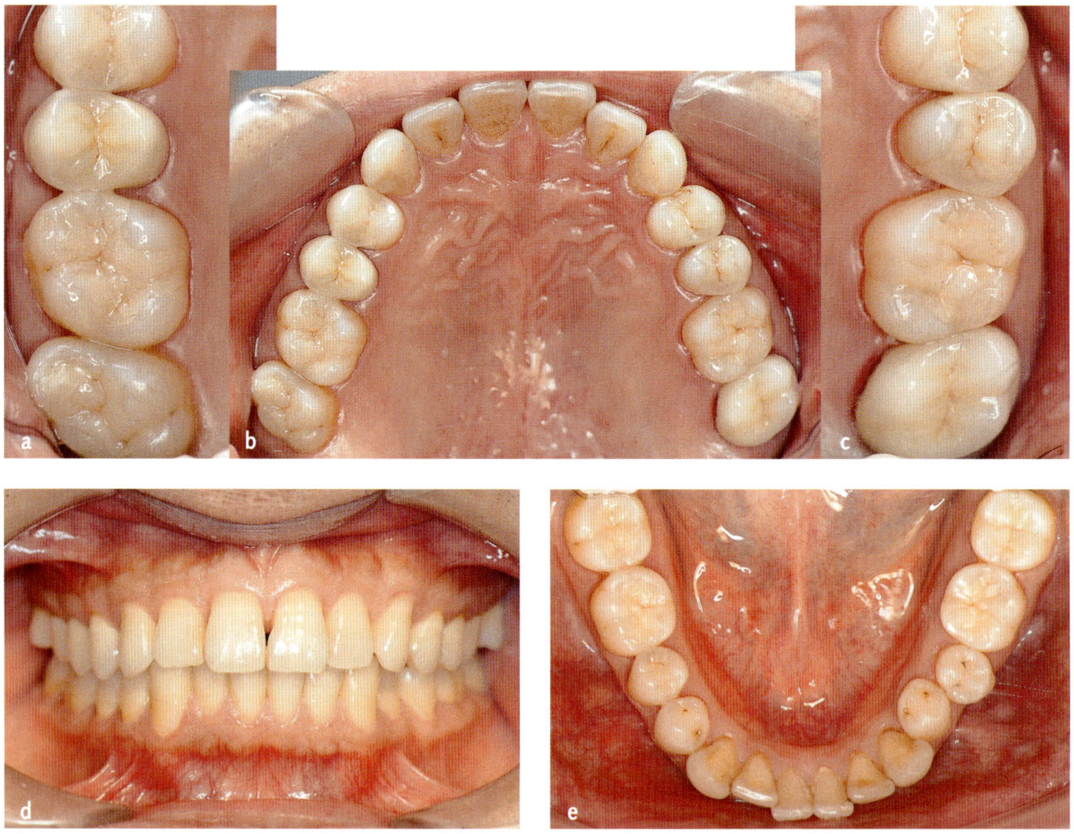

Fig 2-223 (a to e) Photographs taken about 5 months after the first visit. This is the condition achieved through only the reshaping that was conducted at the first visit. Morphologic correction involved mostly grinding of the inner slope of maxillary left canine to provide agreement of the guidance between the right and the left sides. Modest reshaping was conducted for the mesial interior slopes of the lingual cusps of the maxillary right and left first premolars, the mesial marginal ridge of the maxillary left second molar, and the interior slope of the distal buccal cusp of the maxillary right first molar. Gold inlays have been removed and newly replaced with ceramic. The asymmetric tooth axes of the maxillary canines and the rotation of the maxillary left canine are corrected.

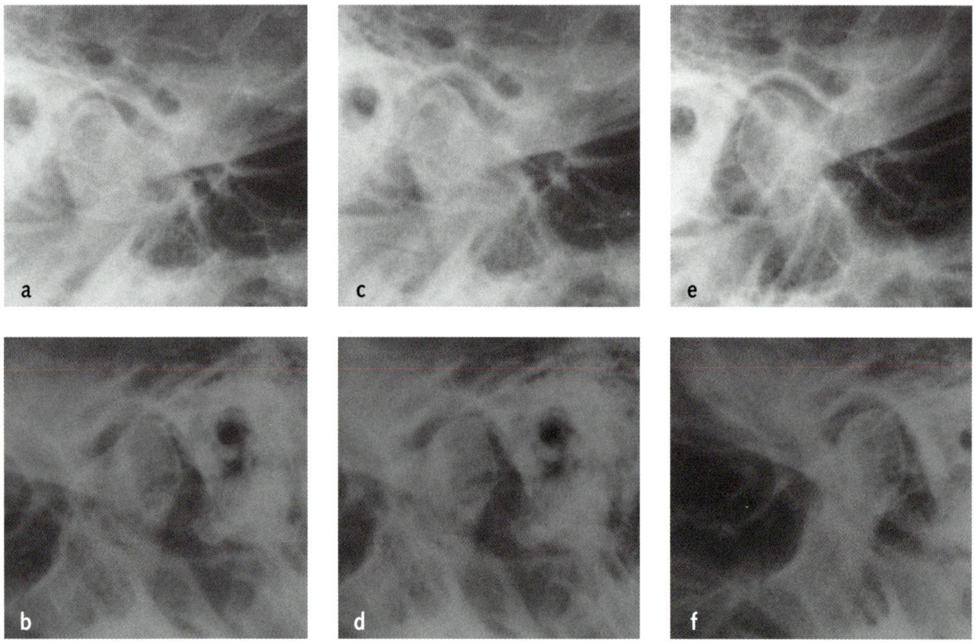

Fig 2-224 Schuller radiographs of the TMJs. (a) Right and (b) left TMJs at ICP at the first visit. The posterior part of the left condyle is somewhat flat and compact bone is lost, indicating that the condyle is pressed backward in the articular space at ICP. (c) Right and (d) left TMJs at the first visit when the splint is worn. The condyle is located anteriorly. (e) Right and (f) left TMJs at ICP after reshaping. The posterior part of the left condyle becomes round and compact bone is regenerated. This indicates that space is secured, clenching is discontinued, and vertical dimension is recovered. Although the change is not as clear for the right condyle, the posterior compact bone becomes clearer.

Case 2-16 Basic strategy to cope with anterior disc displacement without reduction

Patient: *35-year-old woman at the time of first visit in 1995*

Chief complaint: *Pain in the right TMJ (spontaneous pain)*

The patient had clicking of the left TMJ 2 to 3 years previously without pain. She remembered that she could open smoothly after a clicking sound when she moved the jaw left and right. About 1 year previously, she felt heavy dullness in the right TMJ area and visited a university hospital. She received splint therapy, which did not improve the conditions. The discomfort of the right side of her face worsened afterward. Although her chief complaint was about the right side, the vertical dimension of the left side was lower, suggesting that there was a major problem on the left side. The left condyle did not move well at maximal opening. Judging from the case history, this seemed to be anterior disc displacement of the left TMJ without reduction. The patient felt pain in the right side because of myalgia of the right TMJ area. During the interview, it was found that she was in the habit of resting her right cheek on the right hand and biting her lips. First, the patient was instructed to stop the habits and to avoid clenching as much as possible. A repositioning splint in a slightly anterior position was applied, which caused disocclusion of the left molars. After that, orthodontic treatment was planned. The course of treatment is shown in Figs 2-226 to 2-228.

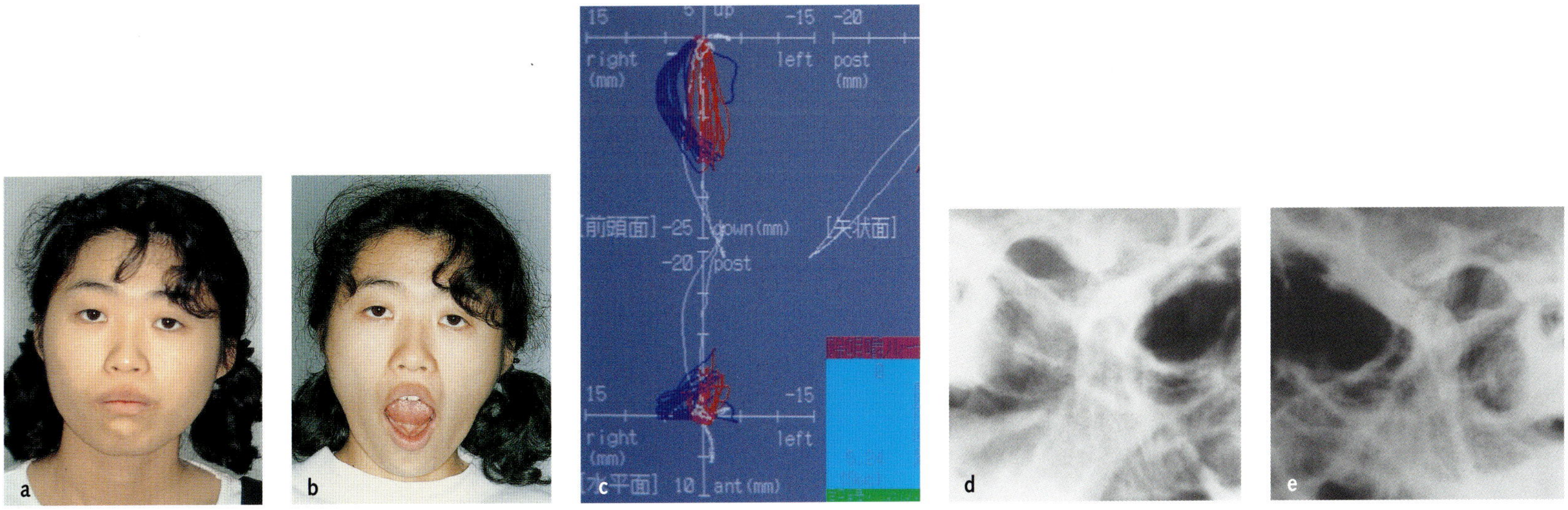

Fig 2-225 Photographs taken at the first visit. (a) The lower face is shifted to the left. The line connecting both eyes is tilted and lower on the left. The left vertical dimension is decreased. It is surmised that the left side also has some problem. (b) The jaw is shifted to the left at opening. The left condyle rotates only without translation. The opening is 4 cm. It is diagnosed as a slightly old anterior disc displacement without reduction. (c) Unconscious chewing on the Sirognathograph indicates right-side chewing. The patient says she chews on the right side because left-side chewing causes premature contacts of the right teeth and is uncomfortable. This has grown into a habit. Radiographs of the (d) right and (e) left TMJs at maximal opening. The left TMJ does not get over the eminence and is locked. Still, maximal opening is 4 cm.

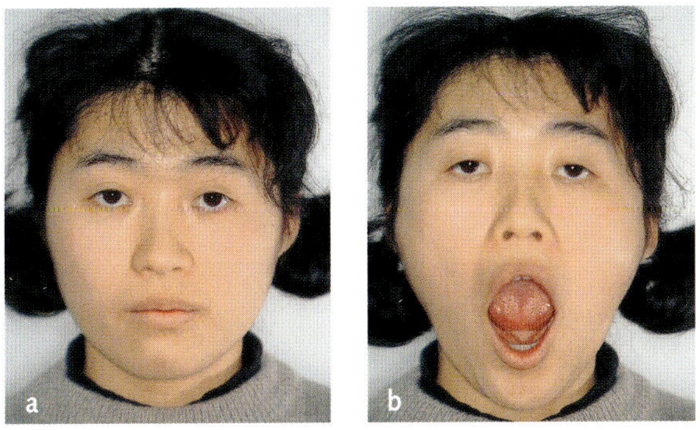

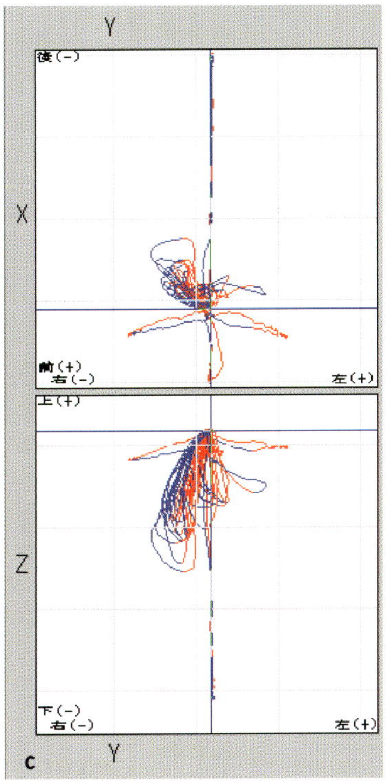

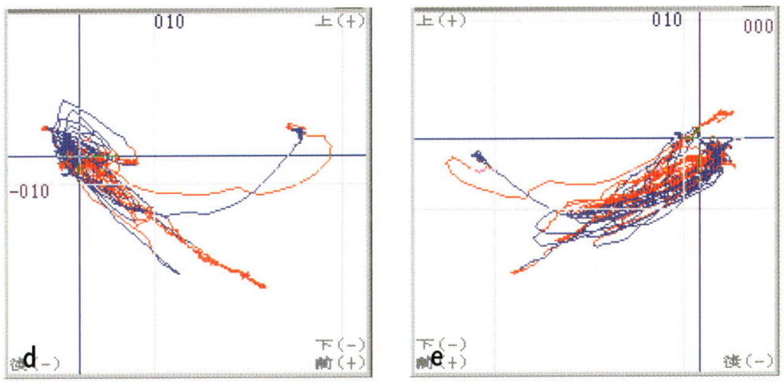

Fig 2-226 Photographs taken after treatment (3 years 4 months after the first visit). (a) Symmetry of the face has been recovered. (b) The condyle is on the disc at opening position, although it is sometimes off the disc during functional movements. (c) Sirognathograph after treatment shows right-side chewing in the transverse plane *(top)* and the frontal plane *(bottom)*. Sirognathographs of condylar movements after treatment show the (d) right condyle and (e) left condyle in the sagittal plane. After treatment, the maximal opening is not pulled to the left and most of the turning points on the masticatory movement paths are on the right side, indicating that the condyle is on the disc.

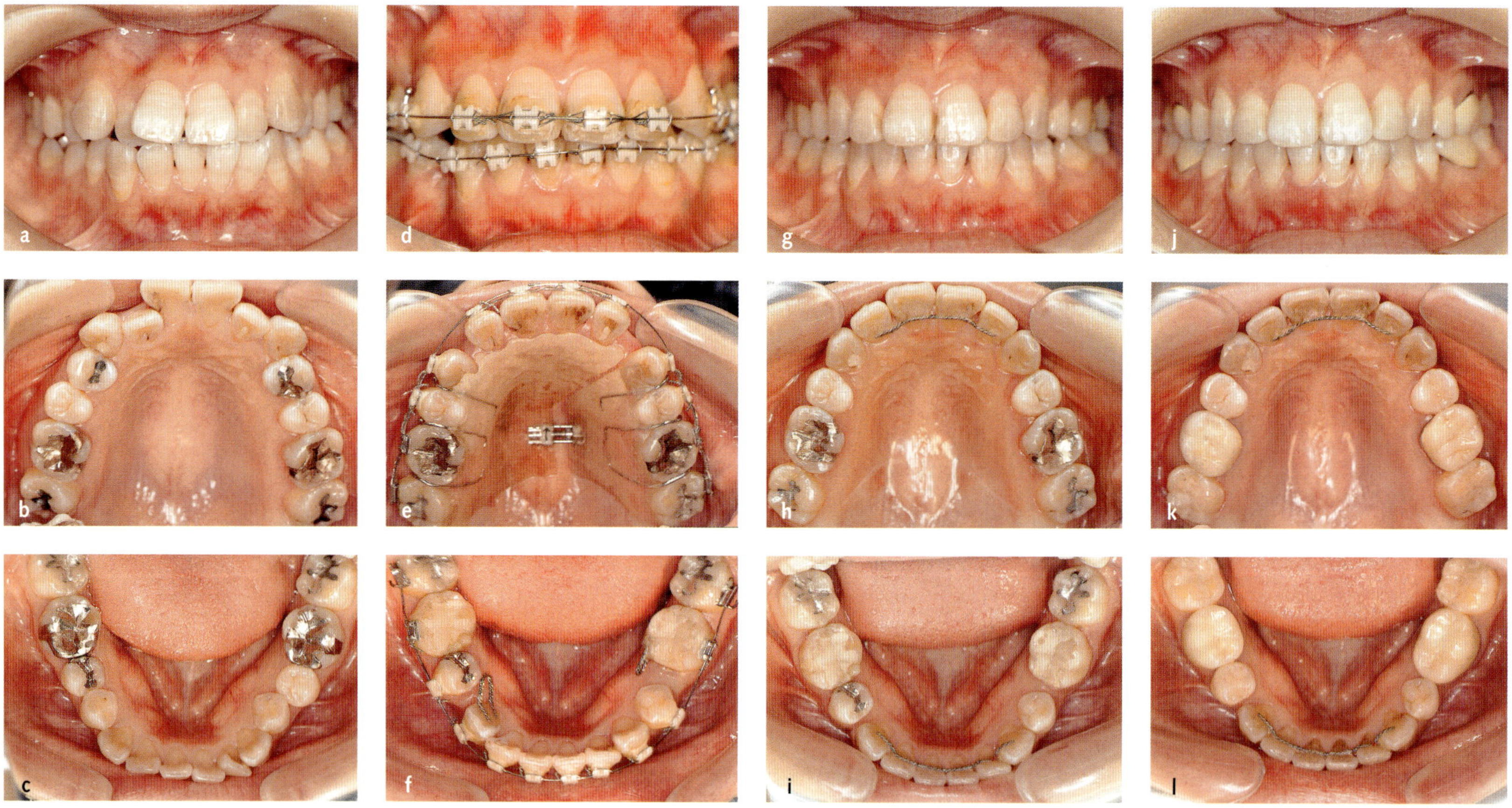

Fig 2-227 Orthodontic tooth movements targeting redistribution of forces. (a to c) Photographs taken at the first visit. After the left molars are disoccluded due to basic occlusal therapy and a repositioning splint, the maxillary right first premolar, maxillary left first premolar, mandibular left second premolar, and mandibular right first premolar are extracted in accordance with the change in the mandibular position. Orthodontic treatment with multibrackets is started (end of 1995). (d to f) Photographs taken at completion of orthodontic treatment. In conjunction with myofunctional therapy, mandibular exercise is also conducted. The load applied in the exercise helps anterior sliding of the left condyle (Box 2-22). A contraction screw is applied to the area of the maxillary left second premolar, first molar, and second molar to reduce the width of the left maxilla (until April 1997). Twisted wire is bonded to the mandibular arch to prevent the tongue from getting into the extraction spaces. (g to i) After 2 years 2 months of active treatment, orthodontic appliances have been removed. Slight clicking remains at this point in time. The maxillary and mandibular midlines agree. The patient is instructed to consciously chew on the right side. (j to l) Photographs taken 4 months after completion of active orthodontic treatment. A repositioning splint is delivered, and crown restoration is provided for the four worn first molars. Hybrid hard resin composite has been used because further change of a mandibular position is expected. Clicking has subsided.

Box 2-22 Mandibular exercise for anterior disc displacement without reduction

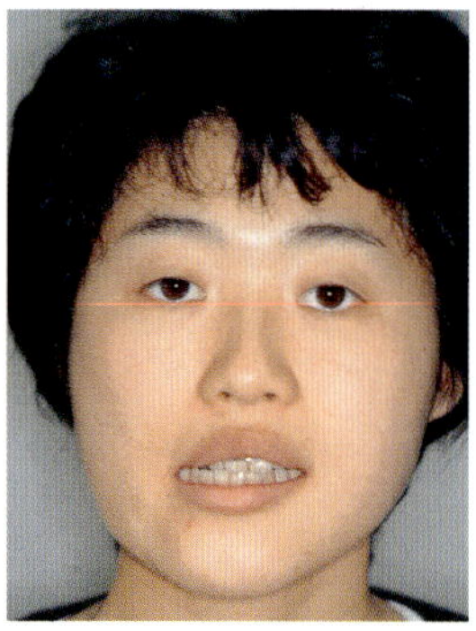

Fig 2-228

This is an exercise to pull forward a condyle that has fallen behind the disc. The mandible is moved to transfer the condyles medially and anteriorly (Fig 2-228). The patient's hands are applied so that translation of the condyles can be felt. This training should be conducted everyday.

- With this exercise, adhesions may be ameliorated.
- The discs will be pushed anteriorly to expand the range of motion.
- If successful, a condyle may get on the disc.

Case 2-17 Degenerative lesion in a condyle

Patient: *49-year-old woman at the time of first visit in 1992*
Chief complaint: *Sensitivity to cold and warm water, mouth pain, and symptoms involving the left ear*
The patient experienced sensitivity to cold and warm water at the maxillary left canine and felt pain in the full mouth. She also had symptoms involving the left ear, including tinnitus and difficulty in hearing as well as dizziness. With suspected Ménière's disease, she visited an otolaryngologist, but the cause was not identified. She had the feeling that the left ear was obstructed and received myringotomy at an otolaryngologist. Figures 2-230 to 2-237 show her treatment.

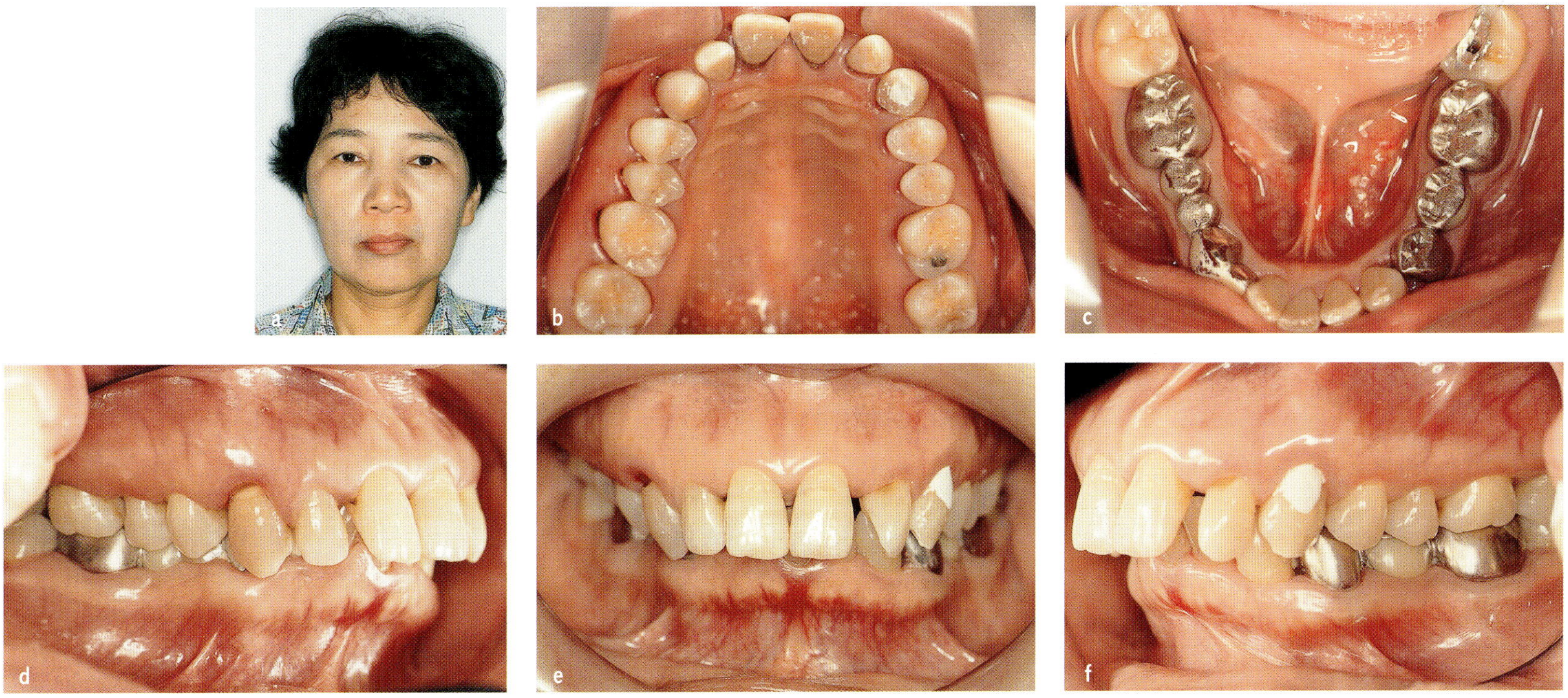

Fig 2-229 At the first visit. (a) It is obvious that the lip line is tilted, the left corner of the mouth is higher, and the lateral angle of the left eye is lower. (b to f) Anterior overlap indicates an extremely deep bite, especially at the maxillary right canine. The maxillary right teeth are lingually inclined. The left TMJ has noise during movement.

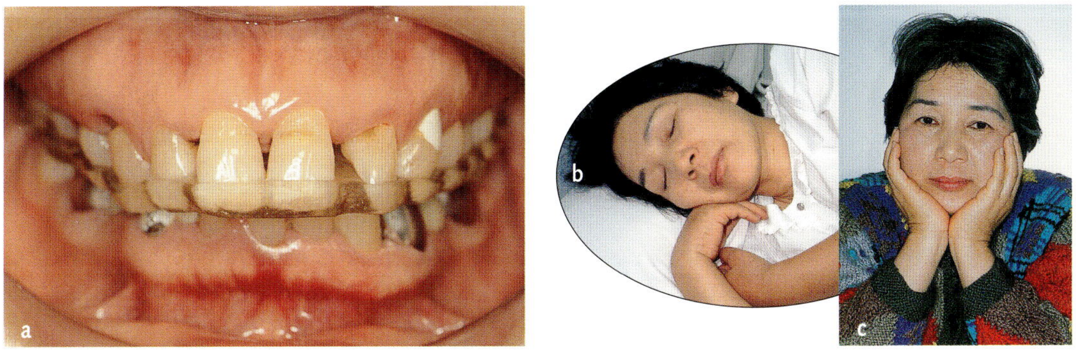

Fig 2-230 (a) The mandibular right central incisor is missing. The lingual inclination of the maxillary right arch seems to have been caused by her sleep posture habit. A stabilization-type bite plane has been applied to the maxillary arch to eliminate muscle spasm. One month after the bite plane was delivered, systemic symptoms, such as tinnitus and dizziness, have disappeared. (b) The patient has been sleeping on her right, pillowing her head on her right arm, since childhood. She tried to sleep in the supine position when she was about 20 years old, but it was too distressing for her to do so. (c) She also has a habit of resting her cheeks in her hands. We encouraged her to stop these habits.

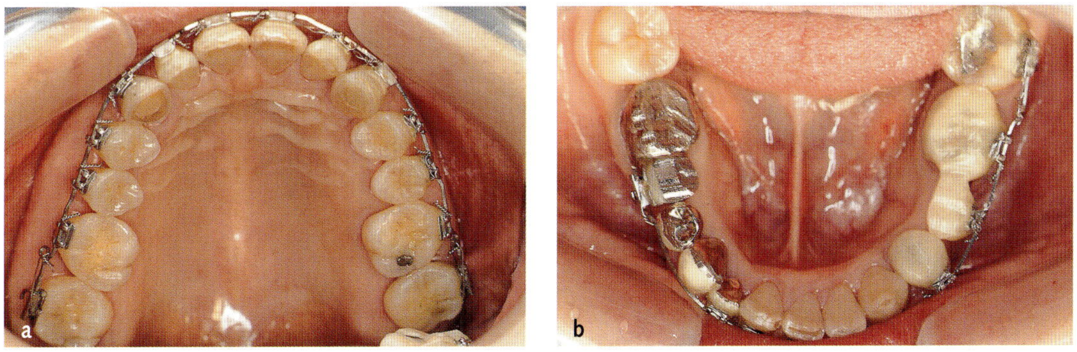

Fig 2-231 (a and b) Improvement of tooth axes and reshaping 1 year 8 months after the first visit. The treatment strategy is to conduct orthodontic treatment to move individual teeth to appropriate positions while correcting the mandibular position. A special effort has been made to improve tooth axes on the right side. Orthodontic treatment is mostly completed.

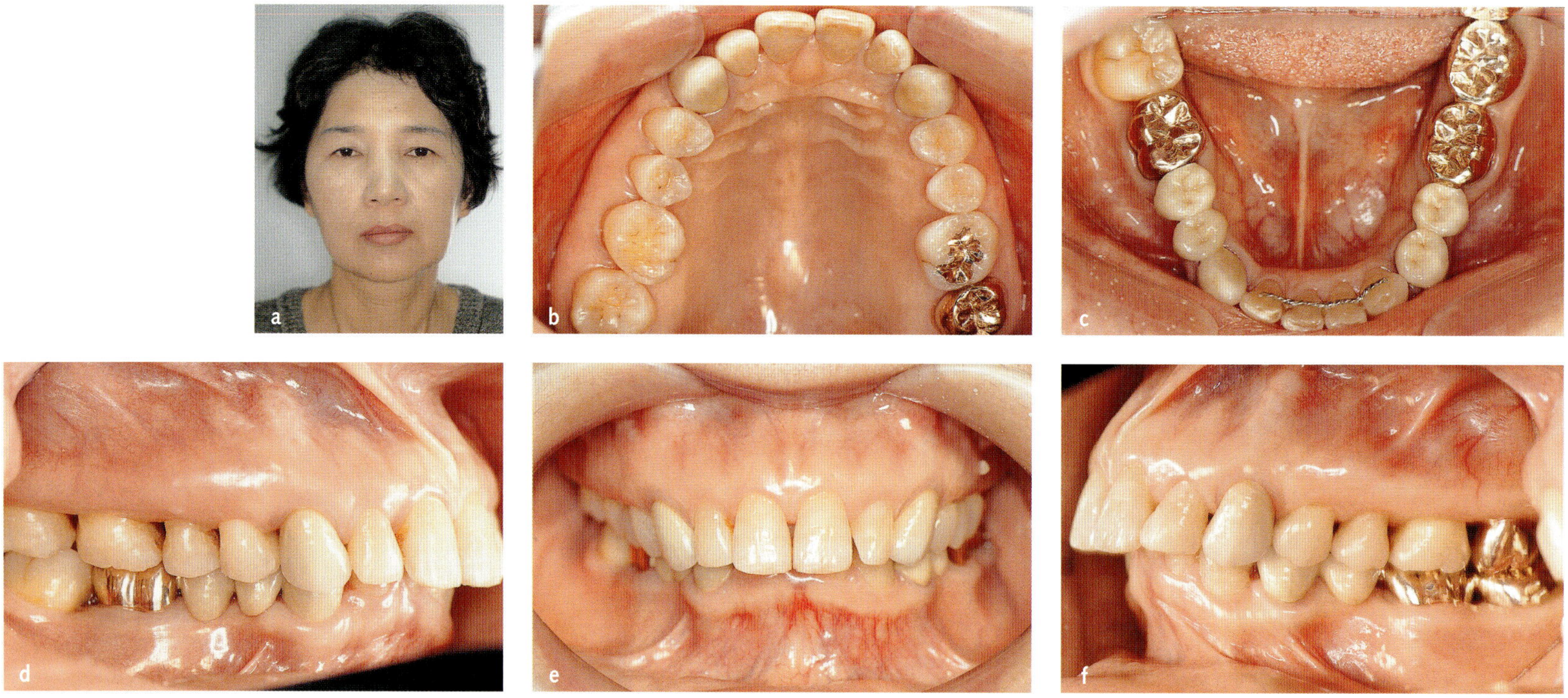

Fig 2-232 After placement of restorations. (a) Photograph taken 2 years 11 months after the first visit. The patient's face has become fairly symmetric and looks peaceful. (b to f) About 2.5 years after the first visit, definitive treatment for improvement of the periodontal environment and crown restoration is started. Reshaping is concomitantly conducted for the maxillary right canine, first premolar, second premolar, first molar, and second molar, which exhibit excessive guidance, to give freedom to the mandible.

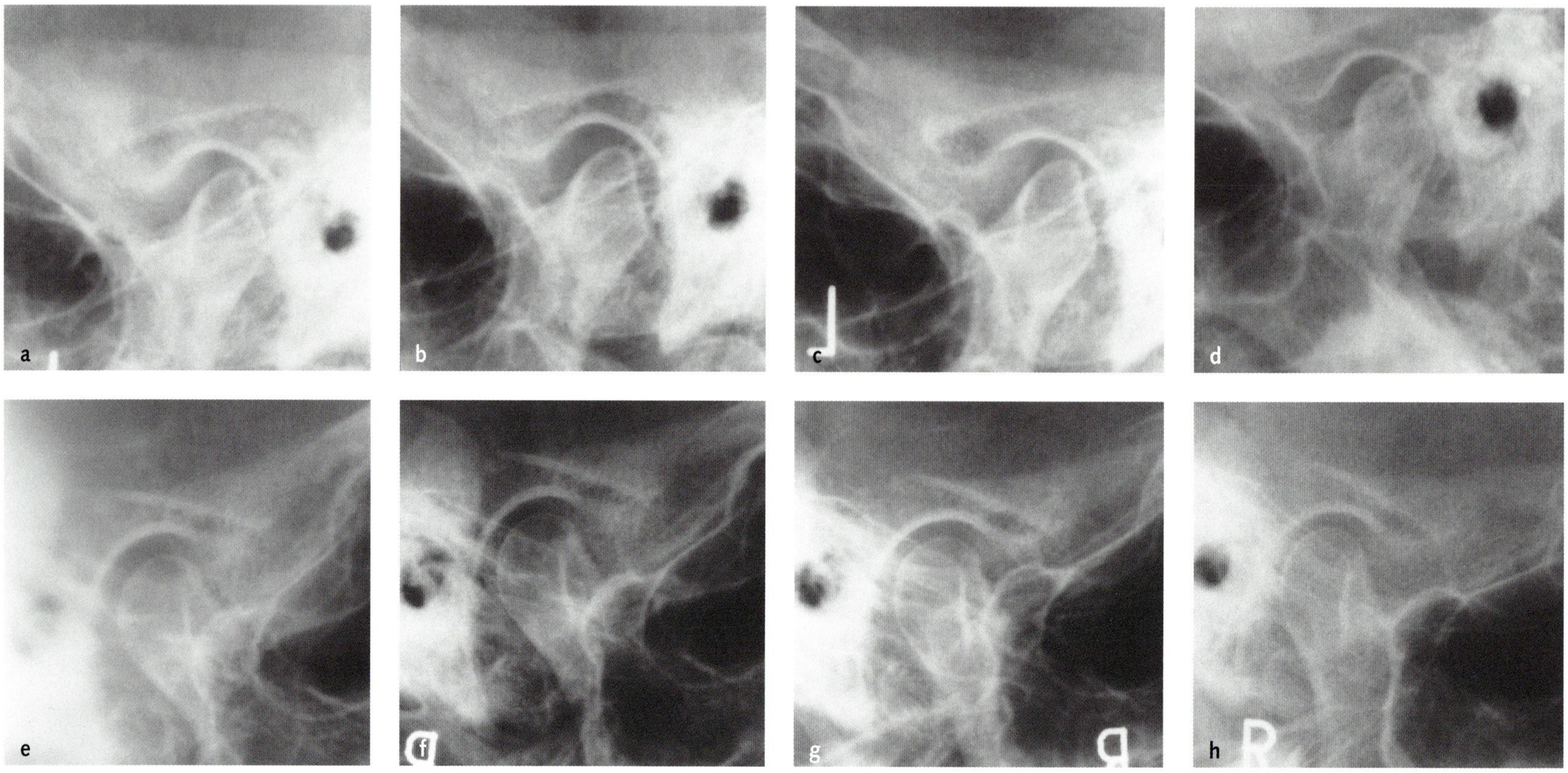

Fig 2-233 Changes in the TMJ areas. The left TMJ at ICP is shown (a) at the first visit, (b) after 1 year 1 month, (c) after 3 years 3 months, and (d) after 10 years 4 months. At the first visit, the condyle is posteriorly located. The posterior part of the condyle has erosion and is deformed flat. There is no displacement between the condyle and the disc. Control of inflammation and function was conducted, and 10 years later, changes in the positions of the right and left condyles are noted as the mandible has returned to the right. As the left articular space has expanded in the posterior area, compact bone has been generated in the posterior area of the condyle. Also, the flat portion has decreased while the rounded area has increased. The right TMJ at ICP is shown (e) at the first visit, (f) after 1 year 1 month, (g) after 3 years 3 months, and (h) after 10 years 4 months.

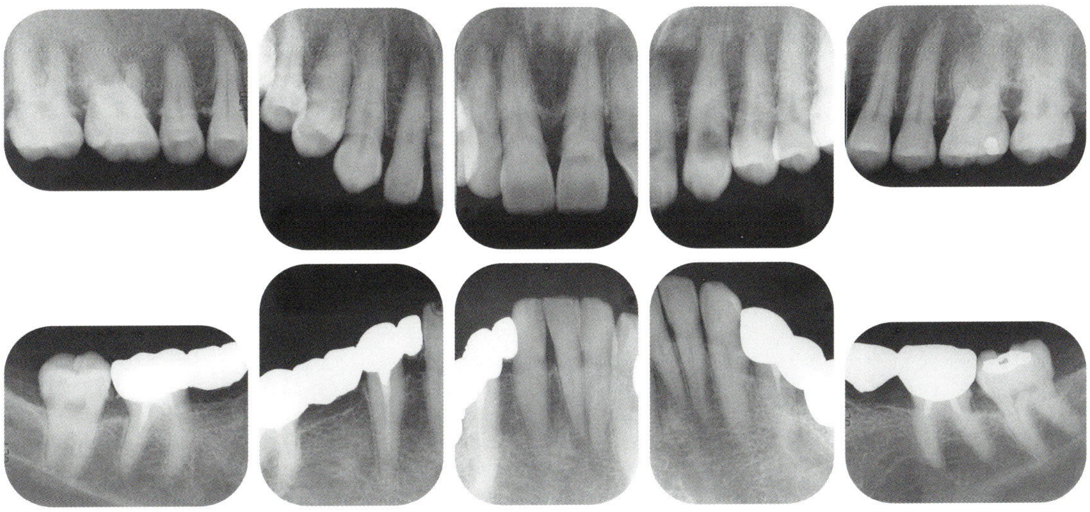

Fig 2-234 Full-mouth radiographs at the first visit (March 1992).

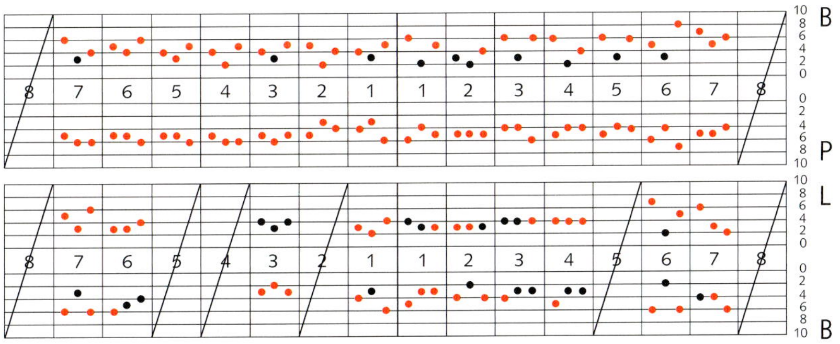

Fig 2-235 Probing chart at the first visit. Red indicates bleeding sites.

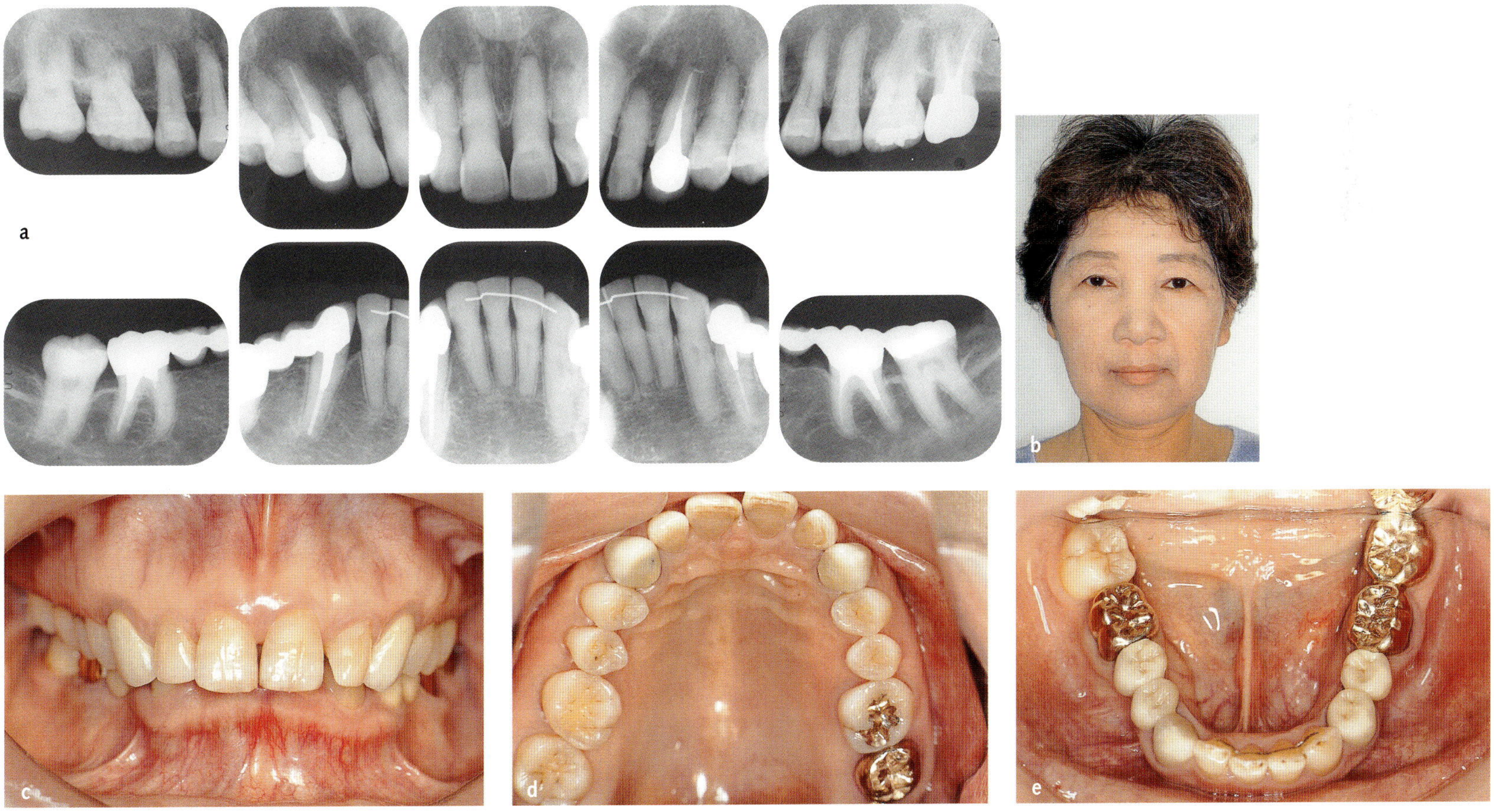

Fig 2-236 (a) Radiographs taken 10 years 4 months after the first visit (July 2002). (b) The frontal view of the face has regained symmetry. (c to e) Intraoral views.

Distortion of Face and Body and Psychologic Stress

Distortion of face and body

Abnormality of the occlusion and the habits that have caused it will invite distortion of the face and body. In a mild case, a patient often is not aware of the problem. Through improvement of the occlusion together with amelioration of habits, myofunctional therapy, and correction of posture, the distortion of the face and body will be resolved (Case 2-18).

"Normal occlusion": Occlusion neglecting functional movements

The idea is dominant that the cause of TMD symptoms in many patients is psychologic stress. This belief is probably derived from an incorrect perspective about normal occlusion. In a case when a clinician says, "There is nothing abnormal detected about occlusion," or "TMD symptoms do not ameliorate although occlusion was improved and is normal," the occlusion almost always was planned without consideration of functional movements.

Also, because many patients with TMD symptoms suffer from distress because people around them do not understand their afflicting symptoms and consequently the patients always feel nervous and frustrated, sometimes their symptoms are mistakenly attributed to psychologic problems. In many cases, however, psychological stress has been caused by an anomaly of occlusion. We have experienced a number of cases in which a patient's unbearable frustration, which had tortured the patient for more than 10 years, was resolved on the same day of treatment after areas with excessive guidance were ground. Through improvement of occlusion, most patients with a strong complaint of TMD symptoms will be psychologically stabilized and become cheerful and calm (Cases 2-19 and 2-20).

"Psychiatric patient"

There may be cases where a patient's TMD complaints have no primary cause related to occlusion and the occlusion issues receive excessive attention because of the patient's psychologic stress. What a dentist can do in such a case is to have sympathy to support the patient and to cope with various oral problems that can be improved. The strong anxiety, irritability, and emotional instability that are often observed in patients with TMD complaints do hinder regular dental treatments. However, these difficulties should be considered to have been caused by abnormality in occlusion. Such patients should not be labeled as "psychiatric patients" and excluded from treatment.

Case 2-18 Treatment of facial deformity caused by habits

Patient: *26-year-old woman at the time of first visit in 1998*
Chief complaint: *TMJ pain*
Although her chief complaint was TMJ pain, a glance at her face clearly shows that the balance between the right and the left is lost. Although her facial deformity is conspicuous, a certain degree of remodeling can be expected if the cause is identified and eliminated (Figs 2-238 to 2-242).
The patient had experienced clicking of the right TMJ at opening and pain for about 2 years. Sometimes she could open her mouth only by half, because the right side was stuck. She searched for a path where her jaw would not get caught when she opened the mouth.
Because of scoliosis (since her high school days), she suffered from pain in the right side of the back when she was tired. She visited an orthopedic surgeon when she was in high school and used a corset for 1.5 years. She was told the condition would not be cured because her growth was completed. She had a habit of resting her cheeks on the hands (for both sides, but especially the right side) and slept on her right because of the scoliosis.
In view of the TMJ symptoms at opening and closing, the condition was diagnosed as slightly old anterior disc displacement of the right TMJ with reduction (old, type III TMD) She exhibited a skeletal Class I occlusion and crowding.

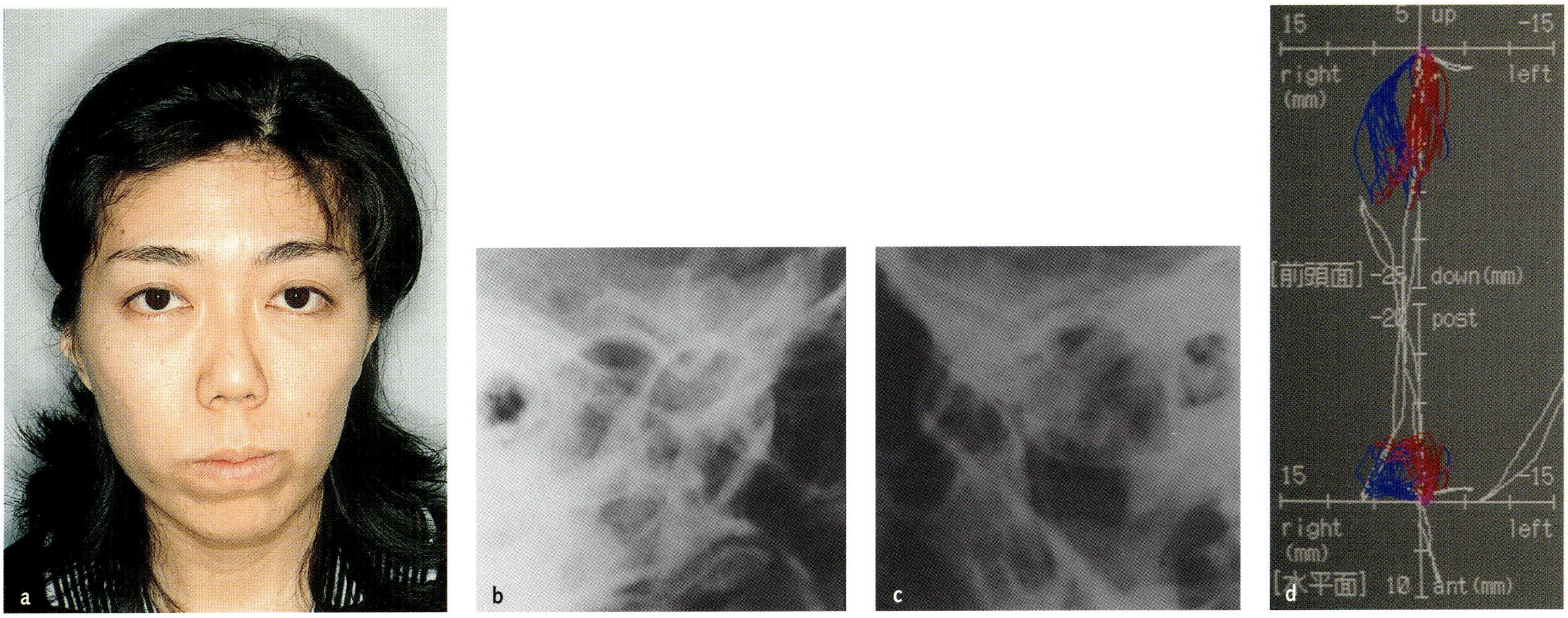

Fig 2-237 Shift of the face. (a) From the middle face to the lower face, there is a shift to the left. Although the patient says she has no chewing habits, the right masseter is hypertrophic (the wrinkly skin on the left cheek is considered hypofunctional), suggesting that she chews on the right side. (b) Right and (c) left TMJs at maximal opening. (d) Unconscious chewing according to the Sirognathograph also indicates right-side chewing. The facial shift to the left suggests the application of some external force. When the patient is allowed to open the mouth to a maximal level while the TMJ areas are palpated, clicking of the right TMJ occurs at about 4 cm of opening.

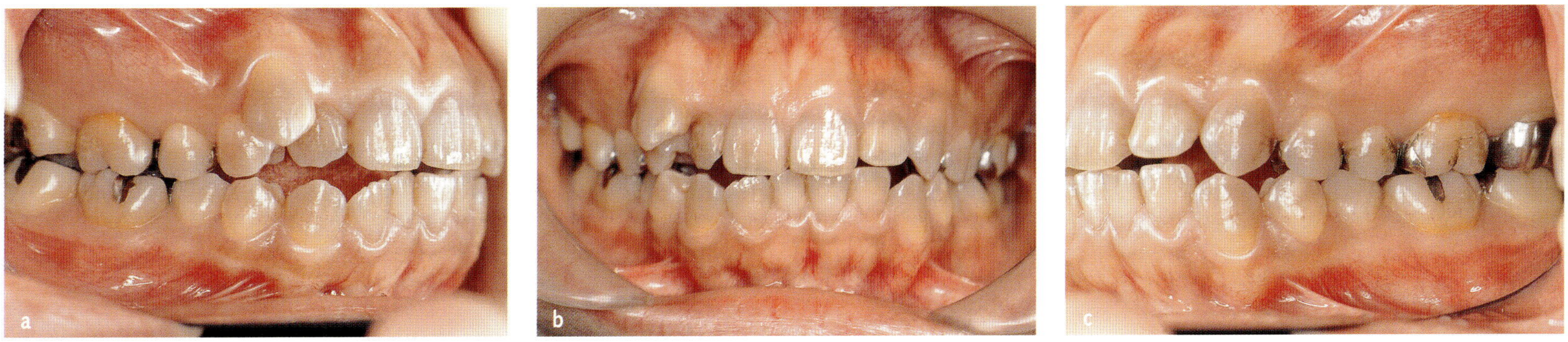

Fig 2-238 Cuspal interference. (a to c) Clinical examination shows crowding due to a discrepancy, a tongue thrusting habit, and open bite at the maxillary and mandibular lateral incisors and canines.

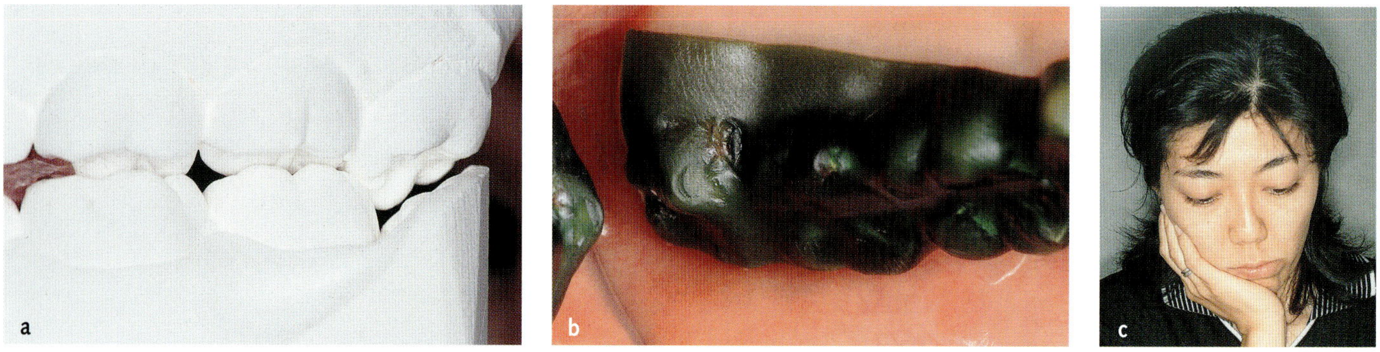

Fig 2-238 (cont) (d and e) It is suspected that the patient has unconsciously tried to avoid premature contact between maxillary left third molar and mandibular left second molar, which has invited the shift to the right. The original mandibular position should be more to the left than is current ICP. With this determination, the puzzle is solved (Box 2-23). (f) The external force applied to the face was found to be the patient's habit of resting her right cheek on her hand and her sleep postural habit.

Box 2-23 Deductive reasoning: Why is the right condyle off the disc while the lower face is shifted to the left?

- The patient chews on the right side.
- The occlusion at the molars is better on the left side.
- Why does she chew on the right side although there is a shift to the left?
- There should be some reason in the mouth that prevents her from chewing on the left side.
- When she is allowed to relax and tap, there is contact between maxillary left third molar and mandibular left second molar.

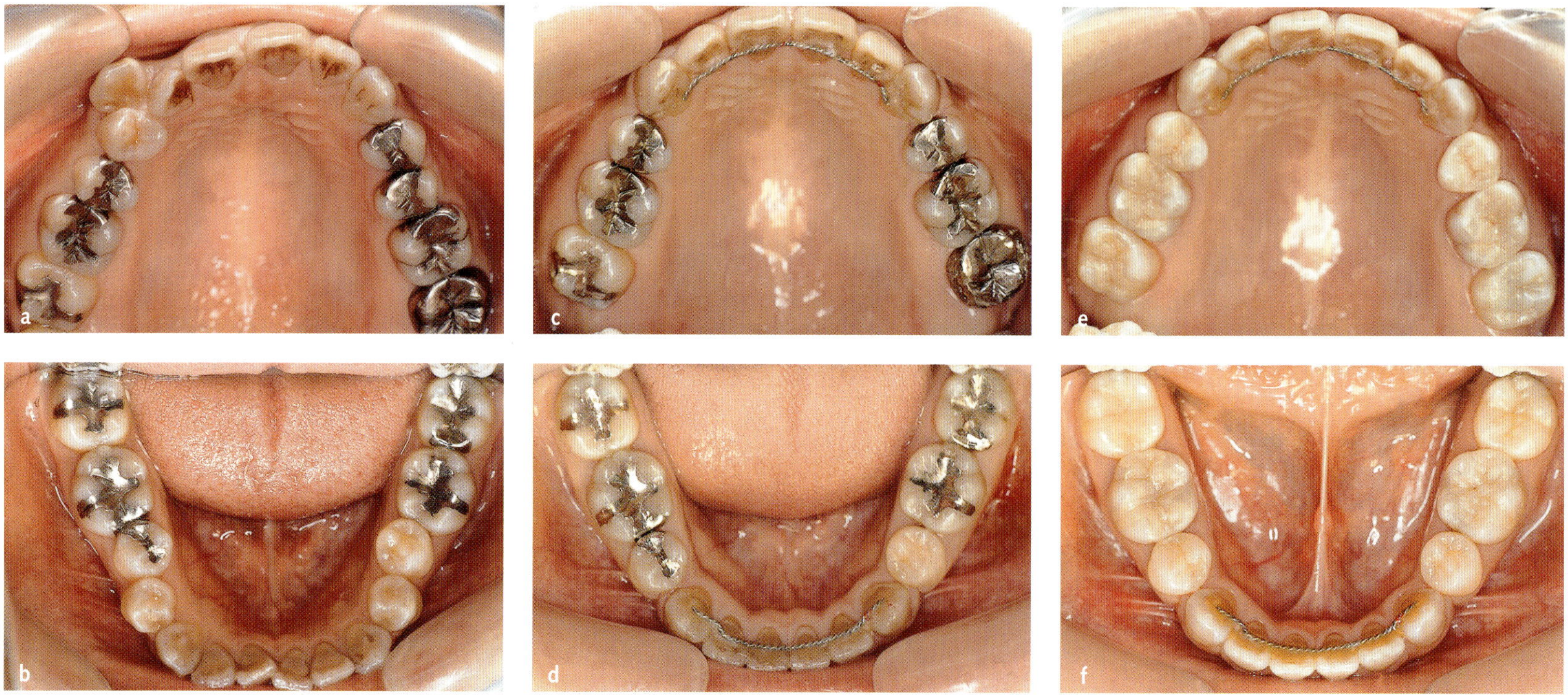

Fig 2-239 After the condyle returned to the disc, irreversible therapeutic intervention was made:
- The maxillary left third molar that caused interference was extracted.
- The patient was instructed to chew on the left side. (Because the right side will be a nonworking side, the right condyle is to be pulled forward.)
- She was instructed to stop her habits.
- She was instructed to consciously place her jaw in a position that does not cause clicking and to open and close in that position.
- A stabilization-type splint was used.

With these treatments, the condyle got on the disc shortly. Then all the first premolars were extracted while myofunctional therapy was conducted, the habits were prohibited, and occlusion was reestablished. (a and b) Occlusal views at the first visit. (c and d) Occlusal views at completion of active orthodontic treatment, 2 years 6 months after the first visit. (e and f) Occlusal views at completion of the restoration of occlusal surfaces, 3 years 5 months after the first visit.

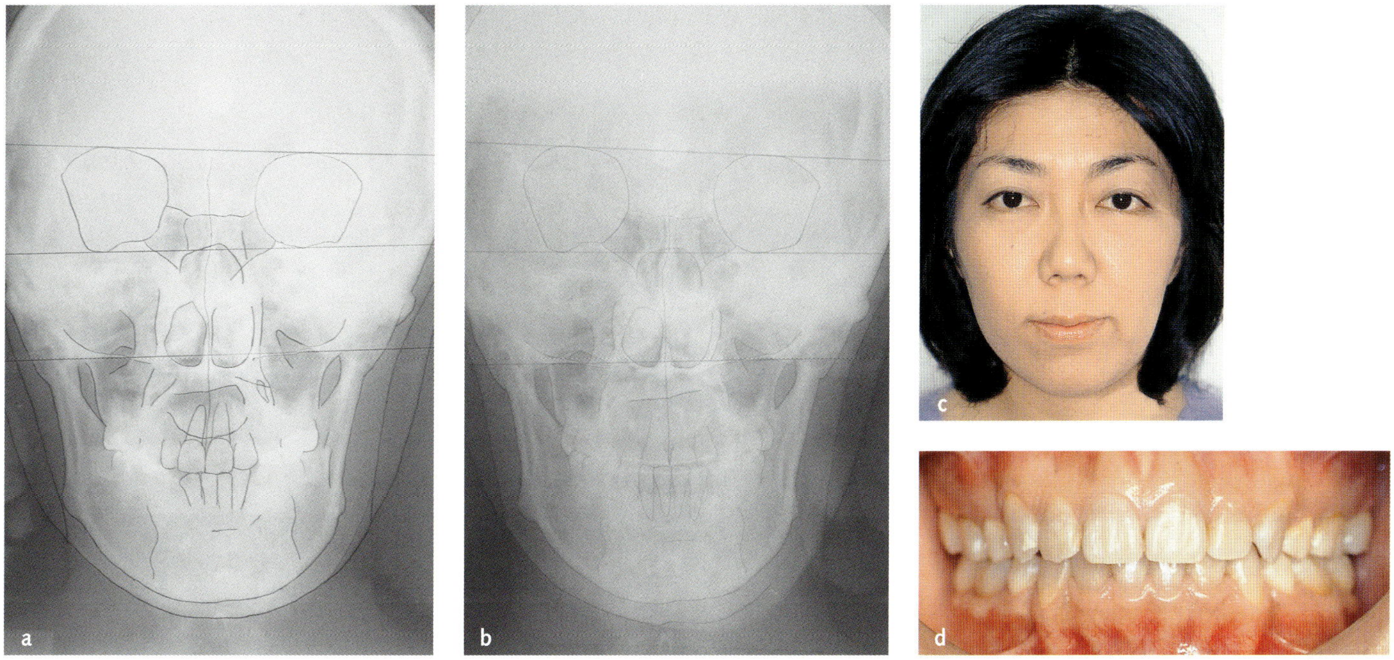

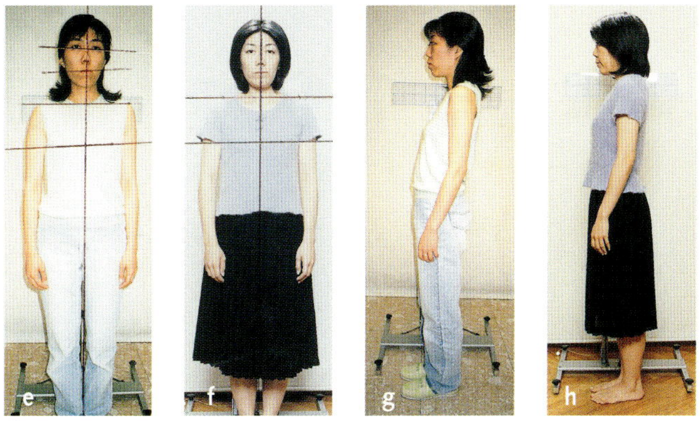

Fig 2-240 Facial deformity resolved by the correction of habits and orthodontic treatment. The skeletal shift of the whole body as well as the face has been ameliorated. A relaxed position and ICP are consistent. Tooth whitening was conducted for the maxillary anterior teeth. (a) Posteroanterior cephalogram at the first visit. (b) Posteroanterior cephalogram 3 years 5 months after the first visit. (c and d) Photographs taken 3 years 5 months after the first visit. (e to h) Her back pain still remains but has been alleviated. She can sleep in the supine position now. She says she feels much better than before. Her posture also has been improved significantly. (e and g) Photographs taken at the first visit. (f and h) Photographs taken after 3 years 5 months.

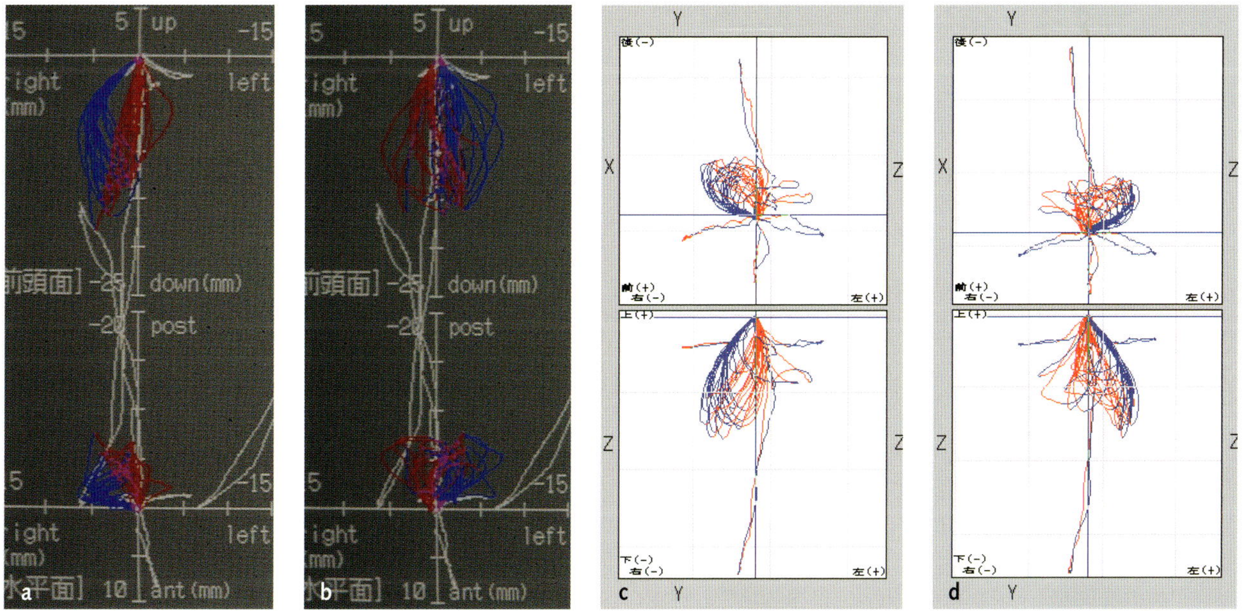

Fig 2-241 Changes in functional movements. (a) Sirognathograph of right-side chewing in the frontal plane *(top)* and the transverse plane *(bottom)* at the first visit. (b) Left-side chewing in the frontal plane *(top)* and the transverse plane *(bottom)*. Because the right condyle is off the disc, at maximal opening the path is pulled to the right to almost 50 mm. Masticatory movement paths have varied turning points on both the right and the left, and the condyle is on or off the disc during mastication. (c) Sirognathograph of right-side chewing in the frontal plane *(top)* and the transverse plane *(bottom)* after 3 years 5 months. Maximal opening has become straight. (d) Left-side chewing in the frontal plane *(top)* and the transverse plane *(bottom)*. Although masticatory movement paths have turning points mostly on the left, sometimes they are pulled to the right and the condyle gets off the disc.

Case 2-19 Patient who believed she had mental disorder

Patient: *42-year-old woman at the time of first visit in 1994*

This patient experienced trismus (disturbance of mouth opening due to pain) 5 months before the first visit to us and visited a university hospital to receive splint therapy. As a result, her right shoulder stiffness and tension in the neck were resolved and she could open her mouth. However, the splint was removed after 4 months and crowns were delivered for mandibular right second premolar and first molar. At that time, various symptoms were manifested again, including tinnitus, restlessness, frustration, and isolated feeling. These symptoms started about 2 years ago. She was told by an otorhinolaryngologist that there was no problem. She visited an internist and a neurologist, and an antidepressant was prescribed. Figures 2-243 to 2-248 show the good results achieved when her complaints were taken seriously.

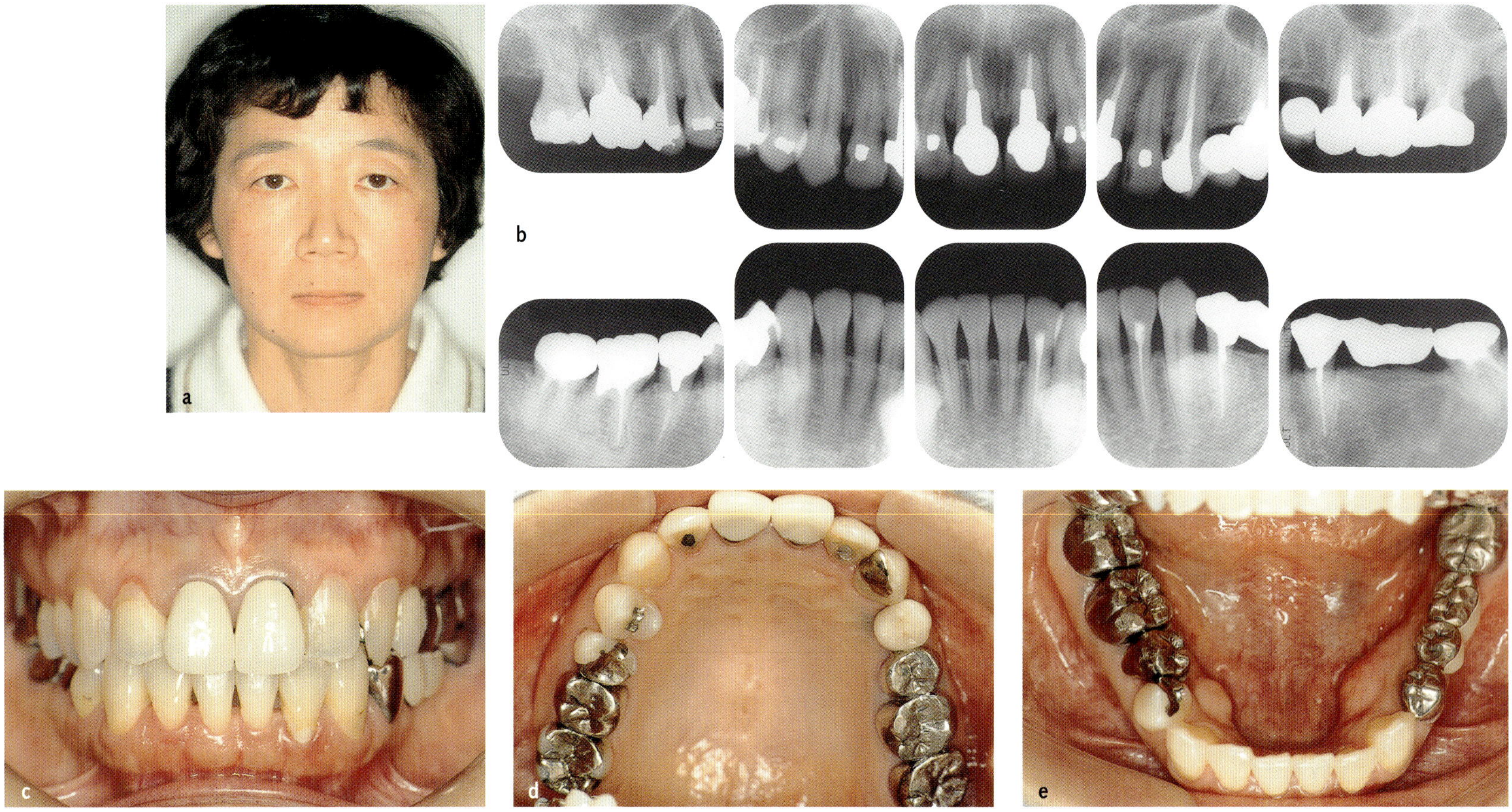

Fig 2-242 At the first visit. (a) Because she habitually uses antidepressants, she has a vacant look. She says she gets terribly irritated. The right masseter is hypertrophic, suggesting right-side chewing or right clenching. Although not clearly shown in this photograph, the right nasolabial fold is deeper. (b) The maxillary right canine, first premolar, and second premolar are extruded. (c to e) Metal-ceramic crowns were placed on the maxillary central incisors 17 or 18 years ago. An inlay was placed on the maxillary left canine 13 or 14 years ago. A fixed partial denture with the maxillary left second premolar, first molar, and second molar as abutments (pontic: maxillary left first premolar) was placed 4 years ago. A fixed partial denture extending from the mandibular left first premolar to the mandibular left second molar (pontics: mandibular left first molar and mandibular left second premolar) was placed some time ago, but she did not remember the exact year. Crowns had been fabricated for the mandibular right second premolar, first molar, and second molar 3 years ago. Although there is some noise during opening and closing, there is no pain in the TMJ areas. Because of the various restorations and distortion of the arches, the occlusion has gradually become tight.

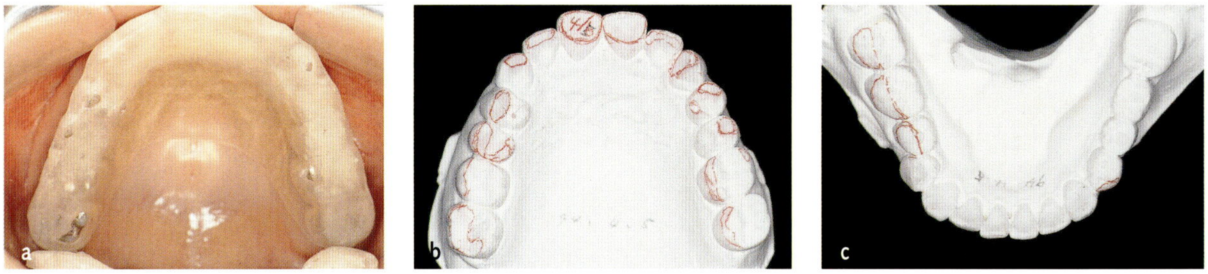

Fig 2-243 Occlusal therapy. (a) A splint is delivered. Symptoms caused by tight occlusion will be immediately reduced by the use of the splint. When the patient was reexamined after wearing the splint for 3 days, she said the throbbing of the heart had disappeared, she could sleep well, she felt much better, and she had no shoulder stiffness. The dose of antidepressant was reduced. (b and c) Guidance is eased. Red areas on the casts are ground to ease the guidance. All the symptoms were resolved except stiffness of the left side of the neck. The use of the antidepressant was discontinued.

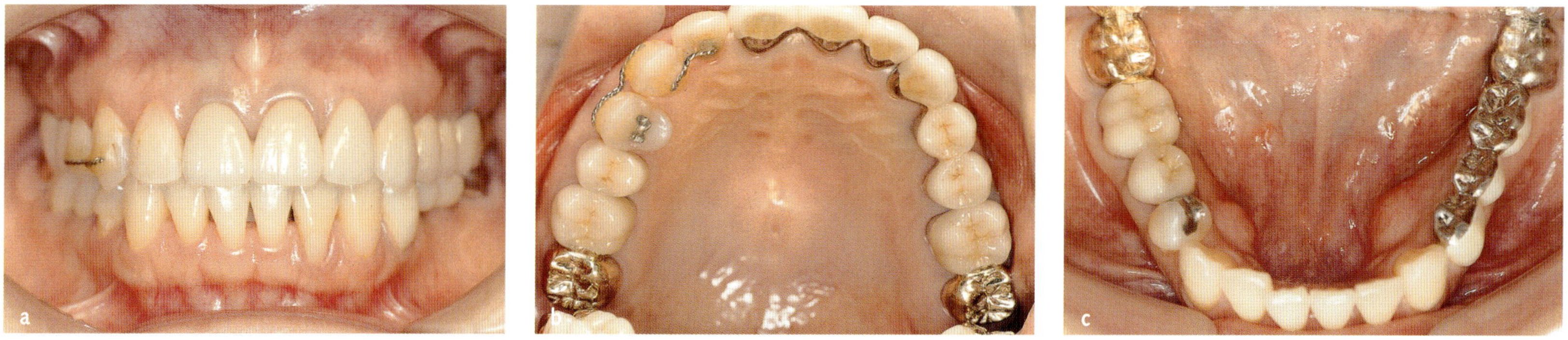

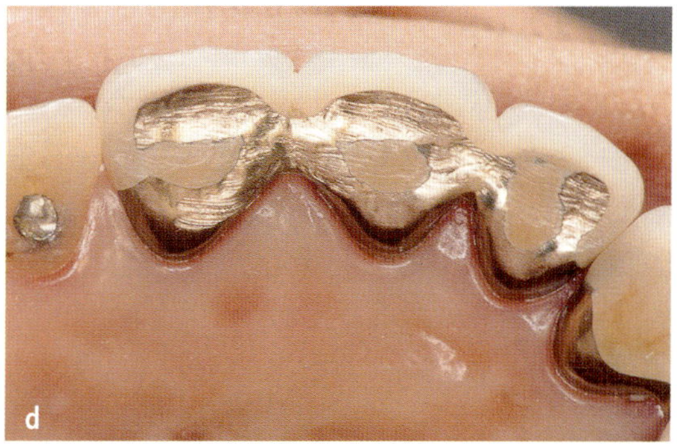

Fig 2-244 (a to c) Photographs taken 2 years 9 months after the first visit. As the molars have become disoccluded, existing crowns have been removed and metal provisional restorations have been delivered. The maxillary right canine, first premolar, and second premolar have been intruded while the occlusion of the remaining teeth has been prosthetically improved. (d) Photograph taken 2 years 3 months after delivery of final prostheses. Remodeling has continued even after delivery of the final prostheses. The lingual side of the maxillary anterior teeth with strong contacts are ground as necessity dictates.

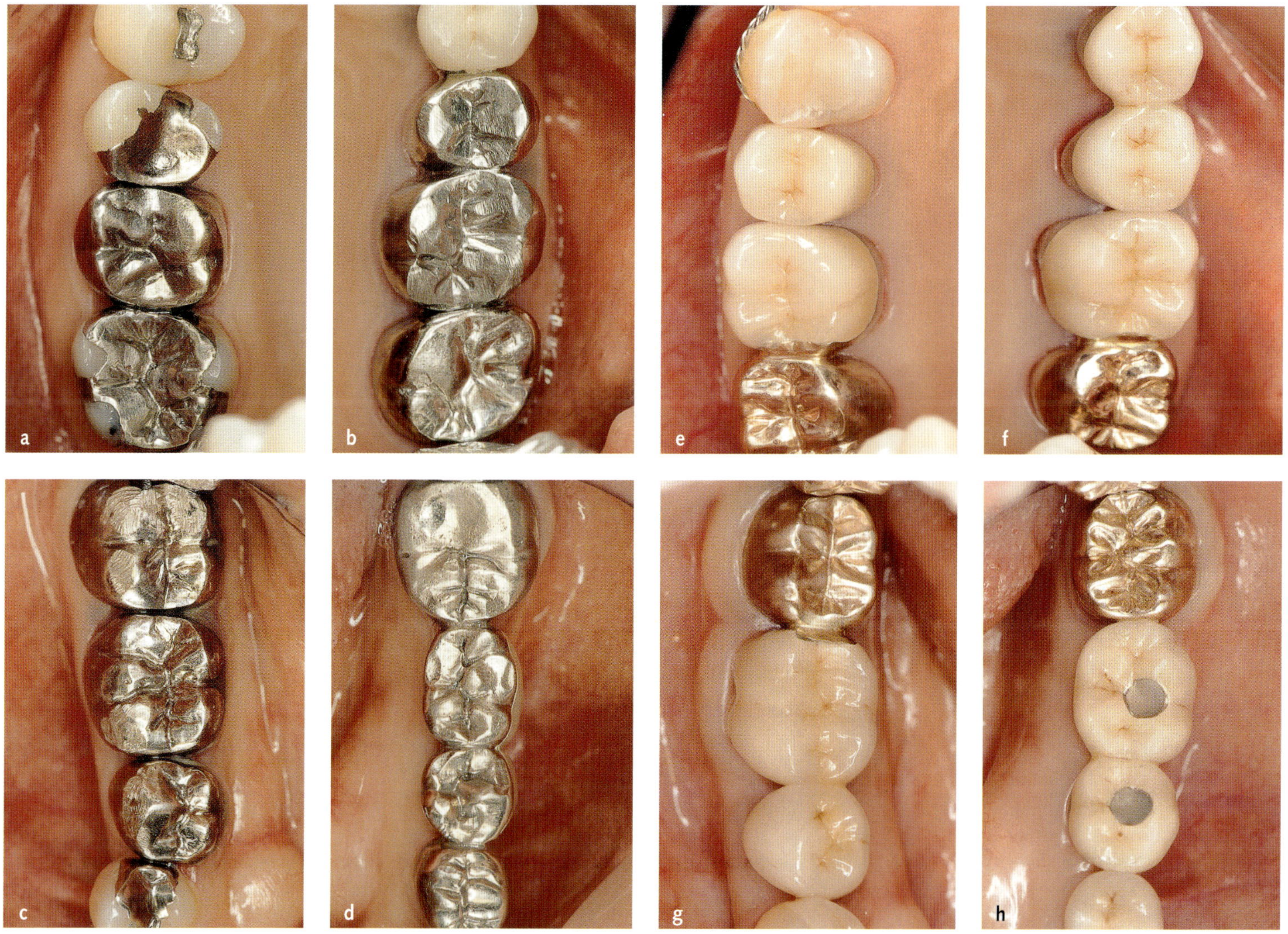

Fig 2-245 Improvement of the occlusal surfaces. (a to d) Photographs taken at the first visit. (e to h) Photographs taken 2 years 11 months after the first visit. (g) Implants have been placed for the mandibular left second premolar and first molar.

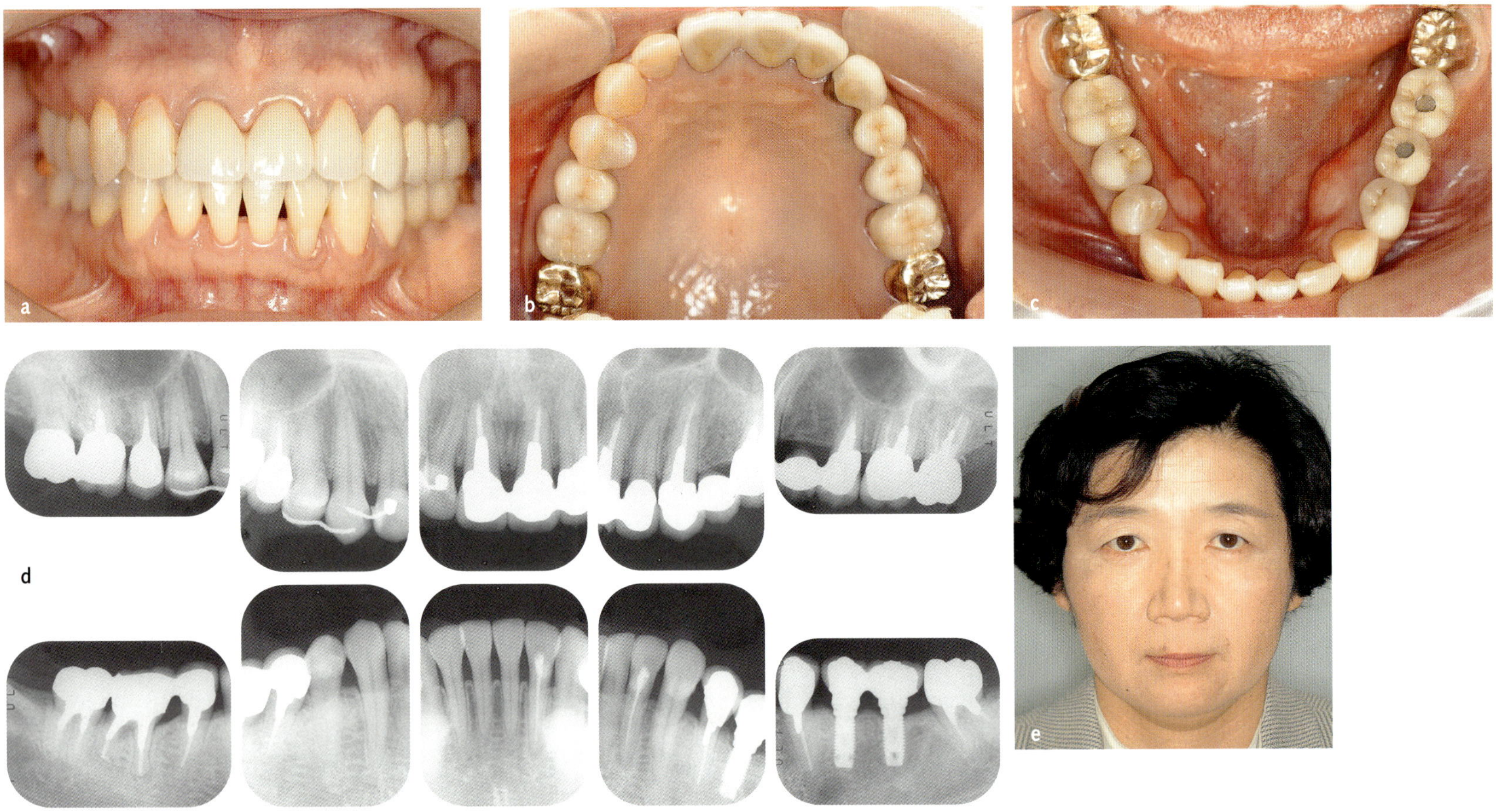

Fig 2-246 Maintenance phase. (a to c) Photographs taken 6 years 7 months after the first visit. Although there is some inflammation in the gingiva, the prosthesis for the maxillary anterior teeth has been newly fabricated according to the change in the mandibular position. The patient is cheerful and happy. It is almost impossible to believe this is the same person whom we met at the first visit. (d) Radiographs taken 2 years 11 months after the first visit. The maxillary right canine, first premolar, and second premolar are intruded. (e) Facial photograph taken 3 years 1 month after the first visit.

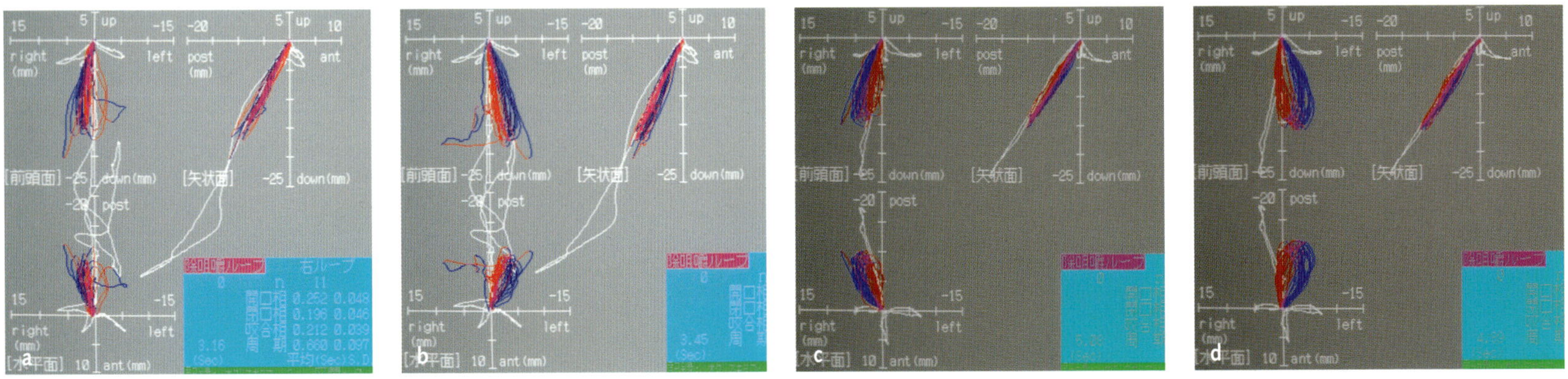

Fig 2-247 Change in mandibular functional movements during (a and c) right-side chewing and (b and d) left-side chewing. (a and b) The mandibular arch is deeply interdigitated in ICP and there is clenching caused by the tight occlusion. Although problems had developed over 10 years, every time partial restoration was repeated, it seems that the mandibular right fixed partial denture and the sleep postural habit triggered symptoms eventually. It was surmised that the right-side opening was delayed and that symptoms such as tinnitus resulted because the right-side clenching was strong. (c and d) Functional movements measured about 4 years after the first visit. The functional movement path that used to converge at ICP in a thin, arrowlike manner now forms fine cycles.

Case 2-20 Abnormality of occlusion causing psychological stress

Patient: *20-year-old man at the time of first visit in 1997*

Chief complaint: *Continuing pain in various sites of the body and distortion of the face*

The patient's maxillary and mandibular right first premolars were extracted when he was 17 years old and started orthodontic treatment for crowding. The orthodontic appliance was removed about 1 year later. From about this time on, he became concerned about a series of symptoms, "feeling the body has been distorted to the right." He received splint therapy, which did not improve the condition. His family and his doctor considered this to be "a psychiatric problem." His orthodontist referred him to us 2 years after the orthodontic treatment. We treated him successfully by paying careful attention to the occlusion in terms of functional morphology(Figs 2-249 to 2-259).

Observations at the first visit

- *Various symptoms that the patient was aware of were concentrated on the left side of the body.*
- *He complained that his body was distorted to the right.*
- *The lower face was shifted to the right, and the maxilla was shifted to the right. The mandible was shifted to the right by the width of one tooth.*
- *He was restless in the dental chair, constantly rubbing his shoulder and twisting his body.*
- *The frontal view of the face showed that the nasal column was shifted to the right and the nasal apex was shifted to the left.*

We considered the possibility that not only the mandible but also the maxilla might be shifted to the right and that the nasal apex might be closer to the original midline.

Inference about onset of the pathologic conditions

A photograph taken when the patient was about 10 years old indicated that the lower face was shifted to the right (see Fig 2-249g). Study casts made before orthodontic treatment also showed that the maxillary left arch was narrowed. The case history indicated the following progression of events:

- *The maxilla was shifted to the right due to his sleep postural habit.*
- *The shift to the right was increased by the extraction of the maxillary and mandibular right first premolars.*
- *The mandible was shifted to the right because of premature contact of maxillary left first premolar and mandibular left first premolar. (Because the patient believed that this had been caused by the orthodontic treatment, habits such as sleep posture could not be elucidated.)*
- *Occlusion was stabilized at a habitual ICP.*
- *Prosthetic treatment took place.*
- *Onset of TMD symptoms followed these changes.*

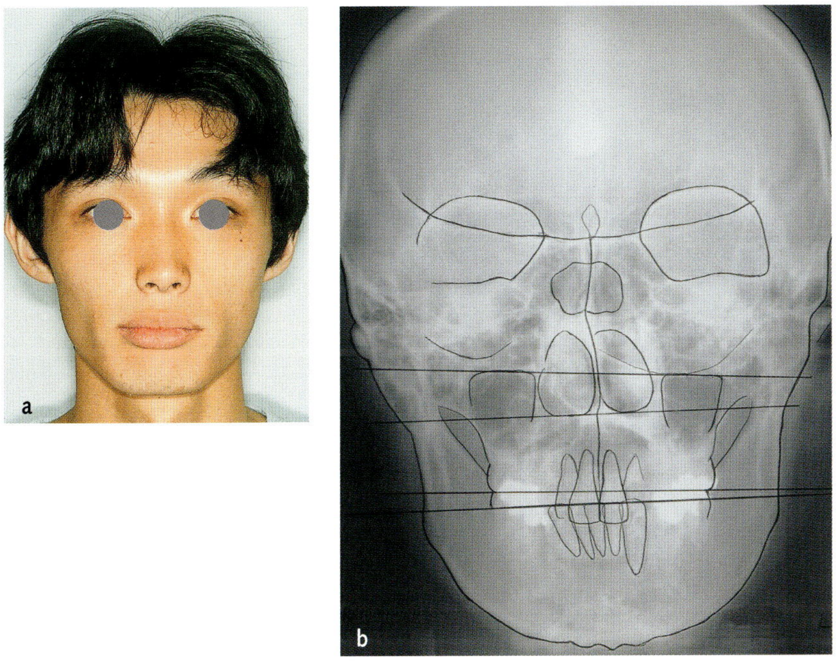

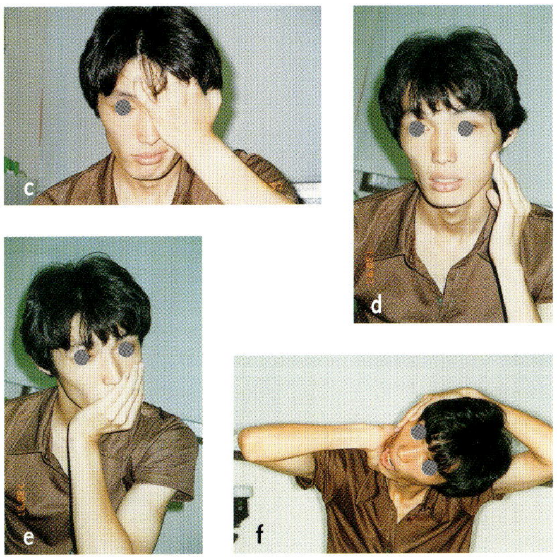

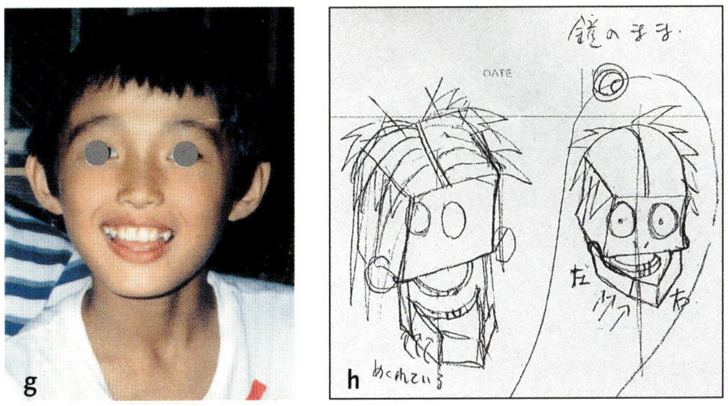

Fig 2-248 At the first visit. (a and b) Observation of the face indicates that, compared to the root of the nose, the apex of the nose is shifted to the left and that the midline of the lips is also shifted to the right. (b to f) When he is in a dental chair, he is restless. (g) A photograph taken when he was about 10 years old shows that the maxilla was already shifted to the right. (h) The patient brought his drawing of distortion of his face, which surprised us because he drew exactly what we surmised from findings of his face.

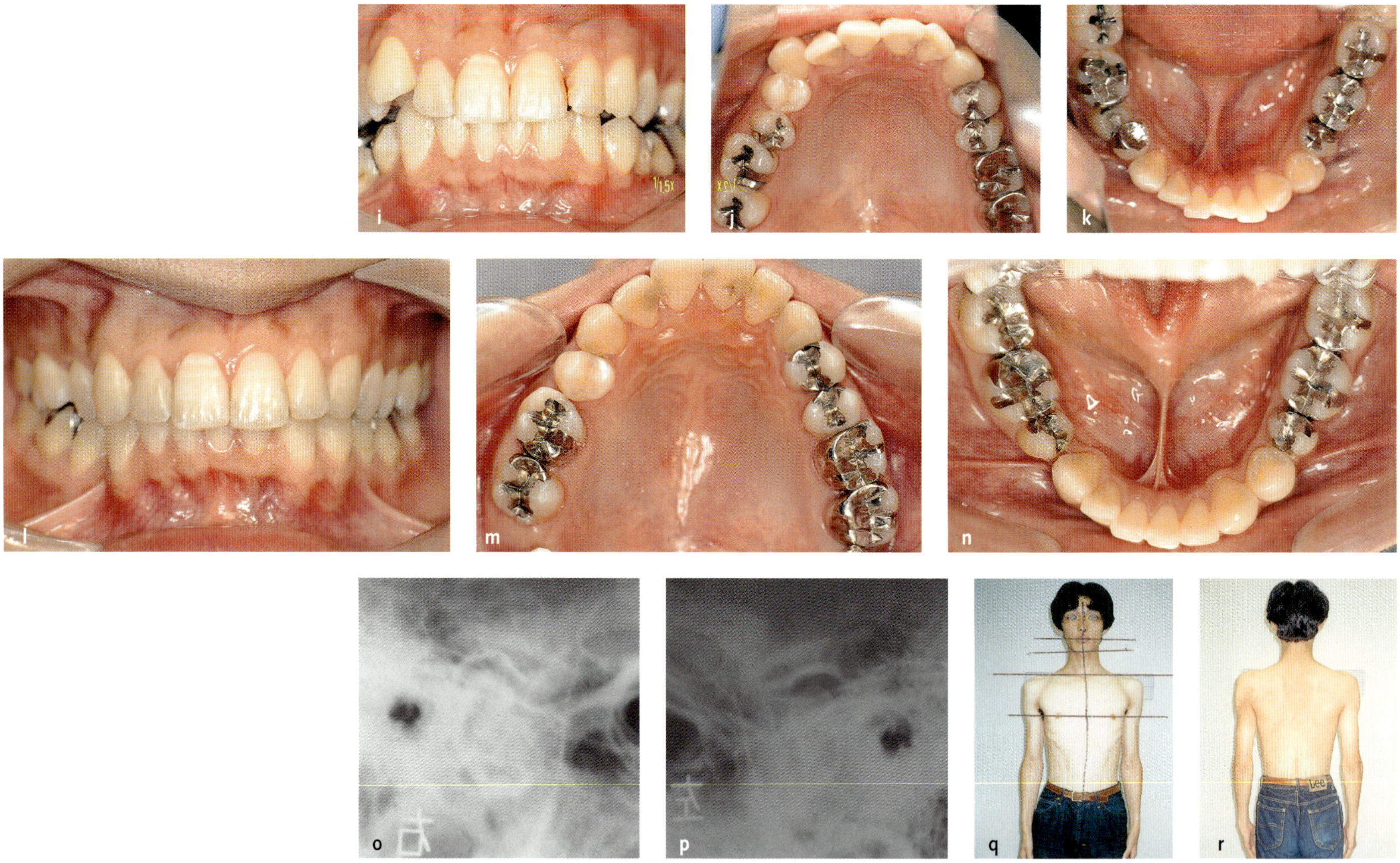

Fig 2-248 (cont) (i to k) Clinical photographs taken before orthodontic treatment was provided by his previous dentist. The maxillary left arch is narrow and the maxillary right arch is wide. (l to n) Clinical photographs taken when he first visited us, 2 years after orthodontic treatment was completed by a previous dentist. Because orthodontic treatment was conducted with full brackets after extraction of the right first premolars, the shift of the maxillary and mandibular arches to the right is conspicuous, especially that of the mandibular arch. At a relaxed position, the mandible is shifted to the right by 1 mm more than is shown in these photographs. (o and p) Because the patient has a brachyfacial-type pattern, the condyles are well developed and less likely to come off the disc, which would have been a cause of serious and unpleasant symptoms. The articular space is wider on the left side. The patient says the left TMJ is slightly painful. (q and r) The patient strains his muscles throughout the body. The midline of the chest is shifted to the left. He says he feels better when his body is rotated to the left.

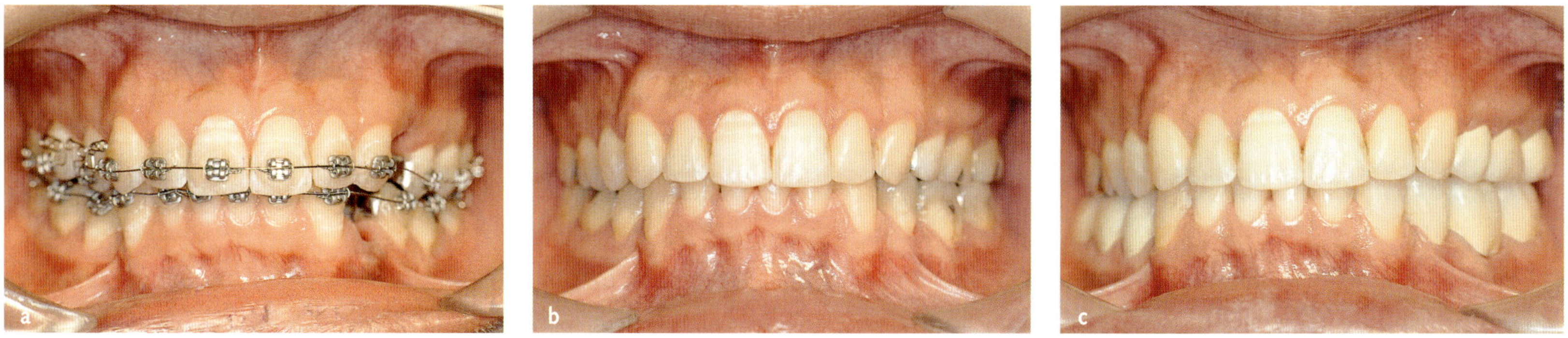

Fig 2-249 Restorative tooth movement. (a) First, we patiently listened to the patient's complaints and encouraged him to correct his habits. A splint was delivered after 2 months. The maxillary and mandibular left first premolars were extracted. Full brackets were attached about 2 months after the first visit. (b) Photograph taken after 3 years 5 months, when orthodontic appliances have been removed. Resin composite is added to disoccluded areas in molars. (c) Estenia superhard hybrid resin crowns are provisionally cemented for the maxillary left second premolar, first molar, and second molar; the mandibular left second premolar, first molar, and second molar; and the mandibular right second premolar, first molar, and second molar.

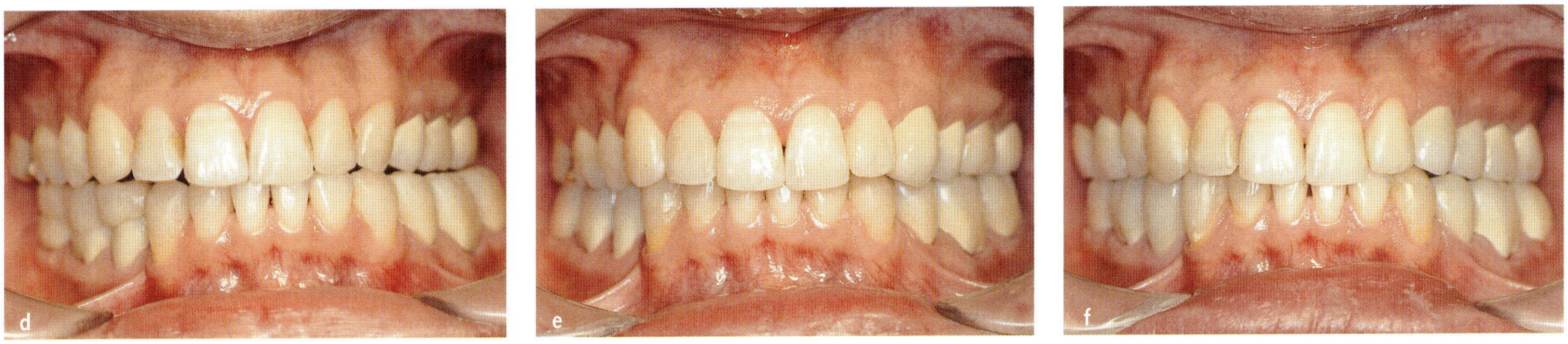

Fig 2-249 (cont'd) (d) At a recall examination after cementation of the provisional restorations, the patient is already chewing at a position shifted to the left by about 3 mm. Resin crowns should be fabricated not only with vertical dimension but also with occlusal surface morphology for chewing. (e) This process of adding resin to disoccluded molars is repeated for about 10 months after provisional cementation, and the restorations are luted as the final prostheses. The patient felt better and became stable psychologically. (f) He went abroad to study, but because of further remodeling that took place, we had to fabricate new prostheses when he returned to Japan. When he was temporarily back in Japan, the lingual side of the maxillary left canine was ground; the A slope was added for the maxillary left second premolar, first molar, and second molar; the A slope was narrowed for the mandibular left second premolar, first molar, and second molar; and the A slope was added for the mandibular right canine, second premolar, first molar, and second molar. After these adjustments, new prostheses were fabricated and delivered for the maxillary right second premolar, first molar, and second molar; the maxillary left canine, second premolar, first molar, and second molar; the mandibular left second premolar, first molar, and second molar; and the mandibular right second premolar, first molar, and second molar. The vertical dimension at the molars has been naturally raised and the midline is meeting. Significant change is not expected to occur even with further remodeling in the future. Crown restoration for the maxillary right second premolar, first molar, and second molar was conducted because of the patient's desire. He reported that final stability was achieved after crown restoration of these teeth.

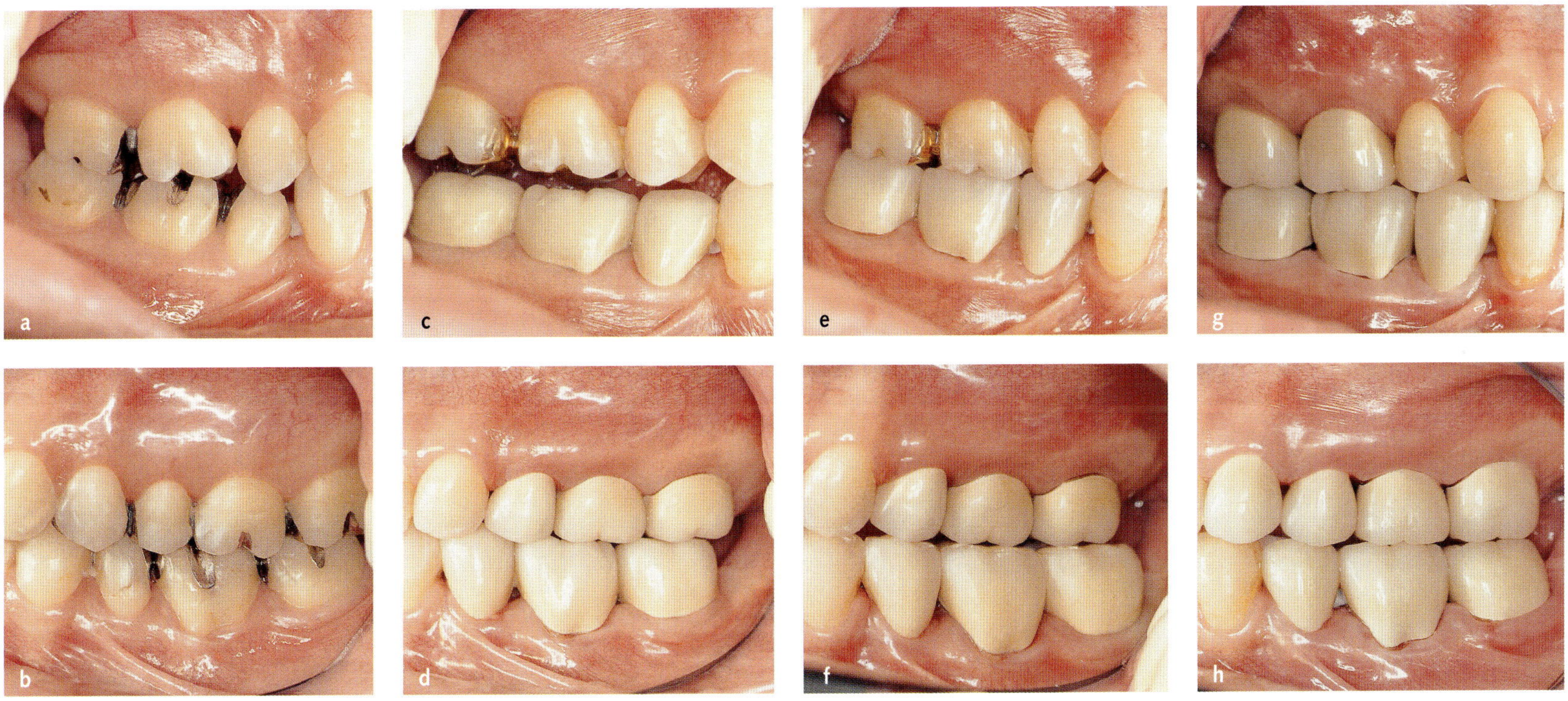

Fig 2-250 Change in vertical dimension accompanying the change in mandibular position. (a and b) Every time the mandible moves forward and to the right or the left, material is added to the molars and the A, B, and C slopes are created repeatedly. When occlusal morphology is provided to stabilize ICP and allow mastication in a mandibular position that the patient expresses, the occlusion will naturally revive. (c and d) After provisional cementation of the final prostheses, the patient has started to chew at a different position. (e and f) As molars are disoccluded, resin is added to the occlusal surface of the Estenia crowns. This process is repeated for 10 months after provisional cementation. (g and h) Appearance at delivery of the newly fabricated final prostheses.

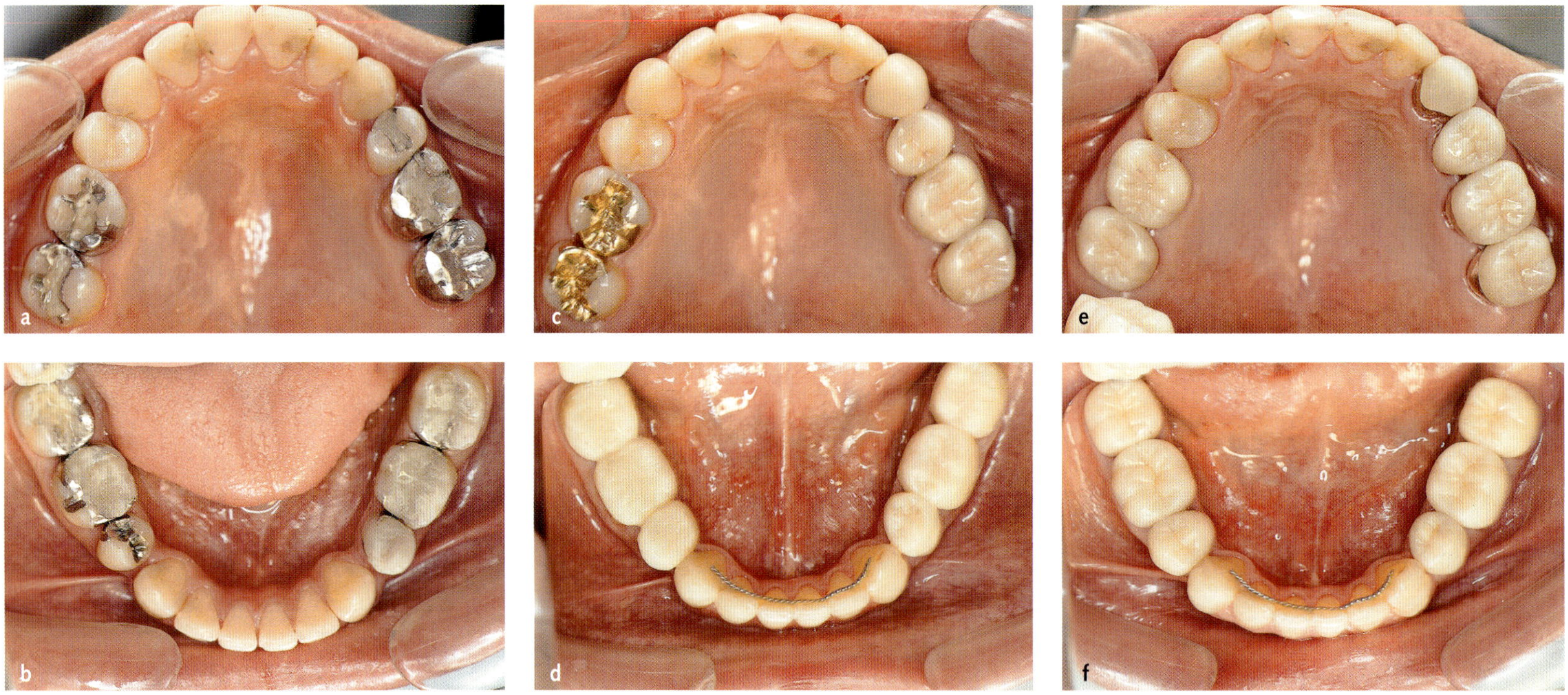

Fig 2-251 Occlusal surfaces after orthodontic treatment. (a and b) As the mandible moves forward due to remodeling and the molars become disoccluded, light-curing resin is added to the occlusal surface for correction. This process is repeated. (c and d) The restorations include Estenia crowns for the maxillary left canine, second premolar, first molar, and second molar; the mandibular left second premolar, first molar, and second molar; and the mandibular right second premolar, first molar, and second molar; an Estenia inlay for the maxillary right second premolar; and gold inlays for the maxillary right first and second molars. (e and f) As the mandible has returned further to the left, the A slope has been increased and the C slope has been reduced on the maxillary left second premolar, first molar, and second molar. Similarly, the A slope has been reduced and the C slope has been increased on the mandibular left second premolar, first molar, and second molar. The A slope has been increased and the C slope reduced on the mandibular right canine, second premolar, first molar, and second molar. As the patient desired, crowns also have been fabricated for the maxillary right second premolar, first molar, and second molar.

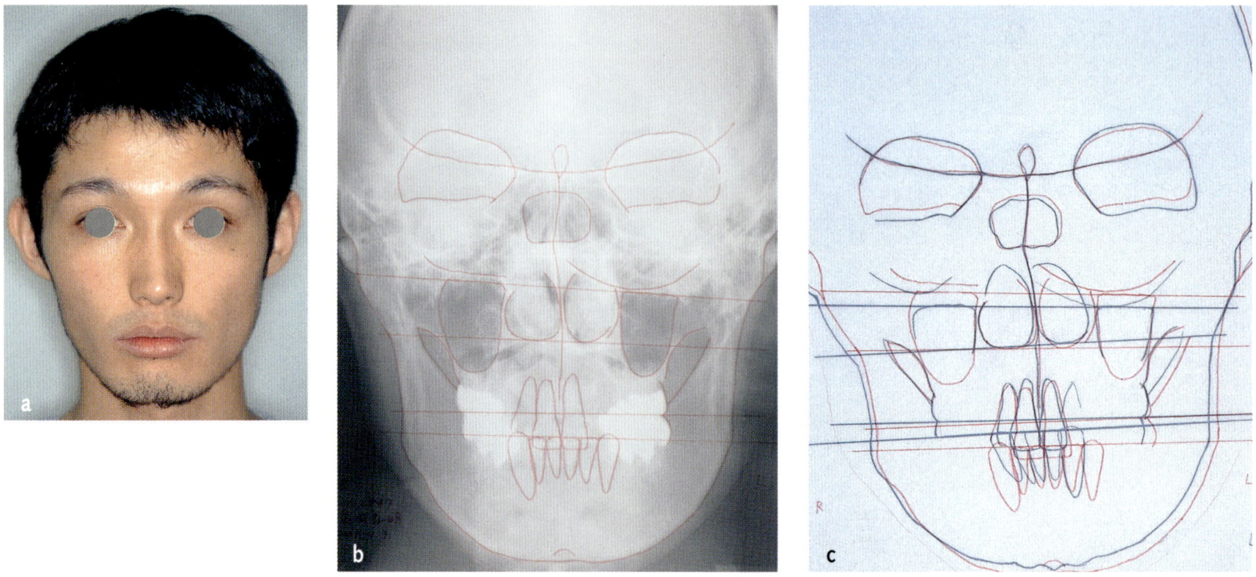

Fig 2-252 (a) After treatment, his face has become full and peaceful. The midline of the face is mostly aligned, and the discrepancy between the apex and the column of the nose is diminished. (b) Posteroanterior cephalogram after treatment. (c) The superimposition of tracings before *(black)* and after *(red)* treatment clearly shows that the shift to the right has been reduced. The parallelism of planes obtained from several reference points is improved. This comparison may indicate the patient's suffering at the time of the first visit.

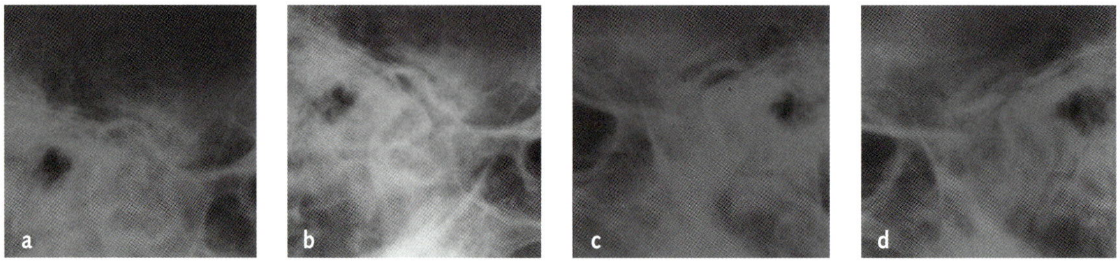

Fig 2-253 Radiographs of the TMJs after treatment. (a) Right TMJ at ICP at the completion of orthodontic treatment. Although the mandible has advanced, the articular space is not expanded much, suggesting movement of the whole temporal bone. (b) Right TMJ 8 months after completion of orthodontics. The right condyle is located quite anteriorly. (c) Left TMJ at ICP at the completion of orthodontic treatment. At the first visit, although the mandible was shifted to the right, the left condyle was posteriorly located and the articular space was expanded. After completion of orthodontic treatment, the right and the left sides are mostly symmetric. (d) Left TMJ 8 months after that completion of orthodontics, when the mandible is further moved to the left.

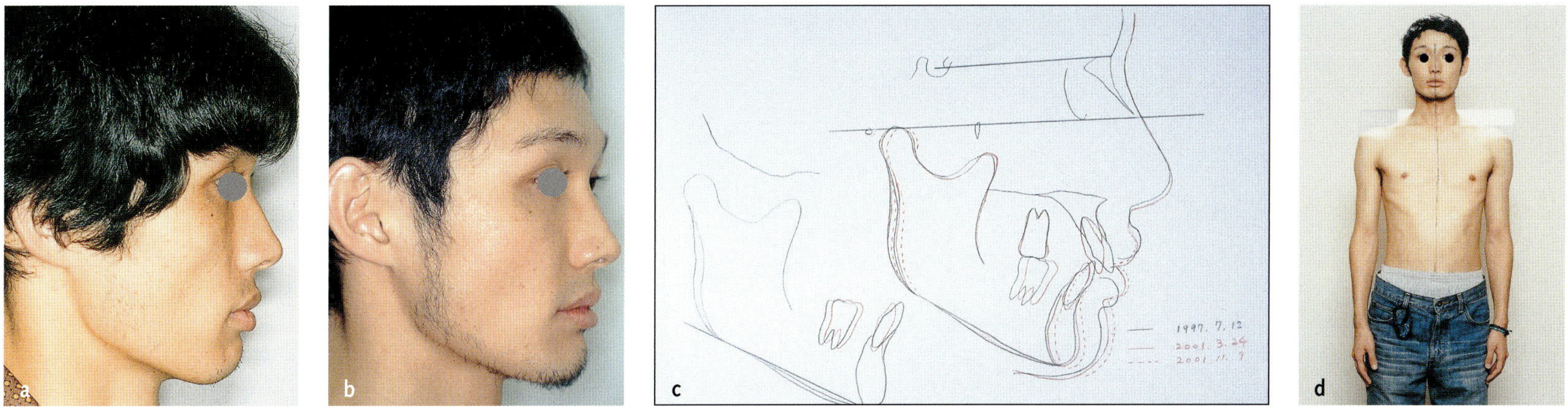

Fig 2-254 Changes in the profile and the whole body. (a) Profile at the first visit. (b) In profile, the lower facial height has increased and it looks as if his nose has become more prominent, 4 years 4 months after the first visit. (c) The superimposition of lateral cephalograms confirms similar changes over time, from 1997 *(black)* to March 2001 *(solid red)* to November 2001 *(dashed red)*. (d) Appearance of the body 4 years 4 months after the first visit. His posture is mostly straight and he has become heavier.

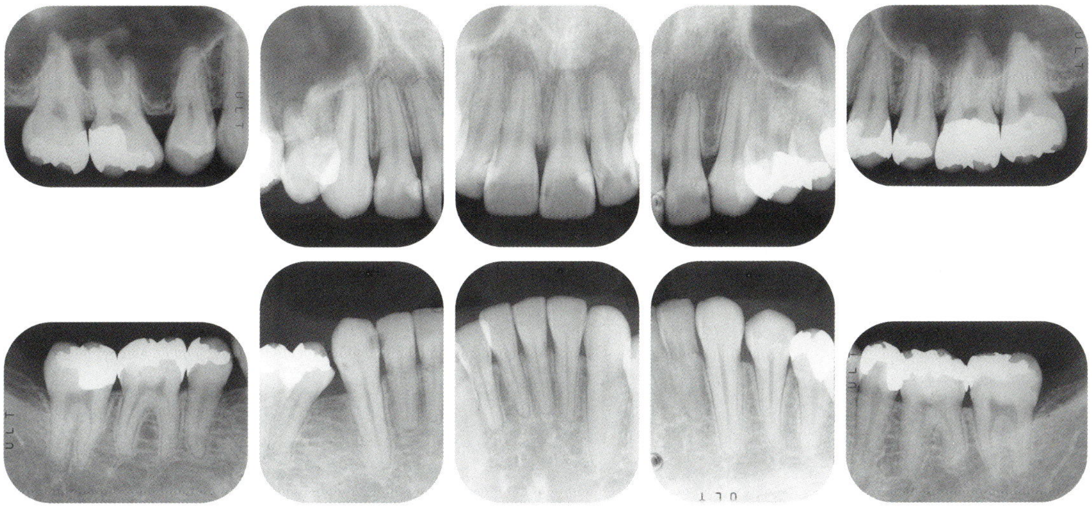

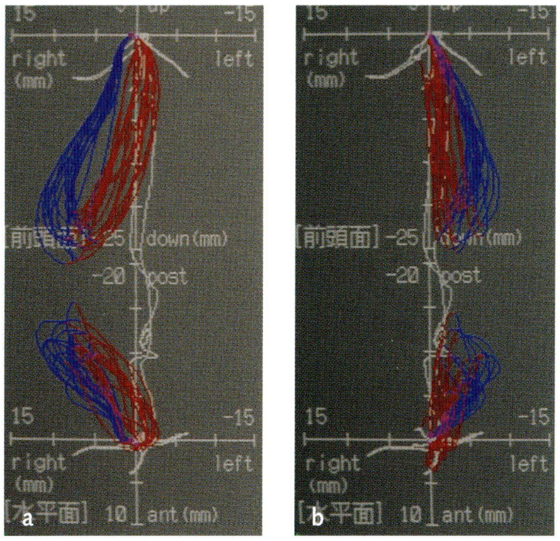

Fig 2-255 Radiographs taken at the first visit.

Fig 2-256 Functional movements at the first visit. (a) At the first visit, right-side chewing is evaluated in the frontal plane *(top)* and the transverse plane *(bottom)*. There is excessive guidance at closing. (b) At the first visit, left-side chewing is evaluated in the frontal plane *(top)* and the transverse plane *(bottom)*. There is interference at opening, and excessive guidance at closing is observed.

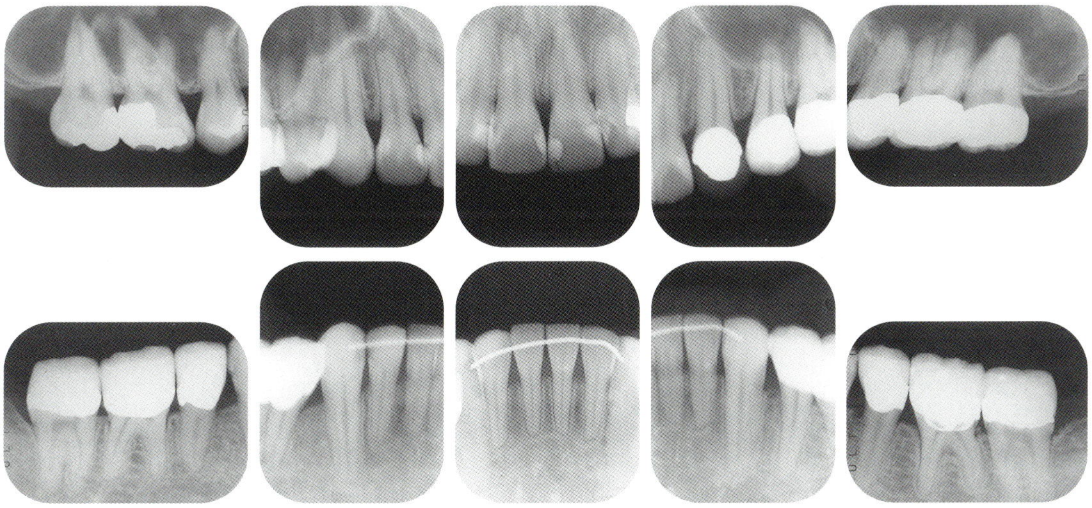

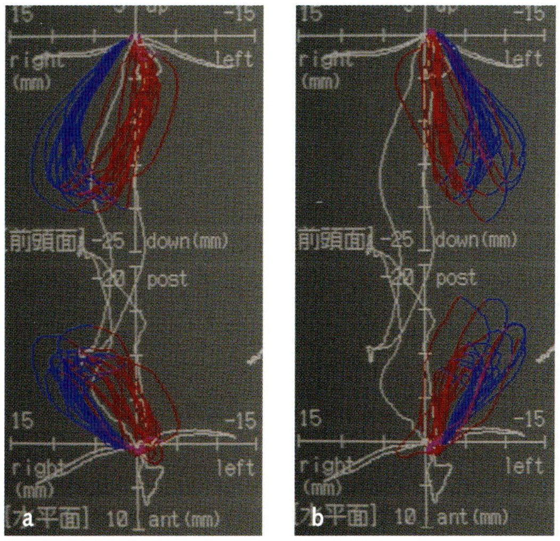

Fig 2-257 Radiographs taken 3 years 8 months after the first visit, at completion of active orthodontic treatment. Although ideally extrusion of molars should be promoted, these molars are buried deeply in the bone.

Fig 2-258 Functional movements (a) Right-side chewing is evaluated in the frontal plane *(top)* and transverse plane *(bottom)*, 3 years 8 months after the first visit. Acceptable chewing cycles are observed. (b) Left-side chewing is evaluated in the frontal plane *(top)* and transverse plane *(bottom)*. Excessive guidance at opening still remains. Although the mandibular position is different, this is not expressed in a mandibular movement analyzer.

Chapter 3

Restorative Tooth Movement

Restorative Tooth Movement

Orthodontic treatment and restorative tooth movement

By actively changing the oral environment, orthodontic treatment corrects and treats imbalances that have been generated during the growth process. In contrast, the authors define *restorative tooth movement* as tooth movement with the therapeutic intention of restoring harmony that originally existed. While conventional orthodontic treatment divides patients into growing and nongrowing categories, restorative tooth movement is characterized by therapeutic intervention to an occlusion that has collapsed. This collapse occurs when occlusion and periodontal status have fallen into a vicious cycle of imbalance caused by a combination of periodontal inflammation and destructive occlusal forces. Tooth movement conducted to rebuild a collapsed occlusion and/or to restore the periodontal environment requires different concepts from those of conventional orthodontic treatment (Fig 3-1).

"Leveling" to adjust bone level

An example of conventional orthodontic treatment would be orthodontic treatment to level an occlusal plane or the height of the proximal surfaces of the teeth, which is based on the premise that, if the vertical height of teeth is normal, the bone level will be arranged, the gingival attachment level will be adjusted, and the depth of the gingival sulcus will be within a normal range. This scenario assumes that the patient is a growing individual without attrition and with a high capacity for adaptation or an individual who has completed growth and has a basically healthy periodontal environment. In restorative tooth movement, which involves teeth with attrition, advanced loss of attachment due to periodontitis, and bony defects, the primary purpose of leveling is to achive flat bony architecture. Only by such therapeutic interventions can the level of the gingival margin as well as the attachment level be adjusted to obtain results that will be satisfactory from the functional, hygienic, and esthetic points of view. Afterward, if necessary, the morphology of the teeth will be adjusted with restorations.

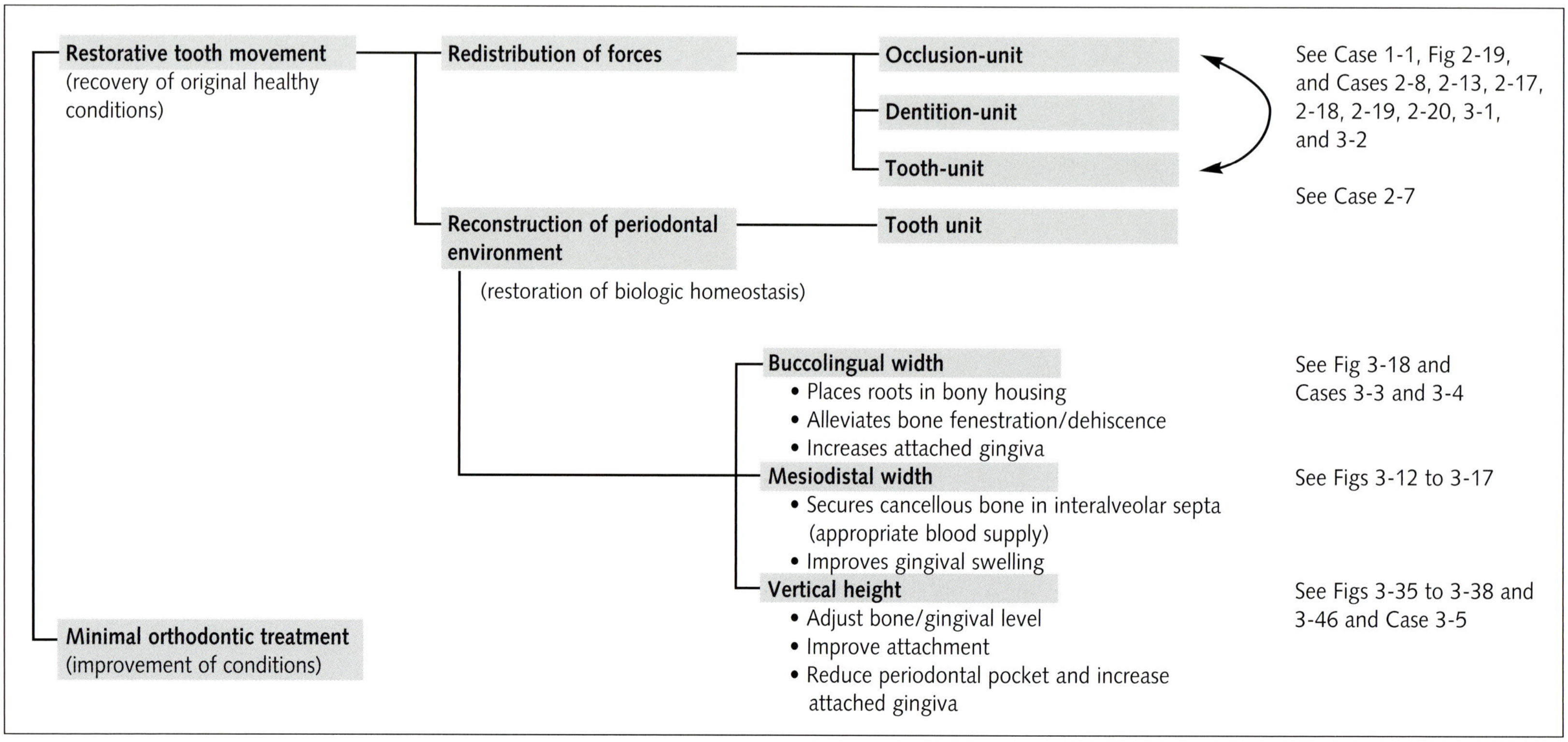

Fig 3-1 Restoration of harmony in the stomatognathic system through tooth movement.

The purpose of restorative tooth movement is, microscopically, to reconstruct the physiologic periodontal environment and to redistribute occlusal forces. Macroscopically, the purpose is to stabilize the position of the mandible in relation to the cranium and the maxilla.

Control of inflammation and trauma

Figure 3-2 shows a patient with dental compression syndrome (DCS) and conspicuous abfraction. Because the molars were compressed, remodeling was postponed while reshaping was conducted. As the vertical dimension of occlusion (VDO) increased naturally, natural extrusion of the mandibular arch and orthodontic extrusion for the maxillary arch were conducted. With this movement, the bone level was gradually adjusted, while deep bony defects were decreased.

Restorative tooth movement is most effective when combined with control of inflammation and correction of the mandibular position in a coordinated manner.

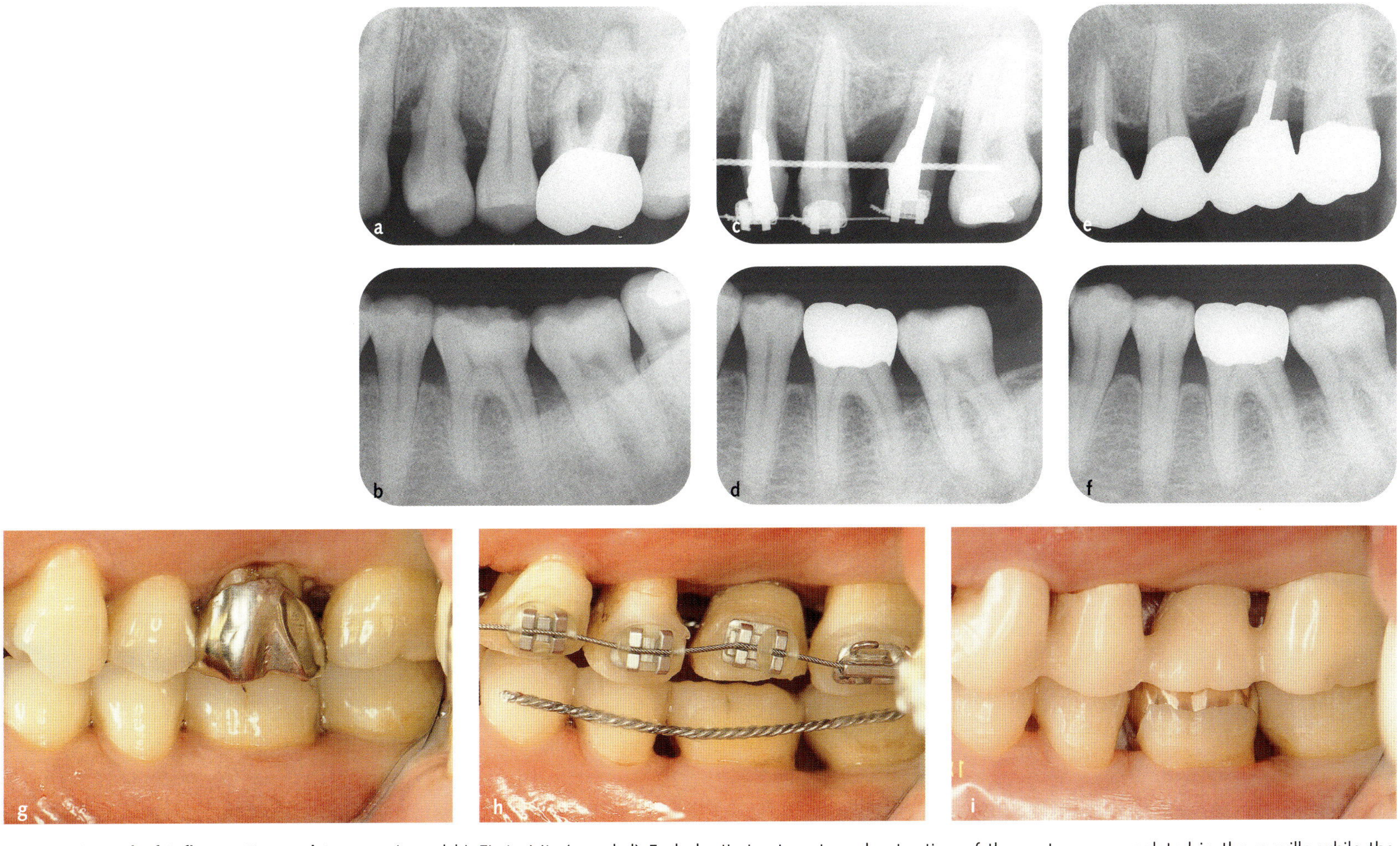

Fig 3-2 Control of inflammation and trauma. (a and b) First visit. (c and d) Endodontic treatments and extraction of the root were completed in the maxilla while the mandibular left first molar was naturally extruded and restored. The mandibular left first molar was also reshaped. (e and f) About 10 years since the first visit. (g) First visit. (h) In the mandibular arch, teeth on the both sides were splinted for natural extrusion of the left first molar, which had deep bony defects. In the maxillary arch, the left first premolar and first molar were extruded orthodontically. (i) Remodeling progressed, and the clinical crown has been elongated.

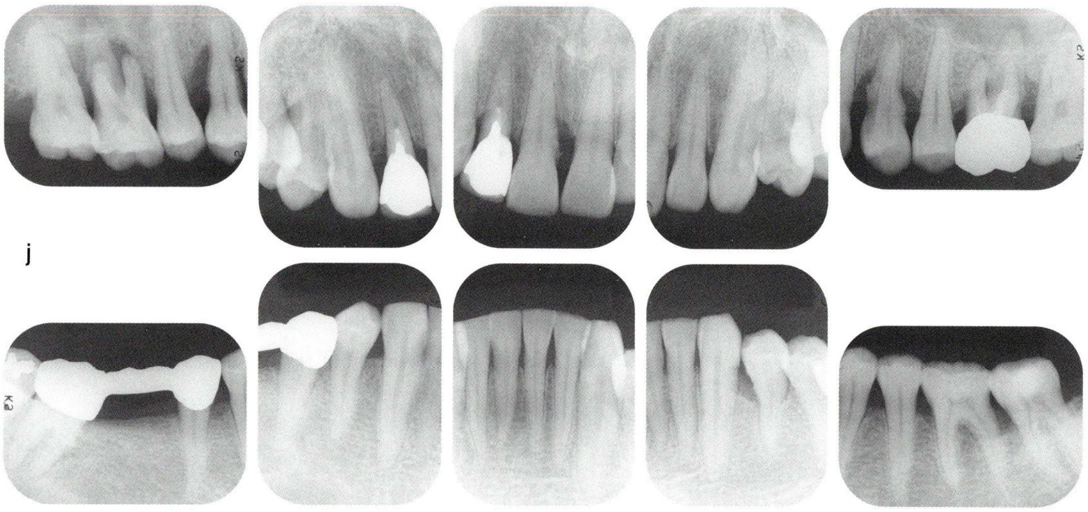

j

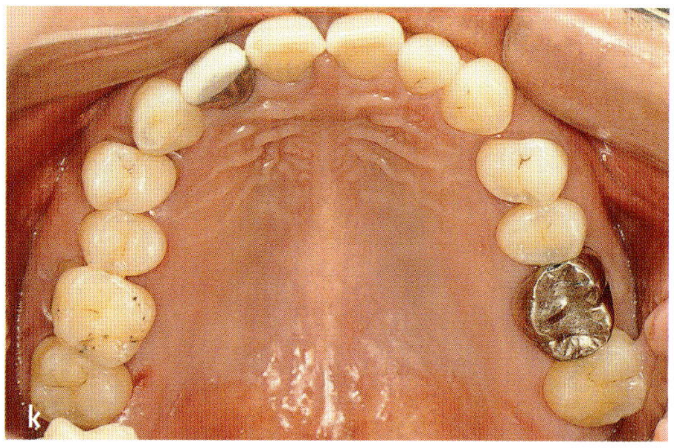

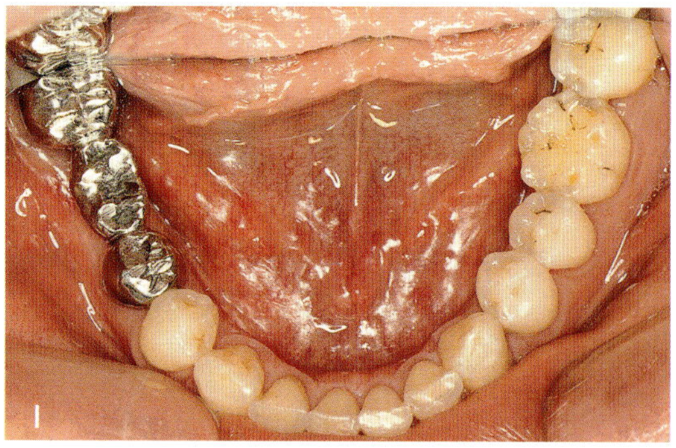

Fig 3-2 (cont) (j to l) Full-mouth radiographs and occlusal views at the first visit (September 1987).

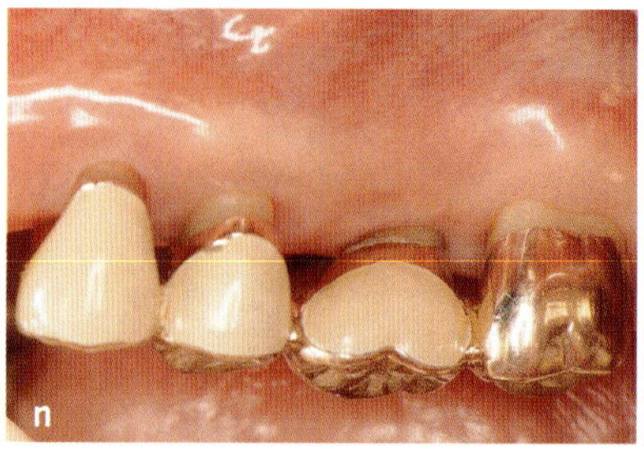

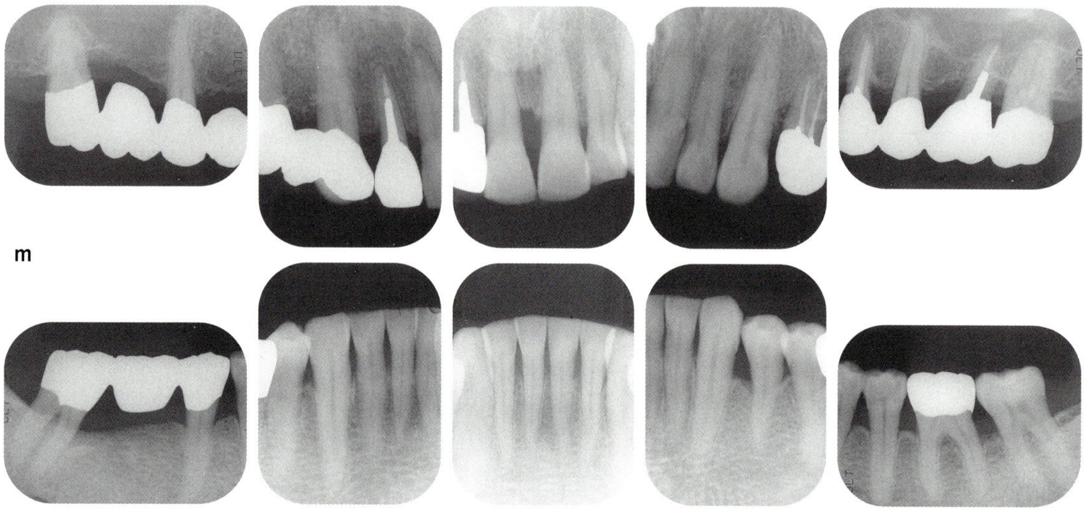

m

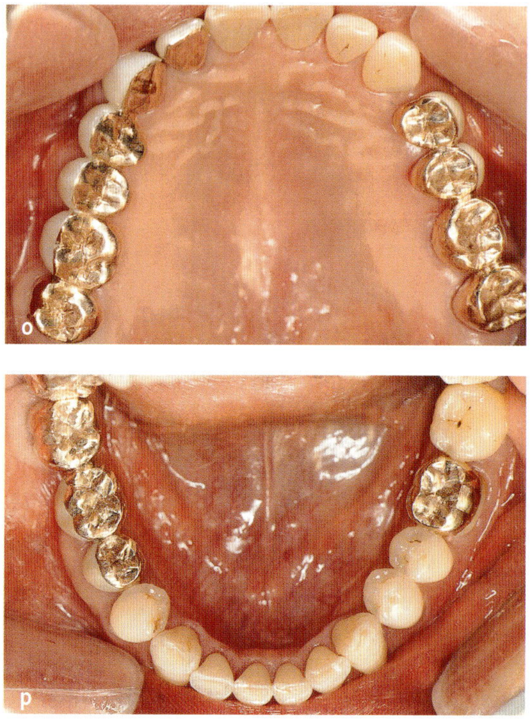

(m to p) Full-mouth radiographs and occlusal views, 11 years 4 months after the first visit (January 1999). The maxillary molar regions shown in g to i exhibit significant gingival recession.

Case 3-1 Tight Occlusion—Arch expansion by restorative tooth movement

Patient: *36-year-old woman at the time of first visit in 1997*
Chief complaint: *Discomfort in the left side of the jaw that had persisted for about 1 month. She felt unbalanced during walking*

This was a temporomandibular disorder (TMD) case, and the patient exhibited a typical "tight occlusion" (Fig 3-3). A tight occlusion is caused by habits. In this patient, as a result of narrowed arches, the movement of the mandible was extremely restricted. The patient related that her body "rocks from side to side," although no remarkable oral symptoms were found. She felt as if her ears were blocked and had discomfort and pain in the left temporomandibular joint (TMJ). She was aware of symptoms such as sounds during movement of the left side of her jaw, headache, and numbness of the right hand, although there were no abnormal findings during a medical examination. Diagnosed as having autonomic imbalance, the patient complained of various physical conditions. When we asked the patient, "Do you feel like you are walking on a narrow balance beam?" she said, "Exactly!"
This patient may be regarded as normal according to conventional viewpoints of occlusion. However, the patient's arches were narrowed and the tongue space was also narrowed. In other words, because the occlusion, or the pivot of the body balance, was narrow, the head and the body were not stabilized.
At the first visit, we evaluated her habitual sleep posture (see Fig 3-3g). Merely abstaining from the habit of resting her cheek on her hand during sleep improved her physical conditions, according to the patient. She wore a stabilization splint, which decreased the sense that her ear was being blocked and the pain in the TMJ area. After she wore the splint for some time, the occlusion on the left side became less tight. In patients with tight occlusion, a stabilization splint may provide significant correction. The treatment is provided in conjunction with myofunctional therapy. In a case such as this, there is no fundamental solution except arch expansion using tooth movement (Figs 3-4 to 3-8).
The patient's complaint of body sway could not be confirmed with stabilometry (Gravicorder) (see Figs 3-7e and 3-7f). We believed that she felt body sway because her center of gravity was located backward. We instructed her to try to maintain her balance on her toes, which improved the conditions of her body sway.
In this patient, leveling was started in the maxilla. Because it takes longer to intrude teeth than to extrude them, the maxillary posterior teeth, which had to be intruded, were treated first. With this treatment alone, the mandibular arch starts to expand naturally. If appliances were delivered to both arches simultaneously, extrusion would be accelerated and the opposing teeth would contact prematurely, which would invite instability.

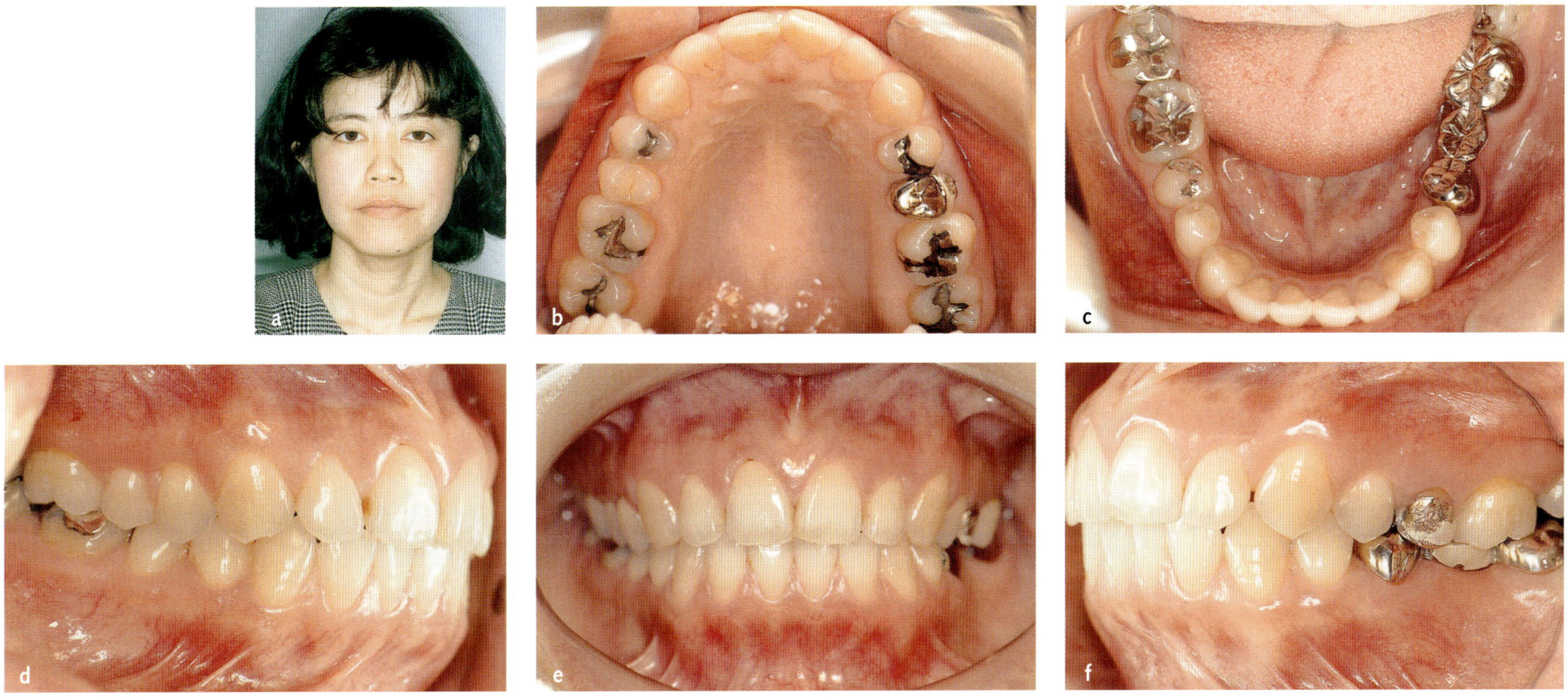

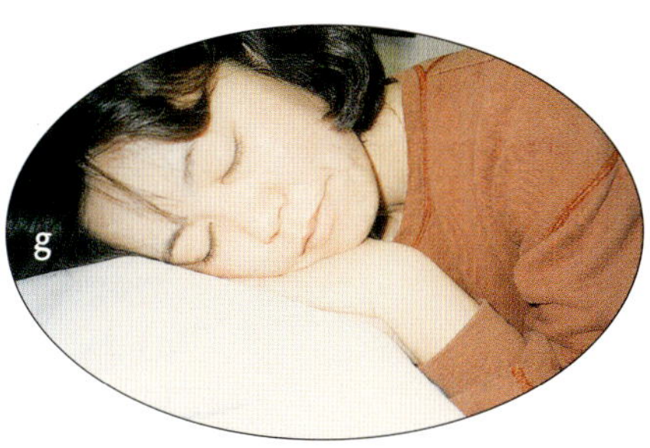

Fig 3-3 At the first visit, the patient stated that she felt "like [she is] walking on a narrow balance beam." (a) Facial photograph showing the mandible's shift to the left. She tends to chew on the right side, because chewing on the left side is difficult due to the tight guidance on the right side. Left clenching is suspected (the left corner of the mouth is raised). Although she stated that her body "rocks from side to side," no remarkable oral symptoms are present. The patient complained of various physical problems. (b to f) The teeth, especially on the right, are lingually inclined. The patient shows signs of parafunctional habits on both sides, but her habits are more conspicuous on the right side. It is inferred that the discomfort of the left TMJ is caused by her habit of pressing the mandible to the left and clenching, which has loaded the joints. (g) She has a habit of resting her cheek on her hand while sleeping.

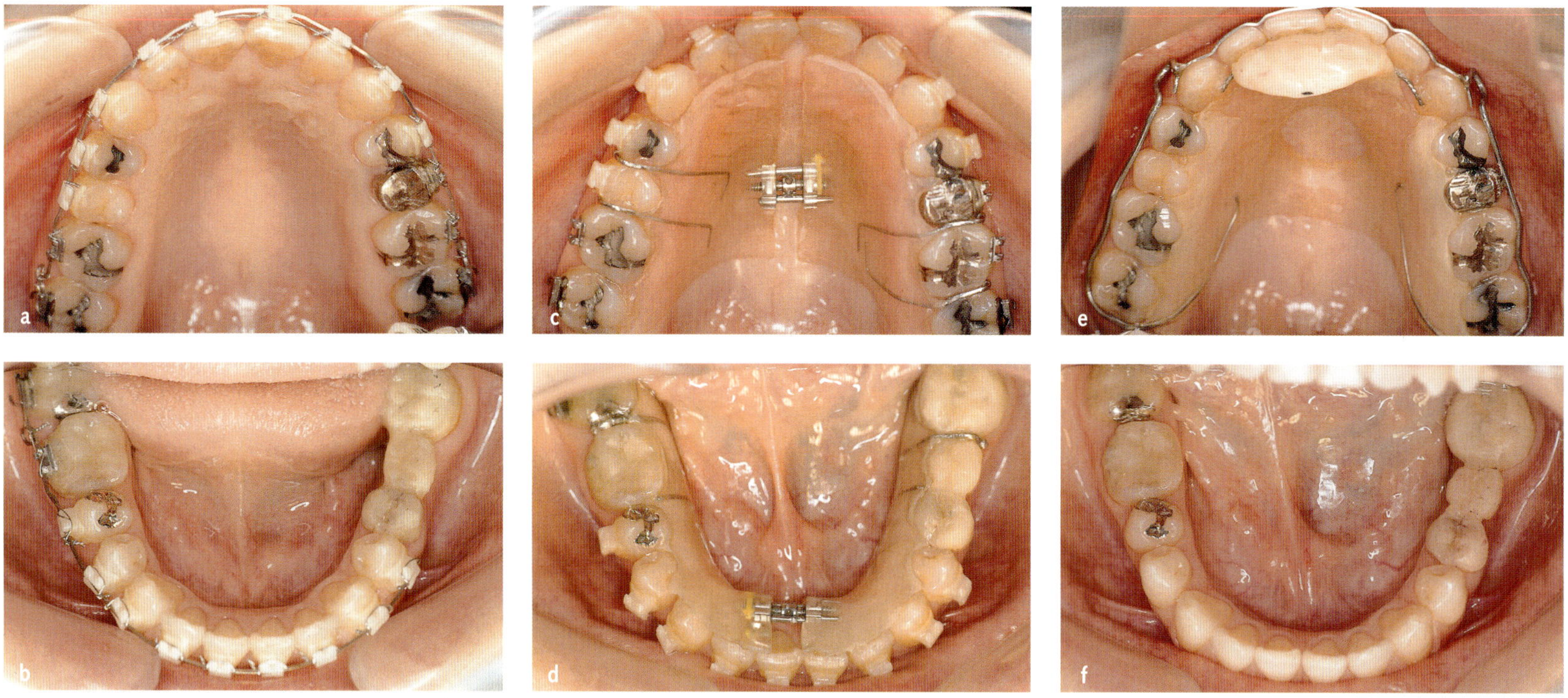

Fig 3-4 Arch expansion. (a) Photographs taken 2 months after the first visit. Brackets are bonded to the maxillary arch. Expansion is conducted first in the maxilla. (b) The orthodontic appliance is delivered to the mandibular arch 7 months after the first visit. (c and d) Photographs taken 1 year 5 months after the first visit. Multibrackets are used for the expansion. However, because the patient still feels tightness in the molar region, plate-type expansion screws are used. Her body weight has increased by 6 kg. The screws are turned once every 5 days to gradually expand the arches. (f and g) Photographs taken 2 years 4 months after the first visit. Expansion was completed 1 year 9 months after the beginning of active treatment. After the appliances were removed, some clenching remained. A splint with an anterior block was used, only at nighttime, to advance the mandible slightly. As expected, the molar regions started to disocclude, especially on the left side. Some light-cured resin was added to the occlusal surfaces. The disocclusion continued for about 3 years.

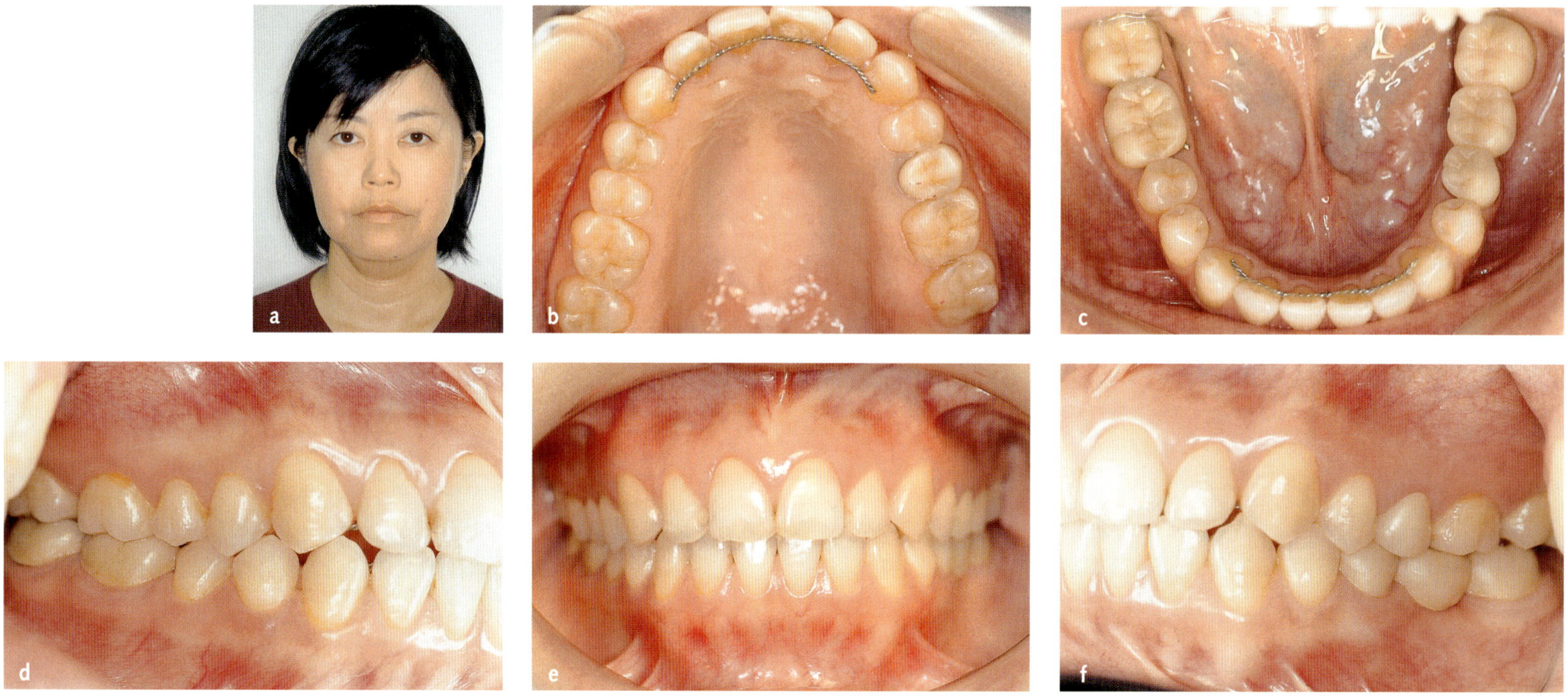

Fig 3-5 Photographs taken 5 years 5 months after the first visit. (a) Facial photograph. The patient's body weight had increased, and her complexion had improved. The tension in the sternocleidomastoid muscles was diminished. (b to f) Restoration of the clinical crowns with a hybrid resin material. Remodeling is expected, and this material is a convenient way to allow addition as necessary. The fixed partial denture replacing the mandibular left first molar is still provisionally cemented, although this is 5 years since the first visit. The arches were expanded 2.0 mm in the maxillary anterior, 3.0 mm in the mandibular anterior, 1.5 mm in the maxillary posterior, and 2.5 mm in the mandibular posterior.

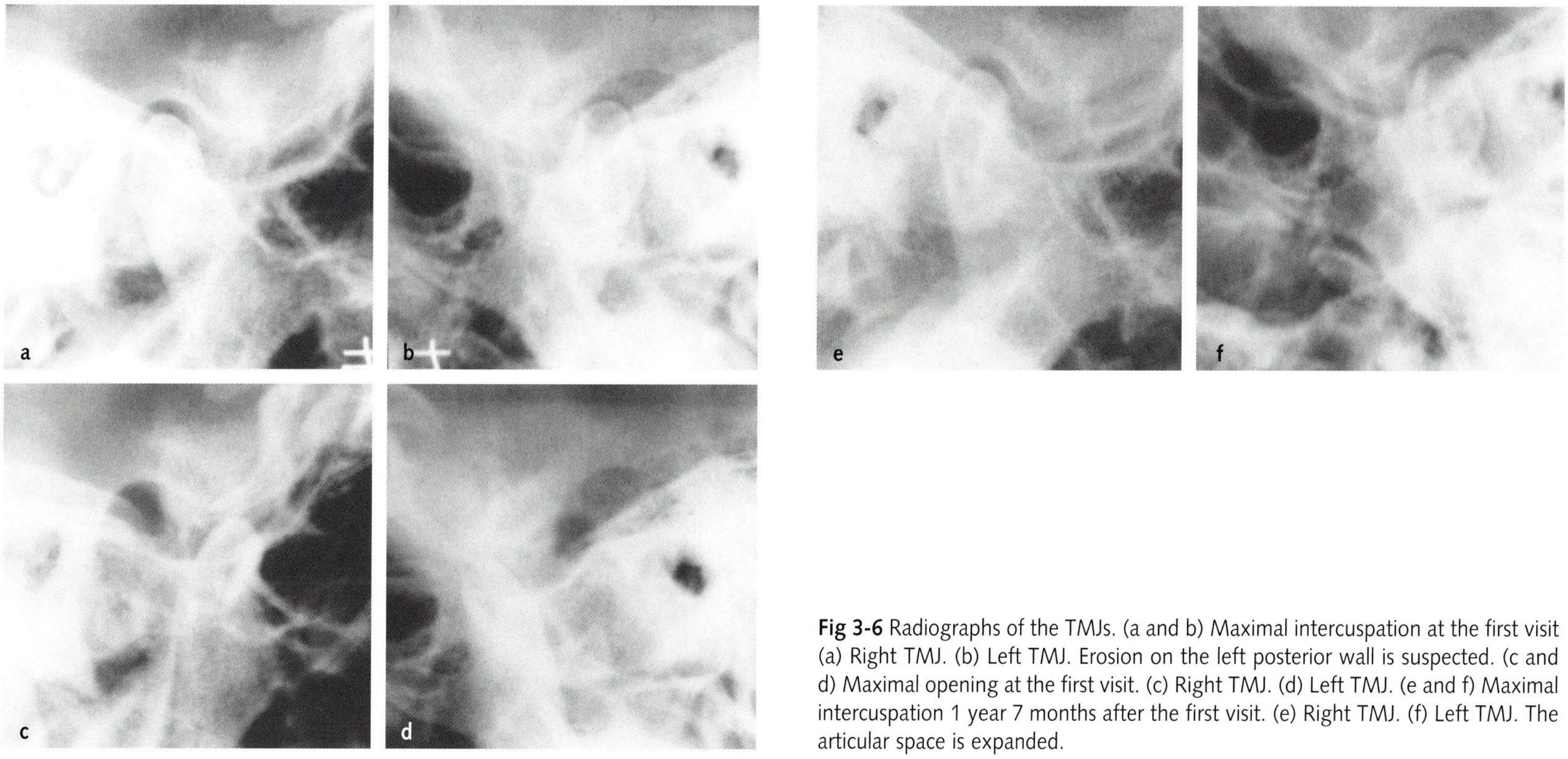

Fig 3-6 Radiographs of the TMJs. (a and b) Maximal intercuspation at the first visit (a) Right TMJ. (b) Left TMJ. Erosion on the left posterior wall is suspected. (c and d) Maximal opening at the first visit. (c) Right TMJ. (d) Left TMJ. (e and f) Maximal intercuspation 1 year 7 months after the first visit. (e) Right TMJ. (f) Left TMJ. The articular space is expanded.

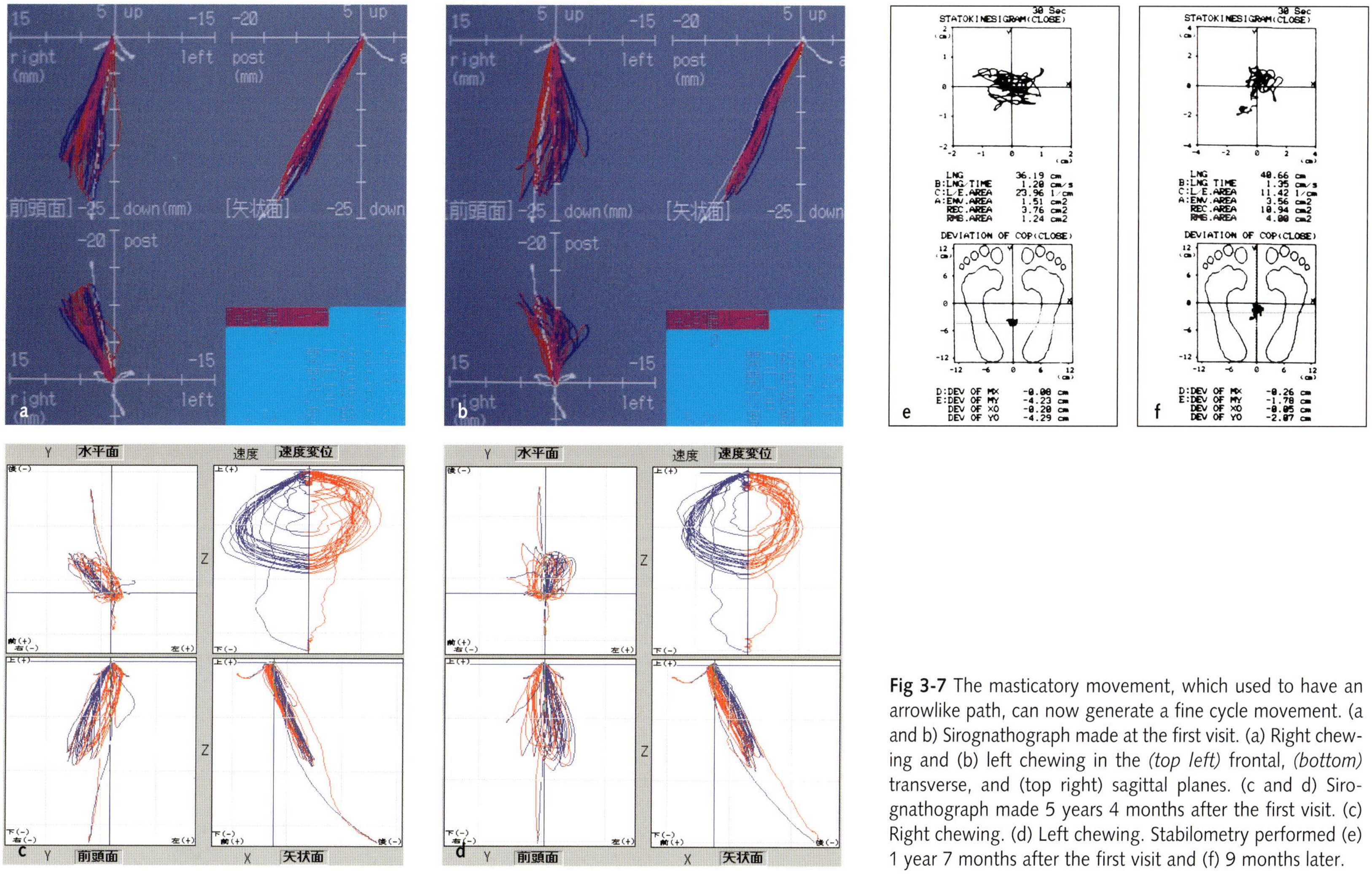

Fig 3-7 The masticatory movement, which used to have an arrowlike path, can now generate a fine cycle movement. (a and b) Sirognathograph made at the first visit. (a) Right chewing and (b) left chewing in the *(top left)* frontal, *(bottom)* transverse, and (top right) sagittal planes. (c and d) Sirognathograph made 5 years 4 months after the first visit. (c) Right chewing. (d) Left chewing. Stabilometry performed (e) 1 year 7 months after the first visit and (f) 9 months later.

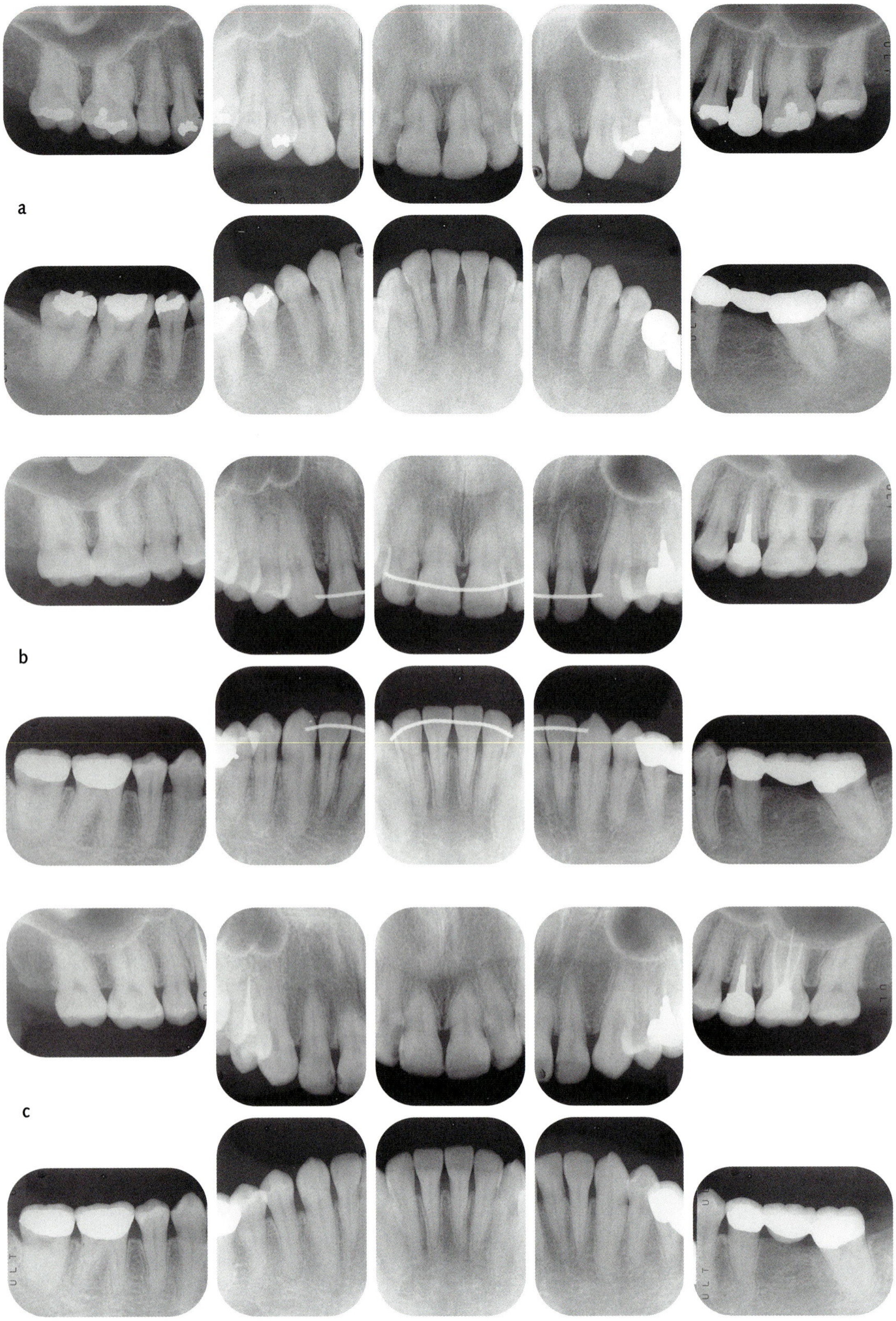

Fig 3-8 Full-mouth radiographs. (a) At the first visit. (b) Radiographs taken 2 years 11 months after the first visit. (c) Radiographs taken 5 years 5 months after the first visit. The bone level is adjusted. Traumatic findings in the molar region have disappeared. The cortical plate line at the crest and bone trabeculae have become clearer.

Case 3-2 Occlusal trauma

Patient: *49-year-old woman at the time of first visit in 1985*
Chief complaint: *Mobility of the maxillary left first premolar. She wondered if it was possible to save the tooth. She exhibited moderate to severe periodontitis with 2- to 8-mm periodontal probing depths.*

The patient was a bruxer. Along with the horizontally reduced bone level, the morphology of the tooth roots was unfavorable. In such situations, when bruxism is intense, the mobility of teeth becomes more pronounced. The teeth on the right side of the mandibular arch were crowded, and the curve of Spee was pronounced. The patient chewed on the right to avoid left-side chewing due to the mobility of the maxillary first premolar, which made the mandible shift to the right. As the tooth position improved, the mandible shifted to the left simultaneously. Furcation involvements were significant, and both the maxillary right second molar and left second molar were impossible to maintain. A root resection for the maxillary right first molar and a hemisection for the mandibular left first molar were performed. Although the mandibular right first molar was difficult to maintain, it was uprighted and restored. Regular maintenance has been performed. The dentition has been successfully maintained for 17 years since the first visit, except for the eventual extraction of the mandibular right first molar (Figs 3-9 to 3-11).

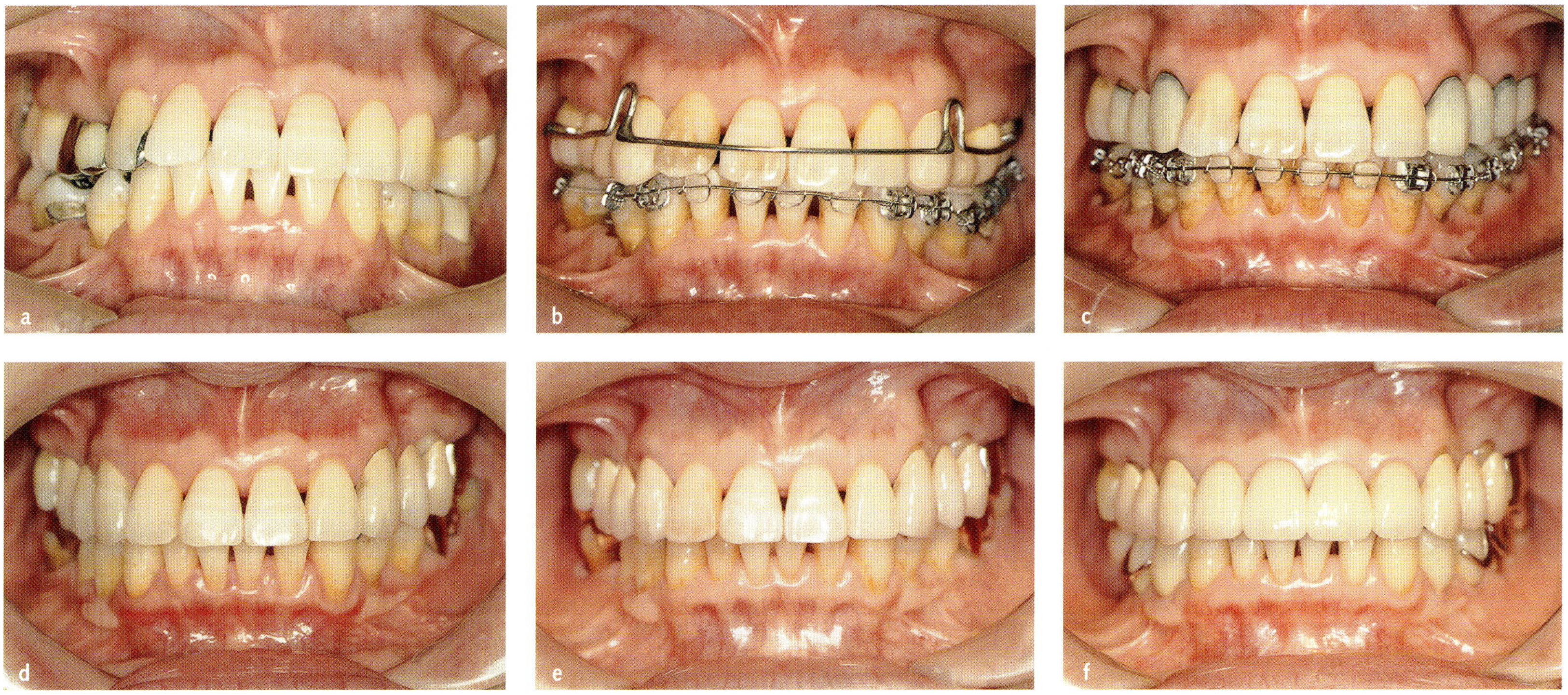

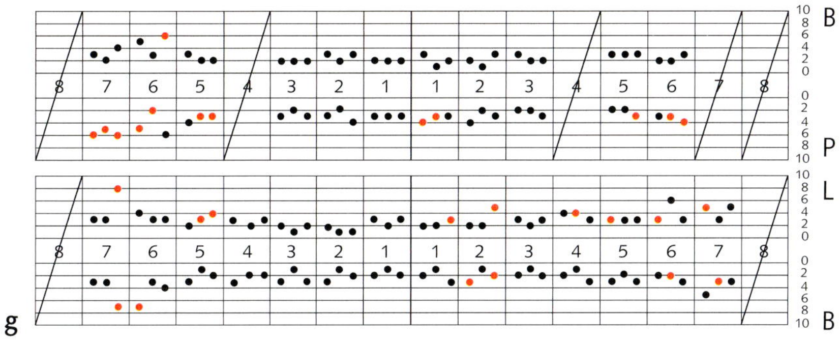

Fig 3-9 Frontal views of treatment progress. (a) Photograph taken at the first visit (1985). The mandibular shift is visible. (b) A stabilization-type splint with a circumferential plate is placed in the maxillary arch. The stabilization splint is designed so that the mandibular position is returned to the left and reciprocation will not allow orthodontic and occlusal forces to be applied to the periodontal tissues. Wires are used to control labial inclination. The mandibular appliance is designed for leveling and alleviation of crowding. (c) Restorative tooth movement is completed (1987). The maxillary molars are provisionally restored with metal backing. (d) Fixed partial dentures have been placed to restore the maxillary molars about 1 year 6 months after the first visit (1987). Although periodontal support is compromised, no splinting was conducted. The photograph was taken in January 1991. (e) Photograph taken about 10 years after the first visit. In the maxillary arch, force is being controlled by contouring the teeth. (f) Photograph taken about 12 years after the first visit. The mandibular right second molar has been extracted. A distal extension removable partial denture has replaced the missing mandibular right molars. The maxillary central and lateral incisors are splinted because of their increased mobility. (g) Probing depths chart made at the first visit (1985). Red dots indicate bleeding points.

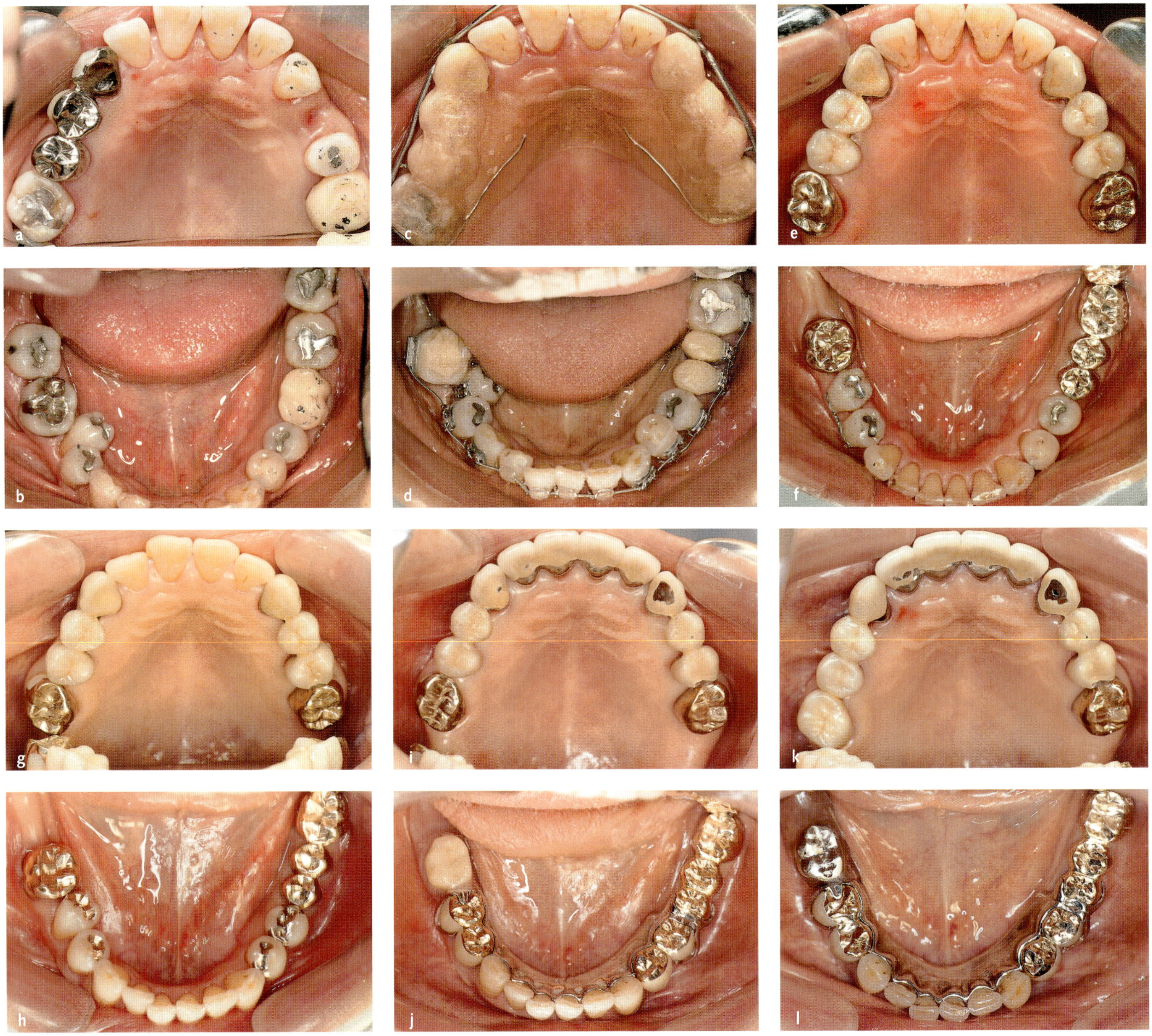

Fig 3-10 Occlusal views of treatment progress. (a and b) Photographs taken 2 months after the first visit (December 1985). (c and d) Photographs taken in 1986. A splint for the maxillary arch and the full brackets for the mandibular arch have been placed to alleviate crowding, upright tooth axes, and restore the occlusal plane. The mandibular right first molar has been uprighted; the crowding of the mandibular second premolar is reduced; a hemisection, space opening, and extrusion have been performed for the mandibular left first molar; and anterior teeth have been intruded. (e and f) Photographs taken in 1988. Fixed partial dentures have replaced the maxillary molars. The mandibular left first molar has been hemisected, and the separated roots are splinted. (g and h) Photographs taken in September 1993. (i and j) Photographs taken in February 1997. The maxillary central and lateral incisors are splinted. The lingual plate of the unilateral distal extension removable partial denture in the mandibular arch has eliminated the mobility of mandibular teeth. (k and l) Photographs taken in August 2002.

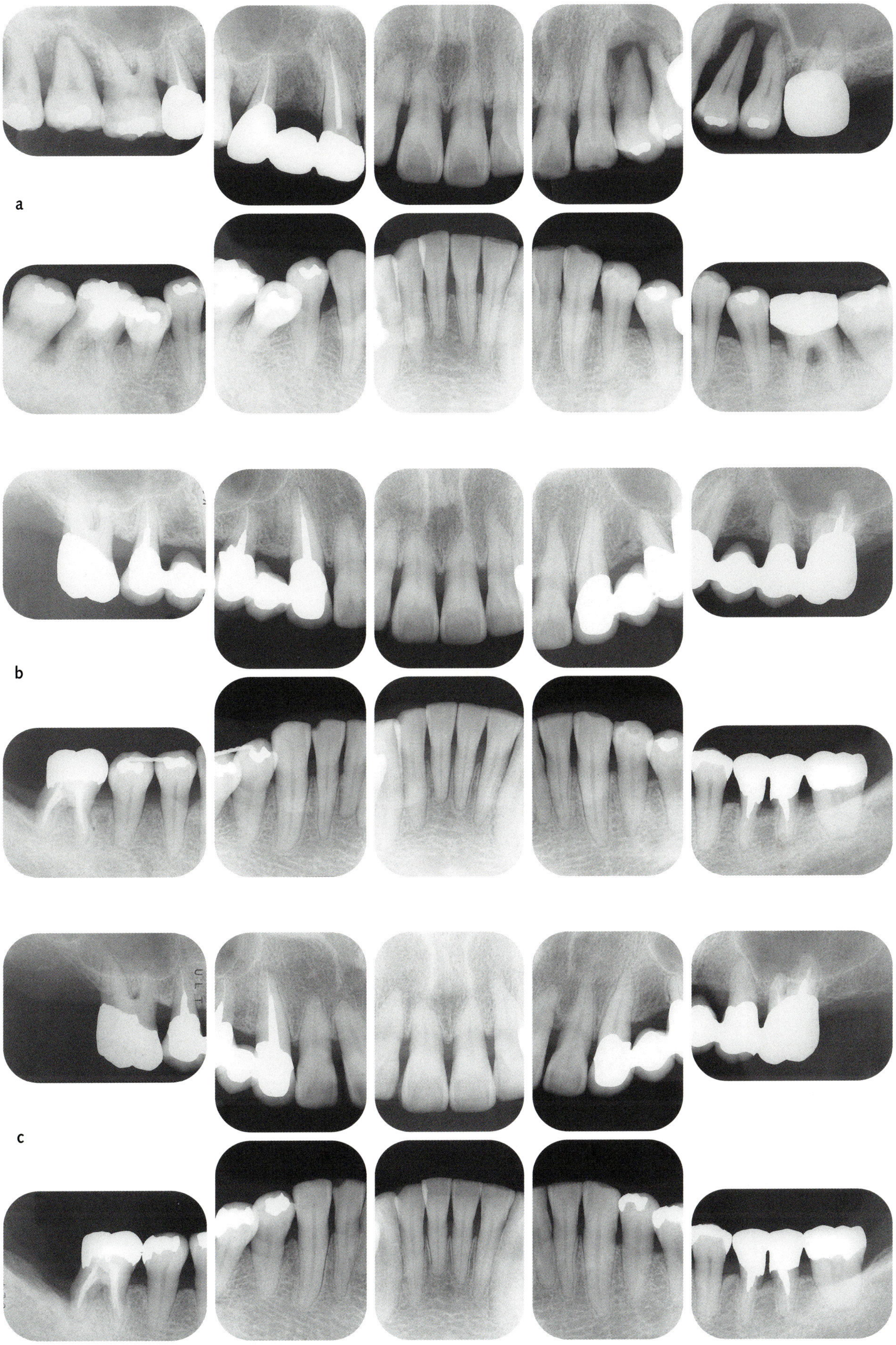

Fig 3-11 Radiographic views of treatment progress. (a) Radiographs taken at the first visit. The maxillary right second and third molars, maxillary left first premolar, mandibular left third molar, and mandibular right second molar have been extracted. (b) Radiographs taken about 2 years after the first visit. First restoration is completed. (c) Radiographs taken in March 1991. The mandibular right first molar had repeated alveolar abscesses and bone resorption around the distal root was considerably advanced. In 1995, the tooth was extracted. Inlays have been fabricated for the mandibular right first and second premolars.

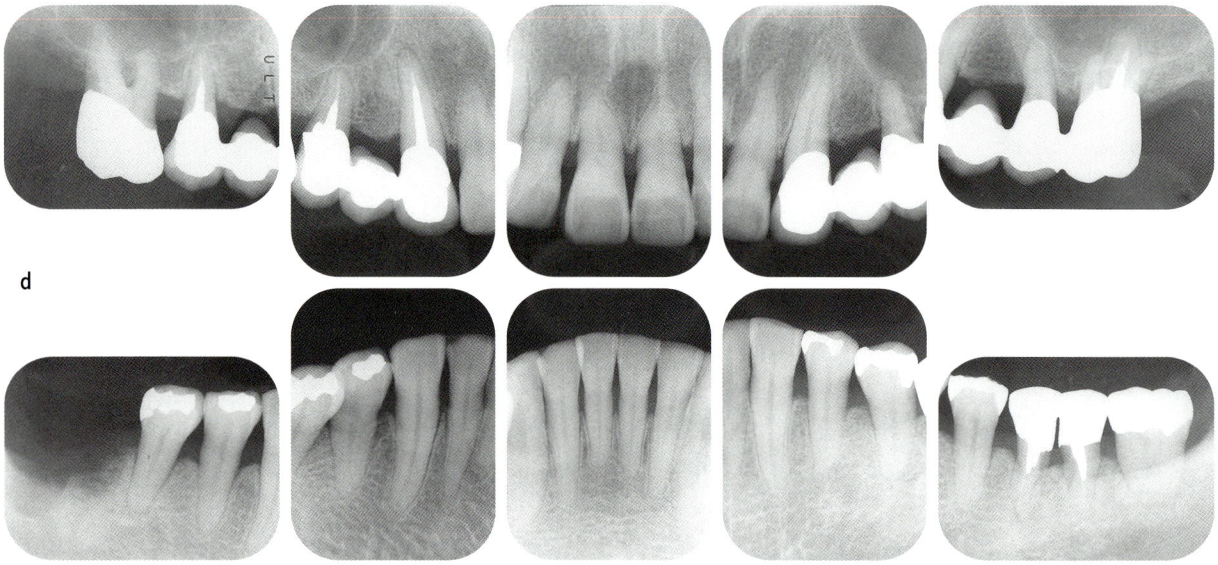

d

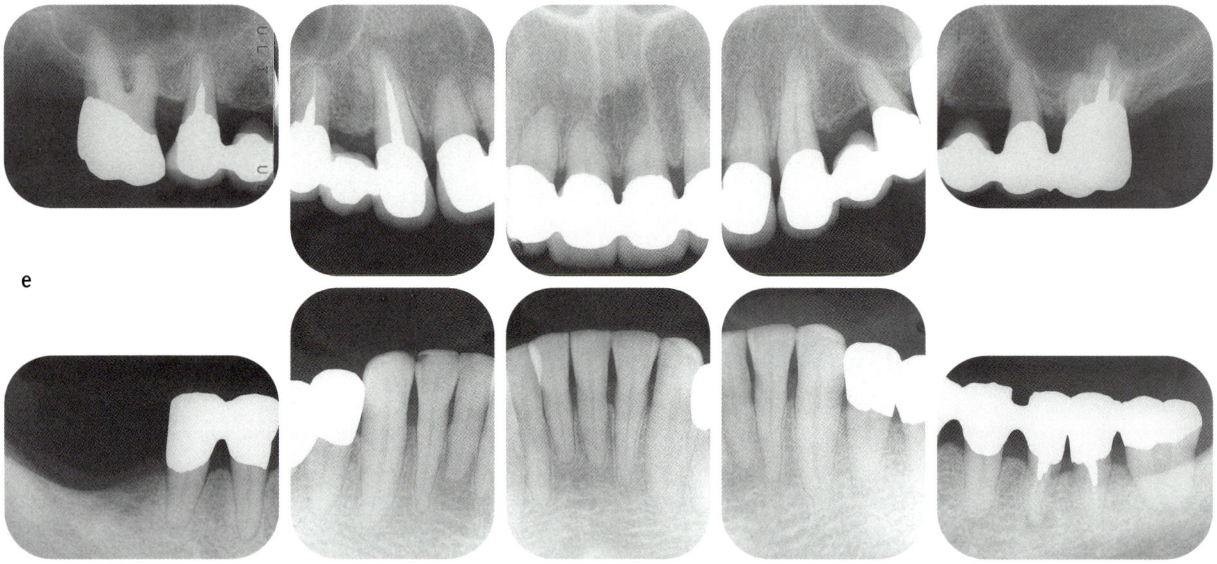

e

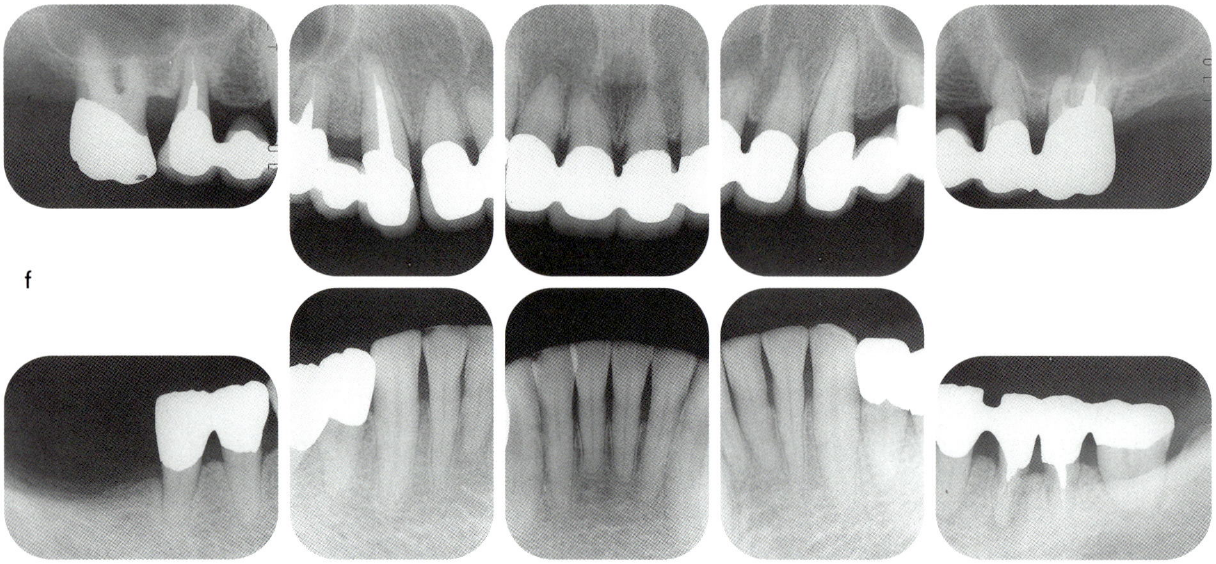

f

Fig 3-11 (cont) (d) Radiographs taken in January 1996. Although such treatment is not ideal, the bite plane was used long-term. In August 1996, splinted crowns were delivered for the mandibular right first and second premolars, which served as abutments for the partial denture. (e) The maxillary incisors were splinted in January 1997. In April 1997, a distal extension removable partial denture was delivered to replace the missing mandibular right molars. (f) Radiographs taken in March 2001. After the completion of treatment, the mandibular right first molar was extracted. The gingival sulcus is within 2 mm in all areas. Periodontal tissues are stable because of the control of inflammation and occlusal forces.

Restoration of the Periodontal Environment: Mesiodistal and Buccolingual Tooth Movement

Bony housing and tooth root

Tooth roots form alveolar bone proper via the periodontal ligament. The tooth root cementum, periodontal ligament, and alveolar bone proper are stabilized in the alveolus. The alveolus consists of cancellous bone surrounded by cortical bone. Tooth roots are stabilized in cancellous bone, conventionally described as a bony housing. Tooth roots that extend beyond the bony housing are located within cortical bone. During tooth movement, these teeth do not move smoothly and often have root resorption. In adults, those teeth that protrude beyond the bony housing are said to have a dehiscence if the condition is described on the basis of bone. Dehiscence is often accompanied by gingival recession. These problems in the periodontal tissues should be solved naturally by bringing the tooth roots back into the bony housing (see Fig 3-18), not by mucogingival surgery or regeneration therapy.

Mesiodistal tooth movement

When the width of a clinical crown is relatively narrow compared with the width of the tooth root, root proximity often arises. When a tooth root is wide, for example, an interdental space is often identified at the clinical crown level; root proximity will result when such a space is orthodontically closed (Fig 3-12). Disking, or limited grinding of proximal surfaces within enamel, is likely to cause similar problems. When tooth roots are too close to each other, there is insufficient space for cancellous bone between them. The blood supply will be insufficient, which is likely to cause a large bony defect, and periodontal disease may develop. In addition, the interdental papillae will swell. In mesiodistal tooth movement as well, thorough consideration should be given to the biologic width.

To apply the same concept in a different situation, we may encounter a clinical case of advanced bone resorption resulting from periodontal disease in a crowded mandibular anterior dentition. In a case such as this, the attachment position is lowered, which increases the interradicular distance. Disking is an effective method to eliminate crowding and improve cleansability in such a case.

Buccolingual tooth movement

Tooth labioversion or linguoversion may occur for a variety of reasons. The causes are not limited to hereditary crowding. Body postures or habits, parafunctions, chewing habits, tongue habits, and circumoral muscle problems are also involved. The morphology of the dental arches is stable, as shown in chapter 2. When teeth are out of the dental arch for some reason, homeostasis of the dental arch will be restored by bringing such teeth back into the dental arch.

Gingival recession and /or root exposure may result when an arch is expanded laterally and/or anteriorly. This seems to occur when labial or buccal pressure exceeds the capability of the alveolar bone to follow the tooth roots.

Widths required between roots

The hypothesis that a certain width is necessary between the mesenchymal tissue and the outside is called the biologic width. Because this concept is frequently discussed with regard to the relationship between a crown restoration and the periodontal tissue, there is sometimes a misunderstanding that the term refers to the width of the attachment. However, this principle of homeostasis is not merely a principle about the width of a healthy root surface required by the attachment; this width is also obtained as a horizontal distance between two roots. The patient shown in Fig 3-12 has a narrow crown width compared to the root width. The diastema in this patient is physiologic.

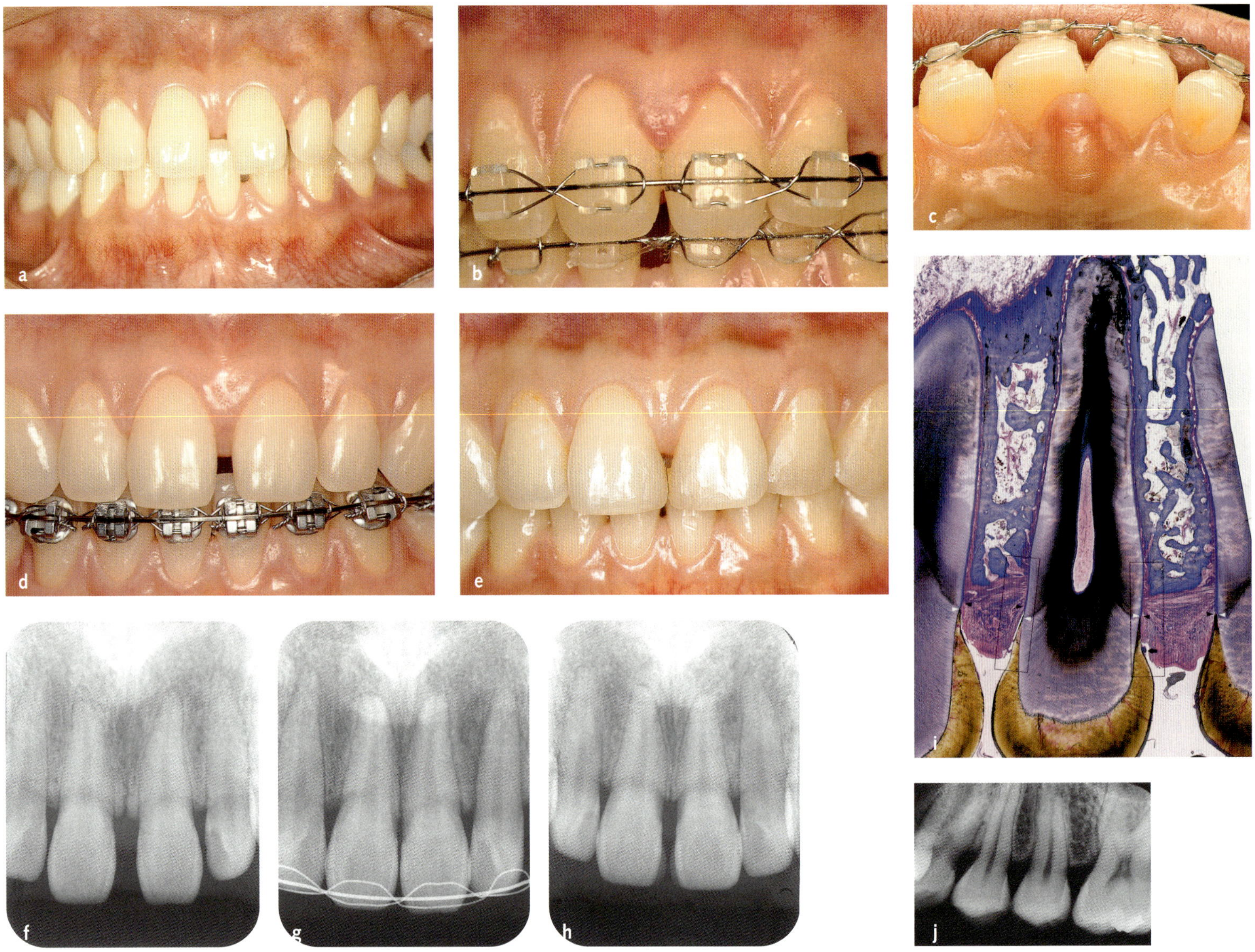

Fig 3-12 (a) A 20-year-old woman demanded improvement where a diastema existed. The space was closed using elastics. (b and c) After the space was closed, the gingiva had swelling on the labial and lingual aspects, which did not resolve with brushing. (d) After the appliance was removed, 1-mm diastema was manifested again, and the gingival swelling healed naturally. (e) Light-cured resin was applied to the mesial aspects of the central incisors (1 year 10 months after the first visit). The direct bonding was repeated 9 years 7 months after the first visit. (f) At the first visit. The crown width is narrow compared to the root width. (g) Radiograph taken 10 months after the first visit. The roots of the central incisors are close to each other, leaving little space for cancellous bone between them. (h) After the appliance was removed, the space appeared again to provide a physiologically stable distance. (i and j) A mesiodistal section of teeth and alveolar bone shows that a certain width between roots is necessary to have sufficient cancellous bone to secure a blood supply. (From Urago. Reprinted with permission.)

Closure of diastema in the presence of anatomic restrictions

In one patient, supernumerary teeth existed between the maxillary central incisors (Fig 3-13). After they were extracted, space closure was attempted but was not successful due to the large incisive foramen (incisive canal). The patient was treated prosthodontically.

In a similar case, prosthodontic treatment was conducted instead of orthodontic treatment to close a diastema because the incisive foramen was large (Fig 3-14).

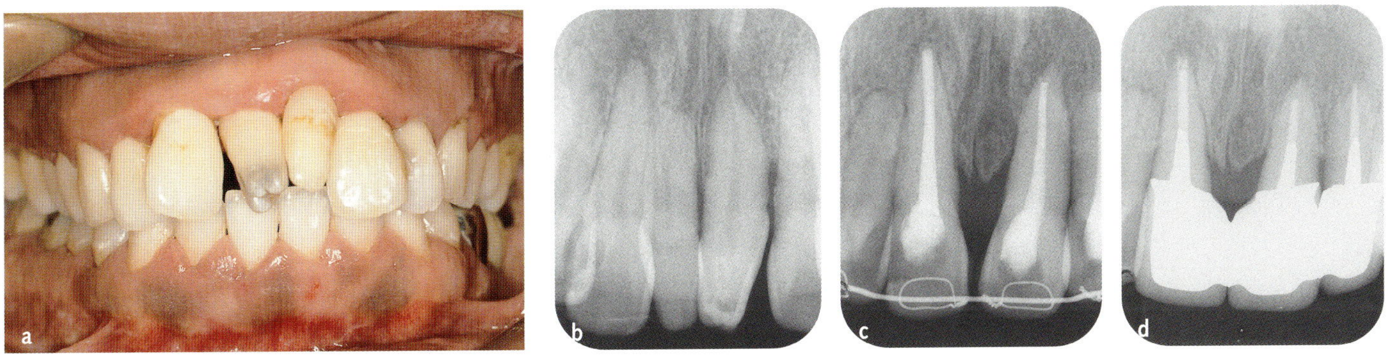

Fig 3-13 Failure to close diastema. (a and b) Supernumerary teeth between the maxillary central incisors (March 1986). (c) After extraction, orthodontic treatment was conducted to close the space; this treatment was not successful. (d) Active treatment was discontinued 1 year 5 months later, while the diastema was still open.

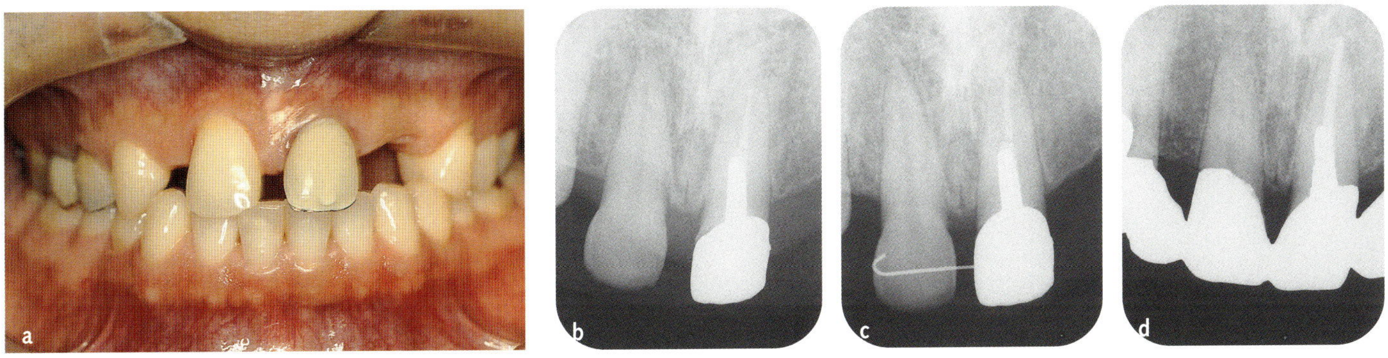

Fig 3-14 A patient with a large incisive canal. (a and b) At the first visit (October 1990), the patient requested closure of the diastema. Radiographic examination revealed that this goal would be difficult to achieve, due to the large incisive foramen. (c) The space was closed slightly, using a simple elastic module. (d) The remaining space was treated prosthodontically.

Periodontal risks of crowding

From the viewpoint of periodontology, the problems of crowding are not limited to difficulty with cleaning. Even more serious is the problem that exists when a tooth root with a labial or lingual axioversion cannot fit into the bony housing (Figs 3-15 and 3-16). Also, because of root proximity, cancellous bone will be missing in some parts of the interradicular space, disturbing blood circulation. Swelling of the gingiva in a crowded area can be the result of inflammation caused by dental plaque and swelling accompanied by congestion. This fact should be easily understood through comparison of conditions before and after the crowding is resolved.

Fig 3-15 (a and b) Lingual axioversion of the maxillary right lateral incisor caused the mandible to shift to the left. To reduce the shift, multibrackets were applied for tooth movement after the extraction of the four first premolars. The patient was instructed in thorough toothbrushing. (c) The result of treatment is healthy marginal gingiva and interdental papillae that are less likely to experience future inflammation.

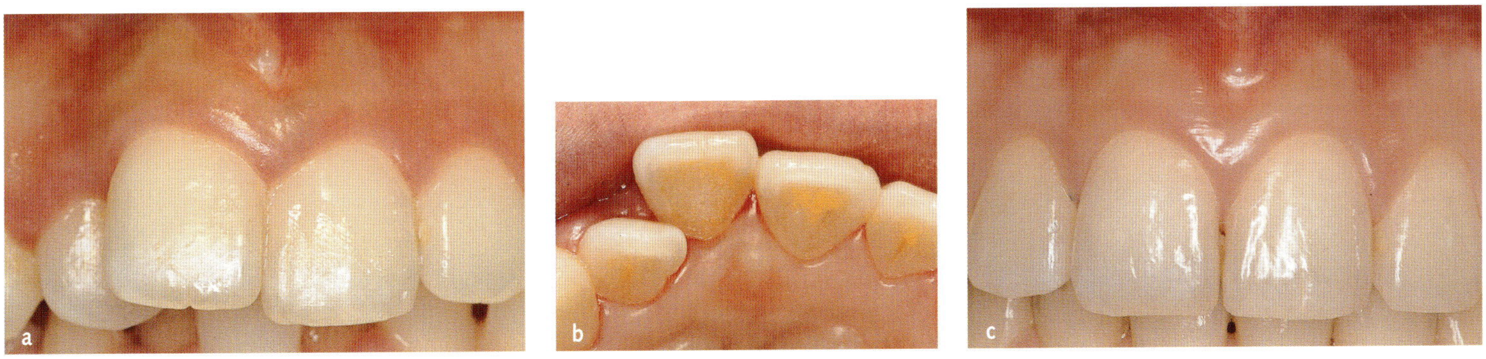

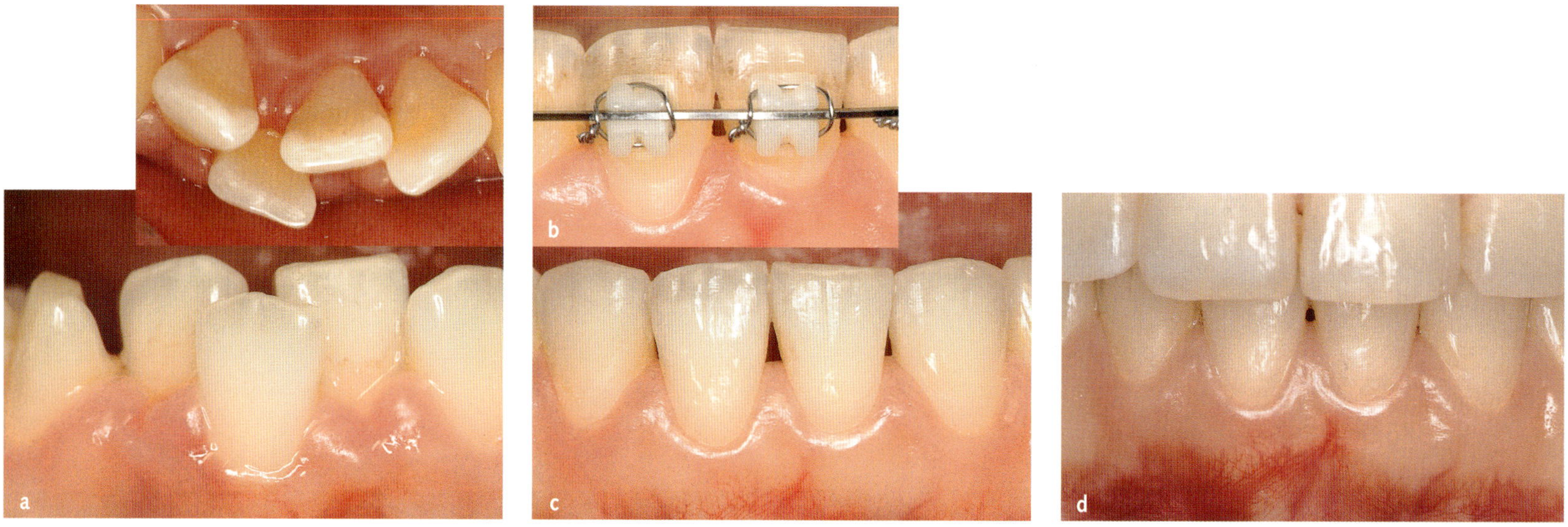

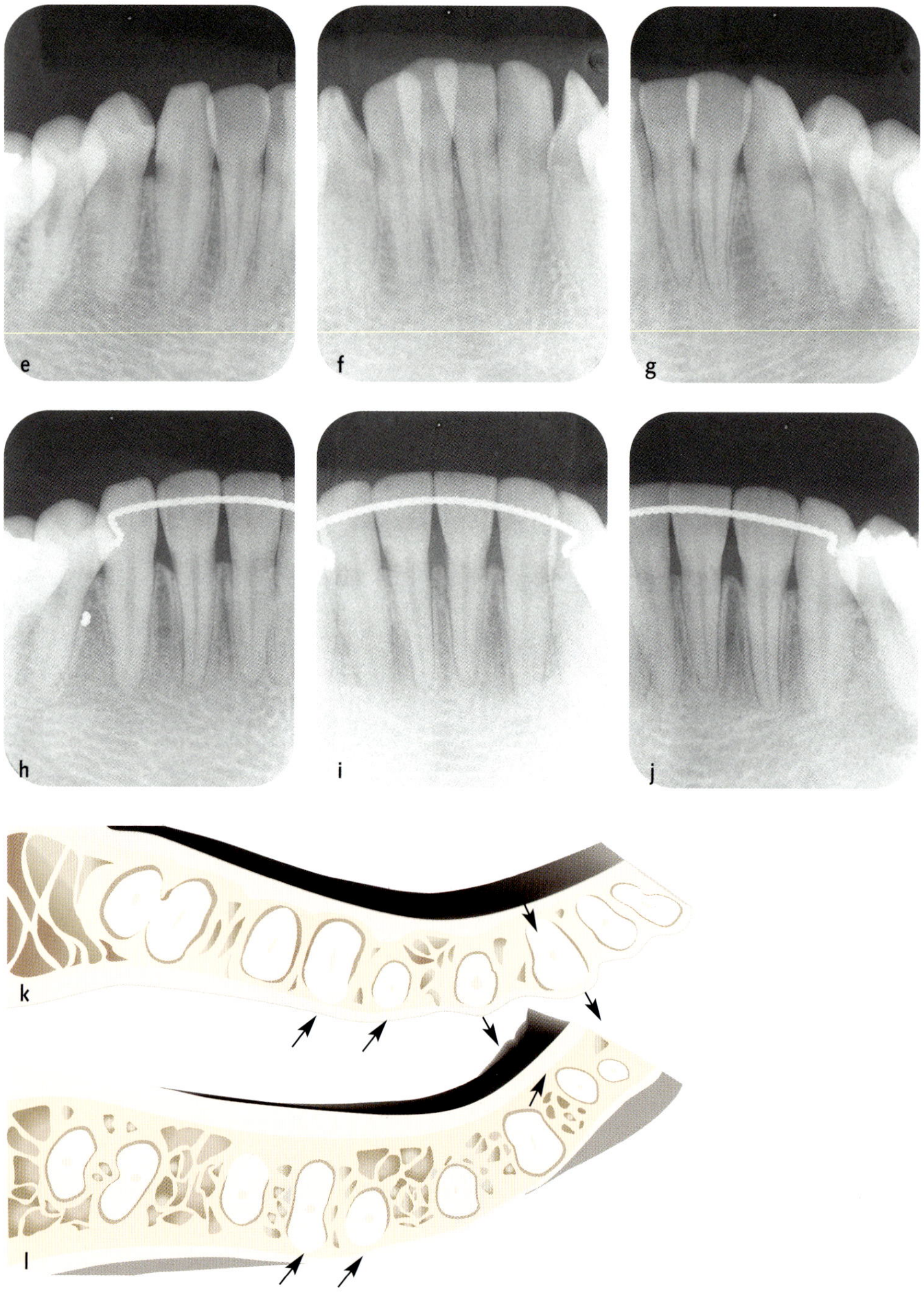

Fig 3-16 (a) At the first visit. (b) Photograph taken 2 years 9 months after the first visit. (c) Photograph taken about 3 years 6 months after the first visit. (d) Photograph taken about 5 years 2 months after the first visit. (e to g) Radiographs taken at the first visit (December 1993). (h to j) Radiographs taken after 3 years 2 months.(k and l) Horizontal section of an adult mandible. Even with an appropriately aligned, healthy dentition, (k) at the coronal one-third, alveolar bone proper is in continuity with compact bone and cortical bone in the alveolar process. (l) At the apical one-third also, alveolar bone proper, which forms alveolar socket walls, is often in continuity with cortical bone (From Lindhe et al. Reprinted with permission.)

Attachment loss and interradicular distance

Disking is a method to eliminate mild crowding and esthetically align teeth. It is not recommended, however, in restorative tooth movement focused on root-periodontal tissue, because it induces root proximity. Tooth crowns may be aligned properly, but the biologic width between tooth roots will be invaded. Having said that, in a clinical case such as that shown in Fig 3-17, where significant attachment has been lost due to severe periodontitis, the apical root width is narrower than the crown width, which eliminates the concern of inviting root proximity when disking is employed. Rather, disking will reduce the interdental embrasure space that is wide open.

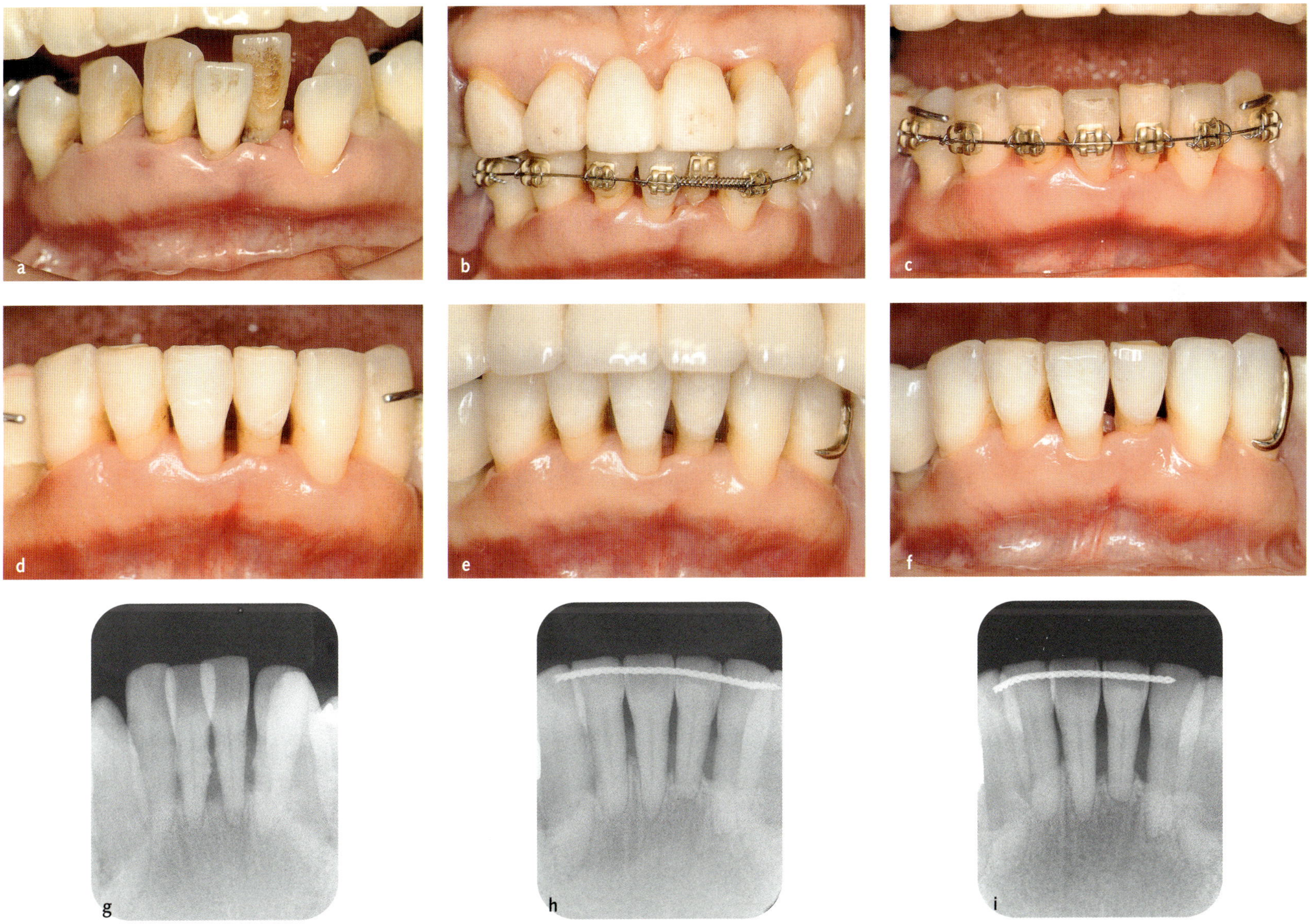

Fig 3-17 (a) The patient is a 41-year-old woman who visited our clinic due to severe periodontitis. Significant bone resorption and swelling are noted throughout the arches, and most teeth exhibit mobility. Periodontal probing depths are 6 to 11 mm, and all the teeth bleed on probing. (b) Initially, a soft toothbrush (Perio B3, Sunstar) was used for plaque control, after which scaling and root planing were initiated. To improve the periodontal environment, disking was done for the crowded anterior region in the mandible. The active treatment period was 2 months. (c) Tooth movement is completed. At this time, pockets were deep and bone resorption was considerable, but no surgery was conducted. (d) Photograph taken 10 months after the completion of active treatment. (e) Photograph taken about 3 years after the first visit. Probing depths have been reduced to 2 to 3 mm. (f) Photograph taken about 8 years after the first visit. (g) At the first visit. The bone level is about at the apical one-fourth. Massive amounts of calculus are present. (h) Radiograph taken about 5 years later. Although the bone level is low, it is stable, even with a long epithelial attachment. No pathologic pockets are found. (i) Radiograph taken about 7 years later.

Importance of bone support

Class III mandibular anterior teeth show the importance of bone support for periodontal tissue (Fig 3-18). In this nonextraction case, the majority of the anterior tooth roots seemed to be outside of the labial cortical bone before treatment, causing a dehiscence or fenestration. The teeth seemed to be pushed labially by the low tongue position and were subjected to pressure from the labial side because of the strong orbicular muscle. Tooth extraction was not conducted in this patient. First, the roots of the mandibular anterior teeth were inclined lingually; this was followed by a surgical setback of the mandible. Attachment was improved after treatment. Tooth root shapes were visible on the labial aspect because of the pressure from the orbicular muscle. We instructed the patient to keep some air beneath the lower lip. Superimposed cephalograms show that the tooth roots were relocated lingually. If a case like this were treated with extraction without surgery, the tongue space would be narrowed, making it difficult to stabilize the teeth.
Case 3-3 demonstrates the use of regenerative periodontal therapy to stabilize improvements in the occlusion.

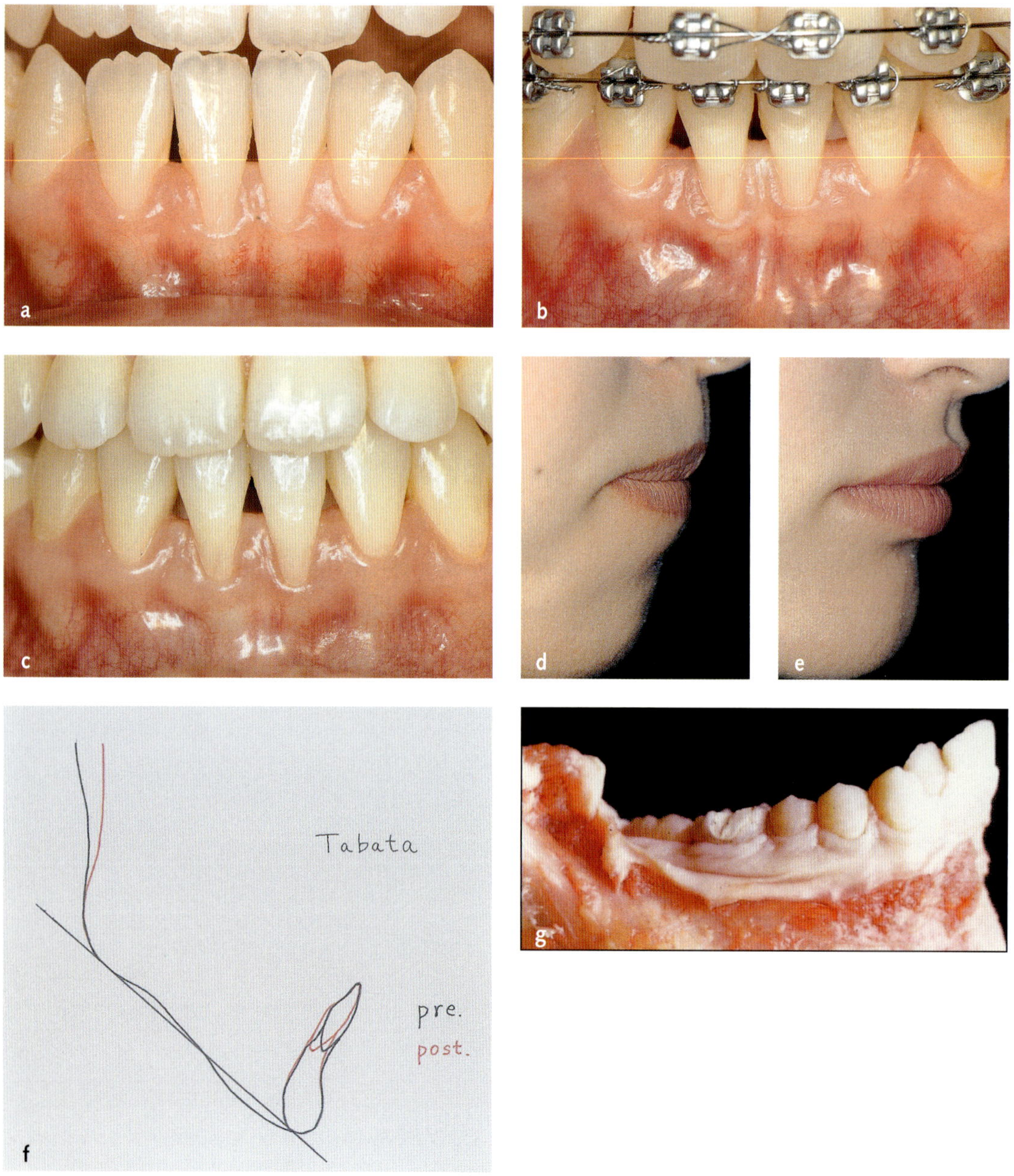

Fig 3-18 (a) At the first visit. (b) After surgery, 2 years 1 month after the first visit. (c) Photograph taken 3 years 3 months after the first visit. Tooth roots that used to be visible are not prominent, suggesting that they are back in the bony housing. A free gingival graft was placed after orthodontic treatment. (d and e) The patient was instructed to keep some air beneath the lower lip (lip buffer). The profile is shown after treatment. (f) Superimposition of cephalograms. (g to i) Even healthy mandibular anterior teeth have only a thin bony wall on the buccal side. (From Urago. Reprinted with permission.)

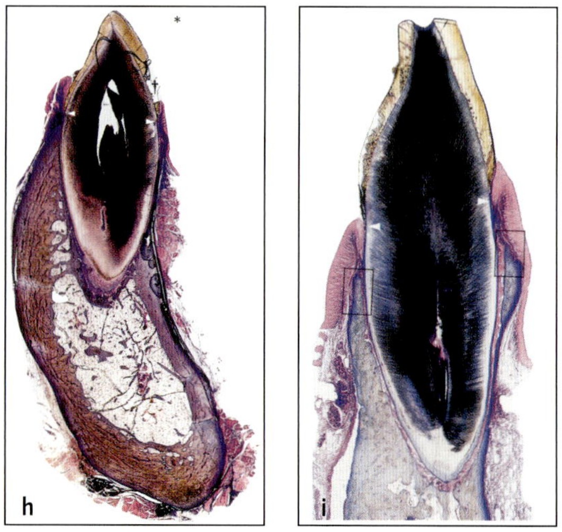

Case 3-3 Restorative tooth movement and regeneration therapy using periosteum

Patient: *44-year-old woman at the time of first visit in March 1996*
Chief complaint: *Dislodgment of a fixed partial denture*
This is a case in which the restorations were completed on a patchwork basis to cope with dental caries, which allowed the advancement toward an occlusal collapse. There were other problems, including the mandibular shift to the left and an irregular bone level. Regenerative periodontal surgery using periosteum, autogenous tooth transplantation, and tooth movement were conducted to improve conditions (Figs 3-19 to 3-26). The occlusion was reconstructed with minimal prosthodontic intervention.

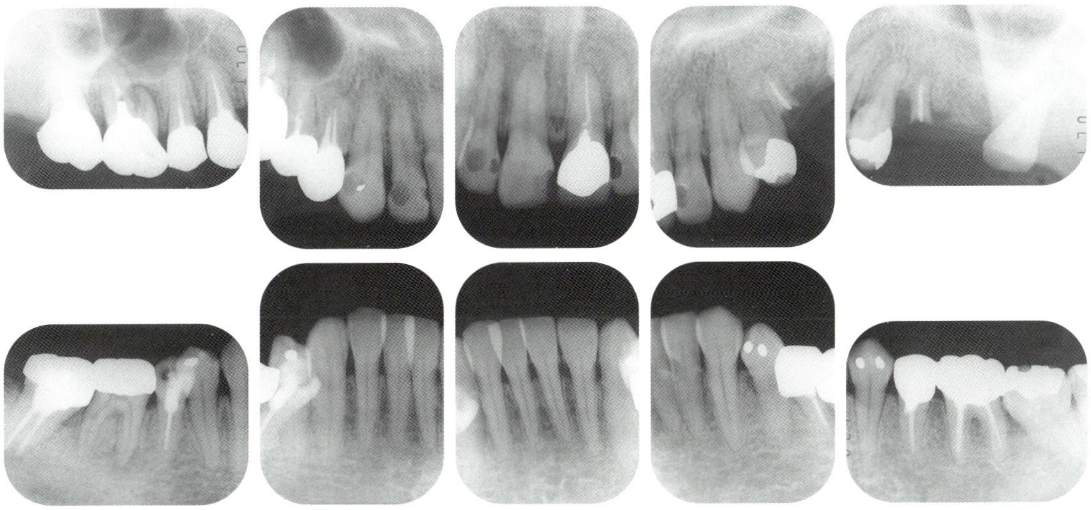

Fig 3-19 Radiographs taken at the first visit (March 1996). The maxillary right first molar, maxillary left second premolar, and mandibular left third molar were extracted (root fractures). Endodontic treatment was conducted for the maxillary right first premolar, second premolar, and second molar; the maxillary left central incisor; the mandibular left second premolar and first molar; and mandibular right second premolar and first molar. Periodontal surgery for regeneration was carried out at the mandibular right first and second molars; crown-lengthening surgery was performed for the maxillary right first premolar, second premolar, and second molar; flap access was created for the mandibular left first premolar, second premolar, and first molar. The mandibular right lateral incisor was extracted and transplanted to the site of the maxillary left second premolar. Most teeth exhibit traumatic lesions.

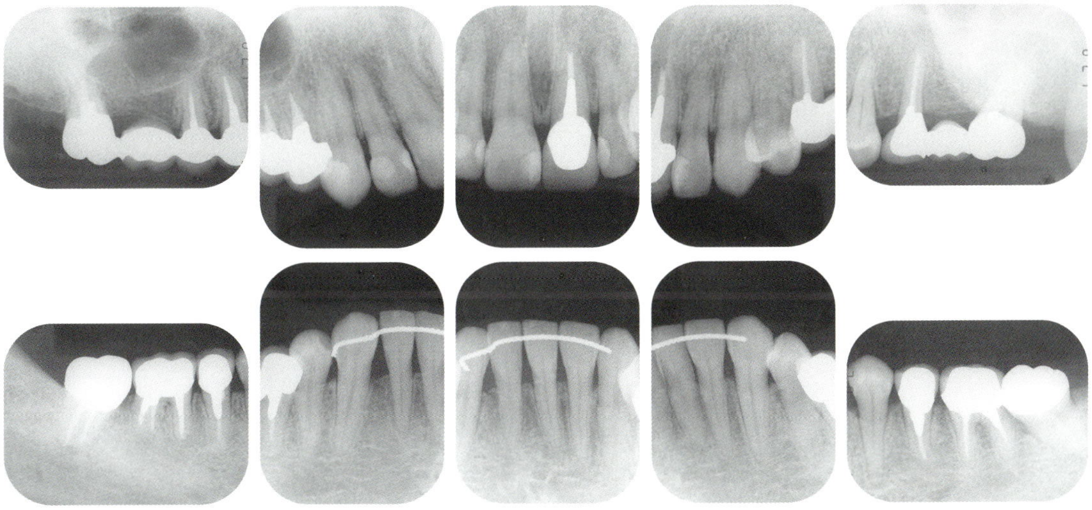

Fig 3-20 Radiographs taken when treatment was completed (March 1999). The mandibular position as well as the alignment of the dentition had improved. Traumatic findings had been reduced.

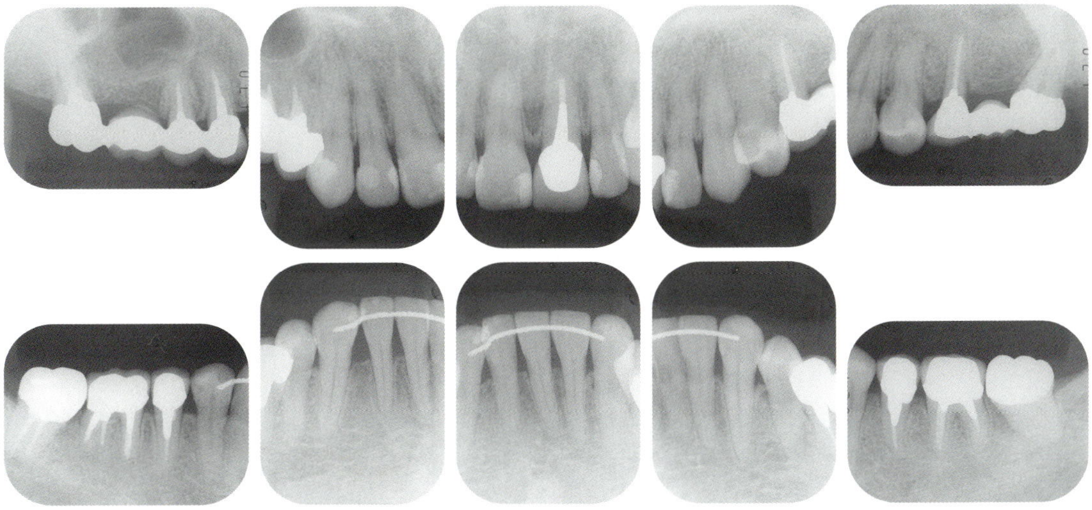

Fig 3-21 Radiographs taken during the maintenance period (September 2001). Conditions are stable.

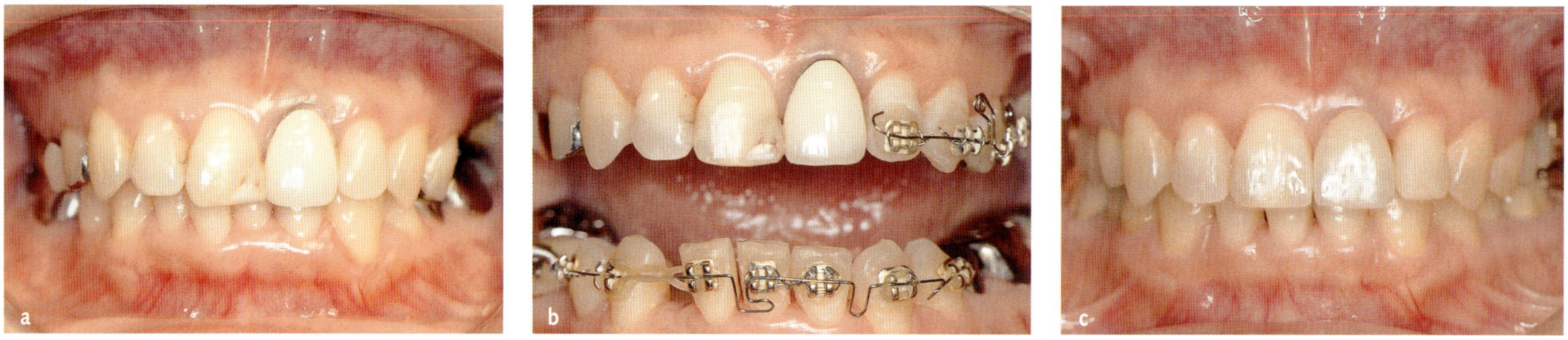

Fig 3-22 Changes in the occlusal plane and the mandibular position. (a) At the first visit. The mandible is shifted to the left. There are no TMD symptoms. (b) Due to the existing crowding, it was decided to have only three incisors. The mandibular right lateral incisor was extracted and transplanted to the site of the maxillary left first premolar, where occlusal support was needed. After that, an appropriate mandibular position was determined using a bite plane. (c) Photograph taken 2 years 4 months (April 2001) after the completion of treatment. The occlusal plane and the mandibular shift are improved.

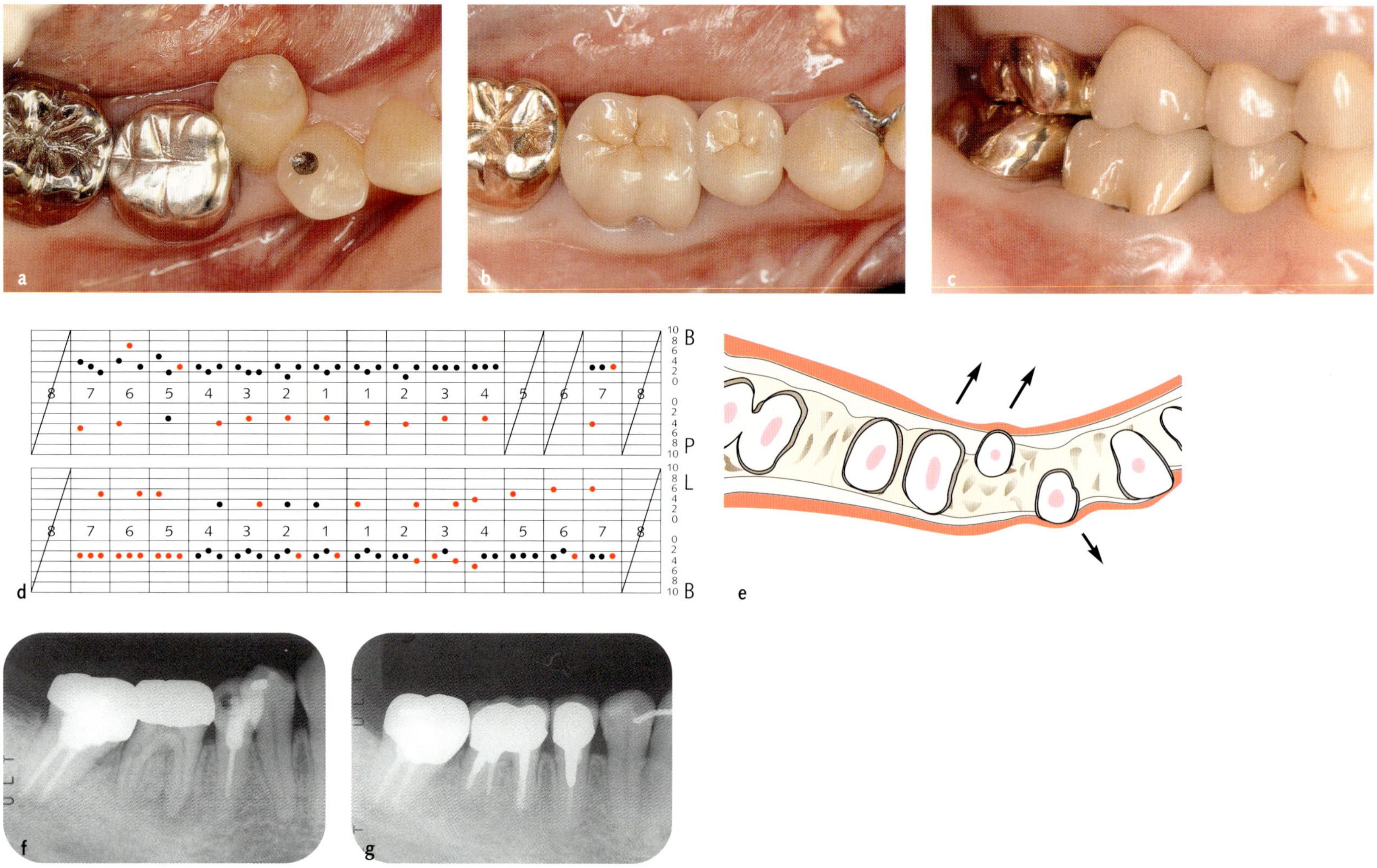

Fig 3-23 Improvement of the arch form using tooth movement and crown restorations. (a) At the first visit. (b) Photograph taken 4 years 6 months after the first visit. (c) Completion of crown restorations, 3 years after the first visit (about 1 year after surgery). Periodontal tissue regeneration using periosteum has been achieved for the right side. Transplantation of the mandibular right lateral incisor to the site of the maxillary left second premolar and crown lengthening were used to restore occlusal support on the left side. (d) Probing chart made soon after the first visit. (e) In a crowding condition, such as that seen at the first visit, premolar roots at the coronal one-third are outside of bone support, resulting in a bony dehiscence. The horizontal biologic width from the bone surface to the buccal or lingual surface of the mucosa and an appropriate width between the roots are lost. (f) Radiograph taken at the first visit. Apical radiolucency, bony defects, and traumatic findings are observed. (g) Radiograph taken 5 years after the first visit.

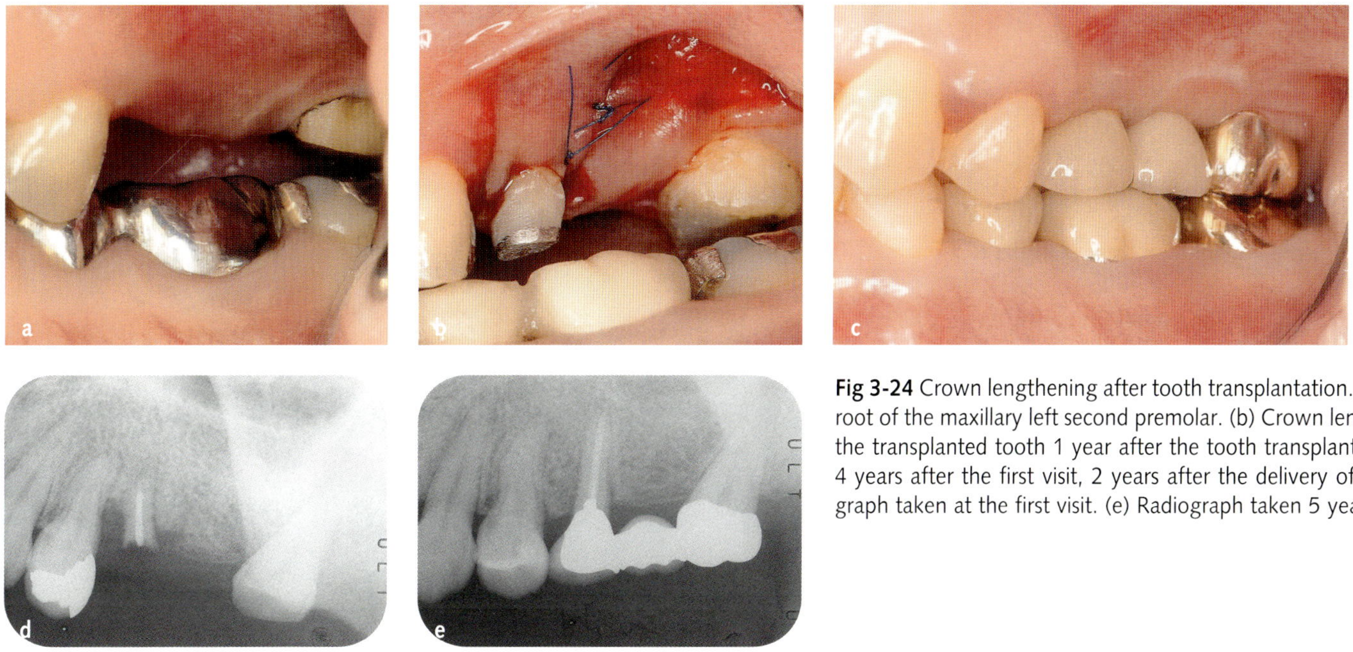

Fig 3-24 Crown lengthening after tooth transplantation. (a) At the first visit. Residual root of the maxillary left second premolar. (b) Crown lengthening was conducted for the transplanted tooth 1 year after the tooth transplantation. (c) Photograph taken 4 years after the first visit, 2 years after the delivery of final prostheses. (d) Radiograph taken at the first visit. (e) Radiograph taken 5 years after the first visit.

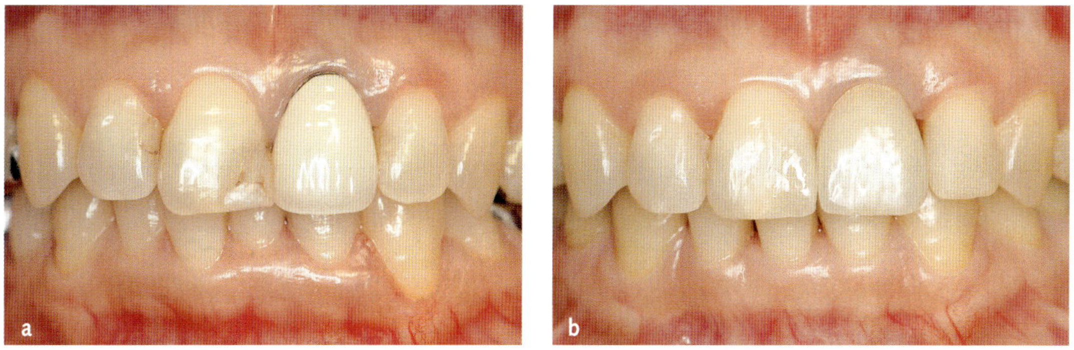

Fig 3-25 Improvement in the anterior teeth. (a) At the first visit, the anterior region shows a metal line at the maxillary left central incisor and a shadow through the gingiva. The root of the mandibular left canine was exposed because of its malposition. (b) A metal-ceramic crown has been placed on the maxillary left central incisor and resin composite restorations have been placed on the maxillary right central and lateral incisors and maxillary left lateral incisor. Note the conformity of the cervical margins of the anterior teeth. To achieve this, the bone level was adjusted both horizontally and vertically, which allowed a normal tooth-gingiva structure. This is the order of priority in treatment.

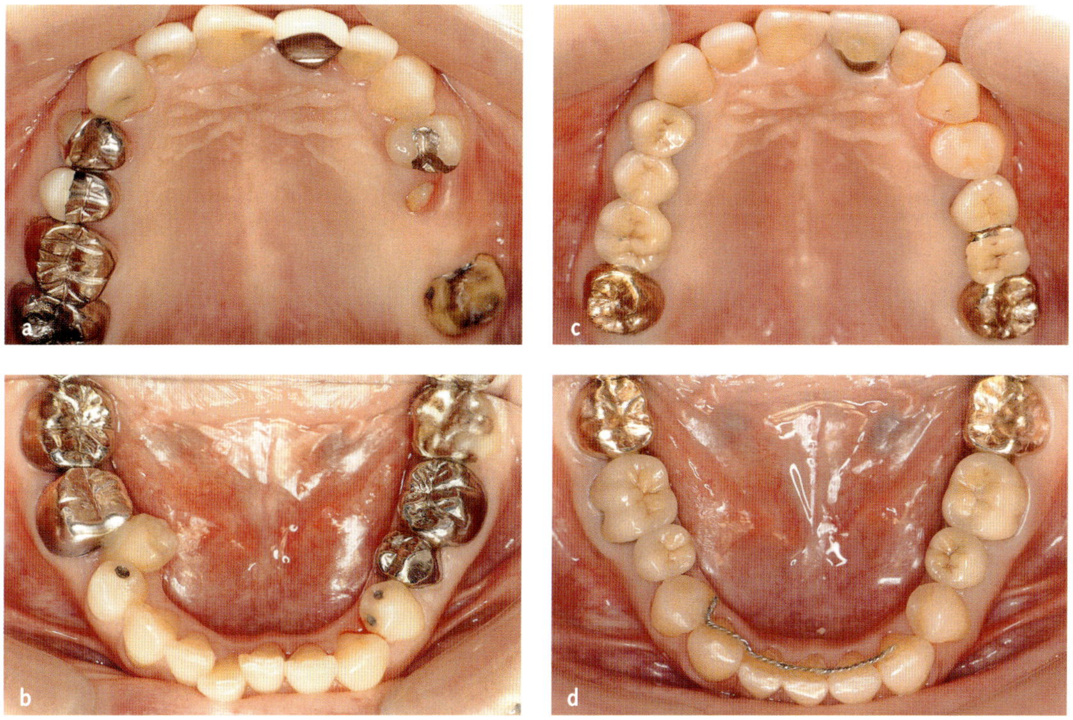

Fig 3-26 Improvement in the arch form. (a and b) At the first visit. In the maxillary arch, the residual root of the maxillary left second premolar and a root-fractured maxillary right first molar were extracted. After the transplantation of the mandibular right lateral incisor to the site of the maxillary left second premolar, myofunctional therapy was conducted, followed by tooth movement to improve the arch form. In the mandibular arch, the mandibular right second premolar, which exhibited lingual axioversion, was moved back in line with the dentition. (c and d) Photographs taken 5 years after the first visit. Restorations included a metal-ceramic crown for the maxillary left central incisor and fixed partial dentures to replace the maxillary right first molar (extending from the first premolar to the second molar) and the maxillary left first molar (extending from the second premolar to the second molar).

Restoration of the Periodontal Environment: Vertical Tooth Movement

Restorative tooth movement to improve the periodontal environment

Teeth are supported by the periodontal supporting tissues, which comprise the root cementum, periodontal ligament, and alveolar bone proper. This periodontal tissue is located in cancellous bone between inner and outer basic lamellar bone (cortical plates), which is covered by connective tissue and epithelial tissue. There seems to be homeostasis in the thickness of connective tissue and epithelial tissue that cover bone tissue. Gargiulo focused on the supracrestal width of the periodontal tissue, proposing a hypothesis that the width is constant. This is the hypothetical concept of the biologic width. It is considered that this width should not be invaded. Indeed, when a tooth without inflammation is orthodontically extruded, the position of the crestal bone is changed as much as the amount of extrusion, and any infrabony defect is eliminated, while the width of the connective tissue and epithelial tissue hardly changes. Extrusion is the most classic and common procedure utilized in restorative tooth movement.

Buccolingual tooth movement

- Crowding [Tooth unit] [Dentition unit] [Occlusion unit] — *See Case 1-1, Fig 3-17*
  To cope with discrepancies, correction of the crown morphology (disking), arch expansion, and tooth extraction are utilized. Conditions that affect diagnosis: (1) Degree of discrepancy; (2) occlusal relationship; (3) skeletal pattern; (4) profile; (5) conditions of circumoral muscles; (6) site of crowding; (7) periodontal tissue conditions; (8) dental caries and nonvital teeth; (9) planning for retention and prosthodontic treatment; (10) treatment period; (11) type of appliances; (12) patient's desire, compliance, age, and financial conditions.
- Buccolingual malpositions are mostly caused by parafunctions. [Occlusion unit] — *See Cases 1-9 and 3-6*
  Tongue habit, lip habits, imbalance between tongue and lip pressures, and other habits
  An adult case of bimaxillary protrusion (low tongue) should be treated with myofunctional therapy.
- Flared-out anterior teeth should be treated in a parallel manner with improvement of posterior occlusion. [Occlusion unit] — *See Case 1-4*

Mesiodistal tooth movement

- Appropriate width between tooth roots is mainly considered in individual tooth units and overall dentition units. [Tooth unit] [Dentition unit]
  Disking is indicated for teeth with lost attachment, etc. It can enhance increases in tissue levels. — *See Fig 3-35*
- Movement is conducted within the bony housing. The bony narrow segment does not move.
- Spaced dentition: Simple closure of a space may be problematic. It is mainly considered in overall correction of the dentition as a whole. [Dentition unit] [Occlusion unit] — *See Cases 1-4, 1-9, and 3-6*
  The cause of spaces is to be identified: (1) Discrepancies between the jaws and the teeth (microdontia, congenitally missing tooth); (2) discrepancy between crown and root widths; (3) large incisive foramen; (4) impacted supernumerary tooth; (5) anomaly of frenulum; (6) narrow bone; (7) muscle dysfunction (tongue); (8) habits (finger sucking, etc); (9) untreated missing tooth; (10) posterior interference of molar teeth; (11) premature contact; (12) unilateral mastication and bruxism; (13) periodontal disease.

Vertical tooth movement

- [Tooth unit]
  - Extrusion — *See Case 3-5, Figs 3-39 and 3-40, and Case 3-3*
    Indications: vertical bony defect, subgingival caries, tooth fracture, impacted tooth, a need for creation of bone or attached gingiva
    An extruded tooth should not make contact with the opposing teeth.
    Extrusion of the opposing tooth must be prevented.
    After extrusion, osseous surgery is conducted.
  - Intrusion
    Indication: teeth that are extruded with bone and without attached gingiva — *See Cases 2-14 and 3-4*
- [Dentition unit]
  - Extrusion
    Indication: improvement of strong curve of Spee (mandibular arch)
  - Intrusion
    Indication: improvement of strong curve of Spee — *See Case 3-2*
    When extrusion and intrusion are indicated for opposing arches, intrusion is prioritized.
- [Occlusion unit]
  - Extrusion — *See Cases 1-4 and 2-9*
    Indication: restoration of vertical maxillomandibular distance

Fig 3-27 Points of consideration for various tooth movements.

The principle in restorative tooth movement is that, in order for a tooth to be stabilized in the periodontal tissue, a certain width must be maintained in the vertical, buccolingual, and mesiodistal directions. Securing this width is the microscopic starting point of the tooth movement. Using this principle, we can change not only the vertical positions and angles of teeth but also the mesiodistal distances between tooth roots and the buccolingual positions of tooth roots in the bony housing through tooth movement, improving the periodontal environment and redistributing occlusal forces (Fig 3-27).

Attachment loss due to periodontal disease and vertical tooth movement

Vertical tooth movement is the most predictable method to control the attachment level of a dentition unit. Attachment level does not change as a single tooth unit. In vertical tooth movement, the dentition-unit attachment level is improved. Vertical tooth movement includes extrusion to move a tooth coronally to heighten the attachment level and intrusion to move a tooth apically to lower the attachment level. Extrusion is conducted for an individual tooth. Intrusion is conducted only for teeth that are not affected by periodontal disease. Often, simultaneous intrusion is conducted in a dentition unit, for example, to improve an excessive curve of Spee. With the development of regeneration therapy, it has become possible to restore attachment that was lost due to periodontal disease. However, there are many prerequisites for success, including the number of bony walls surrounding the defect, the space necessary for regeneration, complete closure of the wound, and time. The predictability of regeneration is not high in patients with a deep, bony defect. In contrast, vertical tooth movement has broad applications and high predictability (see Fig 3-1).

Intrusion of teeth with lost attachment

The first visit of the patient shown in Fig 3-28 was in 1975, when we started our practice. The chief complaint at the first visit was a periodontal abscess at the maxillary right lateral incisor. The patient had a Class II, division 1 occlusion. Orthodontic treatment was started in 1983, when the patient was 43 years old. At that time, we did not have enough experience with periodontally compromised teeth, and inappropriately intruded the lateral incisor, resulting in subsequent loss of attachment. The patient's record at that time indicates that the periodontal probing depth was 7 mm, but it might have been deeper. Because the infected root surface was intruded, not only was the attachment height relative to the bone level lost, but also the periodontal tissue destruction was initiated. We deeply reflected on the procedures completed in this case. Fortunately, the patient is still attending our clinic, and the probing depth of the maxillary right lateral incisor is maintainable at 5 mm.

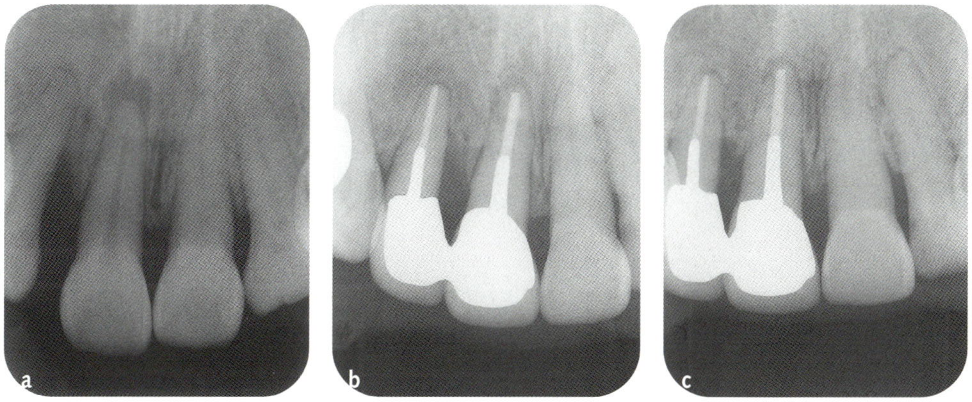

Fig 3-28 (a) Bracket height was determined from the incisal edge, and the maxillary right and left lateral incisors were intruded (March 1983). The maxillary right lateral incisor had a periodontal abscess 8 years before and had been extruded. (b) July 1986. (c) October 1998. (d) Probing chart at the first visit (1975). (e) Probing chart 24 years after the first visit.

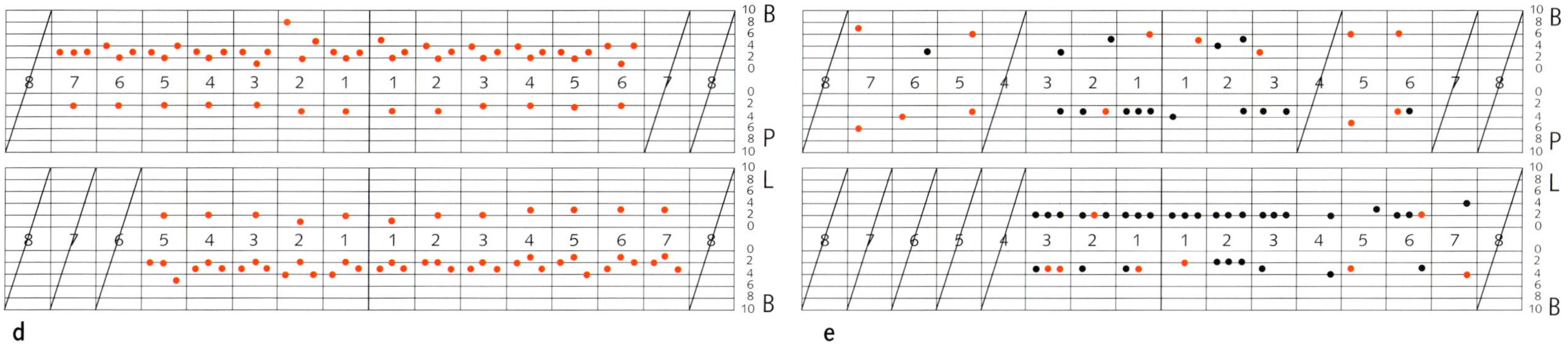

d

e

Vertical tooth movement and improvement of infrabony defects

A vertical movement, or tooth extrusion, utilizes the principle of maintaining a certain width of epithelial and connective tissue while moving a tooth coronally (Case 3-4). It applies the principles for reconstruction of periodontal tissues, including adjustment of the attachment level in a dentition, restoration of the bone level, and restoration of the conformity of the gingival cuff line.

When periodontal disease causes an infrabony defect and attachment level is irregular, extrusion of the affected tooth can eliminate the infrabony defect and readjust the attachment level (see Figs 3-35 to 3-38). This enables restoration of continuity in the height of the bone crest and the height of the gingival margin. In a tooth with subgingival caries, a healthy root surface, which is necessary for the biologic width, is lost. The biologic width can be restored through vertical tooth movement.

Case 3-4 Dentition-unit intrusion and tooth-unit extrusion

Patient: *23-year-old woman at the time of first visit in 1993*

A disturbance in the cervical margins was clearly observed, as were tooth malpositions, which were caused by oral habits (Fig 3-29). Lingual axioversion of the maxillary and mandibular incisors and considerable extrusion of the maxillary incisors were noted. The lips were tight and the area around the lips showed redness, indicating that the patient had a habit of biting her lips. This could also be the direct cause of the gingival recession of the mandibular central incisors as well as the unnatural cervical line. The patient had a habit of resting her cheek on her hand, causing the lingual axioversion and extrusion of the maxillary left first and second premolars. The gingiva exhibited inflammation, but there was no attachment loss from periodontitis.

Treatment was initiated with hygiene instructions and myofunctional therapy to stop the habit of lip biting and to improve the low position of the tongue. In conjunction with this therapy, surgical treatments were conducted, including crown lengthening of the maxillary right central and lateral incisors and left central incisor as well as lateral repositioning of a pedicle flap to cover the exposed roots of both maxillary central incisors (Figs 3-30 to 3-34). In addition, endodontic treatment was performed, followed by provisional restoration. Multiple brackets were delivered, starting with the maxillary arch, 11 months after the first visit. The maxillary right central and lateral incisors and first molar and the maxillary left central and lateral incisors and first and second premolars were intruded, while the mesially inclined molars in the maxillary and

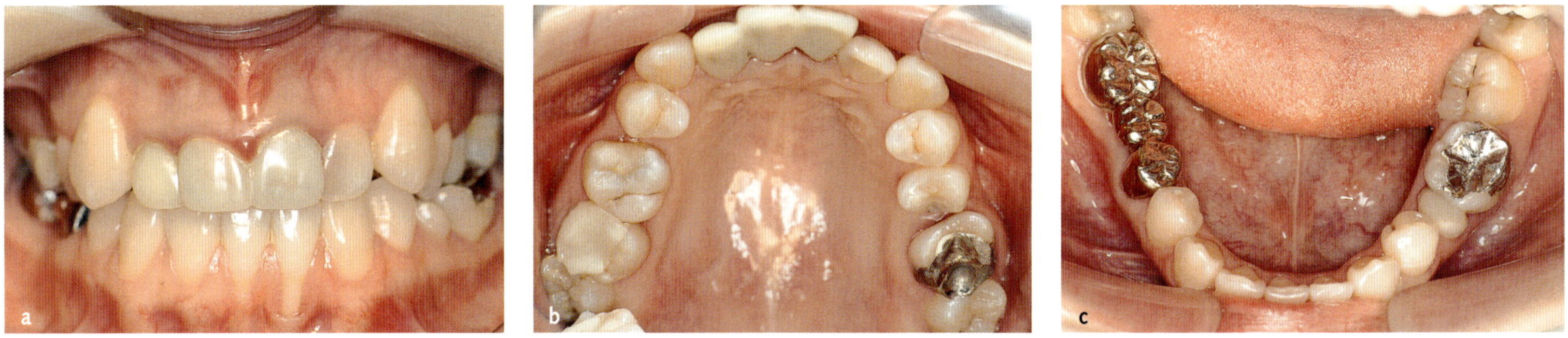

Fig 3-29 (a to c) At the first visit. A disturbance in the cervical margins, lingual axioversion of the teeth, gingival recession, and a disturbance in the occlusal plane are noted during the initial evaluation. The soft tissues show gingivitis, but there is no attachment loss.

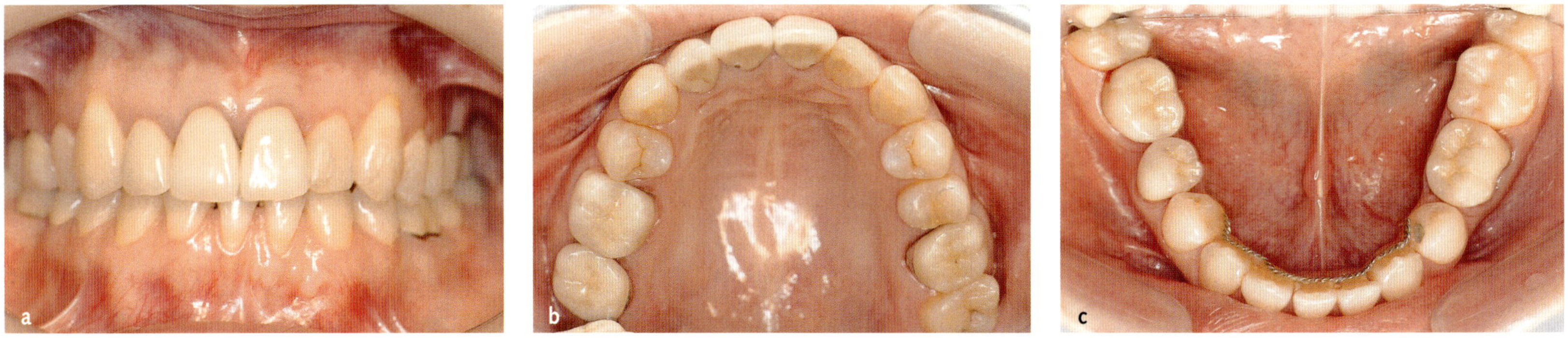

Fig 3-30 (a to c) Photographs taken 4 years 7 months after the first visit. The patient did not continue regular visits, and it took longer than anticipated to complete active treatment. Still, the arch form is improved.

mandibular arches were uprighted. When the disturbance of the occlusal plane is treated by dentition-unit intrusion, intrusion is conducted first, and then extrusion is conducted. Intrusion is more time-consuming than extrusion. Brackets were delivered to the mandibular arch 1 year 6 months after those in the maxillary arch. The roots of the mandibular anterior teeth were outside the bony housing, exhibiting root exposure, and they were moved lingually. Because of the irregular visits of the patient, active treatment took longer than anticipated, requiring 3 years to debond brackets.

The tracing of the cephalogram indicates that, posttreatment, the lips are less tight, the mandibular anterior teeth are in the bony housing, and the molar teeth are uprighted (Fig 3-33a).

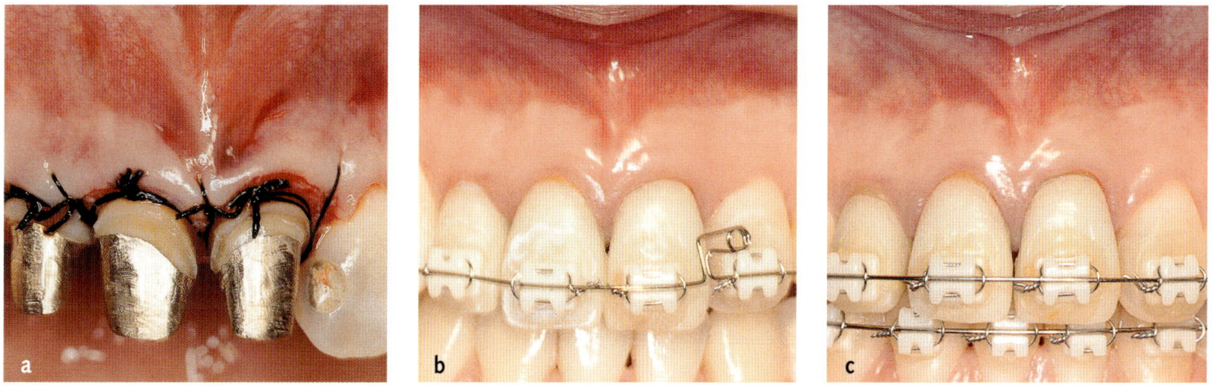

Fig 3-31 Clinical crown lengthening. (a) Initial therapy, 1 year 5 months after the first visit. After the completion of endodontic treatment, clinical crown-lengthening surgery was conducted to secure the biologic width and to obtain some degree of consistency in the cervical margins. (b) After provisional restoration is provided. The maxillary right central and lateral incisors and first molar and the maxillary left central and lateral incisors and first and second premolars are intruded, while the mesially inclined molars in the maxillary and mandibular arches are uprighted. (c) Brackets are delivered to the mandibular arch 1 year 5 months after the surgery.

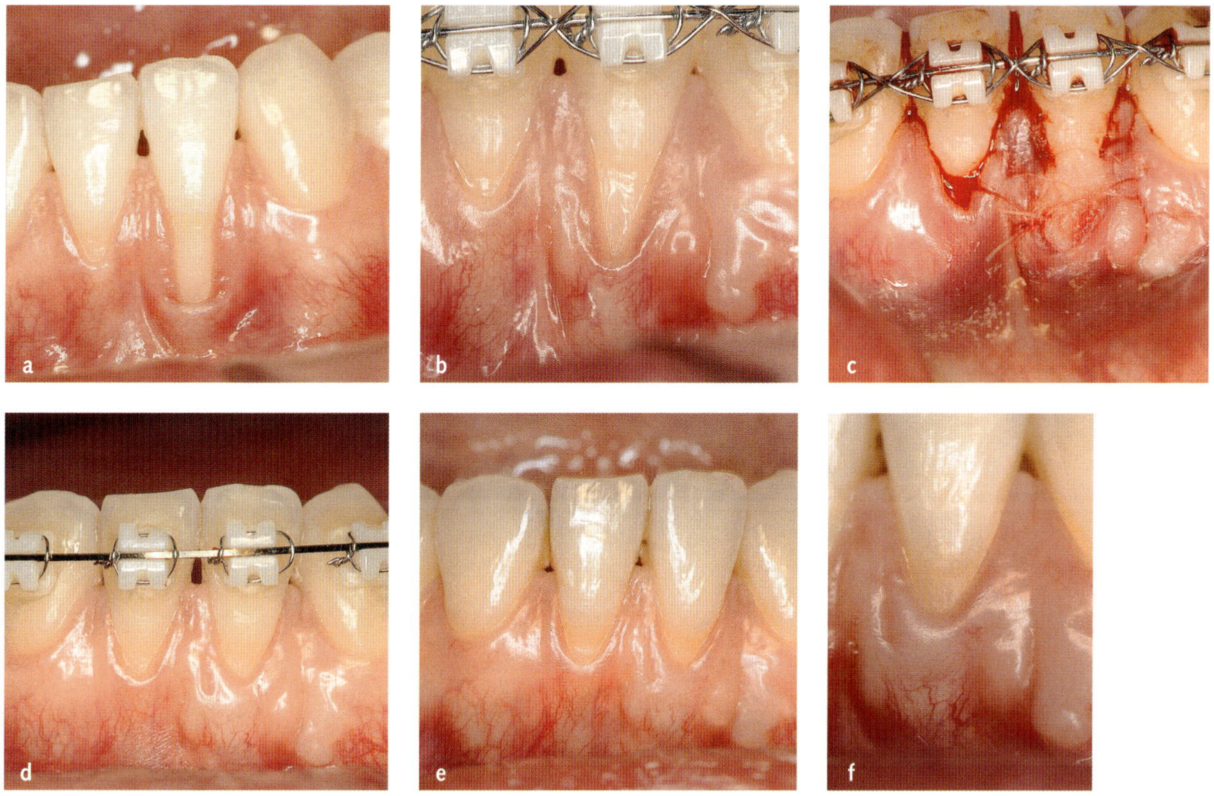

Fig 3-32 Mandibular anterior teeth outside of the bony housing. (a) Completion of initial therapy. Due to the patient's habit of biting her lips, the mandibular anterior teeth are inclined lingually and show significant gingival recession. (b) Photograph taken 2 years 9 months after the first visit. Brackets have been delivered to the mandibular arch. (c) Lateral repositioning of a pedicle flap has been completed to correct the exposed root. (d) Photograph taken 9 months after treatment, prior to debonding of brackets. Active treatment is completed. (e and f) Photographs taken 3 years 8 months after the first visit. The mandibular anterior teeth are in the bony housing, and the gingival recession is reduced.

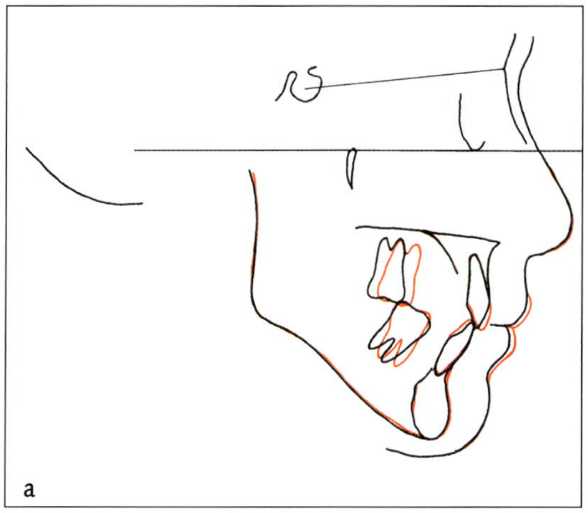

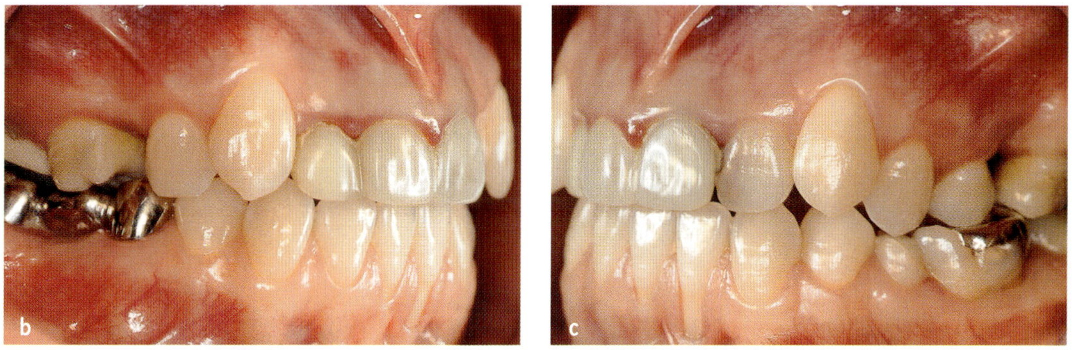

Fig 3-33 Changes in lateral cephalograms and lateral views. (a) Tracings of cephalograms, superimposed on sella-nasion at sella. *(black)* Before active treatment, 24 years 2 months old. *(red)* After treatment, 27 years 11 months old. (b and c) Lateral views at the first visit.

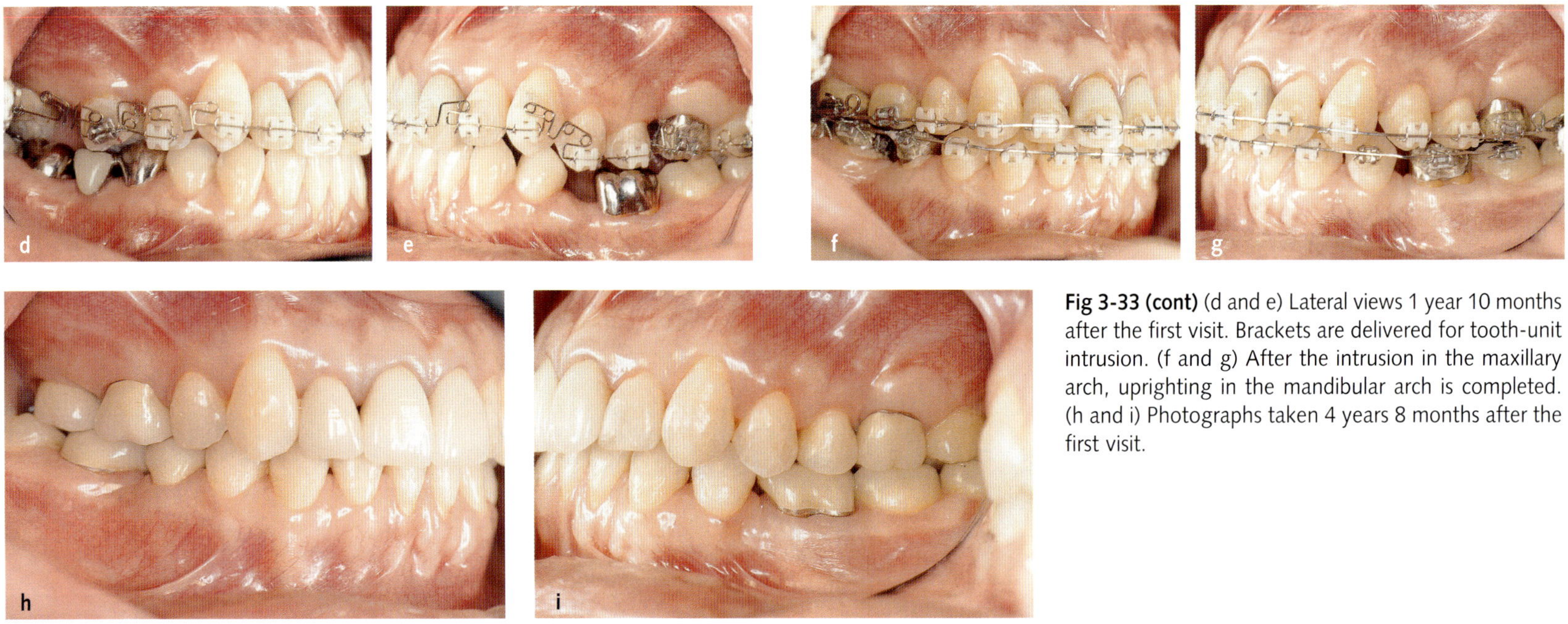

Fig 3-33 (cont) (d and e) Lateral views 1 year 10 months after the first visit. Brackets are delivered for tooth-unit intrusion. (f and g) After the intrusion in the maxillary arch, uprighting in the mandibular arch is completed. (h and i) Photographs taken 4 years 8 months after the first visit.

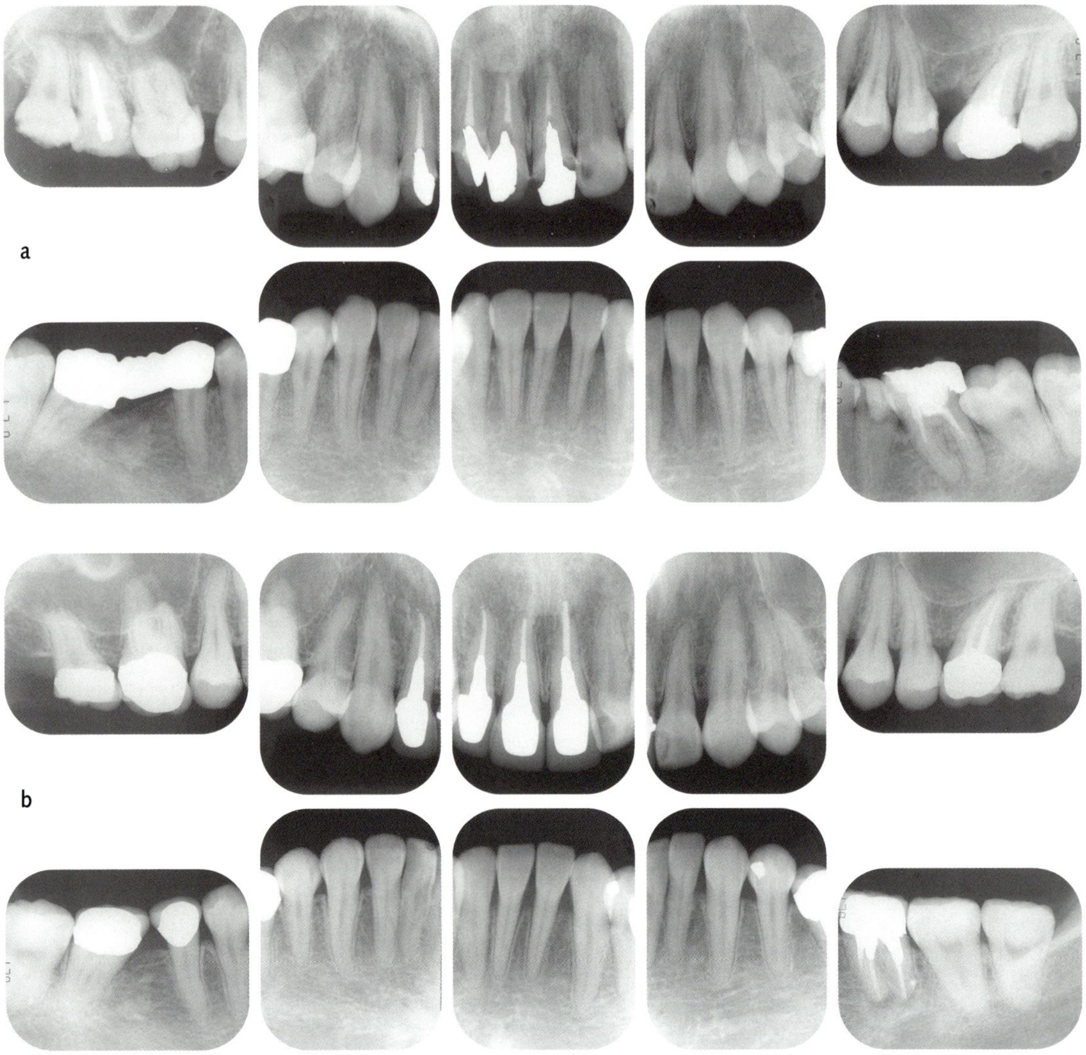

Fig 3-34 Radiographic views of treatment progress. (a) At the first visit. (b) Radiographs taken 8 years 9 months after the first visit. There is still widening of the periodontal space in the mandibular anterior teeth. The patient's lip-biting habit is not completely resolved.

Improvement of the periodontal environment

When molar teeth that are compressed and have local traumatic bony defects are treated, and when crown restoration is needed, the occlusal cusps are reduced in almost all cases to allow a period for natural extrusion. This is because there is a high likelihood that the inflammation around tooth roots will be alleviated at an earlier stage, because the attachment level will be increased by the extrusion, a significant benefit for improvement of infrabony defects. When root canal–associated inflammation is present around the apex of the root, natural extrusion has a positive effect on healing.

The patient shown in Figs 3-35 to 3-38 had a deep infrabony pocket reaching 11 mm on the mesial surface of the mandibular left first molar. The tooth was uprighted and extruded orthodontically to improve the periodontal environment.

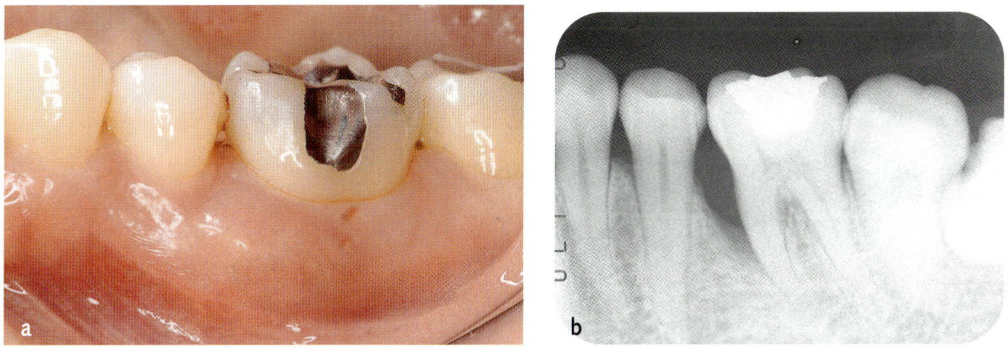

Fig 3-35 (a and b) The patient is a 29-year-old woman. There is an 11-mm infrabony pocket on the mesial surface of the mandibular left first molar.

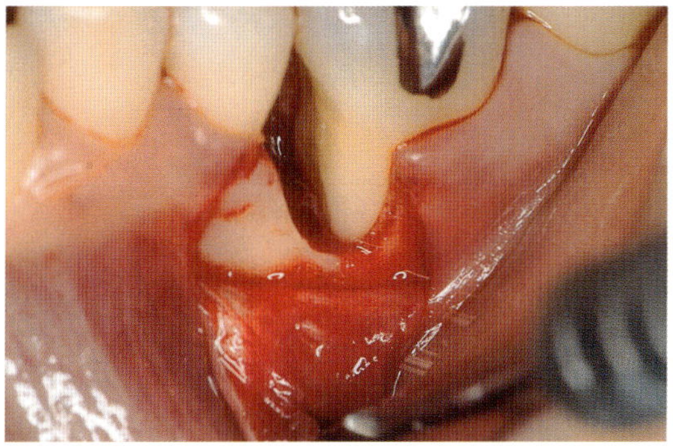

Fig 3-36 The deep infrabony defect is visible after the flap is raised. After thorough debridement, Emdogain was applied.

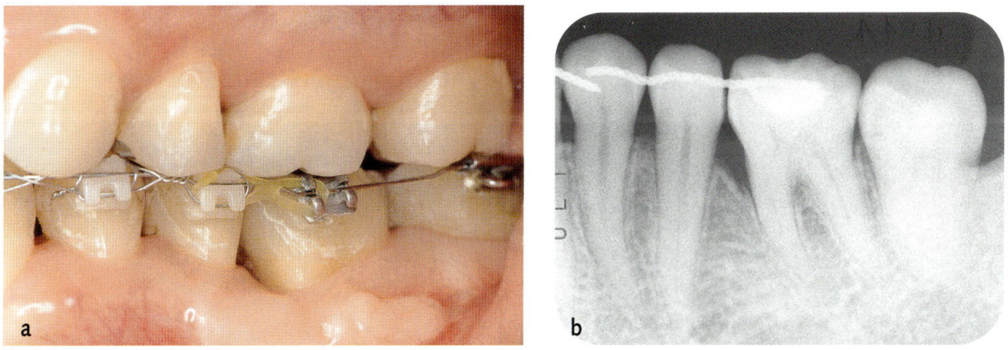

Fig 3-37 (a) Orthodontic treatment was started 3 months later and included uprighting and mesial movement (with disking of the mesial surface). (b) Radiograph taken 2 years after surgery, when orthodontic treatment was completed.

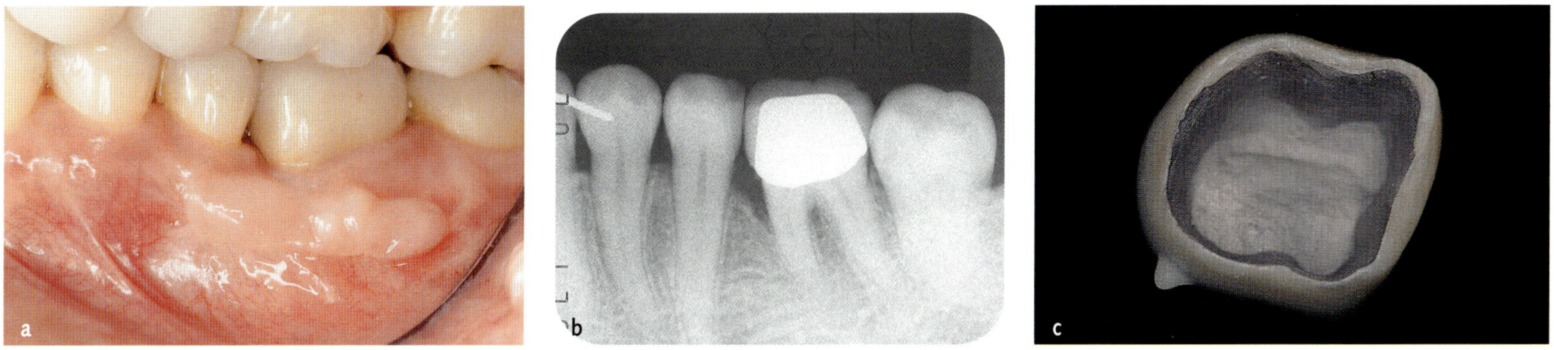

Fig 3-38 (a) After the completion of the tooth movement, a metal-ceramic crown restoration was fabricated (2 years 9 months after the surgery). The mesial probing depth is 2 mm. (b) Radiograph taken 9 months after the completion of orthodontic treatment. (c) The crown contour is designed so that the embrasure space is filled.

Traction of an impacted third molar

When the mandibular second molar is missing or considered impossible to maintain, and if an impacted third molar is present, we orthodontically move the impacted tooth to the position of the second molar so that the third molar is engaged in occlusion (Fig 3-39). This is a useful restorative tooth movement in our patients, many of whom have impacted third molars. Third molars are valuable as a stock of healthy teeth. We do not agree with their routine extraction at the stage of tooth germination.

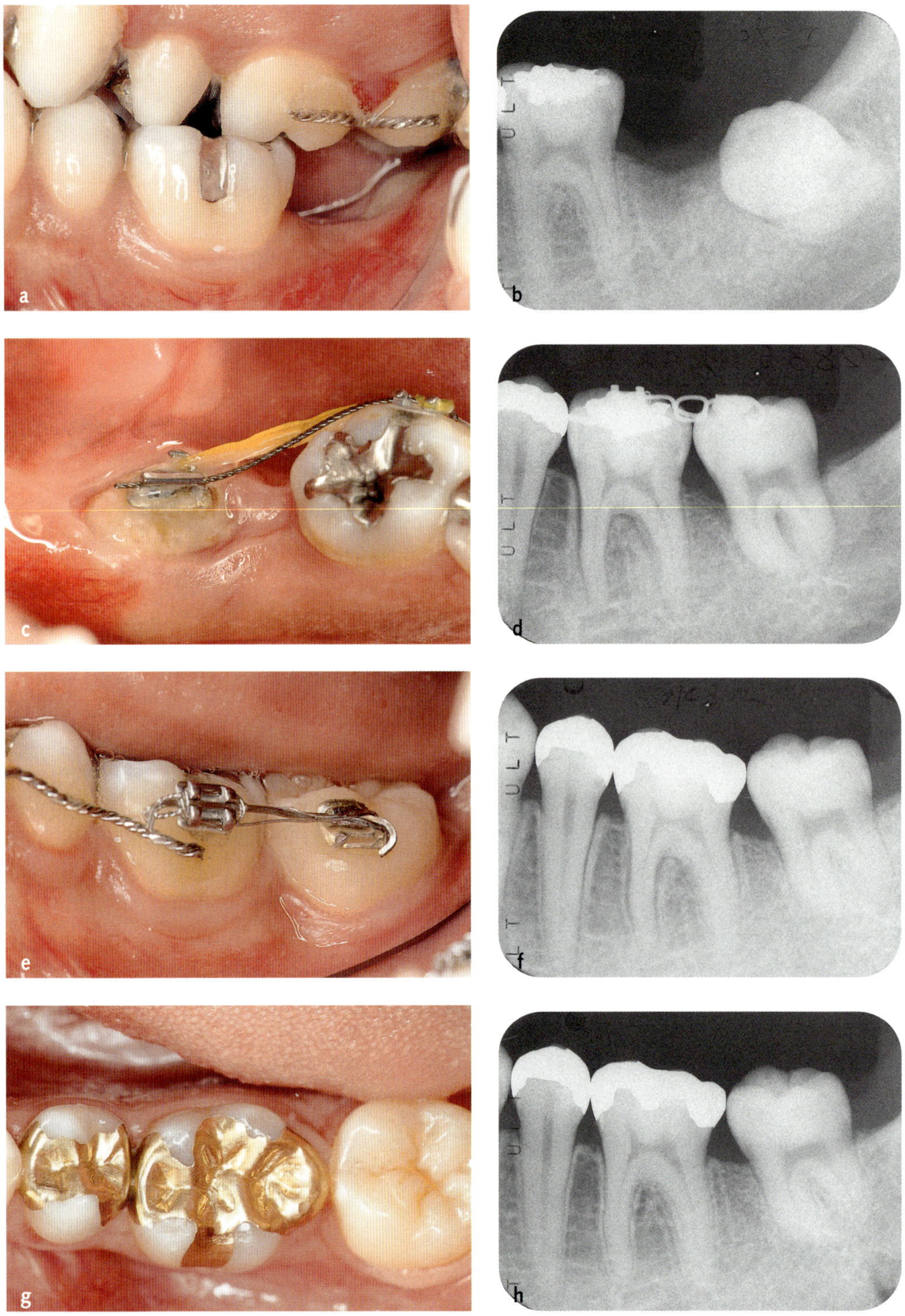

Fig 3-39 (a and b) The mandibular left second molar is missing and the third molar is impacted in mesial axioversion. (c and d) The opposing teeth, the maxillary left first and second premolars, are splinted with twisted wire; the mandibular left canine, premolars, and first molar are splinted, and the third molar is moved mesially. (e) The active treatment period was 1 year 5 months. (f) Radiograph taken about 2 years after the start of active treatment. (g and h) Photograph and radiograph taken about 5 years 2 months after the first visit, about 4 years 11 months after the start of active treatment.

Secondary caries and extrusion during long-term periodontal maintenance

Although maintenance of periodontal disease can be predictable, management of secondary caries is unreliable. Early detection is difficult in the case of nonvital teeth. Even if the caries is detected, intervention is difficult if a large prosthesis has been delivered, as in this clinical case (Figs 3-40 to 3-42). When the prosthesis is finally removed, the teeth may only have residual roots left. Orthodontic extrusion for residual roots to restore the biologic width is a predictable technique among restorative tooth movements.

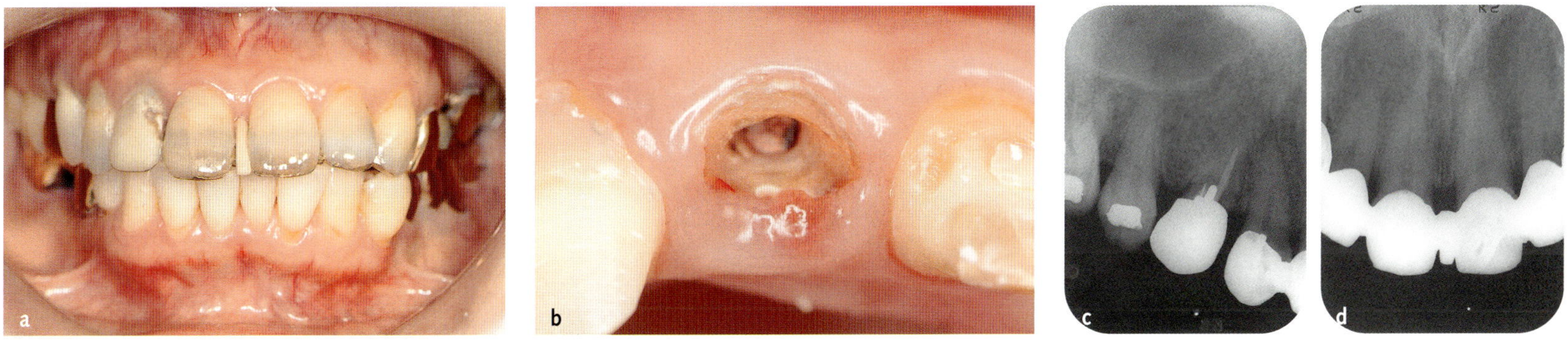

Fig 3-40 (a and b) Periodontal maintenance had been continued since 1977 for this woman (42 years old at the first visit). We did not initiate active intervention. Seventeen years after the start of maintenance, intervention was made as the root caries affecting the maxillary right lateral incisor became serious. (c and d) Radiographs taken at the first visit (1977).

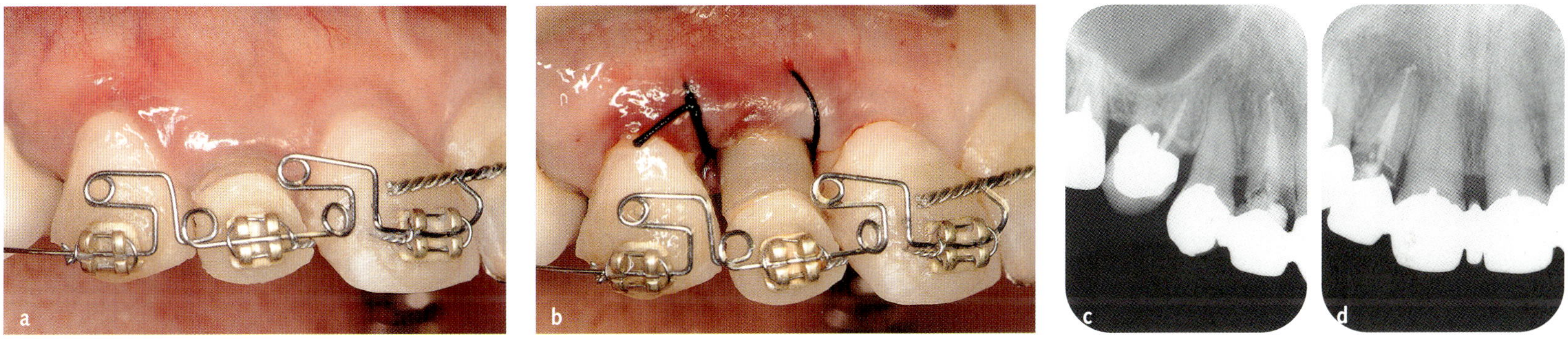

Fig 3-41 (a) Extrusion was conducted for 1 month. (b) The cervical margin is adjusted surgically. (c and d) Radiographs taken at the same time (immediately before the removal of prosthesis).

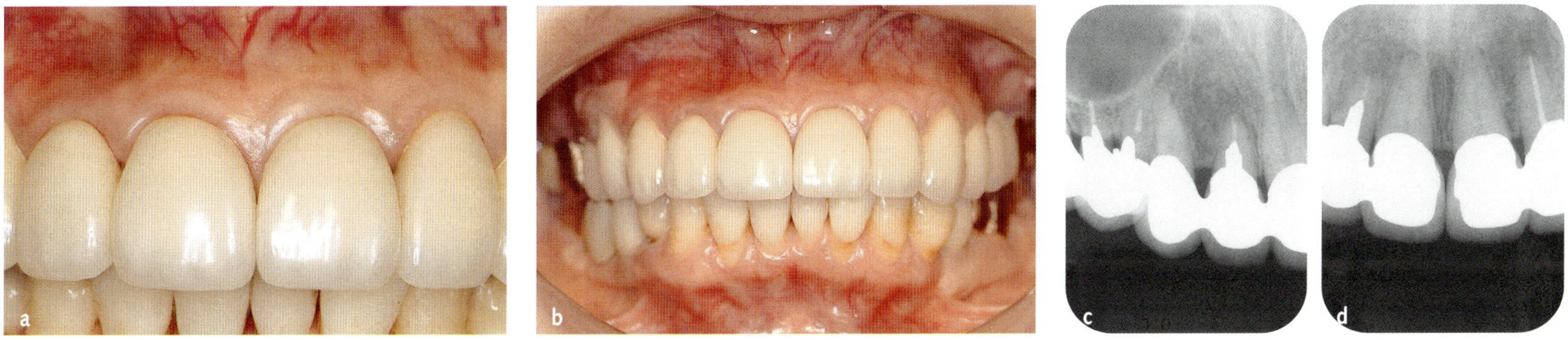

Fig 3-42 (a and b) Photographs taken 21 years after the first visit, 3 years 5 months after the restorative treatment was initiated. (c and d) Radiographs taken 23 years after the first visit, 6 years after the intervention. Although the root of the maxillary right lateral incisor is shortened, the condition is stable.

Tooth Movement as a Part of Comprehensive Treatment

An intricate step in achieving treatment goals

Preprosthetic tooth movement to restore the appropriate tooth axis and to close interdental spaces will reduce unnecessary tooth preparations (Figs 3-43 to 3-46). Because of this, tooth movement is an essential, significant part of comprehensive dental treatment. In comprehensive therapy, the most rational method should be selected to achieve a certain treatment goal. Accordingly, tooth movement, restoration, prosthetic treatment, surgical treatment, myofunctional therapy, and other means are used to complement each other. For example, when an interdental space is to be closed, there are some cases where tooth movement alone does not suffice, as discussed previously (see Figs 3-12 to 3-14). A case like this requires restoration with light-cured resin or a crown prosthesis, the selection of which depends on the occlusal relationship, esthetic conditions, and/or periodontal conditions. When improvement of the occlusal plane is envisioned, consideration should be given, first, to whether or not the VDO should be increased, how intrusion or extrusion should be conducted as a dentition unit, whether or not enameloplasty should be conducted, whether or not a crown restoration should be placed, and whether or not surgical crown lengthening is possible. Only after the necessary treatments are combined correctly can the treatment goals be rationally achieved.

Selective tooth movement

In many cases, except in the presence of full-mouth occlusal collapse, brackets are applied not to all teeth but to some teeth. In such cases, brackets should not be applied to a number of teeth as anchorage. Rather, reinforced anchorage should provided by a lingual arch or plate, twisted wire, and other means, and a sectional arch should be used to move selected teeth only. In tooth movement in adults, imprudent tooth movement in an area with stable occlusion must be avoided.

Limitations of treatment

In restorative tooth movement, a diagnosis has to be established to determine "which parts are collapsed, what caused the destruction, which part of the collapse can be restored, and which part will be difficult to rebuild." The stomatognathic systems of patients with TMD, issues involving bone, muscle, periodontal tissue, tooth crown and root morphology, oral habits, and other issues will also have aspects that can be changed, aspects that can be changed with difficulty, and aspects that cannot be changed. These patients should be identified based on an understanding of the characteristics of each tissue prior to the start of treatment. Some clinicians tend not to make an effort to improve patients' habits of chewing the tongue or the lips, on the pretext of poor compliance of the patients. Such efforts are very important to eliminate the causes of some dental problems. It is necessary also to clarify the responsibilities of the clinician and the patient. It is important for the patient to understand that we as clinicians cannot have everything under our direct control. Often periodontal tissue is compromised, and consideration should be given to control of the inflammation before and during tooth movement as well as to control of orthodontic forces. Natural extrusion methods, such as a combination of selective enameloplasty and a bite plane, may be used. It is necessary to make sure that no excessive occlusal force is exerted. The risk of root resorption is higher in adults than in children. The tolerance range of the TMJs is limited as well.

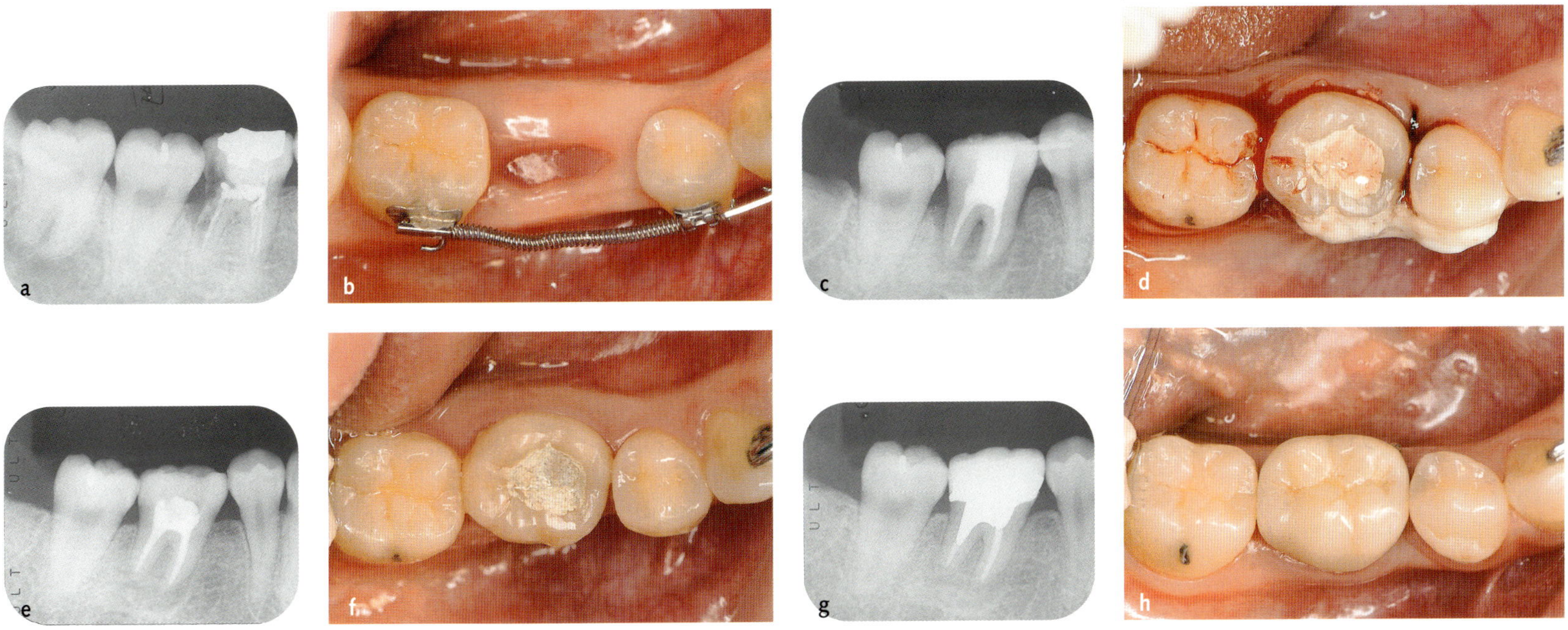

Fig 3-43 Adjustment of an extraction space before reimplantation. (a) The mandibular right first molar has internal resorption, and its distal tooth defect caused a mesial axioversion of the second molar. (b) Transplantation of the mandibular right third molar to the site of the mandibular right first molar was planned. Because the third molar was large and the space for reimplantation was limited because of the mesial axioversion of the second molar, restorative tooth movement was completed before transplantation. (c and d) The third molar was transplanted to the site of the first molar 1 month after active treatment was completed. (e and f) Views 3 months after treatment. (g and h) Appearance 7 months after treatment. The transplanted tooth was prepared and a crown restoration was delivered.

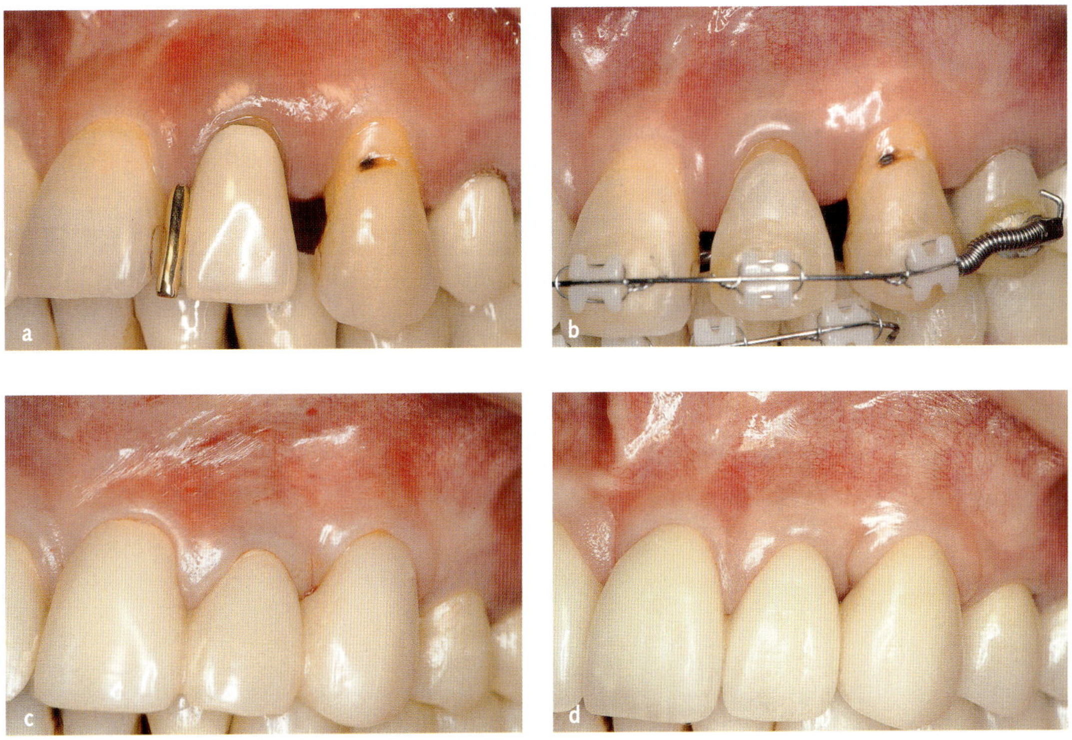

Fig 3-44 Mesiodistal tooth movement before crown restoration. (a) Although this interdental space is conspicuous, mere closure of the space without improvement of the occlusion could be detrimental. Because a crown restoration is inevitable after improvement of the occlusion, tooth movement will be conducted under the assumption that a crown restoration will be placed in the future. (b) A provisional restoration is fabricated to improve the occlusion and the interdental papillae as well as the gingival level via mesial movement of the maxillary left canine and extrusion of the maxillary left lateral incisor. (c) The final provisional restoration after tooth movement (mucogingival surgery is shown in Fig 4-120). (d) Reconstruction of the interdental papillae and balanced cervical gingivae were achieved.

Asymmetry in the cervical gingivae caused by the restoration of the occlusal plane

The patient in Fig 3-45 was a 46-year-old woman at the first visit (1982). The occlusal plane was disturbed because of preexisting crowding, missing maxillary right second premolar and mandibular left first premolar, and inappropriate prostheses, with localized attachment loss. The maxillary right first premolar had subgingival caries and the maxillary left first premolar and mandibular right first premolar had unsuccessfully treated root canals and were extracted, which alleviated crowding and allowed adjustment of the occlusal plane. The scope of the prosthodontic treatment was limited to the anterior regions.

Sufficient consideration was not given to incorporating an improvement of the cervical gingivae into the tooth movement. As a result, an extreme asymmetry existed between the right and left cervical margins of the prostheses in the anterior regions. Subsequently, the patient discontinued visiting the clinic and then later revisited with subgingival caries. This scenario was repeated several times, compelling us to refabricate full-coverage restorations. The subgingival caries involving the maxillary right canine required clinical crown-lengthening surgery, which was conducted for the maxillary right central incisor, lateral incisor, and canine to restore consistency to the cervical gingivae.

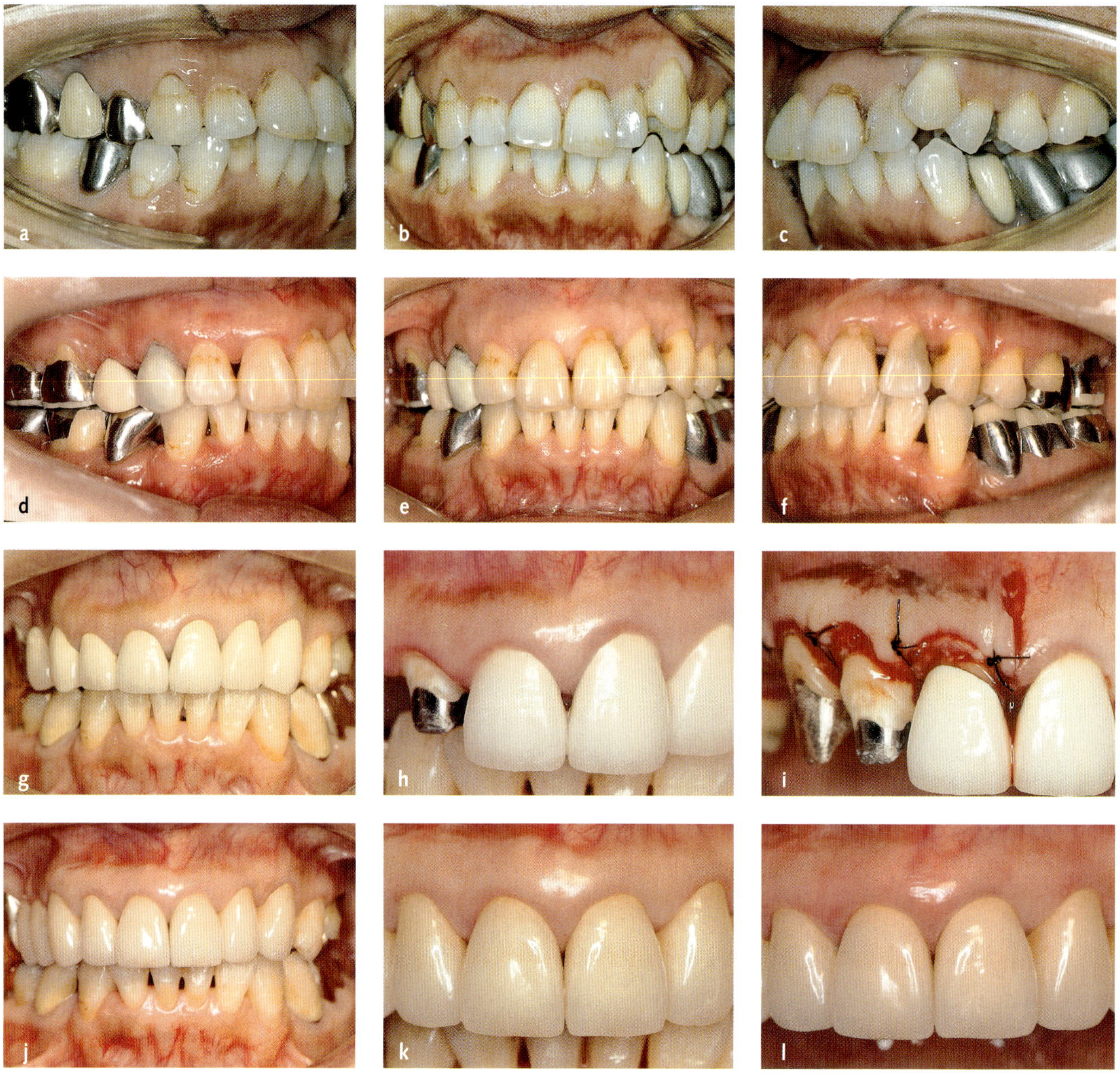

Fig 3-45 (a to c) The first visit (1982). (d to f) The maxillary right first premolar had subgingival caries and the maxillary left and mandibular right first premolars had undergone unsuccessful root canal treatment. These teeth were extracted, after which crowding was alleviated and the occlusal plane was adjusted. The molars have provisional restorations placed with resin on the occlusal surface (1984). There was a bony defect distal to the maxillary left central incisor. If this patient were treated now, we would selectively grind the incisal edge of the central incisor and position the bracket height so that the level of the cervical gingivae at the first visit (see Fig 3-45a) would not be changed. However, at the time, we intruded the incisor, which significantly impacted the treatment afterward. (g) Photograph taken 8 years 8 months after the first visit (1990). Due to attachment loss, the cervical margins were asymmetric. (h) Subsequently, pulpectomy was conducted and the maxillary central incisors were connected with a splinted crown restoration. The patient discontinued visiting us but later revisited when the prosthesis dislodged (1995). (i) Clinical crown lengthening was conducted for the maxillary right central incisor, lateral incisor, and canine. (j and k) After crown lengthening, the prosthesis was refabricated. This is 14 years after the first visit (1996). Harmony of the cervical gingivae is achieved. (l) Photograph taken 16 years 9 months after the first visit (1998). Based on our current principles of treatment, the lack of subgingival contour and congestion in the marginal tissues are a concern.

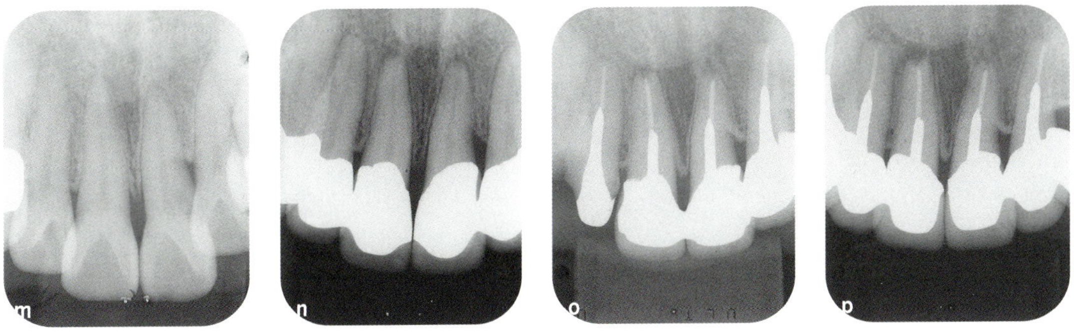

Fig 3-45 (cont) (m) At the first visit (1982). (n) Restoration after tooth movement (1985). (o) Crown restorations splinting the maxillary central incisors. (p) After the crown-lengthening procedure, the prosthesis was refabricated. This is 18 years after the first visit (2000).

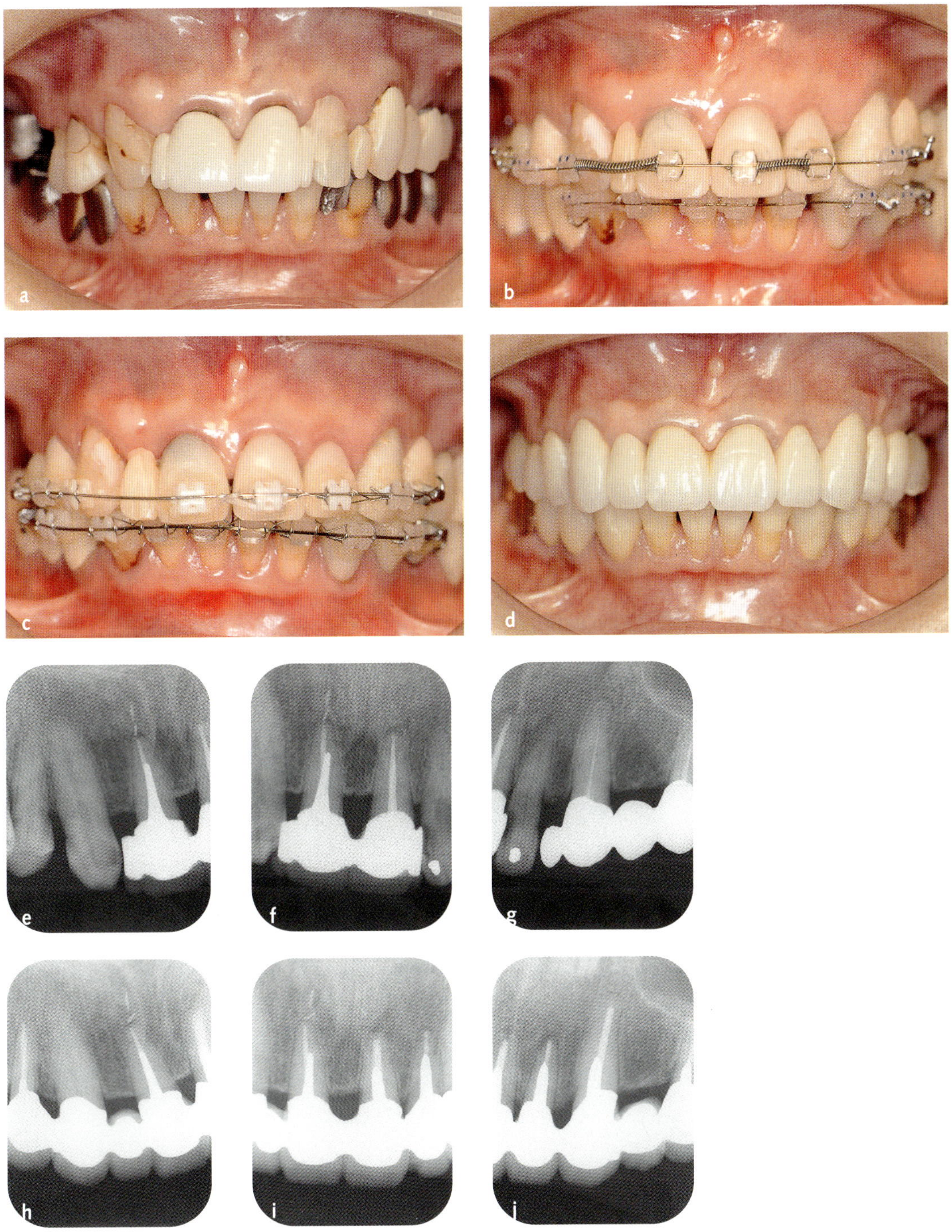

Fig 3-46 Mesiodistal tooth movement to allow an esthetic prosthesis to replace missing teeth. (a) At the first visit, interdental spaces caused by pathologic tooth movement are filled by a prosthesis (between the maxillary right lateral incisor, right central incisor, left central incisor, left lateral incisor, and canine). (b) After the initial therapy, a provisional restoration was delivered, and mesiodistal tooth movement was conducted (1 year 8 months). (c) Active treatment was conducted for about 6 months. Prostheses replacing the missing teeth were envisioned, and teeth were moved to the mesiodistally preferable positions in consideration of the occlusal relationship with the opposing arch. (d) Photograph taken 2 years after the delivery of final prostheses. Interdental spaces are closed, and a consistency of the cervical gingivae has been achieved. (e to g) Radiographs taken at the first visit. (h to i) Radiographs taken after 6 years.

Regeneration of peripheral tissue by tooth movement

Although the predictability of regenerative therapy has been enhanced today, it is still impossible to vertically augment bone tissue without having a basis for regeneration. The basis for regeneration is a healthy periosteum or periodontal ligament. Extrusion of a tooth root is the most predictable way to achieve vertical augmentation of bone and improvement of the vertical attachment level (Fig 3-47). Orthodontic treatment of an alveolar cleft was utilized to extrude the maxillary right lateral incisor (which was treatment planned to be extracted) to guide bone and gingival tissue almost to the same level as that of the adjacent teeth.
Case 3-5 demonstrates another case of combined regenerative therapy and restorative tooth movement.

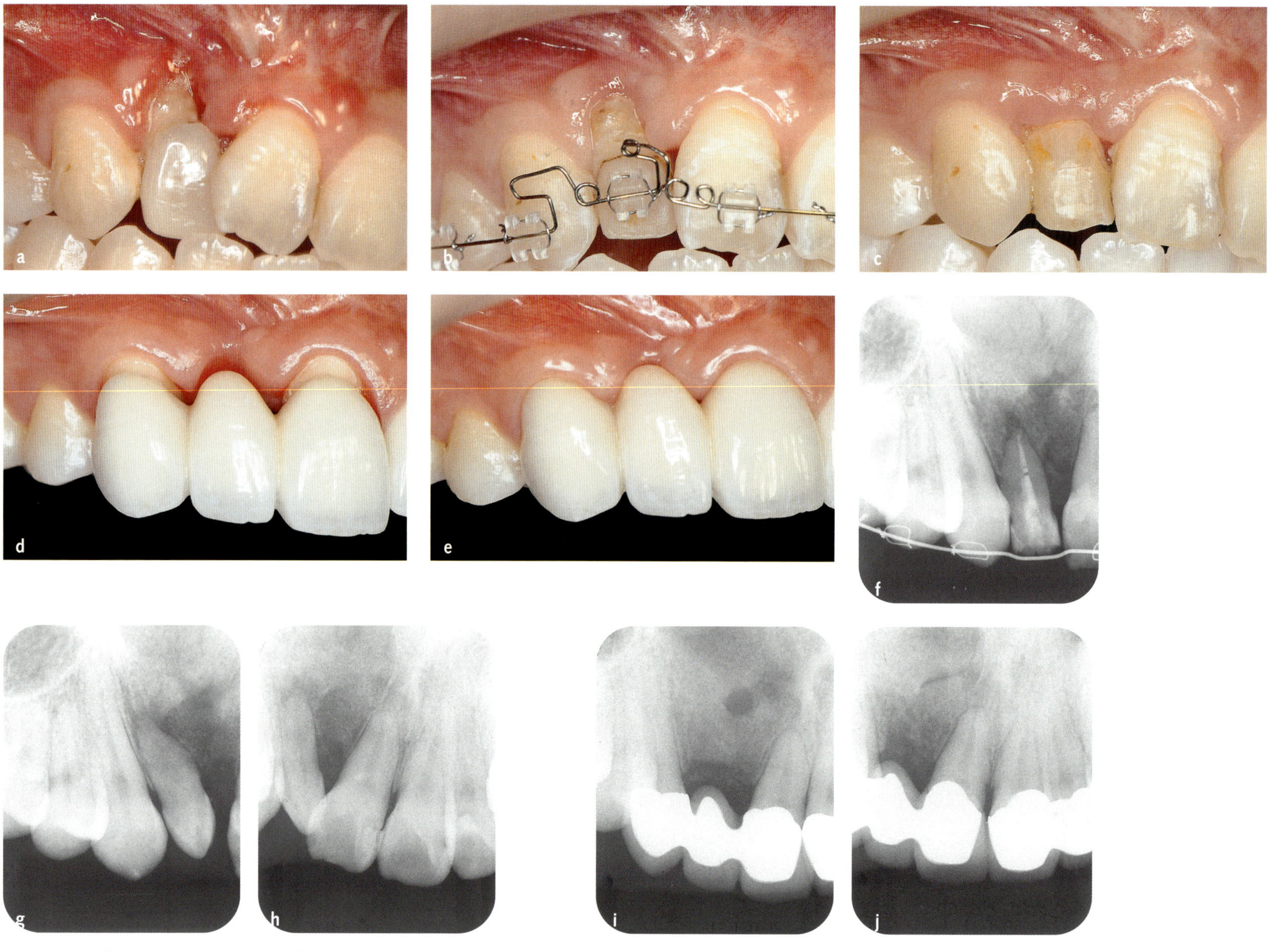

Fig 3-47 (a) The patient was 21 years old. For the right alveolar cleft, periodontal plastic surgery was repeated, including an iliac bone graft to the area between the maxillary right central and lateral incisors, which improved the conditions considerably. Orthodontic treatment was conducted once. (b) The maxillary right central incisor and the mandibular right central incisor are in reverse occlusion. Orthodontic treatment is started before final prosthodontic treatment is initiated. (c) Orthodontic extrusion was successfully conducted to align bone levels and the gingival level. (d) A postimpression technique was used after the extraction of the maxillary right lateral incisor, and a prosthesis with an ovate pontic design has been delivered. (e) The final prosthesis is delivered. (f) After the completion of extrusion, the bone level is adjusted. (g and h) Radiographs taken at the first visit. A conspicuous bony defect is observed around the maxillary right lateral incisor. (i and j) Fixed partial dentures have been delivered 5 months after extrusion.

Case 3-5 Treatment of vertical bony defects by regenerative therapy and restorative tooth movement

With the advancement of regenerative therapy, treatment of vertical bony defects takes on a different appearance today. The presence of multiple severe vertical bony defects is considered to indicate significant involvement of occlusal forces. Even if guided tissue regeneration (GTR) therapy is conducted in addition to procedures to control inflammation, sufficient tissue regeneration is less likely to be achieved in such a case. Control of occlusal force is essential to obtaining good results from regeneration therapy. Shown here is a clinical case in which the combination of therapeutic tooth movement and regenerative therapy produced a satisfactory outcome (Figs 3-48 to 3-57).

Patient: *54-year-old woman at the time of first visit in 1997*

Chief complaint: *Mobility of the maxillary right second and third molars and mandibular left first and second premolars, swelling of the gingiva on the lingual aspect, and periodontal abscess. Severe periodontitis with some periodontal pockets up to 8 mm. Pockets at the maxillary right first and second molar, mandibular left canine, second premolar, and first molar, and mandibular right canine and first premolar were 8 mm. Soon after the first visit, the maxillary right second molar was extracted. At the first visit, the patient was also informed of the planned extraction of the mandibular right canine and first premolar.*

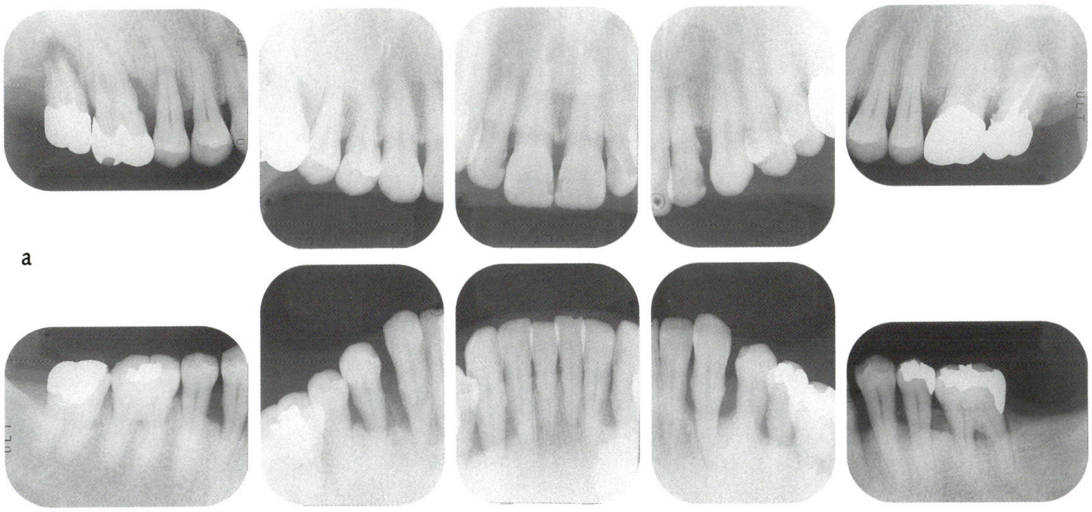

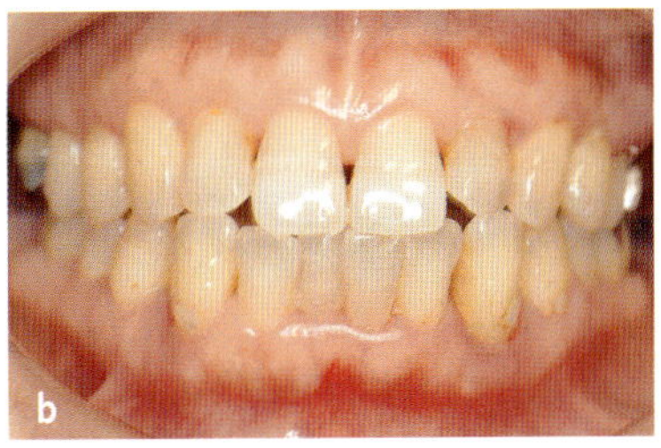

Fig 3-48 (a) Full-mouth radiographs taken at the first visit. Deep bony defects existed at the maxillary right first and second molars, mandibular left canine, second premolar, and first molar, and mandibular right canine and first premolar. (b) The vertical overlap is shallow, and the tongue is in a low position, contributing to occlusal trauma in the molars.

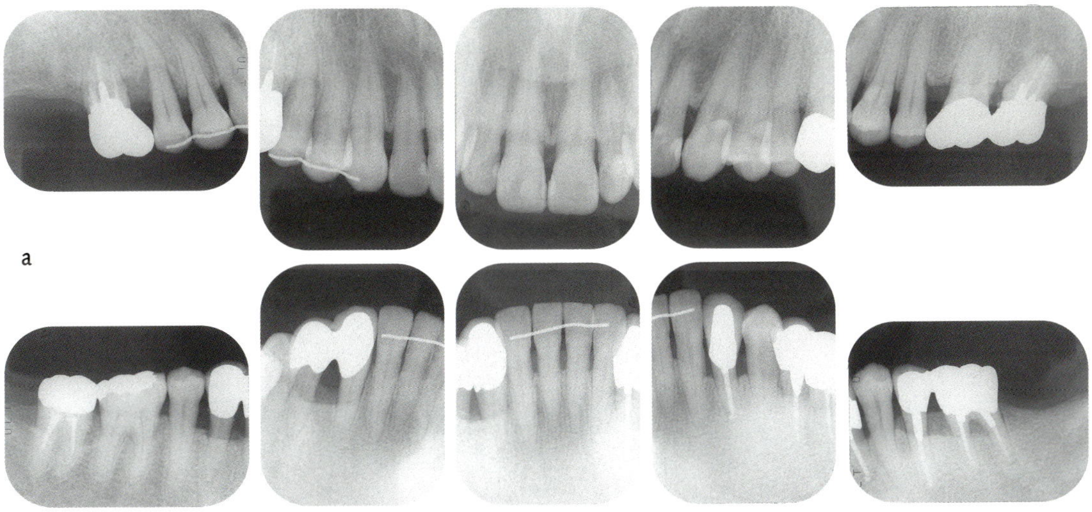

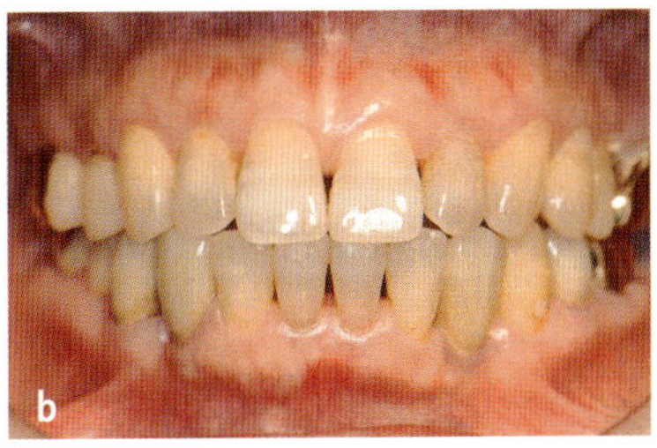

Fig 3-49 (a) Full-mouth radiographs taken 2 years 6 months after the first visit. The goal was natural extrusion of the maxillary right first molar, maxillary left second molar, mandibular left canine, and mandibular left first molar; this was followed by orthodontic extrusion of the mandibular left canine, right canine, and right first premolar. The maxillary right first molar, left first molar, and left second molar, tooth axes were uprighted. Endodontic treatment was conducted for the maxillary right first molar; mandibular left canine, second premolar, and first molar; and mandibular right second molar. (b) Crown restorations have been completed for the maxillary right first molar; maxillary left first molar and second molar; mandibular left canine, second premolar, and first molar; and the mandibular right canine, first premolar, and second molar.

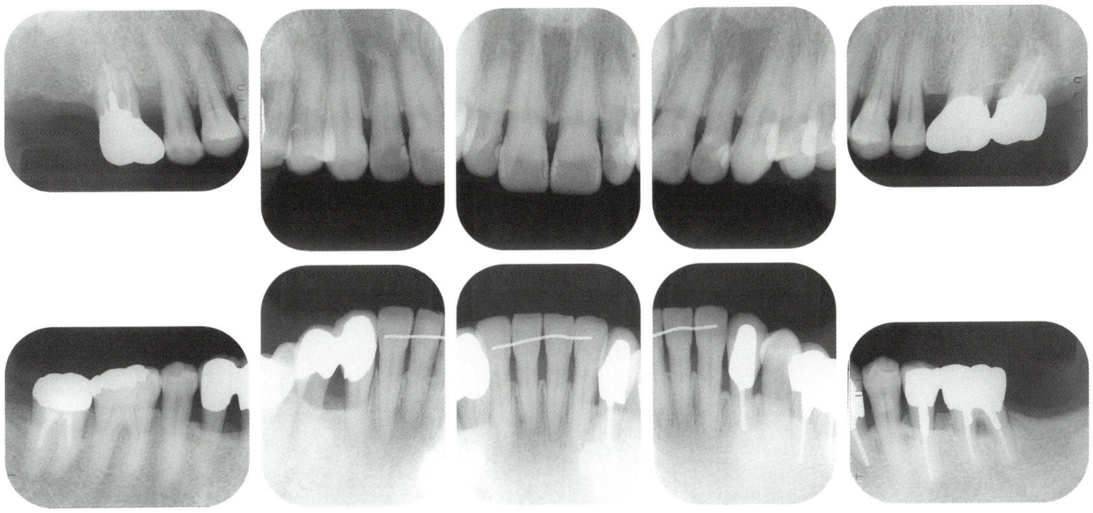

Fig 3-50 Full-mouth radiographs taken 6 years 1 month after the first visit. Periodontal probing depths are maintained at 2 to 3 mm.

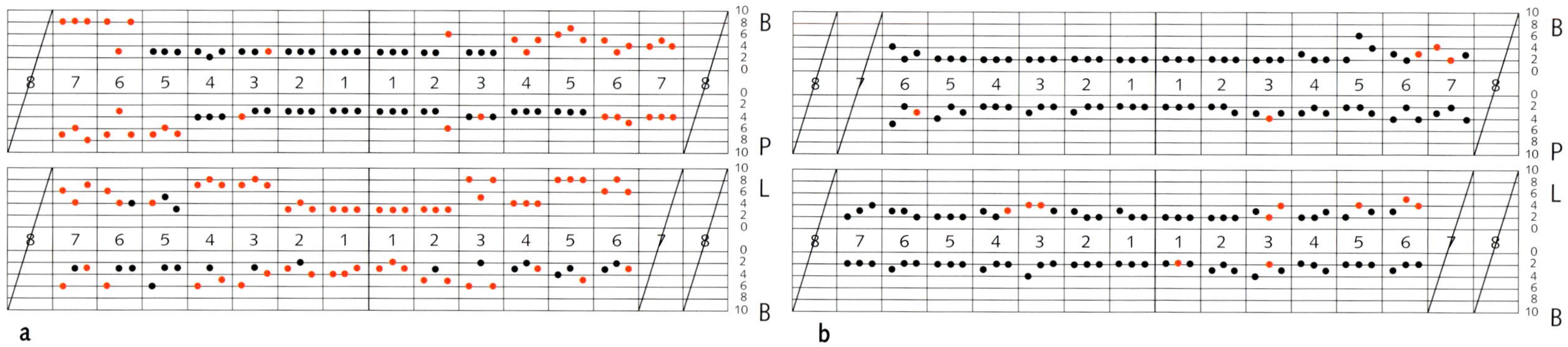

Fig 3-51 (a) Probing chart at the first visit. Red dots indicate bleeding points. (b) Probing chart 10 months after the first visit (August 1996).

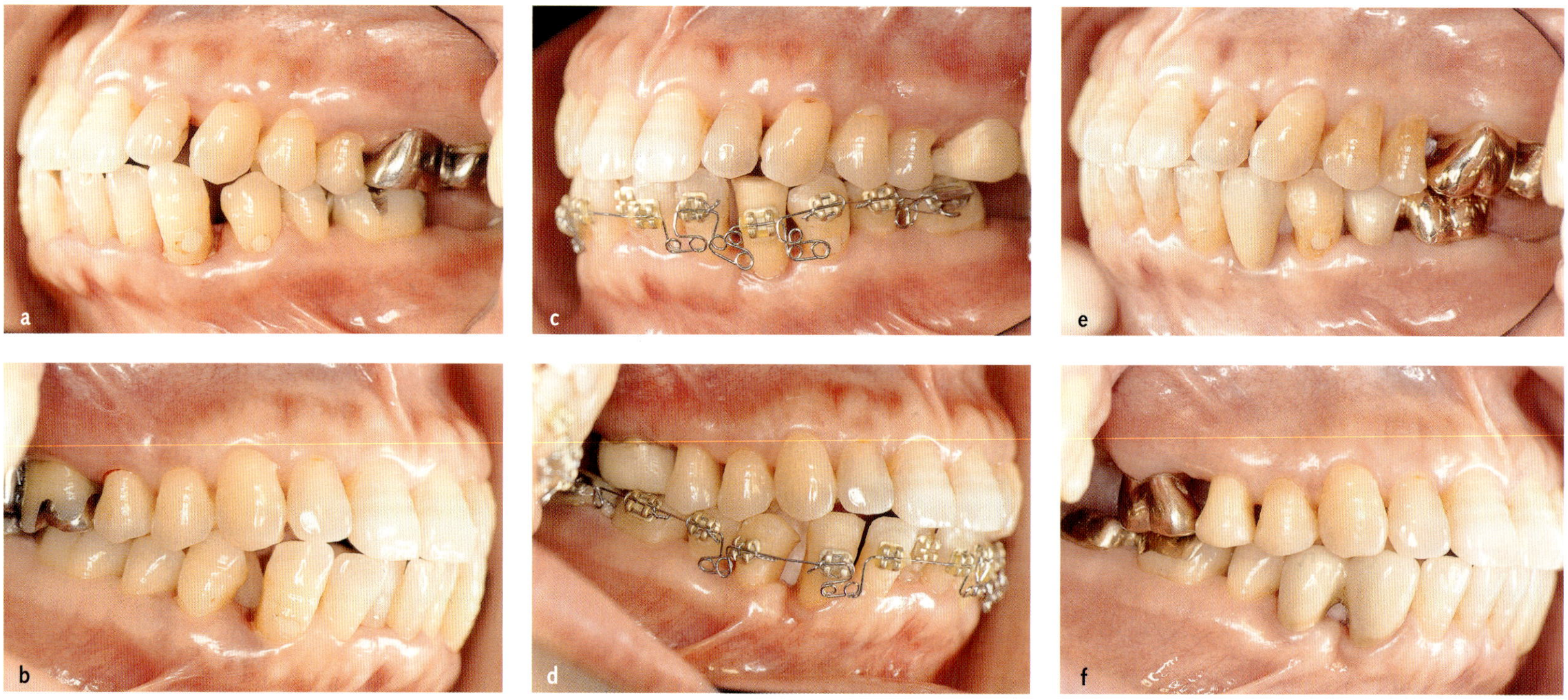

Fig 3-52 Lateral views of treatment progress. (a and b) At the first visit. Mobility of the mandibular left premolars and swelling of the lingual gingiva were noted. (c and d) About 1 year after the first visit. Flap access was completed for the maxillary right premolars and first molar 3 months after the first visit, and for the mandibular right lateral incisor, canine, first premolar, and first molar at 4 months. Full-thickness flaps were raised for the mandibular left lateral incisor, canine, premolars, and first molar, and autogenous bone grafting and GTR treatment were conducted with a resorbable membrane. After natural extrusion of the maxillary right first molar, maxillary left second molar, mandibular right canine, and mandibular right second molar was completed, orthodontic extrusion of the mandibular left canine, right canine, and right first premolar was initiated. (e and f) Photographs taken 1 year 4 months after the first visit. A full-thickness flap was raised again for the mandibular left canine, premolars, and first molar. After bone grafting (harvested from exostosis at the mandibular left first premolar), GTR procedures were performed with a resorbable membrane. Similar treatment was conducted for the maxillary left first premolar, second premolar, first molar, and second molar 1 year 7 months after the first visit. Crown restorations were delivered for the maxillary right first molar, maxillary left first and second molars, mandibular left canine, second premolar, and first molar, and mandibular right canine and first premolar, 2 years and 5 months after the first visit.

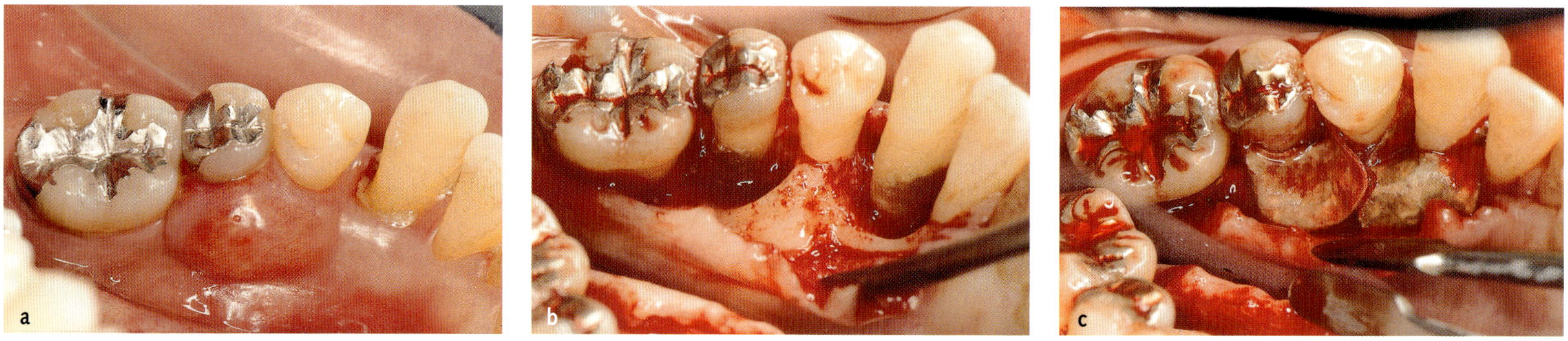

Fig 3-53 Treatment of the mandibular left lateral incisor, canine, premolars, and first molar. (a) Alveolar abscess at the first visit. (b) Status after 3 months. (c) Debridement to remove granulation tissue, followed by autogenous transplantation of a graft harvested from the thick lingual bone and GTR with a resorbable membrane.

Fig 3-53 (cont) (d) The wound is tightly closed. Crowns were recontoured 2 months after treatment, with the expectation that natural extrusion would follow. (e) Photograph taken at the time of second surgery, 1 year after treatment, 4 months after the start of orthodontic extrusion. (f) Because of poor plaque control, calculus accumulated on the mandibular left premolars. Flap access was completed again, along with regeneration therapy. (g) Crown restorations have been completed for the mandibular left canine, second premolar, and first molar, 2 years 4 months after the first visit (10 months after restoration). The periodontal environment is stable.

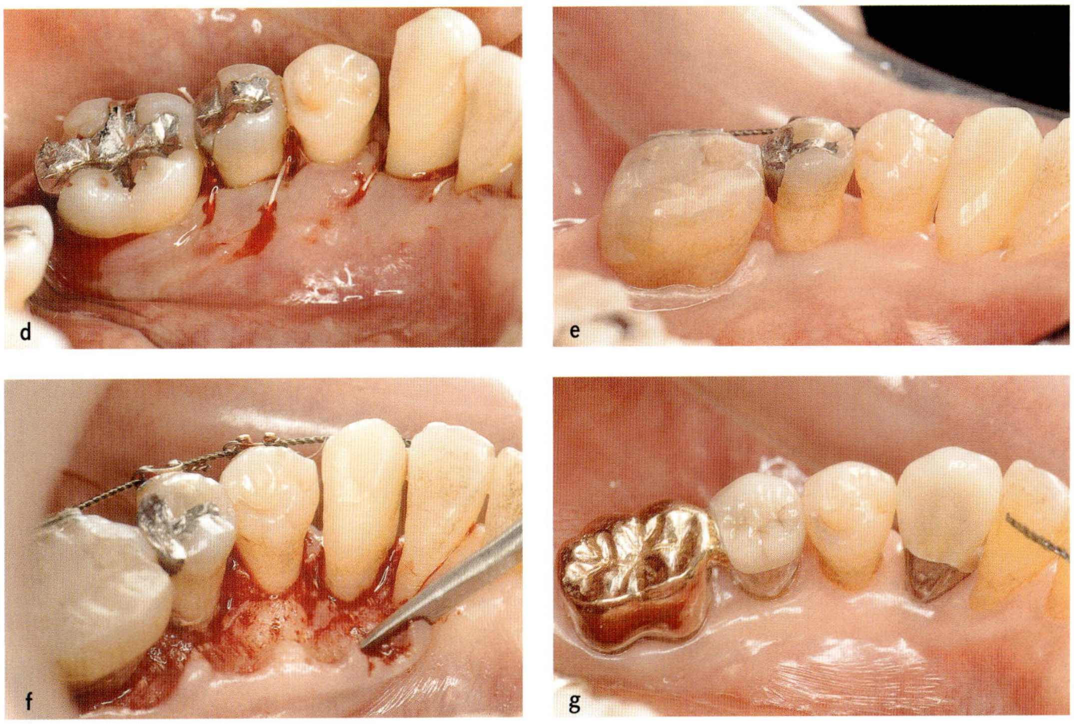

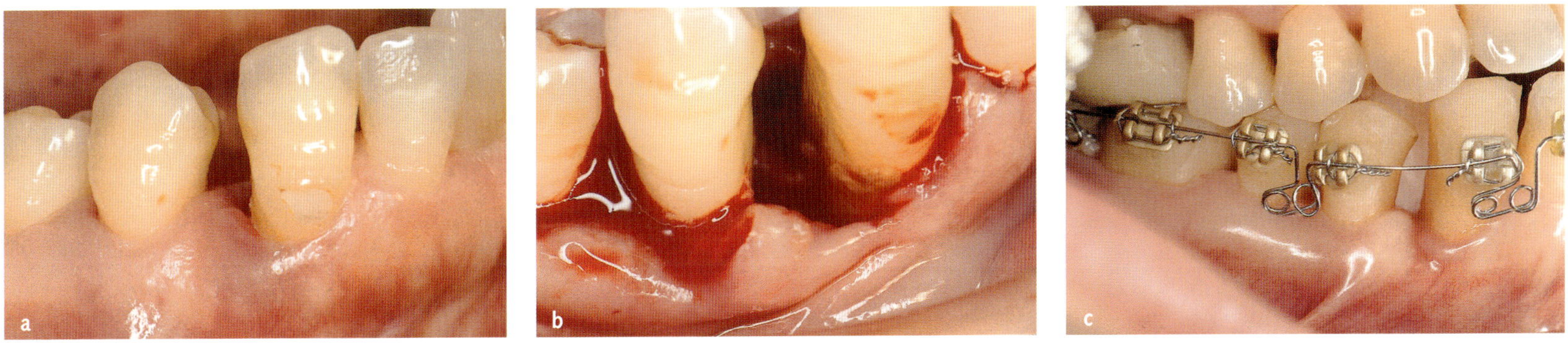

Fig 3-54 Treatment of the buccal aspect of the mandibular right lateral incisor, canine, and premolars. (a) Appearance 3 months after the first visit. The probing depth between the canine and first premolar is 8 mm. (b) A deep bony defect exists between the canine and first premolar. Root surfaces are treated with a saturated solution of tetracycline. (c) Photograph taken 8 months after the first visit. Bracket height was determined based on the pocket depth to start extrusion. Maintained as vital teeth, the canine and first premolar underwent enameloplasty. The tooth movement period was 6 months.

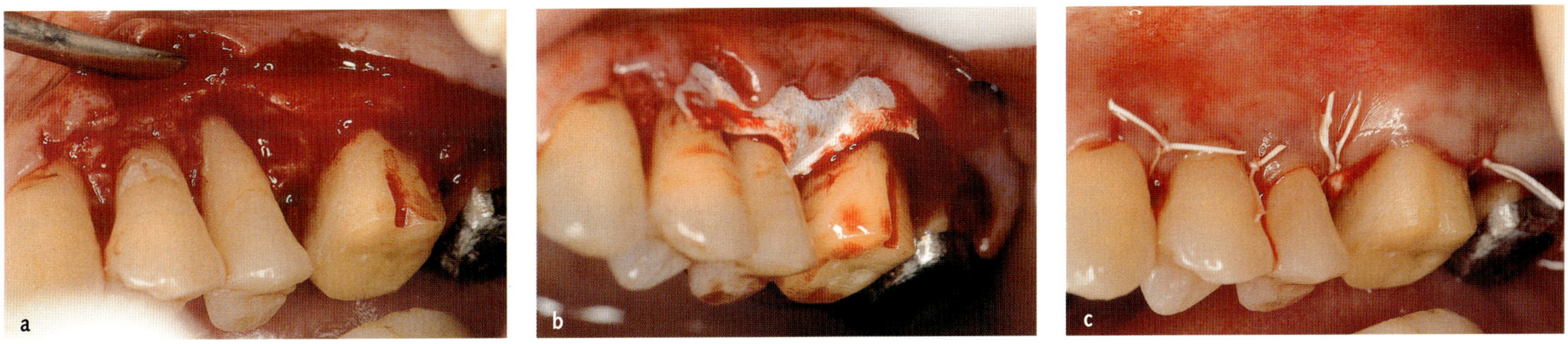

Fig 3-55 Guided tissue regeneration procedure on the buccal side of the maxillary left first premolar. (a and b) Photographs taken 1 year 7 months after the first visit. A full-thickness flap was raised for the maxillary left premolars and first and second molars. (c) GTR was conducted after bone grafting.

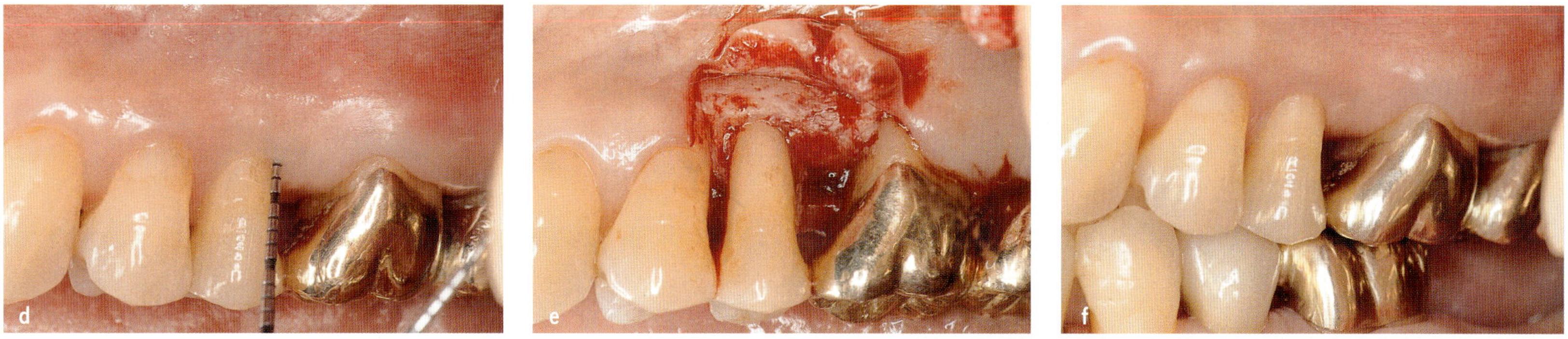

Fig 3-55 (cont) (d) Photograph taken 1 year 10 months after treatment, 1 year after crown restorations were placed. (e) At reentry, bone regeneration was confirmed. (f) Photograph taken 4 years 1 month after the first visit. The interdental space between the maxillary left second premolar and first molar had expanded.

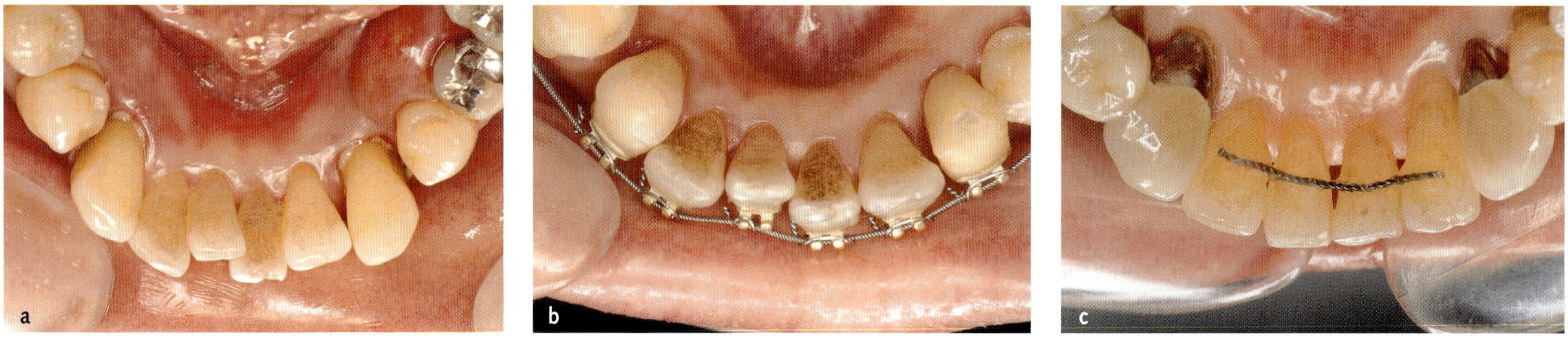

Fig 3-56 Correction of crowding in the mandibular anterior teeth. (a) At the first visit, significant inflammation and degree 2 mobility were noted. (b) Photograph taken after about 1 year. Correction of crowding and extrusion of the mandibular left canine and right canine and first premolar is taking place. (c) The periodontal environment is healthy, 3 years 2 months after the first visit.

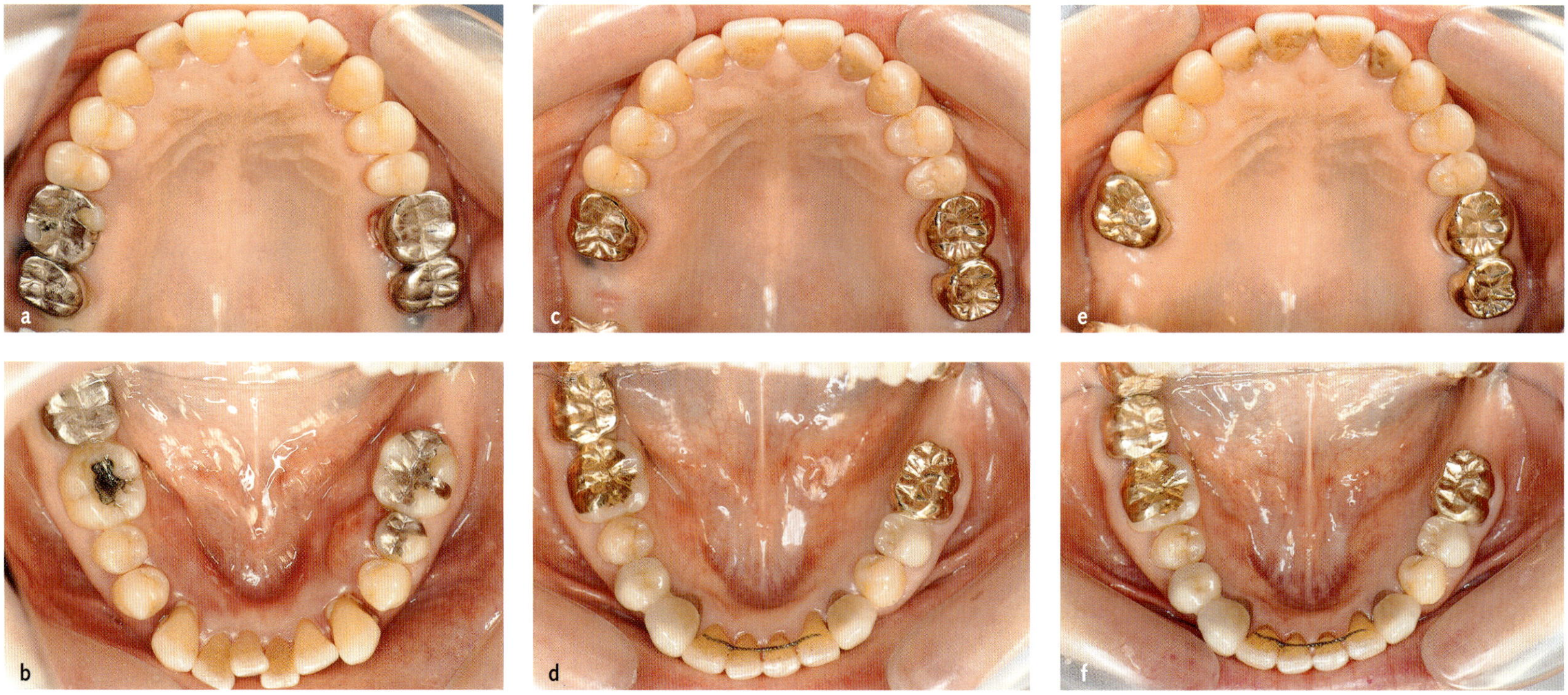

Fig 3-57 Occlusal views of the changes in the arches. (a and b) Photographs taken at the first visit. (c and d) Photographs taken 2 years 7 months after the first visit. (e and f) Photographs taken 4 years 1 month after the first visit. Arch form is improved.

Tooth Movement in the Presence of Occlusal Collapse

Appropriate tooth positions and splinting

In patients with reduced periodontal support and advanced occlusal collapse, full-arch splinting is often applied. Although splinting is a means to restrict tooth mobility and to prevent secondary occlusal trauma, it is merely an auxiliary device for stabilization. Full-arch splinting truly does restrict tooth mobility. Thus, if teeth are splinted in a position different from their physiologic position, the splint may be detrimental to the occlusion. The first consideration should be the development or maintenance of the appropriate occlusal-unit position and the stabilization of the dentition; then the stabilization of the individual tooth becomes possible. The appropriate position of a tooth continues to change minimally, constantly repeating remodeling, to maintain stability. Therefore, even if periodontal support is lost, tooth movement is conducted first to redistribute forces properly, giving priority to preparation of conditions for an individual tooth to be stabilized. Splints are used after such conditions are adjusted. In patients whose occlusal forces are relatively light, splinting should be avoided if possible.

Management of a spaced arch

A spaced arch may arise from a variety of causes. When a dentition has interdental spaces and is in the process of occlusal collapse, control of inflammation and trauma will allow the teeth to return to their original positions in the dentition, restoring the continuity of the physiologic dentition. A spaced arch can develop during the process of occlusal collapse:

- Decreased vertical dimension of occlusion in the posterior region can result in interdental spacing in the anterior region.
- Occlusal interference can lead to single-sided chewing, which allows flaring out of the maxillary arch and interdental spacing around the maxillary canines.
- Tongue habits can result in an unstable occlusion, a habit of anterior chewing, and subsequent interdental spacing in the anterior region.

Because a space in the dental arch may have many different origins, it should not be closed without careful consideration of the situation. When a spaced arch is involved in an occlusal collapse and is accompanied by muscular dysfunction, it may not be possible to improve the condition, even when the causes are clear. To simply close the space may invite trauma in such a case. Before tooth movement is initiated, it is necessary to ascertain the stability of the teeth as well as the occlusion, including functional movements, circumoral muscles, periodontal tissues, and possible discrepancies of the jaws and teeth.

It is not easy to arrest the destruction during the process of occlusal collapse and to restore long-term stability (Cases 3-6 and 3-7). It takes diligent maintenance efforts by the patient and health care professionals, and a clinician who does not overlook subtle changes, to allow the stomatognathic system to continue to function with or without restorations.

Case 3-6 Force redistribution by occlusal reconstruction and long-term follow-up

Patient: *41-year-old woman at the time of first visit in October 1984*
Chief complaint: *Occlusal pain, bleeding, and purulent discharge from the gingiva*
Treatment for a patient with occlusal collapse accompanied by pathologic tooth malpositioning is shown in Figs 3-58 to 3-70. In conjunction with inflammation control by initial therapy, myofunctional therapy (improvement of tongue movement patterns and strengthening of the tongue muscle and lip force) was started. Subsequently, orthodontic appliances were used to correct the pathologic tooth movement. This restorative tooth movement was conducted as an aid to bring pathologically displaced teeth back to their original positions. Pathologically displaced teeth can be moved back to their original position through circumoral muscle control by myofunctional therapy and occlusal equilibration. However, severe pathologic tooth movement, as was seen in this case, exceeds the level that can be restored by such natural approaches. Such severe malpositioning, if left untreated, would invite rapid tissue destruction by secondary occlusal trauma. For this reason, orthodontic appliances were utilized in this clinical case.

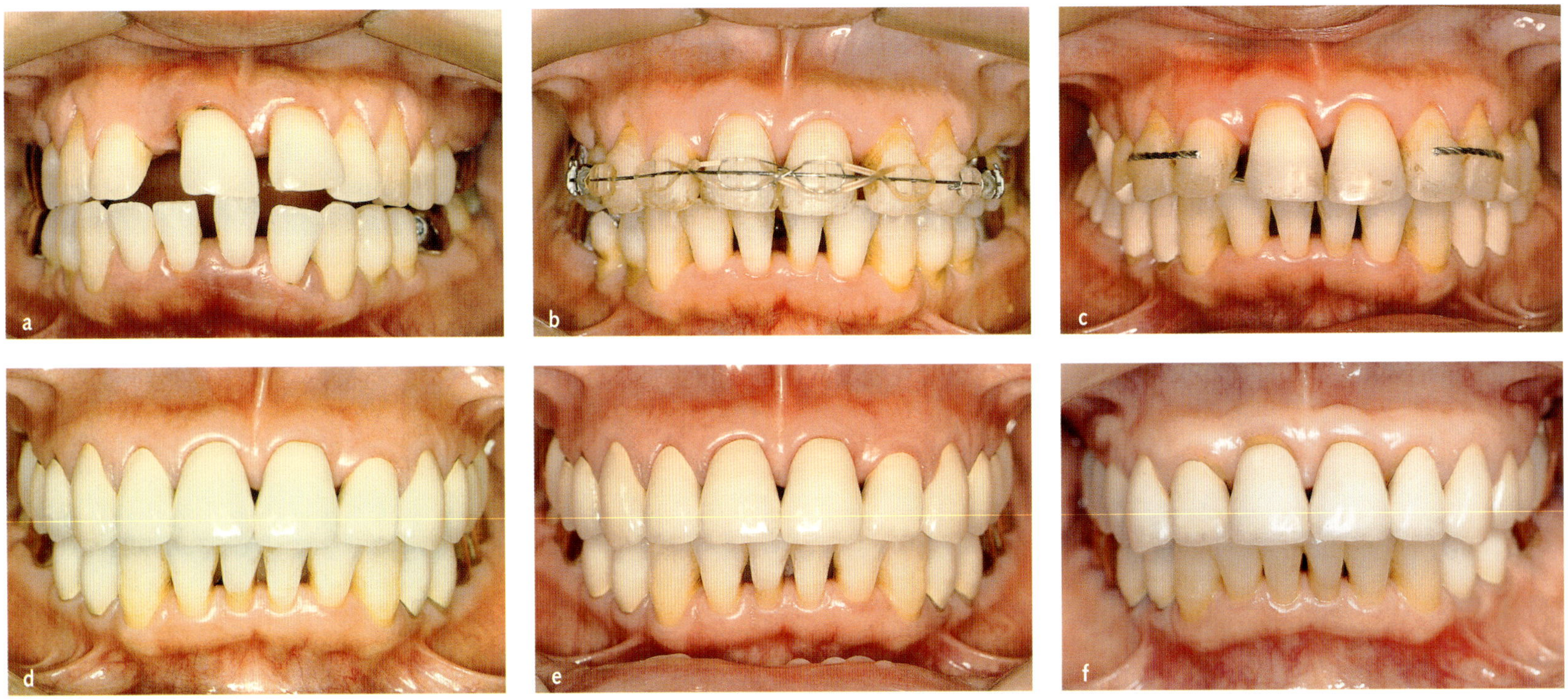

Fig 3-58 Pathologic tooth movement and occlusal reconstruction. (a) The combination of severe periodontitis (adult periodontitis) and traumatic lesions has caused pathologic tooth movement, inviting a full-mouth collapse of the patient's occlusion. The patient has difficulty closing her lips. She also has a tongue thrusting habit (October 1984). (b) After the initial therapy, orthodontic treatment is conducted to close the interdental spaces in the maxillary anterior region. Because of the advanced periodontitis in the molar region, a lingual arch is used for reinforcement, with the right and left first premolars used as anchorage. The six maxillary anterior teeth are bonded. Because cementum has been exposed for some time, no intrusion is conducted, but tipping movements are applied (December 1985). In the mandibular arch, extruded teeth are treated with enameloplasty, and no orthodontic treatment is conducted. Myofunctional therapy alone is used, and continuity is gradually and naturally restored to the dentition. (c) Photograph taken after 4 months of active treatment and 3 months of retention (May 1986). A bonded retainer wire is placed on the labial and lingual sides for the central and lateral incisors. Myofunctional therapy has eliminated the tongue thrusting habit, but the low position of the tongue is not completely controlled. Buccolingual positioning of the dentition is decided only with myofunctional therapy. Tooth movement has been limited to a mesiodistal direction. (d) About 2 years after the first visit. Periodontal prostheses are completed (October 1986). (e) Photograph taken 4 years 7 months after the delivery of final prostheses (May 1991). (f) Photograph taken about 13 years after the first visit (October 1999).

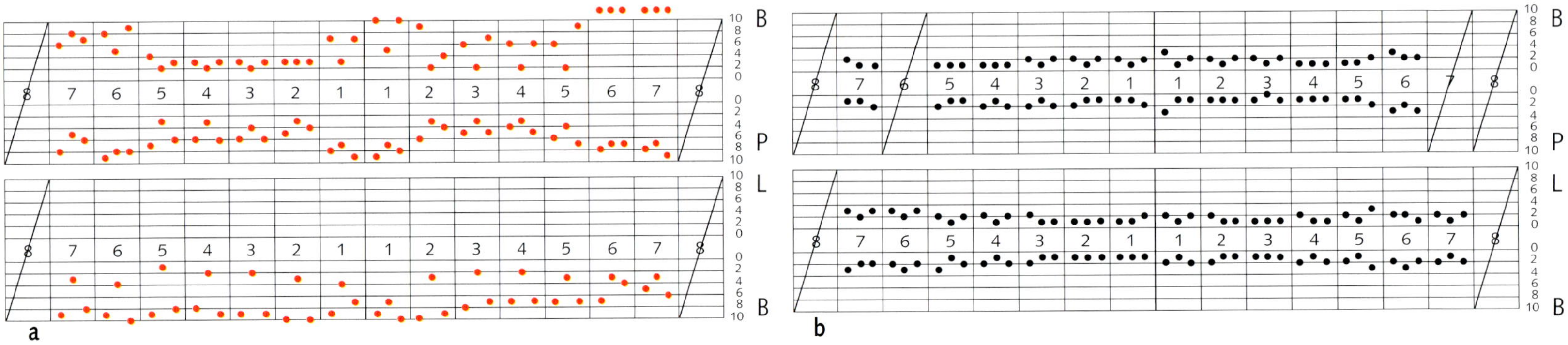

Fig 3-59 (a) Periodontal probing depths at the first visit (12 mm at deepest). There is a degree 2 to 3 tooth mobility. (b) Probing depths in 1986.

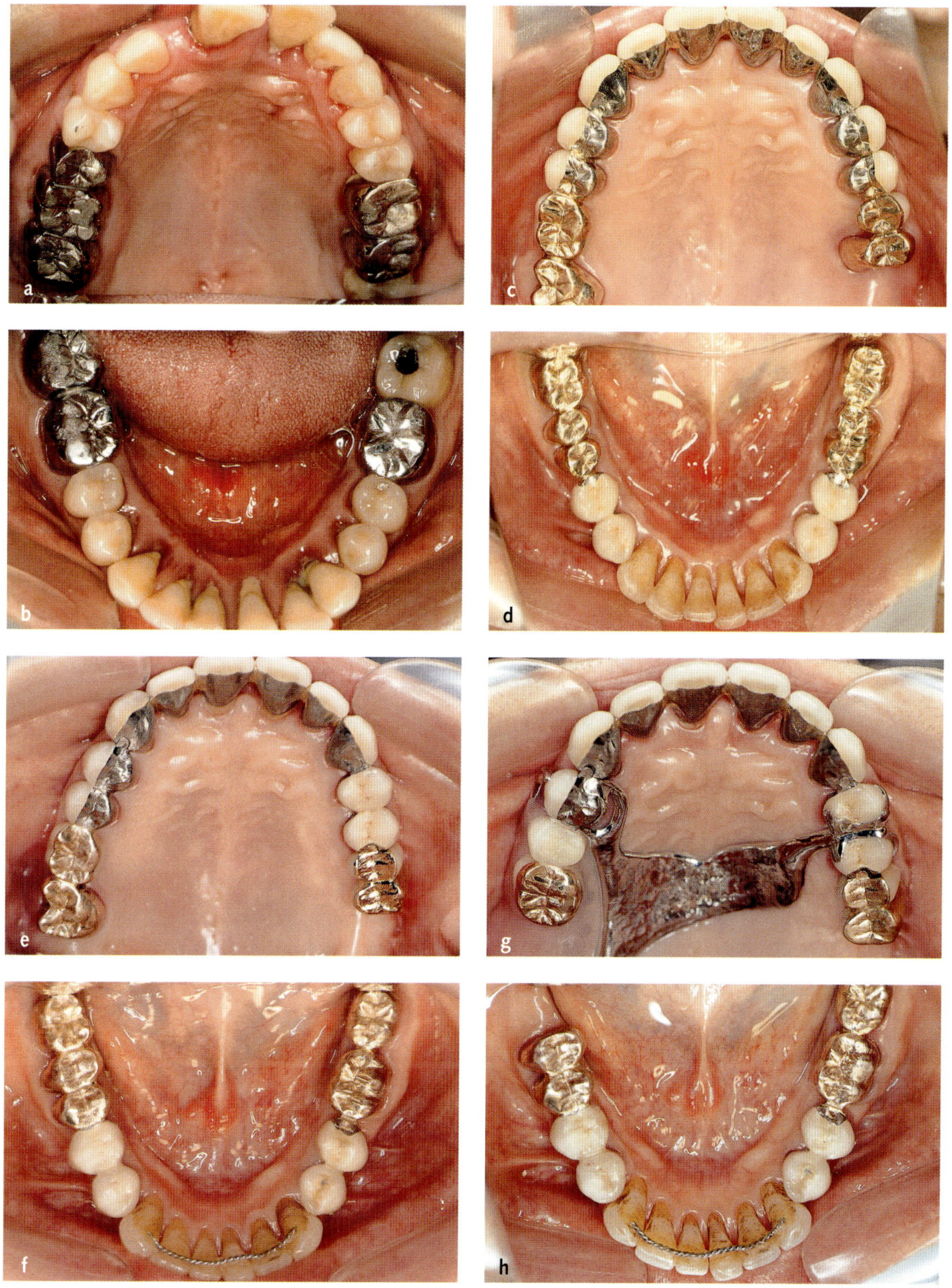

Fig 3-60 Establishment of posterior occlusal support and reduction of anterior flaring. (a and b) At the first visit, severe periodontitis is noted, including remarkable mobility of the teeth and pathologic movement. The anterior teeth are flared, making it difficult for the patient to close her lips (October 1984). (c and d) The completion of periodontal prostheses (October 1986). (e and f) Photographs taken about 13 years after delivery of final prostheses (October 1999). (g and h) Photographs taken about 15 years after delivery of final prostheses and about 17 years after the first visit (August 2002). The mandibular right second molar was lost due to root caries and the maxillary right second premolar and first molar were extracted due to periodontal disease. An I-bar–type removable denture was delivered to replace the maxillary right second premolar and first molar.

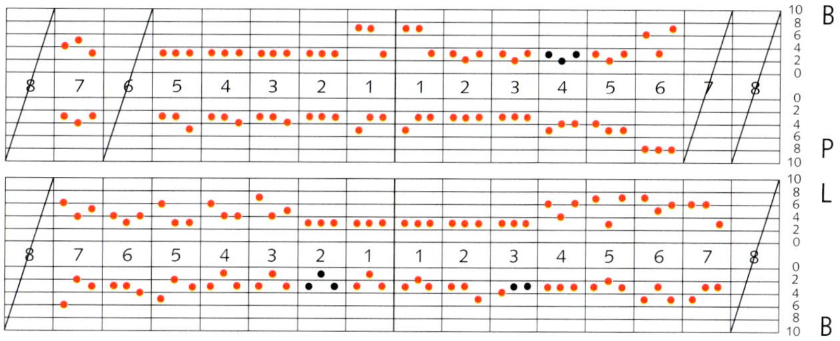

Fig 3-61 In the long-term follow-up period, there were times when the patient discontinued maintenance or showed insufficient plaque control. The probing depths recorded 11 years after the first visit are shown (1995).

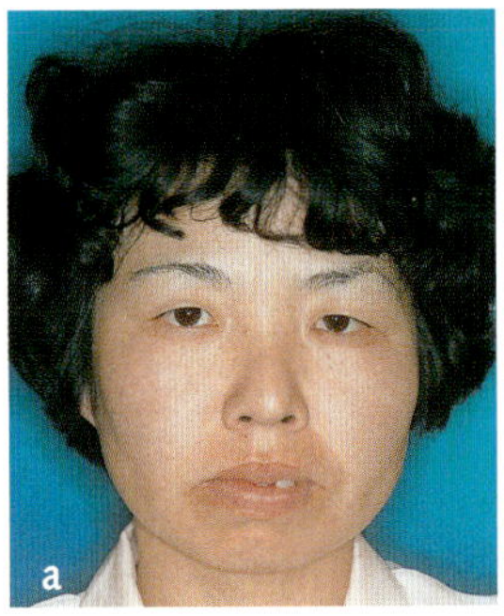

b

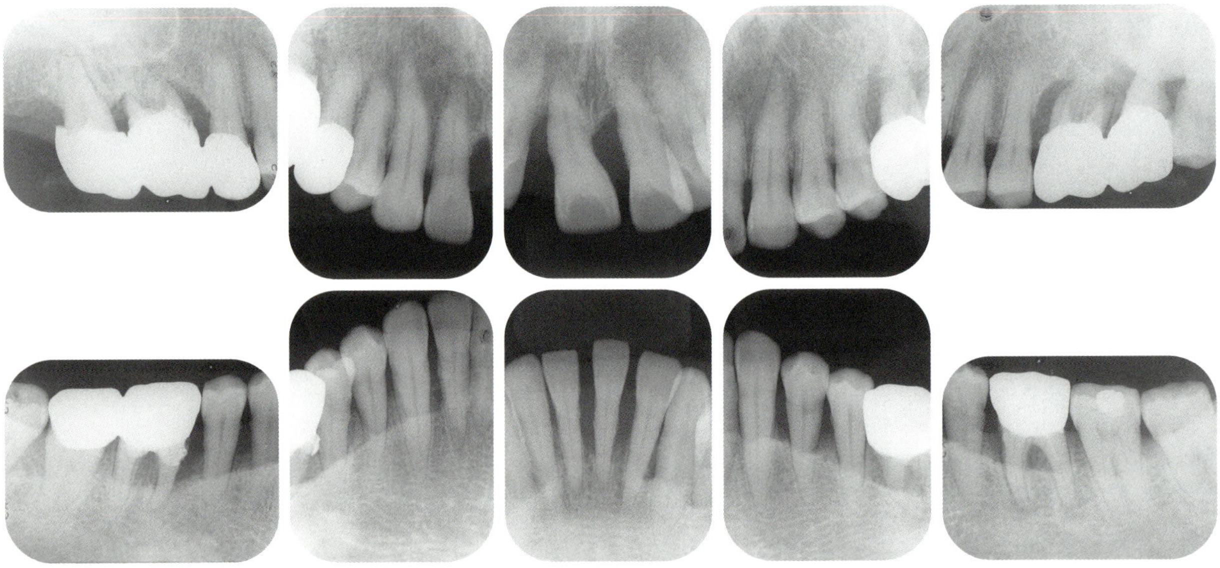

Fig 3-62 (a) Photograph taken at the first visit. (b) Radiographs at the first visit. Conspicuous loss of supporting bone is noted. Molars have been exposed to conspicuous occlusal trauma. This is a case with severe periodontitis where inflammation and traumatic lesions are combined. Class II furcation involvement is observed in the maxillary right first and second molars, mandibular left first and second molars, and mandibular right second molar, and class III involvement is observed in the maxillary left first and second molars and mandibular right first molar (October 1984).

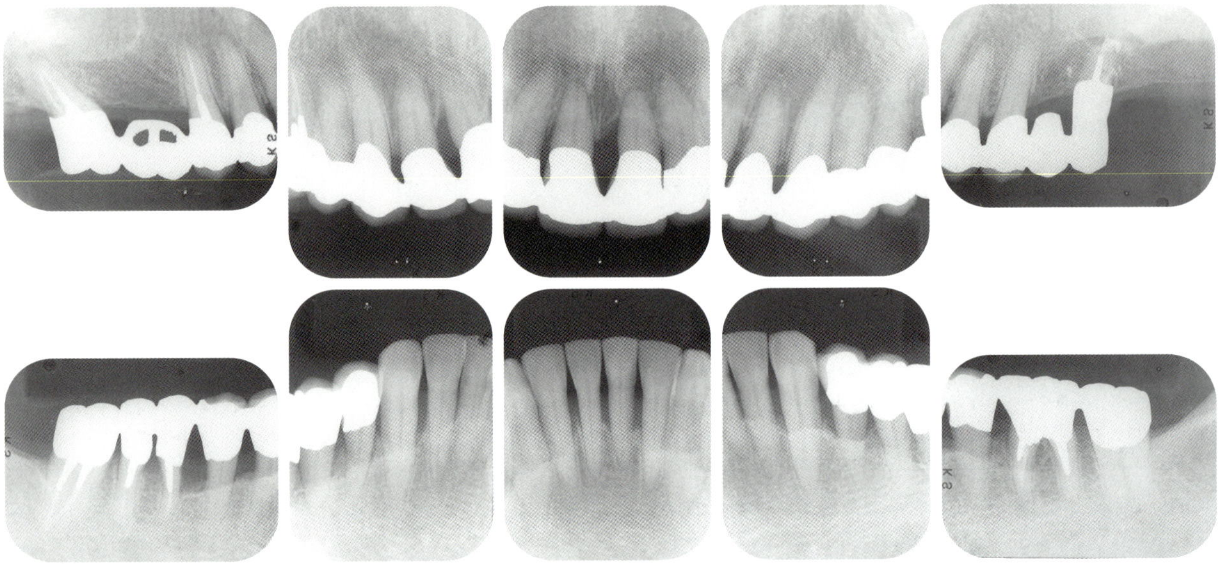

Fig 3-63 Completion of periodontal prostheses. Although the maxillary right first molar and left second molar had to be extracted, efforts were made to maintain other teeth as much as possible. To treat the class II furcation involvement at the maxillary right second molar, apical repositioning and crown fluting were conducted. Because of the deep pocket, the maxillary left first molar underwent mesiobuccal root amputation 12 months after the first visit. A hemisection was conducted for the mandibular right first molar (October 1986).

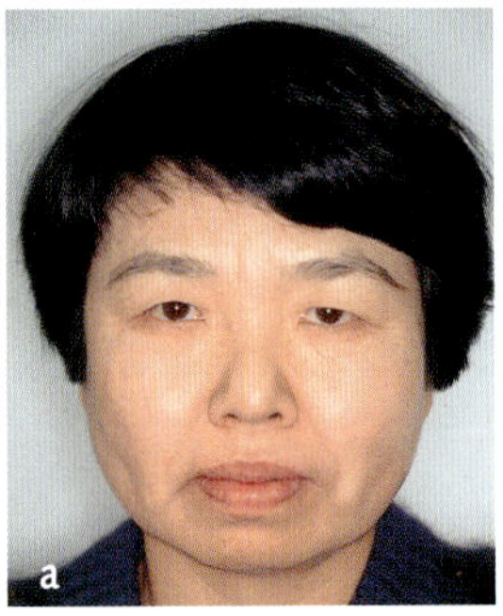

b

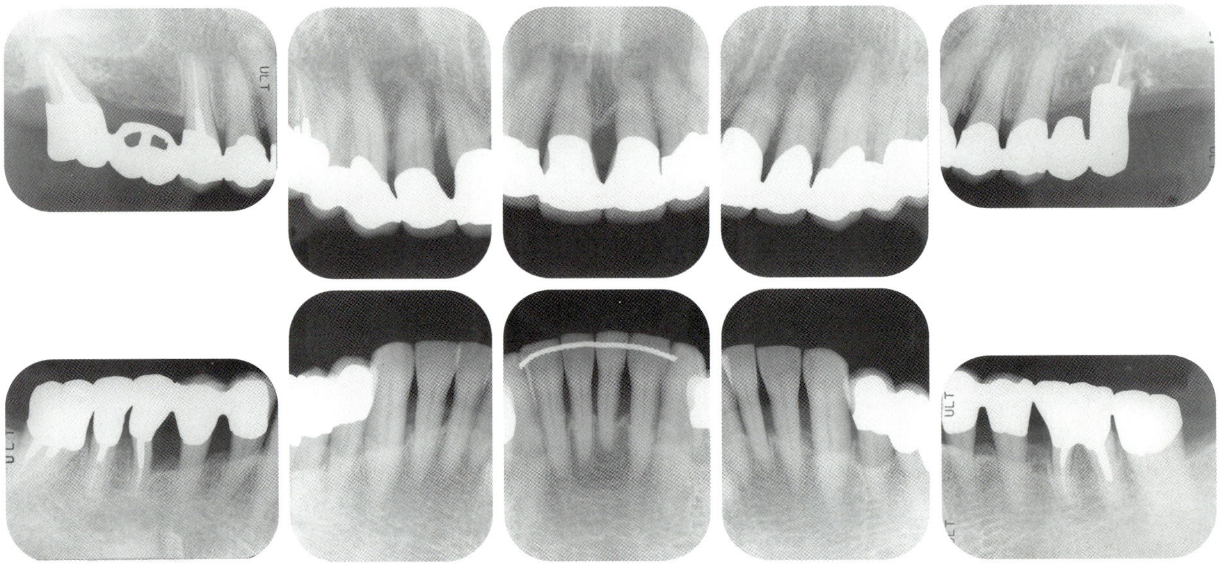

Fig 3-64 (a) Facial photograph taken at the end of 1995. (b) Radiographs taken 9 years after the first visit (May 1993).

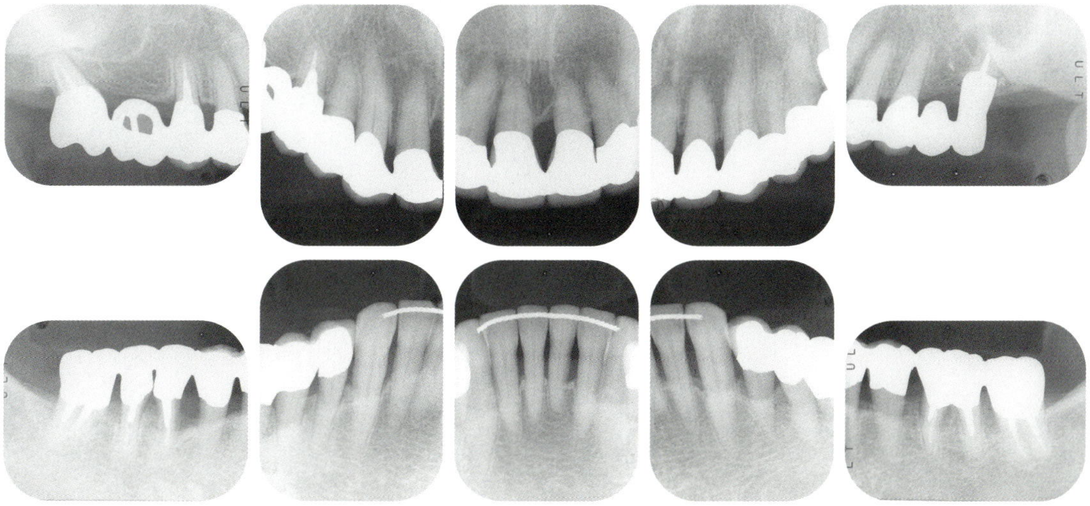

Fig 3-65 Radiographs taken 13 years after the first visit. With widening of the periodontal space of the maxillary right second molar, and problems with the maxillary left first molar and other teeth, it is difficult to determine when to make an intervention.

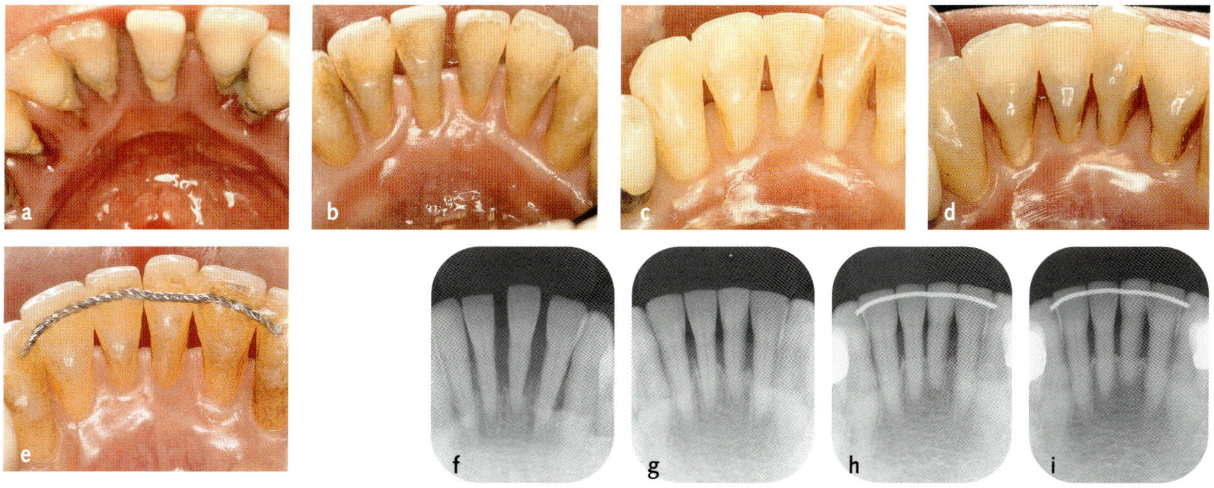

Fig 3-66 Mandibular anterior teeth. (a) The first visit reveals interdental spaces resulting from the tongue thrusting habit and pathologic tooth movement as well as inflammation (October 1984). (b) Photograph taken after 1 year 2 months. Orthodontic appliances have not been used to close the spaces in the mandibular arch. Natural recovery is expected from improvement in the maxillary arch, myofunctional therapy, and enameloplasty. (c) Completion of the final prostheses, 2 years after the first visit. Inflammation is reduced, and the continuity of the dentition is restored. (d) Photograph taken 8 years 7 months after the first visit. (e) Photograph taken 15 years 3 months after the first visit. (f) Radiograph taken at the first visit. (g) Completion of final prostheses, 2 years after the first visit. (h) Radiograph taken 10 years 9 months after the first visit. (i) Radiograph taken 17 years 8 months after the first visit.

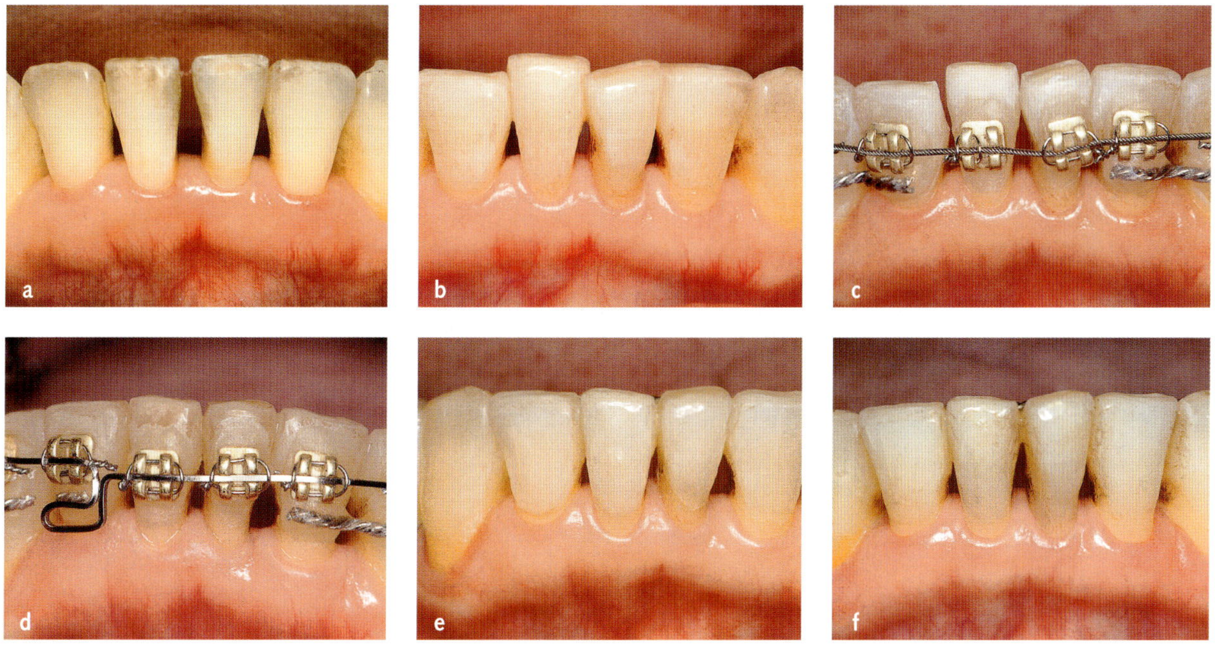

Fig 3-67 Mandibular anterior tooth movement. (a) Photograph taken at the completion of initial therapy, after 1 year 2 months. (b) Photograph taken 10 years 2 months after the first visit. (c) Photograph taken 10 years 3 months after the first visit. Because crowding had developed, orthodontic appliances have been delivered to the mandibular arch. (d) Photograph taken 10 years 6 months after the first visit. (e) Completion of active treatment (May 1995). (f) Photograph taken 17 years 8 months after the first visit.

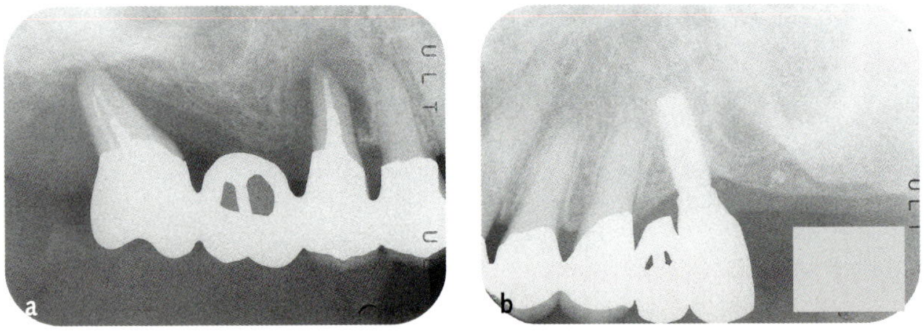

Fig 3-68 Treatment progress of the maxillary molars. (a) Radiograph taken 17 years 1 month after the first visit. Because of the advanced periodontitis accompanied by trauma, the maxillary right second premolar and second molar have been extracted (November 2001). (b) The distal root of the maxillary right first molar, which used to support the occlusion in the left segment, was extracted, and a dental implant has been placed (September 1999).

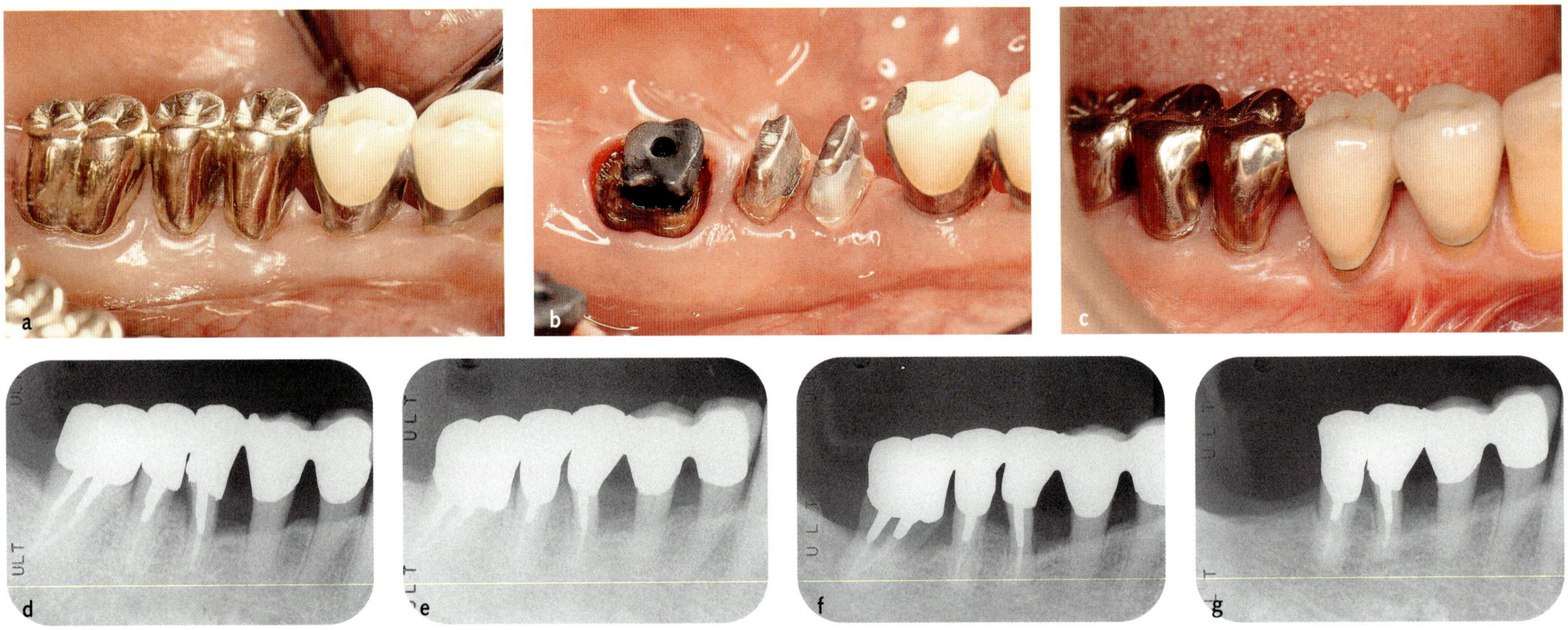

Fig 3-69 Treatment progress of the mandibular right molars. (a) Photograph taken at the time of delivery of the final prosthesis (mirror view, October 1986). (b) Crowns have been refabricated because of secondary caries in the mandibular right second molar (mirror view, July 1993). (c) Delivery of the newly fabricated restoration (April 1994). (d) Secondary caries in the mandibular right second molar (July 1993). (e) Refabricated crowns are delivered after elimination of dental caries (December 1993). (f) Secondary caries has occurred again (November 2001). (g) The mandibular right second molar has finally been extracted (August 2002).

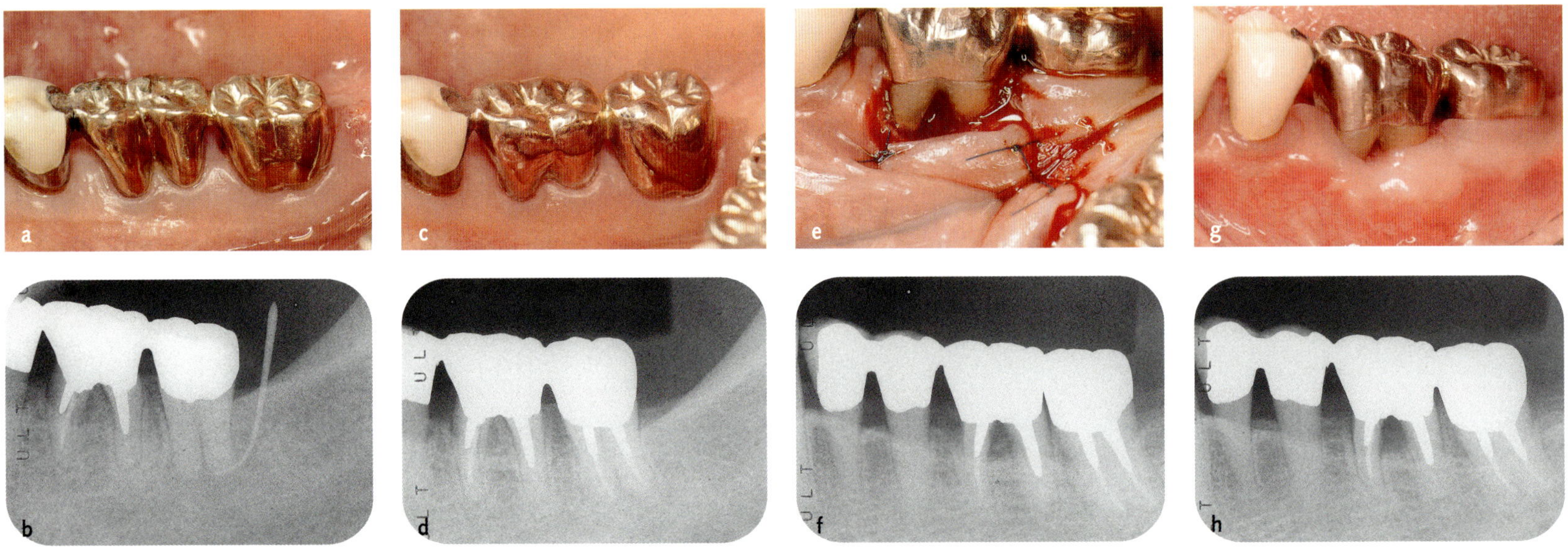

Fig 3-70 Treatment progress of the mandibular left molars. (a) Photograph and (b) radiograph taken 7 years 3 months after the first visit. A fistula was found distal to the mandibular right second molar (January 1994). (c and d) Refabricated crowns have been delivered after endodontic treatment of the infected root canals. (e and f) An apical repositioning flap is completed to treat the recurrence of a furcation involvement (March 1999). (g) Photograph and (h) radiograph taken 4 months after surgery.

Case 3-7 Minimal intervention in a dentition on the brink of occlusal collapse

Patient: *47-year-old woman at the time of first visit in 1995*

Chief complaint: *Mobility and occlusal pain affecting the maxillary right first and second molars, hypersensitivity affecting the right and left molars, and TMD symptoms, including shoulder stiffness and headache*

Facial observation revealed a brachyfacial type with a well-developed masseter muscle, a raised right angle of the mouth, and a deep right nasolabial groove. The interarch distance was shorter on the right, and the right eye seemed smaller. On the other hand, the patient's head was tilted to the left, and her left shoulder was raised. This suggests clenching on the right side.

Oral examination showed there was no ability to release from the tight occlusion on the right posterior quadrants. Lingual axioversion of the maxillary right canine and slight lingual axioversion of the maxillary left canine were noted. In each of the four quadrants, the second molar was trapped in the occlusion.

The dental arches as a whole showed flattening in the right side of the arch and lingual axioversion of the tooth axes. The maxillary left central incisor was pushed outside of the arch, probably because of forces from the right. As a result, the right side exhibited a Class II occlusion and the left side exhibited a Class I occlusion. It was later confirmed during tooth movement that the patient had a habit of sleeping on her right side. Figures 3-71 to 3-83 show the successful treatment and maintenance of her occlusion.

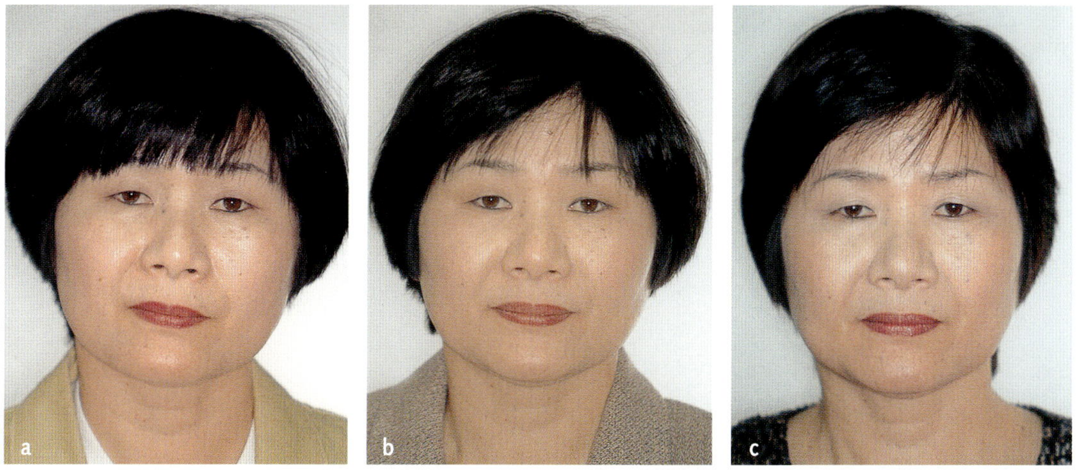

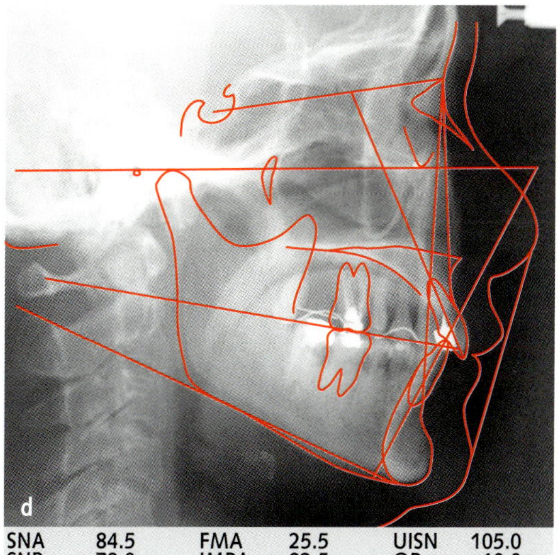

SNA	84.5	FMA	25.5	UISN	105.0
SNB	79.0	IMPA	92.5	OP	10.0
ANB	5.5	FMIA	62.0	II	129.0

Fig 3-71 Facial changes between the first visit and 2 years 10 months later. (a) Facial photograph taken at the first visit. (b) Photograph taken after 2 years 10 months (at completion of restorative tooth movement and restoration). Improvements are noted with regard to the head tilt to the left, the tilted lip line, and smaller interarch distance on the right, showing recovery of symmetry. (c) Photograph taken 7 years 3 months after the first visit. Some signs of relapse are observed. (d) Lateral cephalogram taken at the first visit.

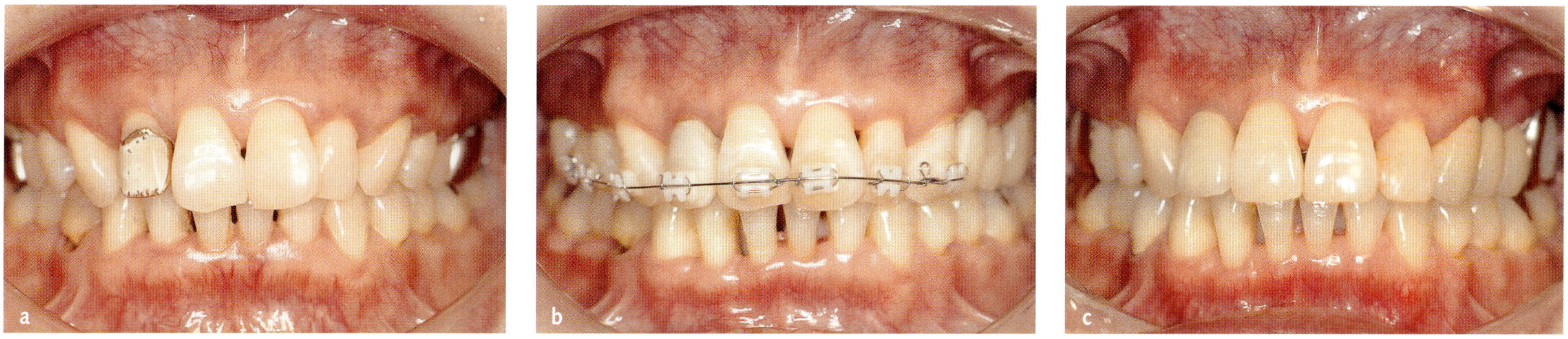

Fig 3-72 Restorative tooth movement in the maxillary arch. (a) At the first visit. Because this is a combined case of periodontal disease and trauma, control of inflammation is initiated before tooth movement. In the meantime, the maxillary right second molar, maxillary left first premolar, and maxillary left second molar were extracted and the maxillary right first molar was naturally extruded. Flap surgery was conducted for the six mandibular anterior teeth as well as the maxillary left second premolar, first molar, and third molar. Provisional restorations were delivered for the maxillary right second premolar, first molar, and third molar (including a pontic to replace the second molar) and the maxillary left canine, second premolar, first molar, and third molar (including pontics for the first premolar and first molar). (b) After morphologic correction of the maxillary central incisors, tooth movement is started, 8 months after the first visit. Brackets have been bonded. Correction of crowding of the maxillary right central incisor and left central and lateral incisors, improvement of rotation of the maxillary right first premolar, uprighting of the axis of the maxillary right canine, and rightward movement of the maxillary right central and lateral incisors and left central incisor are conducted. During tooth movement, arch deformation caused by habits was noted. The patient was instructed to abstain from sleeping on her right side and to chew on the left side. (c) Brackets have been debonded after 5 months of active treatment. Twisted wire is used for splinting the maxillary right central incisor and left central and lateral incisors from the lingual aspect.

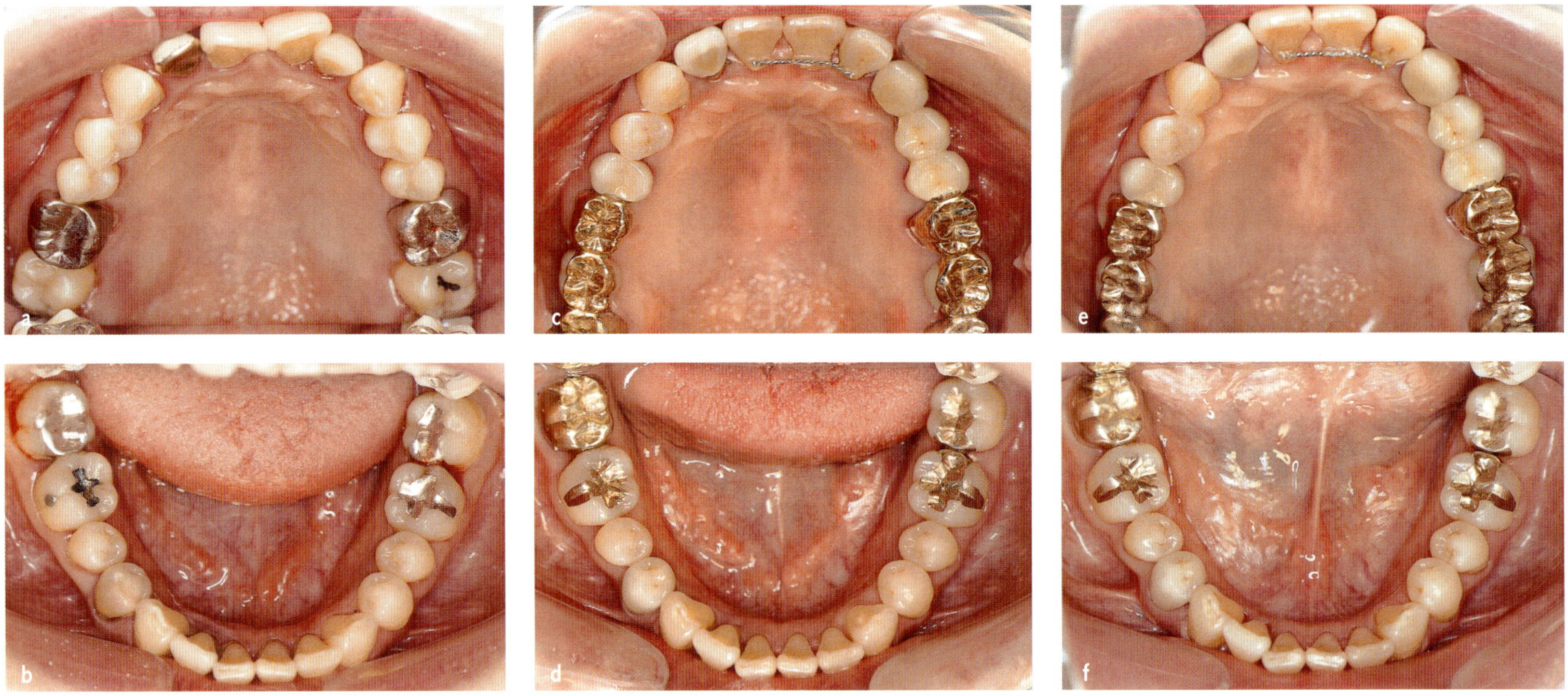

Fig 3-73 Improvement in the dental arches. (a and b) This patient is a brachyfacial type with strong masseter muscle and lips as well as a tight occlusion. When these factors are combined with inflammation, rapid destruction of supporting tissue may be invited. A brachyfacial-type patient is more likely to clench than is a dolichofacial-type patient, making it difficult to control forces. It is effective to provide an appropriate form of the arch and occlusal surfaces that will not induce clenching. (c and d) Although crowding in the mandibular arch at the right central incisor, lateral incisor, and canine has been naturally resolved here (April 1997), it would have been more predictable to use leveling for the mandibular arch as well and have bonding on the lingual aspect. (e and f) Relapse of crowding at the mandibular right central incisor, lateral incisor, and canine is observed. This seems to have been caused by the sleep habit (September 2002). The lingual axioversion of the maxillary right canine became pronounced again. Dental professionals would like dolichofacial-type patients to keep their mouths closed, but their mouths tend to be half open unless they are careful. On the other hand, ideally, brachyfacial-type patients would relax their mouths, but many of them tend to clench with tense lips. It is important to pay attention to a patient's habits during maintenance.

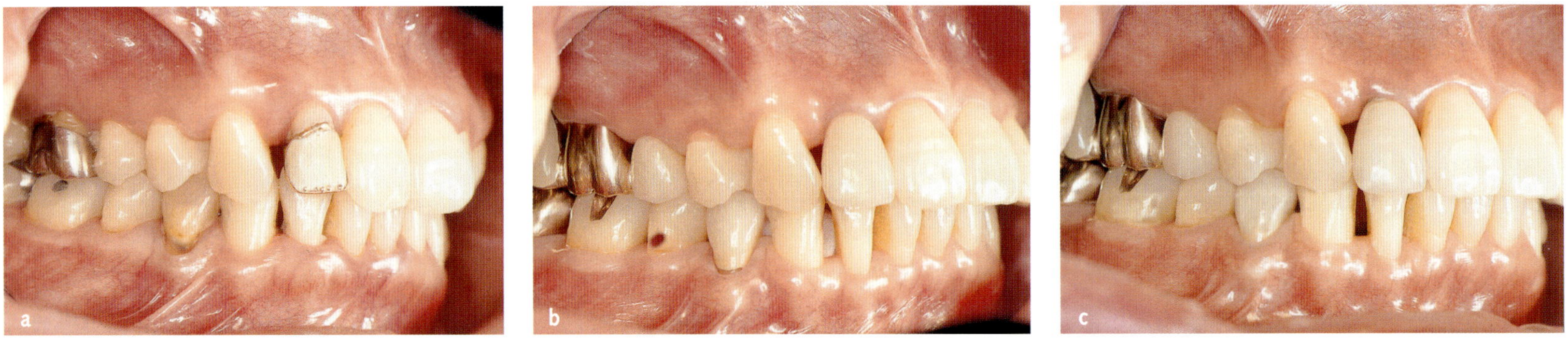

Fig 3-74 The right side. (a) A Class II relationship exists on the right. (b) Photograph taken after 2 years 2 months, 2 months after delivery of the final prosthesis. (c) Photograph taken 4 years 8 months after the first visit.

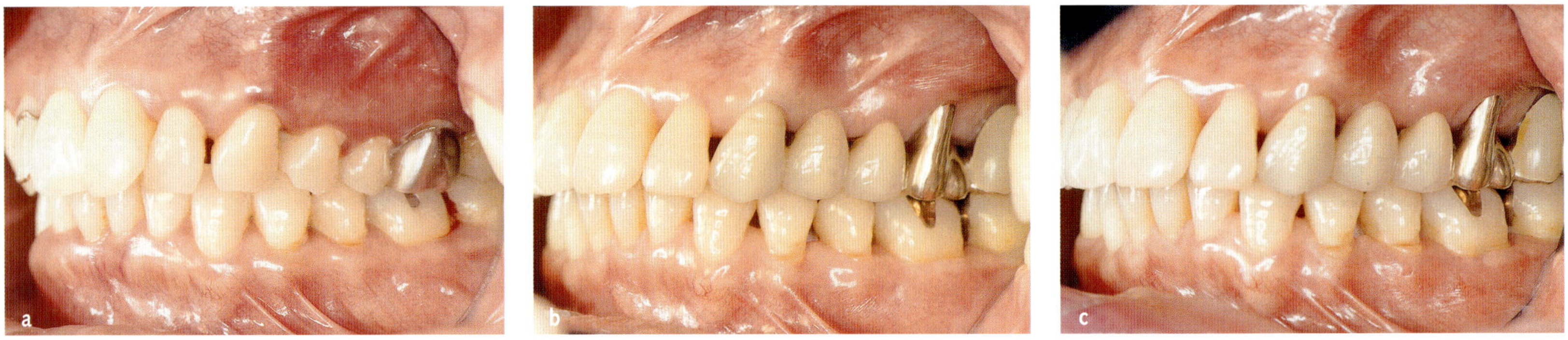

Fig 3-75 The left side. (a) A Class I relationship exists on the left. (b) Photograph taken after 2 years 2 months, 2 months after delivery of the final prosthesis. (c) Photograph taken 4 years 8 months after the first visit.

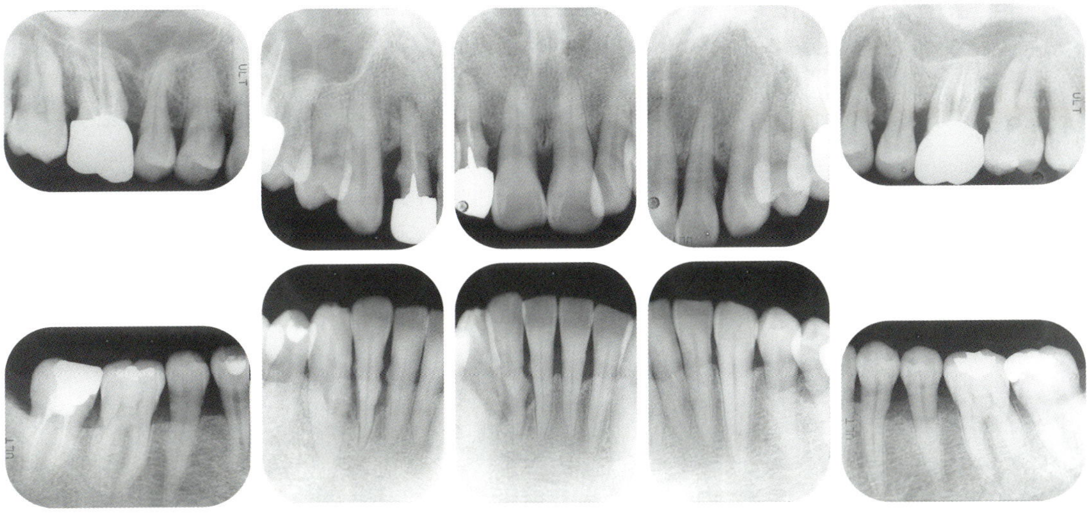

Fig 3-76 At the first visit (April 1995), severe bony defects and secondary occlusal trauma are noted. After the extraction of the maxillary right second molar and left first premolar and second molar, tooth movement was started. Final prostheses were delivered about 2 years after the first visit. During maintenance, Emdogain treatment was conducted for the mandibular left second molar (July 1998). The palatal root of the maxillary right first molar and the distal root of the maxillary left first molar were extracted. Flap access was made for all the mandibular incisors and canines and for the maxillary left second premolar, first molar, and third molar.

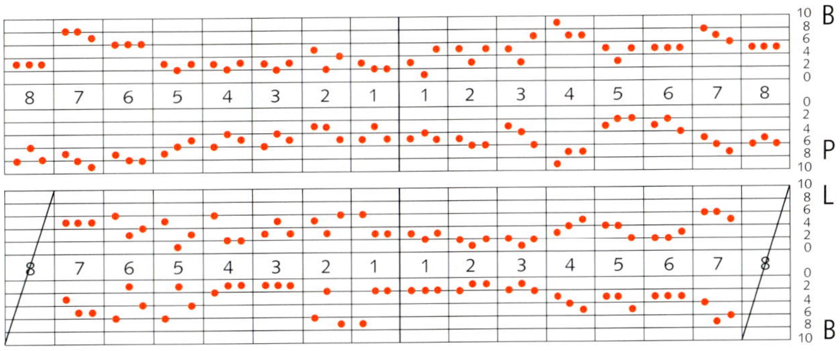

Fig 3-77 Probing chart at the first visit.

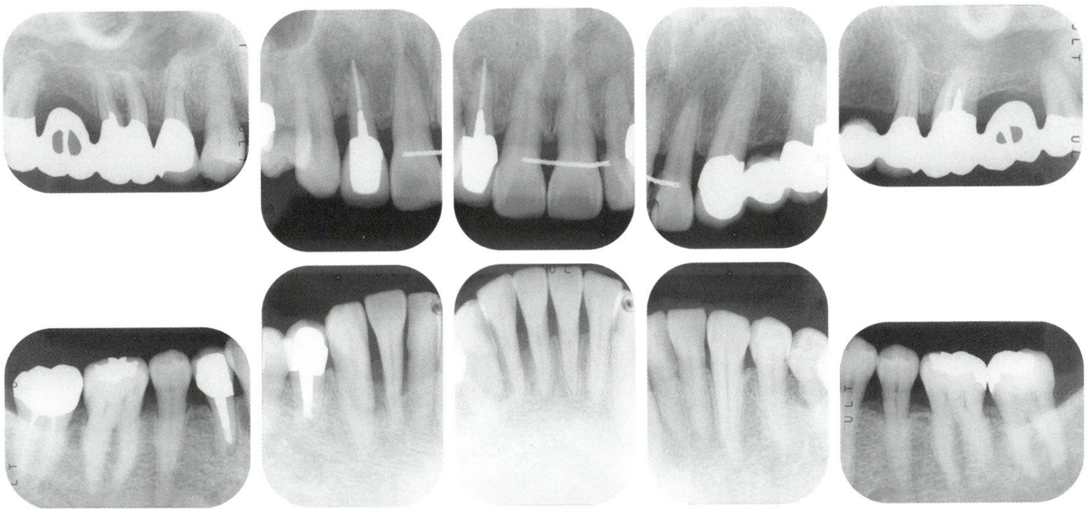

Fig 3-78 Radiographs taken at delivery of the final prostheses.

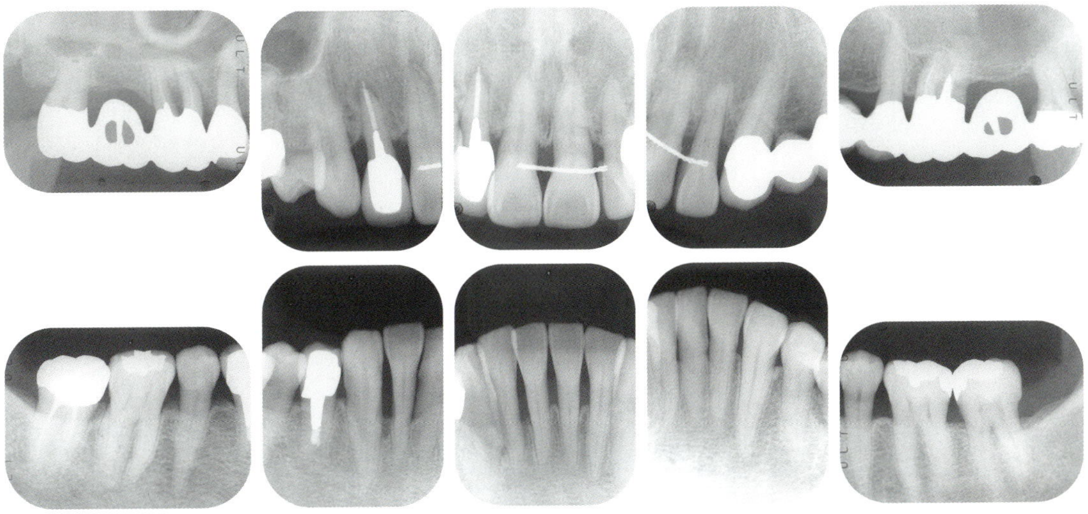

Fig 3-79 Radiographs taken during maintenance, 7 years 3 months after the first visit. Probing depths are maintained within 3 mm, except for two 4-mm sites.

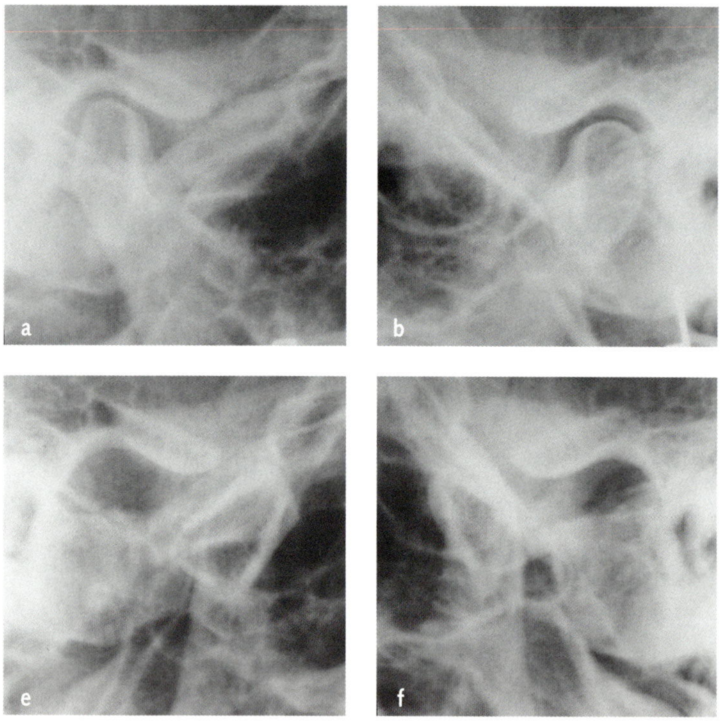

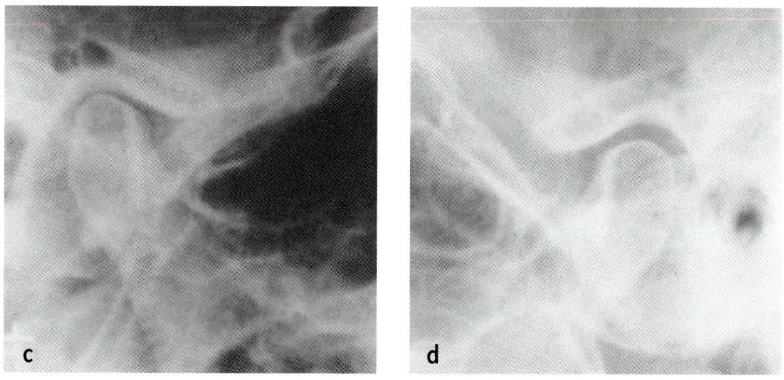

Fig 3-80 Radiographs of the TMJs. (a and b) Maximum intercuspation at the first visit. (a) Right TMJ. (b) Left TMJ. (c and d) Maximum intercuspation 10 months after the delivery of the final prostheses. (c) The right side shows an increase in space at the posterior wall of the condyle. (d) The left side reveals expansion of the articular space. (e and f) Maximal opening at the first visit. (e) Right TMJ. (f) Left TMJ.

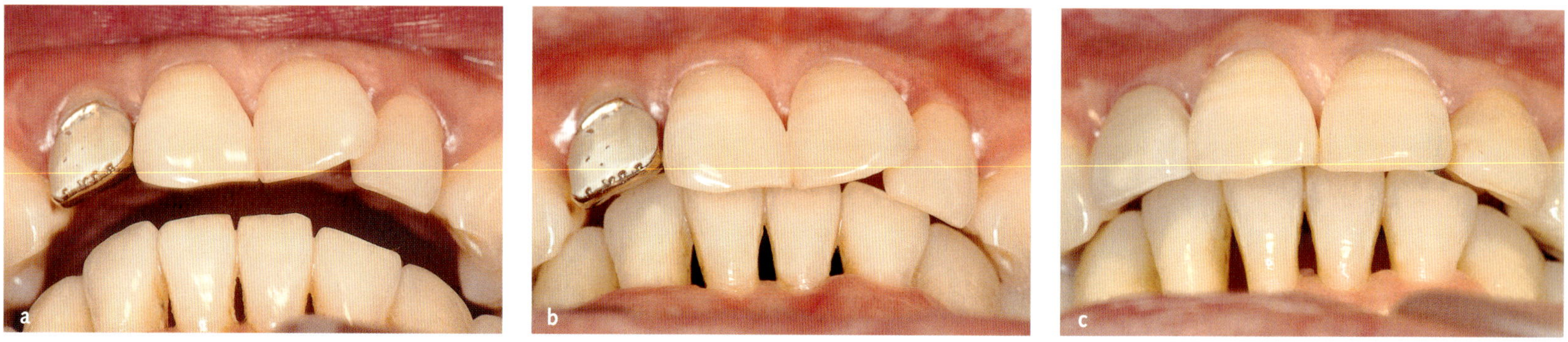

Fig 3-81 Overlapping of anterior teeth. (a) At the first visit. (b) Completion of initial therapy. (c) Completion of tooth movement and restoration. Morphologic correction was made for the maxillary central incisors. A prosthesis for the maxillary right lateral incisor and resin composite restoration for the maxillary left lateral incisor were provided.

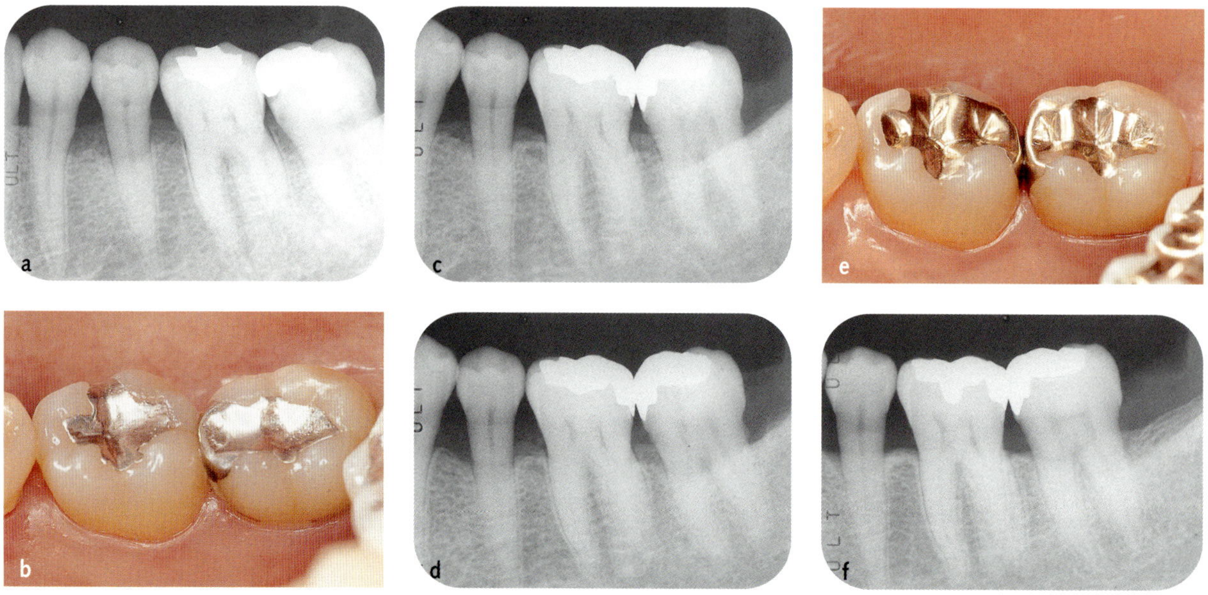

Fig 3-82 Remodeling in the molar regions. Clinical photographs are mirror views. (a and b) Mandibular left molars at the first visit. (c) Final prostheses were delivered after 2 years. (d) Class II furcation involvement is apparent at the mandibular left second molar. Calculus deposits are also present. (e and f) After Emdogain treatment, regeneration at the furcation of the mandibular left second molar is observable, 6 years after the first visit. Along with improvement in the occlusal surfaces, the chewing paths become more vertical, and the axes of molars are being uprighted.

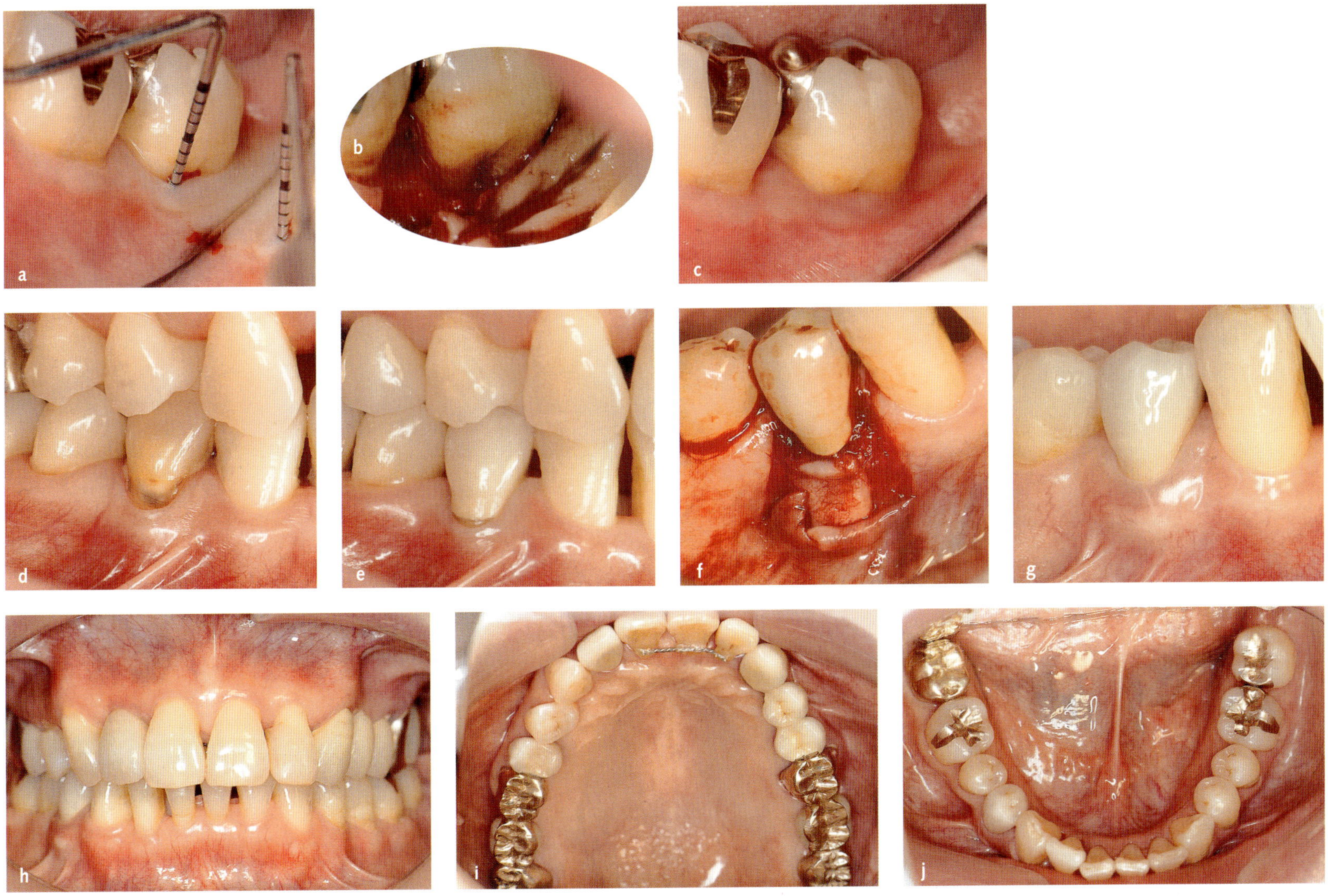

Fig 3-83 Maintenance. (a and b) During maintenance (August 1998), calculus deposits and a class II furcation involvement at the mandibular left second molar are found. (c) Improvement is seen in the furcation involvement, 1 year after Emdogain treatment. (d) Root caries, affecting the mandibular right first premolar, is found at the first visit. (e) Completion of the final restoration. (f) A connective tissue graft is placed to cover the exposed root, correct the frenulum attachment, and increase the attached gingiva. (g) Photograph taken 4 years 5 months after treatment. (h to j) Photographs taken 7 years 5 months after the first visit. With a combination of significant inflammation and brachyfacial-type trauma, the dentition seemed to be on the brink of occlusal collapse. Helped by intensive maintenance therapy and the patient's change in awareness (although her habits are still a matter of concern), almost satisfactory conditions have been maintained with minimal therapeutic intervention.

Chapter 4

Inflammation Control and Establishment of Maintainable Periodontal Tissue

Diagnosis of Periodontal Diseases and Comprehensive Treatment Planning

Initial therapy as a diagnostic tool

What measures should be used to assure elimination of infection and control of inflammation? Even with integration of clinical findings, probing charts, and radiographs, it is difficult to determine treatment policies at an early stage. In periodontal therapy, the final treatment goals and methodology to achieve them are determined through observations of tissue response to initial therapy.

In other words, initial therapy is indispensable to determining the final treatment goals. It has an important diagnostic function in addition to its role as anti-infective therapy.

For the purpose of diagnosis, the clinician's technical skills of subgingival instrumentation have to be excellent, because poor application of basic skills results in misdiagnosis and overtreatment.

Definitive diagnosis via periodontal surgery

In contrast to initial therapy, periodontal surgery is generally regarded as a definitive procedure. However, periodontal surgery also has the objective of gaining instrumental access to ensure anti-infective therapy. Periodontal surgery also has significance as a diagnostic tool (Table 4-1).

In clinical settings, the condition of alveolar bony defects often cannot be determined through probing and radiographs alone. An accurate picture of bone defect morphology often requires direct observation. Hence, the observation of morphology and conditions of alveolar bone with flap elevation is also an important component of the examination of infrabony defects.

Diagnosis and treatment planning

Severe periodontitis is a chronic condition in which the need for tooth extraction has to be decided with the diagnosis. If inflammation can be controlled with continuous maintenance therapy, it has been confirmed that granulation tissue in gingival connective tissue will be healed and support will be restored even in severe cases of periodontitis. Therefore, if it is determined not to extract a tooth, preservative procedures to minimize tissue damage must be selected.

In contrast, for cases of mild to moderate periodontal disease that show no clear response of inflammation control after initial therapy, resective therapy for aggressive pocket reduction and bone modification is recommended. Tissue damage caused by surgery is limited in these cases. Resective surgery aims at reconstruction of maintainable periodontal tissue. For a localized vertical bony defect, it is beneficial to select regenerative therapy to restore attachment. Because the predictability of regenerative therapy has been improved, in a localized vertical bony defect, in two- to three-wall bony defects, or in furcation involvements with an assured scaffold for regeneration, some aggressive procedures should be considered as options.

Table 4-1 Objectives of periodontal surgery

- Assured elimination of etiologic agents
- Definitive diagnosis of periodontal and bony defects
- Elimination and/or reduction of periodontal pockets
- Resection, repair, and/or regeneration of bony defects
- Elimination of granulation tissue
- Establishment of a maintainable environment
- Acquisition of biologic width
- Restoration of esthetic cervical margins

Case 4-1 Severe periodontitis accompanied by secondary occlusal trauma

Patient: *49-year-old woman at the time of first visit in January 1998*
Chief complaint: *Gingival swelling and purulent discharge affecting the maxillary right canine and mobility of maxillary teeth*
The patient exhibited severe clenching, and traumatic factors are considered to be largely involved in bone defects. There were localized vertical bone defects, for which recovery may be expected to a certain degree by regenerative therapy and restorative tooth movement, if forces can be controlled. In this clinical case, force control was challenging, and during initial therapy phase, acute alveolar abscesses repeatedly developed at the maxillary right first premolar and mandibular right first molar. The maxillary right canine had gingival swelling and purulent discharge. The left side had communication with the sinus. The authors routinely apply regenerative therapy for vertical bone defects. Thorough debridement is mandatory. With surgical procedures to allow tight closure of the wound and control of occlusion, regenerative therapy can be highly predictable (Figs 4-1 to 4-13).

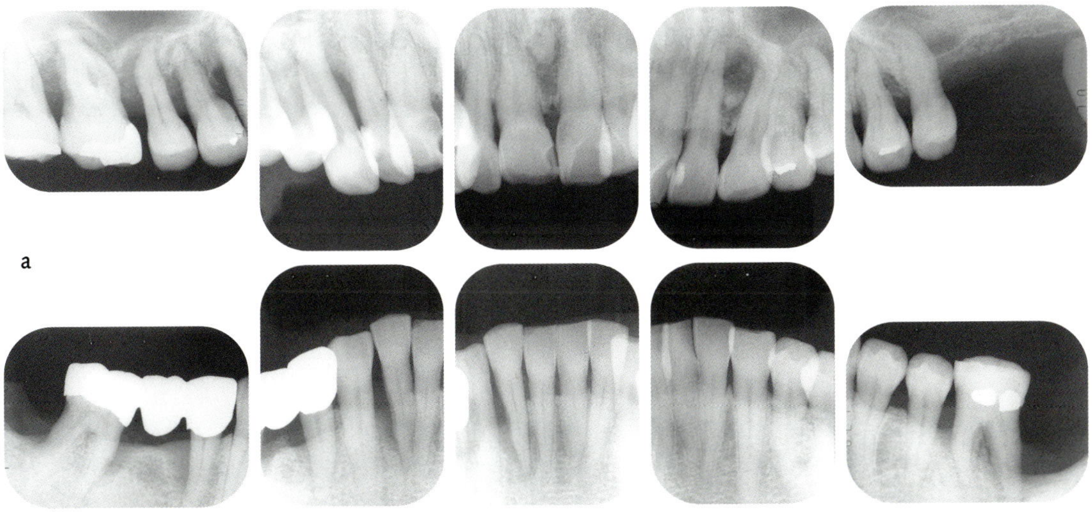
a

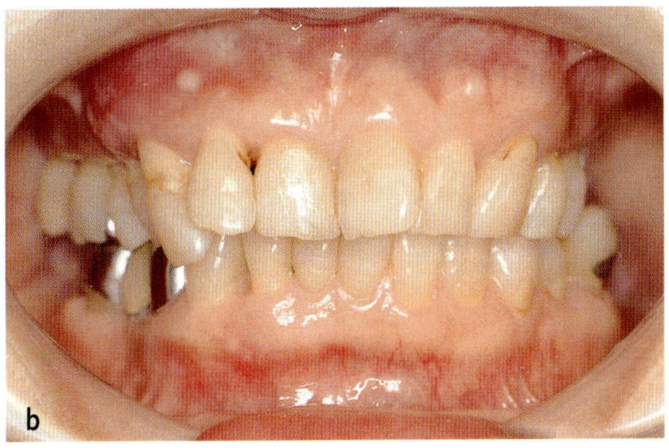
b

Fig 4-1 (a and b) At the first visit, the maxillary left teeth are worn to almost flat buccal cusps. The right side has a deeper occlusion. (c) Probing chart at first visit, showing some localized deep pockets. Red indicates bleeding points.

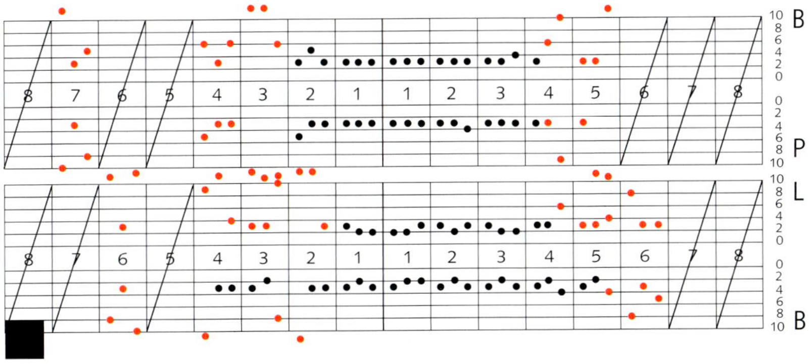

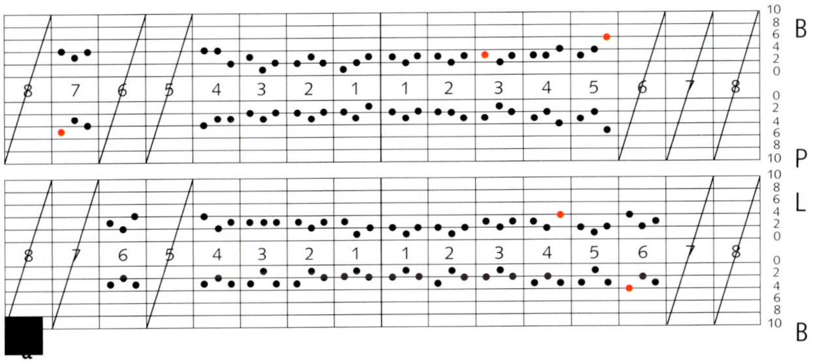

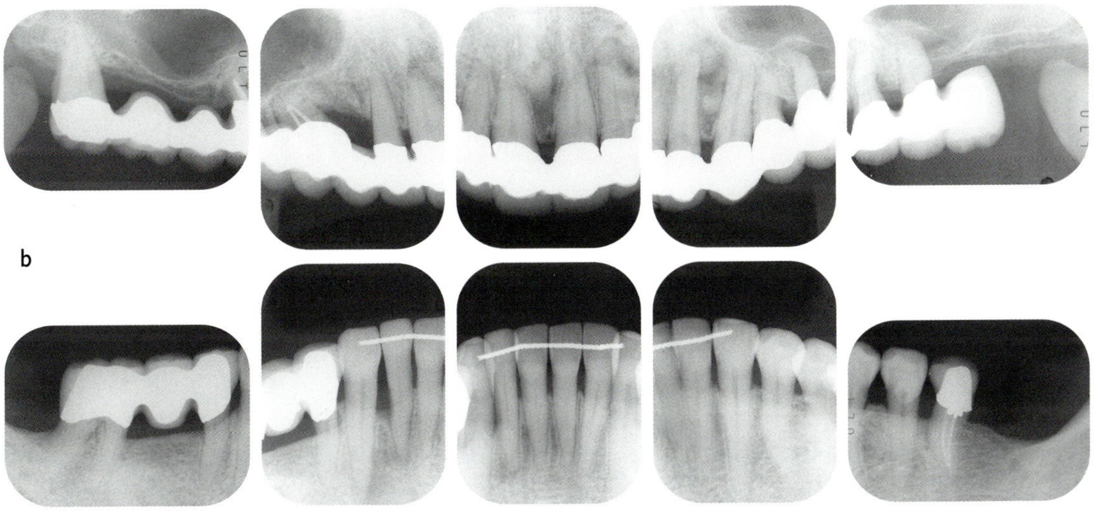
b

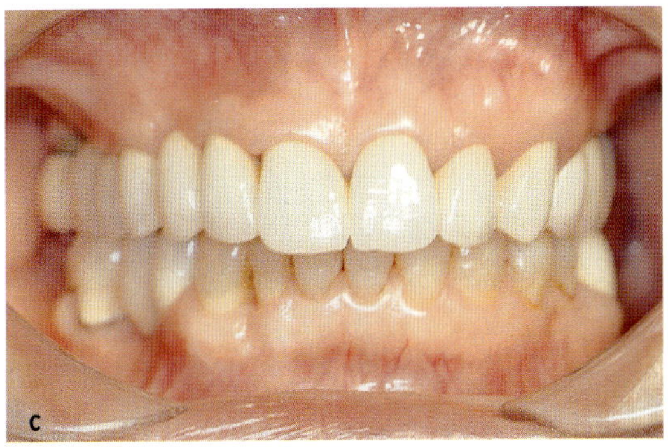
c

Fig 4-2 (a) Probing chart about 4 years 6 months after the first visit. The probing depth is 2 mm or less except at the maxillary right first premolar and second molar and the maxillary left second premolar. (b) Radiographs made 4 years 5 months after the first visit. Regenerative therapy was conducted for the maxillary right first premolar; maxillary left canine, first premolar, and second premolar; and mandibular right first premolar and first molar; and to treat vertical bone loss at the mandibular right lateral incisor. The maxillary right canine and second premolar and the distal root of the mandibular right first molar were extracted. (c) Clinical photograph taken 2 years 6 months after the first visit, at delivery of the final prostheses.

Periodontal treatment goals and treatment plans

In order to restore the normal structure of periodontal tissue after periodontal therapy, it is not sufficient to pay attention only to periodontally compromised tissue. It requires comprehensive diagnosis as well as treatments and procedures that incorporate the immune responses, occlusion, and integrity of the dentition of a patient. Because periodontal surgery has the dual objectives of obtaining diagnostic data and obtaining access for instruments, variations of procedures, including incision design, flap design, handling of periosteum, repositioning of flap, and sutures, should be appropriately used, depending on the objectives.

To improve the internal environment, resection, preservation, or regenerative therapy is to be selected according to pathophysiology. Sometimes surgical procedures are required for improvement of not only the internal environment but also the external environment. These are procedures to establish an environment with good esthetics and/or maintainability, such as mucogingival surgery.

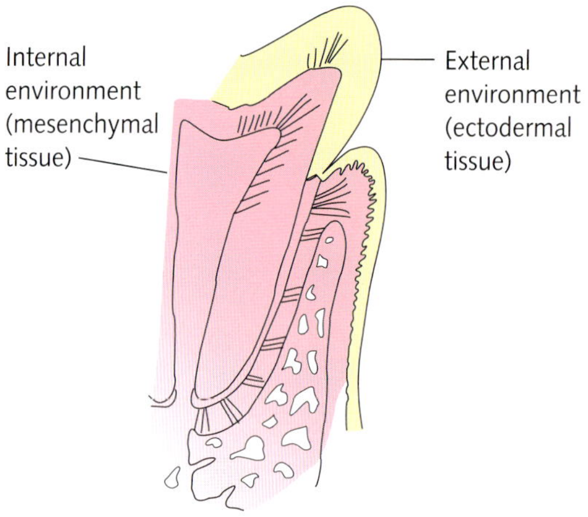

Fig 4-3 Internal and external environment.

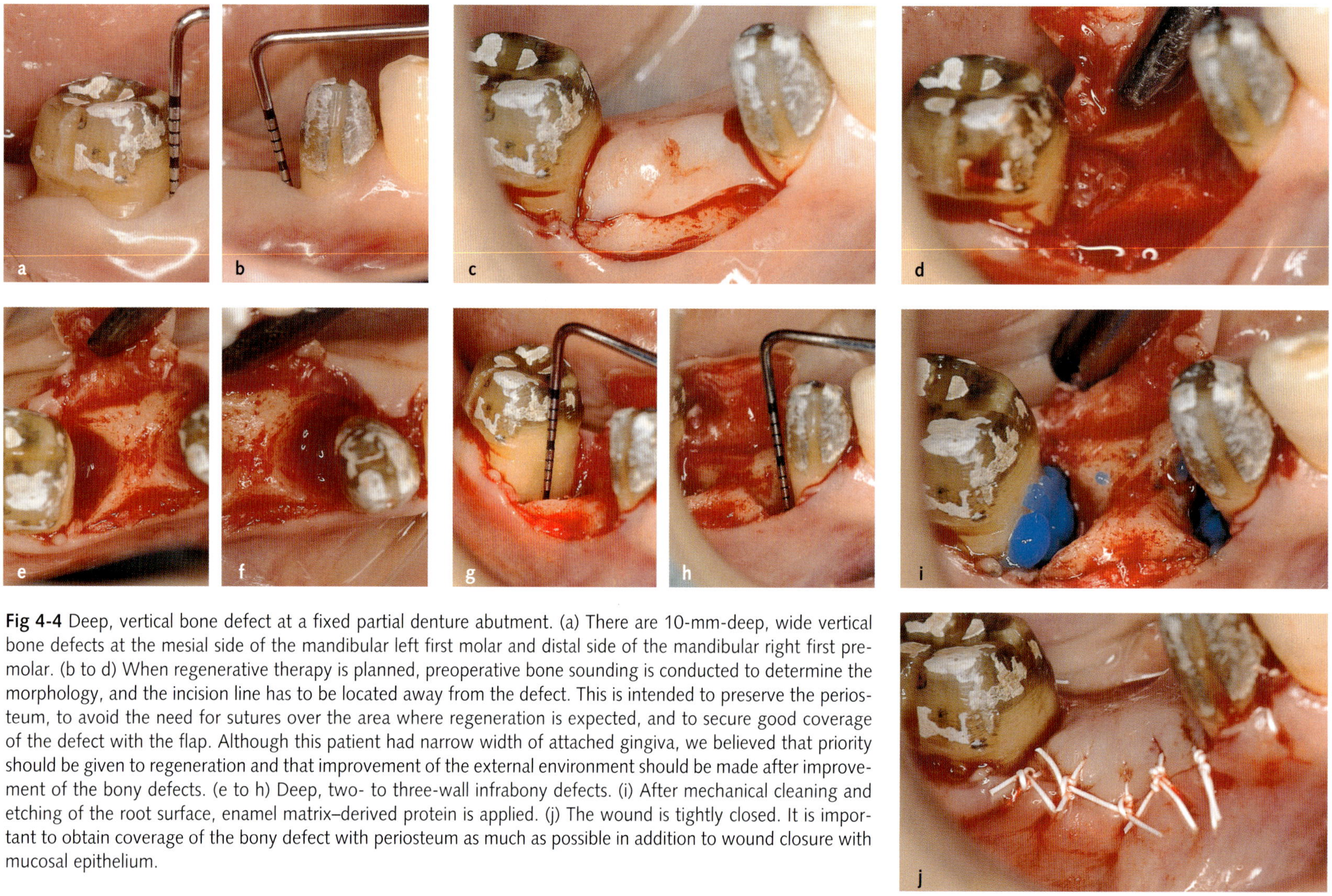

Fig 4-4 Deep, vertical bone defect at a fixed partial denture abutment. (a) There are 10-mm-deep, wide vertical bone defects at the mesial side of the mandibular left first molar and distal side of the mandibular right first premolar. (b to d) When regenerative therapy is planned, preoperative bone sounding is conducted to determine the morphology, and the incision line has to be located away from the defect. This is intended to preserve the periosteum, to avoid the need for sutures over the area where regeneration is expected, and to secure good coverage of the defect with the flap. Although this patient had narrow width of attached gingiva, we believed that priority should be given to regeneration and that improvement of the external environment should be made after improvement of the bony defects. (e to h) Deep, two- to three-wall infrabony defects. (i) After mechanical cleaning and etching of the root surface, enamel matrix–derived protein is applied. (j) The wound is tightly closed. It is important to obtain coverage of the bony defect with periosteum as much as possible in addition to wound closure with mucosal epithelium.

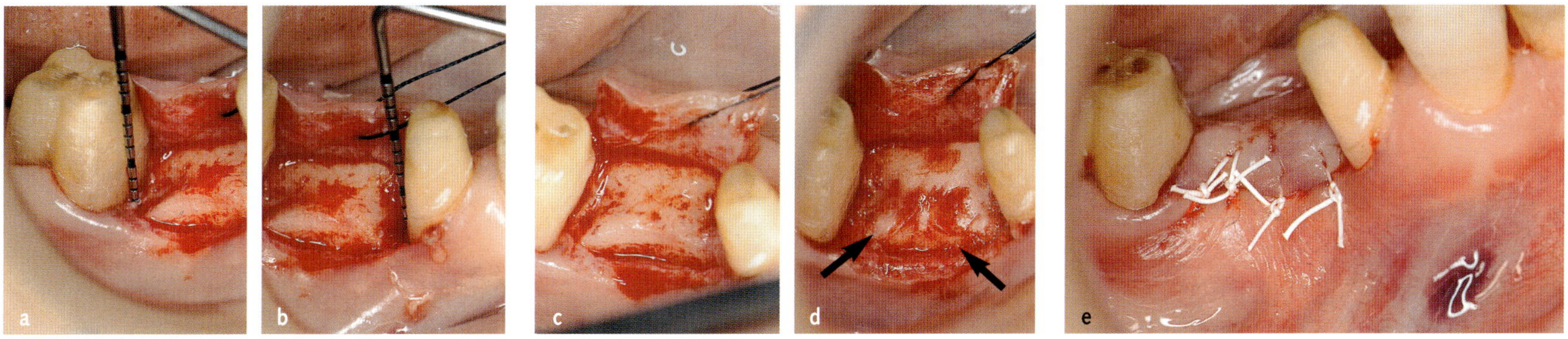

Fig 4-5 Reentry 1 year 4 months after surgery. (a to c) The bone defect mesial to the mandibular right first molar has experienced almost complete bone regeneration. The bone defect distal to the mandibular right first premolar is about 2 mm. (d) Partly for bone modification of the alveolar ridge defect, some autogenous bone is harvested from the area underneath the pontic *(arrows)* and grafted to the distal side of the mandibular right first premolar with some remaining shallow defect. (e) The flap is repositioned after application of Emdogain.

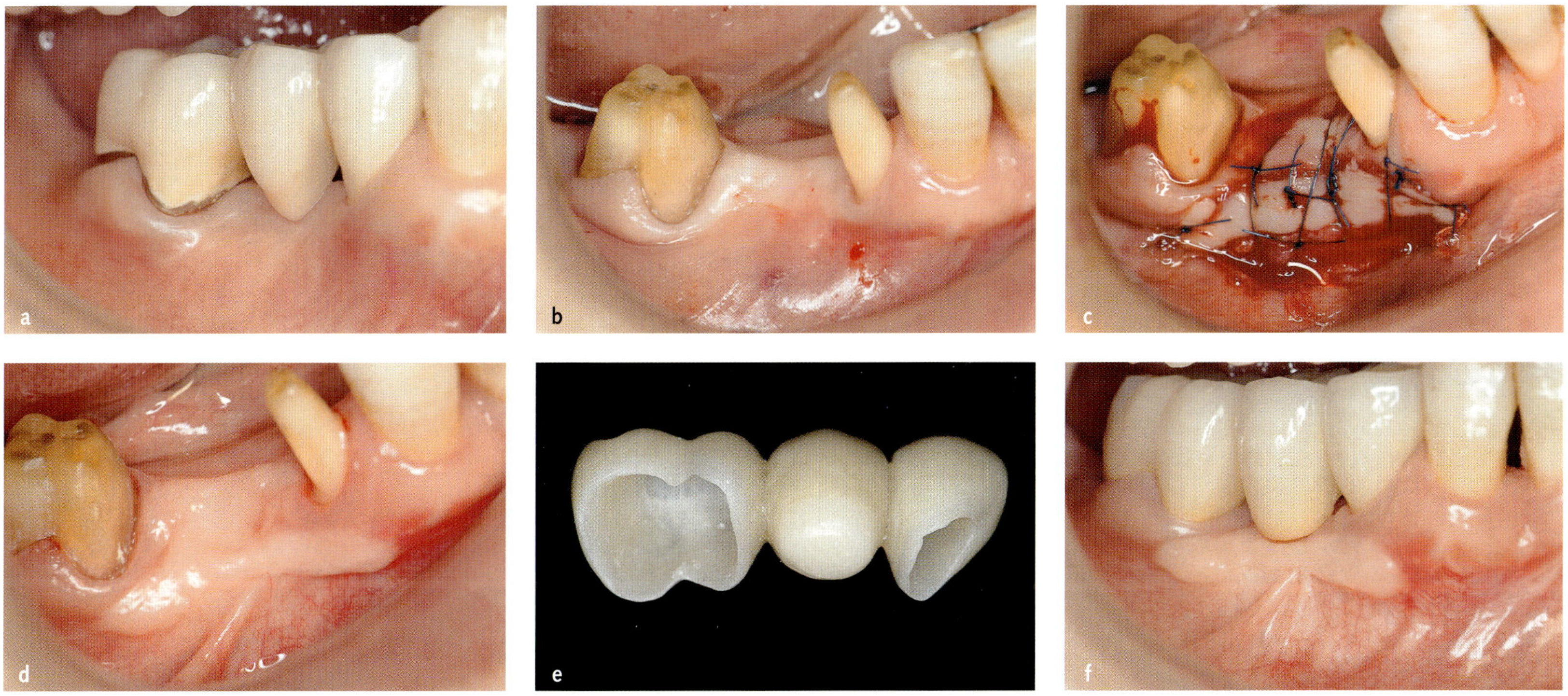

Fig 4-6 (a) Provisional restoration made of metal and resin (with a supragingival margin). (b and c) Because of mobile mucosa on the edentulous alveolar ridge, there were some problems such as food retention. Onlay grafting of two free gingival grafts is conducted to increase the attached gingiva and extend the oral vestibule. (d) Appearance 9 months after free gingival grafting. (e) The provisional restoration was utilized to form a concavity at the pontic site, and an ovate pontic design was selected. (f) The final prosthesis was fabricated, 11 months after free gingival grafting and 4 years after Emdogain application. (Prostheses made by Mr Kiyoharu Takada, RDT.)

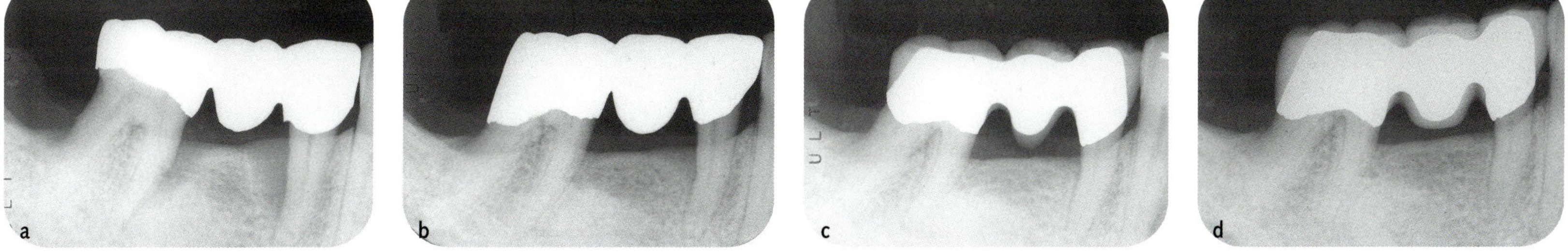

Fig 4-7 Radiographic examinations. (a) At the first visit. (b) Improvement 1 year 7 months after Emdogain application (2 years 1 month after the first visit). (c) Radiograph taken 5 months after (b). The distal bone defect is almost regenerated. (d) Radiograph taken about 4 years after surgery (4 years 6 months after the first visit). Regeneration seems almost complete.

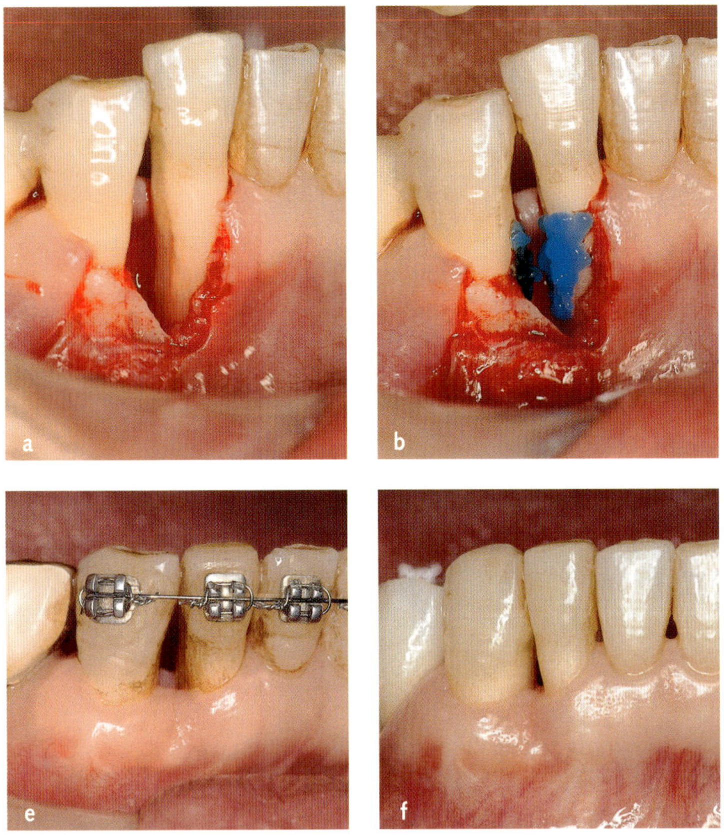

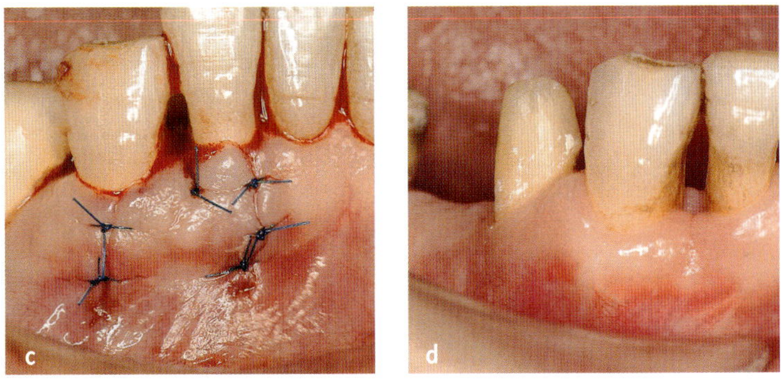

Fig 4-8 Regeneration of deep, crater-shaped, one-wall bone defect at the mandibular lateral incisor. (a) Because a deep infrabony defect was identified, two vertical incisions are made to reflect a full-thickness flap. (b) After mechanical cleaning and root surface etching (36% etching gel), Emdogain is applied. (c) The flap is coronally repositioned and sutured tightly. The incisal edge is reduced, because natural extrusion is expected, and disking is repeated. (d) Photograph taken 4 months after surgery. (e) Leveling. (f) Photograph taken 3 years after surgery.

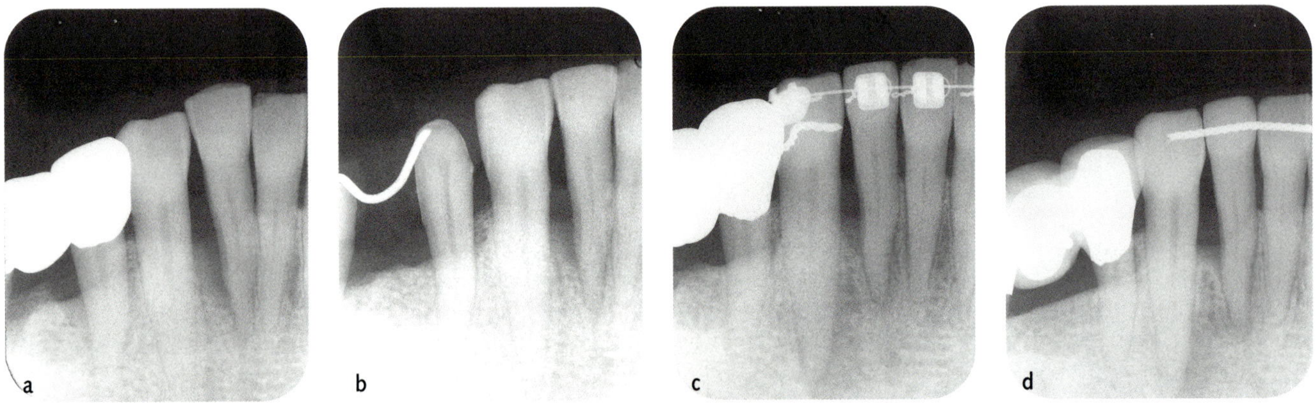

Fig 4-9 Radiographic examination. (a) At first visit. (b) Radiograph taken 3 months after Emdogain application. (c) Tooth movement (about 4 months). The root proximity of the mandibular right central incisor and lateral incisor has been reduced. The mandibular right lateral incisor and canine have undergone disking, and the extruded incisal edge of the mandibular right lateral incisor has been reduced. (d) Radiograph taken 3 years 6 months after surgery. Regeneration is observed.

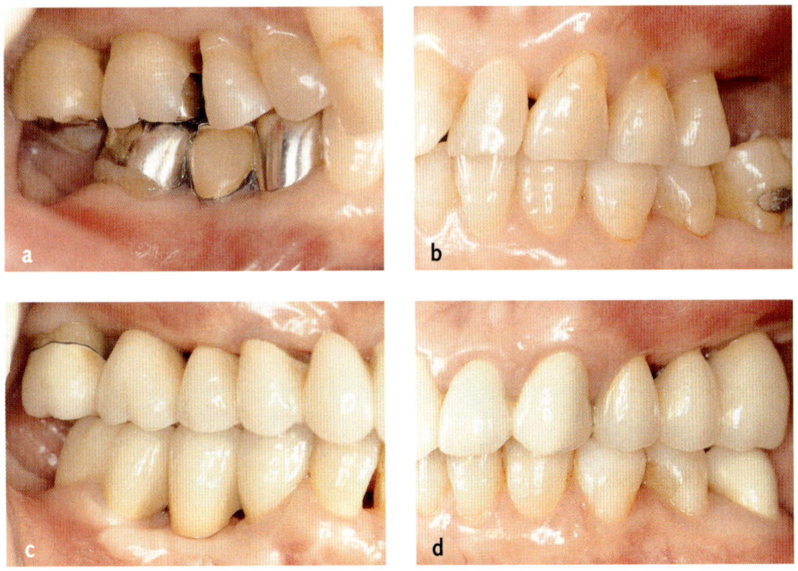

Fig 4-10 Buccal views (a and b) before and (c and d) after treatment. At the first visit, the teeth on the left side are worn away to almost flat buccal cusps. The right side has a deeper occlusion.

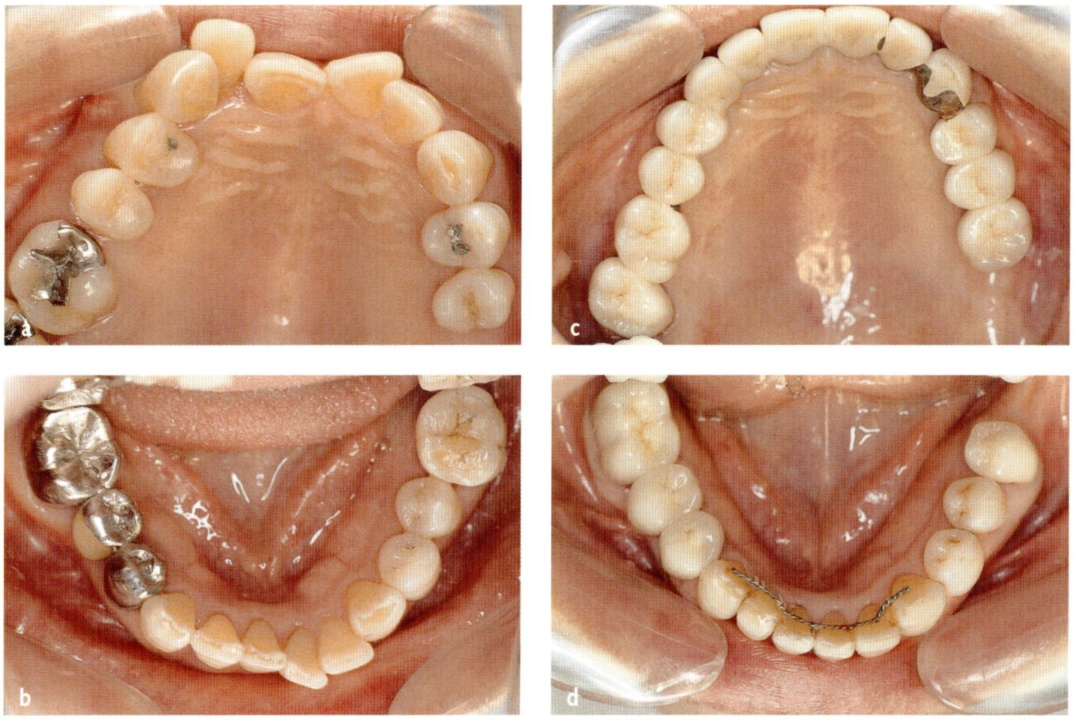

Fig 4-11 (a and b) At the first visit, the teeth on the left are so worn that the buccal cusps are almost gone. (c and d) After treatment, the arch shape, which was externally distorted on the right, is considerably improved.

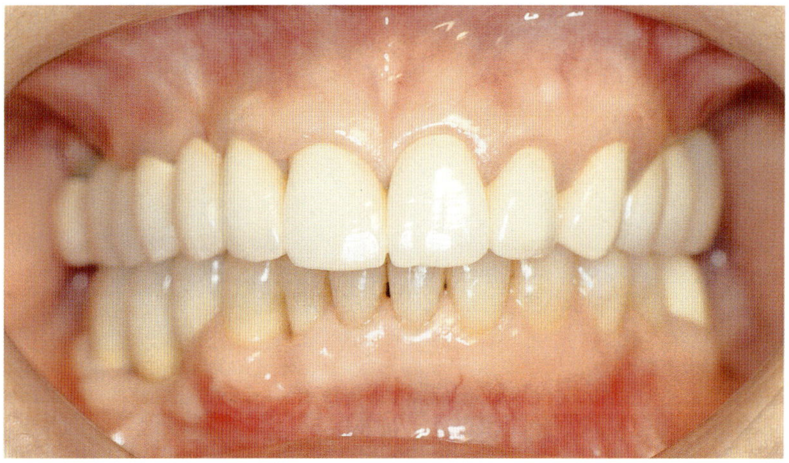

Fig 4-12 Frontal view, 3 years 7 months after the first visit. A cantilever fixed partial denture replaces the maxillary left first molar. The maxillary right first molar, second premolar, and canine are missing.

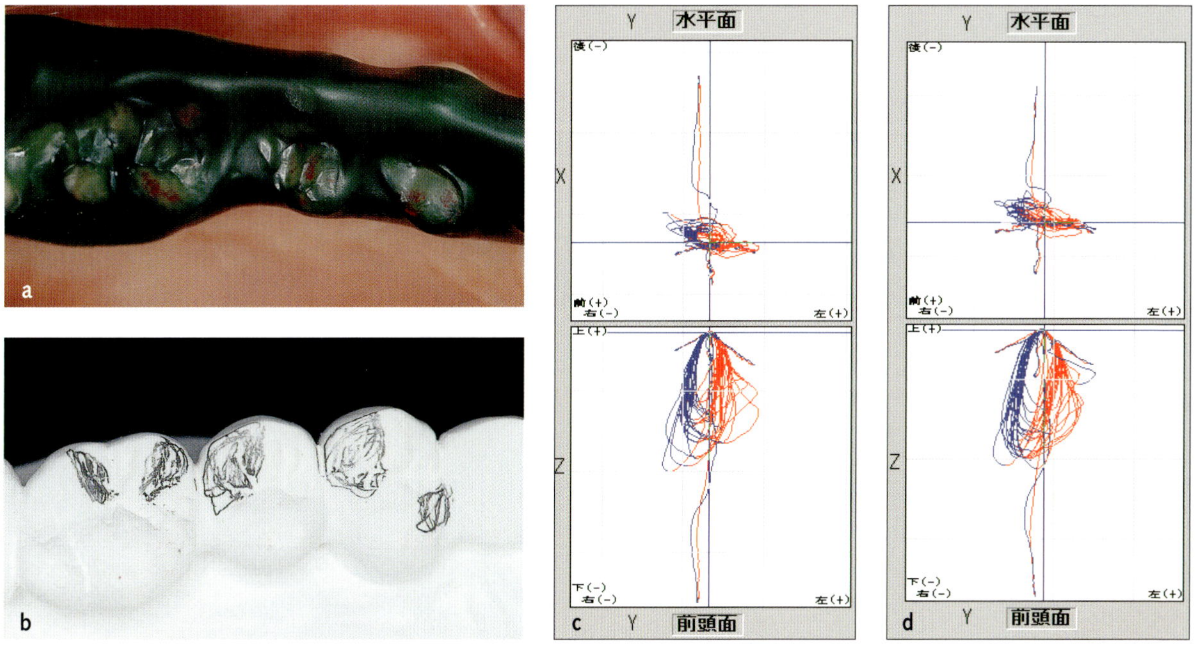

Fig 4-13 Mandibular functional movement before and after enameloplasty. (a and b) Reshaped areas are shown. (c) Horizontal (top) and frontal (bottom) views before reshaping. (d) Horizontal (top) and frontal (bottom) views after reshaping. Chewing has become more vertical.

Objective-Oriented Selection of Periodontal Surgery Procedures

Objectives, conditions, and selection of procedures

Periodontal surgery not only is a means for improving periodontal tissues, but it also has diagnostic significance. It is performed for improvement of the internal environment, such as treatment of infrabony defects and periodontal pockets, when deep periodontal pockets and/or furcation involvements do not exhibit sufficient response to initial therapy (Fig 4-14). There are also procedures for improvement of the external environment, such as an increase of attached gingiva. In addition, various periodontal plastic surgery procedures have been developed, including resective procedures for treatment of subgingival dental caries and improvement of mucogingival tissue. The objectives and conditions of those procedures must be examined closely in the selection of procedures.

Periodontal surgery generally should be conducted after thorough initial therapy is completed. Surgery may be conducted at an earlier stage in a patient with an unstable occlusion or with mild attachment loss, mainly in order to improve the external environment.

Handling of periosteum in periodontal surgery

In periodontal surgery, flaps should be handled properly, depending on the objective of the surgery, such as reduction or elimination of periodontal pockets, enhancement of attached gingiva, or regeneration of periodontal tissue. Flaps can be handled in an objective-oriented manner, mainly depending on the incision, flap formation, and suturing. Although readers are referred to textbooks for details on incisions and suturing techniques, the essential point in flap formation is in the handling of the periosteum. Appropriate procedures, selected on the basis of conditions and objectives, including selection of a full-thickness flap, partial-thickness flap, or a combination flap, will provide the expected outcome of surgery.

Types of periodontal surgery

Procedures can be roughly categorized depending on their objectives. For an access flap or regenerative tissue therapy with the objective of debridement, the incision is made into the pocket along with the tooth axis, reaching the bony crest. A full-thickness flap is formed, reflecting all the tissue from the bony surface. Flaps are sutured back with tight contact to the root surface. Full-thickness flap formation beyond the mucogingival junction (MGJ) is not preferable from the viewpoint of flap stability. When coronal repositioning of a flap is necessary, as in regenerative therapy, releasing incisions are made from the base of the full-thickness flap, extending beyond the MGJ.

Table 4-2 Comparison between full-thickness and partial-thickness flaps

	Periodontal pocket	Bone modification and resection	Acquisition of attached gingiva	Diversity in flap techniques	Techniques and pain	Regeneration therapy	Plastic surgery
Full-thickness flap	○ ○	○	❐	❐	○	○	❐
Partial-thickness flap	○ ❐	❐	○	○	❐	❐	○

The best procedures should be combined for the specific pathosis, to ensure a simple and more accurate procedure.

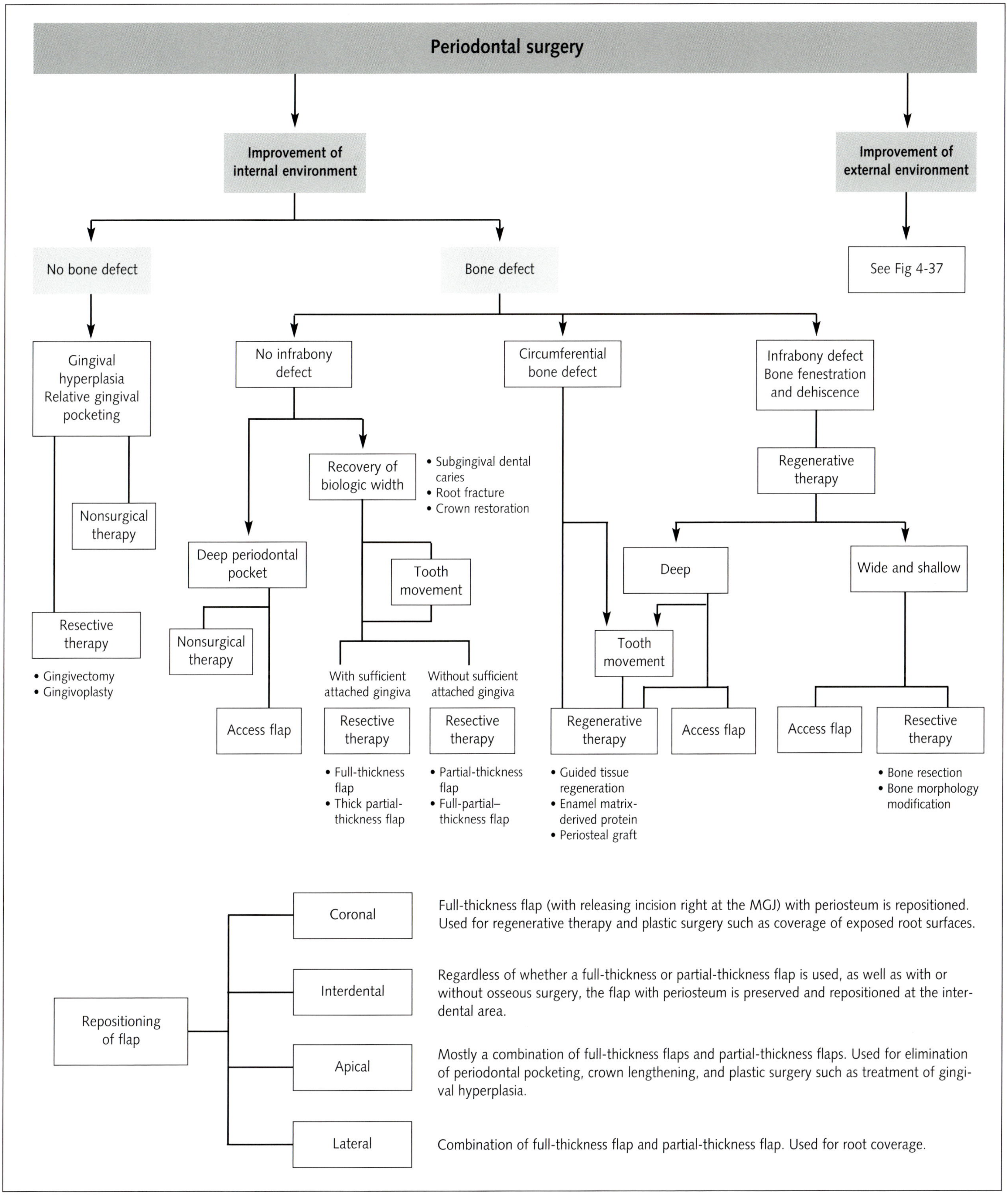

Fig 4-14 Periodontal surgery with the objective of improvement of the internal environment.

In all periodontal surgery procedures, including crown lengthening, periodontal pocket reduction or elimination, resective therapy with osseous surgery, and regenerative therapy, it is essential to envision the morphology of gingival healing, such as the degree of scalloping and especially reconstruction of the interdental papillae, when incisions are designed. Full-thickness flaps and partial-thickness flaps are often combined as necessity dictates (Table 4-2). In alveolar ridge augmentation, especially the roll technique, when the aim is at enhancement of the attached gingiva underneath a pontic, it is useful to have a two-layer flap.

Crown lengthening for preservation of the interdental papillae and enhancement of the attached gingiva

Surgical lengthening of clinical crowns may cause new mucogingival problems if attached gingiva is not sufficient. Because of this, techniques such as free gingival grafts are needed before or after crown lengthening. Because some osseous recontouring is necessary, gingiva over the bony crest is removed in conventional procedures. This technique has a disadvantage, which is the loss of the interdental papillae. The authors have developed a flap design that incorporates both the increase of attached gingiva and preservation of the interdental papillae. In this technique, the flap is raised as a full-thickness flap from the interdental papilla; a partial-thickness flap is then formed, and a horizontal incision is made in the periosteum before the MGJ is reached. The most apical part of the flap is reflected as a full-thickness flap. It has a two-layer structure to ensure release. This technique assures a healthy root surface supragingivally, resulting in interdental papillae with balanced cervical margins and increased attached gingiva.

Periodontal pocket reduction (resective therapy) and interdental papillae preservation using a full-thickness flap

The incision design for elimination of periodontal pockets may vary, depending on whether or not attached gingiva is available. Because there was sufficient attached gingiva in the clinical case shown in Figs 4-15 to 4-22, a full-thickness flap was selected to conduct a pocket reduction procedure with osseous surgery.

Alignment of the bone level with regenerative and resective therapy

Leveling of irregular bone may be achieved by regenerative therapy to regenerate attachment or by resective therapy to eliminate infrabony defects through osseous surgery (Figs 4-23 to 4-35). Both of these methods, however, have limitations, and it is sometimes effective to combine the two approaches. Both regenerative and resective therapy exposes bone, and a full-thickness flap is selected if there is a sufficient width of attached gingiva.

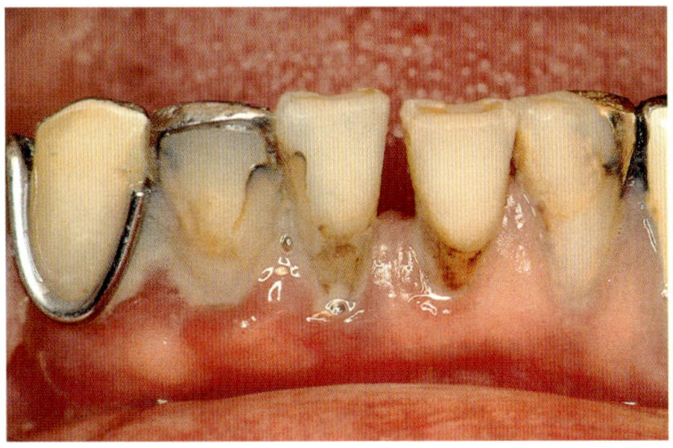

Fig 4-15 The patient was a 60-year-old woman at the first visit (May 1993). Significant plaque accumulation and gingival inflammation are visible. There is a space between the mandibular left and right central incisors. Because of the poor crown-root ratio, splinting of the mandibular anterior teeth was planned to protect the clasped teeth.

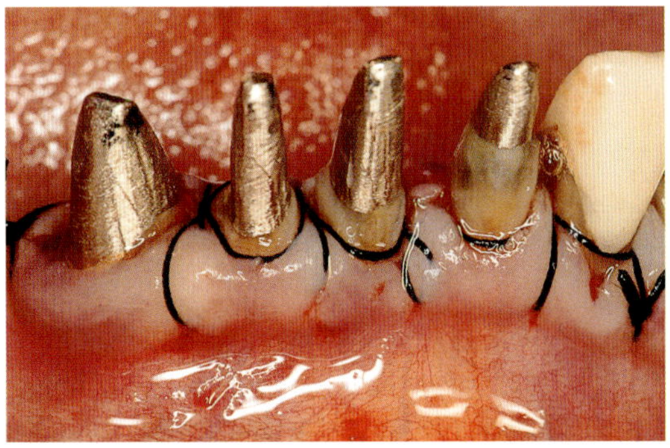

Fig 4-16 A scallop-shaped inverse bevel incision was made to allow configuration of the interdental papillae and to preserve the periosteum. A full-thickness flap was elevated without exceeding the MGJ. Symmetric mattress sutures have been made from the starting points right at the MGJ, which will prevent coronal movement of the flap. It is necessary that buccal and lingual flaps be attached to each other with neither too much nor too little tissue to form the interdental papillae. The flap is apically repositioned.

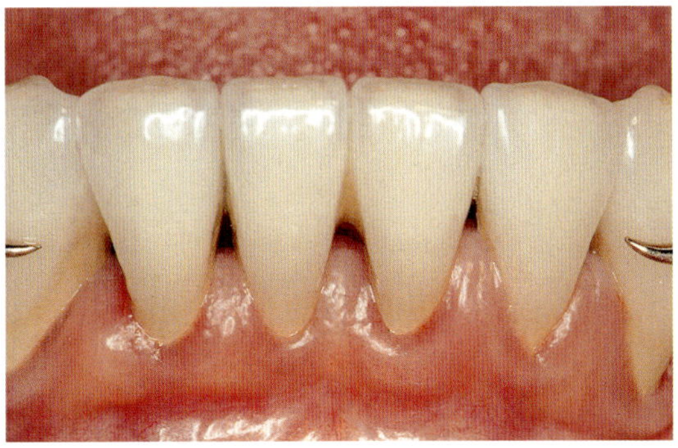

Fig 4-17 Photograph taken 2 years after the first visit. Metal-ceramic crowns have been delivered. Some gingival inflammation is noted. (There are no opposing teeth. The maxillary arch has only one remaining tooth and an overdenture.)

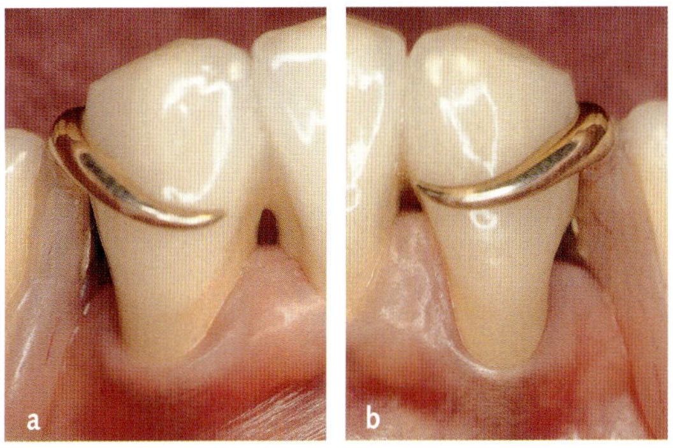

Fig 4-18 (a) Photograph taken 9 months after the delivery of prostheses. Note the profiles and morphology of the connection between transitional areas and gingiva. (b) The left side is shown after 1 year.

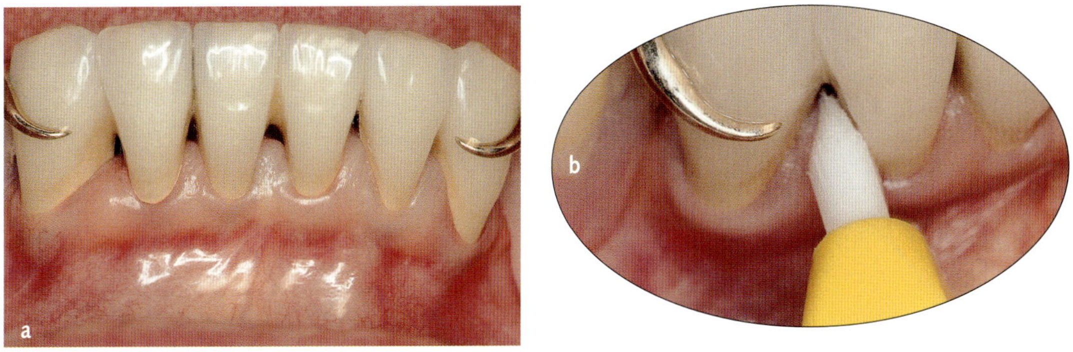

Fig 4-19 (a) Photograph taken 2 years after the delivery of prostheses. Gingival inflammation has been reduced because of good plaque control. For home care, a modified rolling brushing technique and (b) Pocket Cleaner are used to prevent damage of the interdental papillae.

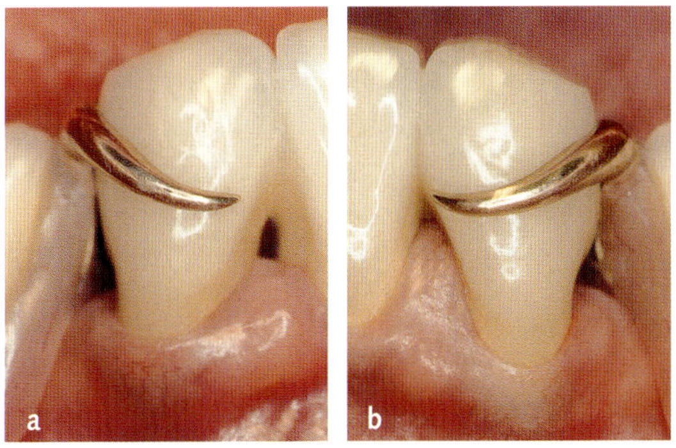

Fig 4-20 (a and b) Photographs taken 2 years 1 month after the delivery of prostheses. Although clasped teeth are likely to be subjected to trauma, an increase in gingival root coverage is observed.

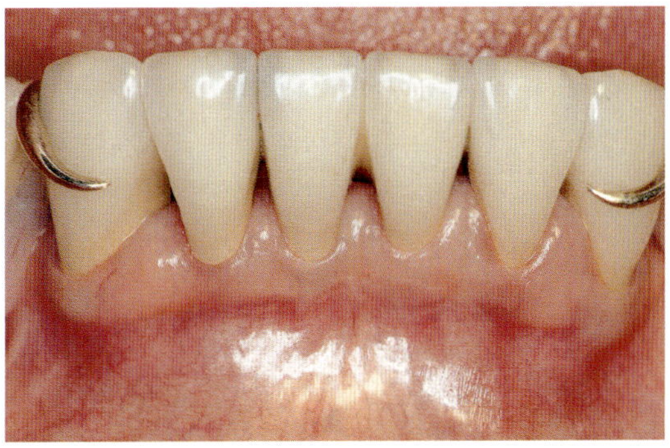

Fig 4-21 Photograph taken 7 years 3 months after the delivery of prostheses. Gingival increases have occurred, and the embrasure spaces at the mandibular canines are nearly filled with healthy gingiva. The mandibular left and right canines have rests and proximal plates to minimize rotation of the denture.

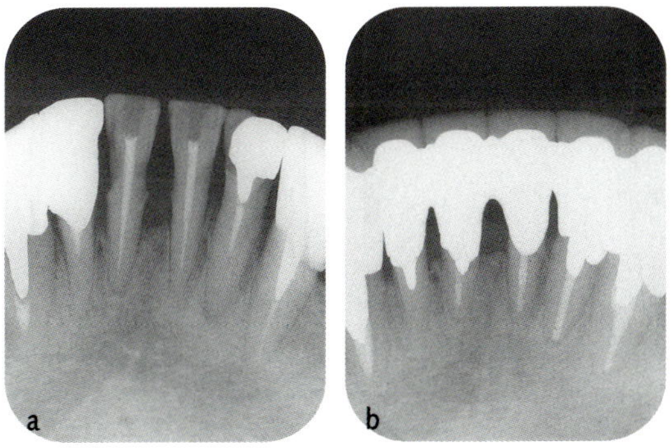

Fig 4-22 Radiographs taken (a) at the first visit and (b) 7 years later.

Figs 4-23 to 4-35 Alignment of the bone level

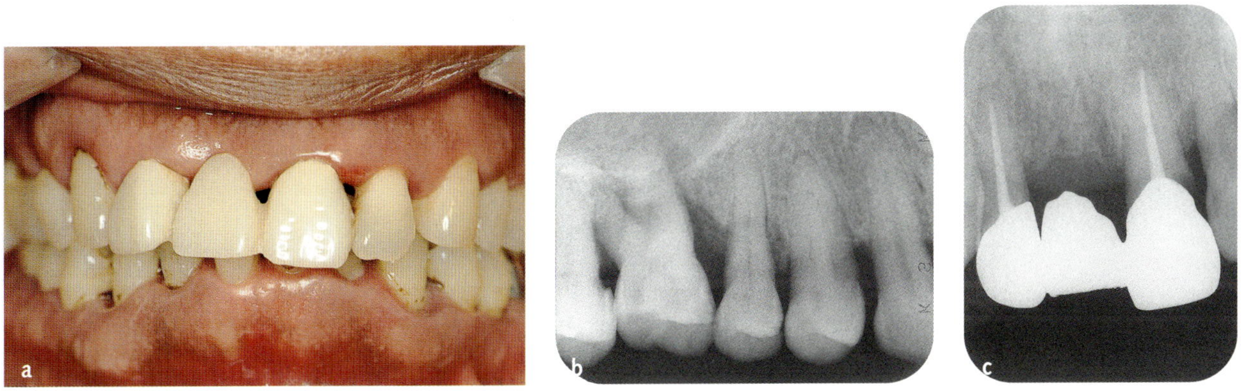

Fig 4-23 (a) Photograph taken at the first visit. (b and c) Radiographs indicate bone defects and an irregular, obscure bone crest due to trauma.

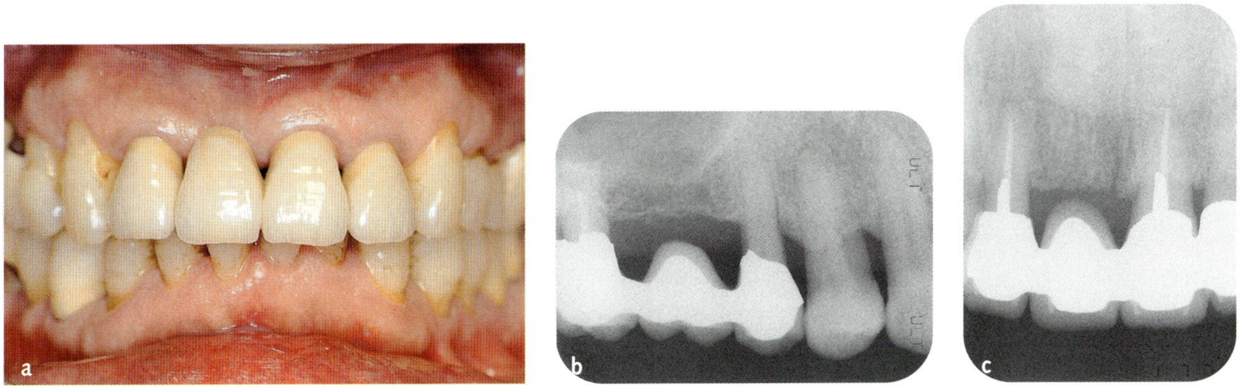

Fig 4-24 (a) Photograph taken 11 years 6 months after surgery (12 years 11 months after the first visit, or 10 years after delivery of prostheses). (b and c) Radiographs suggest regeneration. The bone level is aligned and the laminae dura have become clear.

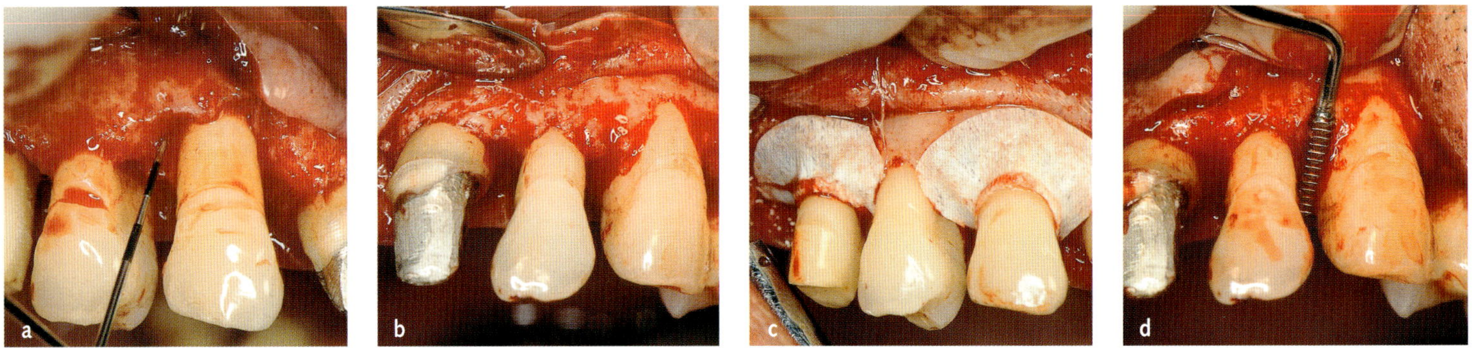

Fig 4-25 Regenerative therapy and resective therapy. (a) A wide bone defect around the maxillary right canine and a narrow defect around the maxillary left lateral incisor are noted. (b) A GTR membrane (wraparound type) is applied to the wide, deep bone defect around the maxillary right second premolar and canine. (c) The bone level around the narrow infrabony defect at the maxillary left lateral incisor and canine is aligned by osseous surgery.

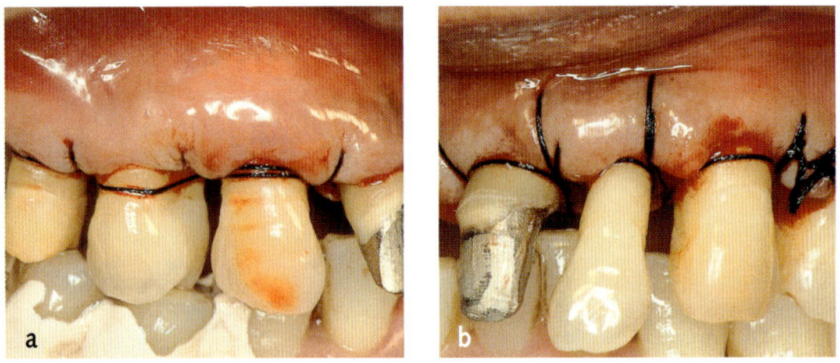

Fig 4-26 A full-thickness flap is tightly sutured with continuous mattress sutures. (a) Coronal repositioning of the flap. (b) Slightly apical repositioning of the flap.

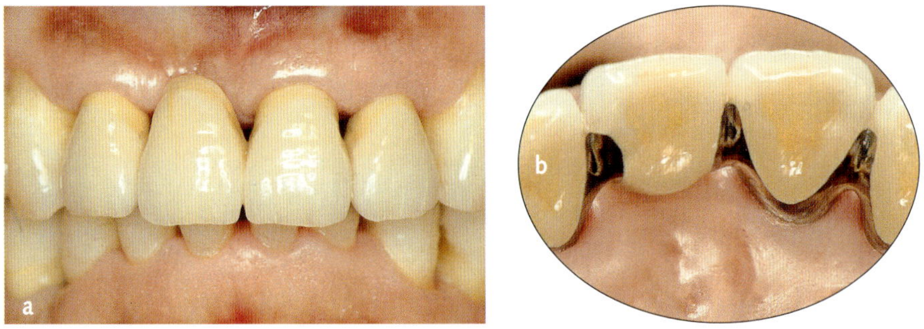

Fig 4-27 (a and b) Photographs taken 1 year 3 months after surgery. A collarless porcelain fixed partial denture extending from the maxillary right lateral incisor to the maxillary left central incisor (pontic: maxillary right central incisor) has been delivered. Because of the clinical crown-lengthening procedure, some concavity is noted at the pontic replacing the maxillary right central incisor. Pontics were not designed as an ovate shape at that time. The interdental space on the buccal side is closed, while the space is wide open on the lingual side. It was difficult maintaining a good balance between the two.

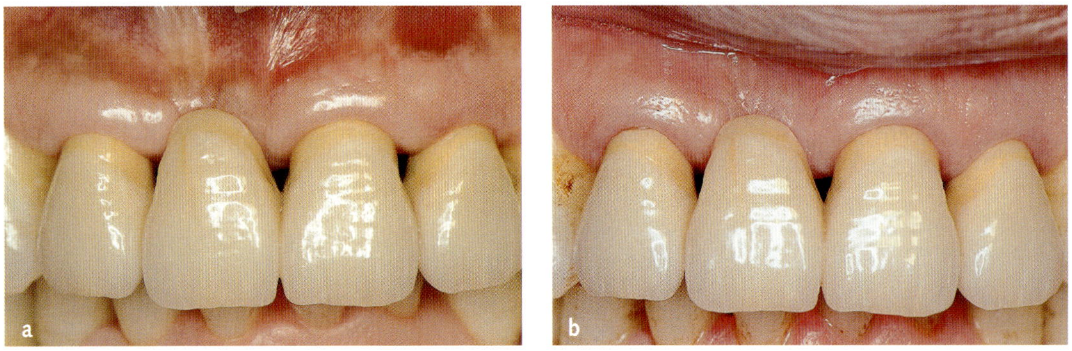

Fig 4-28 Progress of the case. (a) Photograph taken 1 year 3 months after surgery. (b) Photograph taken 11 years 6 months after surgery. Interdental spaces still exist because of the flap design utilized, which led to our later efforts to solve this problem of black triangles.

Figs 4-29 to 4-32 Basic procedures of guided bone regeneration (GBR) (delayed approach): Focusing on flap design.

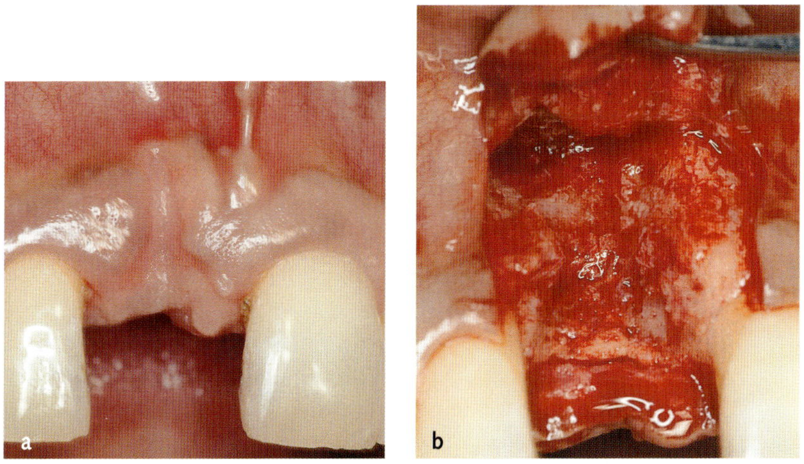

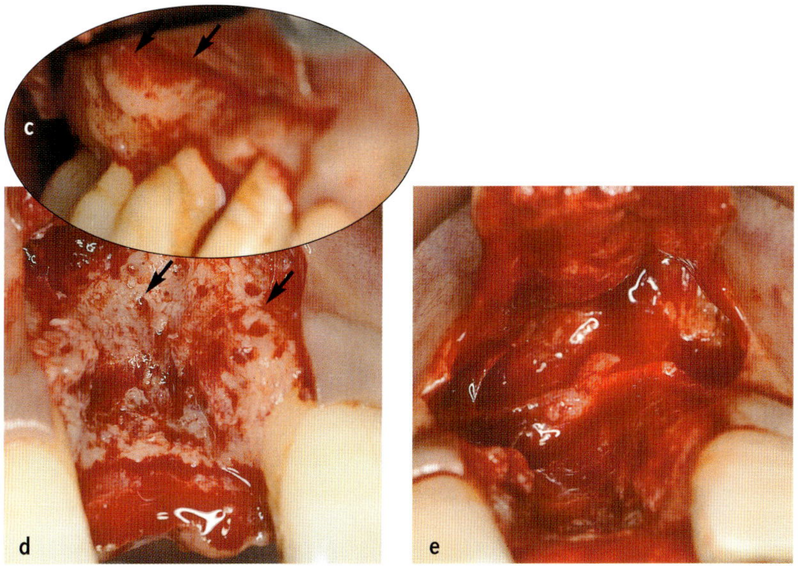

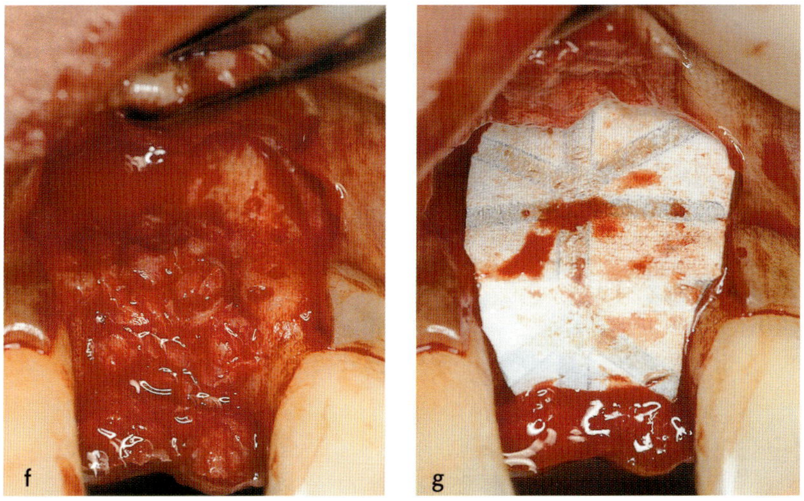

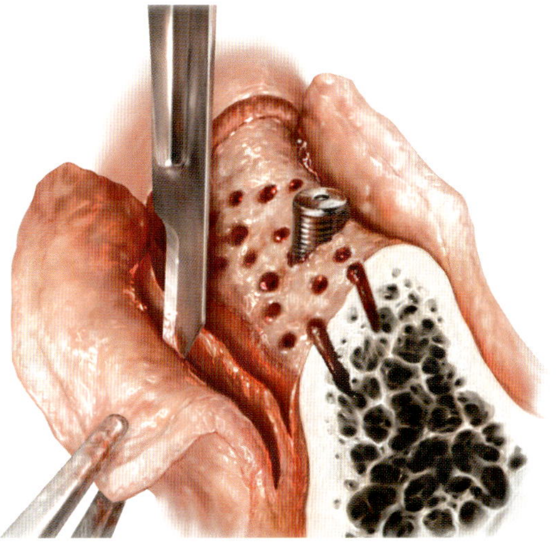

Fig 4-29 Bone augmentation of alveolar ridge defect using GBR. (a) At the first visit. The maxillary right central incisor had been extracted 1 year before. The buccal aspect of the edentulous alveolar ridge is mostly lost, and this site is inappropriate for an implant, unless GBR is used in a combination technique. (b) A butt joint vertical incision is made involving the buccal interdental papillae. Slightly palatal to the alveolar crest, a horizontal incision (slip joint) is made. The flap is reflected almost to the MGJ. (c) After the flap is reflected from the maxillary right second molar to the maxillary right first premolar, bone is collected from the shelflike torus *(arrows)*. (d) Fibrous granulation tissue is removed from the extraction socket, and the cortical bone is well penetrated *(arrows)*. (e) With the intent of creating space, vertical, semilunar incisions are made in connective tissue underneath the MGJ to form one or two additional layers. (f) The harvested autogenous bone is grafted to create a base for regeneration of bone. (g) A titanium-reinforced membrane is trimmed to fit the treatment site and inserted under the multilayered periosteum. The membrane is then tacked into position.

Fig 4-30 When coronal repositioning of the flap is needed, as in regenerative therapy or implant placement, it is useful to utilize semilunar releasing incisions as shown here, right at the MGJ, to form one or two additional layers.

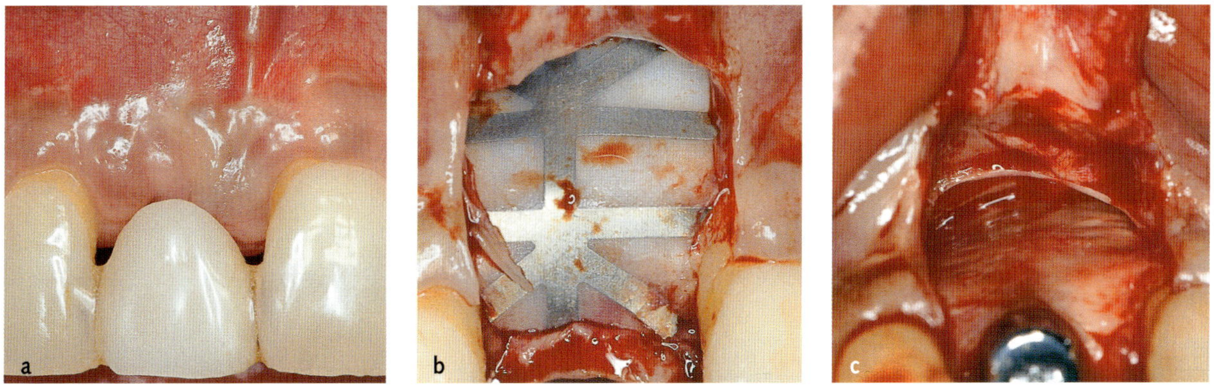

Fig 4-31 Implant placement. (a) Photograph of the site 8 months after surgery. (b) A full-thickness flap is raised, including the interdental papillae of the maxillary right lateral incisor and left central incisor. (c) After the titanium-reinforced membrane was removed, a Frialit-2 cylinder implant was installed utilizing a mallet. The pseudomembranous tissue under the membrane should ideally be removed; here the tissue is preserved. To allow coronal repositioning of the tissue, slitlike releasing incisions have been made at the MGJ to form three layers.

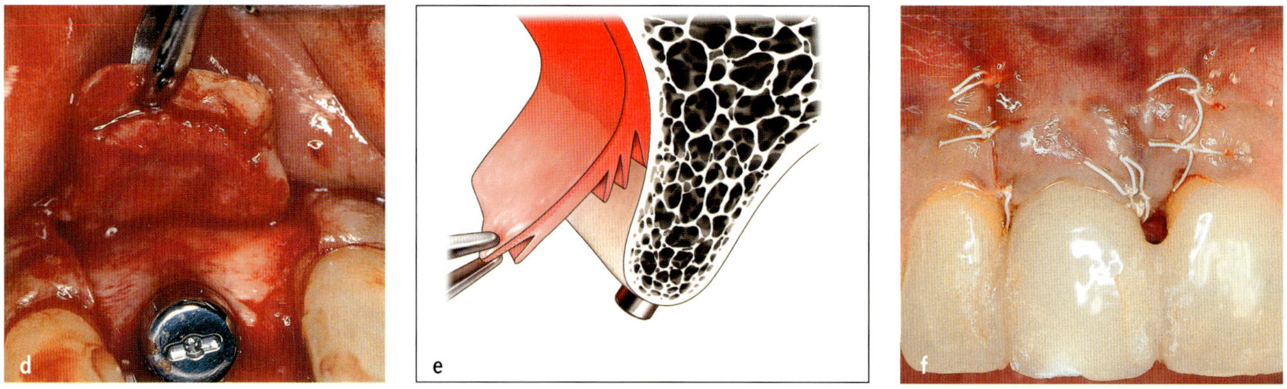

Fig 4-31 (cont) (d and e) To recover a natural emergence profile from the gingiva, slitlike releasing incisions are made at the upper part of the flap, and the coronal end of the flap is placed around the provisional restoration to enhance the harmony of the cervical margins. (f) A sling suture is used to reproduce the interdental papillae.

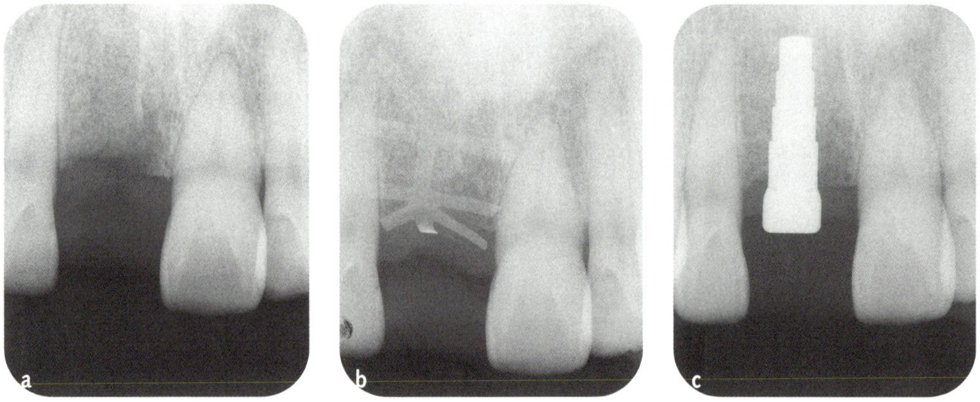

Fig 4-32 Bone changes. (a) At the first visit. (b) Guided bone regeneration with a titanium-reinforced membrane. (c) A Frialit-2 cylinder implant (4.5 × 13 mm) is installed.

Figs 4-33 to 4-35 Crown-lengthening procedure with a full-partial-full–thickness flap technique.

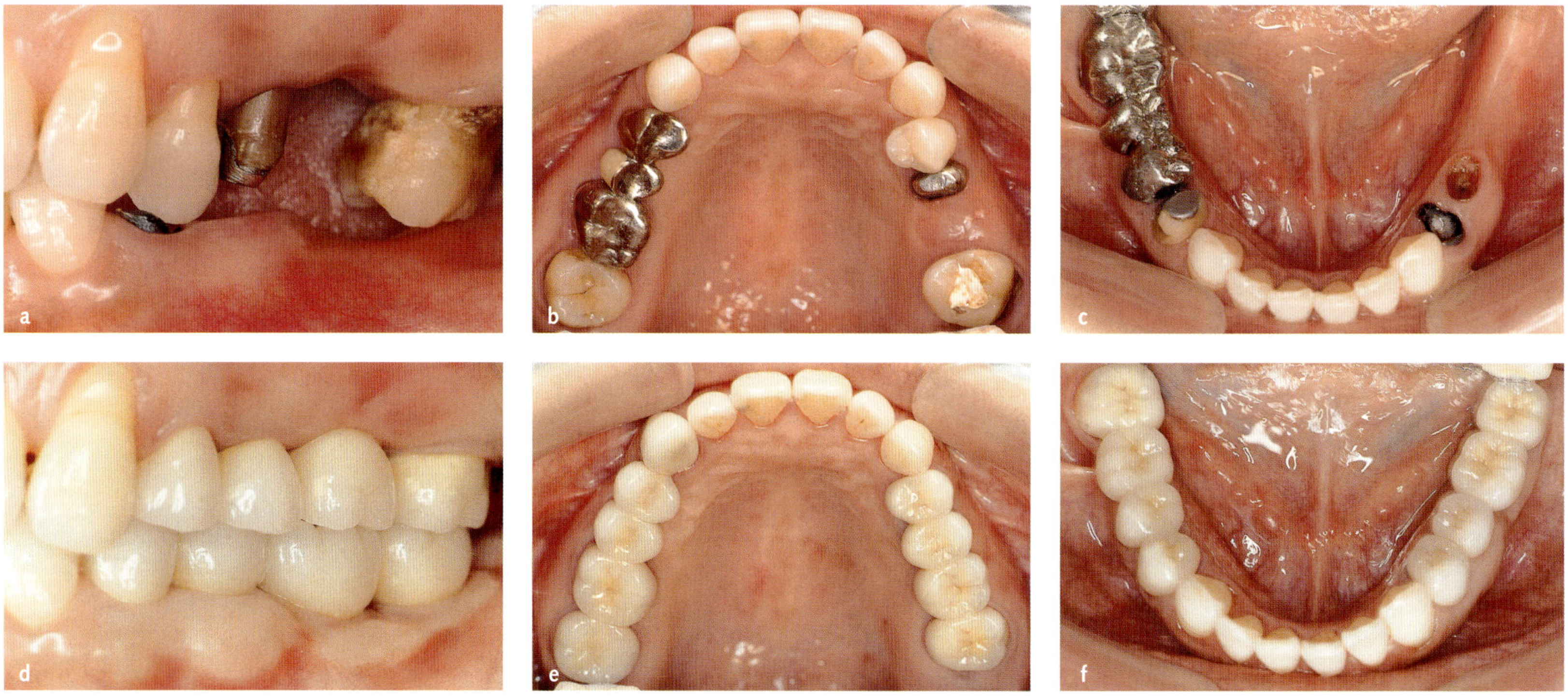

Fig 4-33 (a to c) At the first visit. The mandibular left first and second premolars were only residual roots. The mandibular left first and second molars were missing. (d to f) Photographs taken after 2 years 2 months. The occlusal support has been restored by placement of implants at the sites of the mandibular left first and second molars. Cervical margins are aligned and the interdental papilla-like tissue is restored. (Prostheses were made by Mr Kiyoharu Takada, RDT.)

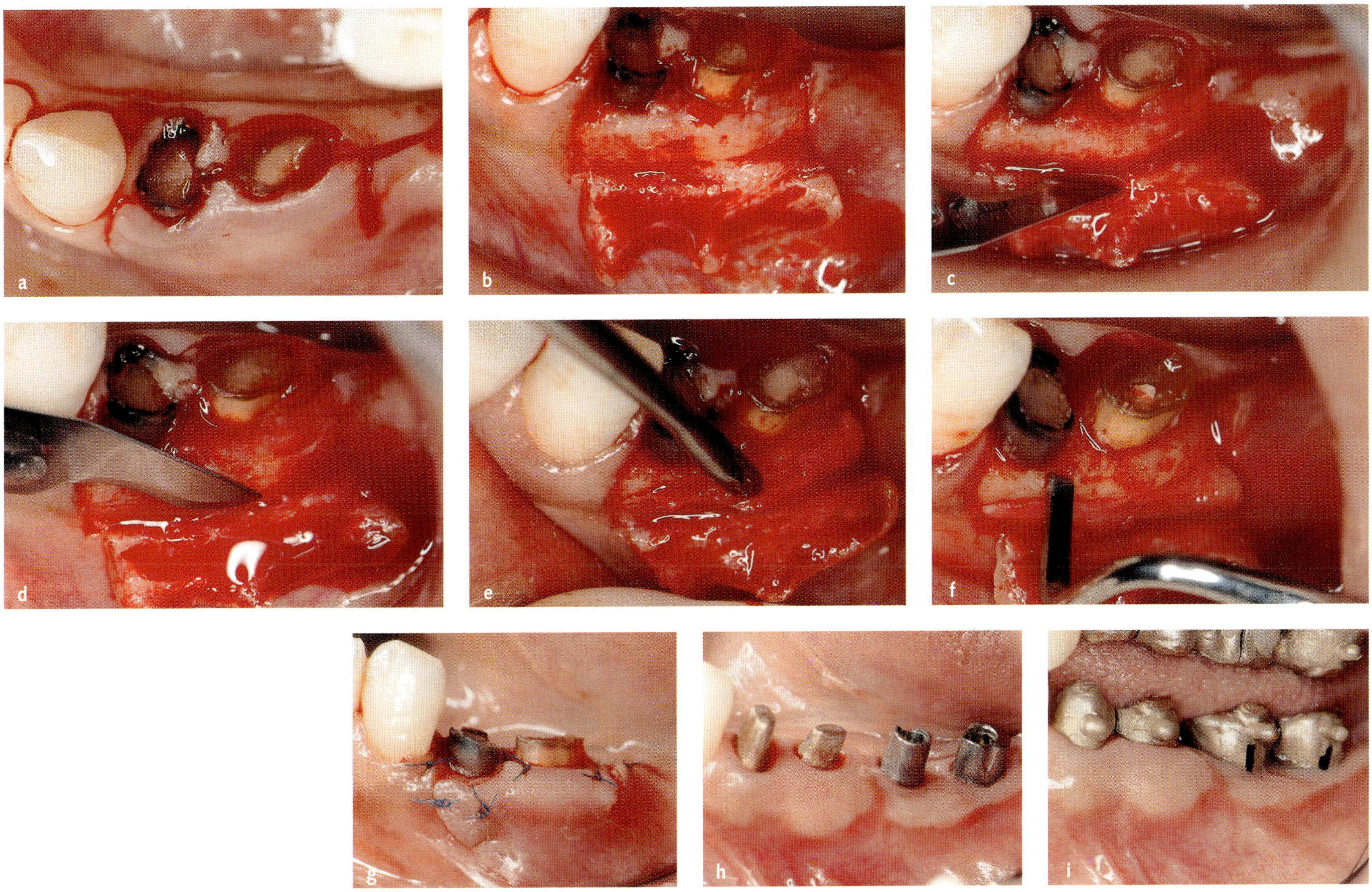

Fig 4-34 Clinical crown lengthening. (a) A vertical incision is made distal to the mandibular left second premolar (3 mm) while preserving the gingiva distal to the mandibular left canine. This vertical incision is not a divergent or widening design and is perpendicular to the bone surface. A sulcular incision reaching the bone surface is made on the buccal aspect of the mandibular left first and second premolars, and an inverse bevel incision is made on the lingual aspect of the mandibular left canine, first premolar, and second premolar to form a full-thickness flap. (b) On the buccal side, a No. 15C surgical blade is used to form a partial-thickness flap from the crest, and dissection is stopped before reaching the MGJ. (c) A horizontal incision is made to the periosteum, perpendicular to the bone surface. (d) A releasing incision is made to the apical aspect to form an additional layer in the full-thickness flap. (e) A raspatory is used to apically reflect the remaining periosteum on the buccal side of the mandibular left first and second premolars; care is taken not to crush the tissue. (f) About 2 mm of bone is removed with a bone chisel. (g) The flap is apically repositioned and sutured in a butt joint manner. (h) The provisional restoration is removed (1 year 8 months after surgery). (i) The metal framework is tried in to check fit. A pick-up impression is taken and appropriate emergence profile and occlusal surface design are created.

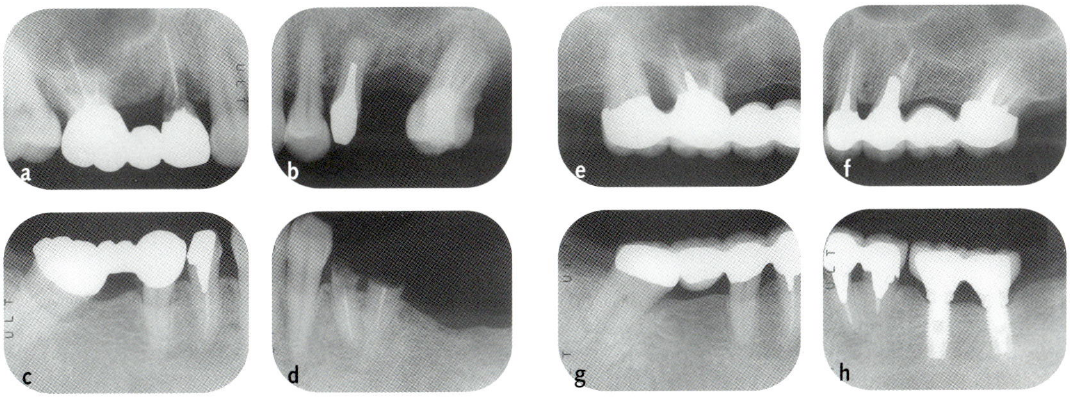

Fig 4-35 Recovery of molar occlusal support. (a to d) Radiographs at first visit. (e to h) Radiographs after 3 years 3 months of maintenance.

Partial-thickness flaps versus full-thickness flaps

A partial-thickness flap is formed by leaving the periosteum on the bone and allowing free repositioning of the flap, which provides options in handling of the flap. It also has the advantages of gaining attached gingiva and controlling horizontal thickness of the gingiva. Soft tissue has to be relatively thick to form a partial-thickness flap with a good blood supply. Inevitably, the periosteum is reflected to form a full-thickness flap in regions where osseous modification or resectioning is required in a large area or for infrabony defects where regeneration is expected. Coverage with periosteum is indispensable, espe-

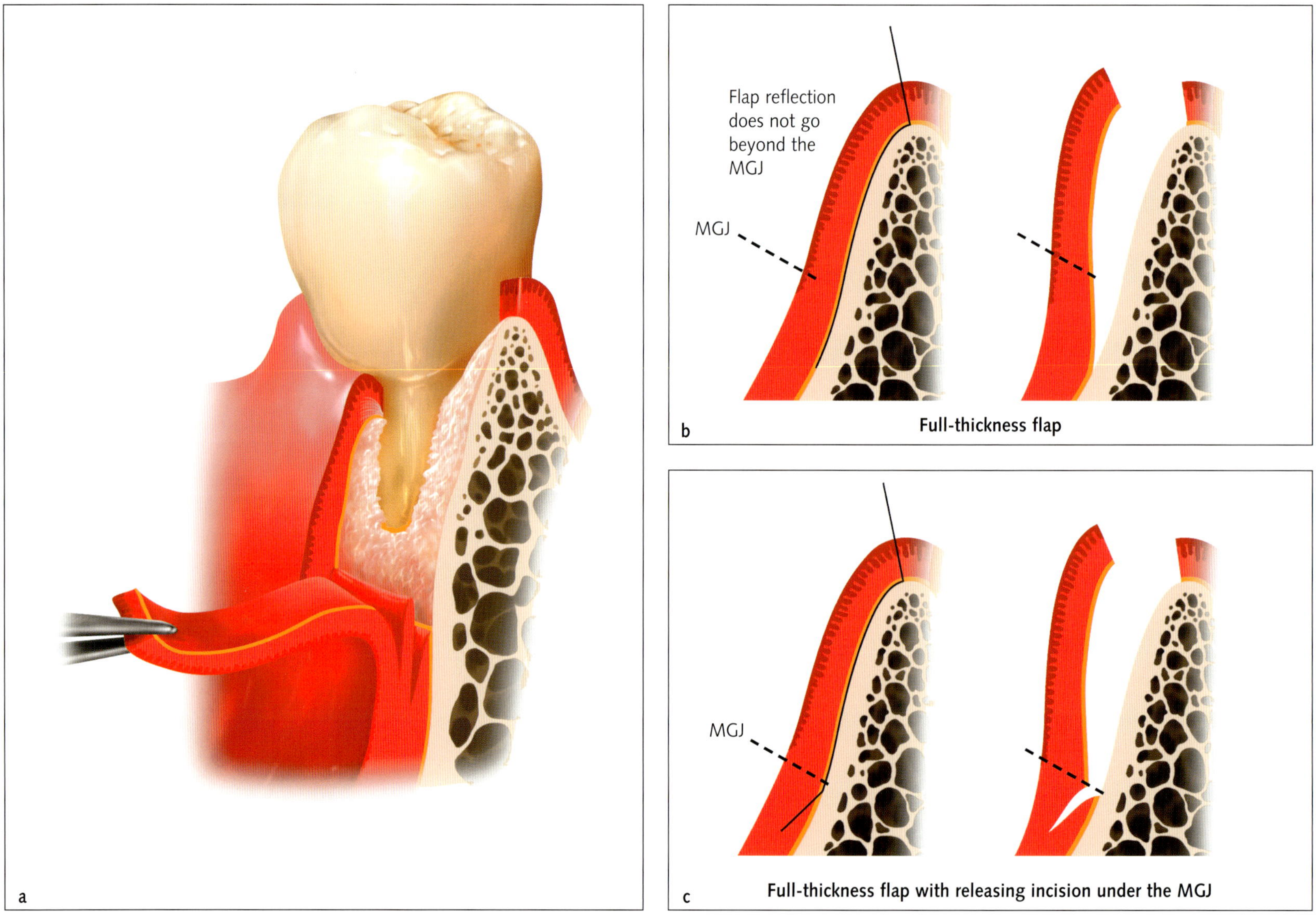

Fig 4-36 Preparation of a mucosal/mucoperiosteal flap. (a) In periodontal surgery aiming at preservation of interdental tissue, handling of the flap, especially the periosteum, in the region should focus on determination of the flap design. A full-thickness flap, or mucoperiosteal flap, has a role in bone regeneration. (b) Although a full-thickness flap is widely indicated, consideration should be given to the bone surface, which is exposed for hours. An inverse bevel incision or sulcular incision is made at the margin of the flap, depending on procedures. When the flap is reflected apically beyond the MGJ, flap stabilization becomes difficult. (c) This procedure is used in regenerative therapy. Vertical incisions are utilized to allow coronal repositioning of the flap. After the full-thickness flap is reflected down to the MGJ, two to three layers are formed with 2- to 3-mm-deep releasing incisions used in the partial-thickness flap preparation.

cially for bone regeneration, and advancement of a pedicle full-thickness flap is also advantageous for this purpose. Because a partial-thickness flap can cause significant pain in some procedures, accurate and delicate techniques are demanded. Postoperative healing is largely affected by the degree of damage to the periosteum. Consequently, selection and possible combination of the two techniques depend on local conditions and objectives; ideally a technique that will maximize the advantages is chosen (Fig 4-36; also see Table 4-2).

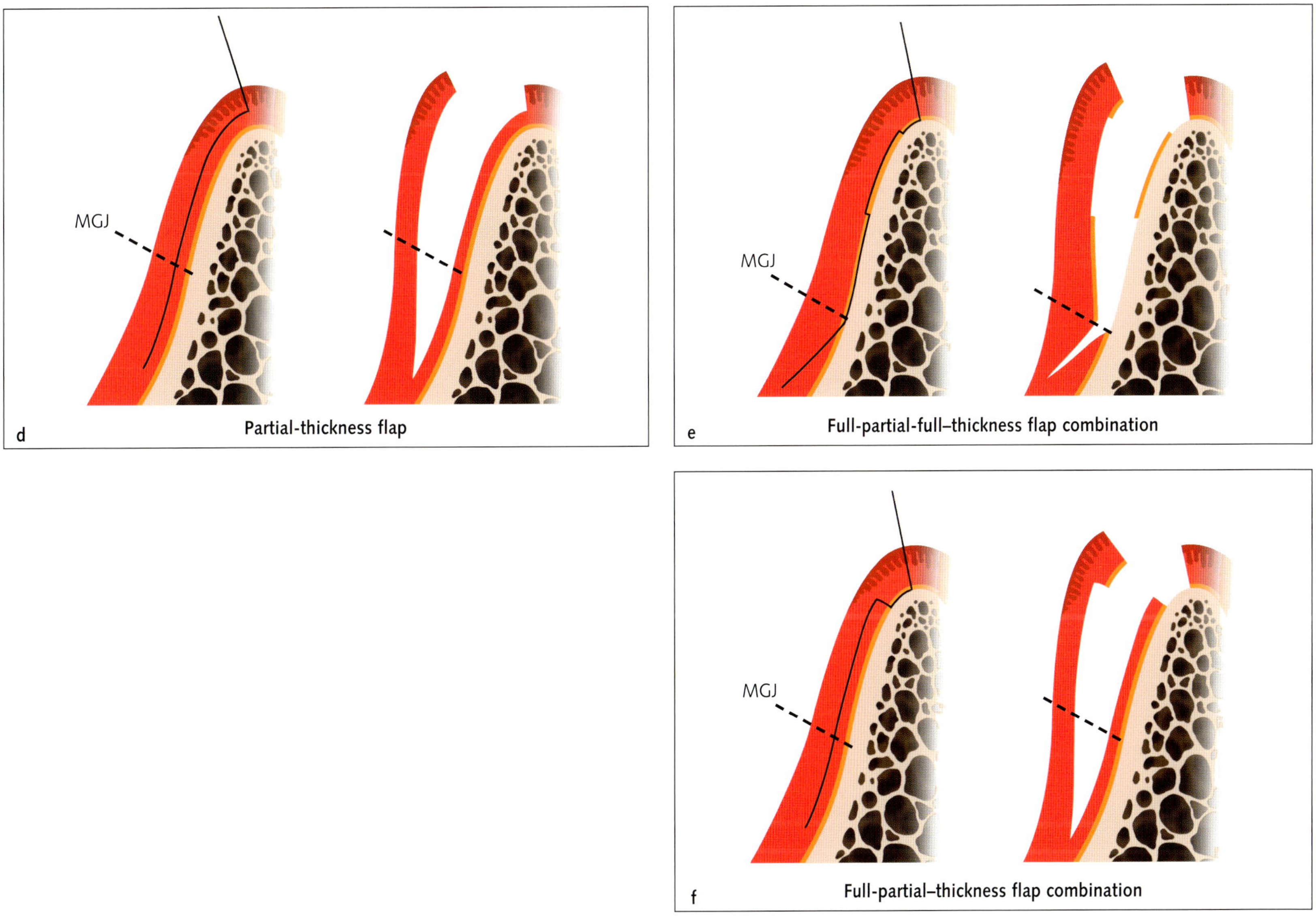

(d) This procedure is used mostly for an apical or lateral repositioning of the flap. Dissection is made from the margin of the gingiva, forming a mucosal layer and a periosteal layer, to extend beyond the MGJ. A vertical incision is essential to enable flap repositioning. In a case of resective therapy with osseous surgery, a partial-thickness flap is formed first, and then the periosteum around the bone crest is carefully reflected. After osseous surgery, the periosteum is replaced. (e) This procedure is used primarily in cases with exostosis or thin mucosa. First, a sulcular incision is made to form a full-thickness flap, then immediately the flap is shifted to a partial-thickness design to allow positioning of the flap. After the design is switched to a full-thickness flap again, a releasing incision is made right at the MGJ. (f) This procedure is used for apical repositioning of a flap involving osseous surgery. A sulcular incision is made to form a full-thickness flap, and an incision is made to shift to a partial-thickness flap, extending beyond the MGJ. Osseous surgery is completed at the full-thickness flap area.

Construction of Maintainable Periodontal Tissue

Restoration of natural tooth–periodontal tissue structure

Clinical treatment goals in advanced periodontal disease include construction of maintainable periodontal tissue (Fig 4-37). A number of ideas, procedures, and thoughts about the morphology of prostheses have been presented, all of which are based on clinical experience and include concepts that are contrary to each other. Should periodontal pockets be eliminated, reduced, or maintained for construction of a maintainable periodontal environment? After much discussion, conclusions have not been reached. Is a minimal amount of attached gingiva necessary? Clinical research data suggest it is necessary, but we cannot agree based on our clinical experience. With regard to crown contour, some clinicians recommend a reverse contour from the viewpoint of plaque accumulation rate, while others maintain that a certain amount of contour is necessary to protect the marginal gingiva. Two different ideas exist concerning interproximal embrasures. The first is to have the embrasures wide open so that an interdental cleaning device can be used, and the second is to close the embrasure with the interdental papilla. In treating class II furcation involvements, a variety of approaches have been tried, from resectioning to eliminate the ledge and improve the instrument access by barreling or fluting to coverage of the ledge by a coronal repositioning flap using regenerative therapy. Despite those efforts, satisfactory outcomes have not yet been achieved.

The meaning of a maintainable environment is different, depending on the pathosis, the region, and the patient. We must admit that we had to go through a trial-and-error process. We have always focused on treatment for the dentogingival complex, aiming at achieving healing close to the natural tooth-periodontal tissue, especially at the bone level.

Loss of interdental papillae

Loss of the interdental papillae cannot be avoided after periodontal surgery, but it can be minimized to a certain degree by adjusting the contour of a prosthesis. For postoperative toothbrushing during pocket maintenance therapy, a rolling technique that is less damaging to the gingiva is recommended. The authors have tried to ensure toothbrush access in periodontal pockets in clinical cases where pocket maintenance is required. We developed a periodontal pocket brush, the Pocket Cleaner, and marketed it. A prosthesis of the appropriate volume and a patient's diligent self-care using the rolling toothbrushing technique and Pocket Cleaners enhance maintenance predictability in many clinical cases, and an increase in the gingival height has been observed.

A Pocket Cleaner does not always need to reach the bottom of the pocket. By inserting the soft brush to the upper part of the pocket, oxygen is believed to be provided to the pocket and the bacterial flora is agitated, allowing maintenance of healthy bacterial flora in a deep periodontal pocket, similar to that seen in a shallow pocket.

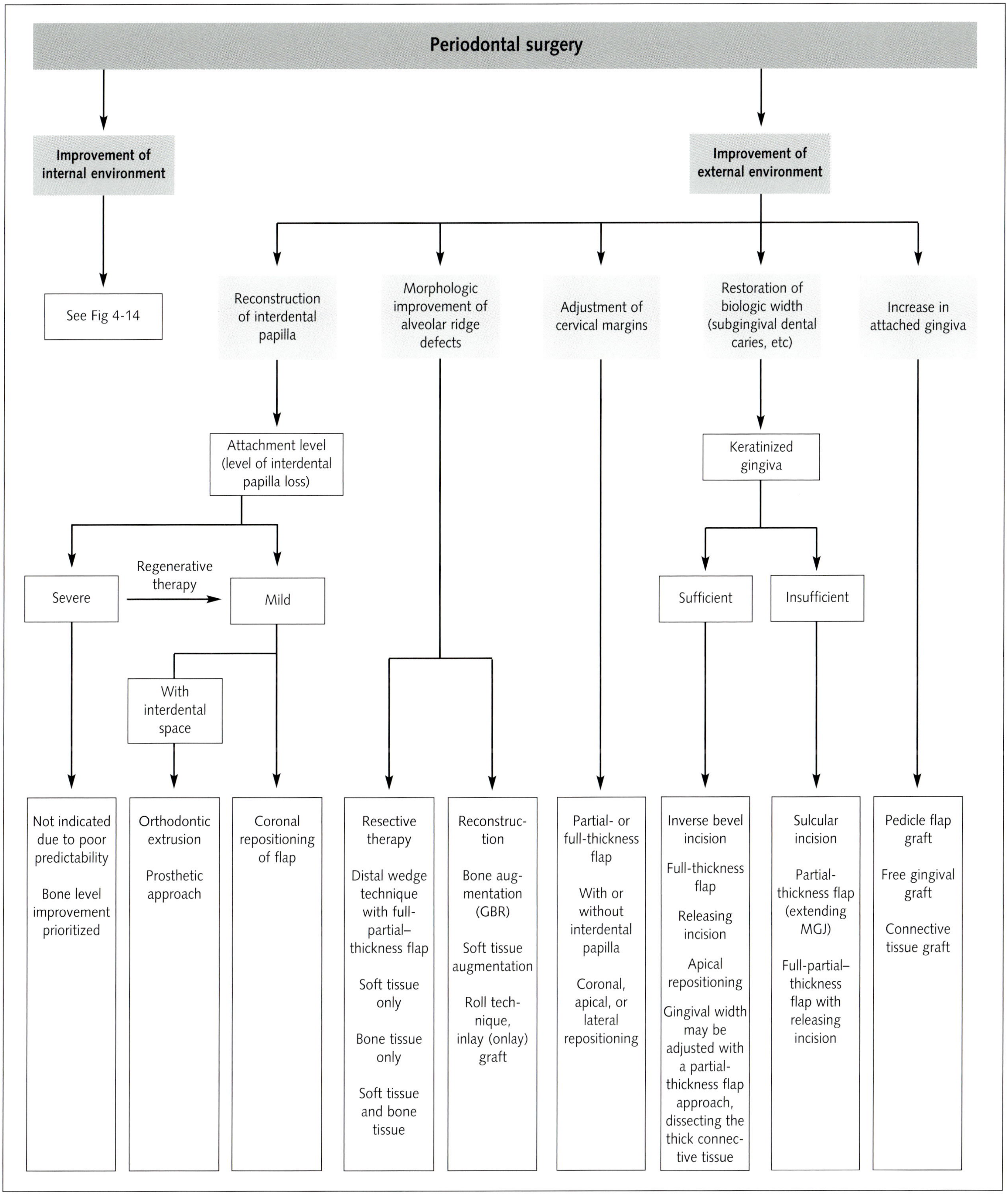

Fig 4-37 Improvement of the external environment.

Subgingival contour

Tooth reduction in the preparation and restoration contour should be adjusted, depending on the progress of the periodontal disease, region, tooth axis inclination, root proximity, and gingival conditions. In regions with advanced periodontal disease, the thickness of the gingiva is increased and the interdental space is enlarged, changing the gingival contour significantly compared to a healthy condition. Consequently, the subgingival contour of a prosthesis has to be adjusted according to local conditions (Fig 4-38). When the tooth is inclined lingually, there is an increase in the thickness of the labial gingiva, and sufficient subgingival contour has to be provided to the labial side. In a case with close root proximity, the required space has to be assured in the interdental area through sufficient tooth reduction and controlled contour.

Figure 4-39 and Case 4-2 demonstrate the benefits of careful gingival preparation before prosthetic intervention.

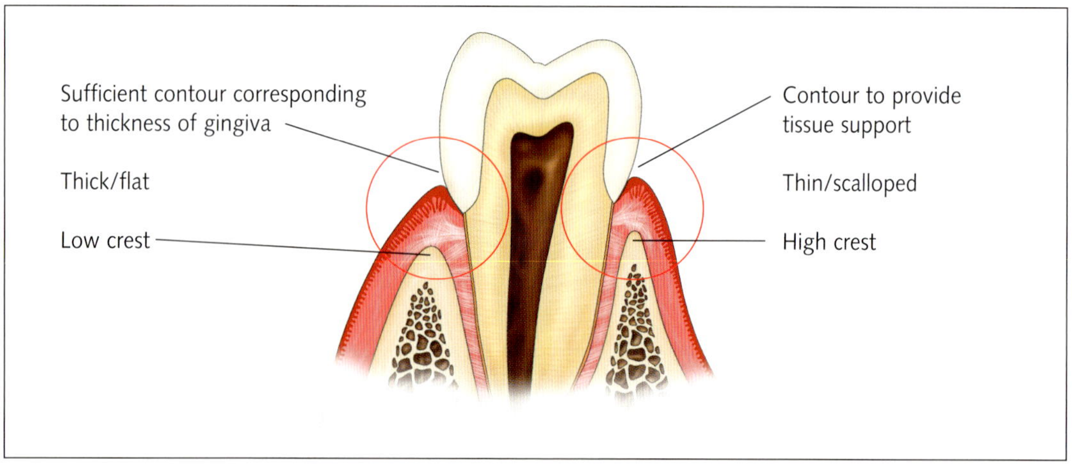

Fig 4-38 Subgingival contouring of the prosthesis is said to have a role in proper support of the gingiva. Relatively strong contours are needed when the gingiva is thick. Consideration should be also given to the inclination of the tooth axis, tooth type, and buccolingual or proximal surface differences. Gingiva becomes thicker in periodontal tissue with attachment loss, for which a relatively stronger contour is required.

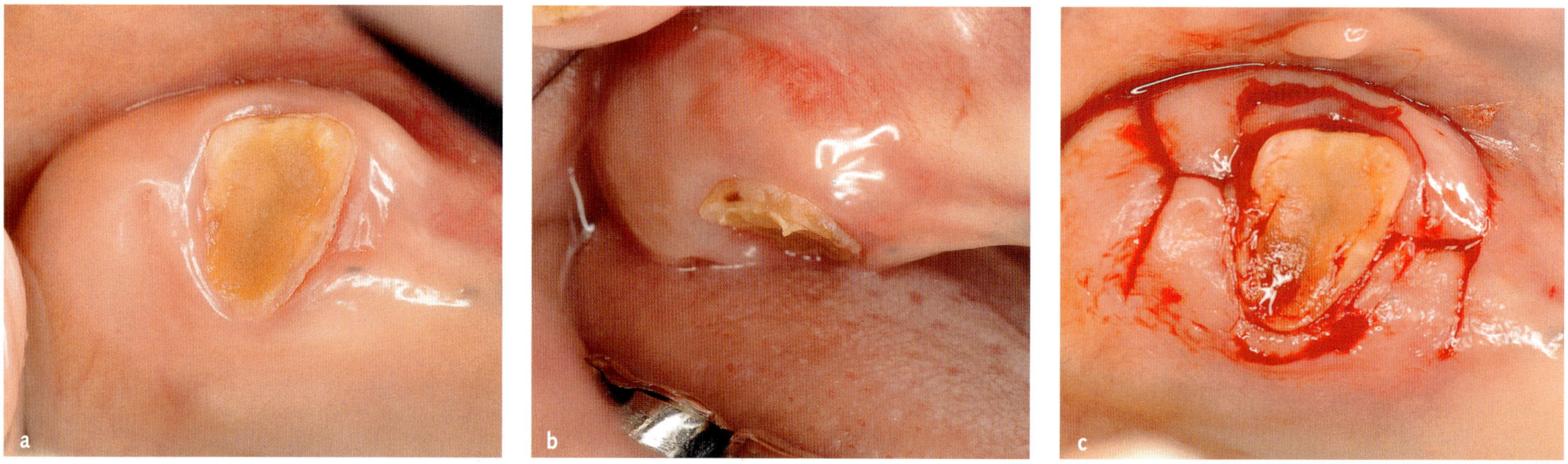

Fig 4-39 Clinical crown lengthening for an isolated residual root of a maxillary molar. (a and b) Residual root of the maxillary right second molar after root canal treatment. (c) An inverse bevel incision and vertical incision are made symmetrically.

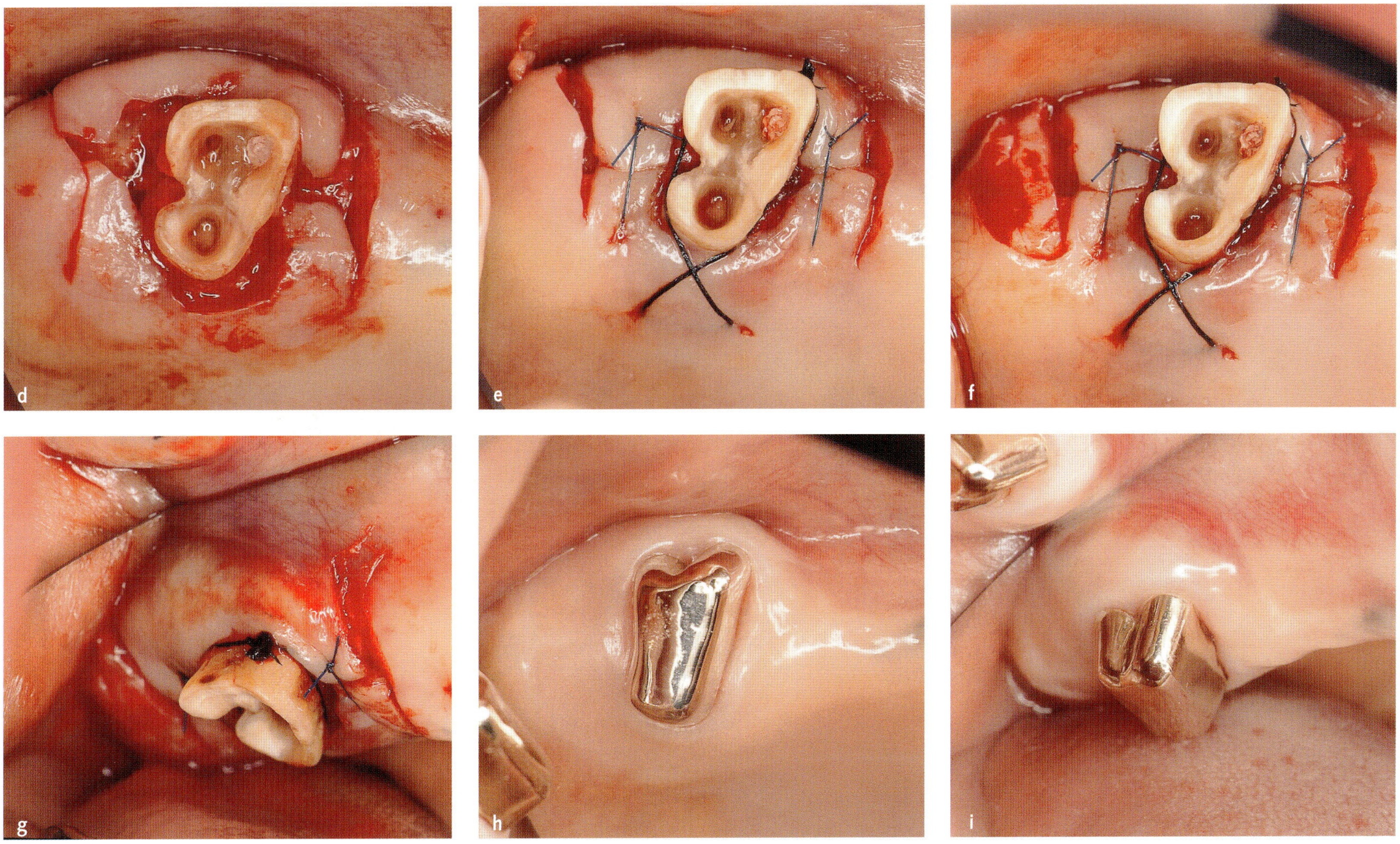

(d) It is important to elevate a full-thickness flap carefully without damaging the periosteum. (e) The connective tissue is dissected, leaving a uniform thickness of the gingiva on the buccal and palatal sides, and removed as one piece to allow bone resectioning. Symmetric simple sutures are made without excessive tension, and cross sutures are made on the palatal aspect. (f and g) Excess gingiva on the palatal aspect is resected to complete the procedure. (h and i) Photographs taken 1 year postsurgery.

Case 4-2 Resective therapy using a partial-thickness flap

Patient: *61 years old at the time of first visit in 1997*
With secondary dental caries, malocclusion caused by restorations, and poorly treated root canals after pulpectomies, this patient seemed to have iatrogenic problems. The conditions almost caused a collapse of the occlusion. The patient exhibited a generally disturbed occlusal plane, deformed dental arches, and tooth migration. Here focus is given to the treatment of the subgingival dental caries of the mandibular right first molar, which exhibited a narrow vestibule and limited attached gingiva (Figs 4-40 to 4-43).

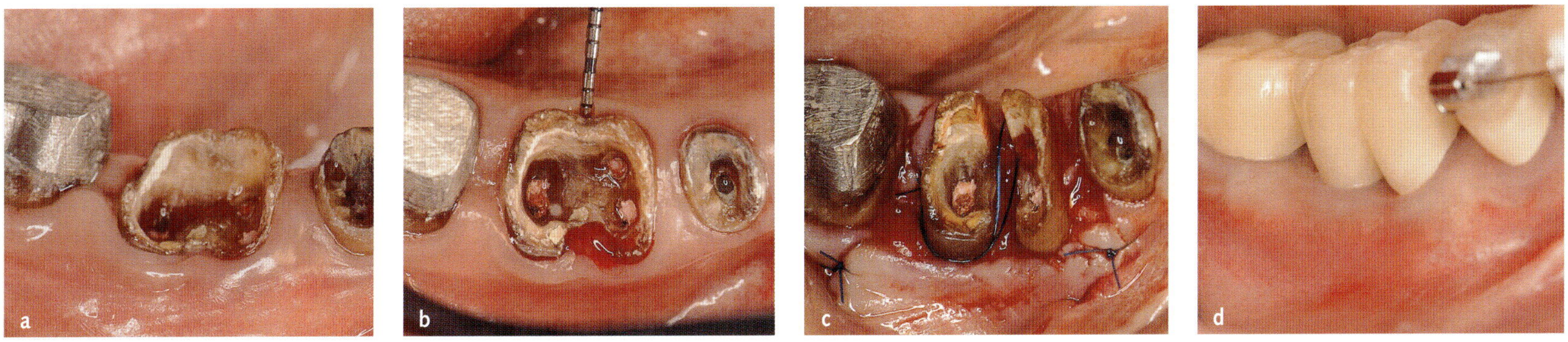

Fig 4-40 Treatment of subgingival dental caries of the mandibular right first molar. (a and b) Photographs taken 1 year 6 months after the first visit. In conjunction with plaque control, a temporary root canal filling is placed. A provisional restoration is placed and orthodontic tooth movement is performed, until the patient is ready for the final stage of treatment. The mandibular right first molar has a class III furcation involvement with subgingival caries and only 1 to 2 mm of attached gingiva. (c) A sulcular incision is made to form a full-partial–thickness flap without loss of the attached gingiva, and the flap is apically repositioned. After osseous surgery, the tooth is hemisected. (d) After a 3-month healing period for the periodontal tissue, orthodontic treatment was restarted. (Photograph taken 6 months after surgery.)

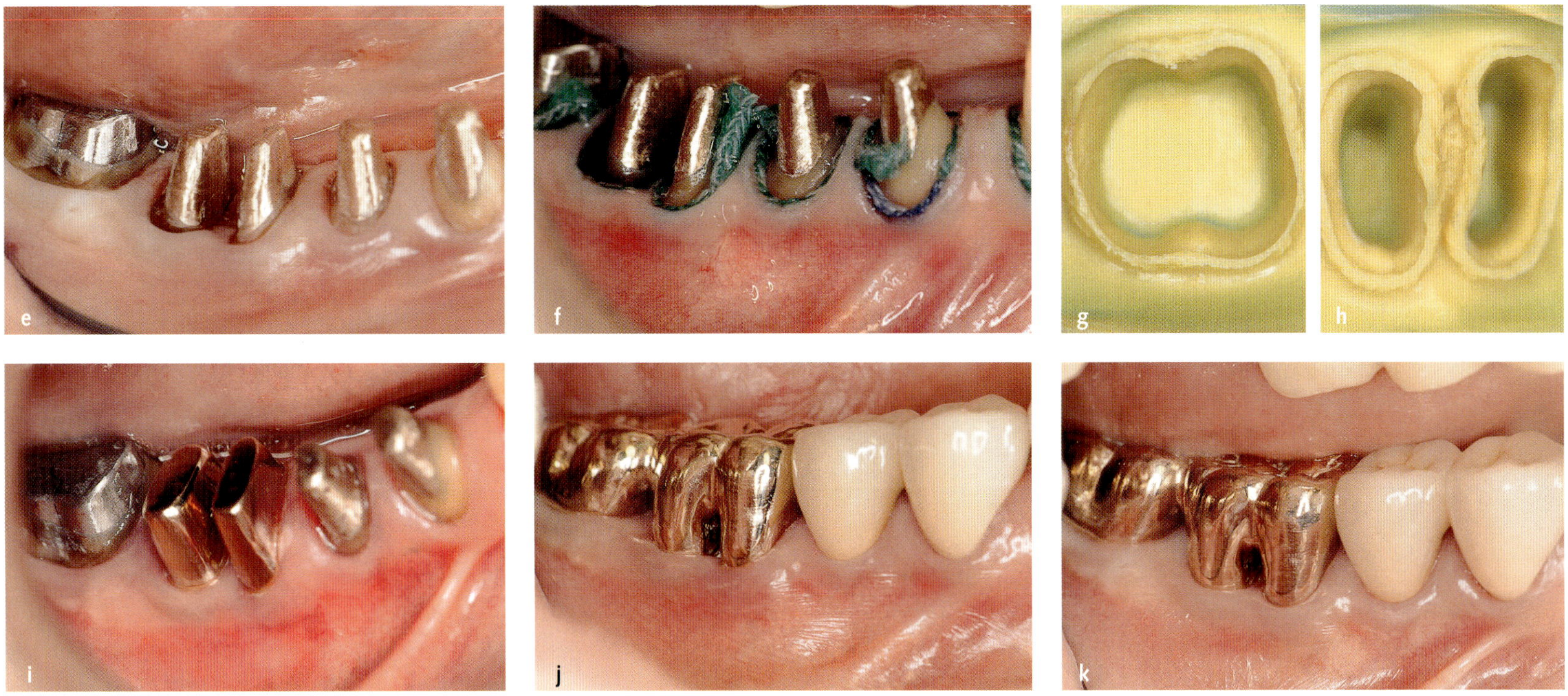

Fig 4-40 (cont) (e) Photograph taken 1 year after surgery. An impression is taken for the final prostheses. (f) The attached gingiva is insufficient, requiring careful and delicate handling of the gingival retraction in using a double-cord technique. A three-cord technique is used for the mandibular right first premolar. (g and h) Distinct margins are reproduced. It is necessary to obtain an impression without tears or voids in the impression material. (i) To maintain parallelism and prevent root fracture, coping crowns are delivered. (j) Delivery of the final prostheses. (k) Photograph taken 1 year 8 months after delivery of the final prostheses.

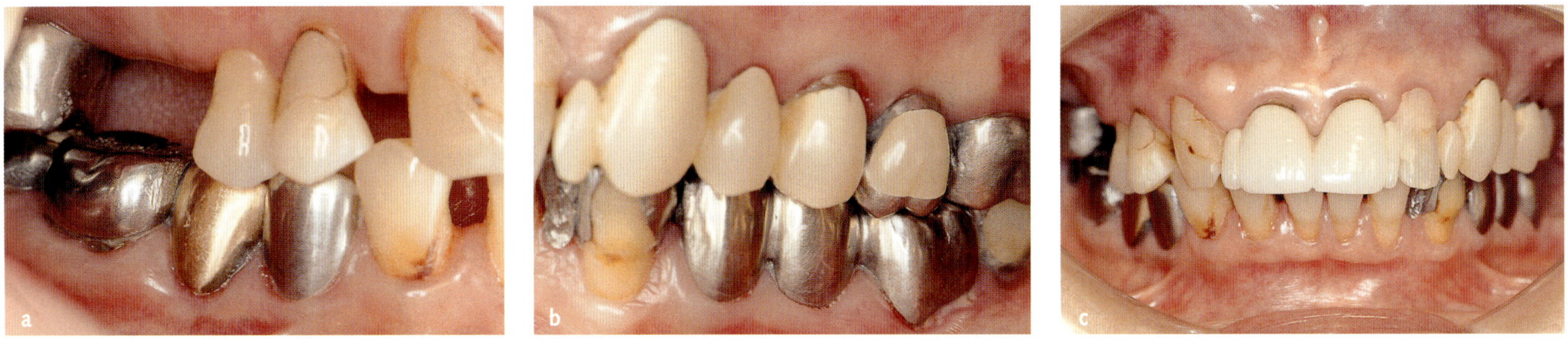

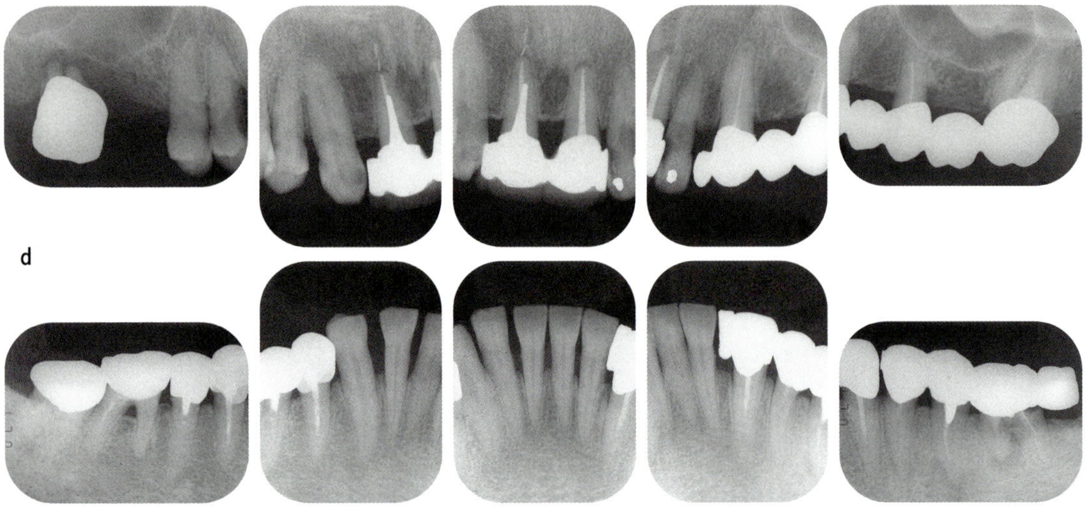

Fig 4-41 (a to c) Clinical photographs taken at first visit, showing the poor occlusal plane and extrusion of the maxillary right first and second premolars. Cantilever pontics are used to fill interdental gaps. (d) Radiographic examination reveals inappropriately treated root canals, extremely poor-fitting prostheses, subgingival secondary caries, and occlusal trauma. The mandibular left first molar presents combined endodontic-periodontal lesions.

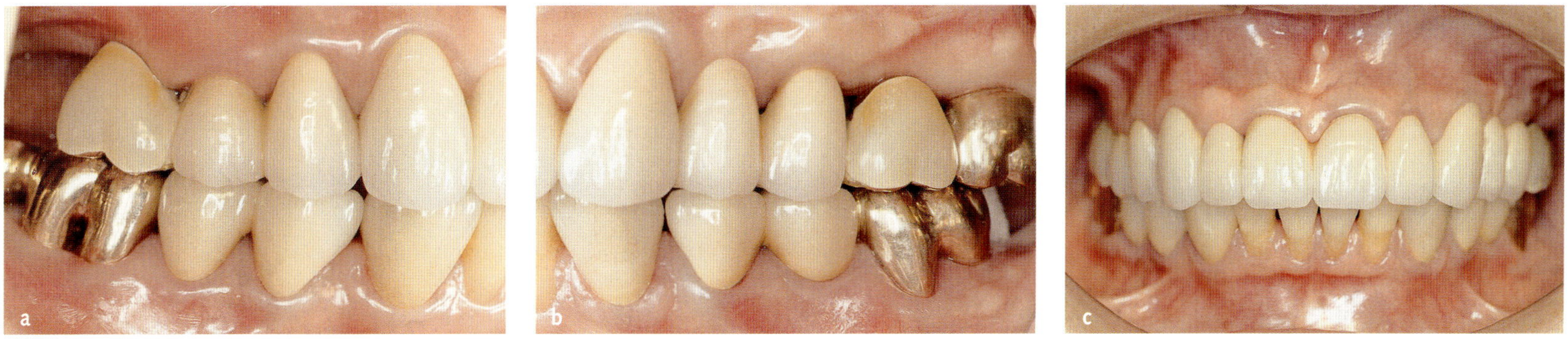

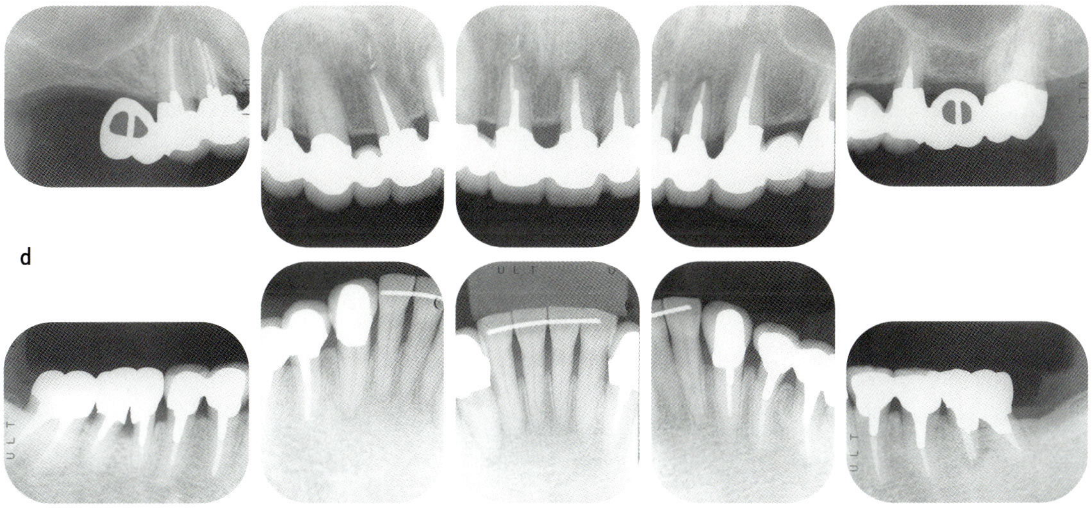

Fig 4-42 (a and b) Lateral views photographed 3 years 3 months after the first visit. Occlusal planes have been improved and harmony of the cervical margins has been restored through tooth movement and restorations. A free gingival graft was conducted for the mandibular left first molar after natural extrusion. (c) Photograph taken 4 years 3 months after the first visit. (d) There is less radiographic evidence of trauma.

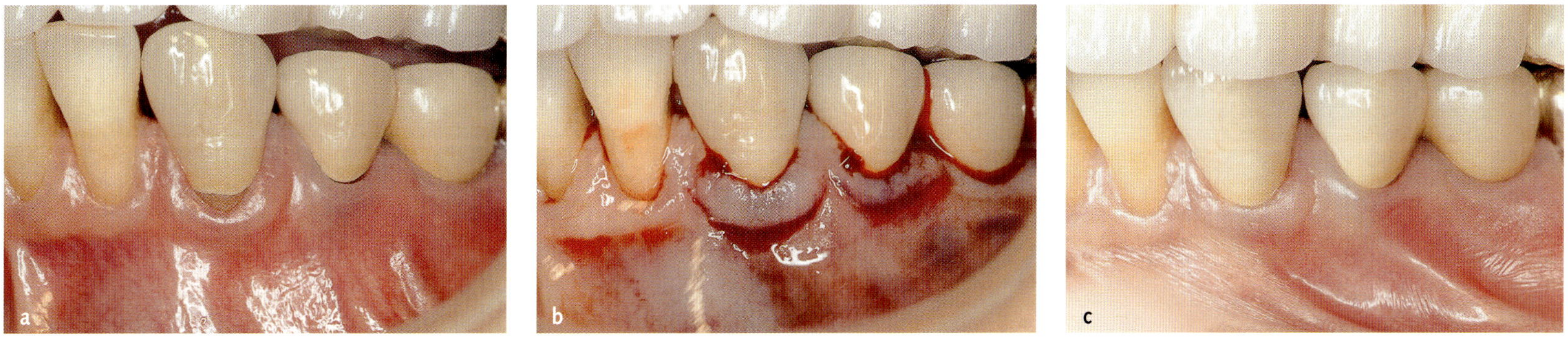

Fig 4-43 Gingival recession during the maintenance phase. (a) A metal collar is exposed because of gingival recession during the maintenance phase. (b) The Turner method (semi-luner incision) is used to improve the gingival morphology. (c) Photograph taken 20 days after surgery. Conditions are improved.

Management of Furcation Involvement

Key challenge of periodontal therapy

Attachment loss in molars may invite furcation involvement. Because of its complicated anatomy, the furcation area is challenging for accurate probing and radiographic examination. Removal of calculus with a curette is difficult. It is impossible to freely insert the blade of the curette into the narrow furcation space. Lesions of endodontic origin often communicate with the periodontal pockets, resulting in so-called endodontic-periodontal lesions. With moderate levels of attachment loss, tooth mobility is not observed. By the time symptoms are subjectively noticed, the disease is generally considerably advanced. As such, even at the tooth-unit level, it is difficult to observe the pathologic conditions, and debridement of the contaminated root surfaces is extremely difficult. In most cases, some traumatic factors as well as an interruption of the dentition's continuity and integrity are combined. Accordingly, the dentition-unit or occlusion-unit approach is required in advanced furcation involvement. It is no exaggeration to say that treatment of advanced periodontal disease boils down to treatment of furcation involvements.

Management of furcation involvement

Advanced furcation involvement does not respond well to initial therapy. During initial therapy, exacerbations of inflammation are often repeated, resulting in rapid destruction of the supporting tissue. Aggressive intervention at a relatively earlier stage is required. Maintenance of the furcation involvement presents many difficulties, as shown here, and the treatment prognosis of the lesion is not at all assured. Because of this, mild furcation involvement should utilize an approach that does not expose the furcation area (Figs 4-44 to 4-48). Aggressive intervention should be limited to Lindhe's class II (one-third or more horizontal loss of supporting tissue, which does not extend to the entire furcation area), Rosenberg's class II (2-mm or greater horizontal probing depth at the furcation), or more advanced lesions.

Conservative treatment of furcation involvement

Even if deep bony defects are identified, acute alveolar abscesses triggered by trauma can be expected to experience restoration of attachment, if contamination of the root surfaces is not advanced. The possibility of conservative therapy should be considered (see Figs 4-44 to 4-48), because maintenance of exposed furcation regions is difficult (Figs 4-49 to 4-55).

Maintenance of exposed furcation regions

About 10 years passed after the previously described procedures to expose the furcation region were completed. Dental caries of the exposed root surface was considerably more advanced 8 years posttreatment (see Figs 4-49 to 4-55). Various restorative measures were contrived, including an increase in the attached gingiva, modification of the crown morphology, and improvement in hygiene methods. Still, the risk for tooth loss is high.

Figs 4-44 to 4-48 Conservative treatment of furcation involvement

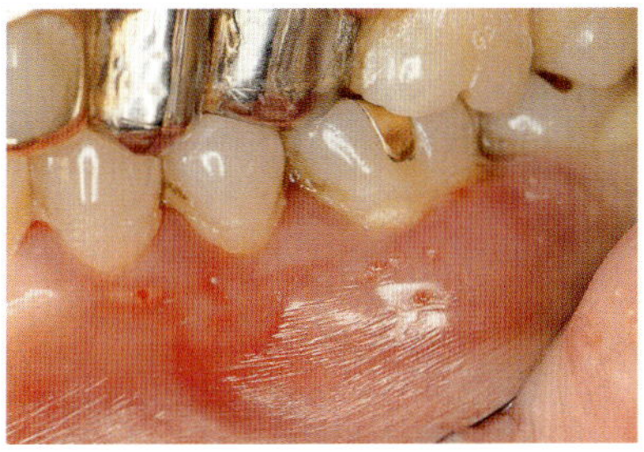

Fig 4-44 At the first visit, an acute alveolar abscess of the mandibular left first molar and signs of clenching are noted.

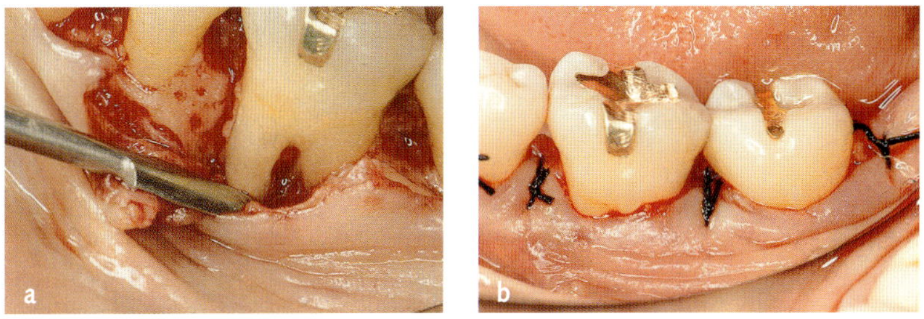

Fig 4-45 (a) After resolution of the inflammation, surgery is performed with a full-thickness flap. Debridement of the root surfaces, removal of the granulation tissue, and root surface treatment with tetracycline-saturated solution are conducted. (b) A flap is coronally repositioned and tightly sutured.

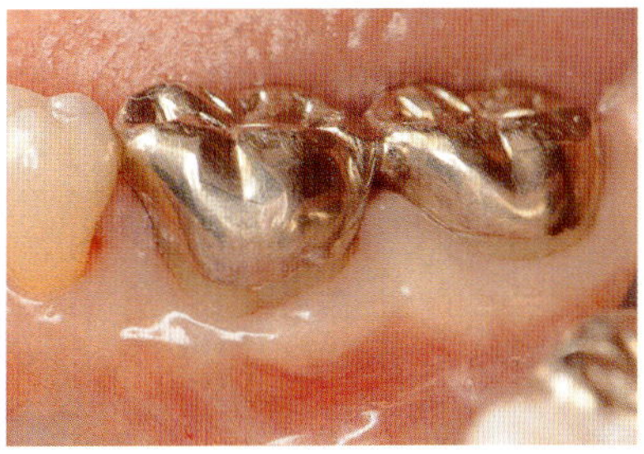

Fig 4-46 Photograph taken 7 years 4 months after the first visit. Crown restoration of the mandibular left first and second molars was conducted to improve the occlusion.

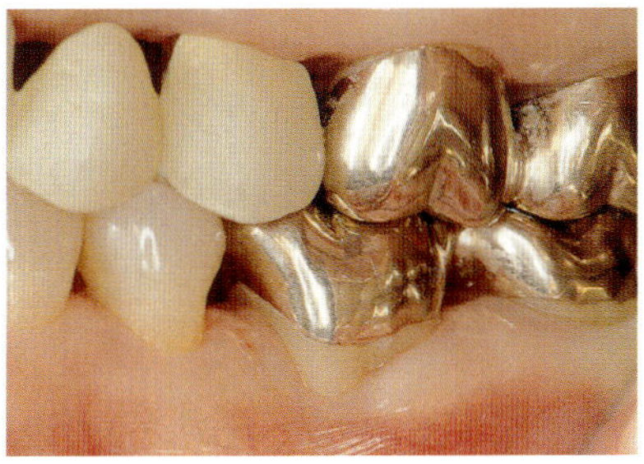

Fig 4-47 Photograph taken 6 years 10 months after surgery (7 years 3 months after the first visit.)

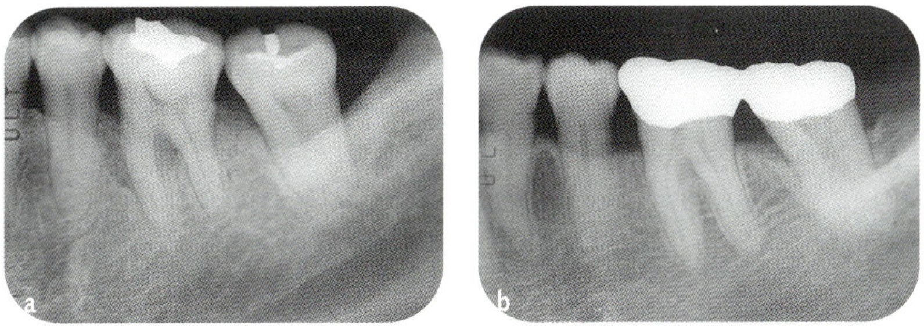

Fig 4-48 (a) At the first visit. (b) Radiograph taken 7 years 4 months after the first visit. Bone regeneration is observed.

Figs 4-49 to 4-55 Maintenance of exposed furcation regions

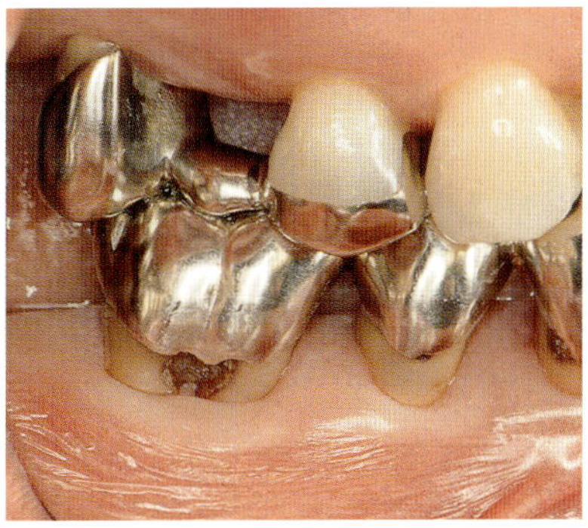

Fig 4-49 Dental caries of the exposed root surface is advanced.

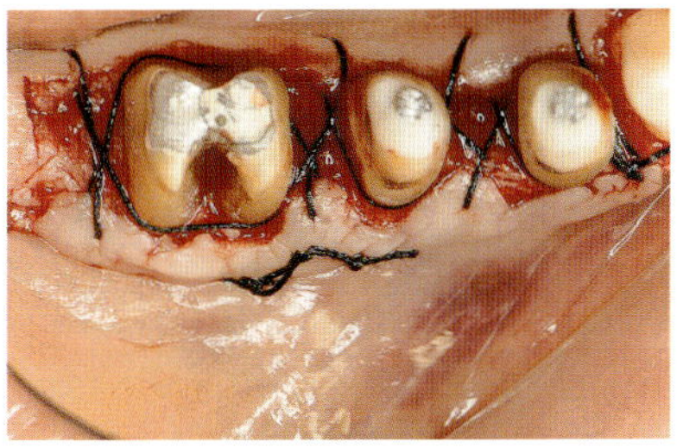

Fig 4-50 Photograph taken 6 months after the first visit. Because of root caries of the exposed furcation area, clinical crown-lengthening and contouring procedures are conducted with an apical repositioning of a partial-thickness flap.

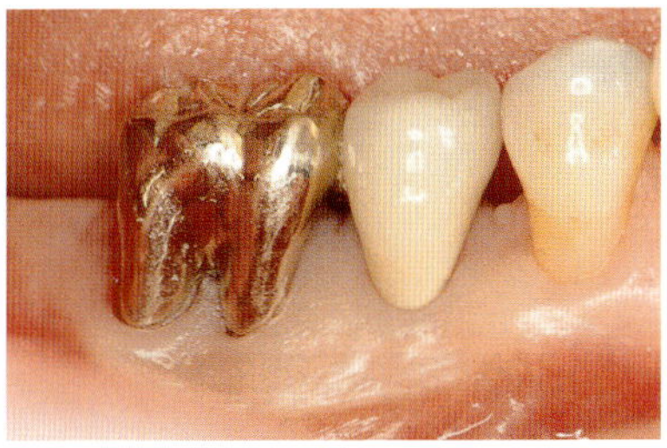

Fig 4-51 Photograph taken 1 year 5 months after surgery. Conditions are stable.

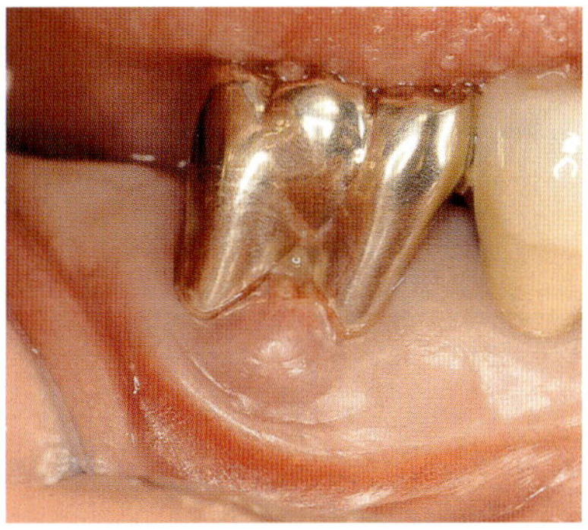

Fig 4-52 Photograph taken 5 years 10 months after surgery. Gingival swelling is visible in the furcation area.

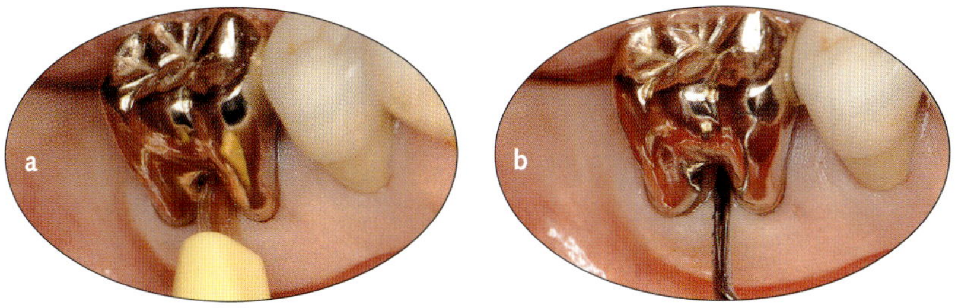

Fig 4-53 (a and b) Photographs taken 6 years 6 months after surgery. Instructions about toothbrushing and the use of an intersulcular brush were given.

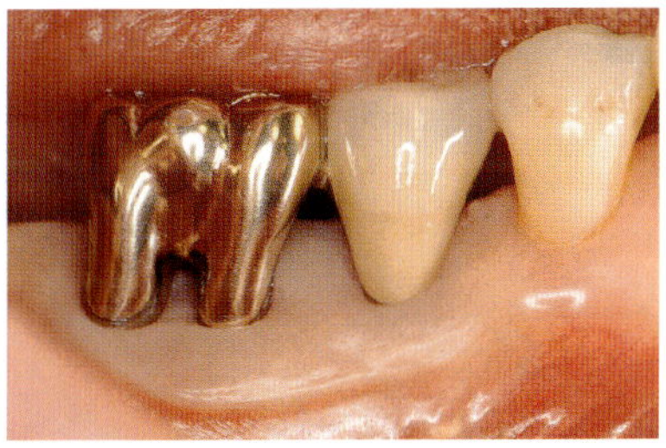

Fig 4-54 Photograph taken 7 years after surgery.

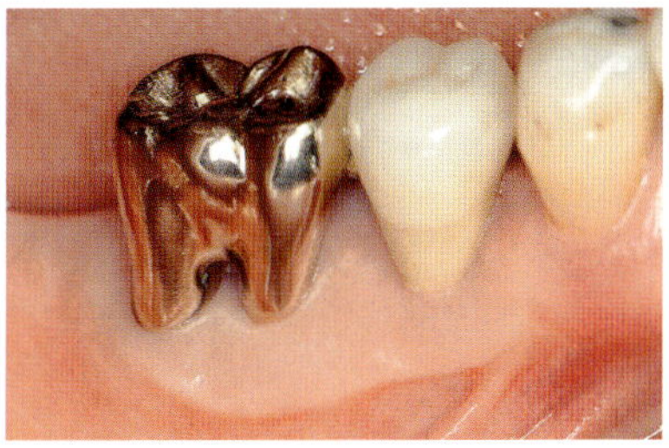

Fig 4-55 Photograph taken 10 years 2 months after surgery. Root caries is noted again in the furcation area, reminding us of the difficulty of maintenance.

From resective therapy to regenerative therapy

Treatments for advanced furcation involvement vary, depending on the morphology of the furcation area and roots, progression of the defects, and prosthodontic conditions. However, the treatment choices are roughly divided into (1) exposure, (2) elimination, and (3) regeneration. Conventionally, general approaches have been exposure via tunneling and elimination of the furcation itself via extraction, root amputation, and hemisection (Figs 4-56 to 4-67). After root amputation and hemisection are completed, orthodontic treatment has to be conducted to adjust a sectional and to align the bony contour in the furcation area (Figs 4-68 to 4-74). A bony contour line can be improved to a certain degree by natural extrusion.

Today, with the improved prognosis of regenerative therapy, it is possible to utilize procedures expecting new attachment at the furcation area via regenerative therapy with a membrane and autogenous bone (or a bone alternative material) and/or regenerative therapy with an enamel matrix derivative (Figs 4-75 to 4-81).

Pocket elimination surgery and maintenance

Although periodontal pockets are removed by pocket elimination surgery, furcation areas will be exposed supragingivally when a deep bony defect exists. In other words, the maintenance challenge is increased in exchange for elimination of the periodontal pocket (see Figs 4-56 to 4-64).

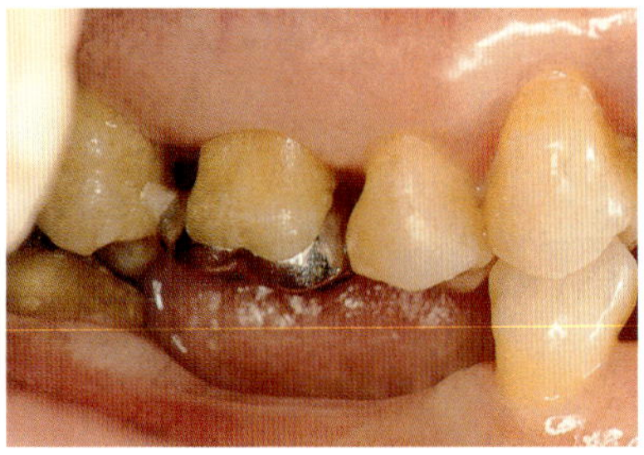

Fig 4-56 At the first visit (July 1989). Missing opposing teeth had been left untreated, causing extrusion of the maxillary right second molar, first molar, and second premolar.

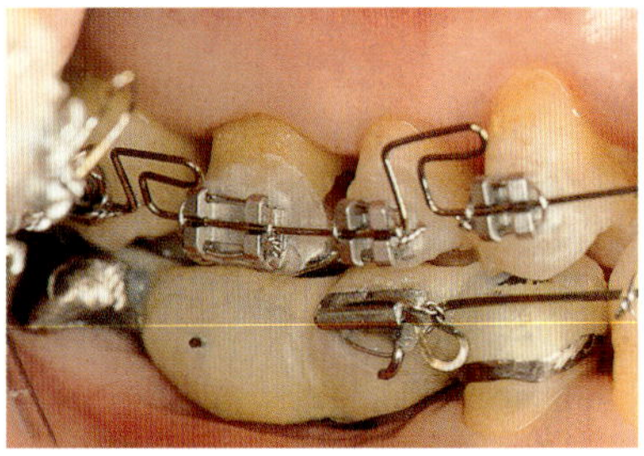

Fig 4-57 To restore the occlusal plane, the maxillary right second molar, first molar, and second premolar are intruded (December 1989).

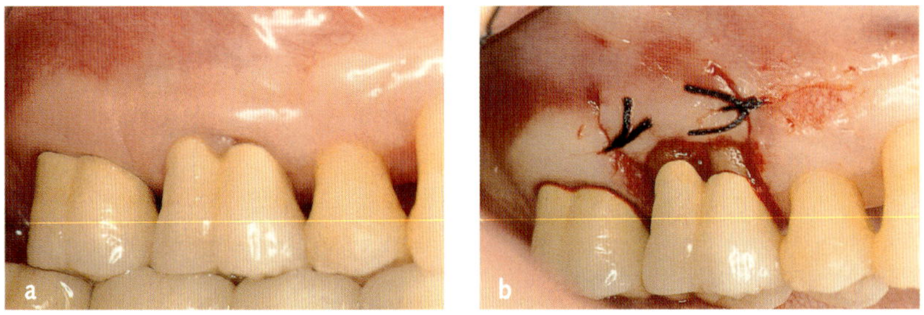

Fig 4-58 (a) After crown restoration of the maxillary right first and second molars (May 1992), inflammation at the furcation region has recurred. The furcation involvement is class II. (b) Pocket elimination surgery has been conducted through apical repositioning of a partial-thickness flap.

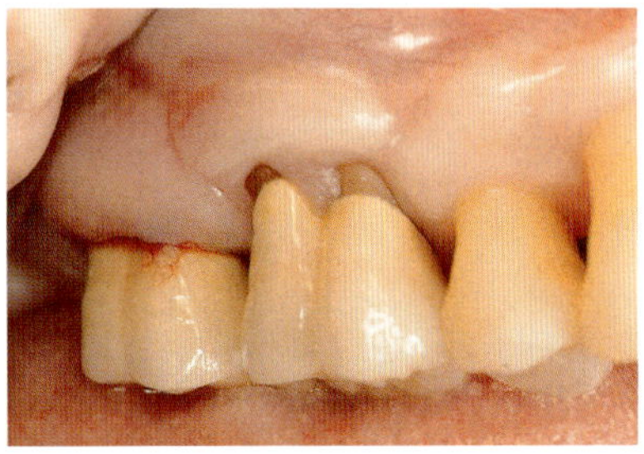

Fig 4-59 Photograph taken 2 months after surgery (July 1992).

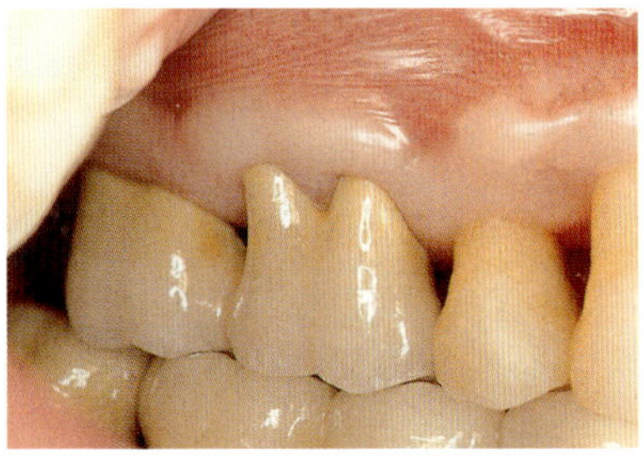

Fig 4-60 New crown restorations were provided after 5 months (December 1992). The opposing teeth, the mandibular right second premolar and first molar, are implants.

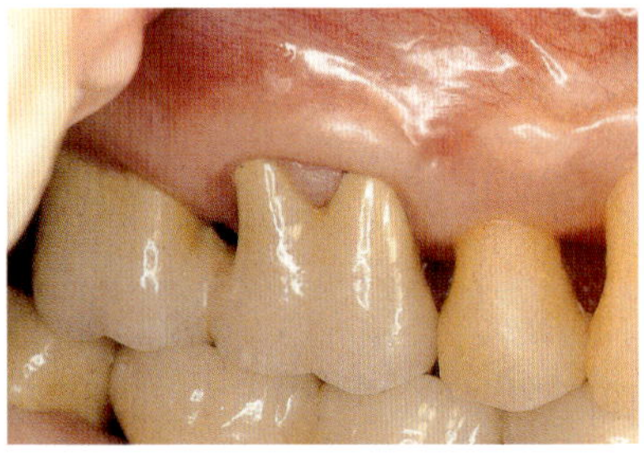

Fig 4-61 Photograph taken 2 years 6 months after pocket elimination surgery. Inflammation at the furcation area has recurred. Although sufficient attached gingiva had been obtained, maintenance was made more difficult when the furcation involvement was hidden (November 1994).

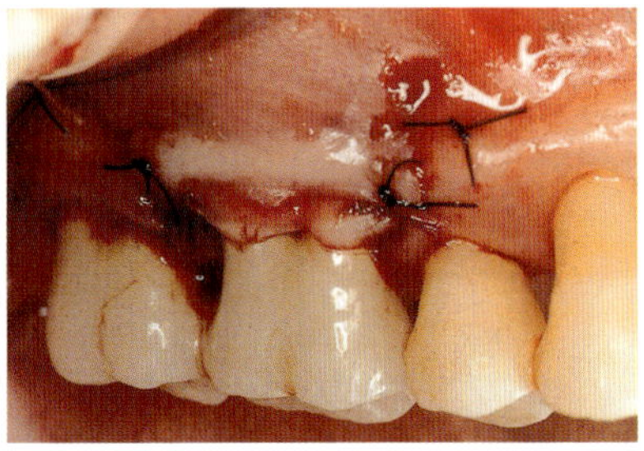

Fig 4-62 To increase the thickness of the gingiva and attached gingiva and enhance the generation at the furcation area, gingival connective tissue with the periosteum is grafted (February 1996).

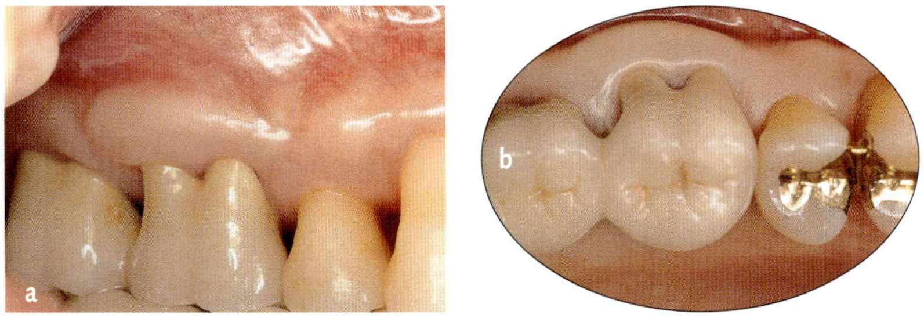

Fig 4-63 (a) Photograph taken 3 years 2 months after surgery, 10 years after the first visit. Although the furcation area was covered with gingiva to obtain the desired outcome, the thick gingiva poses a challenge in maintenance. However, the attachment is further secured and stabilized. (b) The occlusal view was photographed about 11 years after the first visit (June 2001).

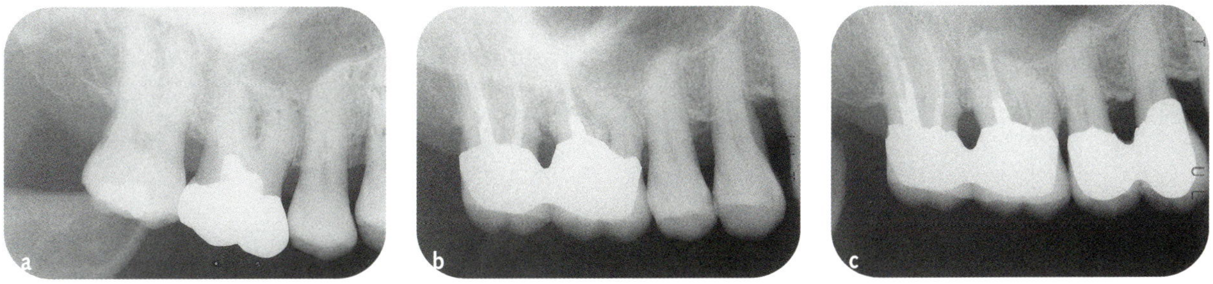

Fig 4-64 Radiographs taken (a) at first visit (June 1989), (b) after 3 years, and (c) after 10 years.

Figs 4-65 to 4-67 Hemisection for Class III furcation involvement.

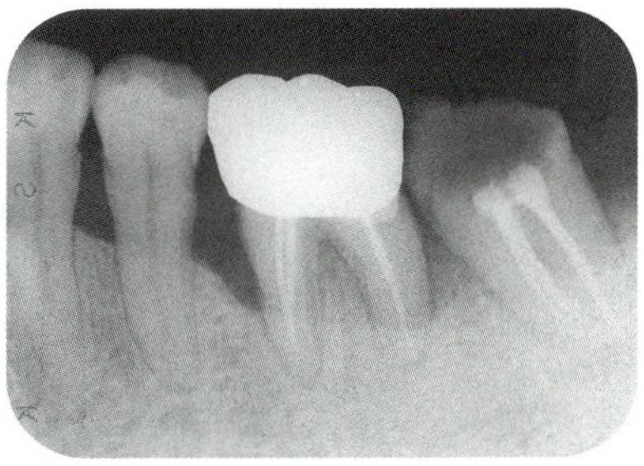

Fig 4-65 At the first visit, an infrabony defect of the mesial root of the mandibular left first molar and nearly a class III furcation involvement are noted.

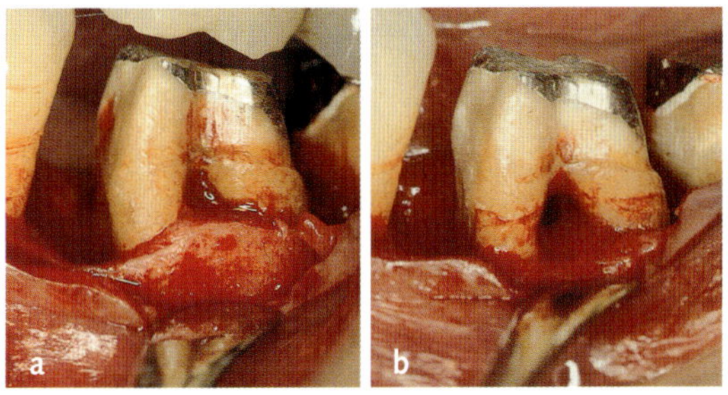

Fig 4-66 (a and b) The mandibular left first molar is hemisected and splinted to the mandibular left second molar. Hemisection is conducted after osseous surgery. The occlusal plane is improved.

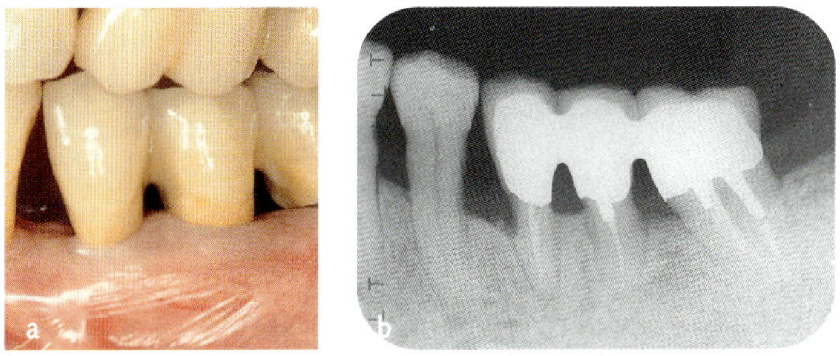

Fig 4-67 (a) Photograph taken after 4 years. (b) Conditions after 5 years.

Figs 4-68 to 4-74 Nonsurgical elimination of the furcation involvement: Natural extrusion and hemisection.

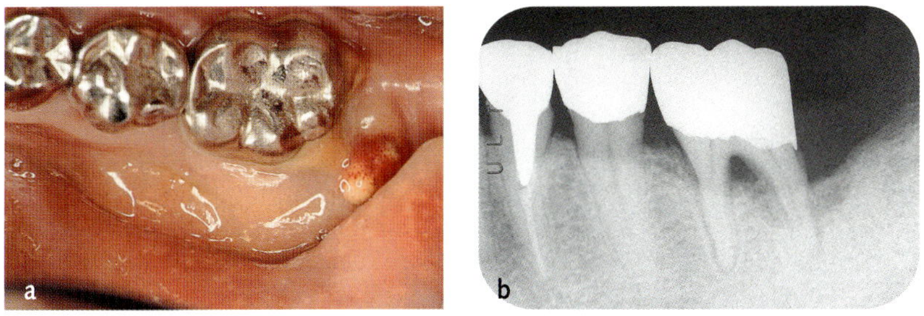

Fig 4-68 (a) The patient was a 58-year-old man at the first visit (1991). An acute alveolar abscess is visible. (b) The radiograph shows a deep infrabony defect around the distal root, from which the lesion seems to have extended to the furcation area.

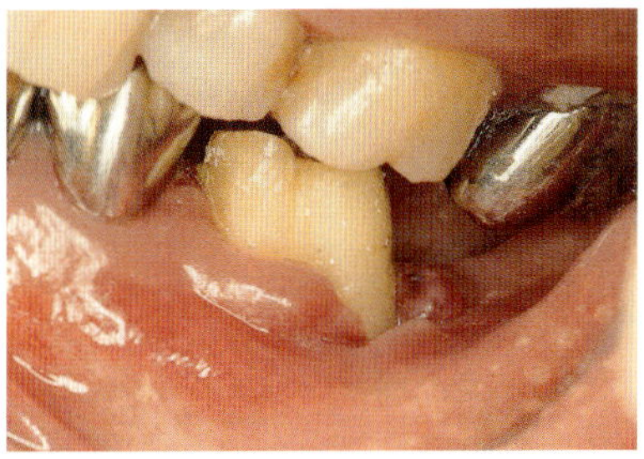

Fig 4-69 After crown removal and resolution of the inflammation, the vertical height of the crown was repeatedly reduced, in anticipation of natural extrusion.

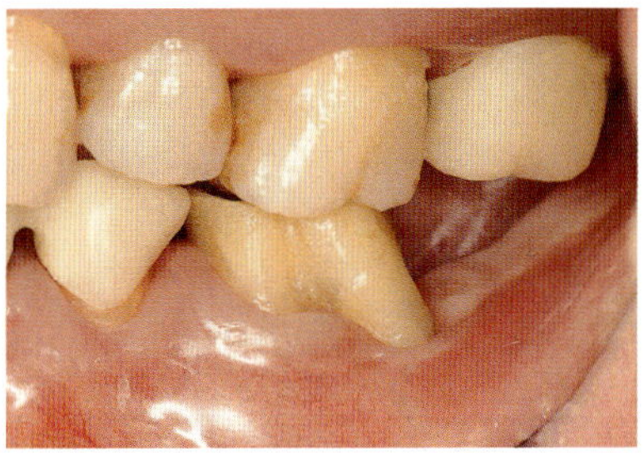

Fig 4-70 Natural extrusion took place in a relatively short period. This photograph shows conditions after 3 months.

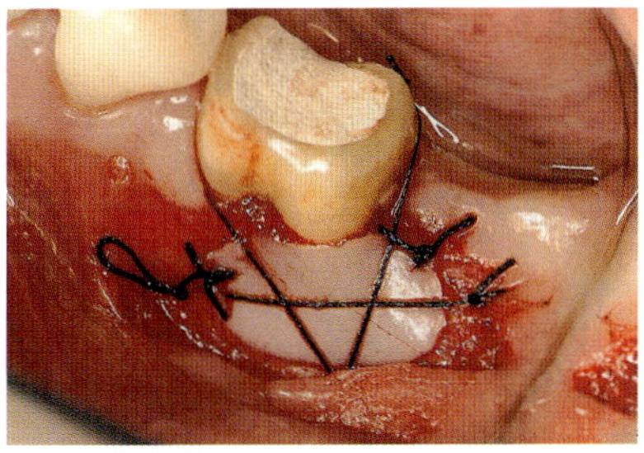

Fig 4-71 A free gingival graft was completed with the intent of expanding of the vestibule and providing distal root coverage. Gingival harmony is improved.

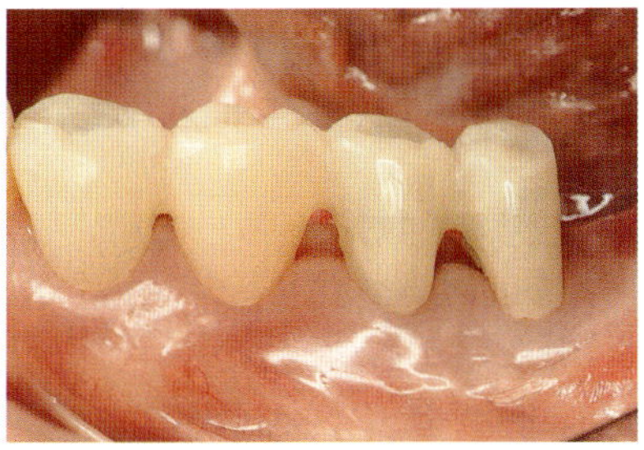

Fig 4-72 The mandibular left first molar was premolarized 3 months after surgery. This photograph shows the conditions 6 months after premolarization. The mandibular left first premolar, second premolar, and first molar are splinted.

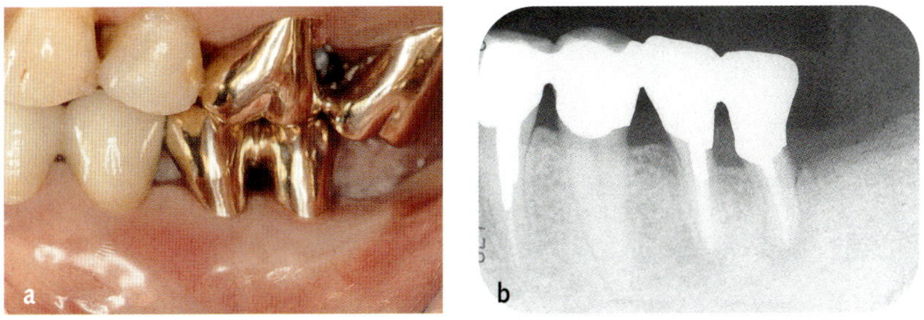

Fig 4-73 (a and b) Conditions 1 year 4 months after the first visit. The gingival margin is regular and stabilized.

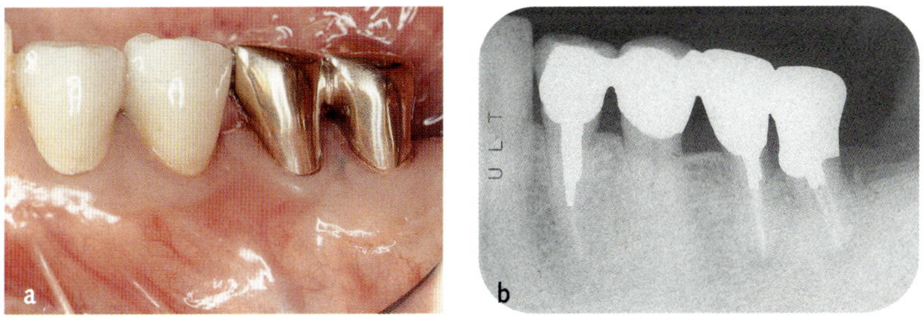

Fig 4-74 (a and b) Conditions 11 years 7 months after the first visit. Slight redness of the gingiva is noted.

Conventionally, the furcation area was exposed supragingivally in conjunction with periodontal pocket elimination; subsequently, modification of crown morphology, such as recontouring, was conducted. Because regenerative therapy is now possible, the prosthodontic treatment has changed, and exposure of the furcation area is limited as much as possible. By creating a more positive crown contour subgingivally, regenerative therapy compensates for the lost supporting tissue at the furcation and supports the gingiva, resulting in considerable improvement in maintainability (Figs 4-82 to 4-87). However, there is no definitive treatment approach that can be applied uniformly.

Resection of the furcation involvement by regenerative therapy

With a certain degree of predictability established for regenerative therapy, treatment options have been increased for class III furcation involvement in the maxilla, where it is difficult to maintain the area after root amputation (see Figs 4-79 to 4-81).

Regenerative therapy for class III furcation involvement

The patient was a 57-year-old woman at her first visit in April 1996. Both the mandibular left first molar and mandibular right first molar had interferences at the lingual cusps, and acute inflammation resulted from the occlusal trauma. Even after the crown morphology was corrected, she had a strong desire to avoid enameloplasty of her teeth because of her experiences with this acute inflammation. Consequently, it was difficult to complete recontouring the crown in this clinical case. Although radiographs revealed that lingual bone was lost because of the class III furcation involvement, and bone regeneration might not be expected, regenerative therapy was tried (see Figs 4-82 to 4-87).

Figs 4-75 to 4-78 Resection of the furcation involvement by hemisection.

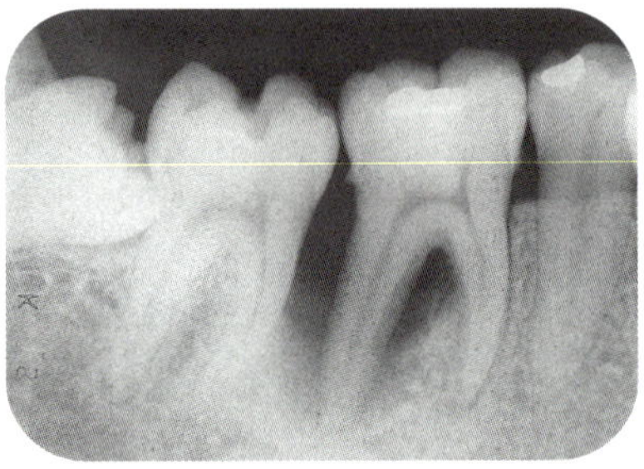

Fig 4-75 The patient was 24 years old at the first visit (1984). A localized, significant bone defect is noted, suggesting juvenile periodontitis.

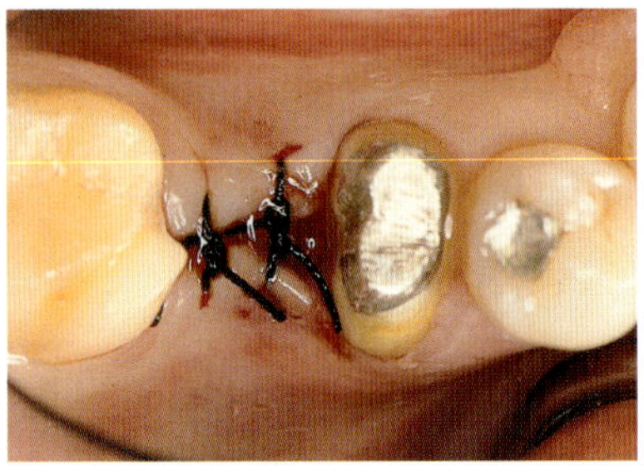

Fig 4-76 After hemisectioning of the distal root, natural extrusion was anticipated. Hemisectioning was followed by a flap operation for odontoplasty of the furcation area.

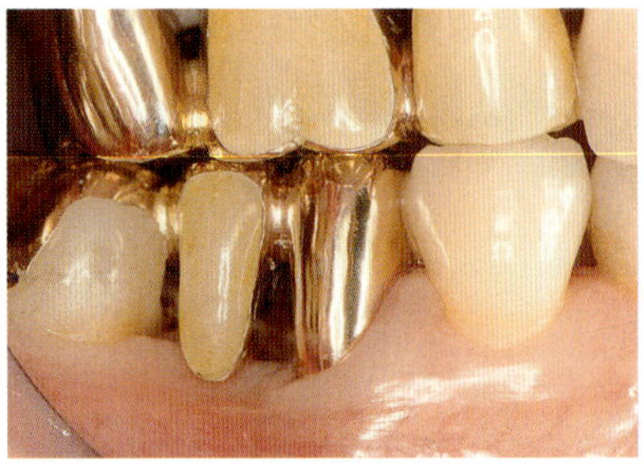

Fig 4-77 Photograph taken 2 years 6 months after surgery.

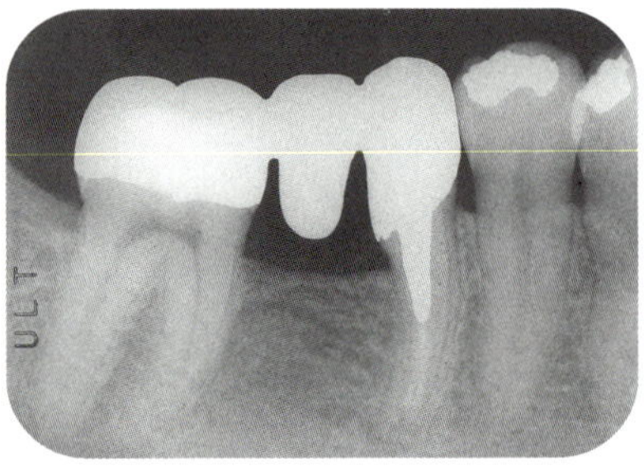

Fig 4-78 Photograph taken about 10 years after the first visit.

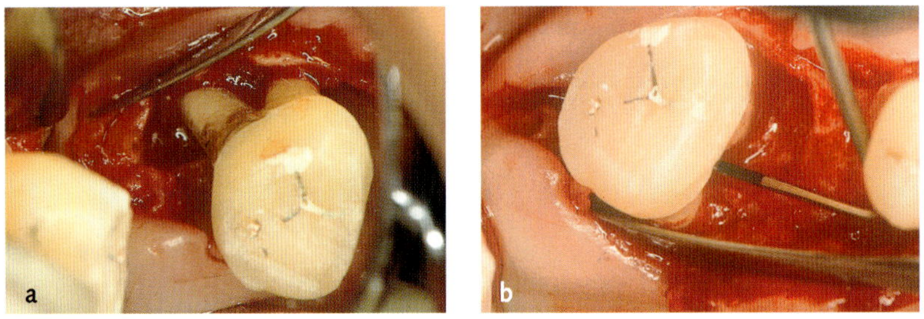

Fig 4-79 (a and b) The patient was a 39-year-old woman. After initial therapy, a class III circumferential furcation involvement was noted. A full-thickness flap was raised so that regenerative therapy could be completed (January 1991).

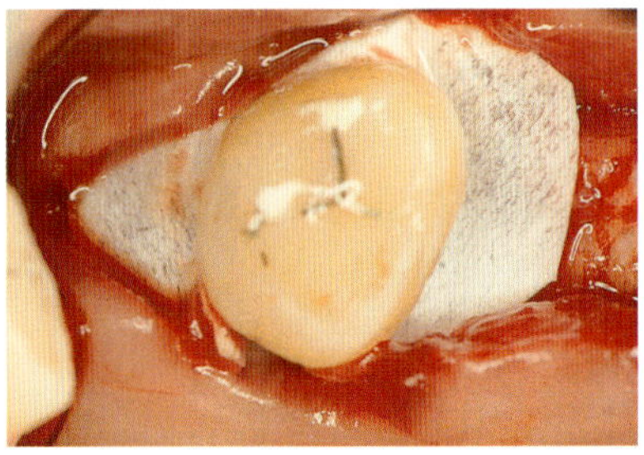

Fig 4-80 Although the tooth was considered almost hopeless, the GTR method was tried. After thorough debridement to remove granulation tissue, the root surfaces were treated with a tetracycline hydrochloride–saturated solution.

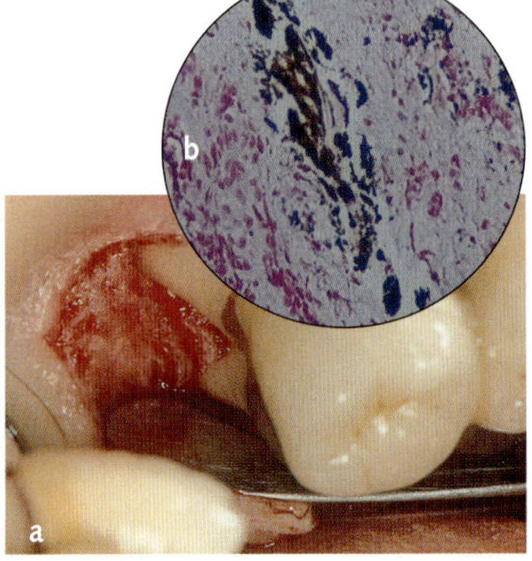

Fig 4-81 The membrane was removed after 2 months. (a) At reentry 1 year 6 months after the removal of the membrane, the furcation area is filled with osteoid tissue. (b) Light microscopic image of the tissue within the furcation area at reentry. Close to bone, a number of calcification areas are noted (dyed black with von Kossa stain).

Figs 4-82 to 4-87 Regenerative therapy for Class III furcation involvement

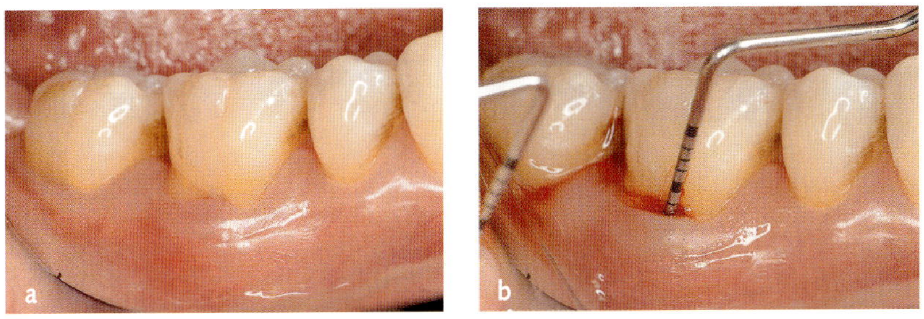

Fig 4-82 (a and b) An acute inflammation occurred during periodontal maintenance therapy. The pocket is 8 mm deep.

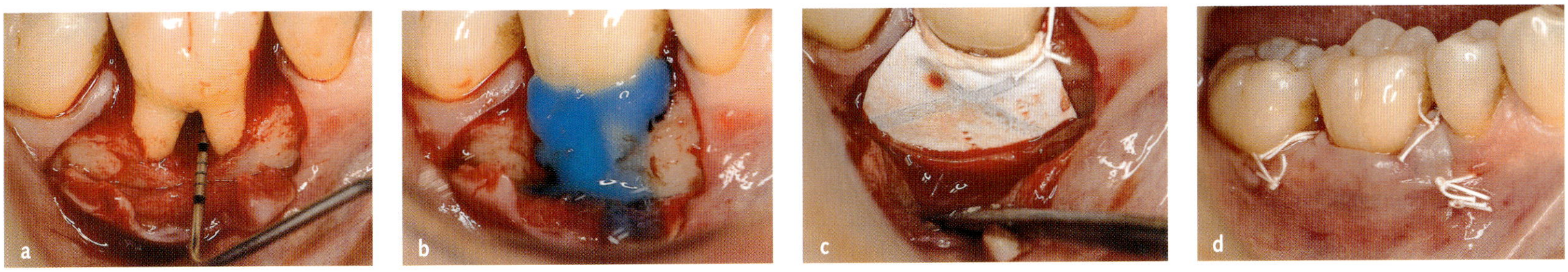

Fig 4-83 A deep class III furcation involvement is present. After (a) debridement, (b) the root surface is etched with 36% phosphoric acid gel, and (c) a GTR membrane is placed over the mixture of bone graft material and Emdogain (enamel matrix). A full-thickness flap is raised, and two to three arch-shaped releasing incisions are made toward the MGJ, with which the lower end of the membrane is fixed to prevent migration. (d) With releasing incisions, the periosteal flap can be coronally positioned as necessary.

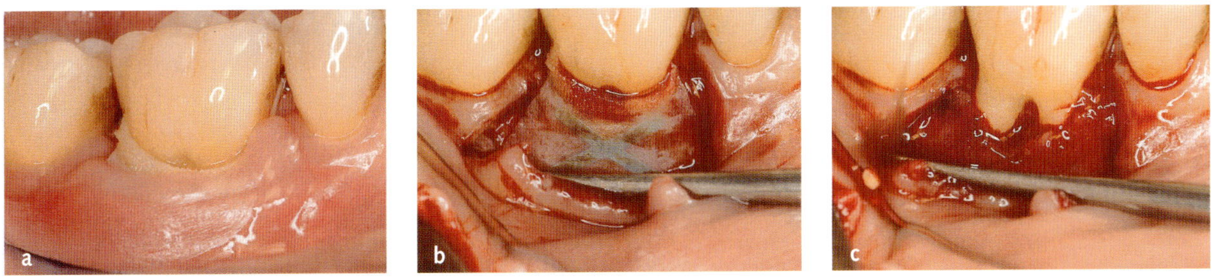

Fig 4-84 (a to c) Photographs taken about 1 month after surgery. Because the membrane was exposed, a flap operation is conducted. Abundant granulation tissue already has been obtained. The purpose of the flap operation is to obtain fresh granulation tissue.

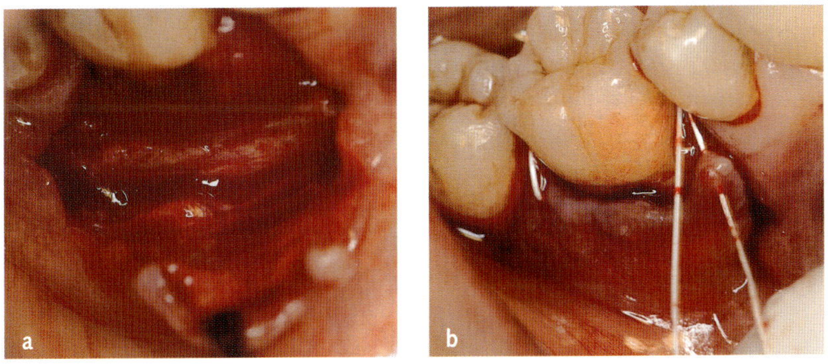

Fig 4-85 (a) At removal of the membrane, Emdogain is applied again, to obtain new attachment. Again, two to three arch-shaped releasing incisions are made under the MGJ. (b) A vertical mattress suture is placed after coronal repositioning of the periosteal flap.

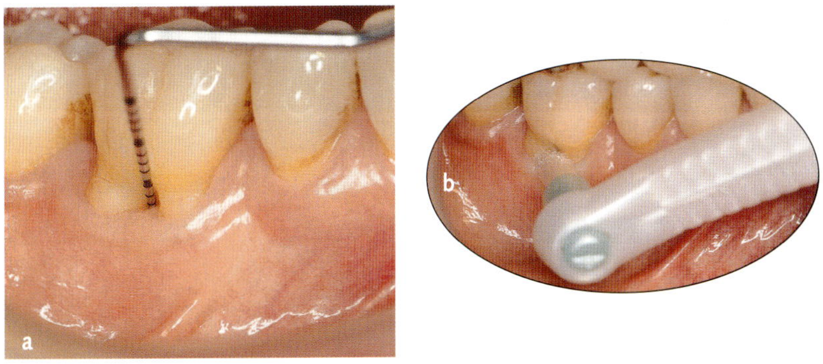

Fig 4-86 (a) Photograph taken 2 years 2 months after surgery. Probing depths are 2 mm (a 6-mm gain in clinical attachment). (b) The concavity at furcation area is cleaned with an intersulcular brush.

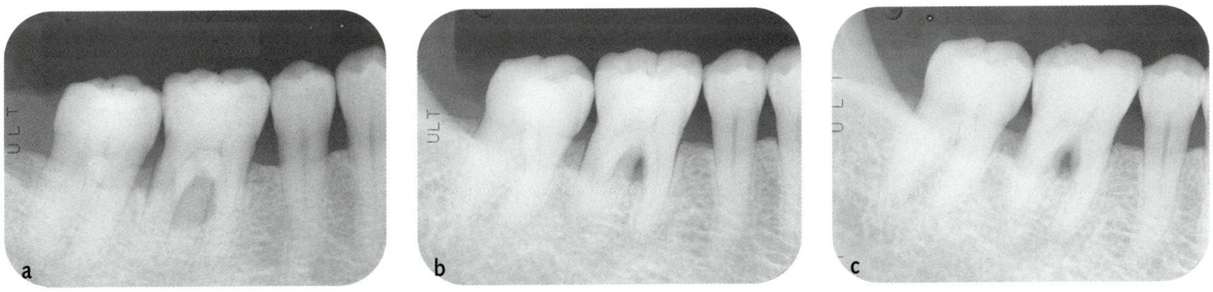

Fig 4-87 (a) At the first visit, a class III furcation involvement is noted. (b) About 1 year after surgery. (c) About 2 years after surgery. Bone regeneration is confirmed in two-thirds of the furcation area.

Support of the gingival morphology of the furcation area by subgingival contouring

We try to provide a concave transitional morphology to the furcation area and crown for easier cleaning. In a patient with a deep furcation involvement, however, this caused a significant gap between the gingiva and the crown that was difficult to fill (see Figs 4-49 to 4-55). Therefore, in the following case, we intentionally created a positive contour in the furcation area of the Procera all-ceramic crown and tried to produce a smooth transition zone at the emergence profile (Figs 4-88 to 4-94).

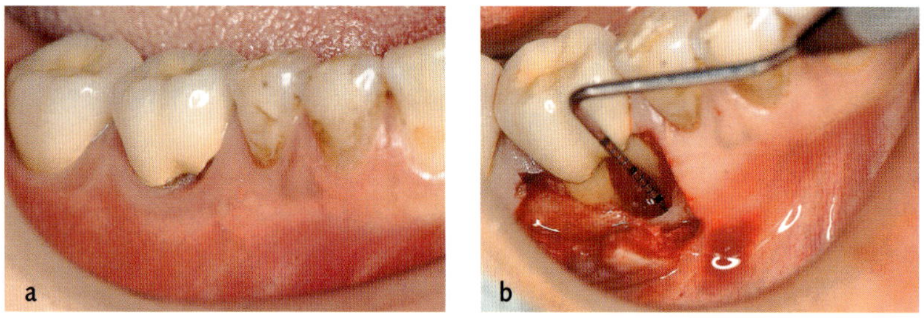

Fig 4-88 (a and b) Photographs taken after 4 years 5 months of maintenance after periodontal pocket elimination surgery for the mandibular right first molar, which had a class II furcation involvement and delivery of the final prostheses. A relapse of the furcation involvement is noted.

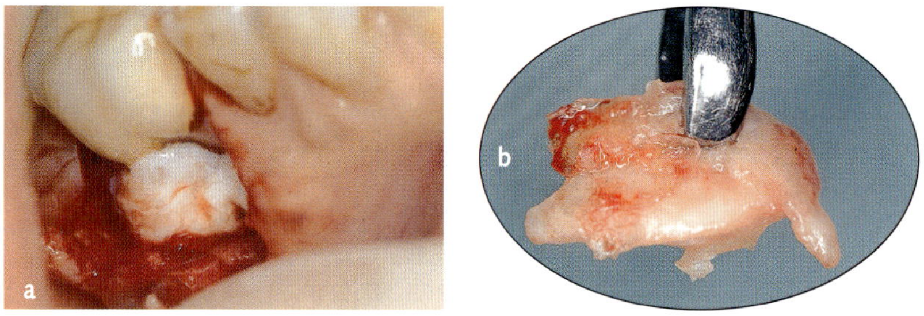

Fig 4-89 (a and b) A connective tissue graft with periosteum is harvested from the palate and grafted to cover the bone surface and furcation area. Emdogain is applied to encourage tissue regeneration.

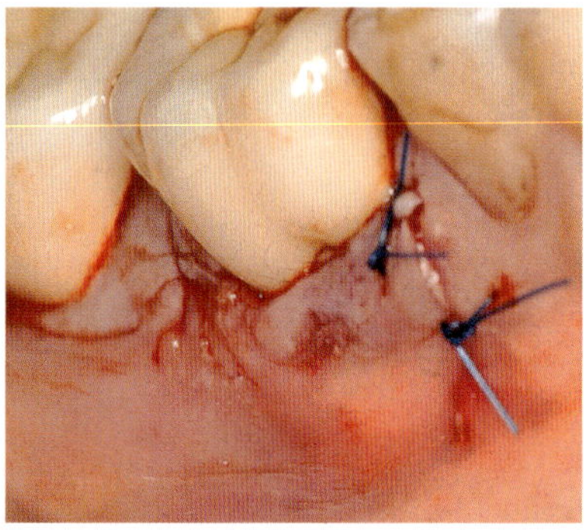

Fig 4-90 The wound is closed tightly with sufficient releasing incisions.

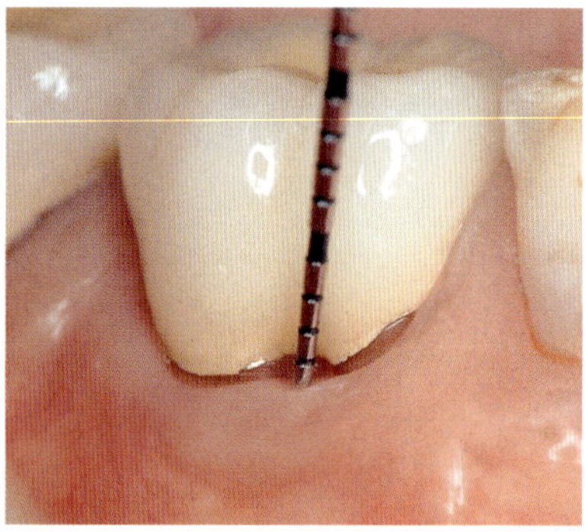

Fig 4-91 Photograph taken 5 months after surgery. Periodontal pocketing is eliminated.

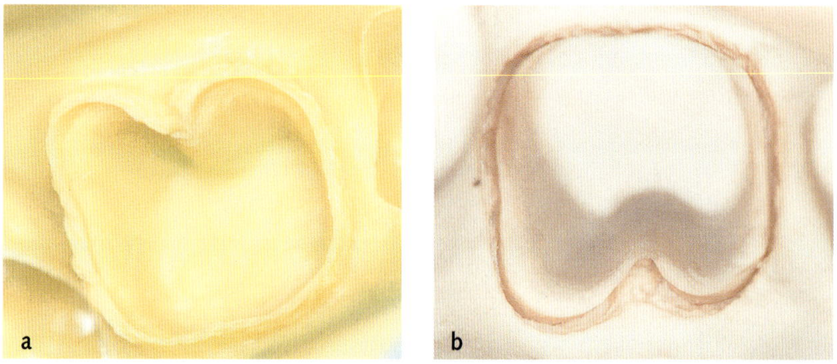

Fig 4-92 (a and b) The crown preparation is made and impressions are taken. The preparation has sufficient fluting.

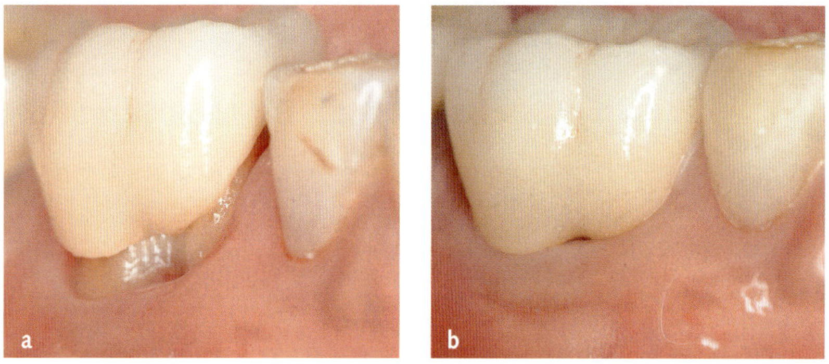

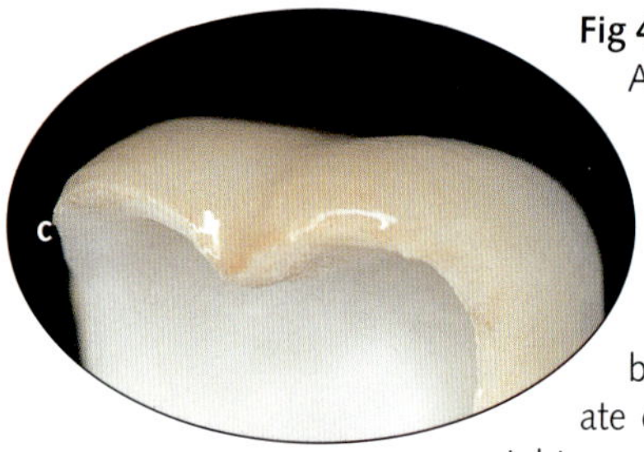

Fig 4-93 Subgingival positive contour. (a and b) At crown delivery. An intentionally positive contour has been given to the Procera crown to allow a smooth transition of the emergence profile. (b) About 1 month after crown delivery. With the good emergence contour, it is difficult to see the deep bone defect at the furcation area. Appropriate contour has been given to the mandibular right second premolar with a resin composite restoration. Compared to the status at crown delivery, the emergence profile has become smoother and more transitional, without a red margin that suggests inflammation.

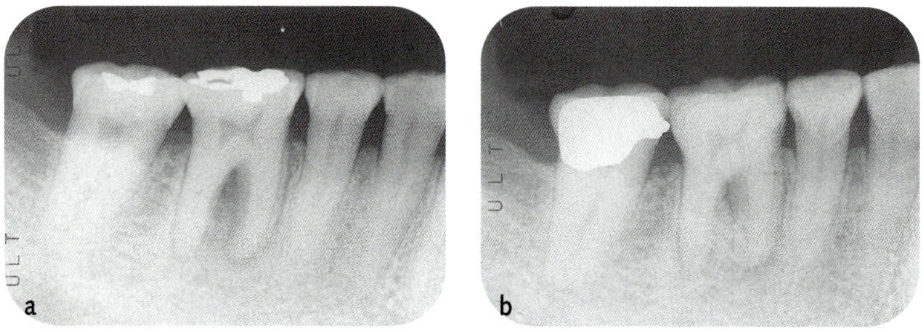

Fig 4-94 (a) At the first visit. (b) At delivery of the Procera final prosthesis.

Vertical Bony Defects and Regenerative Therapy

Clinical application of the GTR method

For many years, regeneration of lost periodontal tissue was an unrealized goal for clinicians. Clinical application of a series of periodontal tissue regeneration therapies is now making this dream a reality. To obtain the expected outcomes, appropriate initial therapy has to be conducted and followed by reevaluation of the situation and proper selection of procedures (Fig 4-95). Decisive diagnostic capability and skills as well as comprehensive clinical expertise are required for successful regenerative therapy. In other words, without an understanding of the individual differences related to inflammation and factors of occlusal forces, which are aspects of periodontal disease, the clinician will find ideal regeneration impossible to attain. Regenerative therapy cannot be discussed without control of inflammation and occlusal forces.

Criteria for case selection

The periodontal tissue most important to the success of regenerative therapy is the periodontal ligament, and how to initiate its regeneration is the secret of success with this technique. The successful acquisition of new attachment supported by bone regeneration is decisively affected by the presence or absence of a base filled by granulation tissue that can differentiate and grow. Namely, the presence of such a basis for regeneration is an indication for this procedure. In determining case selection, priority should be first given to instrument accessibility to the contaminated root surfaces, and then the conditions of the alveolar bony defect, the degree of cementum contamination, and the gingival conditions.

Basis for periodontal regeneration

The pathologic nature of furcation involvement varies widely. Even with similar probing values and radiographic images, the three-dimensional conditions of bony defects are affected by bone housing, root volume, root trunk, and degree of cementum contamination, and the accompanying gingival conditions are complicated with a variety of pathologies. Healing of molar furcation involvement in Japanese patients seems more difficult to achieve than reported in Western studies, probably because of unfavorable conditions, including fragile alveolar bone, poor crown-root ratio, root trunks in high position, and shallow vestibules. With regard to GTR, it has been said that healing is favorable in class II furcation involvement or challenging class III furcation involvements. This, however, seems to be a misdirected view of the theory of tissue regeneration. The indication is dependent not on the degree of bony defect in the furcation involvement but on the three-dimensional morphology of the bony defect surrounding the root surfaces as well as the conditions and volume of the gingiva that can cover the GTR membrane.

For tissue regeneration to occur, there has to be a basis for regeneration. The base is determined by various conditions, such as (1) the morphology and residual volume of external alveolar bone surrounding the defect, (2) the width and volume of the bony defect, (3) the depth of the bony defect, (4) the contaminated root surface, (5) the volume and conditions of the gingiva (Table 4-3).

Table 4-3 Factors affecting periodontal regeneration

1. Degree of inflammation (severe or mild; acute or chronic)
2. Depth and activity of the periodontal pockets (mild, moderate, or severe)
3. Morphology (shallow or deep, narrow or wide) and degree (internal resorption and morphology of external alveolar bone) of the bony defects and volume of the surrounding bone
4. Gingival conditions (fibrous or edematous; thick or thin; morphologic variations, including cleft, festoon, flat, scalloped; quality and quantity of the attached gingiva or keratinized gingiva)
5. Morphology of the furcation
6. Presence or absence of a healthy periodontal ligament
7. History of exposed cementum and root surface treatment
8. Anatomy and position of the tooth and root
9. Resistance and regeneration capability of the body (periodontal tissue)
10. Patient's plaque control, lifestyle management, and values
11. Clinician's accurate diagnosis and skills
12. Degree of occlusal trauma
13. Pathologic status of the occlusion unit and dentition unit
14. Circumoral muscles
15. Systemic health conditions
16. Patient's age and affected time course

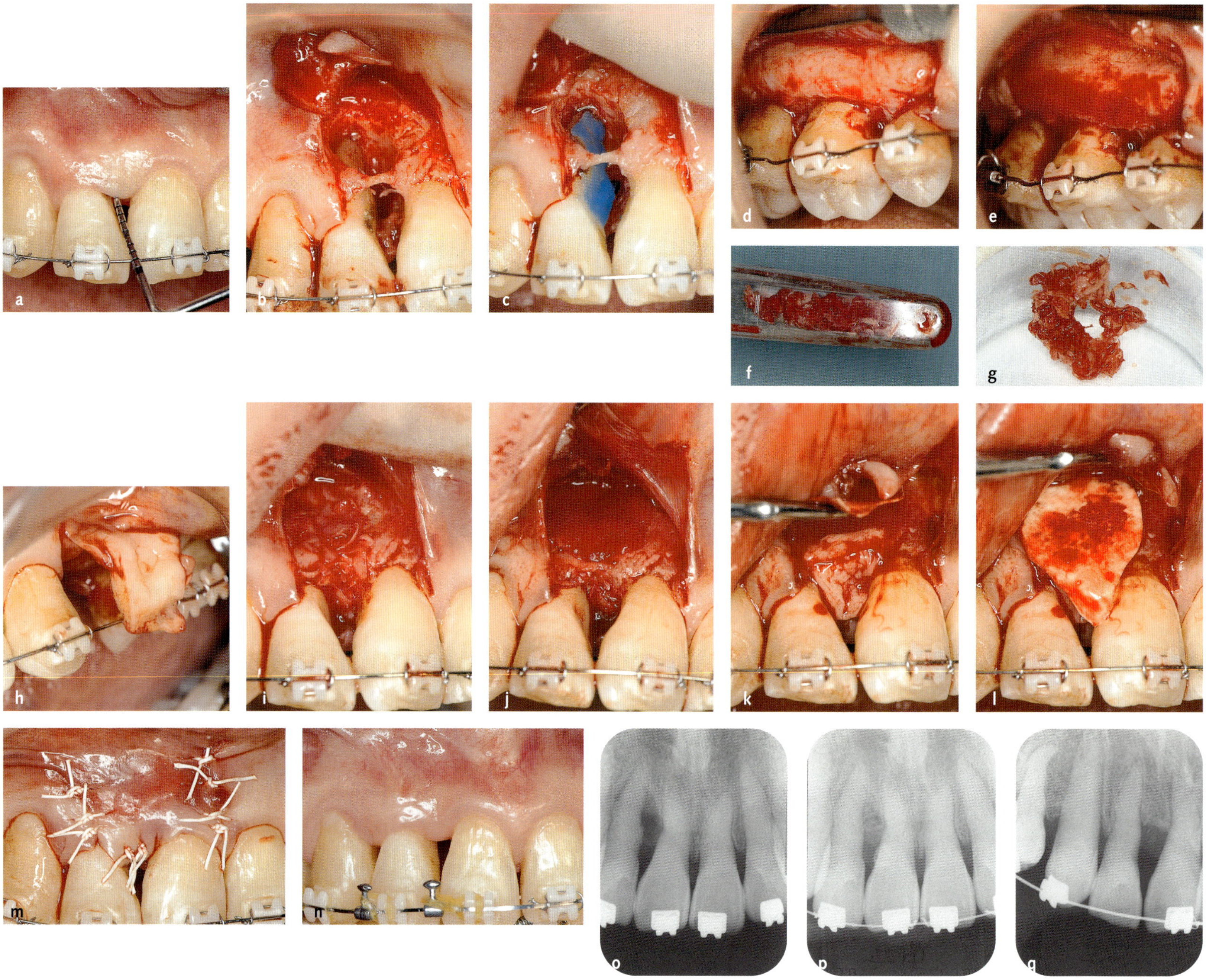

Fig 4-95 Basic procedures of GTR. (a) In this orthodontic case with severe crowding, careful scaling and root planing were conducted before tooth movement, but a 6-mm periodontal pocket has been generated mesial to the maxillary right lateral incisor. (b) After transmucosal sounding of the bone defect area, butt joint–design vertical incisions are made at the limits of the defect. Reflection is started from the mesial aspect of the maxillary right central incisor to assure a base for regeneration. The nondefect area of the lateral incisor is not reflected. (c) After thorough removal of the granulation tissue and debridement, the root surfaces are etched with gel, and Emdogain is applied. (d to g) Autogenous bone is harvested from the buccal shelf of the maxillary right second premolar, first molar, and second molar. (h) A connective tissue graft with periosteum is harvested from the area of the missing maxillary left first premolar. (i) Autogenous bone is packed tightly into the defect, on top of which Emdogain is applied again. (j) CollaTape is used to stabilize the grafted bone. (k) The connective tissue graft is placed, and eventual regeneration of the interdental papilla is expected. (l) A resorbable membrane is trimmed and placed in the area to securely cover the defect. (m) After a releasing incision is made at the bottom of a full-thickness flap, the flap is coronally repositioned and tightly sutured to cover the membrane and close the wound. (n) Photograph taken 7 months after surgery. The teeth have been orthodontically moved to reconstruct the lost interdental papilla. (o) Radiograph taken before surgery. Significant bone loss is noted. (p) An autogenous bone graft, a resorbable membrane, and Emdogain have been applied. (q) Radiograph taken 6 months after surgery indicates that bone regeneration has been achieved.

Regeneration of a deep hemiseptal bone defect with significant traumatic factors

After initial therapy, deep periodontal pockets were noted in the patient shown in Figs 4-96 to 4-98. Judging from the attrition of the maxillary left canine, it was supposed that the adjacent maxillary left first premolar had started to receive considerable occlusal forces. The buccal cusp had a deep overbite. After the flap was elevated, a deep, two-walled, hemiseptal bone defect was noted.

Regeneration of a deep, circumferential bony defect with Emdogain

The clinical case in Figs 4-99 to 4-103 showed a deep, circumferential bone defect palatal to a premolar. Coronal repositioning of the flap cannot be easily conducted on the palatal aspect of teeth.

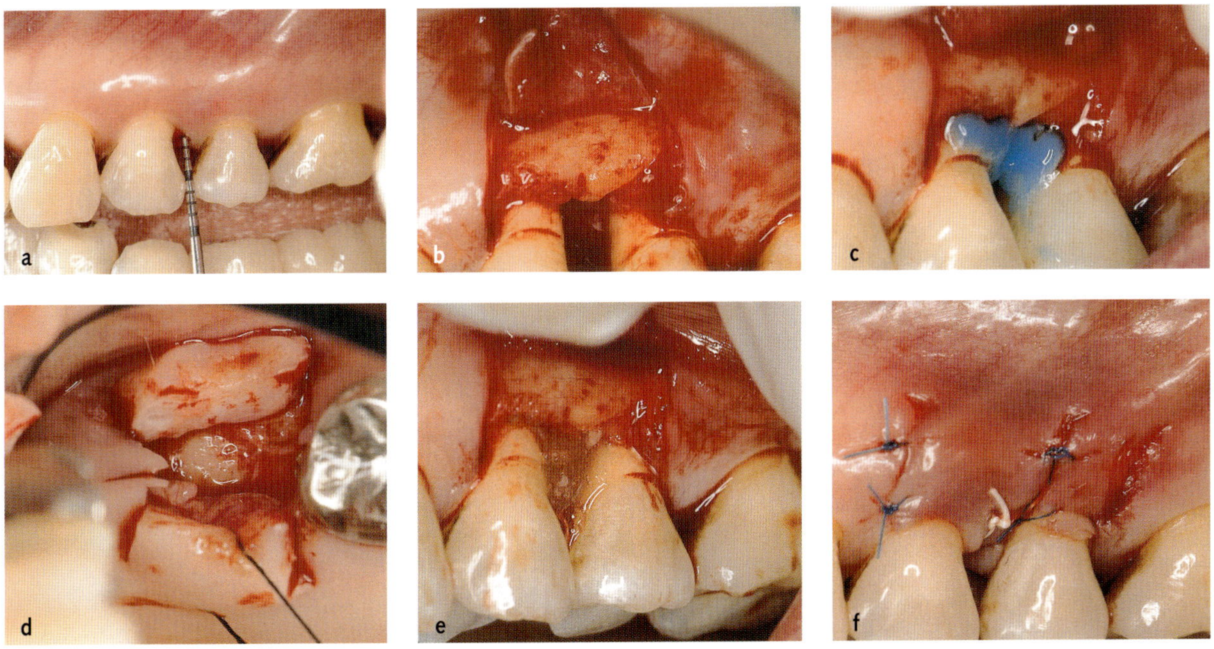

Fig 4-96 (a) After initial therapy, deep periodontal pockets are noted. (b) A two-walled, hemiseptal bone defect is noted. (c) After mechanical cleaning and root surface etching, Emdogain enamel matrix–derived protein is applied. (d and e) Autogenous bone is harvested from the maxillary tuberosity and grafted to the defect. (f) A releasing incision has been made at the bottom of the full-thickness flap to form two layers. The flap is then coronally repositioned and tightly sutured.

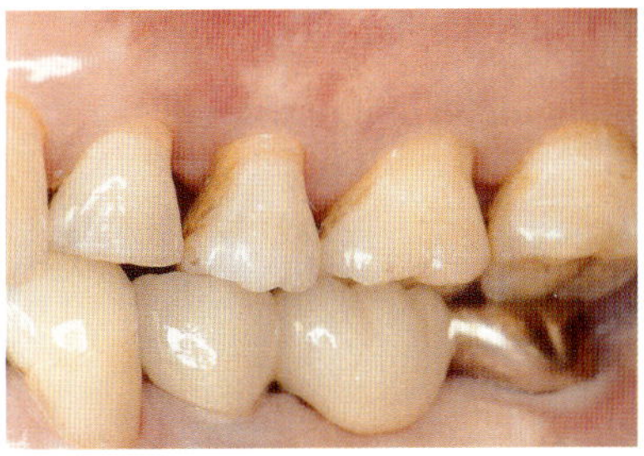

Fig 4-97 Photograph taken 1 year 1 month after surgery. The area with the deep overbite has reshaped.

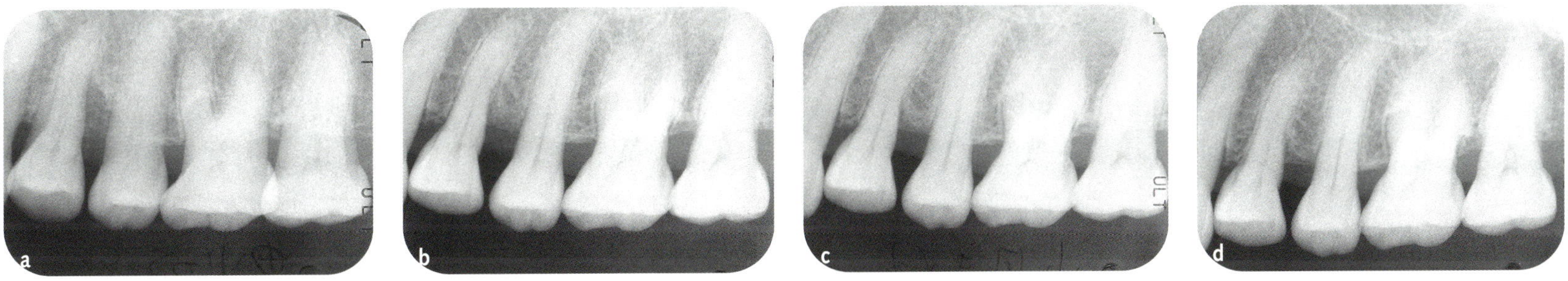

Fig 4-98 Radiographic observations. (a) At the first visit (October 1997), a significant hemiseptal bone defect is noted distal to the maxillary left first premolar. (b) Radiograph taken about 1 year after surgery (February 1999). (c) Radiograph taken May 2001. (d) A radiograph taken in March 2002 reveals bone regeneration.

Fig 4-99 (a) The patient was a 57-year-old woman at the first visit. After initial therapy, an infrabony defect deeper than 8 mm is noted palatal to the maxillary right second premolar, which is splinted to the molar. (b) A large, deep, circumferential defect is noted. (c) After mechanical cleaning and root surface etching, Emdogain enamel matrix–derived protein is applied.

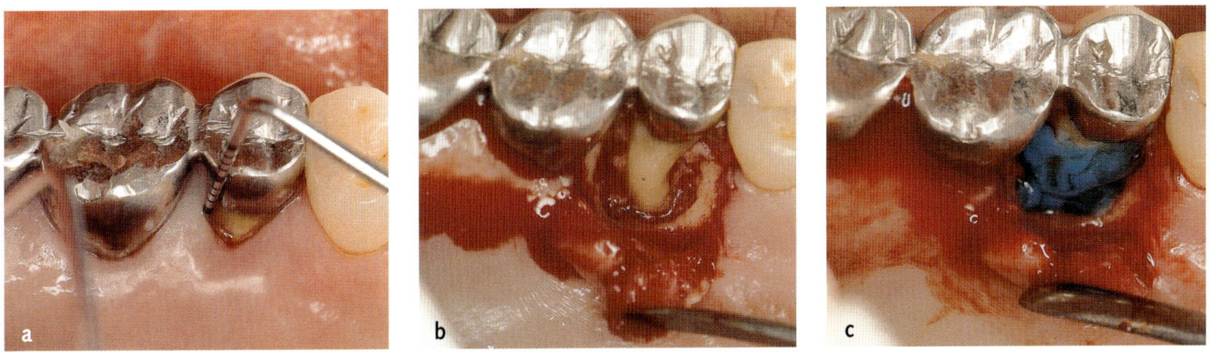

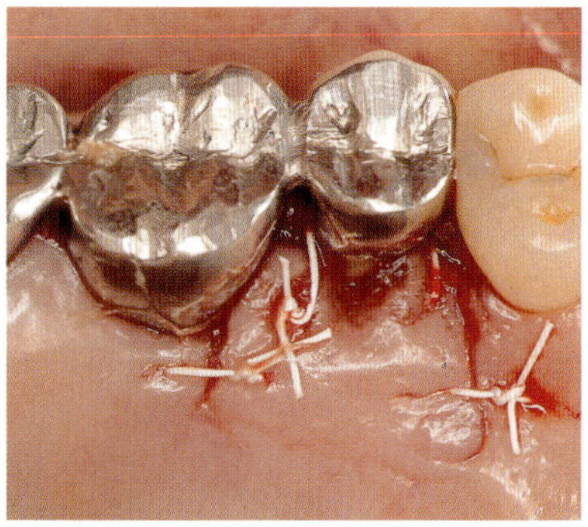

Fig 4-100 In regenerative therapy, the flap has to be coronally repositioned and tightly sutured to ensure closure of the wound. Coronal flap repositioning on the palatal side, however, is difficult. A vertical incision is made on the buccal aspect, with releasing incisions at the base of the reflected flap, and the periosteum is coronally repositioned as much as possible.

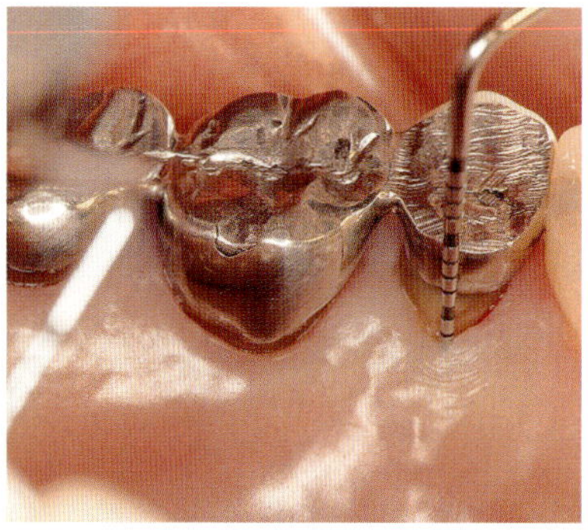

Fig 4-101 About 6 months after surgery, occlusal surfaces have been adjusted to decrease trauma. Probing depths have dramatically improved.

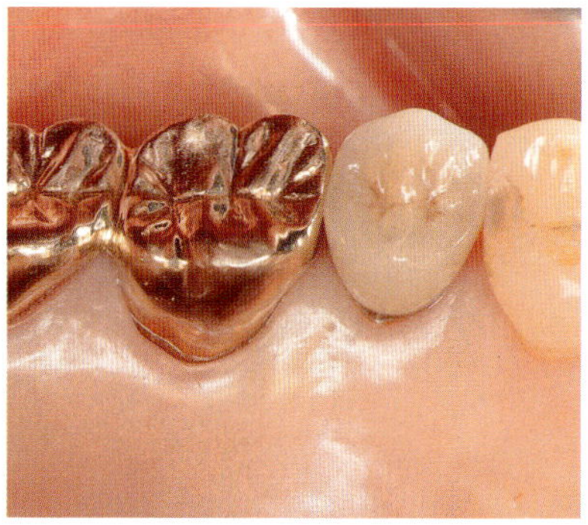

Fig 4-102 About 11 months after surgery, conditions are stable.

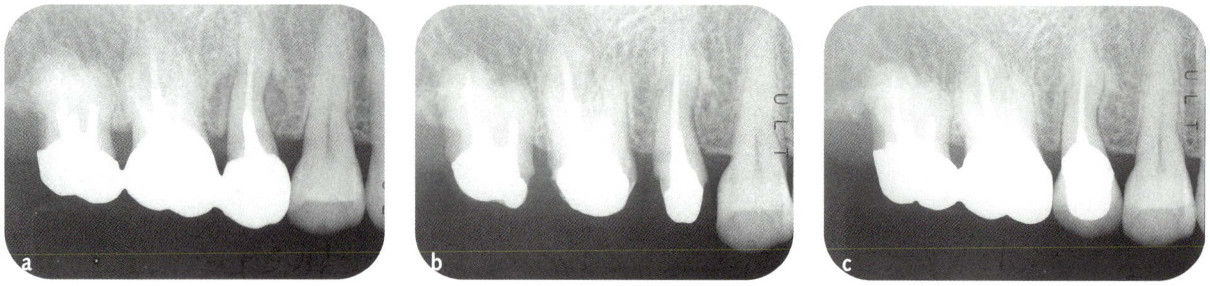

Fig 4-103 (a) At first visit, a circumferential bone defect is noted, radiographically suggesting trauma. (b) Radiograph taken 11 months after surgery. (c) Radiograph taken 1 year 2 months after surgery. Conditions are stable.

Regenerative therapy using periosteum

Periosteum prevents deep proliferation of the epithelium and enhances bone regeneration. In that sense, it is the most suitable material for regenerative therapy if it is possible to reposition the periosteum as a pedicle flap. Although indications are limited, this procedure is worth considering (Figs 4-104 and 4-105). More traditional regenerative procedures are shown in Figs 4-106 to 4-109 and Case 4-3.

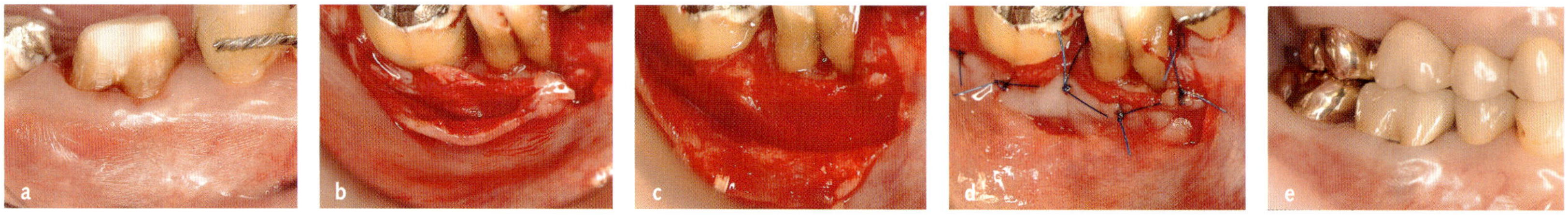

Fig 4-104 An attempt at periodontal tissue regeneration using periosteum. (a) Photograph taken about 2 years after the first visit. After scaling and root planing, orthodontic tooth movement of the mandibular right second premolar with linguoversion was completed. Mesial to the mandibular right second molar, a 5-mm infrabony defect is noted. (b) Vertical incisions are made mesial to the mandibular right first molar and distal to the second molar, and a partial-thickness flap is reflected. (c) A periosteum pedicle flap is grafted from the area of the mandibular right first molar and fixed at the upper part of the bone defect at the second molar with resorbable suture material. Because periosteum prevents deep proliferation of epithelium, effects similar to those obtained with GTR procedures are expected. (d) The flap is repositioned slightly closer to the cervical region at the mandibular right second molar and relatively apically at the mandibular right first molar to eliminate the class II furcation involvement. (e) Crown restorations have been completed 3 years after the first visit (about 1 year after surgery). After tooth movement, the periosteum was used to regenerate the periodontal tissue.

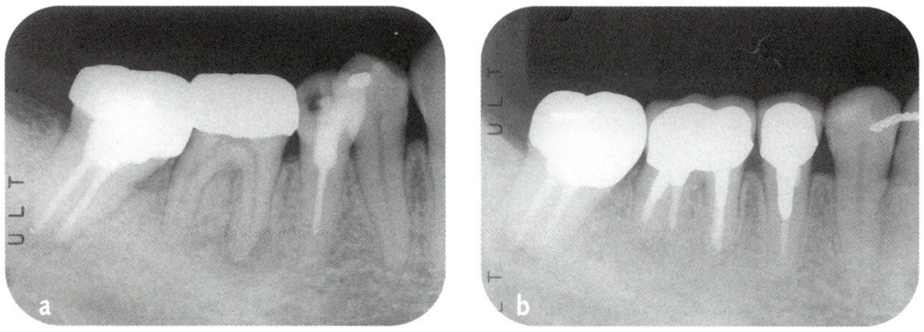

Fig 4-105 (a) Radiograph taken at the first visit. A periapical radiolucent lesion, bone defect, and traumatic findings are noted. (b) Radiograph taken 5 years after the first visit. Improvements are noted.

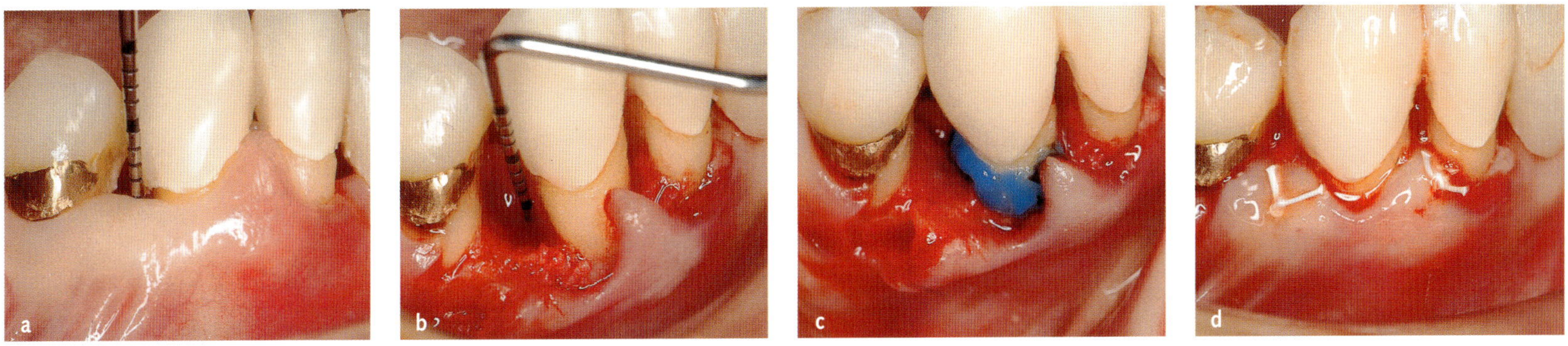

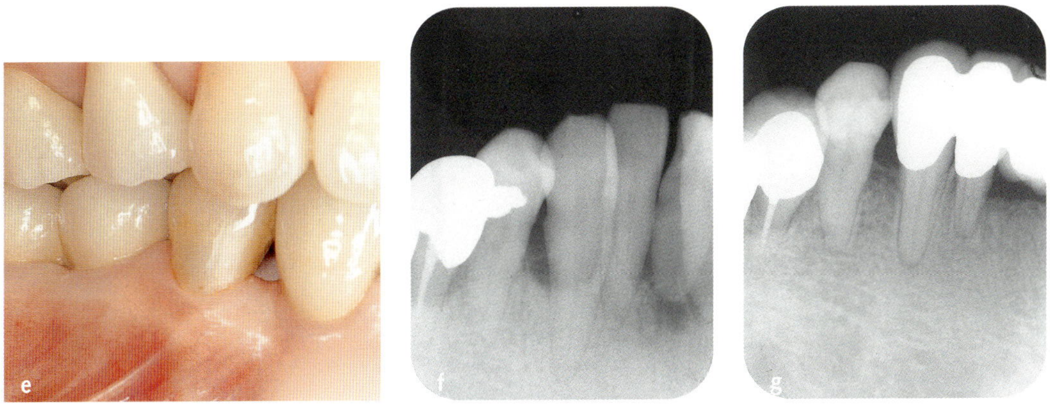

Fig 4-106 Emdogain application for a deep three-wall bone defect. (a) After initial therapy, a 6-mm-deep, three-wall bone defect is noted distal to the mandibular right canine (September 1998). (b and c) The root surface is thoroughly planed, and enamel protein is applied to promote regeneration. (d) After an incision is made in a butt joint manner, the flap is coronally repositioned at the interdental papilla. (e) Photograph taken 2 years 5 months after surgery (March 2001). (f) Radiographic view of the three-wall defect (September 1998). (g) Radiographic verification of bone regeneration (March 2001).

Figs 4-107 and 4-108 Regenerative therapy with GTR.

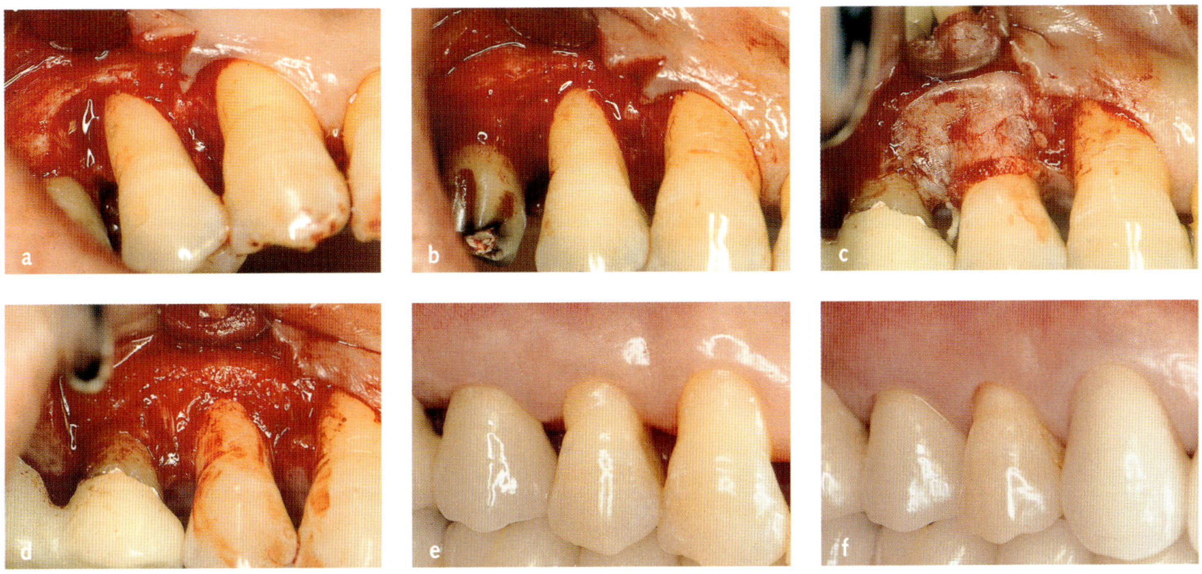

Fig 4-107 Regenerative therapy with a nonresorbable membrane. (a) A cup-shaped bone defect distal to the maxillary right first premolar is noted. (b) Autogenous bone is grafted. (c) A nonresorbable expanded polytetrafluoroethylene (e-PTFE) membrane is applied. The membrane was removed after about 1 month. (d) Granulation tissue has formed under the membrane. (e) Photograph taken 1 year 2 months postsurgery. The prosthesis has been delivered. (f) Photograph taken 9 years after delivery of the prosthesis, 10 years 7 months after surgery. A vertical increase in the attachment has been obtained.

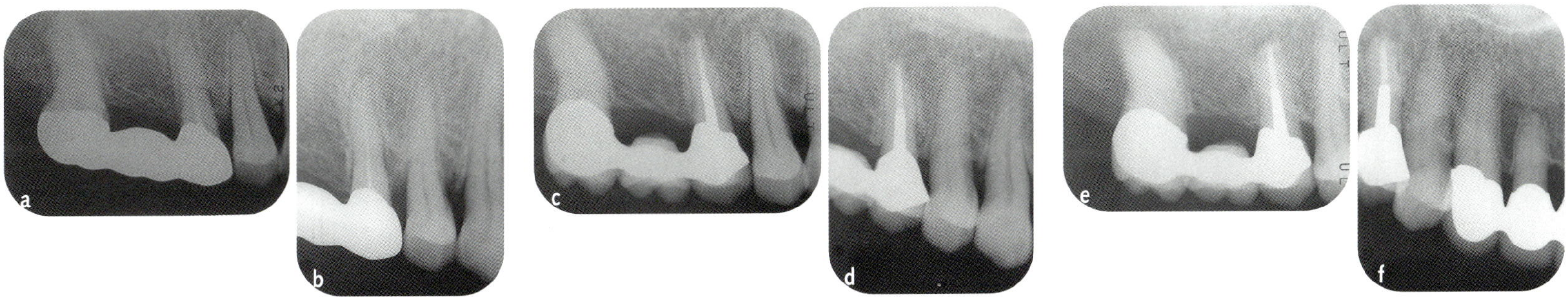

Fig 4-108 (a and b) At the first visit, the bone defect is accompanied by findings of occlusal trauma. (c and d) Radiograph taken 2 years 6 months after the first visit. The bone defects are improved. (e and f) Radiograph taken about 13 years after the first visit.

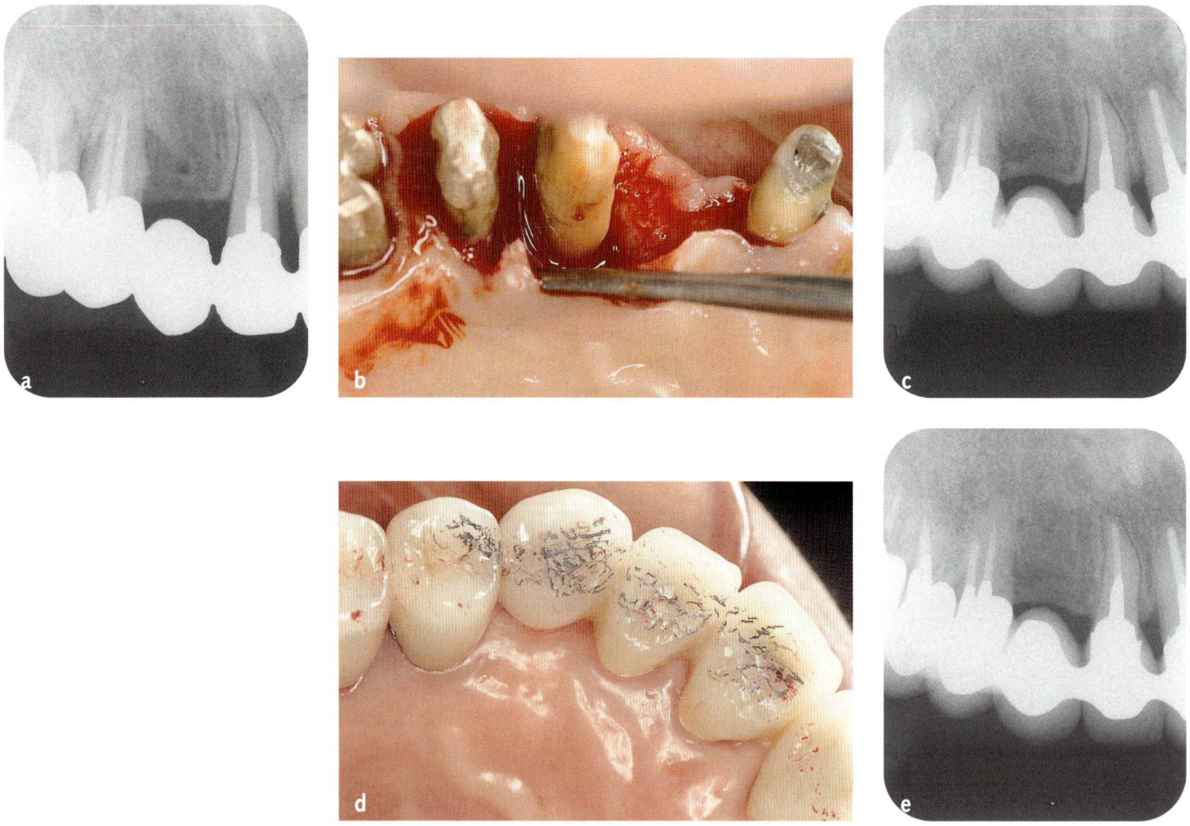

Fig 4-109 Regenerative therapy and force control. (a) At the first visit, a deep bone defect is noted mesial to the maxillary right first premolar. (b) Photograph taken 11 months after the first visit. Regenerative therapy with Emdogain is conducted. (c) Radiograph taken 2 years 9 months after regenerative therapy. Final prostheses are provisionally cemented. Bone regeneration is observed. (d) Occlusal adjustment of provisionally luted final prostheses is conducted. Areas to be adjusted are marked with pencil. (e) Radiograph taken 10 months after delivery of prostheses. The widened periodontal space is improved and stable.

Case 4-3 Advances in regenerative therapy: Changing the possibilities for tooth preservation and prosthetic planning

Patient: *52-year-old man at the time of first visit in June 2000*
Chief complaint: *Difficulty in chewing*
This is a case of severe periodontal disease complicated by tooth luxation caused by occlusal trauma. It was difficult to determine the final treatment goals. The maxillary arch was not considered for implants because of the poor condition of the bone. After regenerative therapy, a telescopic denture was placed. For the mandible, a full-arch fixed splint was used. A premolar was luxated during the periodontal surgery and reimplanted with application of Emdogain. Radiographically, significant bone regeneration was noted. Although further follow-up is needed, this case indicates that improvements in the predictability of regenerative therapy are drastically changing the possibilities for tooth preservation and prosthetic planning (Fig 4-110).

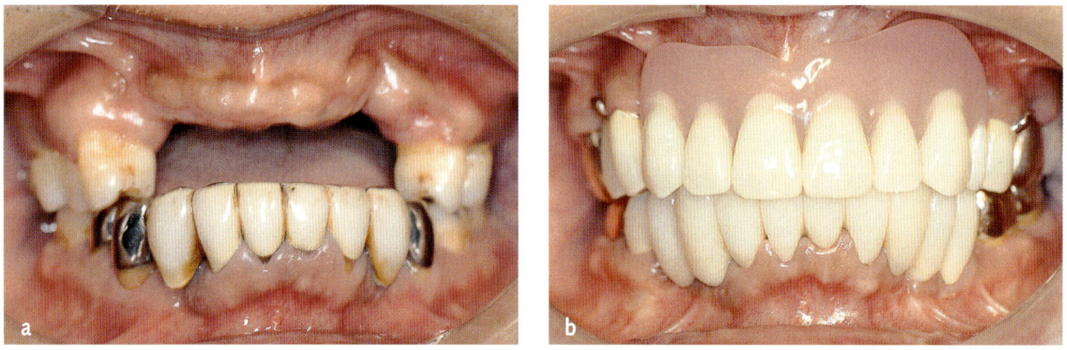

Fig 4-110 (a) At the first visit. Seven teeth, from the maxillary right canine to the maxillary left first premolar, are missing due to trauma. Generalized severe periodontal disease (periodontal pockets of 7 to 8 mm) is noted. (b) After regenerative therapy with Emdogain is conducted for the maxillary right first and second premolars and first and second molars, as well as the maxillary left second premolar and first molar, a telescopic denture is delivered. The area from the maxillary right canine to the maxillary left first premolar has significant bone loss and is not suitable for implant treatment.

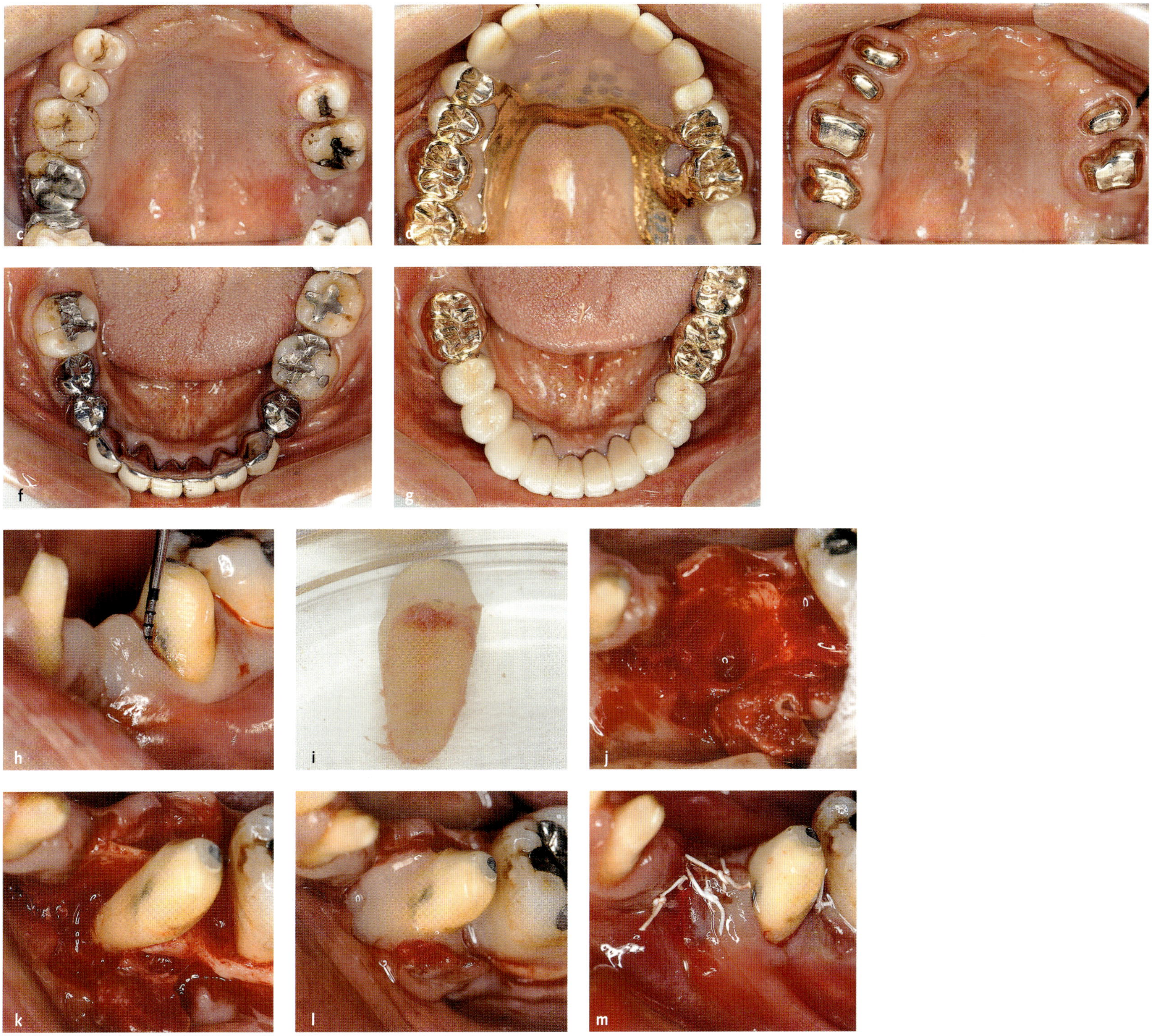

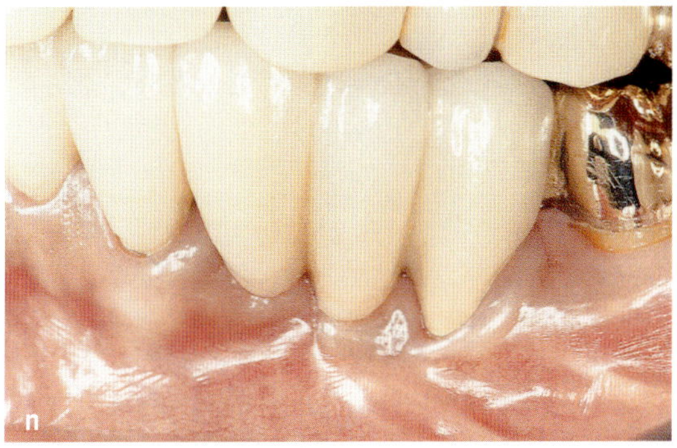

Fig 4-110 (cont) (c) Occlusal view at the first visit. (d) A removable denture with an open palate design, supported by Konus crowns, has been delivered. (Prostheses made by Mr Takahisa Tashiro, RDT.) (e) Inner crowns are delivered to the abutment teeth. (f) At the first visit. The mandibular right first premolar was extracted. Regenerative therapy with Emdogain is conducted for the mandibular left second premolar, first molar, and second molar. (g) Fixed periodontal prostheses extending from the mandibular left second molar to the mandibular right first molar (pontics: mandibular left first premolar, mandibular left canine, mandibular right canine, and mandibular right first premolar) have been delivered. (Prostheses made by Mr Kiyoharu Takada, RDT.) (h) The periodontal pocket at the mandibular left second premolar was 11 mm (5 months after the first visit). (i) During surgical root planing, the tooth was luxated. (j) The socket has minimal bone on the distal side. (k and l) Although the predictability is very low, the tooth is reimplanted in the socket with an application of Emdogain. (m) Suturing. (n) Periodontal prostheses 2 years after surgery.

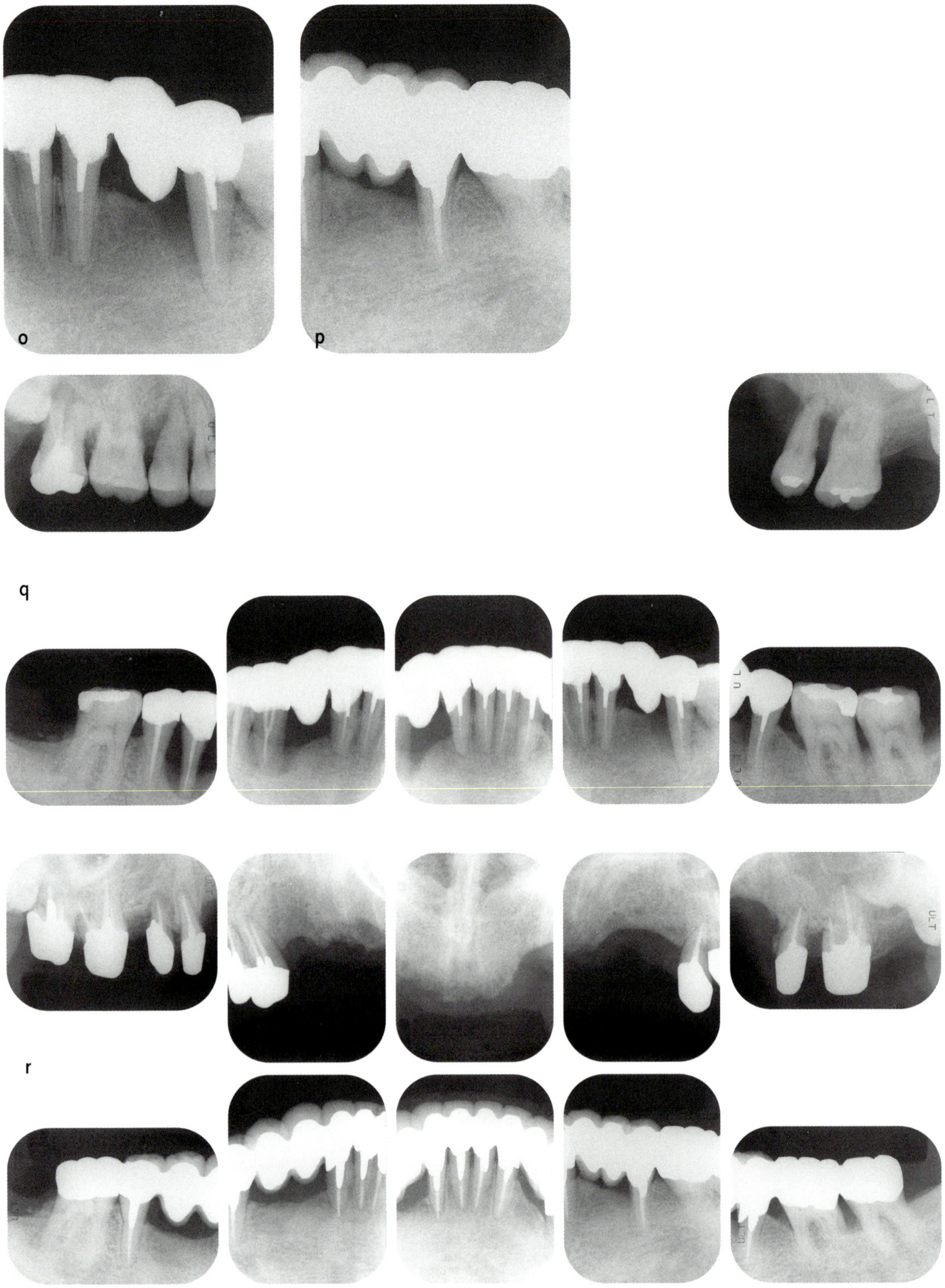

Fig 4-110 (cont) (o) Radiograph of the mandibular left premolar region at the first visit. (p) Bone regeneration is clearly observed at the mandibular left second premolar. Careful follow-up is required. (q) Radiographs at the first visit (June 2000), showing severe periodontal disease. (r) Telescopic crowns have been placed in the maxillary arch and a periodontal prosthesis has been placed in the mandibular arch (October 2002). Bone improvement is observed.

Improvement of Esthetics by Periodontal Plastic Surgery

Periodontal plastic surgery

Periodontal surgery has various objectives, including access for debridement of the root surfaces and improvement of the periodontal environment for enhanced maintainability. Periodontal surgery involving the gingiva and alveolar mucosa and focused on the improvement of esthetics rather than the prevention of disease or maintainability is called periodontal plastic surgery. Mucogingival surgery is clinically considered to have a value of increasing maintainability, a claim that has not been necessarily confirmed in objective evaluations. Consequently, mucogingival surgery should be conducted on the conditions that the patient demands the procedure and there is a high esthetic value.

Indications for and selection of procedures

Periodontal plastic surgery is not limited to conventional procedures such as an increase of attached gingiva or a frenectomy. A variety of procedures have been developed primarily for the improvement of esthetics, including procedures for reconstruction of interdental papillae, coverage of exposed root surfaces, and alignment of irregular gingival draping. Grafts of gingiva and alveolar mucosa are divided into pedicle grafts and free grafts. Pedicle grafts are highly predictable because the blood supply to the graft is ensured. Free grafts include free gingival grafts and connective tissue grafts. The latter can be applied for root coverage, recovery of gingival harmony, and gingiva–alveolar ridge augmentation. The recipient site is well blended with the neighboring tissue, and good esthetics is achieved.

Coverage of exposed root surfaces is one of the more important objectives in periodontal plastic surgery. Miller developed a classification of indications, indicating that 100% coverage can be expected in cases where gingival recession does not exceed the mucogingival junction and there is no loss of interdental bone or soft tissue. Because appropriate indications have been clarified and a variety of procedures are available, clinicians should select the least invasive and most predictable procedure depending on each case (Figs 4-111 to 4-115).

Connective tissue graft effective for small-scale root coverage

Connective tissue grafting using an envelope flap is less invasive and the esthetic outcome can be predictable. It is recommended for small-scale coverage of exposed root surfaces (see Fig 4-111).

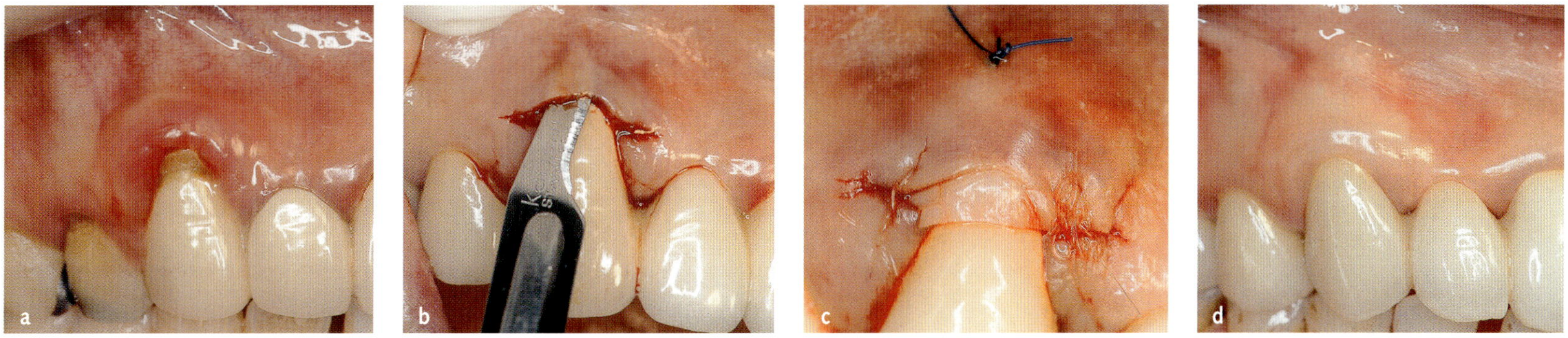

Fig 4-111 (a) Gingival recession with inflammation at the maxillary right canine is noted. (b) A surgical knife with a replaceable blade is used to form an arc-shaped envelope flap. (c) A free connective tissue graft with epithelium is harvested from the palate and grafted to the site. Emdogain is applied in combination with the graft. (d) The postoperative result shows good esthetics and an easily maintainable morphology.

Figs 4-112 to 4-115 Recovery of attachment on an exposed root surface.

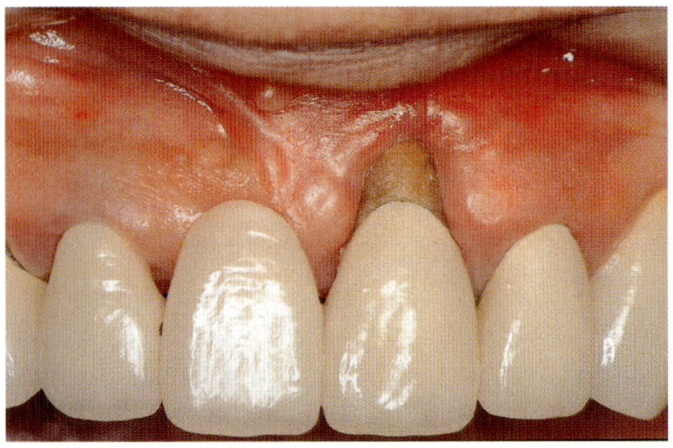

Fig 4-112 The patient was a 51-year-old woman at her first visit. Extreme root surface exposure is noted at the maxillary left central incisor. The exposure seems to have been caused iatrogenically by surgery. The maxillary right central incisor is missing.

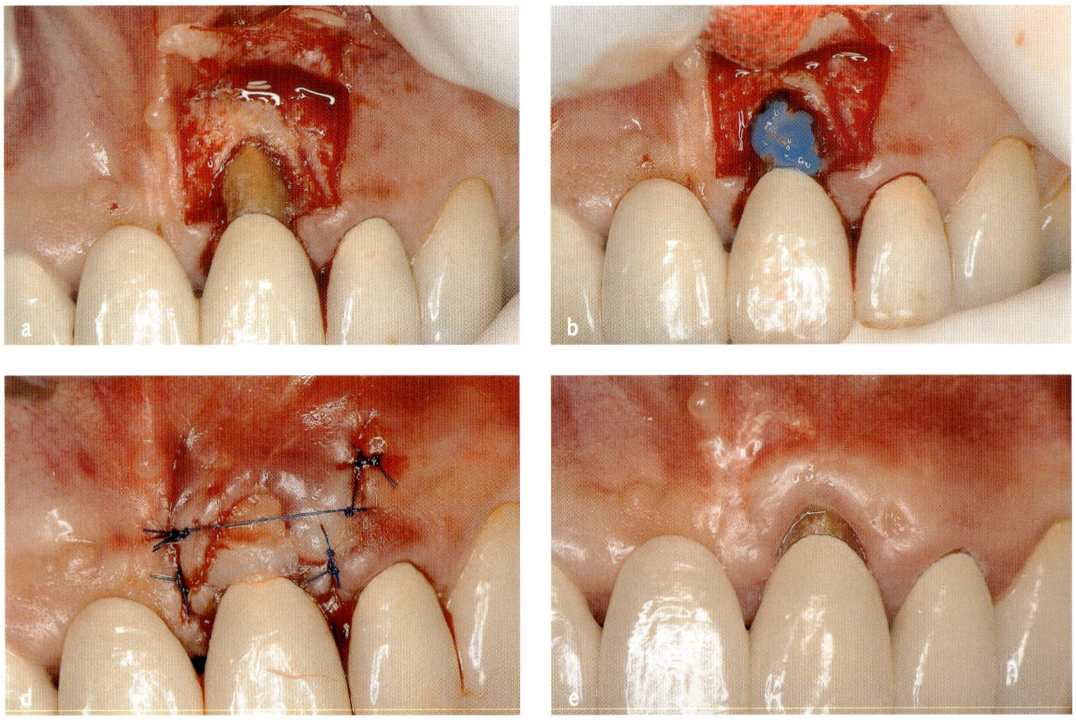

Fig 4-113 Use of the Langer and Langer method of root coverage surgery. (a) Horizontal incisions are made to preserve the interdental papillae, and a partial-thickness flap is raised. (b) After etching, Emdogain is applied to the root surface. (c) The connective tissue harvested from the palate is grafted. (d) A sling suture is made to closely approximate the wound. (e) About 2 months postsurgery. Although the exposed root surface is not sufficiently covered, attached gingiva has been obtained.

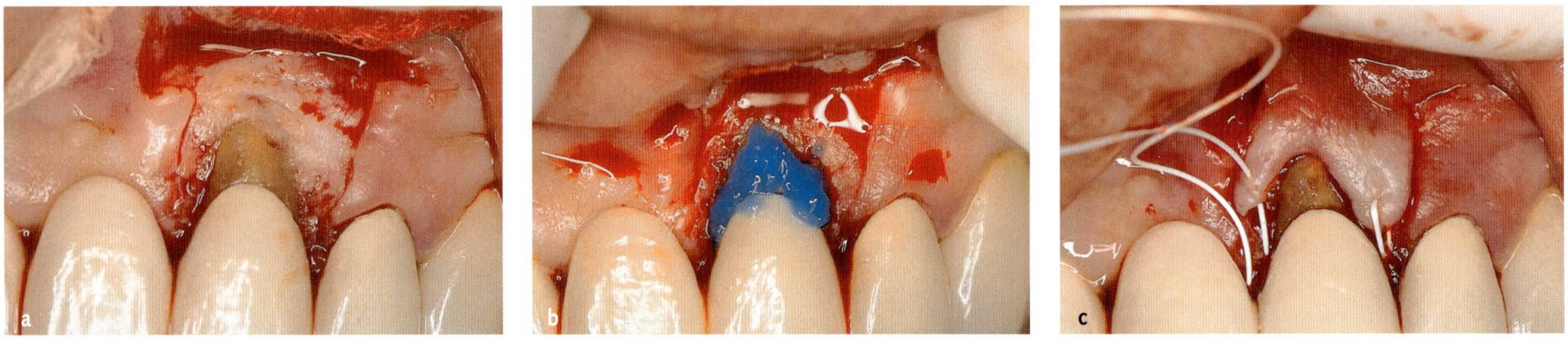

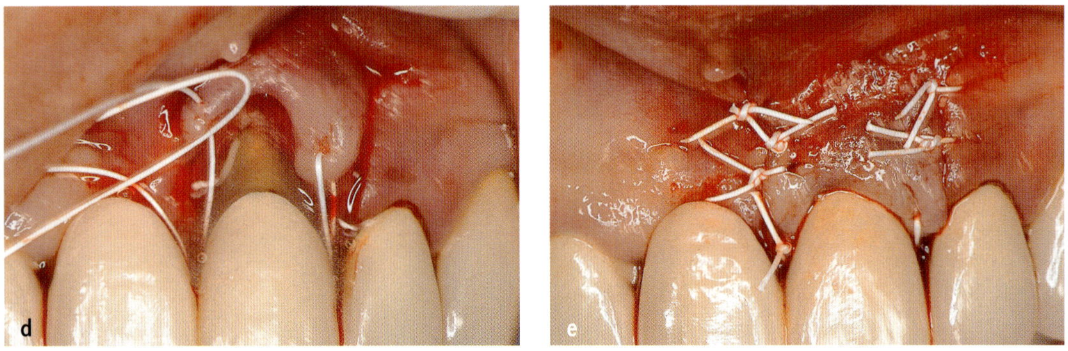

Fig 4-114 Recovery of attachment with Emdogain. (a) Bevel incisions are utilized in the interdental papillae, and butt joint–like vertical incisions are used to expose the root surfaces. Long bevel incisions in the interdental papillae allow margins for suturing. (b) Acid etching. (c) A semilunar releasing incision is made at the bottom of the flap to form two layers. Sling sutures are utilized. (d) When suturing is almost complete, the Emdogain solution is injected. (e) The periosteal flap is coronally repositioned and sutured tightly to enhance regeneration.

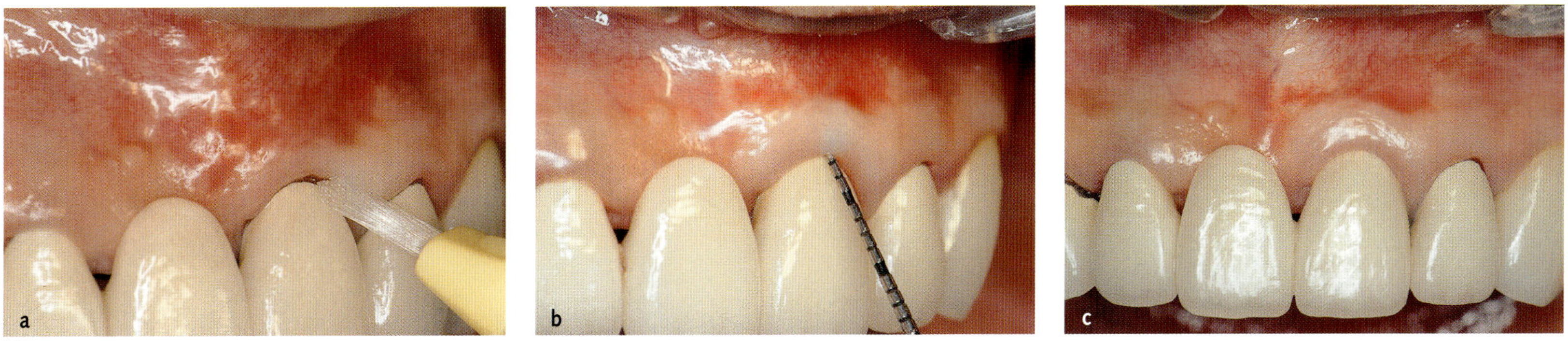

Fig 4-115 Postoperative maintenance. (a) Regardless of the type of regenerative therapy, a patient should not be allowed to take care of the intersulcular area until wound healing is achieved. The patient should visit the clinic frequently to receive professional cleaning. For home care, a soft toothbrush is used alone with a rough rolling technique. Continuation of careful cleaning improves the regenerative therapy results. (b) The first probing is conducted 10 months postsurgery. The labial depth is 1 mm. (c) About 2 years after surgery, a slight increase in gingival height is observed. Because root caries has developed, the prostheses (maxillary right canine and maxillary left lateral incisor) should be removed for re-treatment. This is the same patient as in Case 4-4.

Root coverage with a pedicle flap

For the patient in Figs 4-117 to 4-119, a large area of the exposed root surface of the maxillary right central incisor was covered with lateral and coronal repositioning of a pedicle flap. The key point in this procedure is that a pedicle (with a blood supply) mucoperiosteal flap (regeneration tissue) is used. Grafting of a pedicle full-thickness flap is, in a sense, periosteal grafting with a blood supply, which has a high predictability of success.

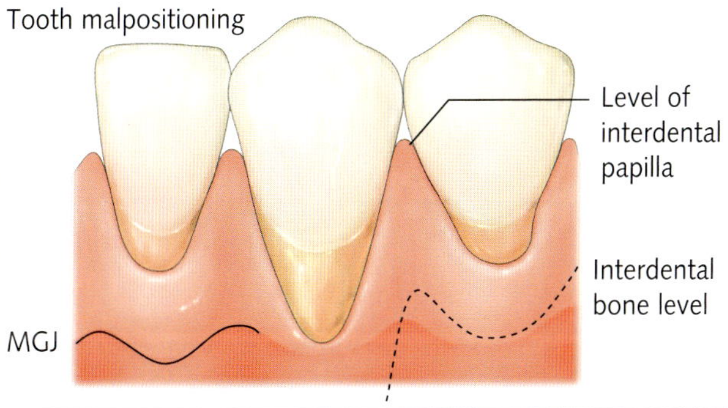

	MGJ	Bone	Soft tissue	Malpositioning	Predictability of root coverage
Class I	Not extended to MGJ	No loss	No loss	No	100%
Class II	Extends to or beyond MGJ	No loss	No loss	No	100%
Class III	Extends to or beyond MGJ	Loss or	Loss or	Yes	Partial
Class IV	Extends to or beyond MGJ	Significant loss	Significant loss	Yes	No

Fig 4-116 Predictability of root coverage. Miller described categories of recession-type defects and their effects on the predictability of root coverage. The predictability in each category depends on the following factors: (1) whether or not gingival recession extends beyond the MGJ; (2) possible loss of interdental bone; (3) possible loss of soft tissue; and (4) whether or not the recession is accompanied by tooth malpositioning.

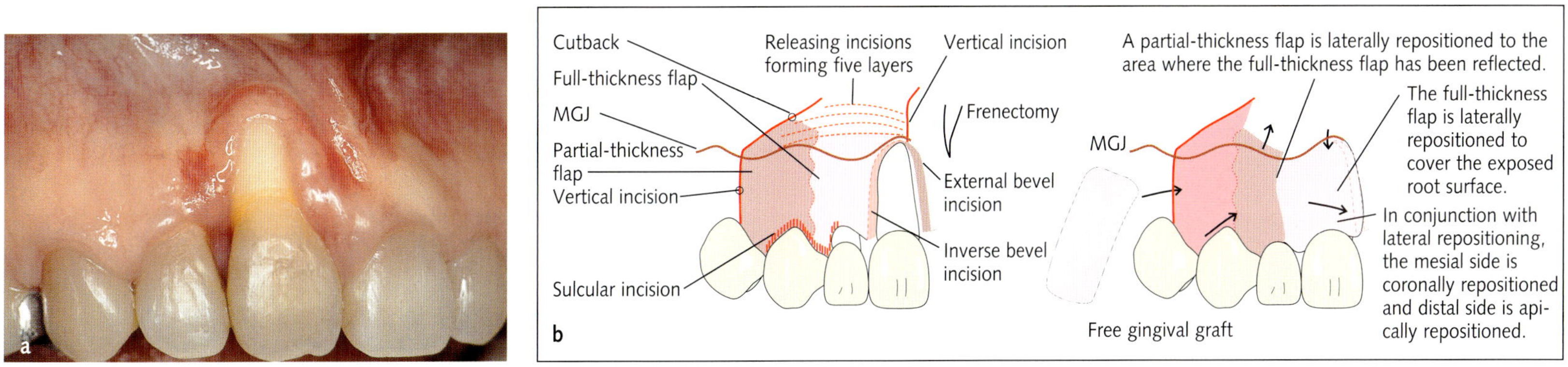

Fig 4-117 (a) Photograph taken before surgery. The patient was a 20-year-old woman. (b) The coronal repositioning design of the pedicle flap is shown. Scallop-shaped releasing incisions are made to the apical base of the flap. There should be no extra tissue or tension of the grafted flap.

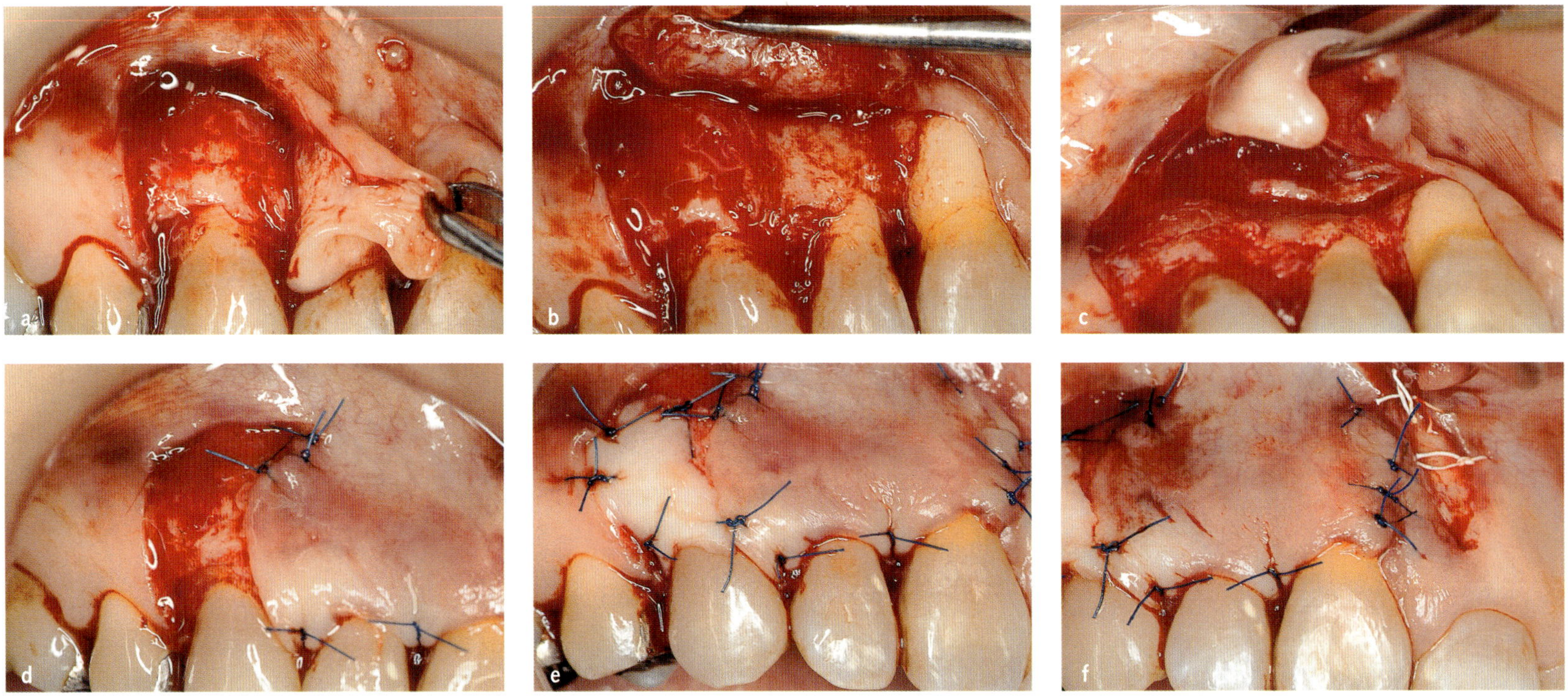

Fig 4-118 Lateral repositioning of a pedicle flap. (a) Vertical incisions are made, preserving the mesial papilla of the maxillary right first premolar. A partial-thickness flap is raised from the maxillary right canine area toward the mesial direction. (b) The incision reaches the bone surface at the mesial side of the maxillary right canine to form a full-thickness flap. A vertical incision is placed at the apical part of the maxillary right central incisor. (c) Cutback is completed, and 1 to 2 mm of shallow releasing incisions are placed at the bottom of the reflected mucoperiosteal flap at the maxillary right canine and the maxillary right lateral incisor, in an apical direction. The flap is moved mesially and laterally, and further releasing incisions are created to release the flap tension. (d) The pedicle flap is mesially rotated and coronally repositioned in a tight manner so that the periosteum at the healthy maxillary right lateral incisor will cover the exposed root of the maxillary right central incisor. The mesial aspect of the exposed root of the maxillary right central incisor is externally beveled, and the distal aspect is internally beveled. (e) The exposed surface of the maxillary right canine is covered with a free gingival graft. (f) With a frenectomy, the surgery is completed. Orthodontic brackets will be bonded to the maxillary right central incisor, lateral incisor, and canine for retention of the surgical pack.

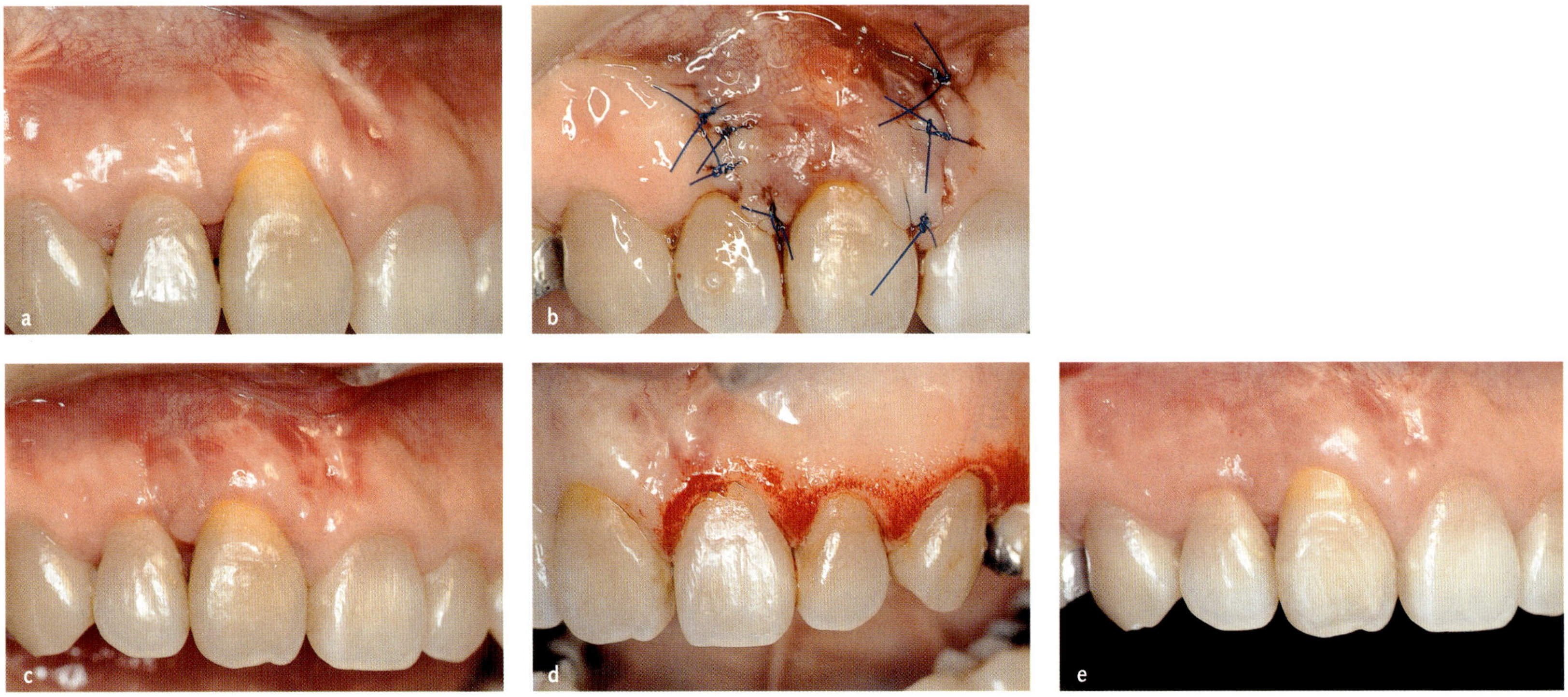

Fig 4-119 Coronal repositioning of the pedicle flap. (a) Photograph taken about 3 months after lateral flap repositioning. (b) A pedicle flap is coronally repositioned to recover the remaining exposed root surface of the maxillary right central incisor. (c and d) Photographs taken 1 month postsurgery. A gingivoplasty is conducted to restore symmetric gingival margins. (e) Photograph taken 1 month after the gingivoplasty; about 6 months after the first lateral repositioning of a pedicle flap. The objective has been achieved to a high level.

Leveling of irregular gingival margin

For correction of the gingival margin in mildly irregular cases, a gingivoplasty will suffice. When large-scale correction is required, exposed root surface coverage and clinical crown-lengthening procedures are combined to reposition the connective tissue (Fig 4-120). In the anterior region, it is mandatory to preserve the interdental papillae regardless of the technique used. In a crown-lengthening procedure in which the marginal gingiva is apically repositioned, butt joint–like vertical incisions are made without including the interdental papillae. When the marginal gingiva is coronally repositioned, the incision should involve interdental papillae. A beveled incision should be made in the interdental papilla. When thick gingiva is apically repositioned, the flap is raised from the gingival sulcus and the inner surface is trimmed so that the tissue thickness is well blended with the surrounding gingiva in a transitional manner.

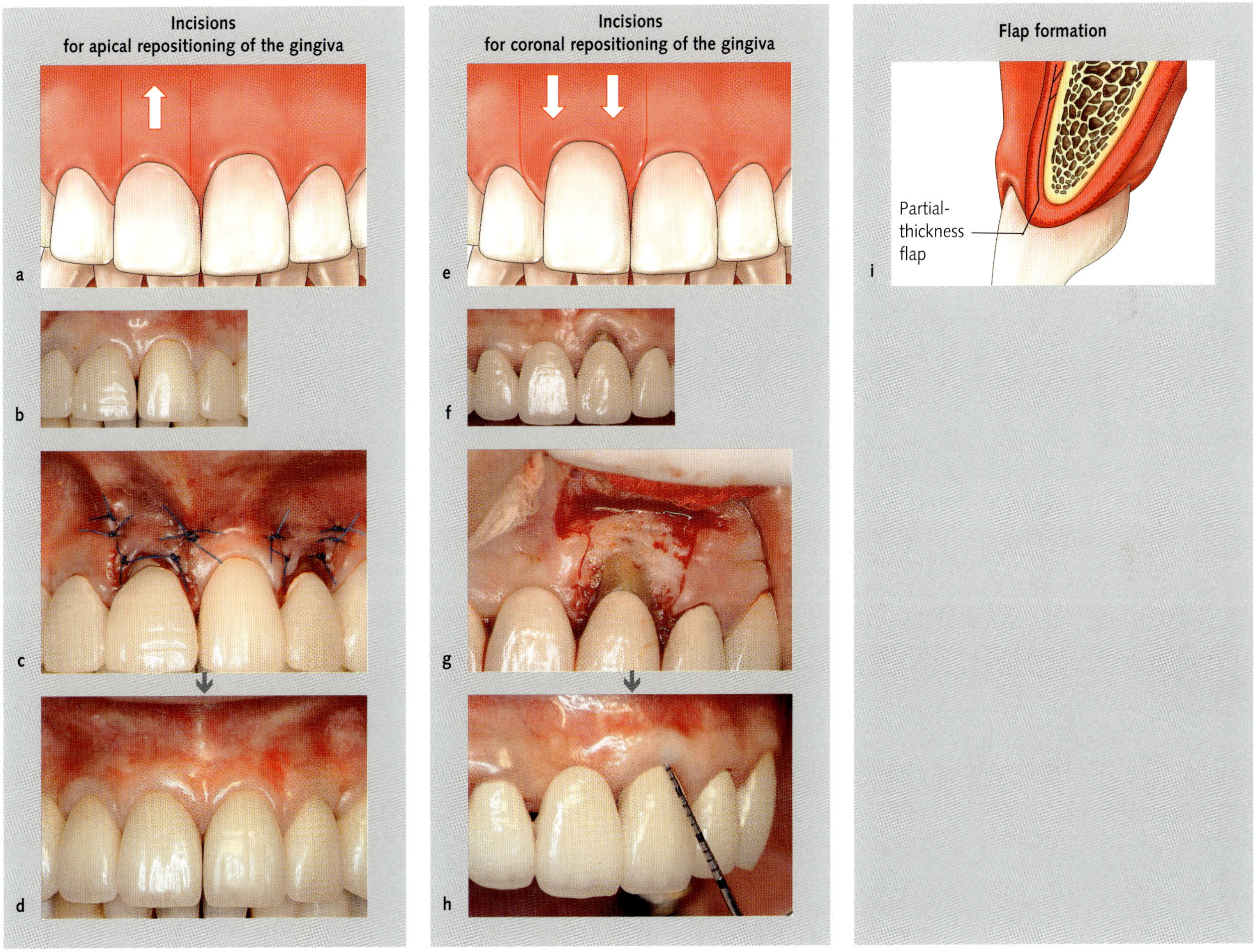

Fig 4-120 (a to i) Techniques for leveling an irregular gingival margin. (f to h) For this clinical case, a full-thickness periosteal flap is coronally repositioned to provide root coverage (new attachment). For esthetic considerations, beveled incisions are made in the interdental papillae to preserve the papillae.

Leveling of the gingivae—Apical repositioning of the marginal gingiva

To level an irregular gingival drape while preserving the interdental papillae, there is sometimes a need to reposition the marginal gingiva apically. Here, the marginal gingiva of the maxillary right central incisor and maxillary left lateral incisor are repositioned apically (Fig 4-121).

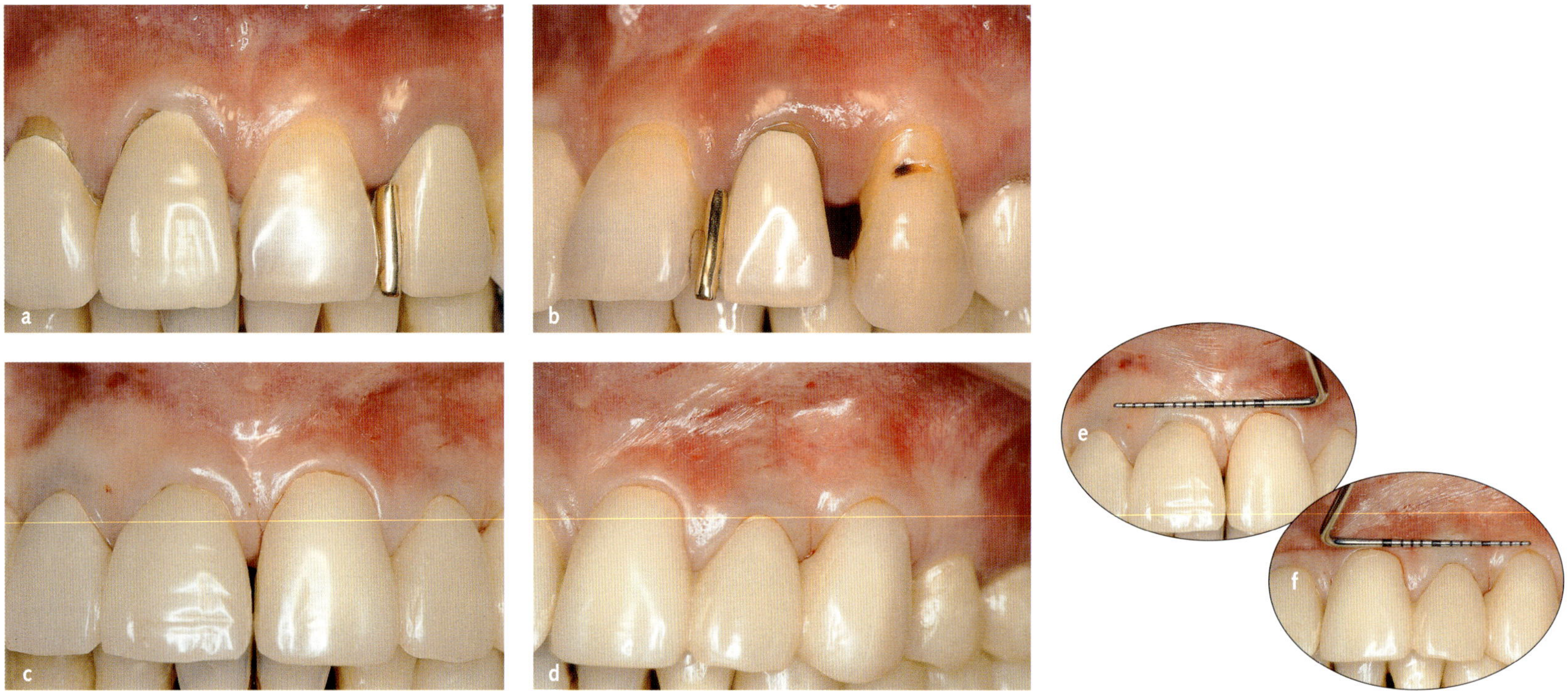

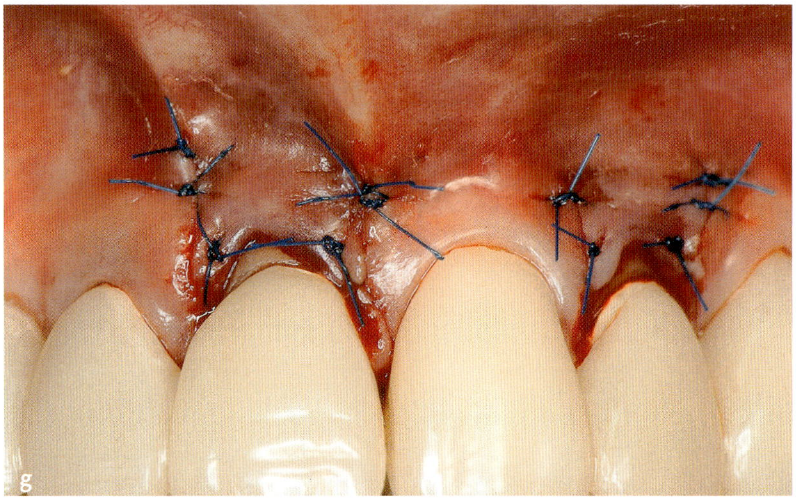

Fig 4-121 (a and b) In patients with loss of attached gingiva, it is preferable to level the attachment or bone crest uniformly. Moderate periodontal disease is noted at the first visit. (c to f) Extrusion and mesial movement were conducted to reduce the periodontal pocket of the maxillary left lateral incisor and restore the interdental papillae; this has resulted in an irregular gingival drape. (g) The attached gingiva is insufficient, so a full-thickness flap is raised with a sulcular incision and converted to a partial-thickness flap from directly under the bone crest. Releasing incisions are made at the bottom of the flap to level the gingiva. (h and i) At delivery of the prostheses, 1 year postsurgery, marginal continuity of the natural teeth has been restored. (j) Photograph taken 2 years after surgery (see Fig 4-109 for radiographs).

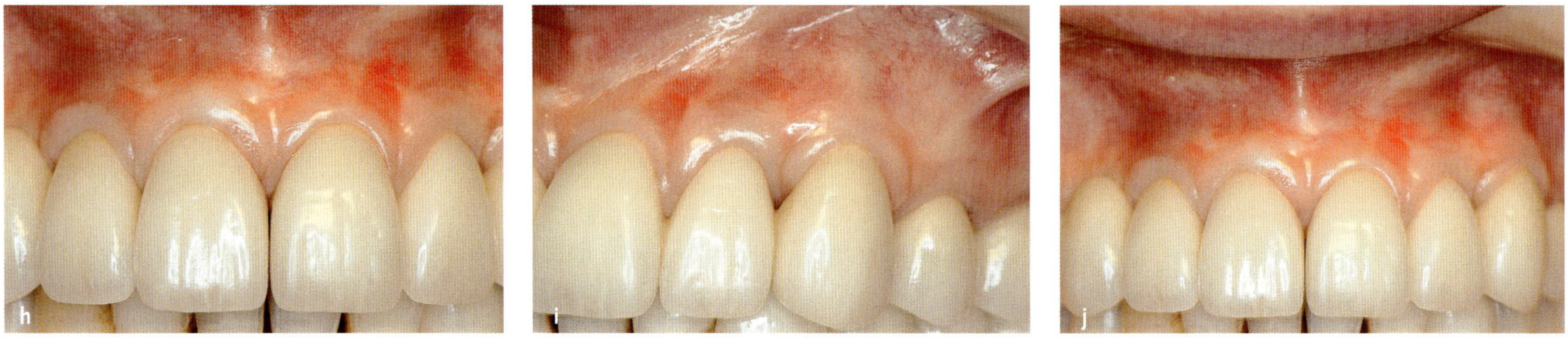

Restoration of asymmetric gingivae through apical repositioning with a full-partial–thickness flap

Handling of the periosteum in periodontal plastic surgery for preservation of the interdental papillae, endodontic treatment methodology, and impression techniques have remained the same since we began practice. The concept we utilize now with regard to controlling the thickness of the gingiva and the contour of the provisional restoration (discussed earlier in this chapter and in chapter 5) had not been established when the patient in Figs 4-122 to 4-124 was originally treated. Because of poor contouring of the provisional restoration, this patient presented with a band of redness at the marginal gingiva, which suggested inflammation arising from inadequate space, especially at the maxillary left central incisor (Figs 4-122 to 4-124).

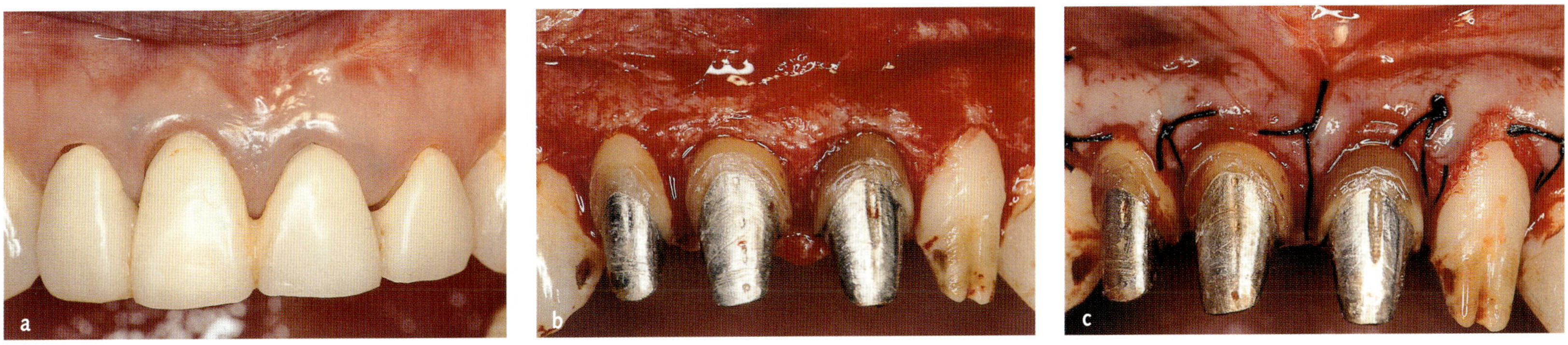

Fig 4-122 Apical repositioning. (a) After orthodontic treatment (1995), an uneven gingival drape is noted. (b) A partial-thickness flap is raised. The periosteum is carefully reflected with a raspatory from the interdental papilla toward the marginal area, and osseous surgery is conducted to adjust the marginal bone level. (c) The gingival margins are positioned at the interdental areas to reposition the periosteum of the interdental area.

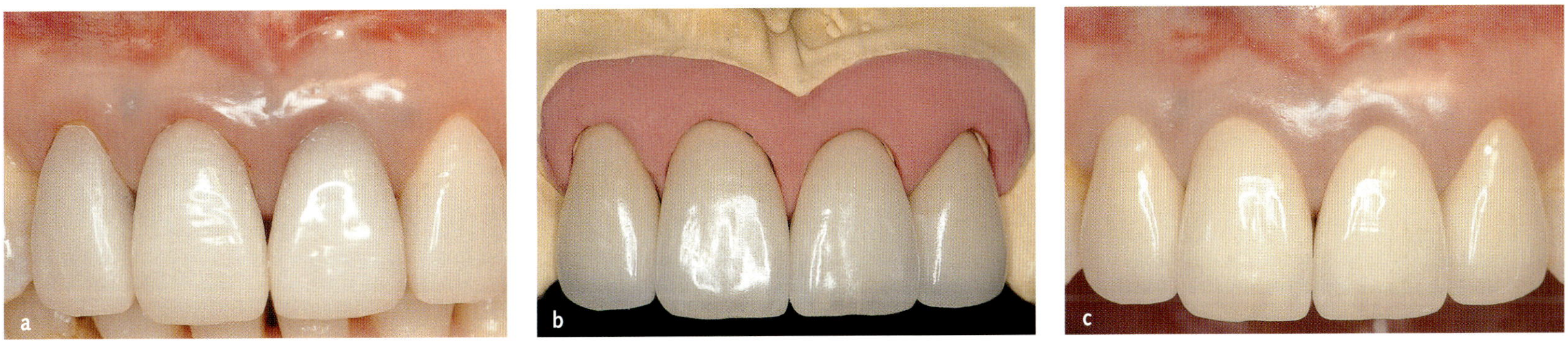

Fig 4-123 Problems with crown restorations. (a) Because of the thick gingiva and poor contour of the provisional restoration, a band of redness is noted, suggesting pressure against the tissues. (b) Although the tissue was correctly prepared, little attention was paid to the therapeutic contour of the restoration. (c) Photograph taken 3 years after surgery. Although contour was added, a band of inflammation remains.

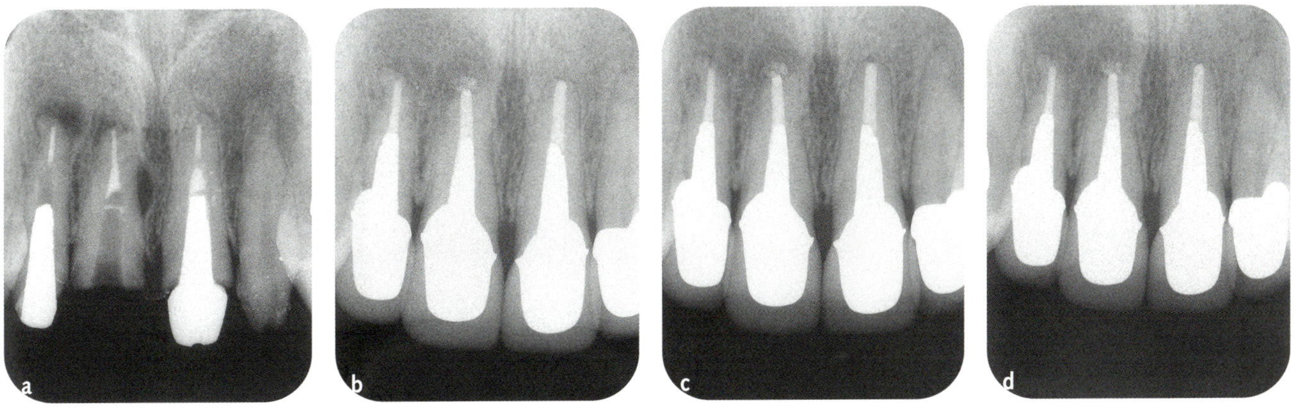

Fig 4-124 Follow-up of endodontic treatment. (a) At the first visit (May 1992). (b) About 6 years posttreatment. (c) About 7 years 7 months posttreatment. (d) About 9 years posttreatment.

Crown lengthening with preservation of the interdental papillae: Full-partial-full-partial–thickness flap

In the patient shown in Figs 4-125 to 4-130, subgingival caries developed at the margins of the metal-ceramic crowns, and crown-lengthening procedures were conducted for the maxillary anterior teeth, from the right lateral incisor to the left canine. The maxillary right canine did not have subgingival caries, and was not included in the

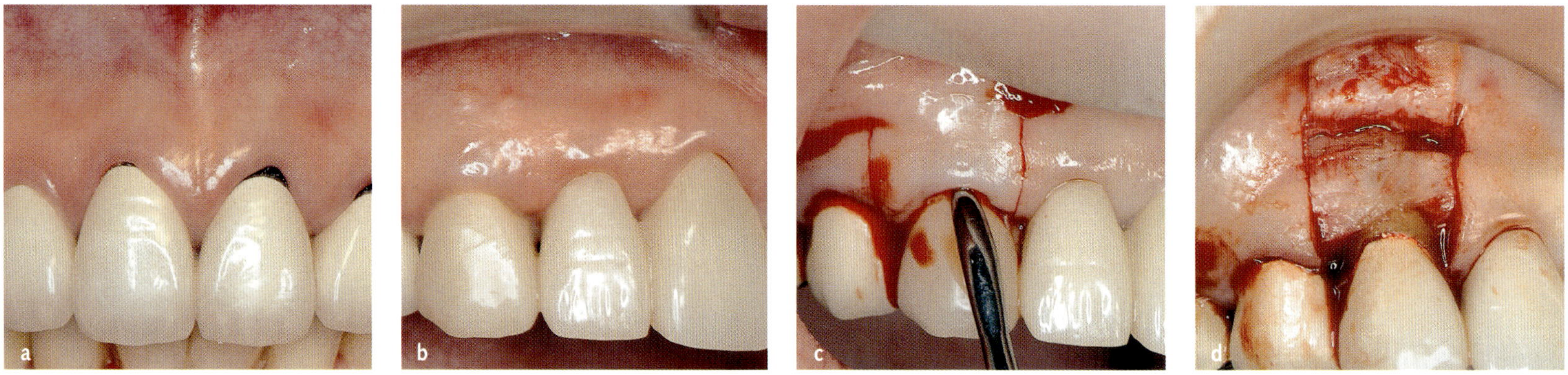

Fig 4-125 Flap design for crown lengthening. (a) Photograph of 13-year-old metal-ceramic restorations with subgingival dental caries at the maxillary right central and lateral incisors and left central incisor, lateral incisor, and canine. (b) Photograph taken 5 months after crown-lengthening procedures. There is an irregularity of the gingiva at the maxillary right canine. (c) Parallel vertical incisions are made without extending beyond the MGJ. After a sulcular incision is made, a raspatory is used to elevate a full-thickness flap only in the gingival sulcus. (d) After the gingival sulcus is elevated, the flap is immediately converted to a partial-thickness design, and the apical portion is made into a full-thickness flap again. The connective tissue preserved on the periosteum is used for plastic surgery in the cervical area. This is a full-partial-full–thickness flap combination.

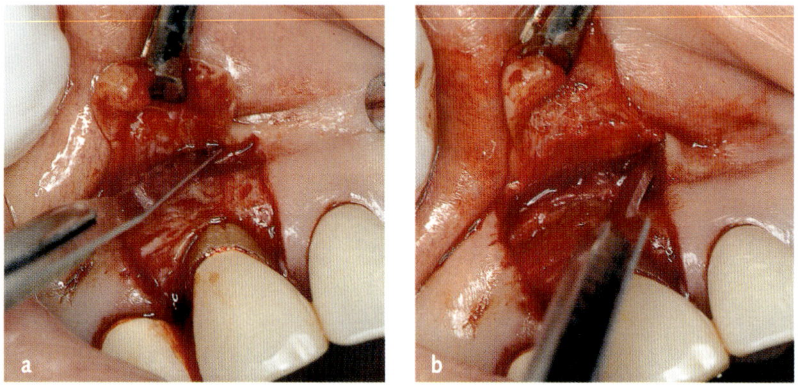

Fig 4-126 Releasing incisions under the MGJ. (a) A semilunar releasing incision is made under the MGJ. (b) A releasing incision is also made at the base of the flap. An incision is made at the coronal side at 45 degrees.

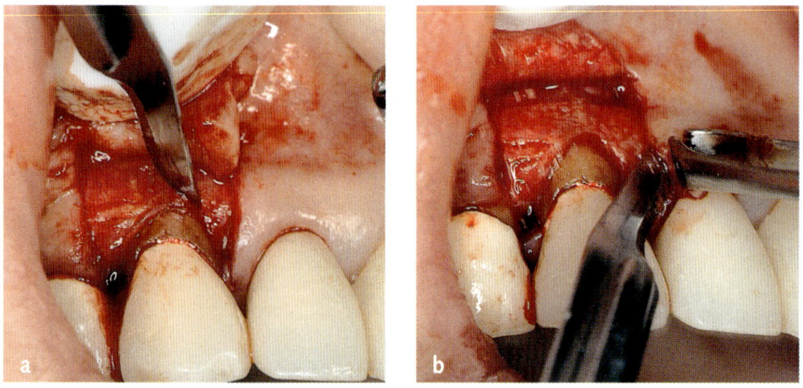

Fig 4-127 Preparation of the cervical connective tissue. (a) Connective tissue on the periosteum is resected in a scalloped form that is slightly larger than the target. A scaler is used to remove the resected tissue as one piece. (b) A surgical knife is used to trim the thickness of interdental area.

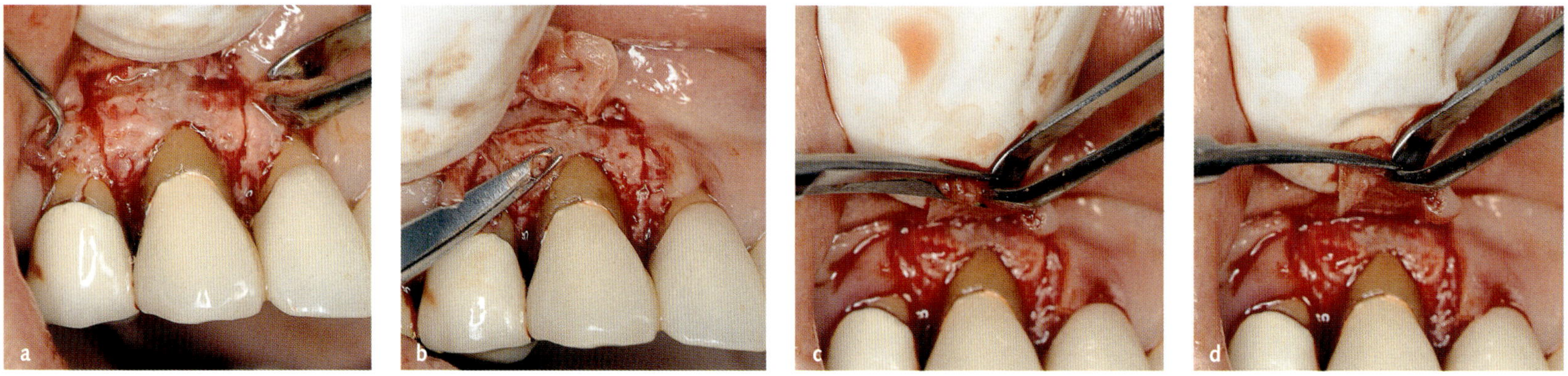

Fig 4-128 Preparation of the interdental area and flap design. (a) The thickness of both of the interdental papilla areas has been adjusted to the appropriate shape and thickness. (b) The thickness of the cervically scalloped area is further adjusted. (c) Delicate trimming is conducted for the interdental papilla areas. (d) The thickness of flap is reduced with Castro Viejo scissors for the plastic surgery. The flap is trimmed in a scalloped shape while being held with forceps.

procedure. The gingiva of the maxillary right canine was positioned coronally to that of the maxillary right lateral incisor, causing an irregular gingival drape. Although gingivoplasty with electrosurgery would have been possible, gingivoplasty cannot change the inner connective tissue attachment to achieve a biologically scalloped form.

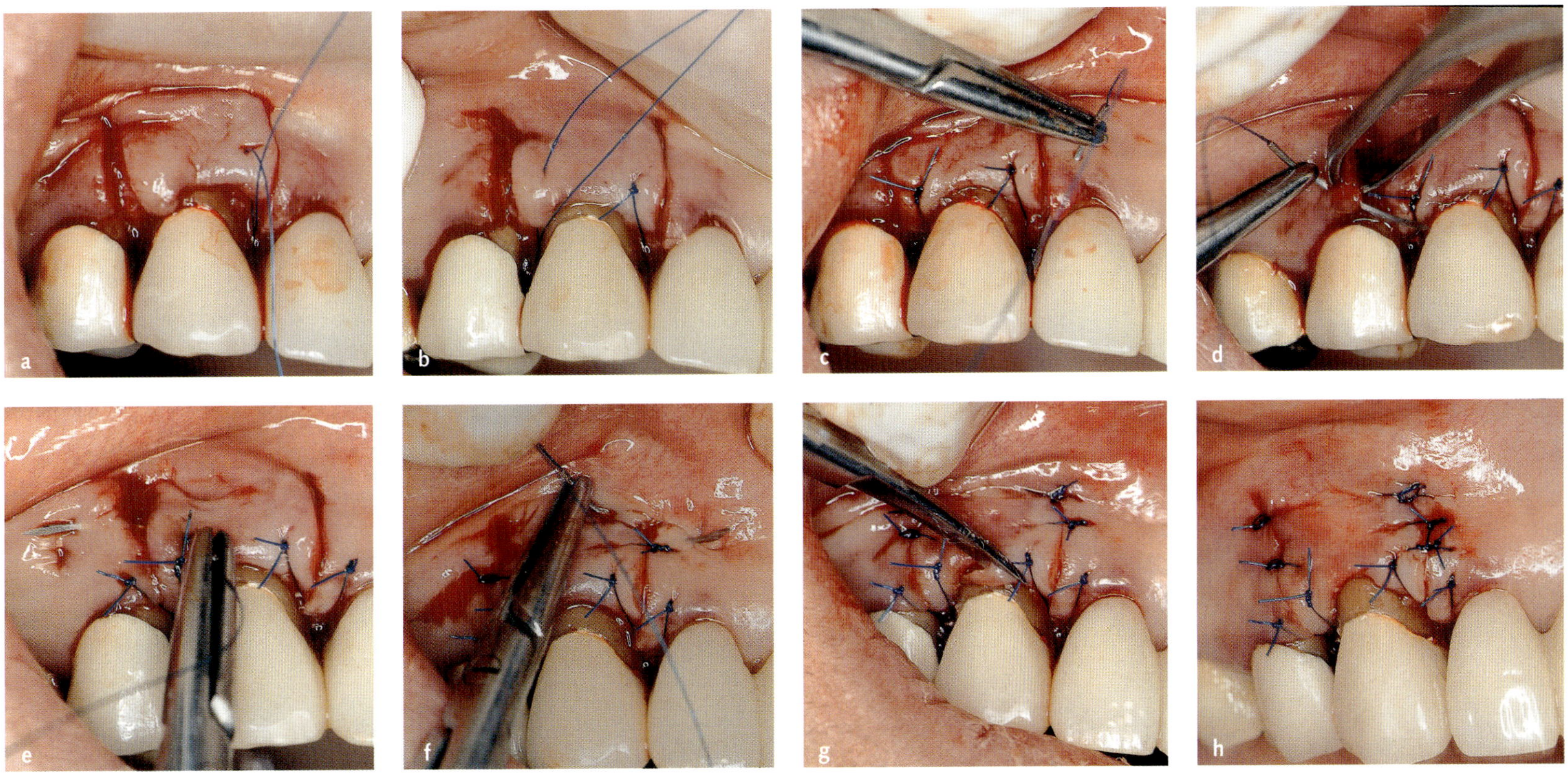

Fig 4-129 Suturing. (a) The needle is inserted 2 mm into the interdental papilla, penetrating the periosteum to form a figure-eight suture on the palatal aspect. A nylon suture designed for plastic surgery is used. (b) A similar suture is made on the opposite side. (c) Again, the needle is inserted 2 mm into the interdental papilla. (d) The needle is inserted in a symmetric position on the other aspect of the flap, while the flap is held with forceps. (e) The vertically incised areas are sutured. Note that needle is pointed downward for the apical repositioning of the flap. (f) The flap is sutured so that the dead space will be eliminated at the MGJ, where the releasing incisions are made. (g) The marginal gingiva is adjusted to a scalloped shape. (h) Final suturing.

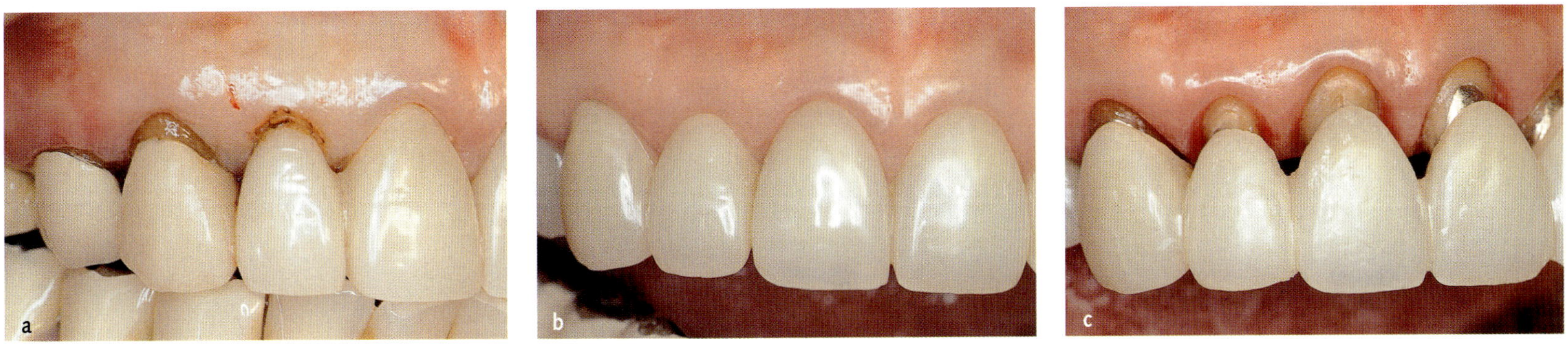

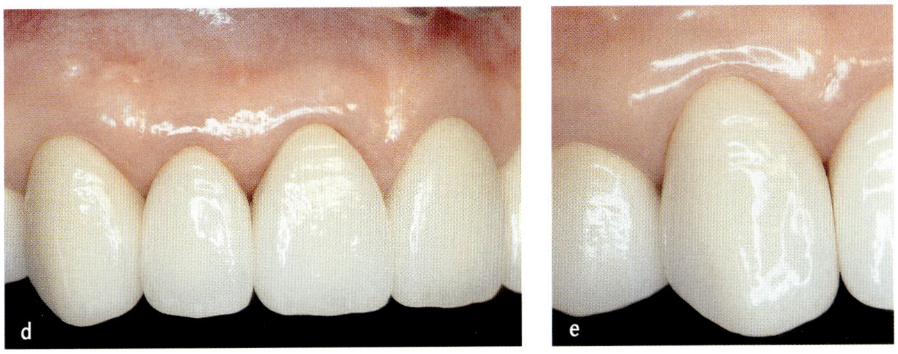

Fig 4-130 Crown restoration. (a) Photograph taken 1 month after crown lengthening at the maxillary right canine. (b) The provisional restoration is shown after 7 months. (c) After 9 months, addition of self-curing resin to the marginal areas is repeated, based on the appearance of the provisional restoration. (d and e) Photographs taken 1 year after surgery, or 1 year 6 months after the clinical crown lengthening that was necessary due to secondary caries. A gingival morphology with high esthetics and maintainability has been achieved (see Fig 1-53 for radiographs).

Tissue Reconstruction of Alveolar Ridge Defects

Classification of alveolar ridge defects

Tooth roots are supported by the surrounding alveolar bone, and at the same time, alveolar bone proper is supported by the tooth roots that receive physiologic loads. Because of this, after teeth are lost, bone is lost and gradually the alveolar ridge itself is resorbed over time. Resorption of the edentulous alveolar ridge is particularly significant in the anterior maxilla, and it results in serious damage to esthetics. The volume of edentulous alveolar ridge has to be increased to maintain the vertical height of the original dentition and to restore a crown morphology that is reasonable and close to that of the natural teeth.

Seibert classified ridge defects into three categories, based on the height and width of the deformity (Table 4-4 and Fig 4-131). When the prosthetic environment and procedures for alveolar ridge augmentation are considered, attention should also be paid to the amount of keratinized mucosa and presence or absence of immobile mucosa as well as the degree of bone resorption (Figs 4-132 and 4-133).

Table 4-4 Classification of alveolar ridge defects (Seibert)

Class I	Ridge defects have a normal apicocoronal height and involve a loss in the buccolingual width only.
Class II	Ridge defects have a normal buccolingual width and involve a loss in the apicocoronal height only.
Class III	Ridge defects involve a combination of buccolingual and apicocoronal loss.

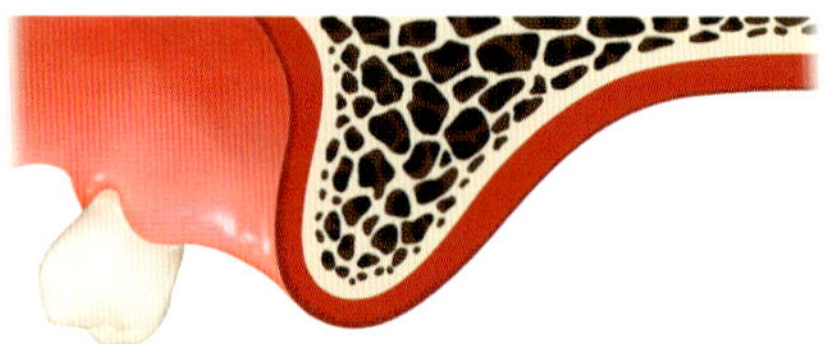

Alveolar ridge of sufficient width and height
It is rare that alveolar ridge defects maintain sufficient width and height. Some augmentation procedure for ridge defects is required for esthetic prostheses. Seibert described classification of ridge defects. The outcome of procedures is affected by the thickness of the palatal (lingual) mucosa and width of the keratinized mucosa as well as the morphology of the defects.

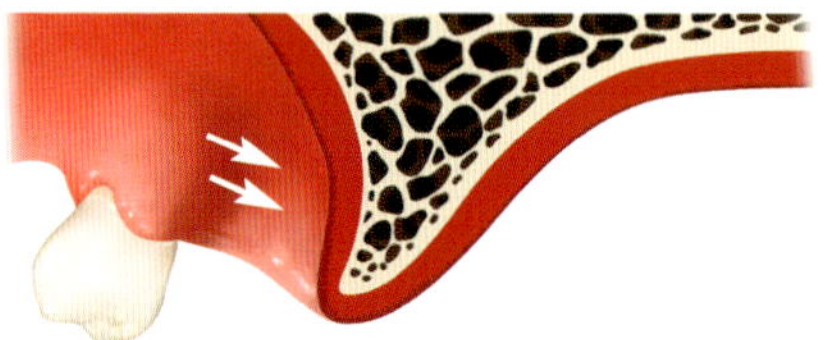

Seibert class I
Loss in the buccolingual width of the ridge, manifested as a concavity. The condition can be treated with a connective tissue graft or roll technique. The indications for ridge augmentation procedures are based on the width and volume of the buccal keratinized gingiva.

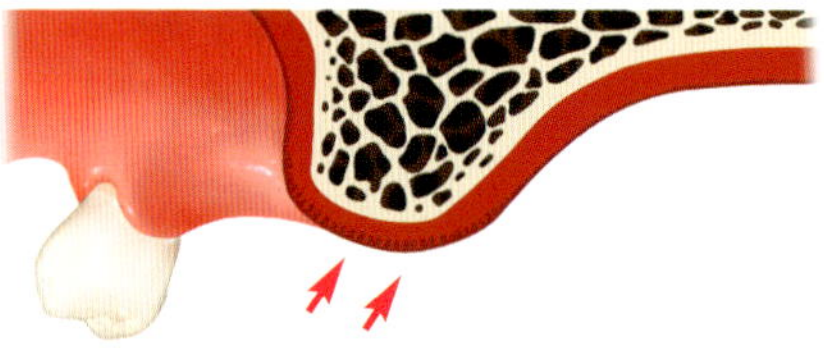

Seibert class II
Loss in the apicocoronal height of the ridge. In class II and class III cases with sufficient connective tissue at the alveolar crest, and when a scalloped form around implants or an ovate pontic is covered, keratinized gingiva cannot be established with a distal wedge technique, and a double roll technique is more suitable.

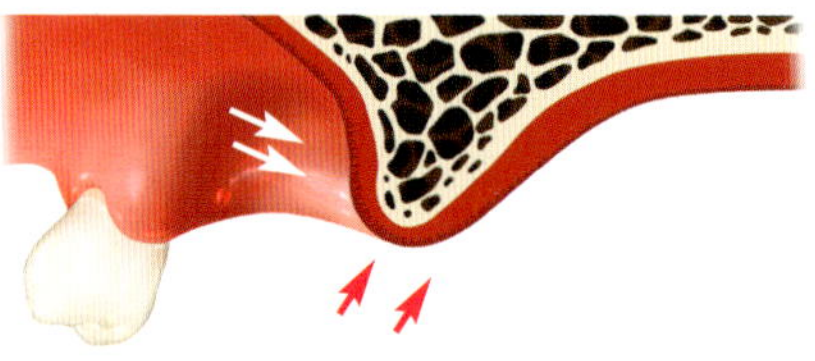

Seibert class III
Combination of buccolingual and apicocoronal loss. In class III cases, a combination of a bone or connective tissue graft and the roll technique is often used. It is essential to have sufficient thickness of the palatal mucosa or lingual gingiva.

Fig 4-131 Augmentation of alveolar ridge defects in the anterior maxilla.

Box 4-1 Augmentation procedures for ovate pontics

① Gingivectomy
② Inlay method (pouch method, sandwich method)
③ Onlay method
- Direct method: epithelialized free gingival graft
- Indirect method: subepithelial connective tissue graft

④ Roll technique
- Normal roll
- Modified normal roll
- Reverse roll
- Double roll (double slide)
- Modified roll

⑤ Bone graft
⑥ Guided bone regeneration method

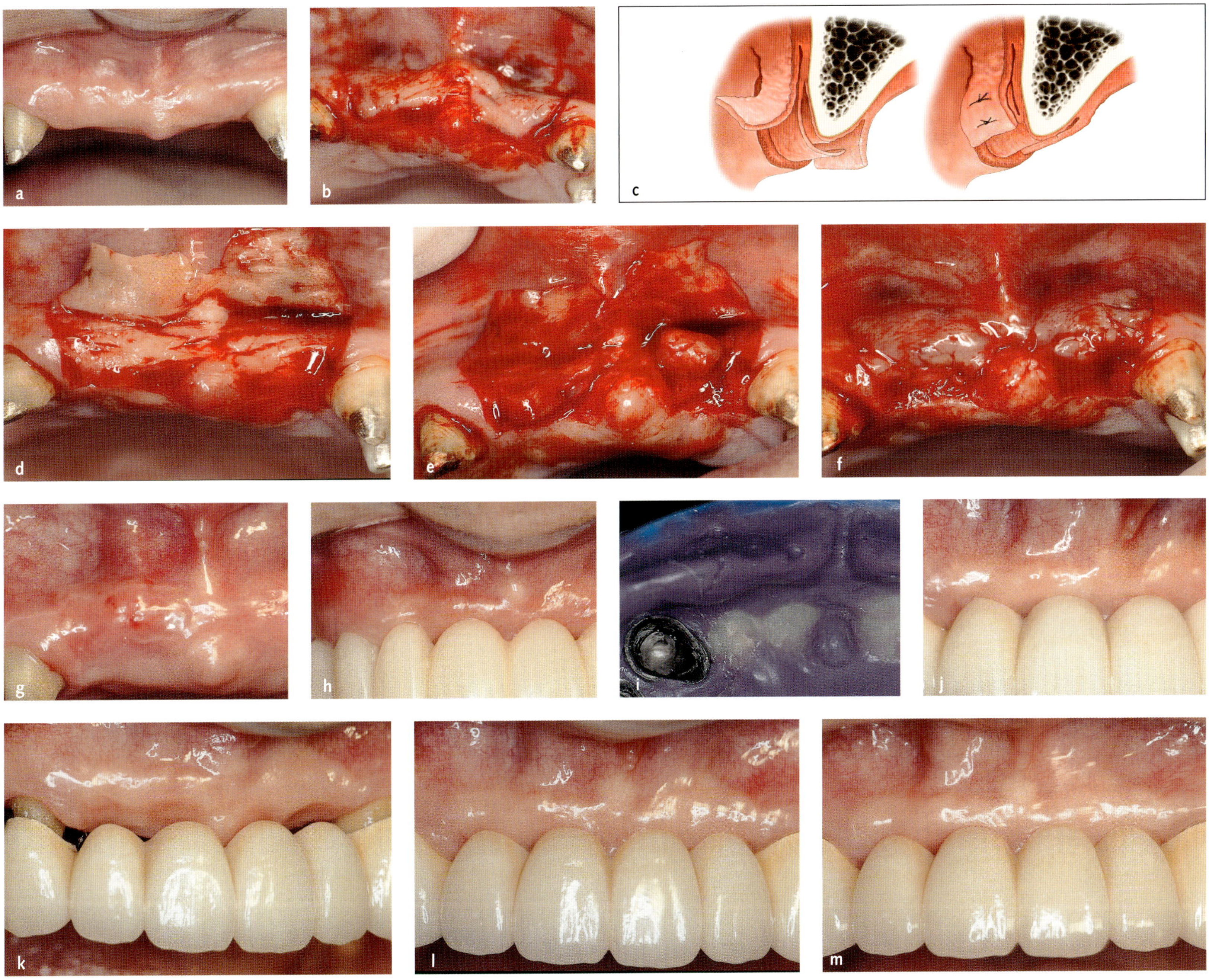

Fig 4-132 Augmentation of alveolar ridge defects in the anterior maxilla. (a) Although the alveolar ridge defect resulting from the extraction of the maxillary right lateral incisor to the maxillary left lateral incisor has reasonable height and width remaining in the area for the pontic, the gingivae will be in movable mucosa. (b) Attention is paid to preserving the interdental papillae mesial to the maxillary right canine and left canine. Vertical incisions are made on the buccal aspect in a perpendicular manner and slip joint beveled incisions are completed on the palatal side. The incisive papilla is preserved, without being included in the buccal flap. A vertical, perpendicular incision is less likely to generate a scar, even after apical repositioning of the flap. (c) Reverse roll technique. (d) A partial-thickness flap is raised and some releasing incisions are made to the connective tissue. The palatal connective tissue is repositioned buccally, and the partial-thickness flap is repositioned (laterally and coronally) so that the keratinized mucosa can be augmented by 2 to 3 mm buccal to the cervical margin of the pontics. (e) Because the palatal mucosa is thick in this case, the palatal connective tissue is sectioned and inserted under the buccal pontic area with a reverse roll technique. (f) The rolled connective tissue is sutured with a resorbable suture, and covered by the pedicle connective tissue graft. The ligature suture is completed with resorbable sutures. (g) Apical repositioning of a sufficient width of keratinized immovable mucosa is achieved along with the alveolar ridge augmentation. This sets the conditions for fabrication of ovate pontics (1 month after surgery). (h) Self-curing acrylic resin is added to the gingival aspect of the provisional pontics to give them an ovate form (2 months after surgery). (i) A pick-up impression is taken for soldering of the metal framework for the metal-ceramic restoration. Slight pressure is placed against the pontic area during impression taking. The emergence profile impression is simultaneously taken for the areas of the maxillary right second premolar and second molar and left canine and first premolar (4 months after surgery). (j) To finalize the ovate shape with appropriate contours, adjustments are made during the bisque bake try-in at the areas that caused ischemia in the gingiva because of pressure. (k) Delivery of the final fixed partial denture. Harmony in the gingival contours as well as the interdental papilla-like tissue is obtained (6 months after surgery). (l) Photograph taken postcementation. (m) Photograph taken 1 year after surgery, or 6 months after delivery of prosthesis.

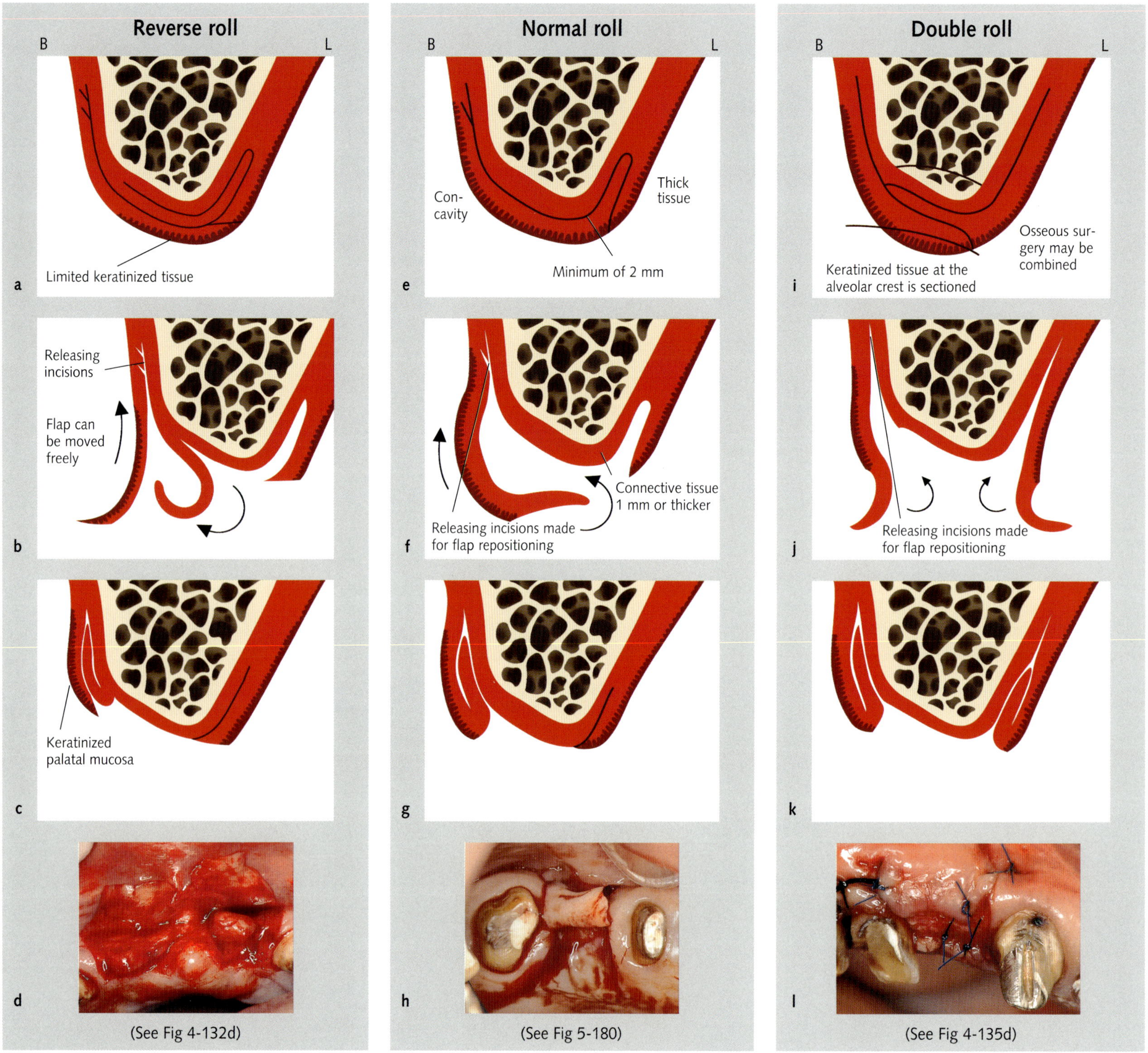

Fig 4-133 Soft tissue augmentation for alveolar ridge defects.

Reverse roll: (a to d) Indications for this procedure are soft tissue augmentation in Seibert class II and class III cases. Even when limited keratinized gingiva is available on the alveolar crest, the mucosa can be moved freely because the buccal flap is movable mucosa. Because of this, vestibular extension and the increase of keratinized gingiva can be conducted simultaneously. Unlike the inlay method, this procedure can not only achieve augmentation of the alveolar soft tissue but also increase the amount of keratinized tissue.

Normal roll: Indication for this procedure is a Seibert Class III with thick lingual soft tissue. (e to h) This is a basic procedure to augment the buccal soft tissue with a pedicle flap graft. It is essential to have thick palatal mucosa and keratinized buccal gingiva. The modified normal roll technique is useful; in this procedure, the buccal connective tissue is sectioned to form a pedicle flap and a scalloped form is established around the implant abutment or pontic regions.

Double roll: (i to l) In cases with sufficient connective tissue at the alveolar crest, when the scalloped form around implants or pontics cannot be established, this technique is indicated. Depending on the case, not only is resectioning of the connective tissue at alveolar crest completed, but osseous surgery is also conducted.

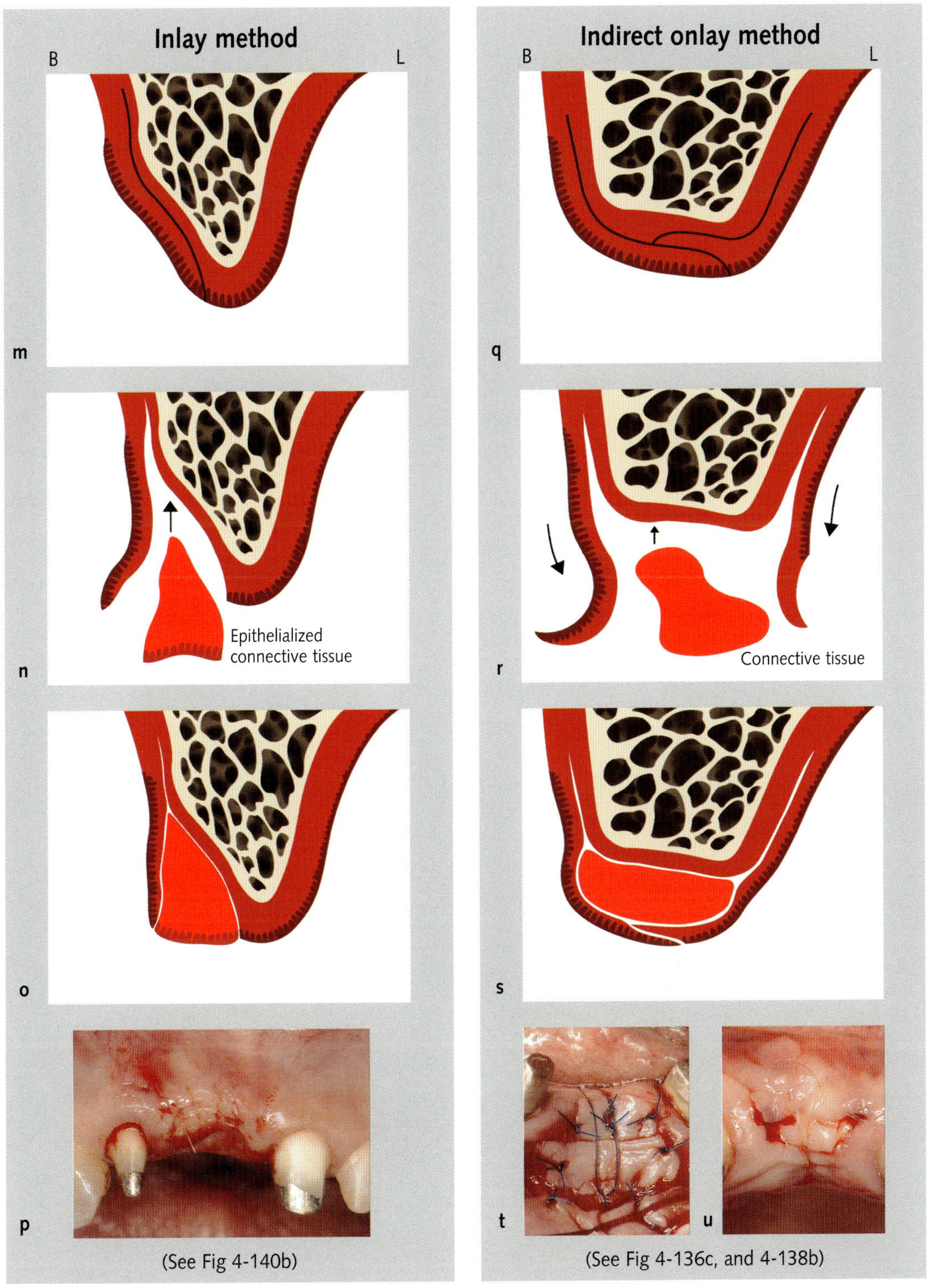

Fig 4-133 (cont)

Inlay method: (m to p) Epithelialized connective tissue is grafted to the buccal defect. The indication for this technique is Seibert Class I situations.

Indirect onlay method: (q to u) Connective tissue harvested from the palate is grafted mostly for vertical augmentation of the alveolar crest. The indication for this technique is Seibert Class II cases. For onlay methods, an epithelialized connective graft (direct method) is usually recommended. A subepithelial connective graft (indirect method) is recommended from the viewpoint of esthetics.

Connective tissue graft for esthetic zone (inlay graft)

Because the maxillary right first premolar was the area that needed regenerative therapy in this clinical case, a minimally invasive connective tissue graft procedure was used (Fig 4-134). There was insufficient keratinized buccal gingiva.

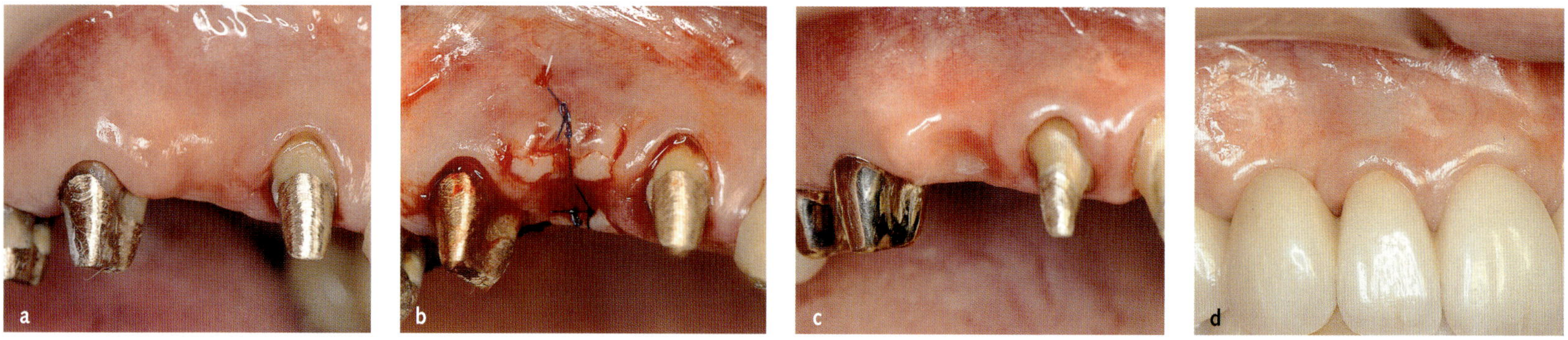

Fig 4-134 (a) A significant concavity exists where the maxillary right canine had been extracted (Seibert Class III). (b) Epithelialized connective tissue is inlay grafted with a modified roll technique. (c) Photograph taken 1 year 8 months after surgery. Ovate form is prepared into the tissue. Telescopic crowns are delivered to the maxillary right first and second premolars to assure parallelism and prevent fractures. (d) Photograph taken 2 years after surgery. Esthetic gingival margins have been achieved.

Augmentation of alveolar ridge defects (double roll)

The double roll technique was applied to the ridge defect shown in Fig 4-135. There was sufficient gingiva at the alveolar crest of the missing maxillary right first premolar (Seibert Class I).

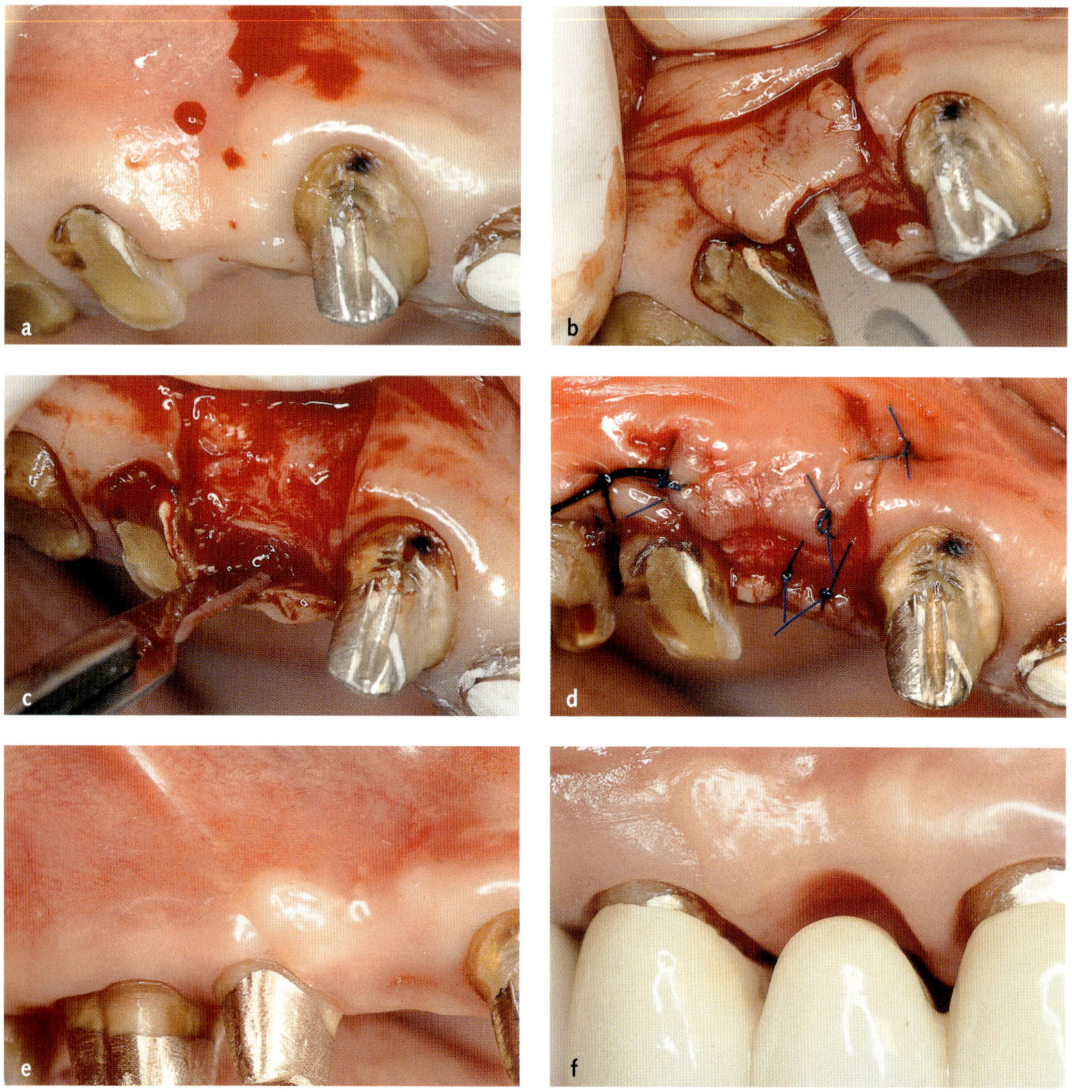

Fig 4-135 (a to d) The gingiva is repositioned buccally and lingually because a gingivoplasty alone will cause loss of the buccal attached gingiva. (e) Photograph taken 2 months postsurgery. Sufficient attached gingiva has been obtained. (f) At delivery of the final prosthesis, good transitional morphology from the buccal papilla to the col and the lingual papilla have been obtained.

Onlay technique for nonesthetic

The fixed partial denture abutment, the mandibular left second premolar, was under evaluation following GTR regenerative therapy (Fig 4-136). The onlay graft technique was adapted to suture a free gingival graft to the alveolar ridge, avoiding the invasion of a roll technique. Because the onlay graft is not the same color as gingiva, the technique can be indicated only for areas where esthetics is not a concern. Buccal grafting was conducted with the intent of increasing the vestibular extension.

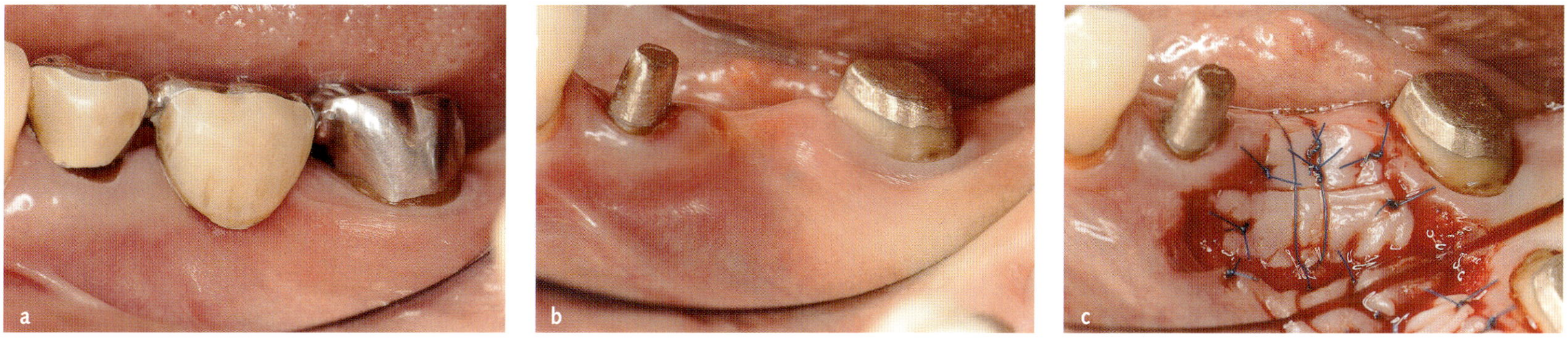

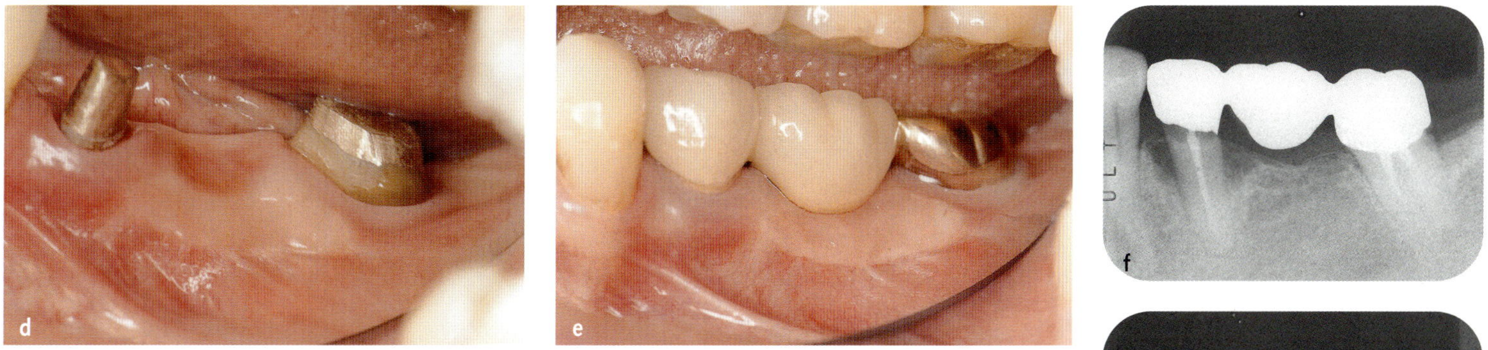

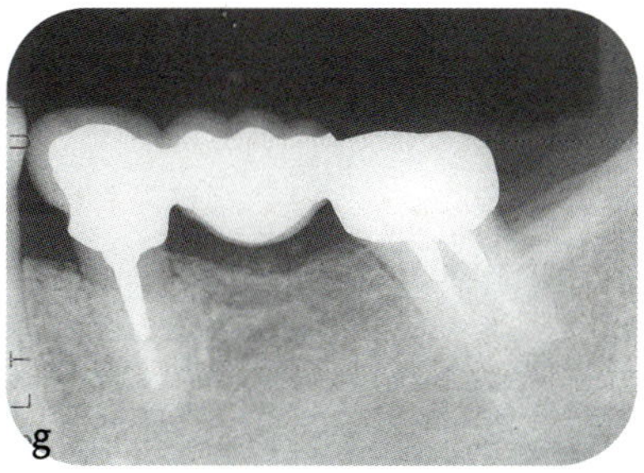

Fig 4-136 (a) Subgingival caries and a cup-shaped bone loss are noted at the area of the fixed partial denture abutment, the mandibular left second premolar. (b and c) After connective tissue regeneration using GTR with a nonresorbable membrane, free gingival tissue is onlay grafted to increase the keratinized gingiva in the pontic area and vestibular extension. (d) Photograph taken 3 months after surgery. An ovate form is placed in the tissue. (e) Photograph taken 5 years after delivery of prostheses. (f) Radiograph taken at the first visit. After debridement, bone is grafted to the defect, the root surface is treated with tetracycline, and regenerative therapy is conducted with an e-PTFE membrane. (g) Radiograph taken 5 years 7 months after surgery.

Figs 4-137 to 4-144 Soft tissue augmentation of alveolar ridge defects and ovate pontic areas

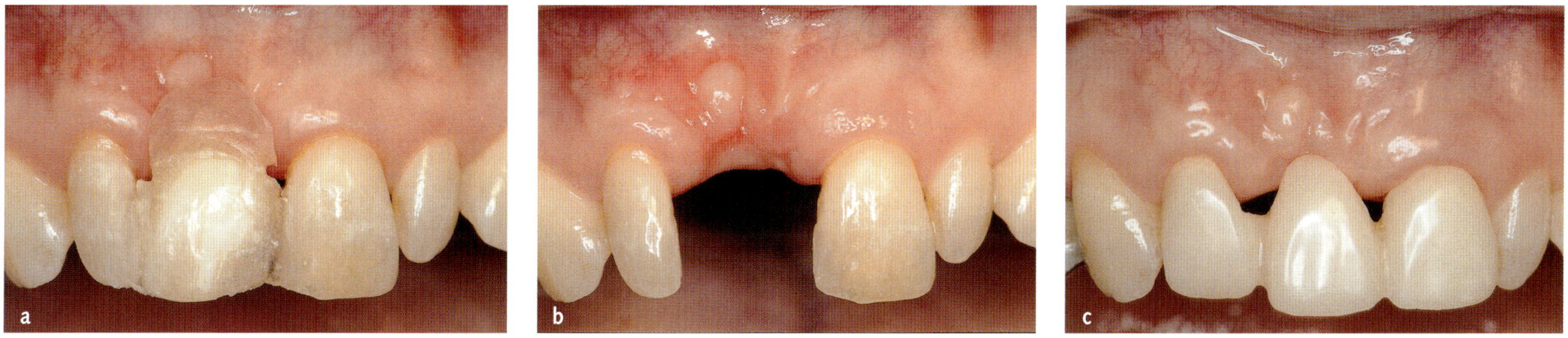

Fig 4-137 Alveolar ridge defects. (a) The patient was a 45-year-old woman at her first visit. She came to us wearing an emergency transitional appliance to replace the extracted maxillary right central incisor. Pink acrylic covers the alveolar ridge defect. (b) There is large concavity on the buccal aspect of the ridge. The maxillary right and left lateral incisors are microdonts. (c) After 7 months, including the initial therapy, it is possible to estimate the amount of soft tissue augmentation necessary.

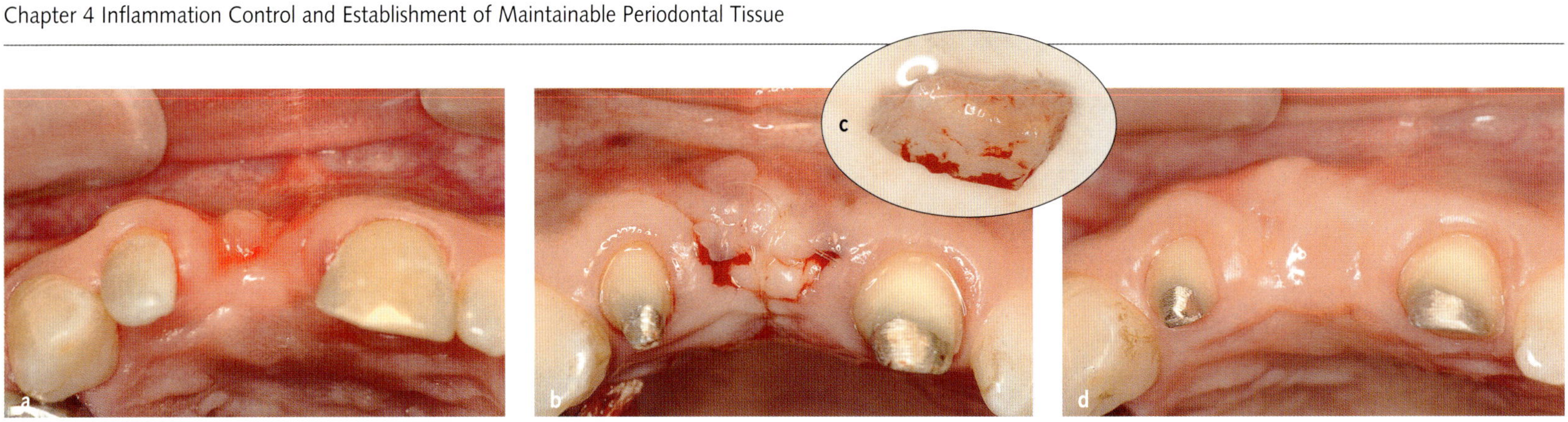

Fig 4-138 Augmentation of the alveolar ridge defects. (a) A significant concavity exists on the buccal aspect of the ridge. (b and c) A large connective tissue graft (6 mm wide × 12 mm long) is harvested from the palate and subepithelially grafted. (d) Photograph taken 4 months postsurgery. The buccal concavity has improved considerably.

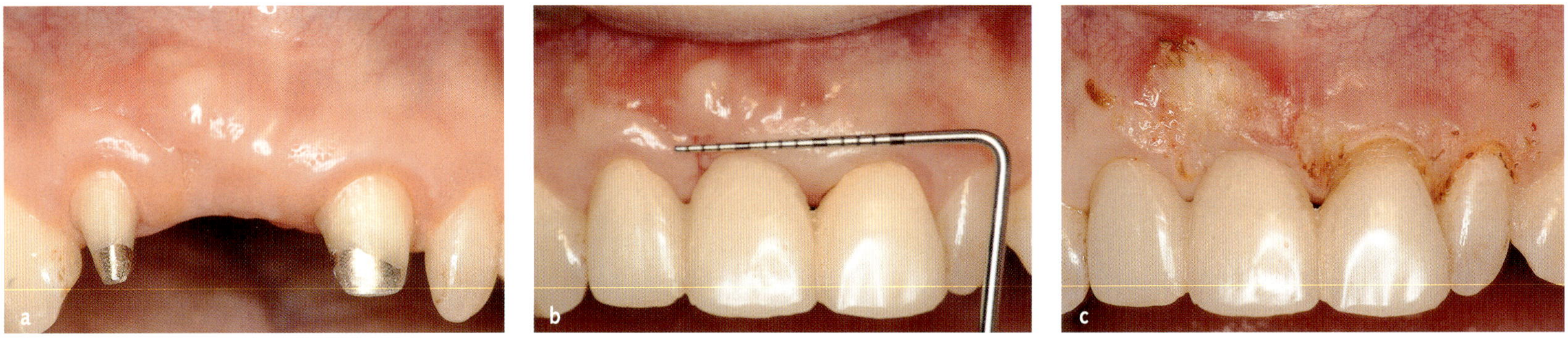

Fig 4-139 Aligning the gingival margin. (a) Photograph taken 4 months postsurgery. The gingival margin is irregular. (b and c) The gingiva is leveled by electrosurgery.

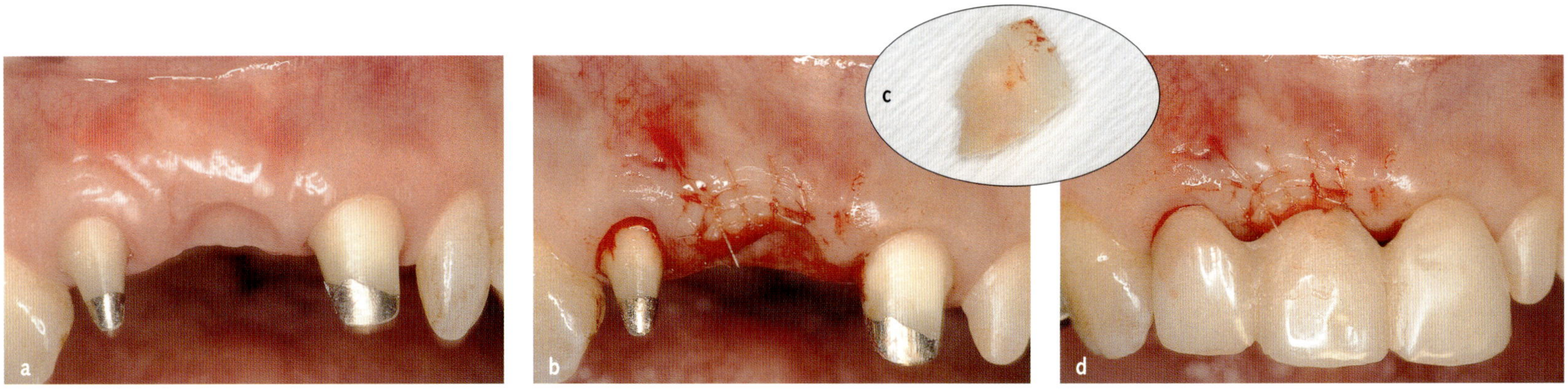

Fig 4-140 Second augmentation. (a) Photograph taken 6 months after augmentation of the alveolar ridge defects. (b) Compared to the left side, the interdental papilla between the maxillary right lateral incisor and central incisor remains flat, with an asymmetric gingiva. There is also a concern about the concavity between the maxillary right lateral and central incisors. (c and d) An envelope is formed to communicate with the mesial sulcus of the maxillary right lateral incisor. A wedge-shaped connective tissue graft is harvested from the area distal to the last molar and grafted to the mesial aspect for regeneration of the interdental papilla.

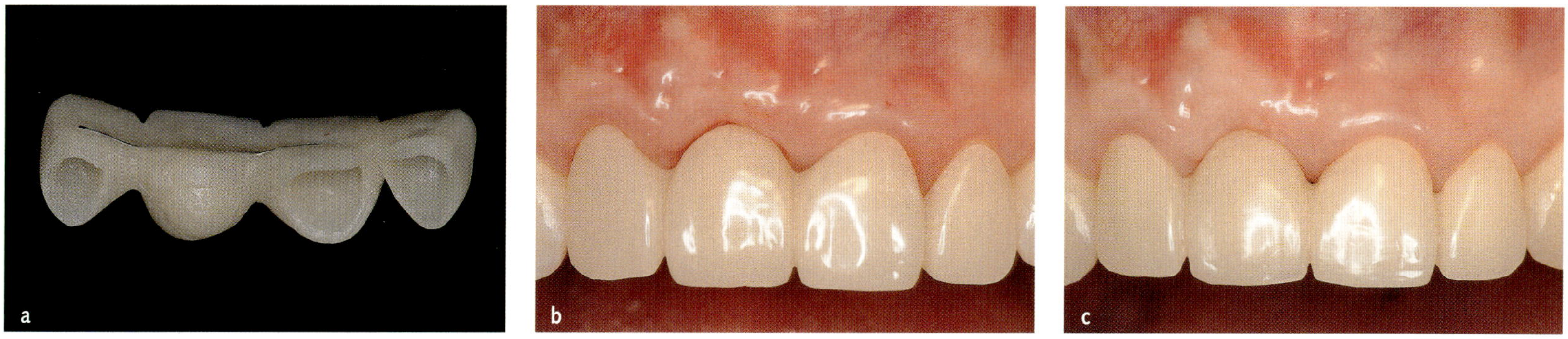

Fig 4-141 Ovate pontic. (a) A provisional pontic is fabricated to be symmetric to the maxillary left central incisor. (b) At each visit, self-curing acrylic resin is added to the pontic to further adjust the pontic shape. (c) The final provisional restoration. Correct gingival margins and interdental papillae have been obtained.

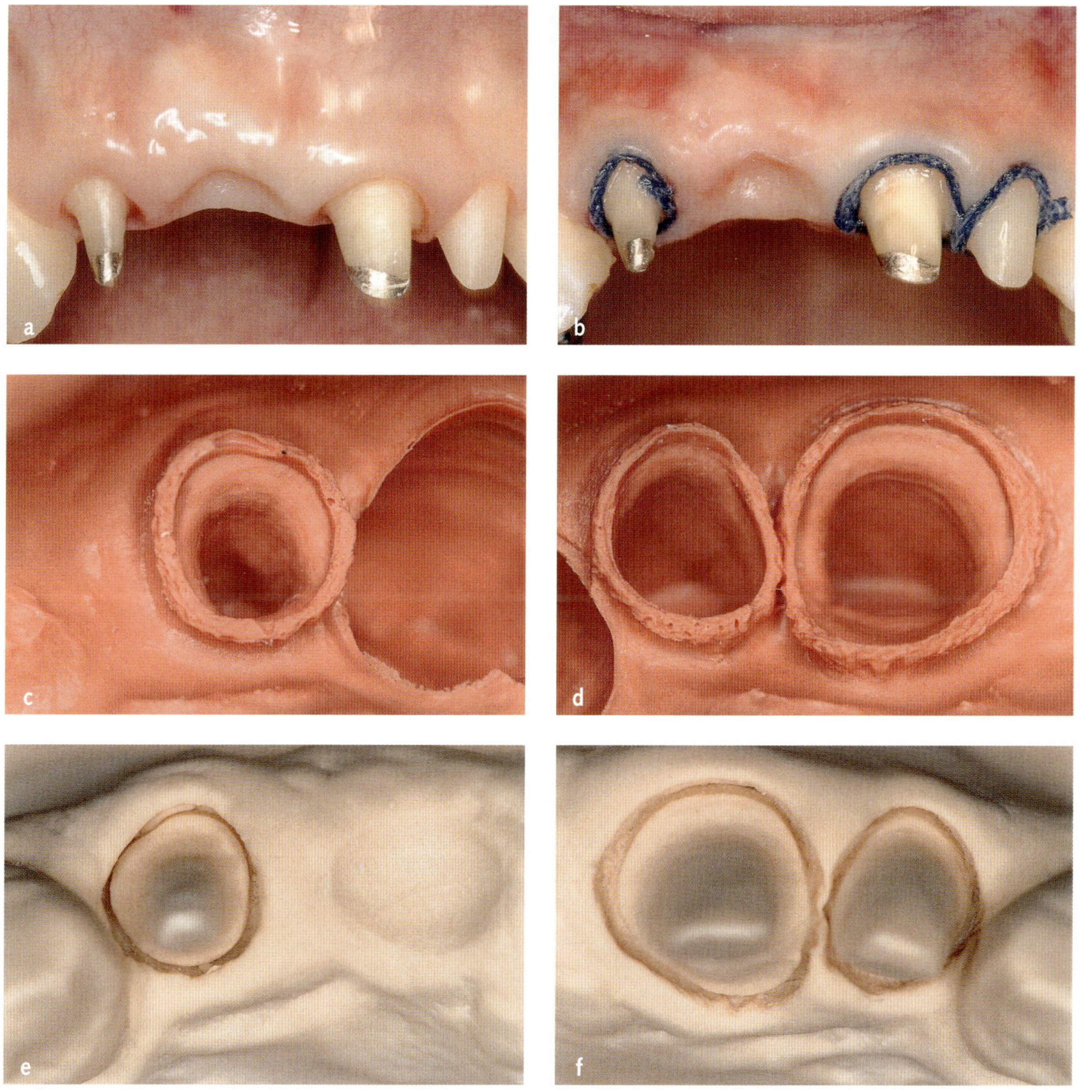

Fig 4-142 Impression taking for final prostheses. (a) Ovate pontic area after preparation. (b) Gingival retraction is completed carefully. To avoid damage to the gingiva, retraction cord must not be left in place longer than 10 minutes. (c to f) HIT impression showing clear preparation margins. (g) Gingival surface of the ovate pontic.

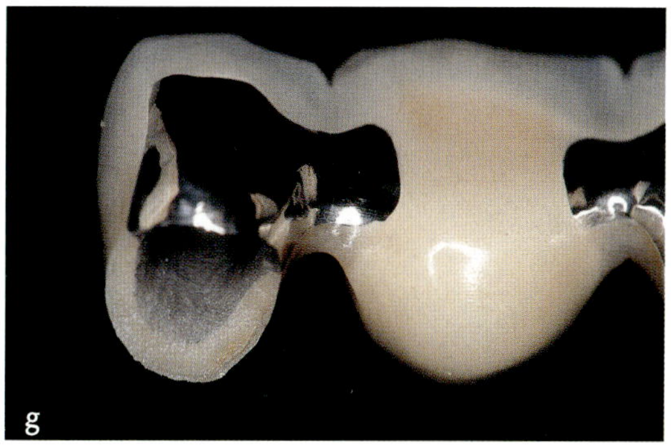

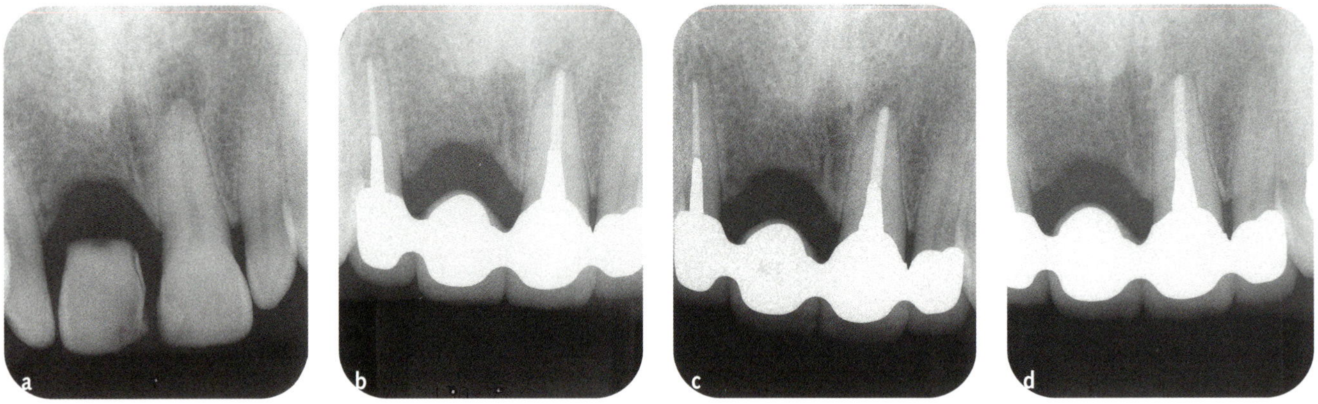

Fig 4-143 Radiographic evaluation. (a) At the first visit. (b) At delivery of the final prostheses, a good fit is confirmed. (c) At delivery of the final prostheses, a periapical lesion is noted. (d) Radiograph taken 2 years 5 months after the first visit, or about 10 months after delivery of the final prostheses.

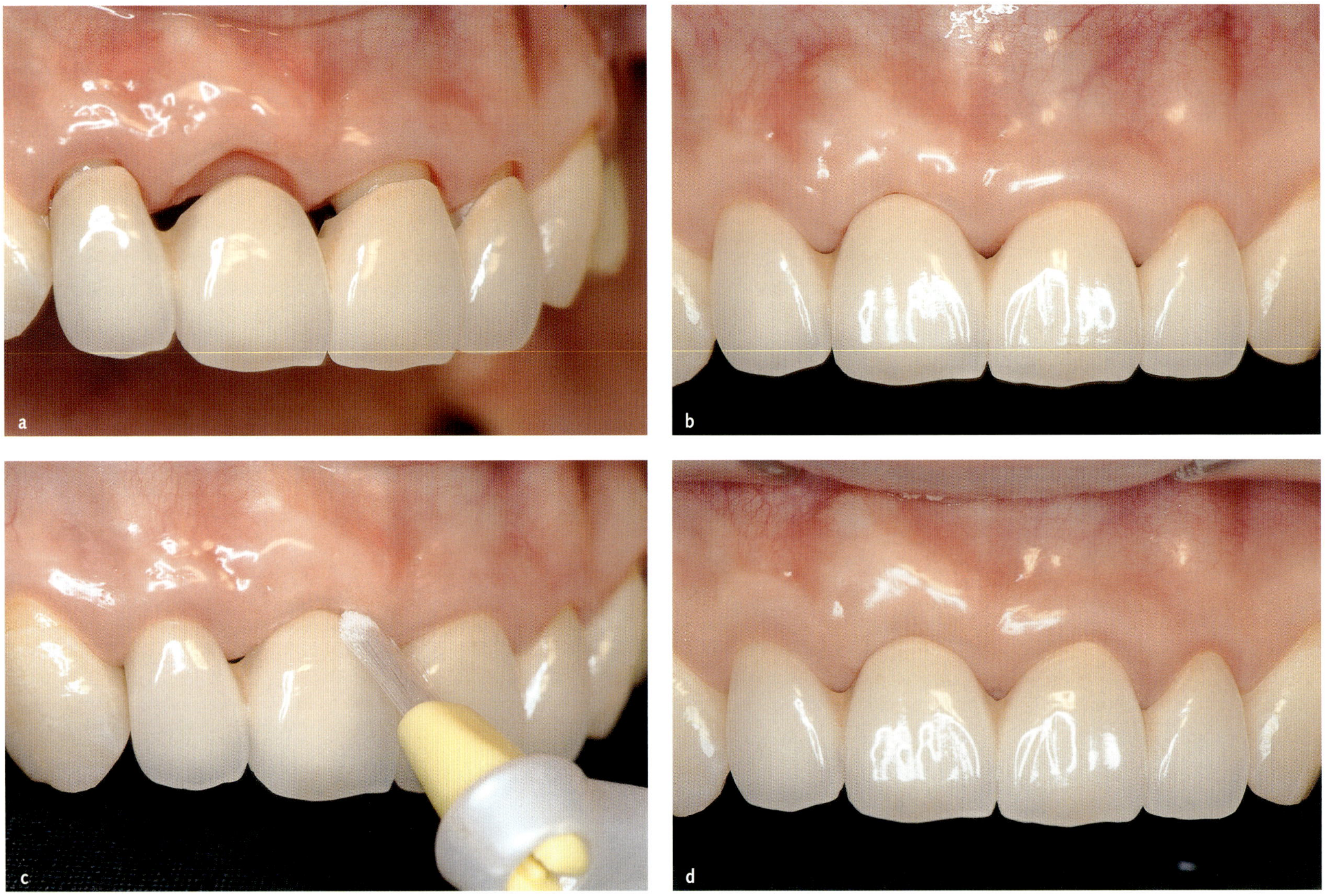

Fig 4-144 Morphology of the interdental papillae. (a) Final prostheses are provisionally cemented. Interdental papilla-like tissue has been established. (b) Photograph taken about 30 days after provisional luting. (c) A Pocket Cleaner (Morimura) is used for cleaning around the pontics. (d) Photograph taken 2 years 5 months after the first visit, or about 10 months after delivery of the prostheses. The contour is mostly symmetric. Tissue crowding is noted distal to the maxillary left central and lateral incisors, but there is no inflammation.

Case 4-4 Crown lengthening and an ovate pontic in a patient with subgingival caries

Patient: *38-year-old woman at the time of first visit in 1985*
Visit after patient was lost to recalls: *About 16 years after the first visit*
The patient completed a full-mouth rehabilitation treatment and continued with her maintenance therapy. She discontinued visits for 2 years. At her last visit, subgingival caries was discovered; however, she did not revisit us for 1 and a half years and returned only due to dislocation of the prosthesis (Figs 4-145 to 4-153).

Fig 4-145 (a) The patient has returned because of dislocation of the fixed partial denture. (b) Photograph taken about 1 month later.

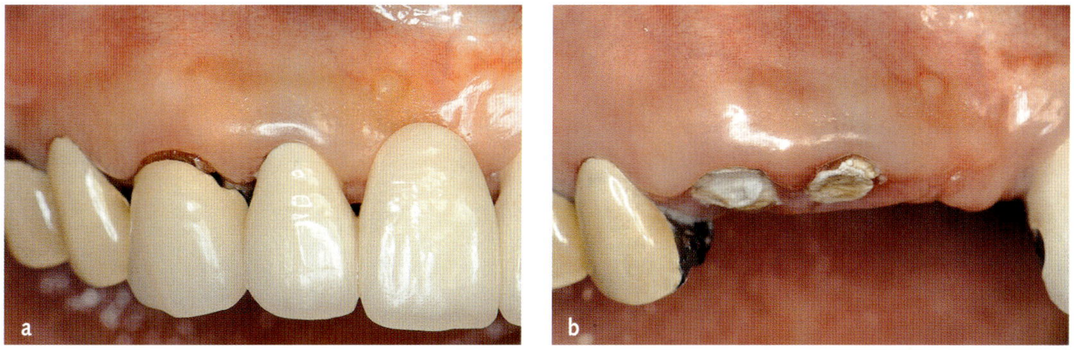

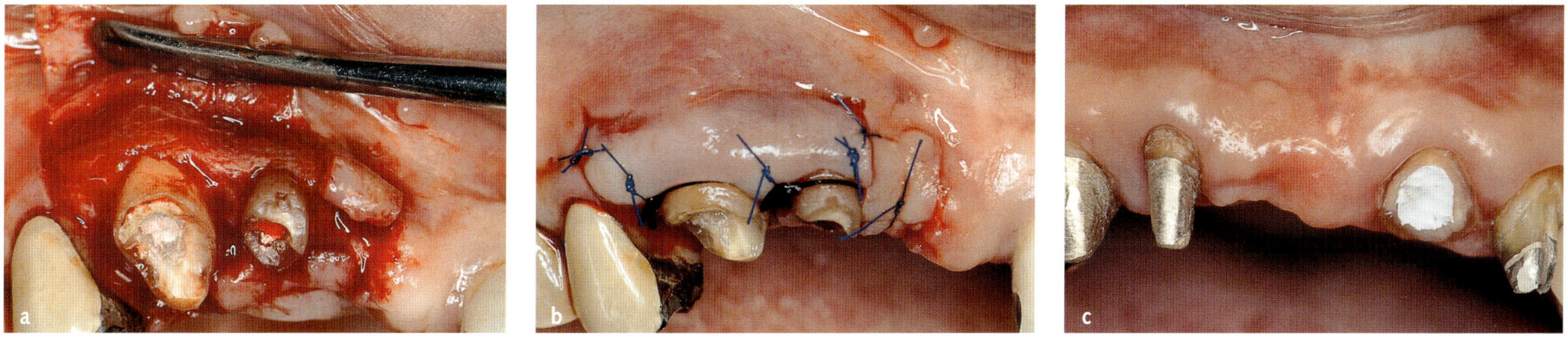

Fig 4-146 Clinical crown lengthening. (a) A flap is to be coronally repositioned in the defect area to increase the keratinized gingiva, and the attachment position is to be apically repositioned in the area of the maxillary right central and lateral incisors, which are residual roots. This will generate a difference in thickness between the apically repositioned tissue at the central and lateral incisor areas and the coronally repositioned defect area. Therefore, the connective tissue in the cervical gingiva is trimmed with a surgical knife, and Castro Viejo scissors are used to adjust the thickness of the gingiva so that the transitional contour of the cervical gingiva will not collapse. To allow sufficient coronal repositioning at the defect area, semilunar releasing incisions are made apically from the MGJ area to form three layers. The palatal aspect is shown after the connective tissue is sectioned to give a thickness similar to the buccal flap and the periosteum is carefully raised with a raspatory. (b) After osseous surgery is completed, the preserved periosteum is sutured back to the wound. (c) Photograph taken 3 months after surgery. While we waited for healing to be completed, endodontic treatments were completed and post and core restorations were fabricated and delivered. The gingival margin is leveled and keratinized gingiva is increased.

Fig 4-147 (a) The gingiva and alveolar mucosa of the ridge defect are trimmed with electrosurgery and a provisional restoration is pressed against the tissue (preimpression technique). After the impression is taken, a plaster cast is trimmed so that the gingival surface of the provisional pontic can be shaped with convexity. At each visit, self-curing acrylic resin is added little by little with a brush to establish an ovate shape (postimpression technique). (b) Photograph taken 5 months after surgery. Interdental papilla-like tissue and convexity for the gingival surface of the pontic are developed by the provisional restoration.

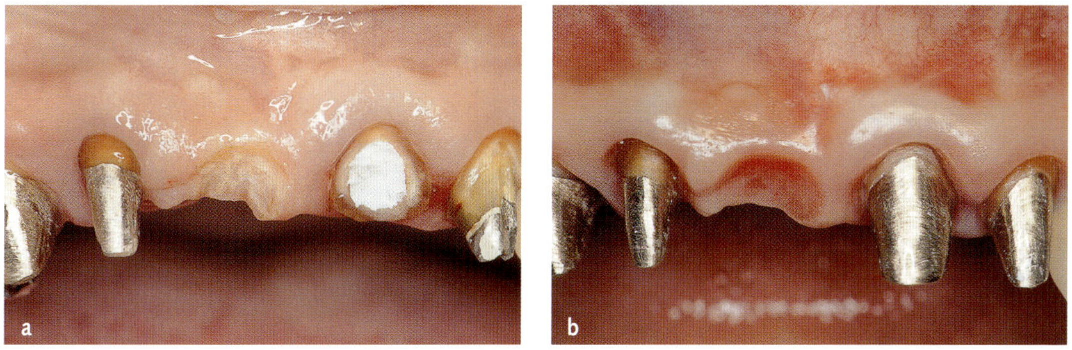

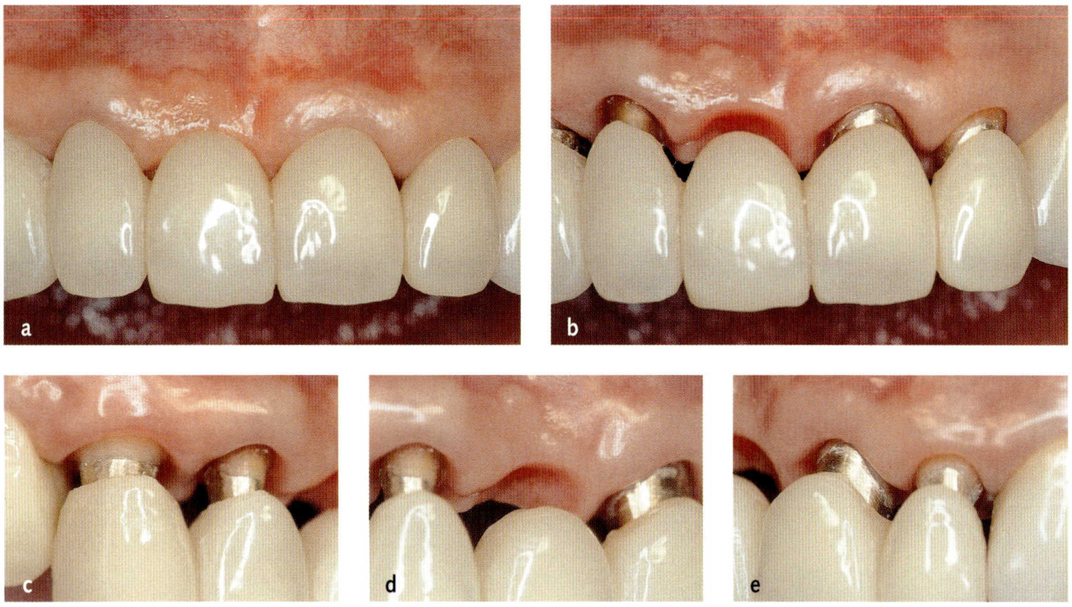

Fig 4-148 (a to e) Marginal adjustment of the final provisional restoration. Attention should be paid to marginal correction with self-curing resin on a provisional restoration. If the margin is appropriately maintained, a better gingival adaptation is more likely to occur. The subgingival marginal contour is carefully adjusted, and crowding and ischemia in the gingiva are noted. The emergence contour established here must be accurately reproduced in the final prosthesis. These clinical photographs of the provisional restorations provide important information to send to the laboratory together with a pick-up impression for the final prosthesis, a centric relation record, and a facebow transfer.

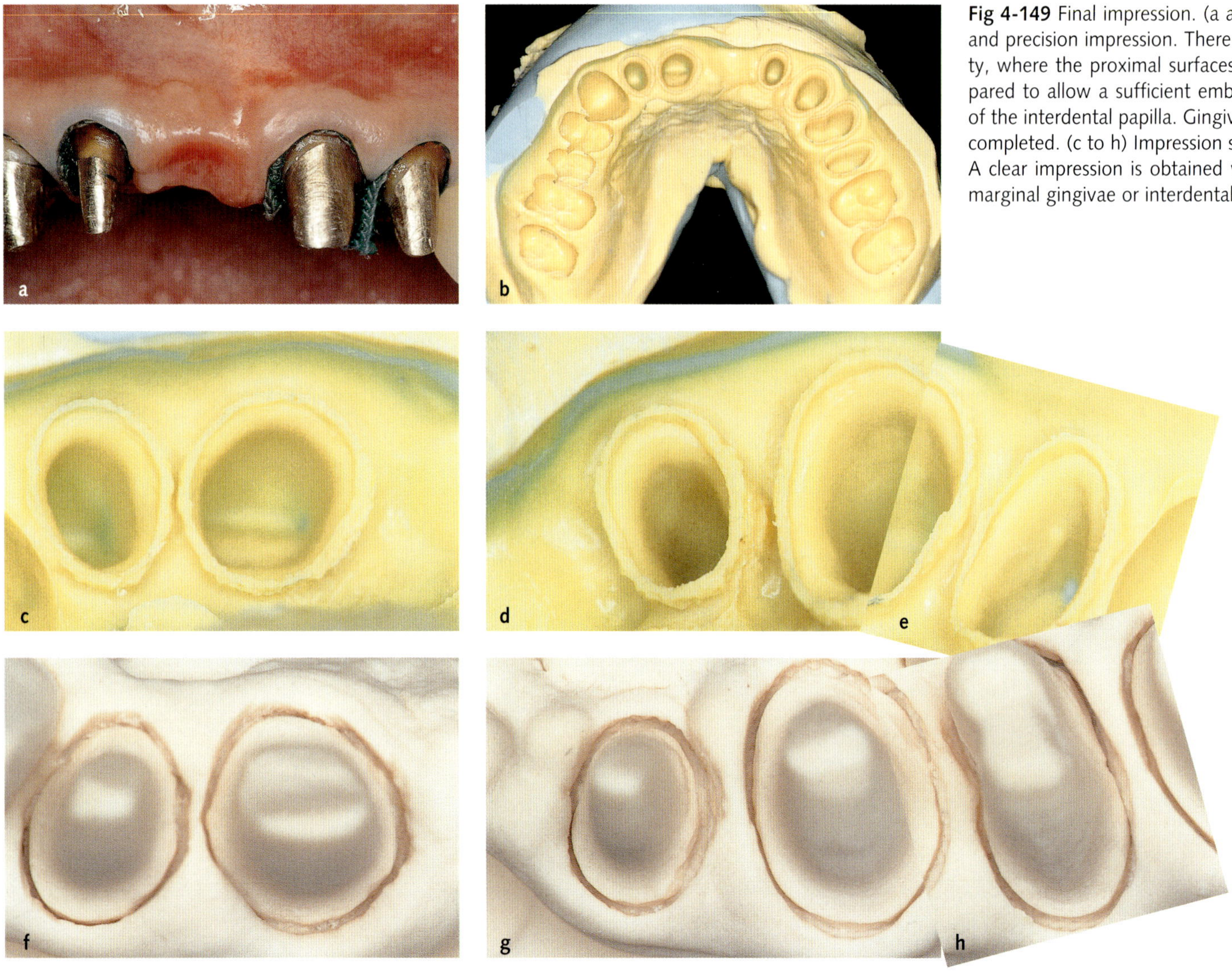

Fig 4-149 Final impression. (a and b) Final preparation and precision impression. There is a close root proximity, where the proximal surfaces are rather deeply prepared to allow a sufficient embrasure for regeneration of the interdental papilla. Gingival retraction is carefully completed. (c to h) Impression surface and plaster cast. A clear impression is obtained without damage to the marginal gingivae or interdental papillae.

Fig 4-150 Three-dimensional record of incisal overlap. Casts of the final provisional restorations are mounted on an articulator. Silicone body putty is pressed against the incisal edge of the provisional restorations to record the three-dimensional incisal overlap relationships between the maxillary and mandibular arches. This information will be important so that the dental technician can transfer the three-dimensional overlap relationships of the provisional prosthesis to the final prosthesis. The incisal overlap is significant to speech, the smile line, and other functions, such as lip support.

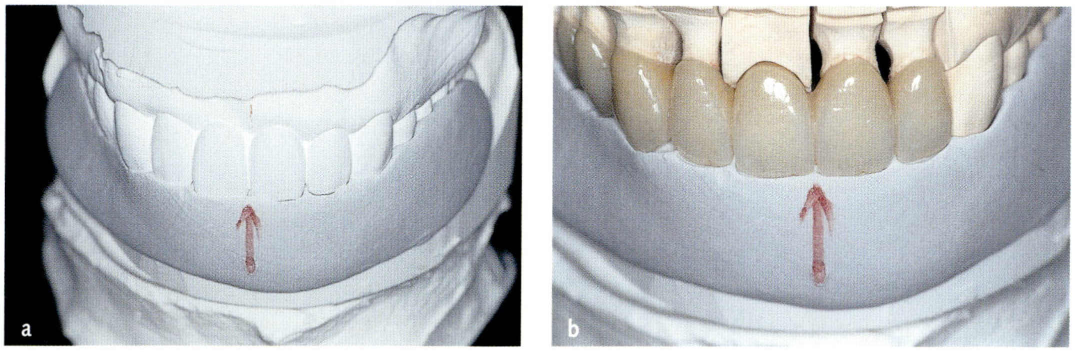

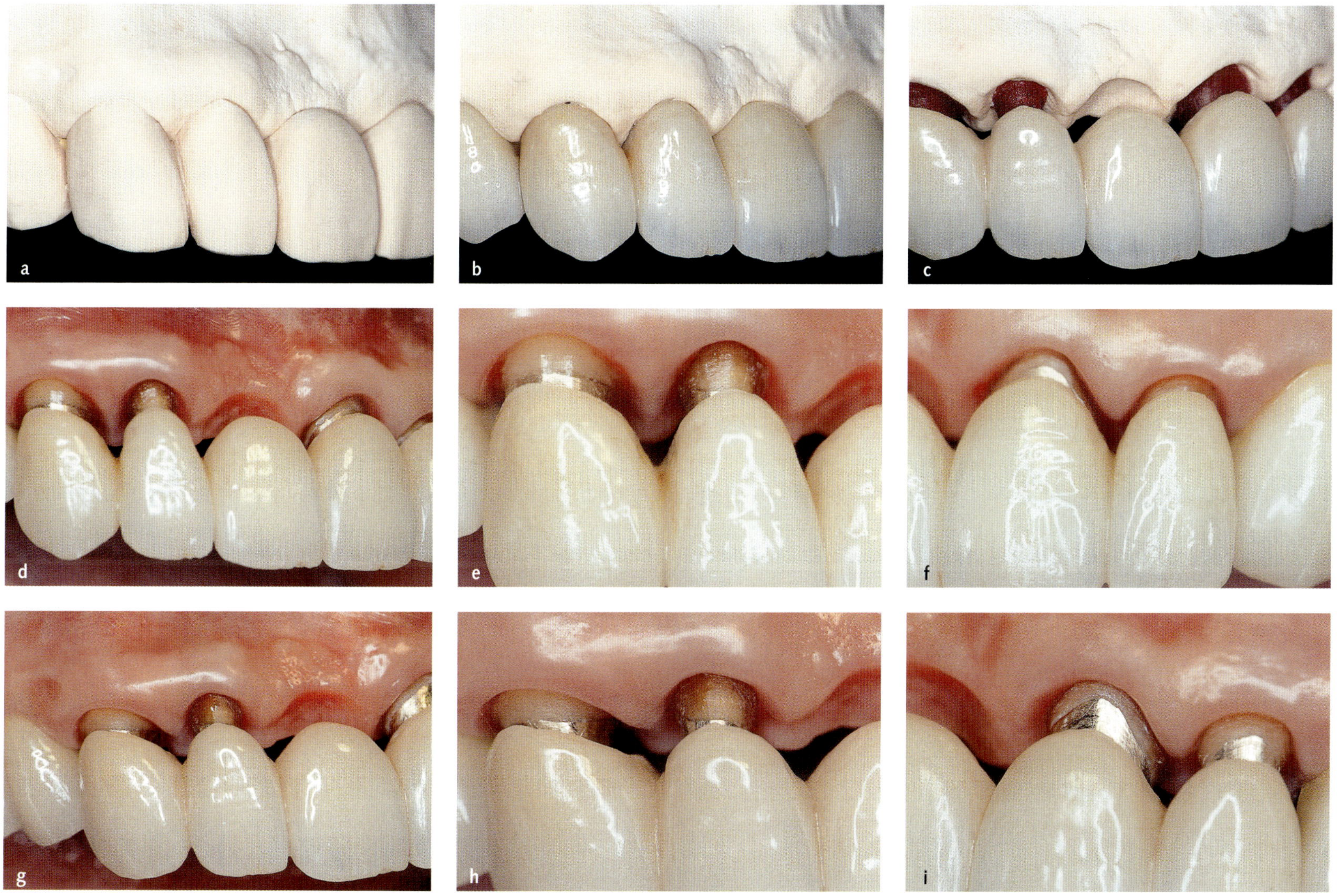

Fig 4-151 Adjustment of the final prosthesis. (a) Full-mouth impression of the final provisional restoration. (b and c) A pick-up impression is taken, and the contour is adjusted with porcelain repair material. (d to f) The fabricated porcelain fixed partial denture is tried in the mouth and picked up in a full-mouth impression to communicate information to the laboratory regarding contour, from the supragingival to the subgingival areas. Although the shape of the natural gingiva of the final provisional restoration is communicated to the laboratory via a pick-up impression, it is not easy to match the contour of the provisional restoration to the final prosthesis. Adjustment of the emergence contour is repeated at this stage. Usually two exchanges of information are conducted with the laboratory. This particular case required three back-and-forth communications. (g to i) Collarless porcelain fixed partial denture with the completed adjustment.

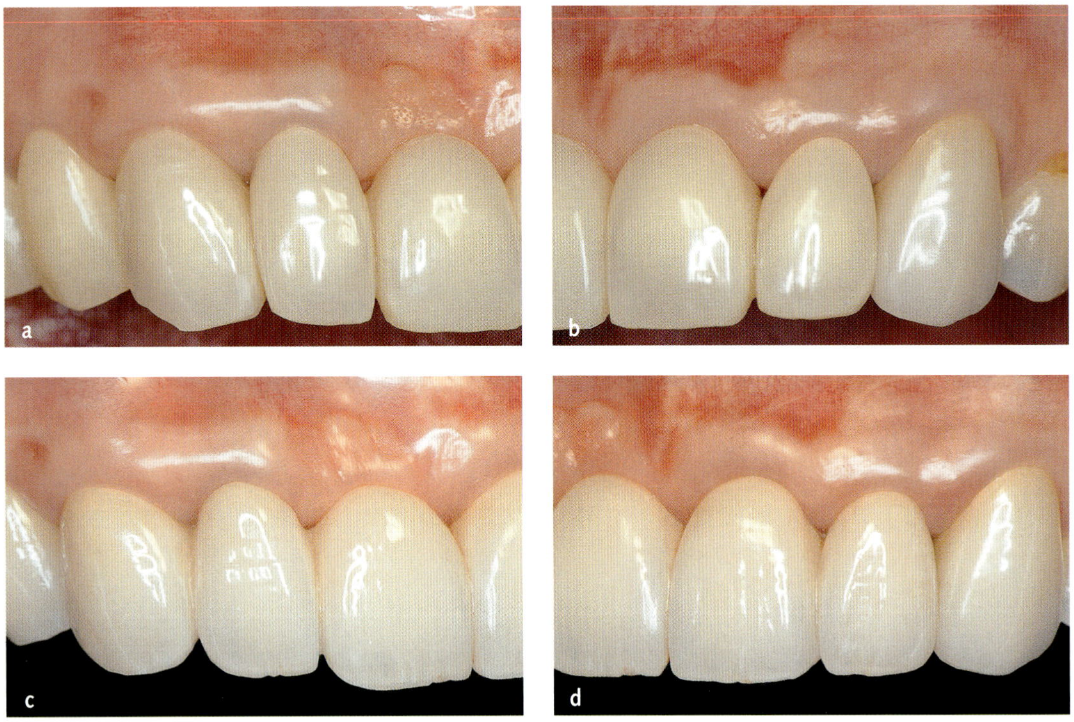

Fig 4-152 Final provisional restoration and collarless porcelain fixed partial denture. (a) Final provisional restoration, 5 months after crown lengthening. (b) The collarless porcelain fixed partial denture is delivered. The gingival morphology, which is very similar to that of the provisional restoration, has been reproduced, 7 months after crown lengthening. (Prostheses made by Mr Kazunari Ohata, RDT.)

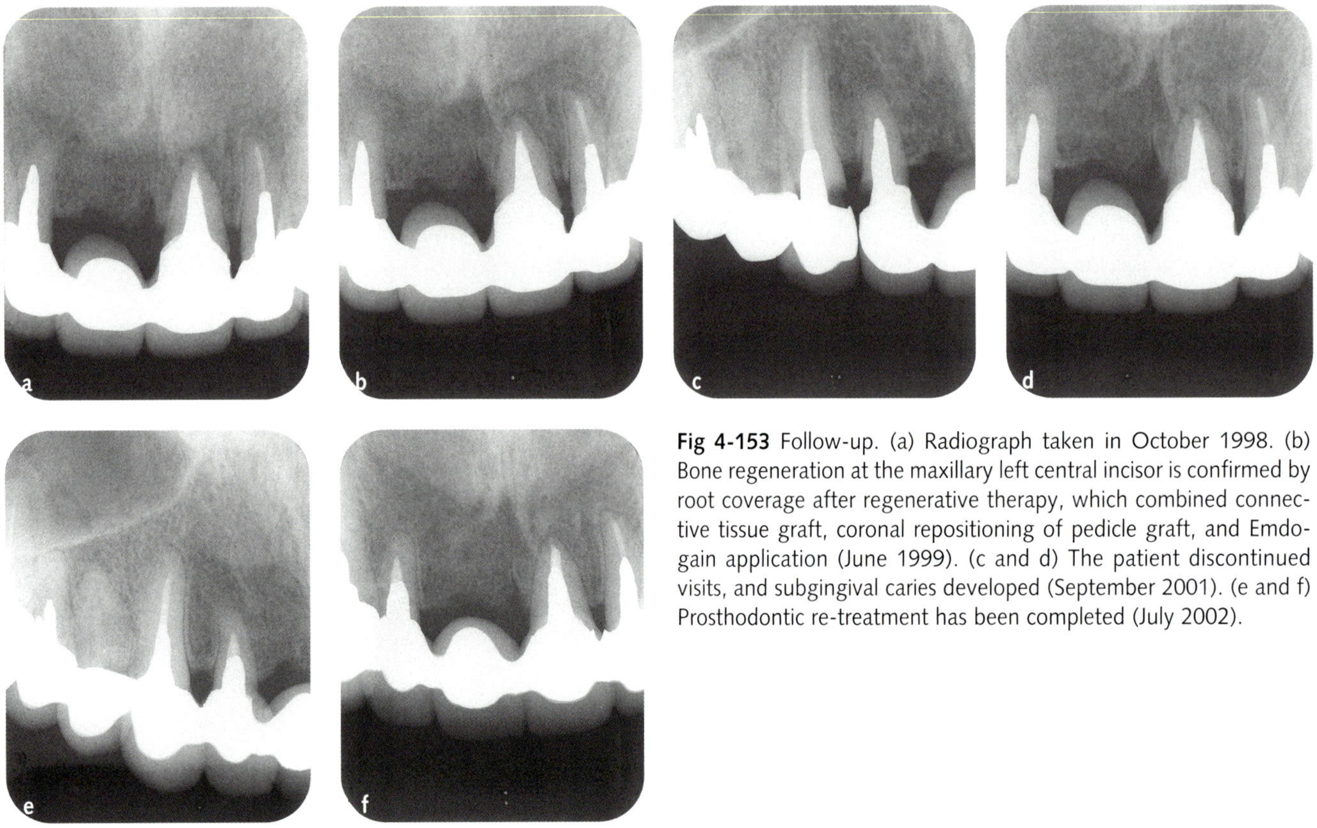

Fig 4-153 Follow-up. (a) Radiograph taken in October 1998. (b) Bone regeneration at the maxillary left central incisor is confirmed by root coverage after regenerative therapy, which combined connective tissue graft, coronal repositioning of pedicle graft, and Emdogain application (June 1999). (c and d) The patient discontinued visits, and subgingival caries developed (September 2001). (e and f) Prosthodontic re-treatment has been completed (July 2002).

Clinical Practice of Periodontal Prostheses

Prosthodontic treatment as a part of periodontal therapy

In severe, advanced cases of periodontal disease, even if inflammation control is exhaustive, it does not mean that the therapy is completed at this stage. Because of existing pathologic tooth movement and loss of teeth secondary to occlusal trauma, the mandibular dentition may be malpositioned when the occlusal support in the molars has been lost. In such a case, initially the continuity and integrity of the dentition must be restored, and a therapeutic occlusion must be built, along with inflammation control. The restoration of function and esthetics for patients is paramount. To achieve the treatment goals, prosthodontic treatment must be a part of the periodontal therapy.

Restoration of maintainable morphology

Amsterdam presented long-term clinical cases and proposed the term *periodontal prostheses* for such comprehensively treated cases. Such diagnosis and treatment covering areas of periodontics, orthodontics, endodontics, occlusion, and prosthodontics must have been an inconceivable challenge under the divided specialist systems, requiring keenly enthusiastic practitioners. Periodontal prostheses required a multidisciplinary team approach involving highly specialized clinicians. Long-term follow-up inspired clinicians to establish a style in which they learn from their own clinical cases. Provisional restoration, a trial-and-error approach in prosthodontics that is now the mainstream in treatment, resulted from the efforts of Amsterdam et al.

In rehabilitation of cases with occlusal collapse, prosthodontic treatment is required as a device for periodontal therapy, where periodontal therapy and prosthodontic treatment are utilized not merely to solve immediate problems but to restore maintainable morphology to allow long-term stability after treatment. Because of this, in the past, efforts were made to obtain maintainability while sacrificing esthetics to a certain degree. Today, however, thanks to regenerative therapy, periodontal plastic surgery, and technological innovations in prosthodontics, it is possible to provide treatments to reconcile maintainability and esthetics.

Restoration of morphologic harmony from the occlusal surface to the alveolar crest

In cases with occlusal collapse accompanied by severe periodontal disease, maintainable morphology of tooth and periodontal tissue has to be reconstructed when good prospects are established in inflammation control (Cases 4-5 to 4-7). This, however, is not limited to restoration of a certain width of attachment (biologic width). Because attachment has already been lost and teeth are malpositioned, even though periodontal tissue is restored without periodontal pockets or infrabony pockets, restoration of health in the stomatognathic system is not complete without restoration of the occlusal surfaces (cusp to fossa), crown-root ratio, occlusal plane, occlusal vertical dimension, and mandibular position. In periodontal prostheses, equitable interocclusal space has to be restored from the occlusal plane to the bone crest line that healthy adults have.

Case 4-5 Severe occlusal collapse accompanied by periodontal disease and a periodontal prosthesis

Patient: *56-year-old woman at the time of first visit in 1989*

As shown in the radiographic comparison of the first visit (Fig 4-154) and completion of the periodontal prosthesis (Fig 4-155), the interocclusal space between the occlusal plane and bone crest, which was significantly disturbed at the first visit, was almost evenly restored. Because the anterior teeth were not restored to preserve the healthy enamel, some problems remained, including partial disturbance of the gingival drape, interdental spaces, and elongated clinical crowns. Prosthetic treatment was added to the maxillary anterior teeth 7 years later, which improved the relationship between the teeth (crown prostheses) and the gingiva (Fig 4-156). Filling of the embrasures by postoperative gingival growth reminds us of the importance of the relationship between the teeth and the gingiva (Figs 4-157 to 4-165).

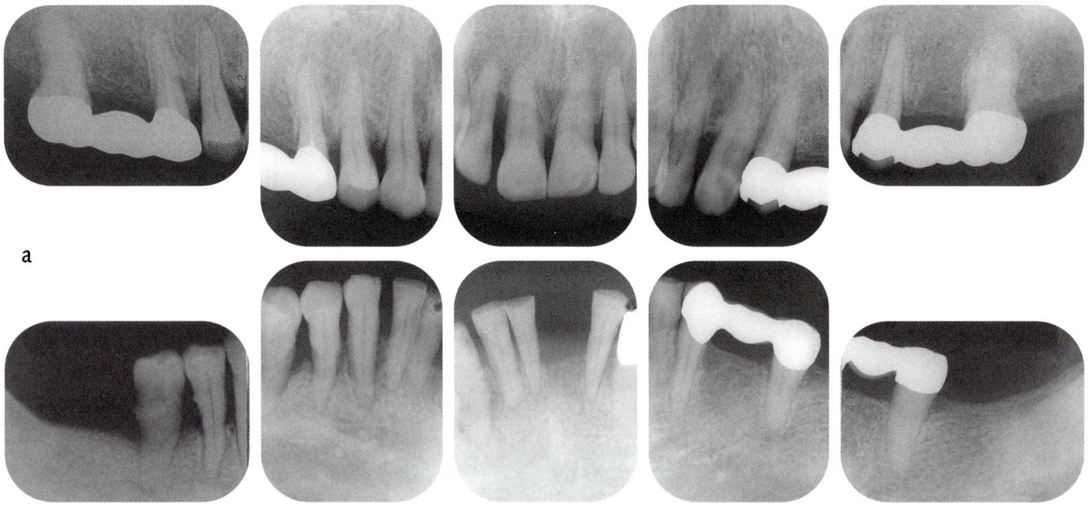

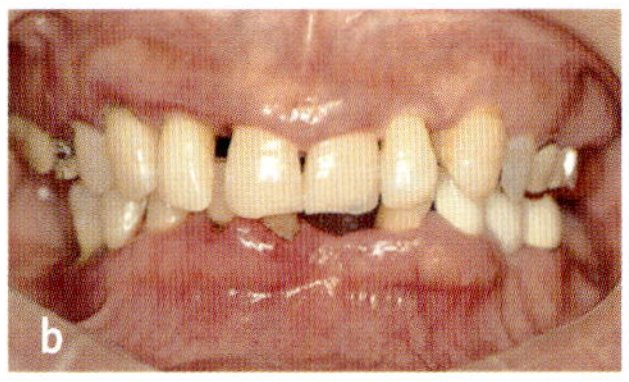

Fig 4-154 (a) Radiographs taken at the first visit. Infrabony defects are noted at the maxillary right first premolar, right lateral incisor, left lateral incisor, and left first premolar and the mandibular right canine and first premolar, where stress is concentrated. Secondary occlusal trauma and interdental spacing is observed for most of the teeth. (b) Frontal view at the first visit, showing severe periodontal disease and a deep overbite.

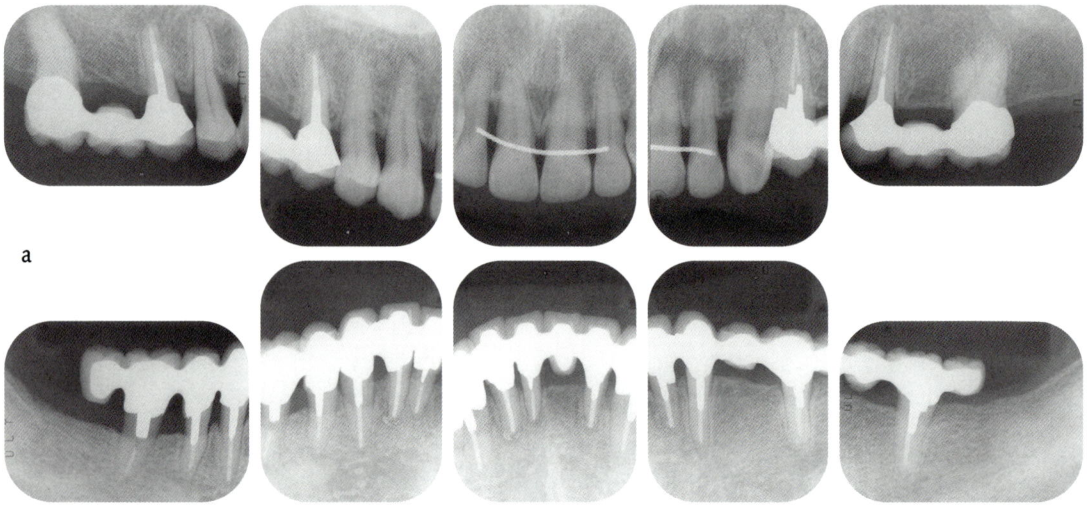

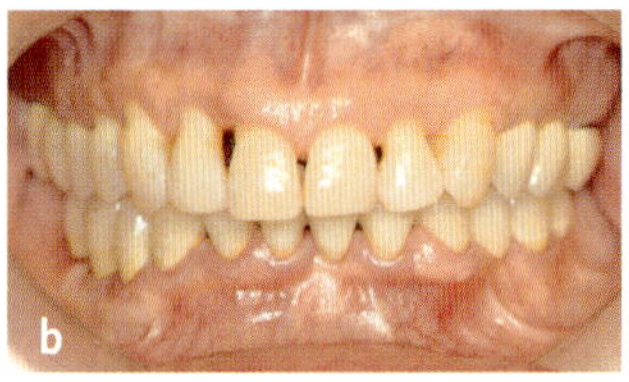

Fig 4-155 After completion of the periodontal prostheses. (a) Radiographs taken 2 years 6 months after the first visit. The reduction in bone defects is notable. The mandibular left second premolar to the mandibular right second premolar are splinted with cantilever pontics for the mandibular left first molar and mandibular right first molar. Fixed partial dentures have been delivered for the maxillary right second premolar to the second molar and the maxillary left first premolar to first molar. (b) Photograph taken 2 years 8 months after the first visit.

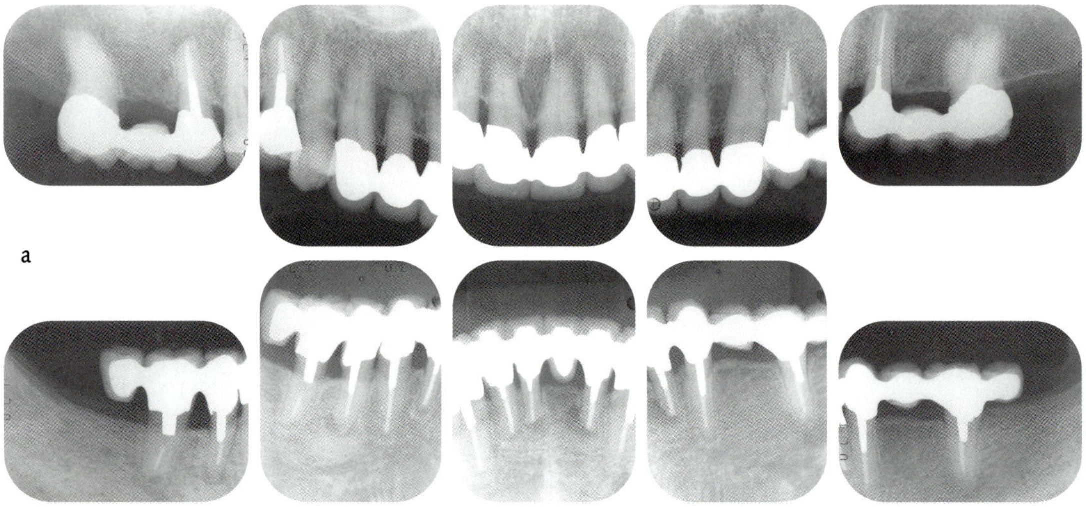

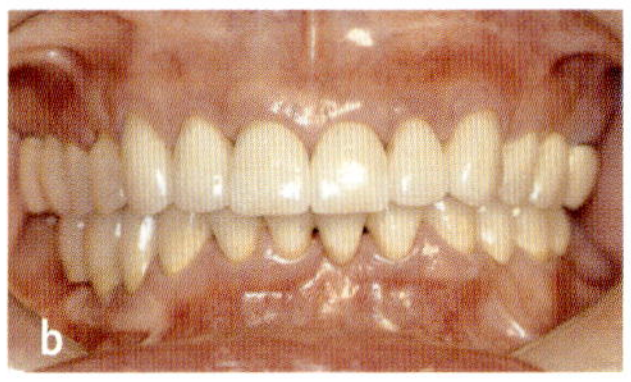

Fig 4-156 (a) About 7 years after the first visit. Splinted anterior crowns were delivered, extending from the maxillary right canine to maxillary left canine. There were suspected cementomas around the apices of the mandibular left lateral incisor and mandibular right central incisor. (b) Good harmony in the gingival drape and a well-balanced occlusal plane between the right and left have been achieved. Photograph taken about 6 years after delivery of the maxillary anterior prosthesis, or 13 years after the first visit.

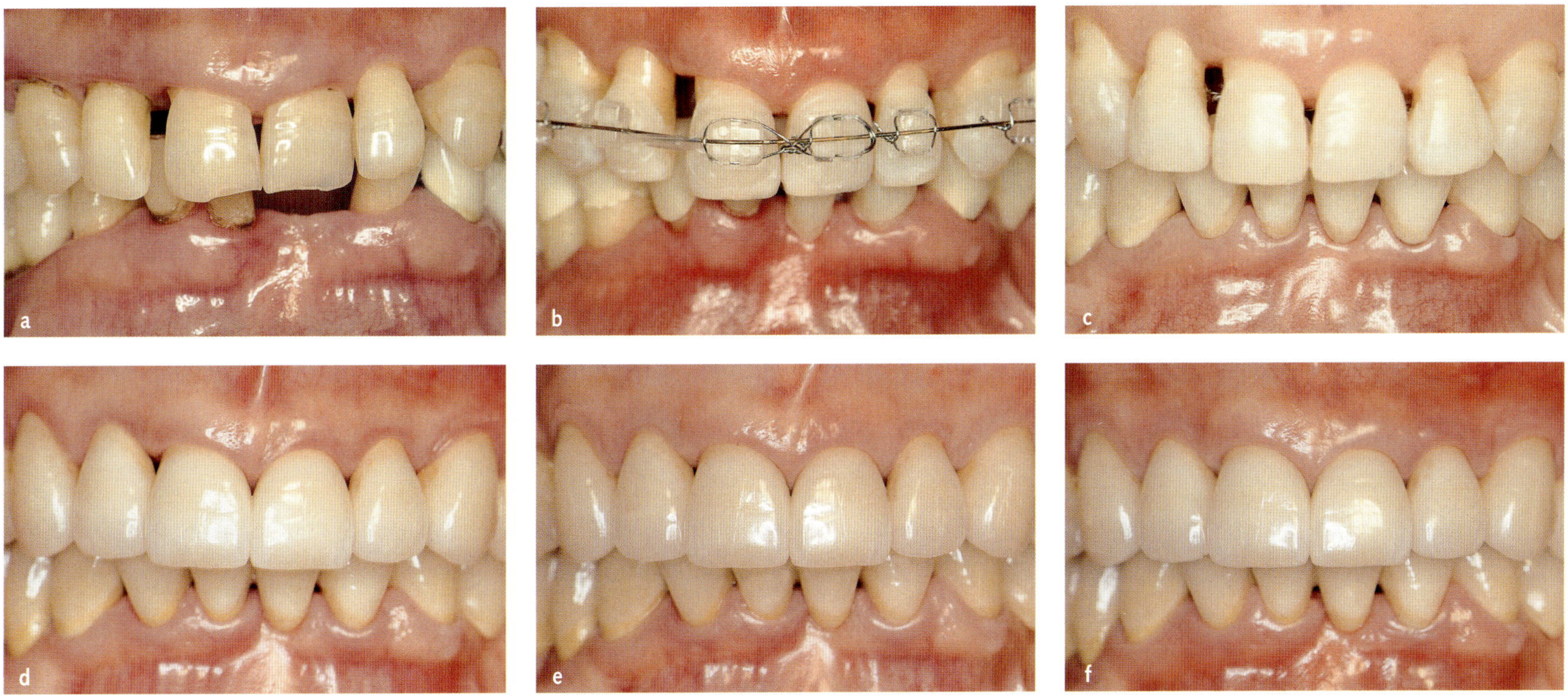

Fig 4-157 Frontal views. (a) At the first visit. (b) After initial therapy. Regenerative therapy (with a nonresorbable GTR membrane) was conducted for the maxillary right lateral incisor and mandibular right canine. The vertical height of the molars is increased by the use of provisional restorations and restorative tooth movement. (c) After completion of the periodontal prostheses (January 1992). The maxillary anterior teeth are not involved in these prostheses. (d) Photograph taken 6 years after the first visit (about 3 years after completion of the periodontal prostheses). Because the maxillary anterior teeth, from right canine to left canine, had severe attrition, splinted collarless porcelain crowns have been delivered to these anterior teeth to restore anterior guidance. (e) Photograph taken 2 years after restoration of the anterior teeth. (f) Photograph taken 7 years later. After crown restoration, tissue gradually increased, establishing a maintainable periodontal environment.

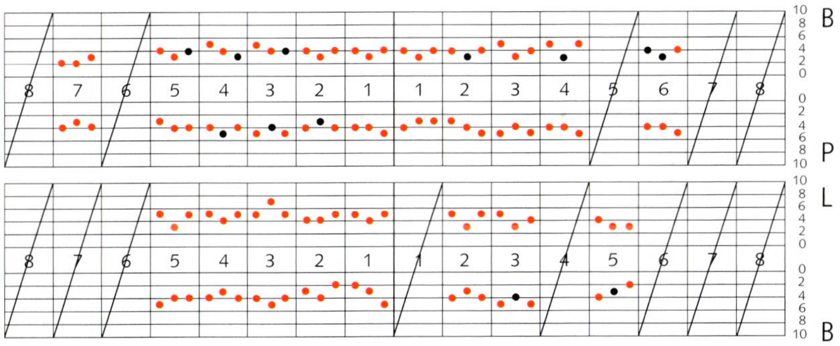

Fig 4-158 Probing depths at first visit. Currently, after 13 years, probing depths are maintained within 2 mm.

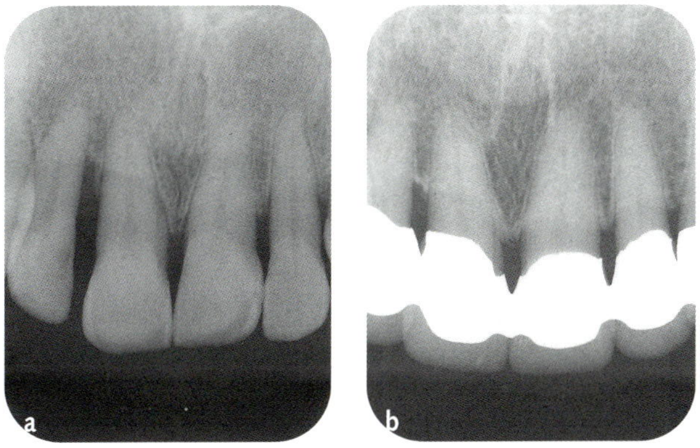

Fig 4-159 Comparison of the maxillary anterior teeth over 13 years. (a) At the first visit, periodontal disease and traumatic findings are obvious. (b) After 13 years, the bone trabeculae and lamina durae have become clear, and the bone crest has been improved. The distance between the finish line of the crown restorations and the bone crest has been improved to be mostly uniform.

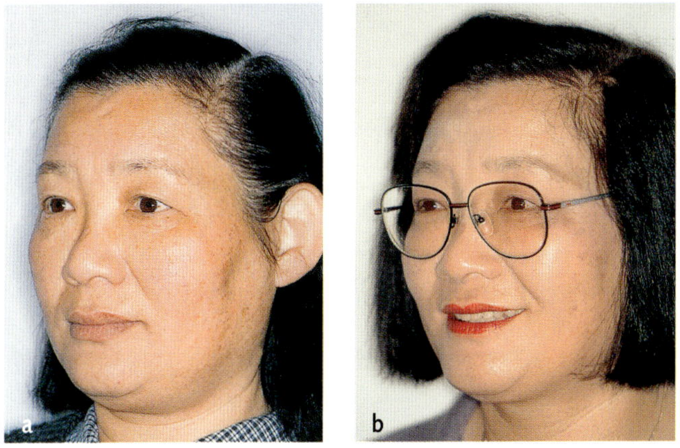

Fig 4-160 Changes in patient's face over the course of treatment. (a) At the first visit. (b) After about 10 years.

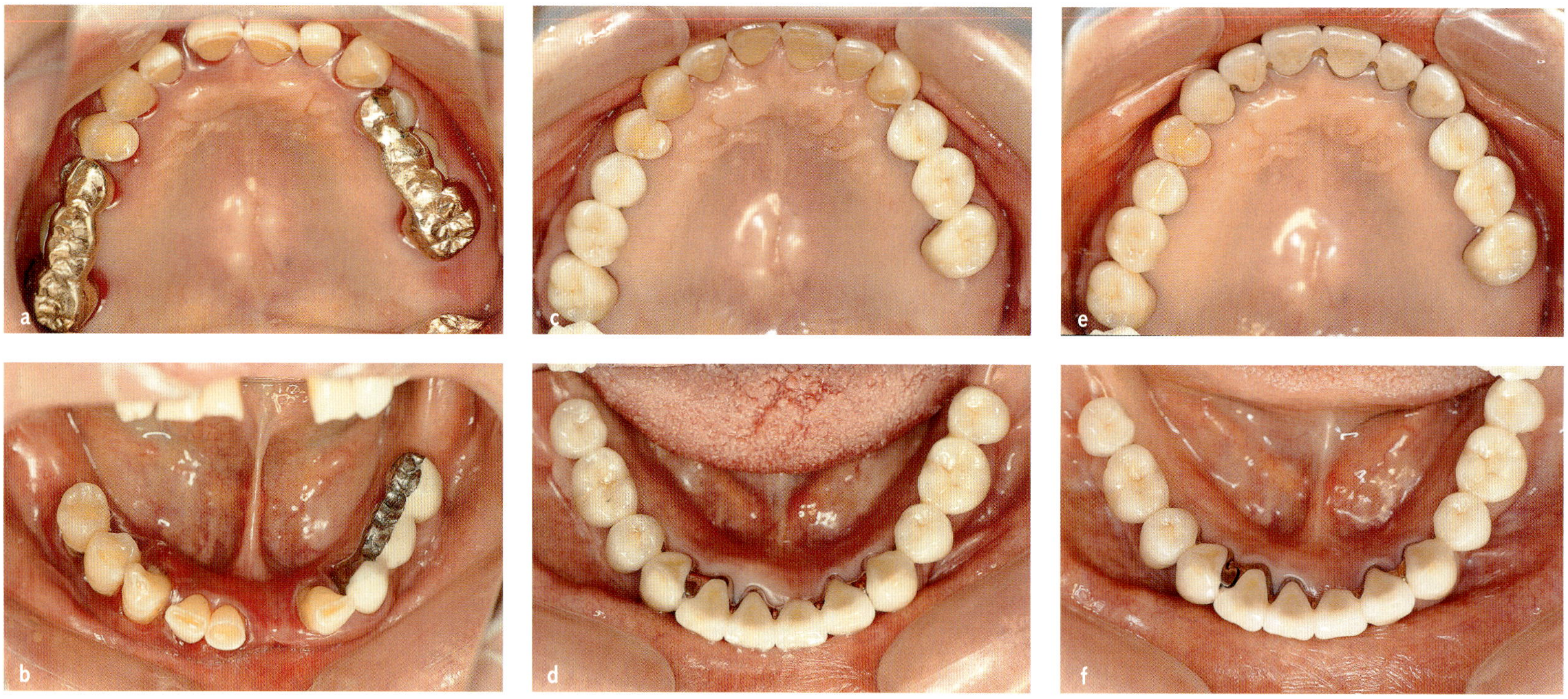

Fig 4-161 Comparison of maxillary and mandibular dental arches (occlusal views). (a and b) At the first visit, the maxillary canines are flared out labially. The mandibular left central incisor, first molar, and second molar and right first and second molars are missing. Worn occlusal surfaces caused by bruxism are conspicuous. There is degree 1 to 2 tooth mobility. (c and d) At completion of the periodontal prostheses. GTR therapy has been conducted for the maxillary right lateral incisor and first premolar. Osseous surgery has been performed for the maxillary left first premolar. This is 1 year after delivery of the fixed partial dentures for the maxillary right second premolar to second molar and the maxillary left first premolar to first molar, following orthodontic tooth movement. Arch forms have been reconstructed. Horizontal and vertical determinants are established that are in harmony with functional movements. (Prostheses made by Mr. Tsugumichi Kawasaki, RDT.) (e and f) Photographs taken after about 12 years, or 10 years after delivery of the original prostheses. With the prostheses for the anterior teeth (delivered about 7 years after the first visit), arch form has been improved and is symmetric. A keyway joint in the mandibular arch is slightly lifted. (Although we suppose that there was a slight change in mandibular position due to attrition of maxillary anterior teeth, no change has been observed in the last 6 years.) The patient visits the clinic monthly to receive hygiene and occlusion examinations.

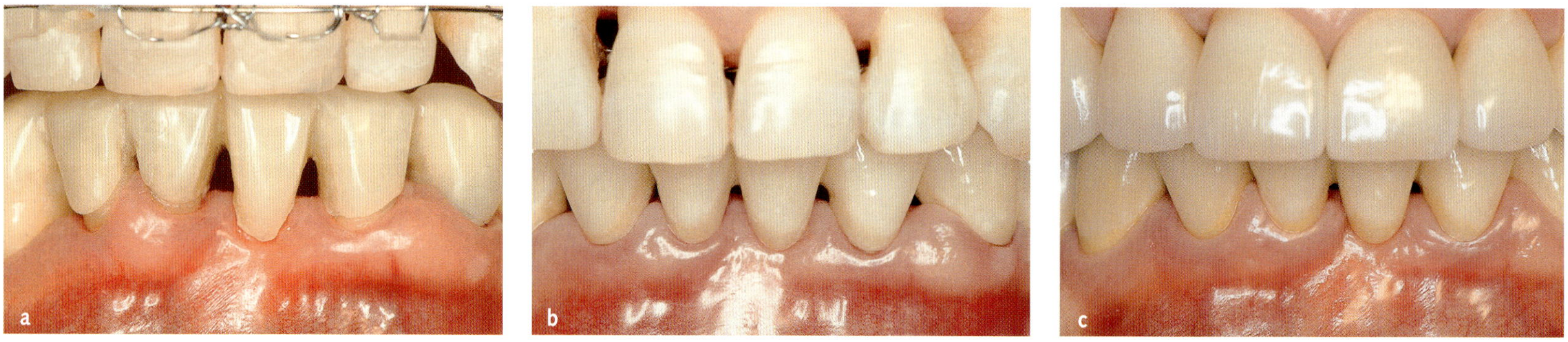

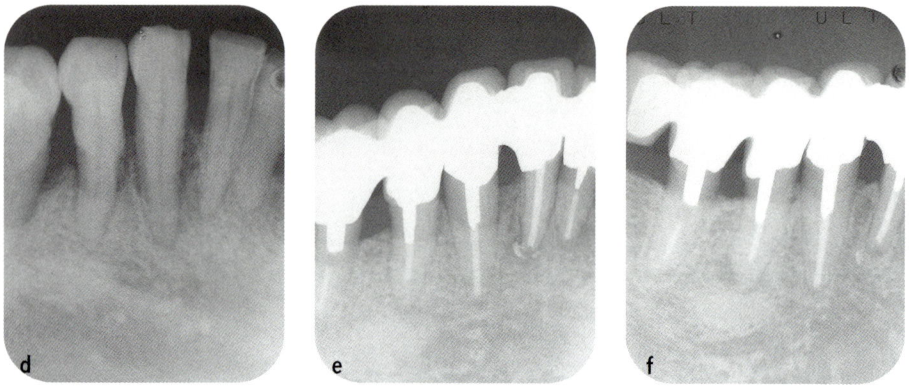

Fig 4-162 Comparison of the mandibular anterior teeth over 12 years. (a) Soon after the first visit. The concavity in the alveolar ridge at the mandibular left central incisor is remarkable. (b) A limited osseous surgery has been conducted to reduce the periodontal pockets and gingival irregularity. Collarless porcelain fixed partial dentures have been delivered, establishing a maintainable morphology. (c) About 9 years after delivery of the prostheses, or about 12 years after the first visit. Stable conditions as well as harmony in the gingivae have been maintained. (d) Radiograph taken at first visit. (e) Radiograph taken at delivery of prostheses. (f) After 13 years, secondary traumatic occlusion and bone defects have been diminished.

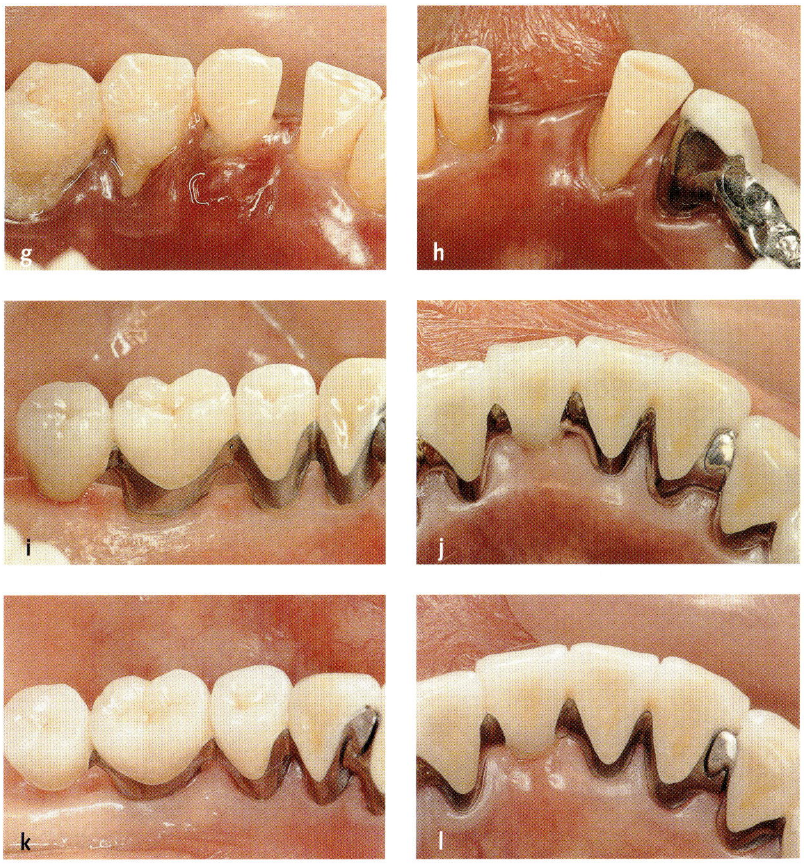

(g and h) Lingual views at the first visit. Note the severe gingivitis and worn occlusal surfaces. (i and j) The keyway joint is fabricated between the mandibular right lateral incisor and canine. Regenerative therapy with GTR procedures has been conducted for the mandibular right canine. (k and l) The keyway joint is slightly lifted after 9 years. (m and n) Relatively shallow canine guidance is developed.

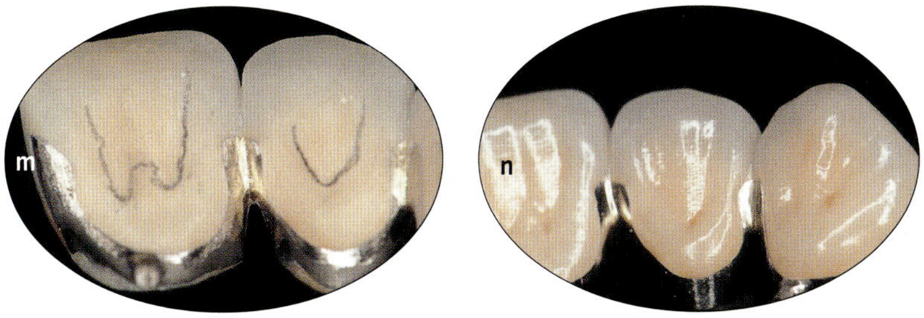

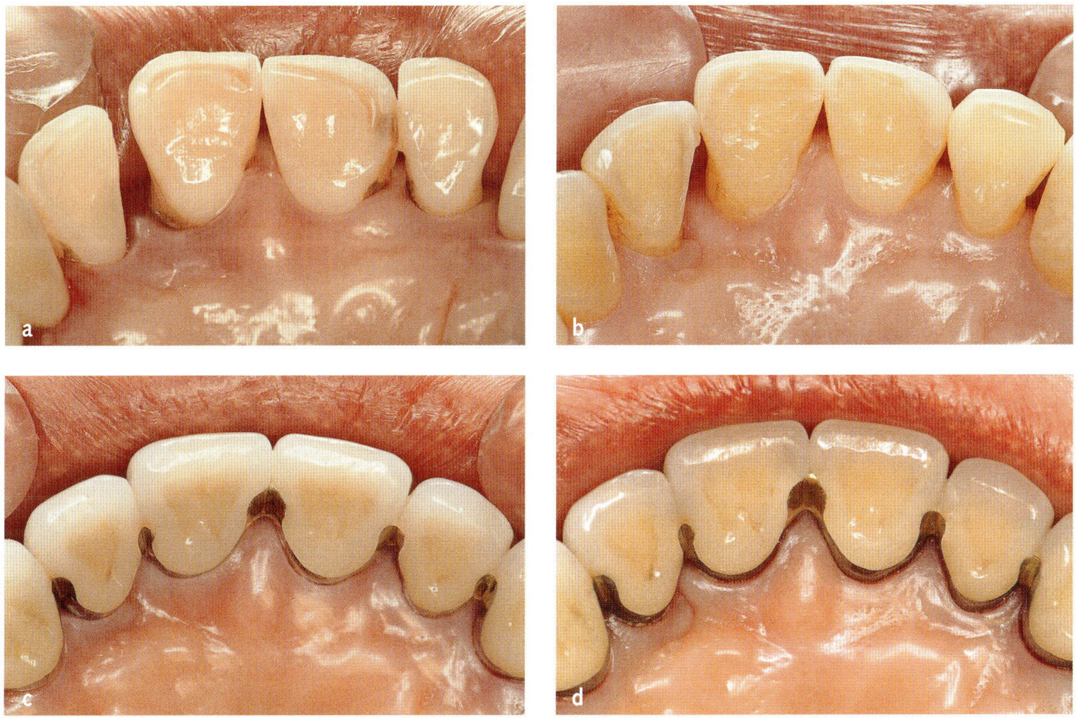

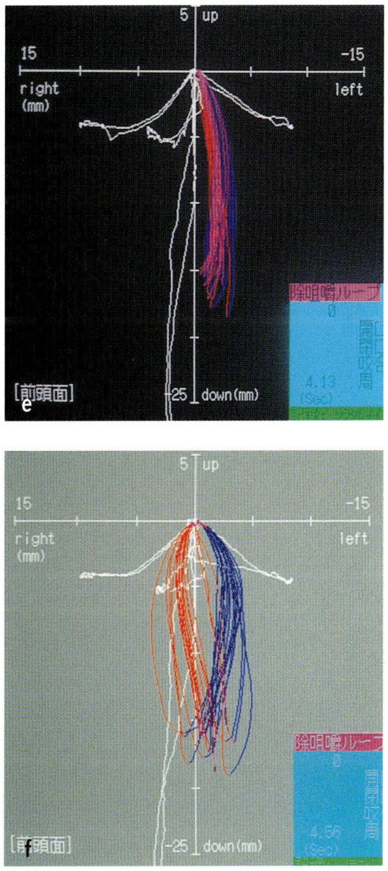

Fig 4-163 Lingual views of the maxillary anterior teeth. (a) At the first visit. Pathologic tooth migrations are noted. (b) After initial therapy. (c) Photograph taken 6 years after the first visit. After periodontal surgery and therapeutic tooth movement, collarless porcelain crown restorations that occlude with the opposing arch have been delivered, partly due to the complaint of temporomandibular disorder symptoms. Note the emergence profile. (d) Twelve years after the first visit, the occlusion is stable. Marginal ridge morphology is fabricated so that the masticatory functions are fully exhibited. (e) Sirognathograph (Siemens) showing left chewing motions on the frontal plane, 2 years 11 months after delivery of periodontal prostheses. Attrition has been caused by abnormal masticatory movement. (f) Sirognathograph showing left chewing motions on the frontal plane 4 years 3 months after delivery of the original periodontal prostheses, or 7 years after the first visit. Reintervention improved the masticatory movement.

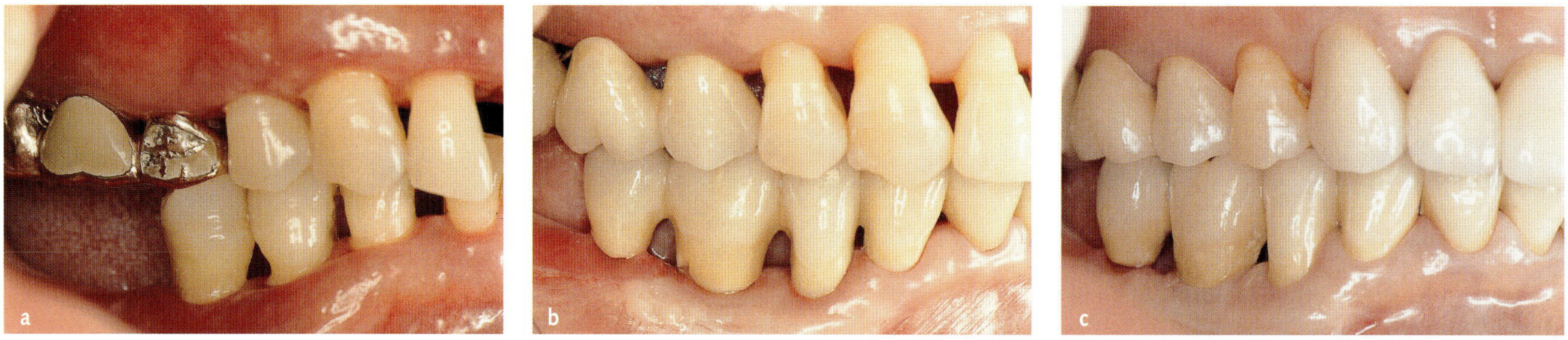

Fig 4-164 Right lateral views. (a) At the first visit. (b) After completion of the periodontal prostheses (January 1992). (c) After 6 years (12 years after the first visit). After crown restorations were placed, the gingivae gradually developed.

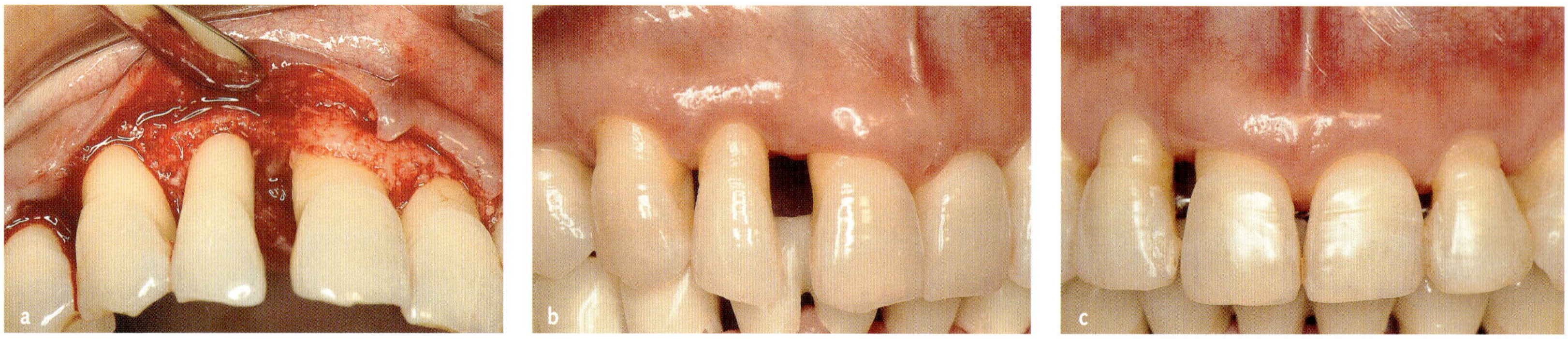

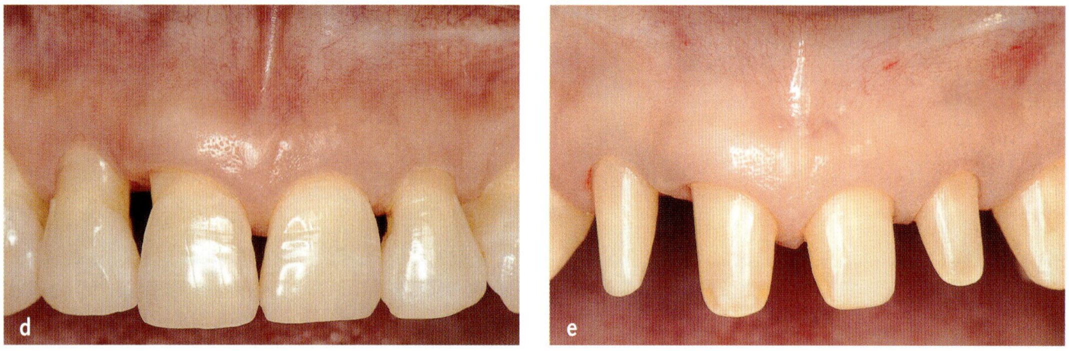

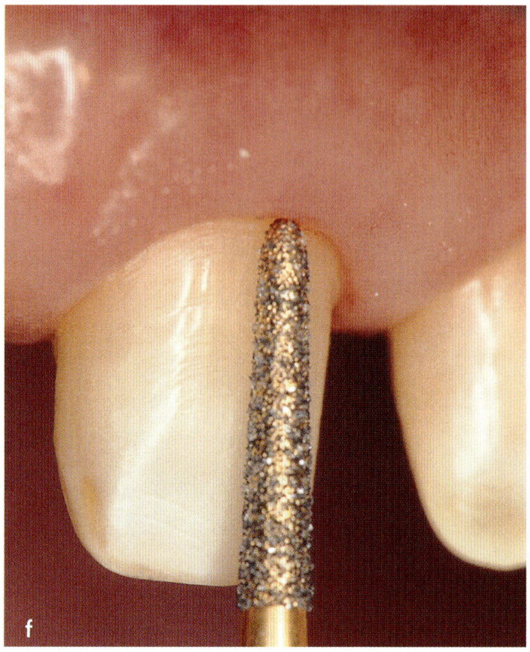

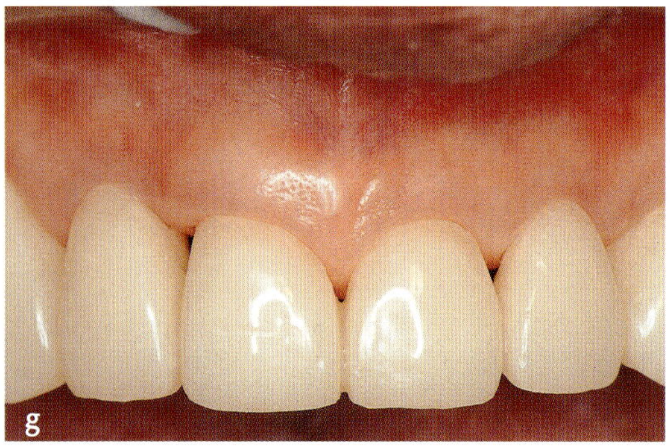

Fig 4-165 Progress of treatments for the right anterior teeth. (a) About 1 year after the first visit. The bone defect between the maxillary right central and lateral incisors is deep (May 1990). (b) Although periodontal pockets are reduced, gingival recession has developed and the embrasure spaces are extremely wide. (c) After orthodontic tooth movement, fixed partial dentures for the molars are delivered (November 1991). A direct resin composite restoration is applied to the maxillary right lateral incisor for morphologic correction. (d) Since symptoms of temporomandibular disorder have been alleviated, restoration of the anterior teeth is started (July 1995). (e and f) Three-surface preparation for vital teeth. (g) The provisional restoration is utilized for adjustment of the emergence profile.

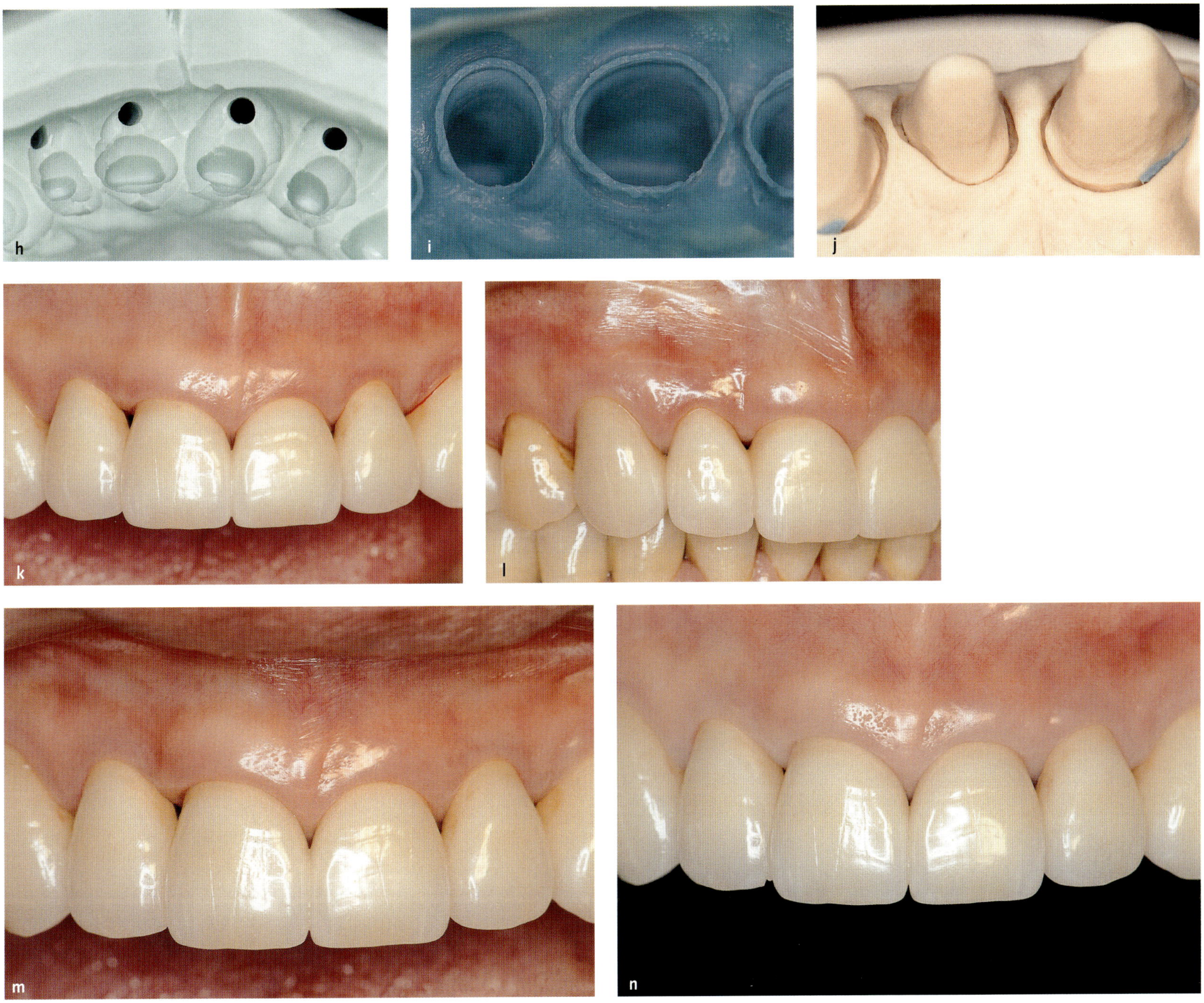

(h and i) Drilled body of the HIT impression and final impression. (j) Note different reduction volume at subgingival level and concentric circle preparation. (k) The metal framework is picked up, and the contour is adjusted on a gum model. The collarless porcelain restoration has been delivered. (l) Photograph taken 6 years after delivery of the prostheses. (m) Photograph taken 2 years after delivery of the prostheses. (n) Photograph taken 6 years after delivery of the prostheses. Gingival morphology has been improved. It is our opinion that the increase in gingival attachment became possible because of the development of appropriate emergence profiles and the use of a modified rolling toothbrushing technique, in which the gingiva is not irritated from the coronal direction. Gentle sulcular access was obtained with a Pocket Cleaner.

Case 4-6 Severe occlusal collapse accompanied by periodontal disease and a periodontal prosthesis: Maintenance of high-risk patients

The patient in Figs 4-166 to 4-177 exhibited advanced periodontal disease and flared-out anterior teeth, for which intervention was made just prior to occlusal collapse of the molars. Because of root fractures, which took place about 9 years after the first visit (5 years 6 months after delivery of final prostheses), regenerative therapy and implant treatment were provided. Currently the case has been maintained for 12 years since the first visit.

Patient: *52-year-old man at the time of first visit in June 1989; the actual start of treatment was June 1990*

Characteristics: *A heavy smoker with brachyfacial skeletal type. He discontinued treatments after the initial therapy and revisited us after about 1 year.*

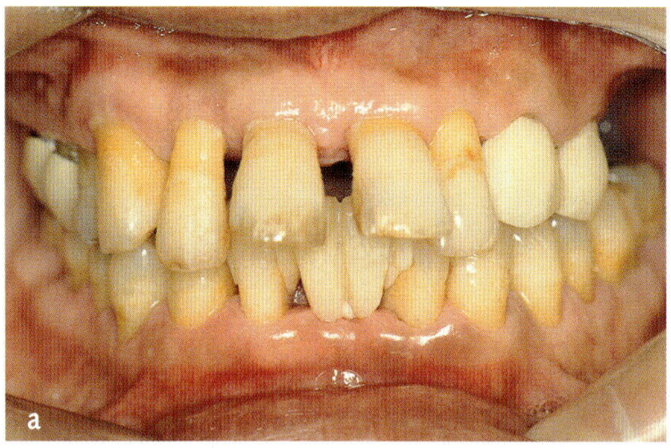

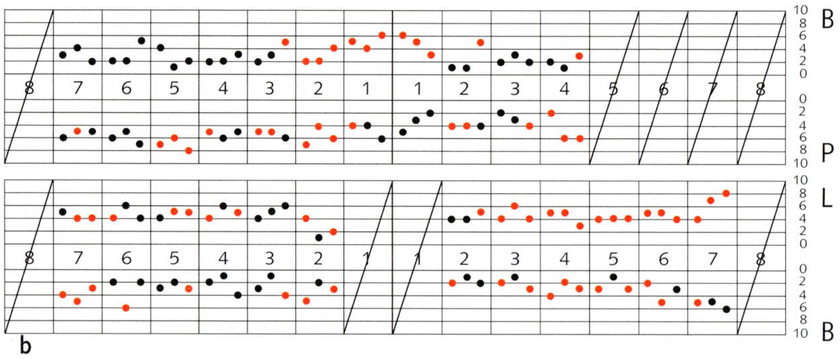

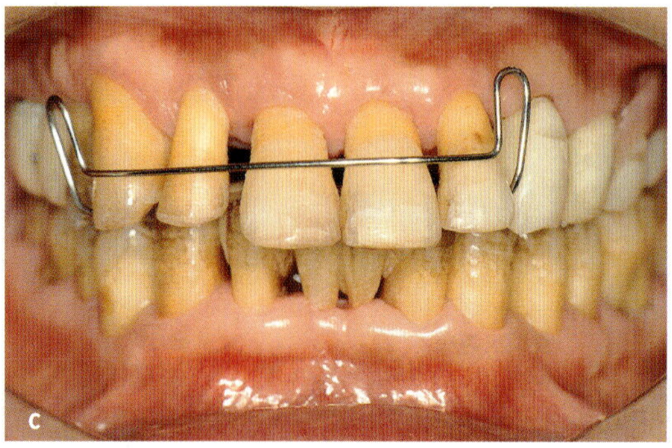

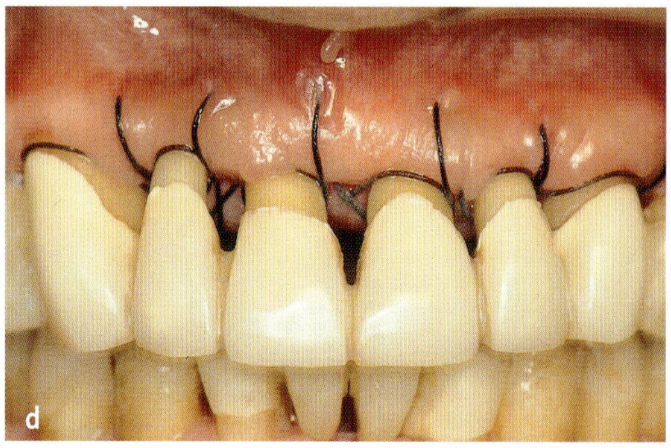

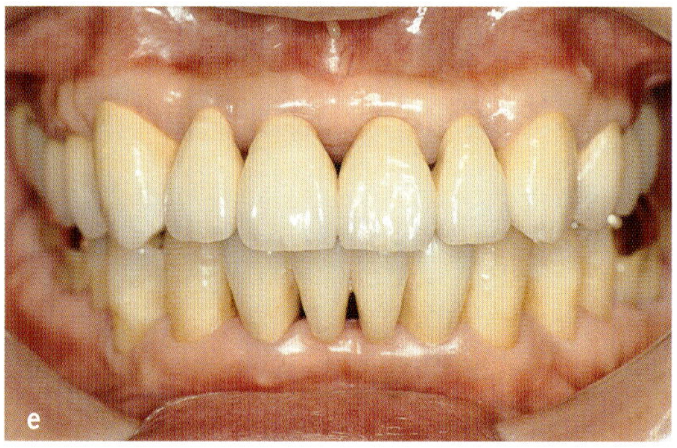

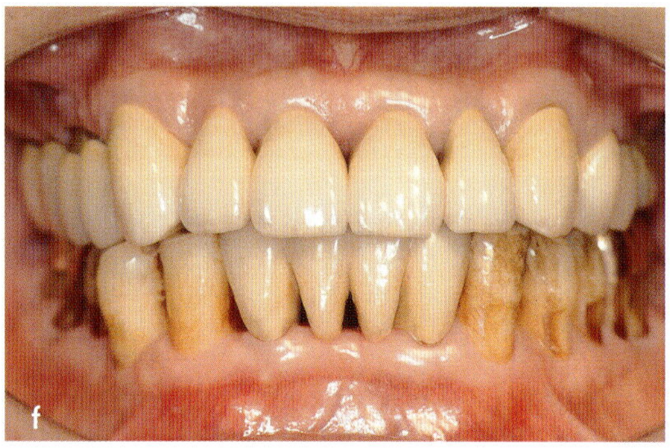

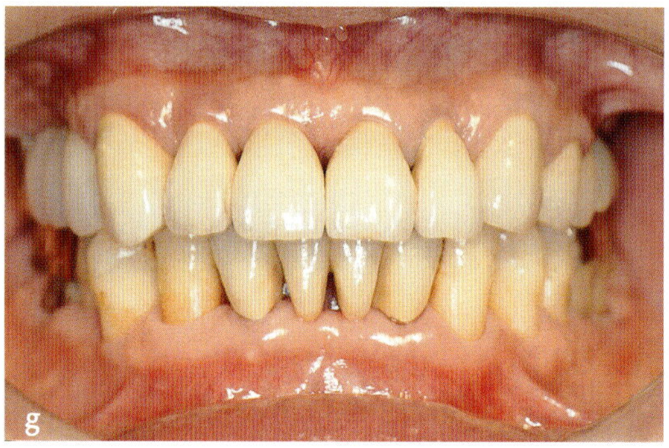

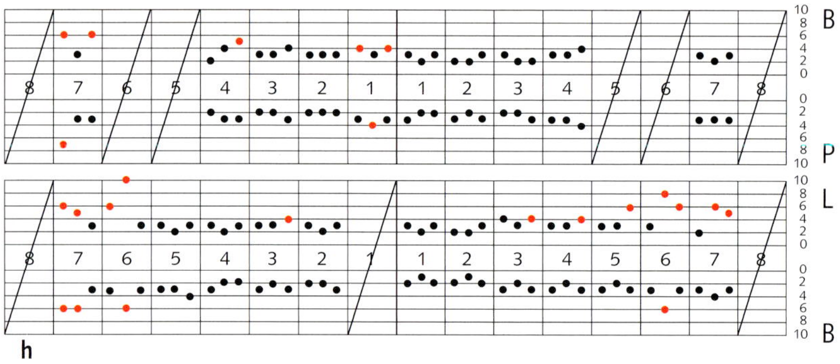

Fig 4-166 From first visit to present status. (a) At the first visit, significant pathologic migration of the maxillary anterior teeth is noted. There are furcation involvements in the molars. Mandibular anterior teeth and the maxillary left second premolar, first molar, and second molar are missing. (b) Probing chart soon after the first visit. (c) After initial therapy (March 1991), an orthodontic plate is used for lingual movement of the flared-out maxillary anterior teeth. (d) Periodontal surgery is conducted for reduction of periodontal pockets (July 1991). (e) The final prostheses have been delivered (October 1992). Key and keyway joints distal to the maxillary right canine and maxillary left canine and a fixed partial denture supported by an implant at the maxillary left second molar are included. Attention was paid so that the crown restorations would not overload the occlusal surfaces, which were flattened by attrition of the mandibular first and second molars. (f) Photograph taken 5 years 5 months after delivery of the final prostheses (March 1998). Probably because of bruxism or unilateral (right-side) mastication, the mandible has shifted to the right. The mandibular right first premolar has migrated buccally. (g) Nine years after the first visit, the maxillary right second premolar had been lost due to a root fracture. After GBR and a sinus lift, an implant was placed to recover occlusal support on the right. The patient is now under monthly maintenance (July 2001). (h) For 4 years 4 months after completion of the periodontal prostheses, the periodontal probing depths had been maintained within 3 mm. Maintenance visits were discontinued as he had to relocate. When the patient returned home in March 1998, several areas of concern were observed.

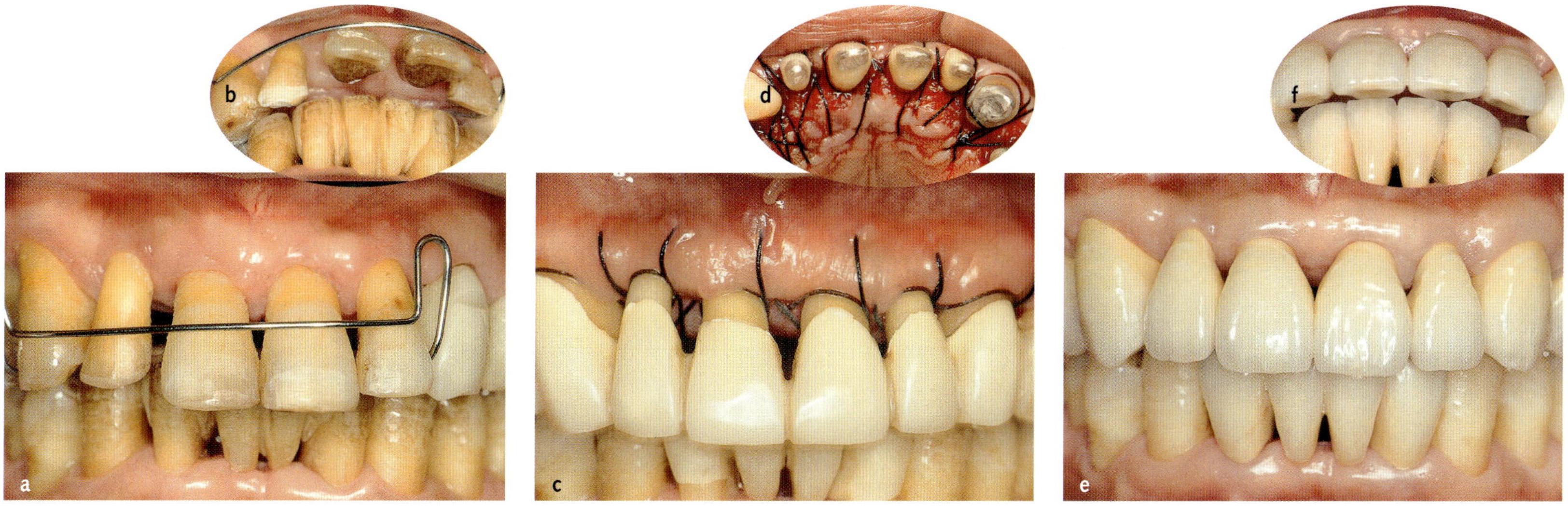

Fig 4-167 Treatments for anterior teeth. (a and b) An orthodontic plate is used to tip the teeth lingually. (c and d) A full-thickness flap is raised and limited osseous surgery is conducted. Based on our current thinking, there should have been more focus on the esthetic elements and the interdental papillae should have been preserved during treatment (incision lines, combined with a partial-thickness flap, and regenerative therapy). (e and f) Completion of the periodontal prostheses. A collarless porcelain fixed partial denture has been delivered from the mandibular left lateral incisor to the right lateral incisor (pontics: mandibular left and right central incisors). Although horizontal and vertical guidances are in harmony with function, the overbite is designed relatively shallow in this case, and it eventually resulted in severe bone defects and a poor crown-root ratio.

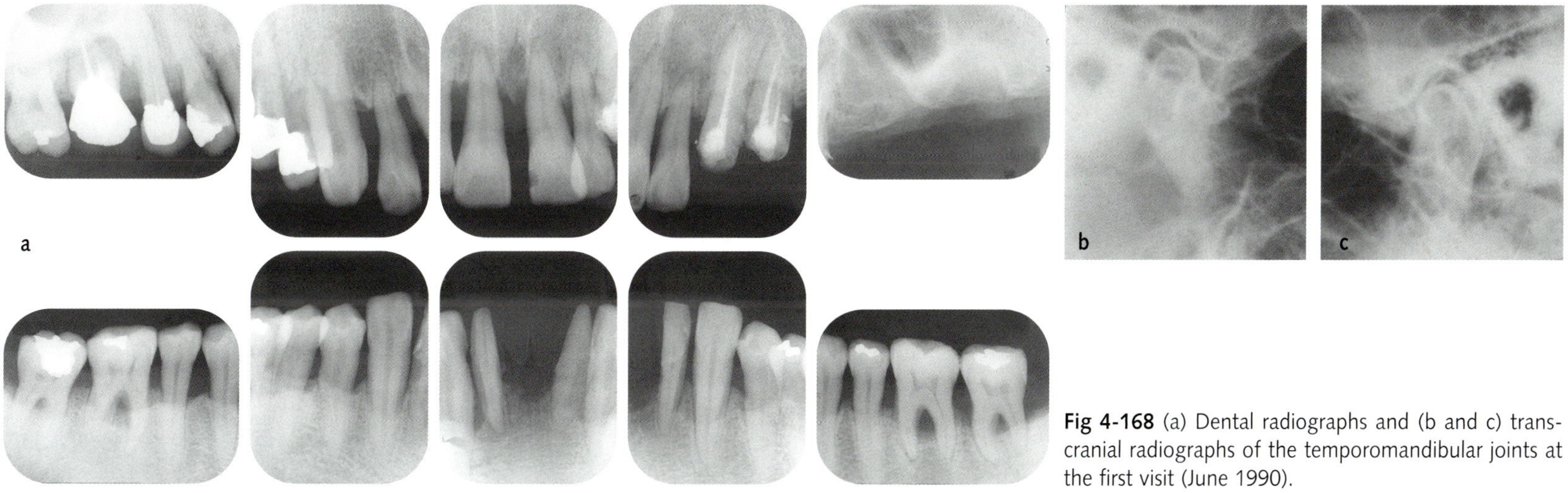

Fig 4-168 (a) Dental radiographs and (b and c) transcranial radiographs of the temporomandibular joints at the first visit (June 1990).

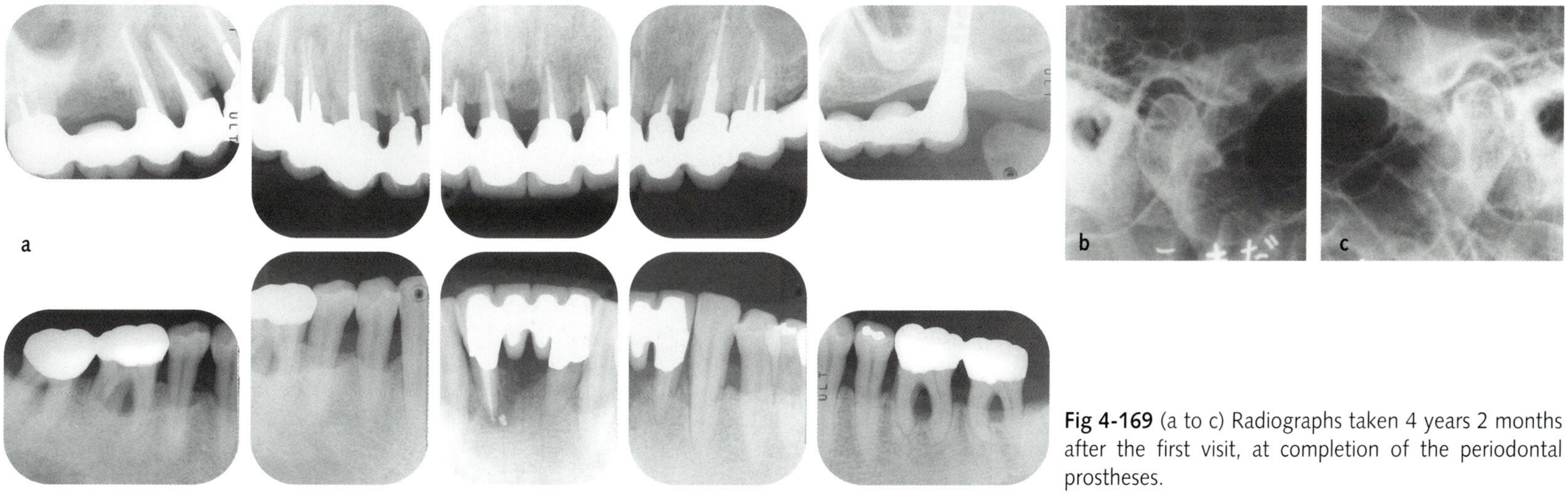

Fig 4-169 (a to c) Radiographs taken 4 years 2 months after the first visit, at completion of the periodontal prostheses.

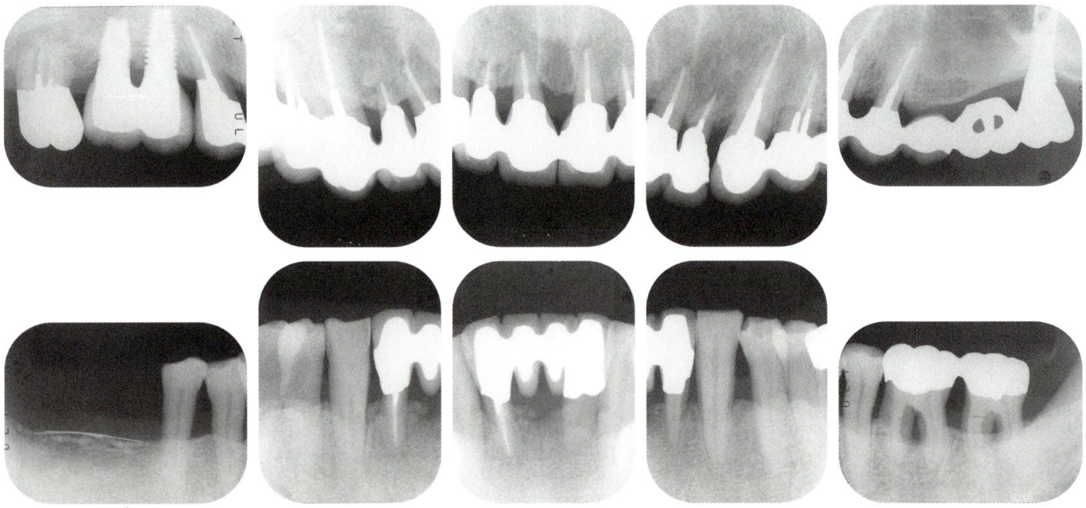

Fig 4-170 Dental radiographs taken about 12 years after the first visit. The severe periodontal disease and the maintenance involved risks to start with. As the patient discontinued visits during his overseas stay, a number of problems surfaced promptly. In 1998, the root of the maxillary right second premolar fractured, and implants were placed for the maxillary right first molar and second premolar in the following year. Crowns on the maxillary left canine and first premolar were removed because of secondary caries and were refabricated. In April 2002, the mandibular right first and second molars were extracted because of periodontal disease and secondary caries, for which GBR treatment is ongoing prior to implant placement.

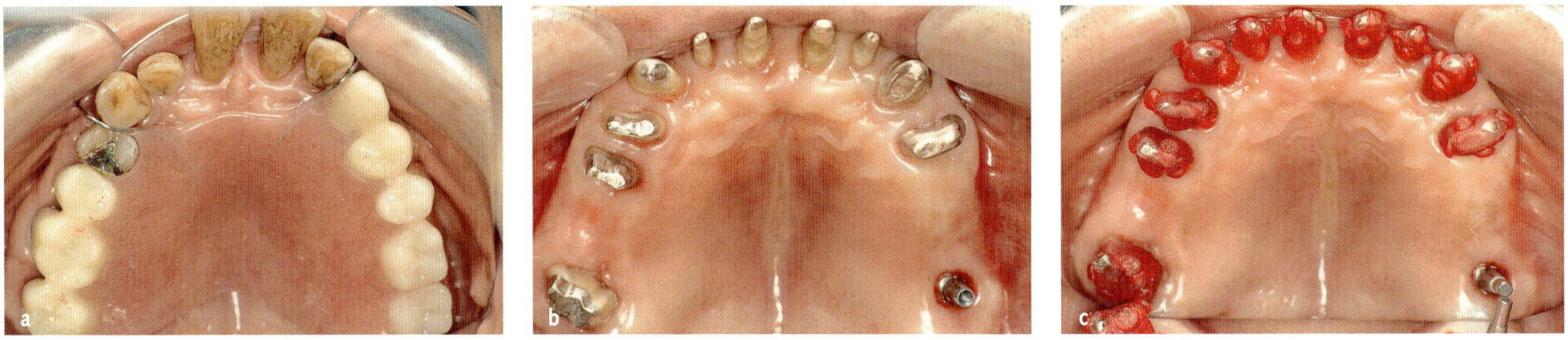

Fig 4-171 Improvement of the maxillary arch. (a) A telescopic denture, in which the maxillary right second premolar, first molar, and second molar and left canine and first premolar serve as abutments, is used for tooth movement in conjunction with initial periodontal therapy and endodontic treatment. (b) An implant has been placed for the maxillary left second molar. Pulpectomies have been conducted for the maxillary right central incisor, lateral incisor, canine, first premolar, and second molar and the left central incisor and lateral incisor, and endodontic re-treatment has been conducted for the maxillary right second premolar, left canine, and left first premolar. The maxillary right first molar was eventually extracted due to a class III furcation involvement. Dowel posts and cores have been created of type IV gold. Double crowns have been fabricated for the maxillary left first premolar (March 1992). (c) Reversible hydrocolloid impression material is used to take impressions of the individual teeth, and pattern resin is used to make copings for the full-arch impression (May 1992).

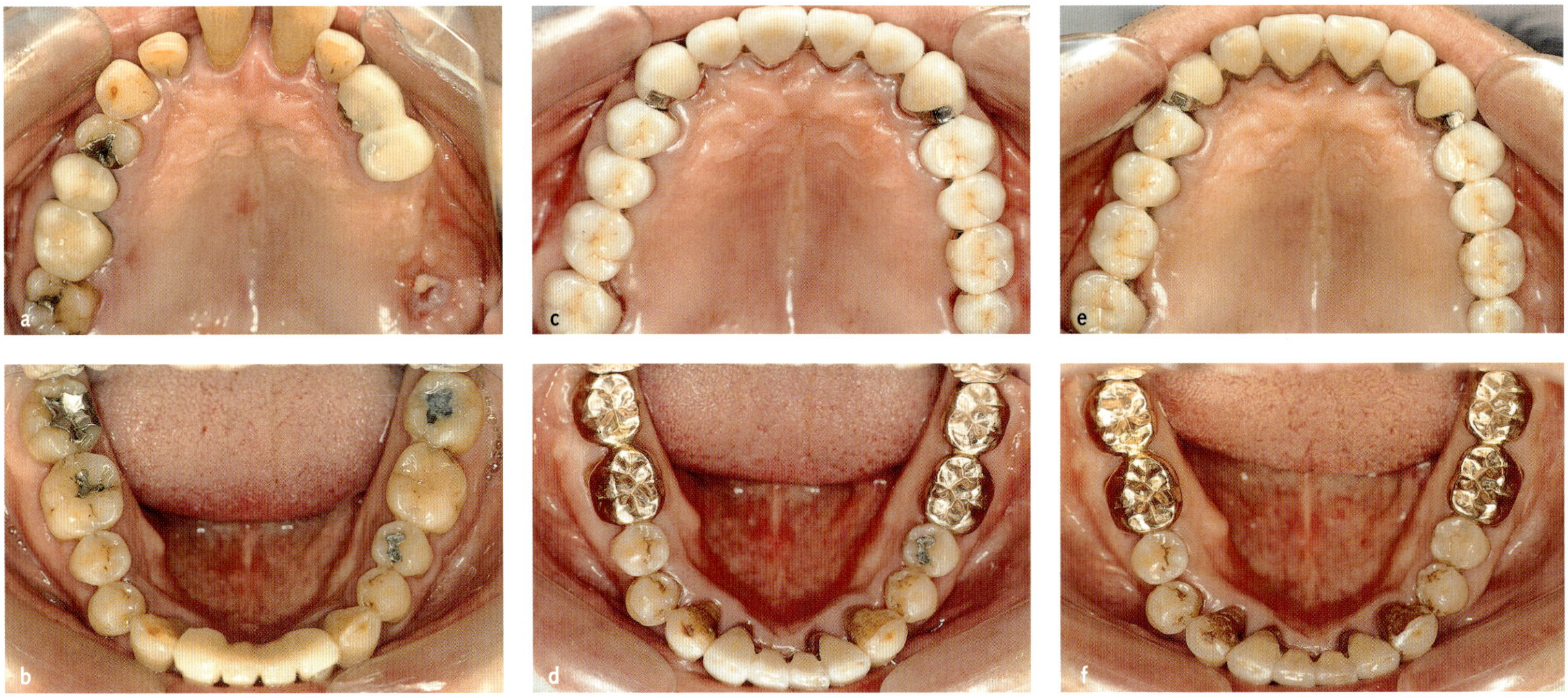

Fig 4-172 Reconstruction of a stable arch form in morphology and function. (a and b) At the first visit. (c and d) Photographs taken at completion of the periodontal prostheses. Taking into consideration the advanced attrition and furcation involvements, the morphology of the occlusal surface is reconstructed by crown restorations, aiming principally at avoidance of occlusal trauma (October 1992). (e and f) Photographs taken 2 years 7 months after delivery of prostheses. There had been no specific problems except for conspicuous tobacco staining (May 1995).

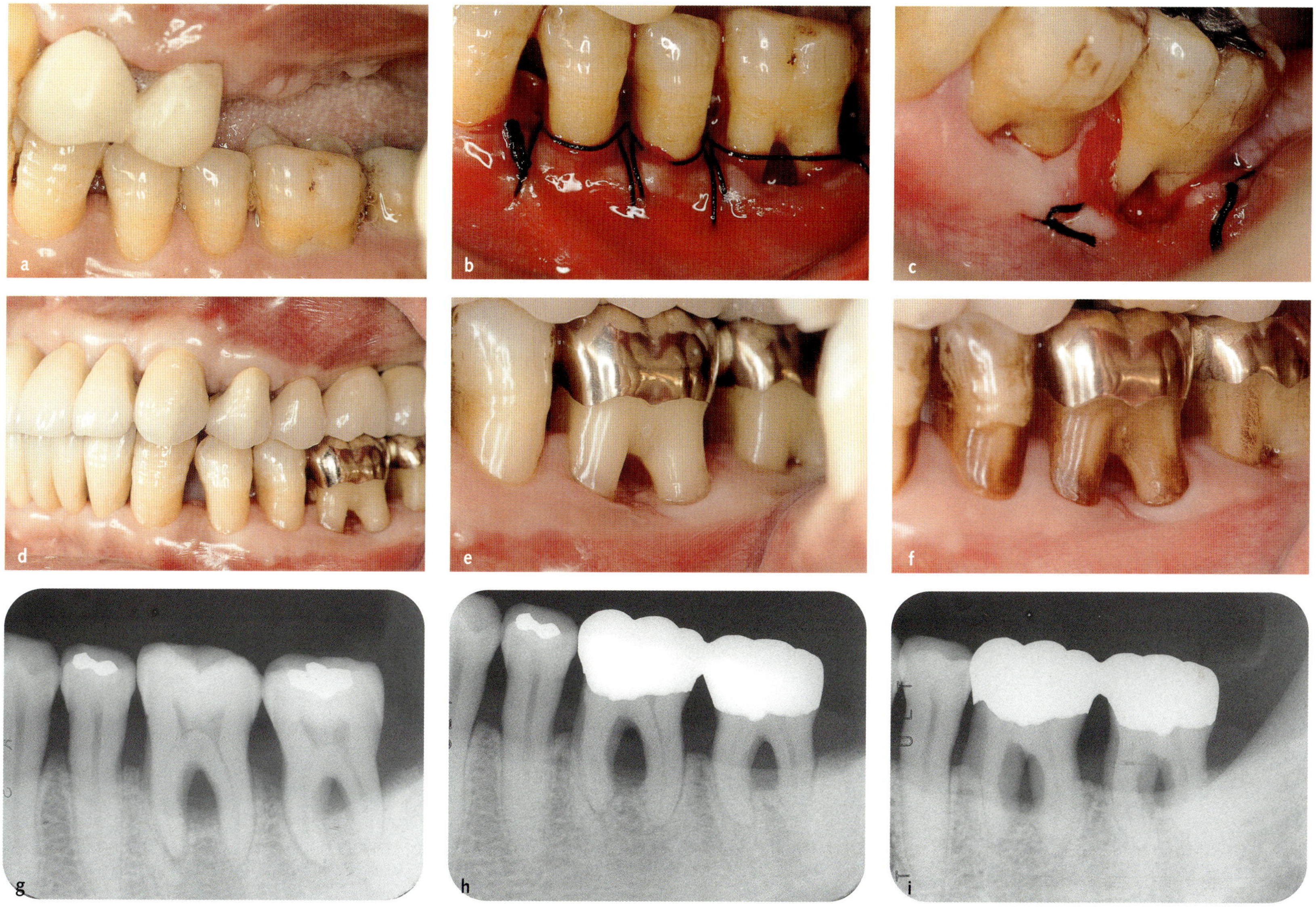

Fig 4-173 Progression of treatment of the left molars. (a) At the first visit. (b) Because there are deep periodontal pockets, a gingival flap is reflected to obtain access (September 1990). (c) For tunneling purposes, a partial-thickness flap is apically repositioned in the furcation area. (d) In the maxillary arch, an ITI implant is placed for the maxillary left second molar, and occlusal support is restored by a fixed partial denture with the maxillary left first premolar and second molar as abutments (pontics: maxillary left second premolar and first molar) (October 1992). (e) Photograph taken 6 years after the first visit (October 1996). An interdental brush is used to clean furcation areas of the mandibular left first and second molars. (f) Photograph taken 10 years after the first visit. Tobacco staining is conspicuous. (g) At the first visit, the mandibular left first and second molars have furcation involvements. (h) Teeth are vital and crown restoration is conducted with tunneling to avoid pulp involvement and root fracture due to dowel post placement. Because the caries risk is high for the exposed furcation areas, it is essential to maintain the sensitivity of the teeth. (i) Although there is some abrasion on the root surfaces because of interdental brush use and professional mechanical tooth cleaning, function has been maintained (July 2002).

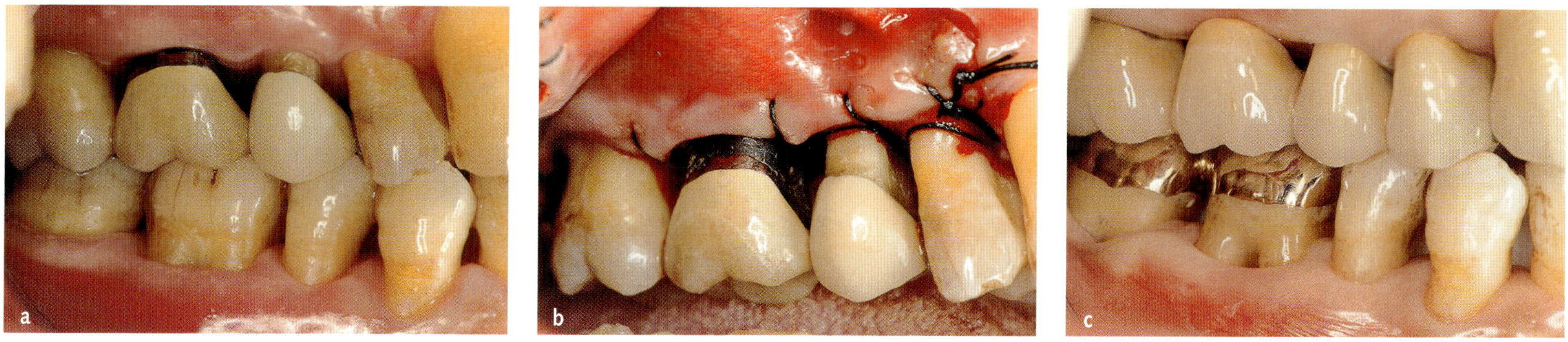

Fig 4-174 Progression of treatment of the right molars. (a) At the first visit. (b) Because there are deep periodontal pockets, periodontal flap surgery is completed (September 1990). (c) Photograph taken after 3 years.

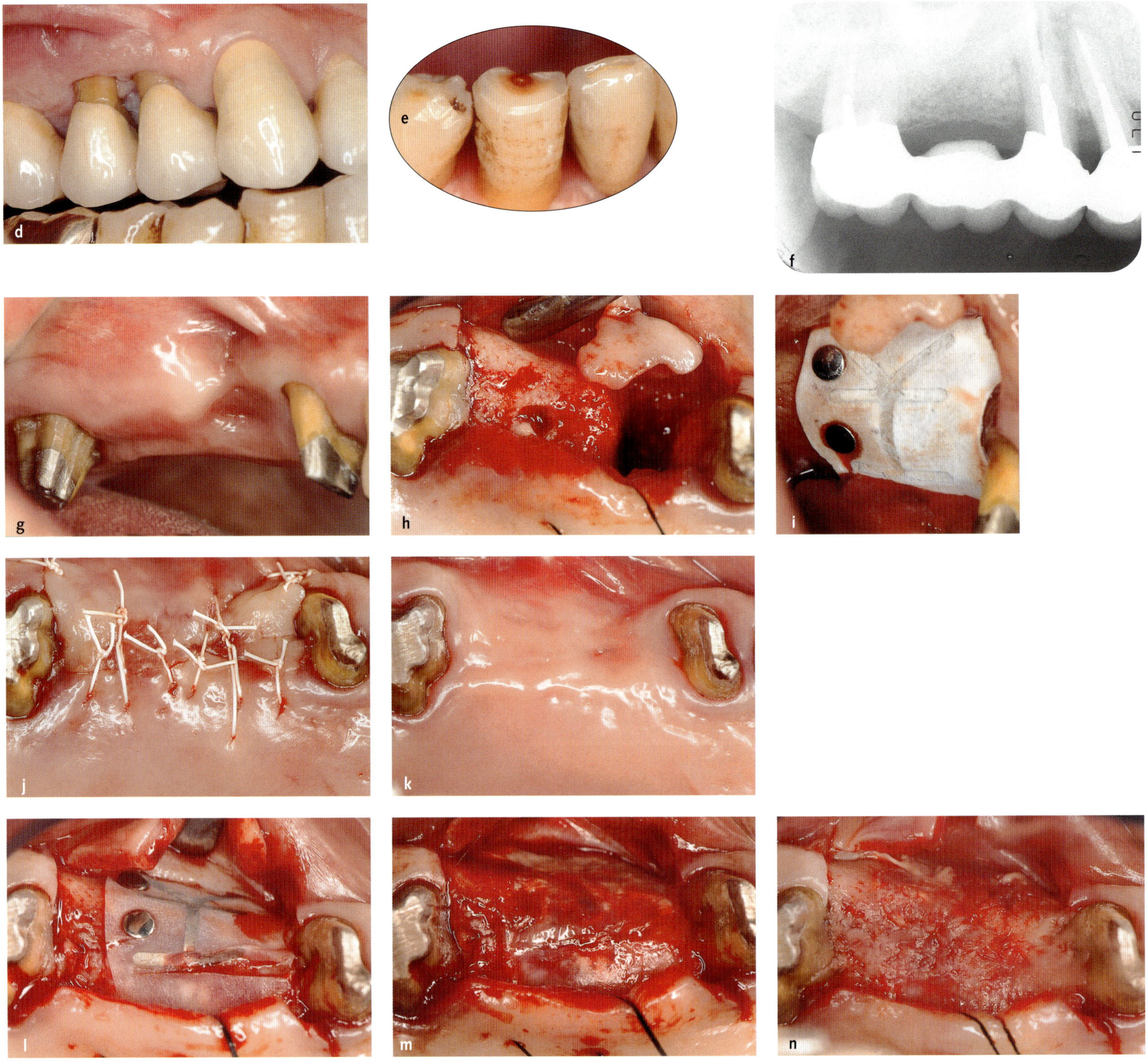

Fig 4-174 (cont) (d to f) Eight years after the first visit (April 1998), the maxillary right second premolar has a root fracture. The luting cement for the dowel core has dissolved. The severity of the bruxism is indicated by the attrition of the canine and buccal migration of the first premolar. (g) Photograph taken 2 months after extraction. (h) The loss of the buccal plate of the extraction site is mostly due to a dehiscence. A full-thickness flap is raised for GBR. (i) A titanium-reinforced nonresorbable membrane is fixed with pins. (j) On top of the alveolar crest, a beveled incision is made in a split manner from the palatal side. Mesially and distally, vertical incisions are made, extending to the MGJ, and releasing incisions are added to form two to three layers. Close attention is paid to the vertical mattress sutures so that no tension will be applied. (k) Appearance 6 months after surgery. (l) Flap surgery is conducted to remove the membrane. A clean membrane is confirmed. (m) The membrane is removed, and the hard tissue is covered by thin film. (n) The film is removed, and newly formed bone is confirmed. The bone level necessary for a healthy emergence profile of the implants has been obtained.

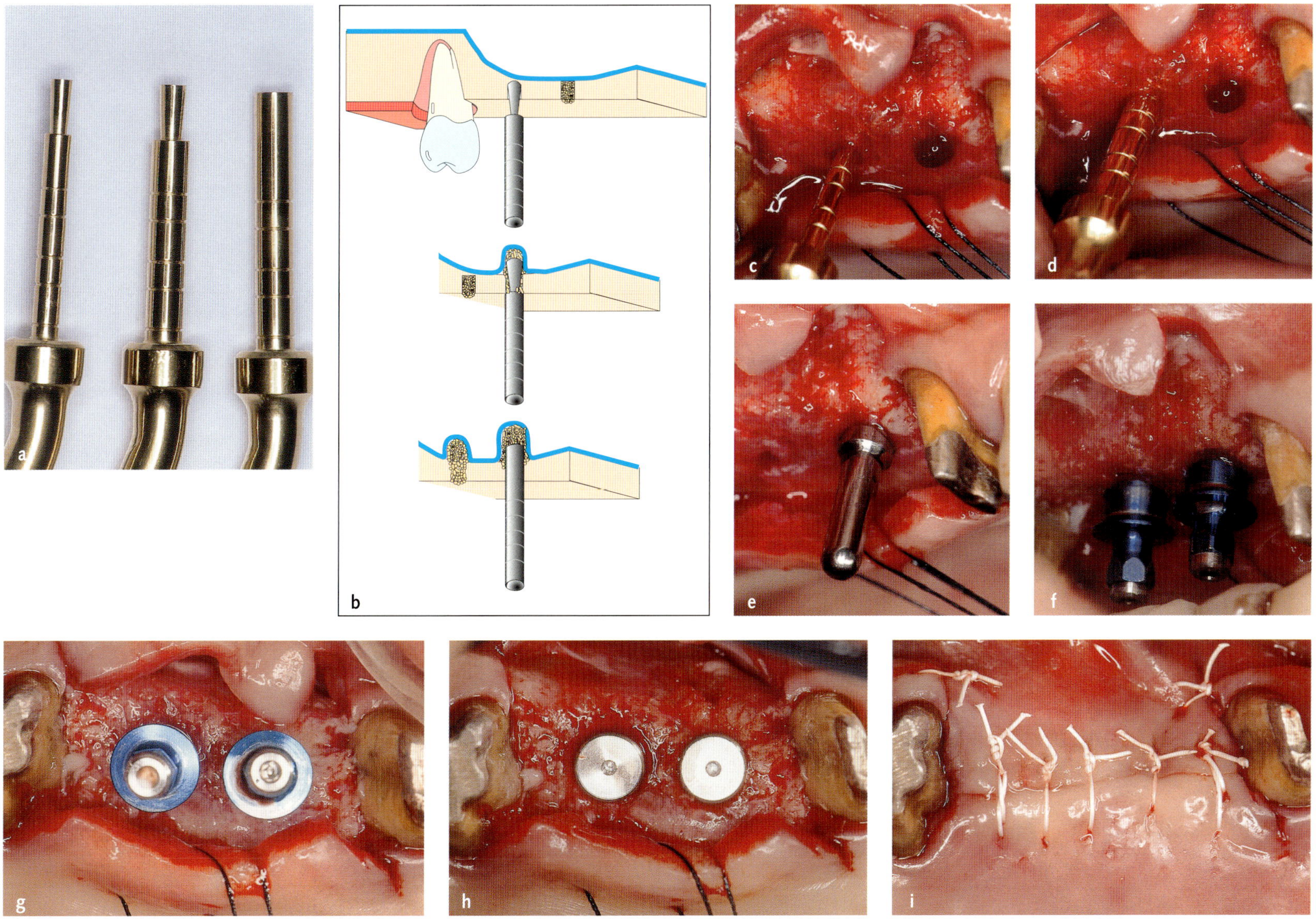

Fig 4-175 Sinus elevation with an osteotome and implant placement. (a) Because the sinus floor is close to the maxillary right first molar (about 5 mm), a sinus lift osteotome is used for the sinus elevation procedure. (b) Principle of osteotome use (modified from Summers). (c) Autogenous bone is grafted, and a mallet is used carefully. (d) Gradually, osteotomes of larger diameters are used to expand the bone to elevate Schneiderean membrane and to secure a place for implant placement. (e and f) A direction indicator is used to confirm the position, direction, and depth of the osteotomy site, and the implants are placed. (g) Two implants, 5.0 × 8.5 mm and 5.0 × 10.0 mm in diameter, are placed. (h and i) Cover screws are placed, and a releasing incision is made to form two layers. Butt joint–like flaps are accurately replaced and sutured.

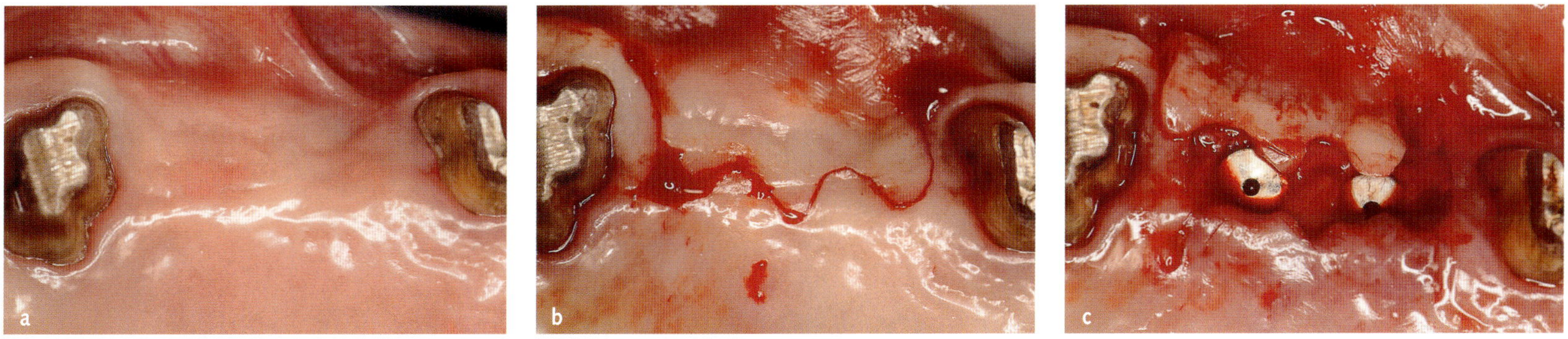

Fig 4-176 Second surgery for the implants. (a) Photograph taken 4 months after implant placement. (b) A scallop-shaped incision is made to establish papilla-like tissue at the healing abutments. (c) A partial-thickness flap is reflected up to the MGJ. The interdental papillae at the maxillary right premolars are preserved.

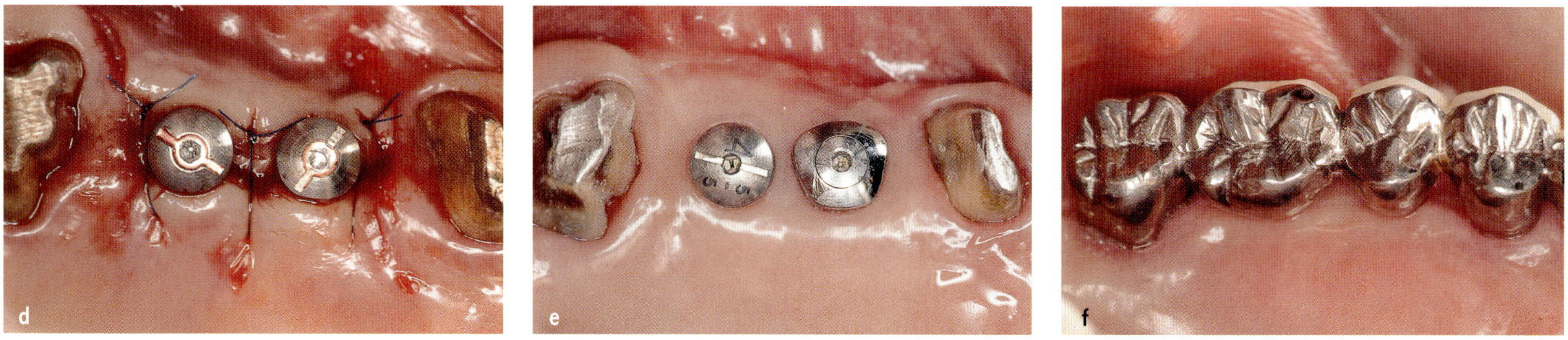

Fig 4-176 (cont) (d) Flaps are tightly sutured. (e) Occlusal view of the provisional restoration during the healing period. It is essential to secure the occlusal support. (f) Final prosthesis.

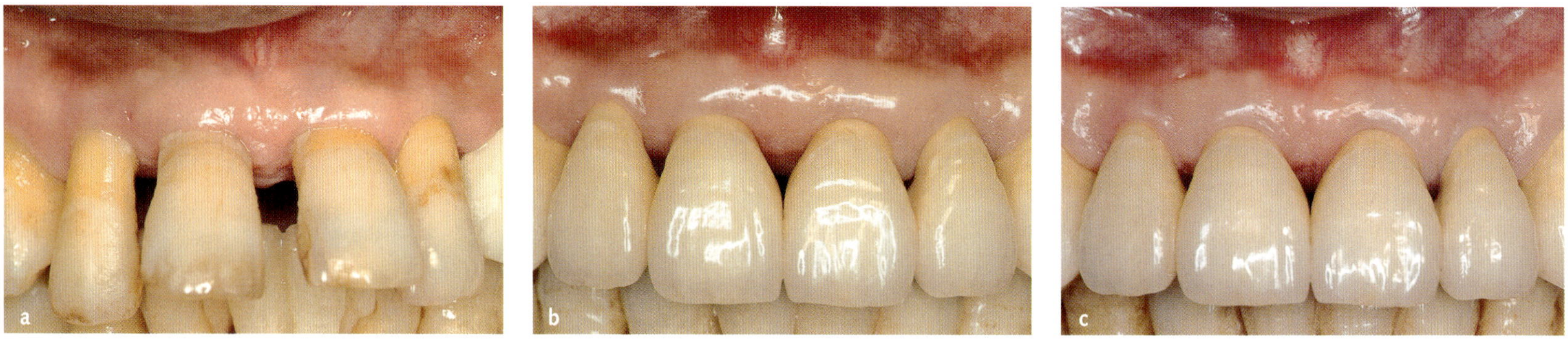

Fig 4-177 Treatment progress of the maxillary anterior teeth. (a) Photograph taken at the first visit. (b) Crown restorations with collarless porcelain are delivered. Although preservation of the interdental papillae was envisioned, we were not as conscious of the esthetics as we are now. We are not sure yet whether it would be appropriate to completely close embrasures in this case. (c) Photograph taken after 8 years. (d) Condition after 12 years. (e) Radiograph taken at the first visit. (f) Radiograph taken after 3 years. (g) Radiograph taken after 10 years. An endodontic-periodontal complication is observed. (h) Radiograph taken 12 years after the first visit. After periapical curettage, regenerative therapy was conducted.

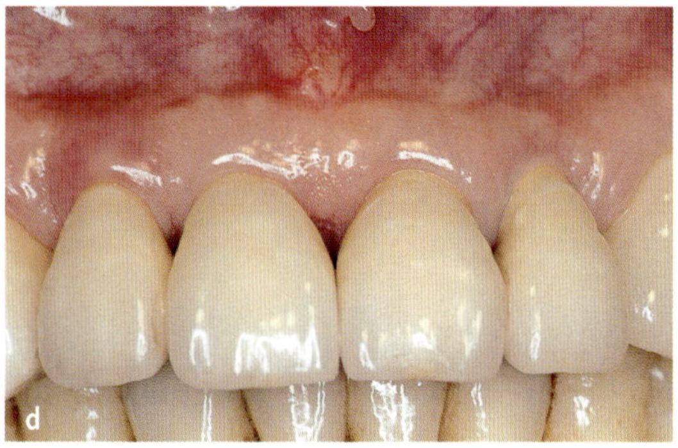

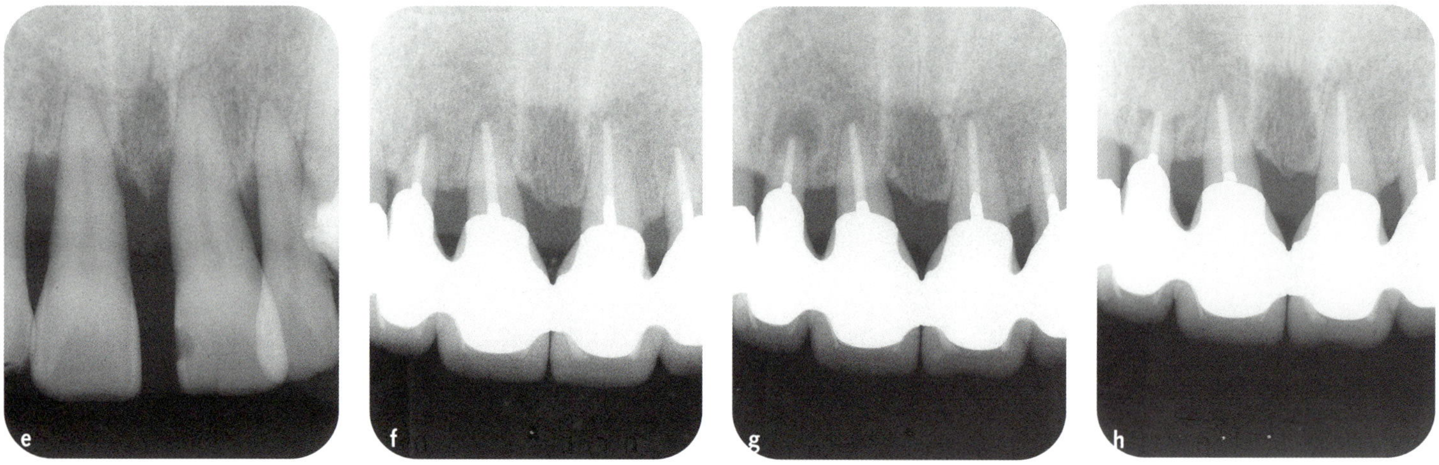

Devices for periodontal therapy: Artificial organs

Periodontal prostheses are devices for periodontal therapy and, at the same time, are artificial organs to support the stomatognathic system as an organ that enables basic life support activities, including mastication, speech, and swallowing. Localized loss of attachment may be recovered to a certain degree by improvement of the periodontal environment. Cases with occlusal collapse accompanied by severe periodontal disease, however, cannot expect maintenance and recovery of the attachment with certainty without stabilization of the occlusion, restoration of the integrity of the dentition, and mechanical stabilization of the individual tooth (see Case 4-7).

Case 4-7 Severe occlusal collapse accompanied by periodontal disease and a periodontal prosthesis in a younger patient

Patient: *33-year-old man at the time of first visit in 1987*

Chief complaint: *Spontaneous pain of the maxillary right lateral incisor*

When the patient visited us with a chief complaint of spontaneous pain of the lateral incisor, he did not seem to be conscious of the symptoms of occlusal collapse, the level of which was almost too advanced to be imagined at his age. Because fixed partial denture dislodgment had been left untreated, the vertical dimension of the molars decreased and the mandibular position was disturbed, which seem to have accelerated the occlusal collapse. Because the patient was still young, extraction was avoided as much as possible and even unpromising teeth were preserved. A case like this has to be approached conservatively while the problems are fixed (Figs 4-178 to 4-186).

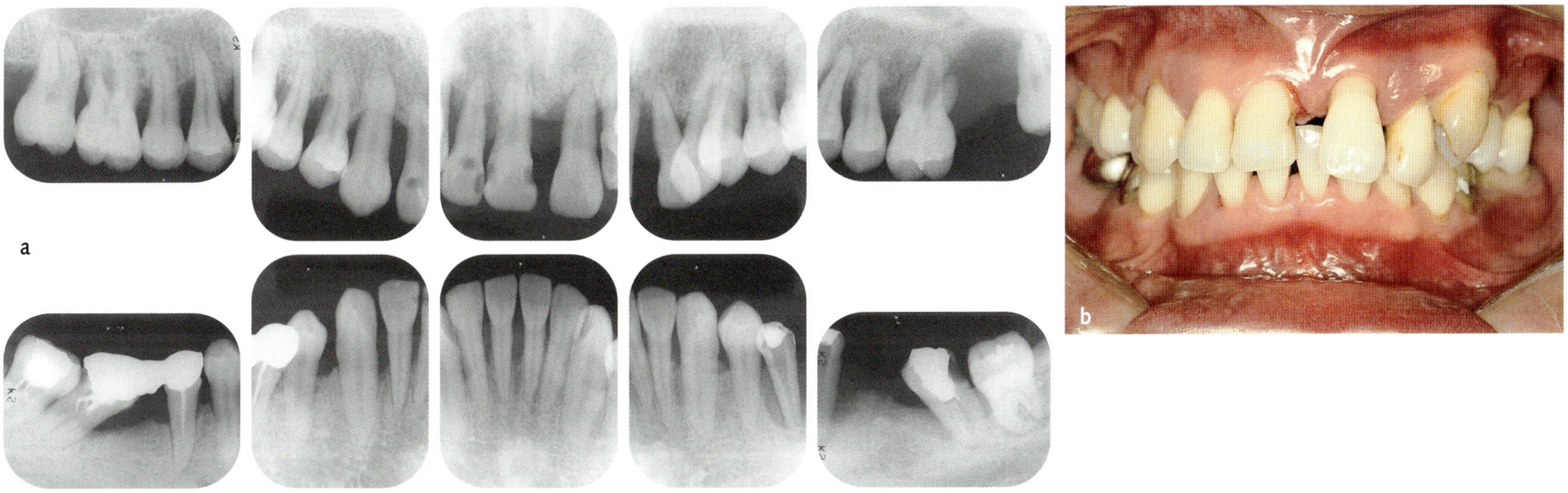

Fig 4-178 (a and b) Radiographs and frontal view at the first visit. The periodontal disease is severely advanced. The dislodged fixed partial denture, which had the mandibular left second premolar and second molar as abutments, is left untreated. This has initiated a decrease in the vertical dimension and distortion of the occlusal plane. As a result, the maxillary left central and lateral incisors flare out labially.

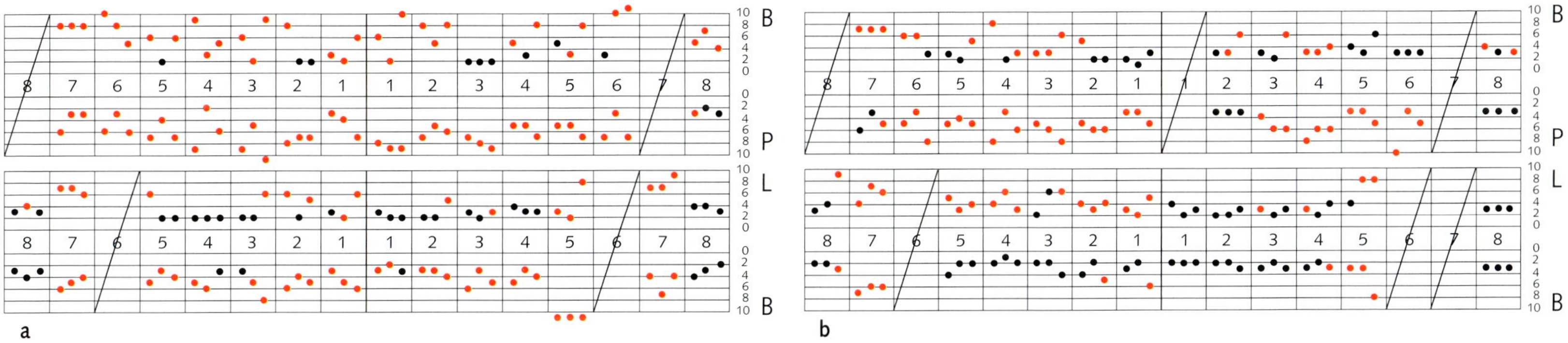

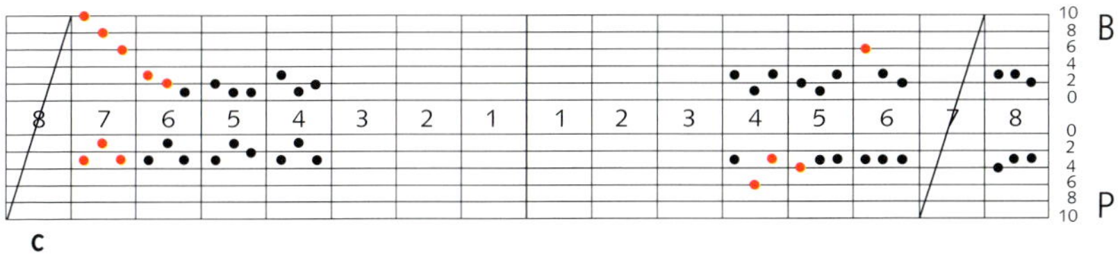

Fig 4-179 Probing charts. (a) Chart made at the first visit. (b) At reevaluation, deep periodontal pockets (9 to 11 mm) and degree 2 to 3 mobility are noted. (c) During maintenance, 2 years 10 months after the first visit, an endodontic-periodontal complication affecting the maxillary right second molar developed, and the tooth had to be extracted.

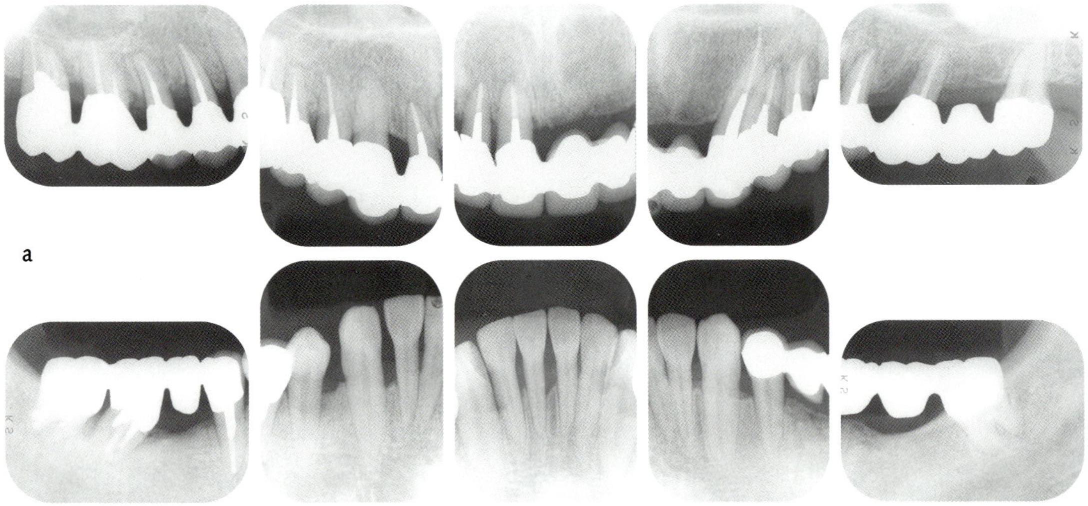

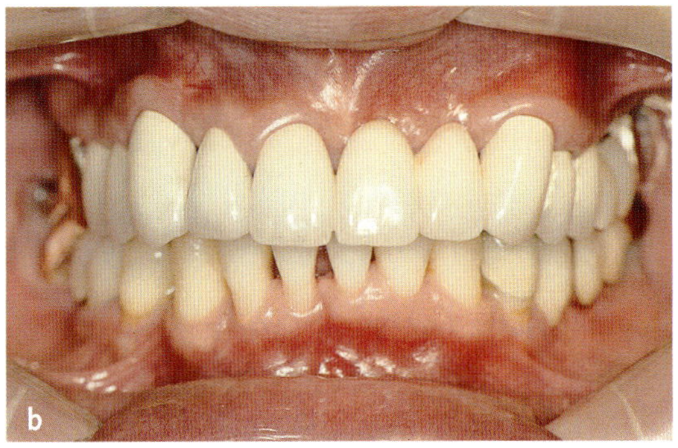

Fig 4-180 (a) Radiographs taken 2 years after the first visit. The periodontal prostheses have been delivered. After initial therapy (the maxillary left central and lateral incisors and mandibular left first premolar and second molar were extracted), an access flap was completed for the maxillary and mandibular anterior regions. General tooth movements with an orthodontic plate were completed about a year after the first visit, followed by tooth axis control and leveling using brackets. After a trial-and-error process with provisional restorations, the case proceeded with an increase of the VDO and an improvement of the mandibular position. (b) Photograph taken 5 months after delivery. For the maxilla, the distal buccal roots of the right first and second molars as well as the buccal roots of the left first molar were amputated. A full-arch splint has been completed, extending from the right second molar to the left third molar (pontics: left central incisor, lateral incisor, and second molar). For the mandible, fixed partial dentures with the left third molar and first premolar as abutments (pontics: left second premolar, first molar, and second molar) and the right second premolar and third molar as abutments (pontic: right first molar) have been delivered. All restorations are metal-ceramic except the molars, which are full-coverage gold.

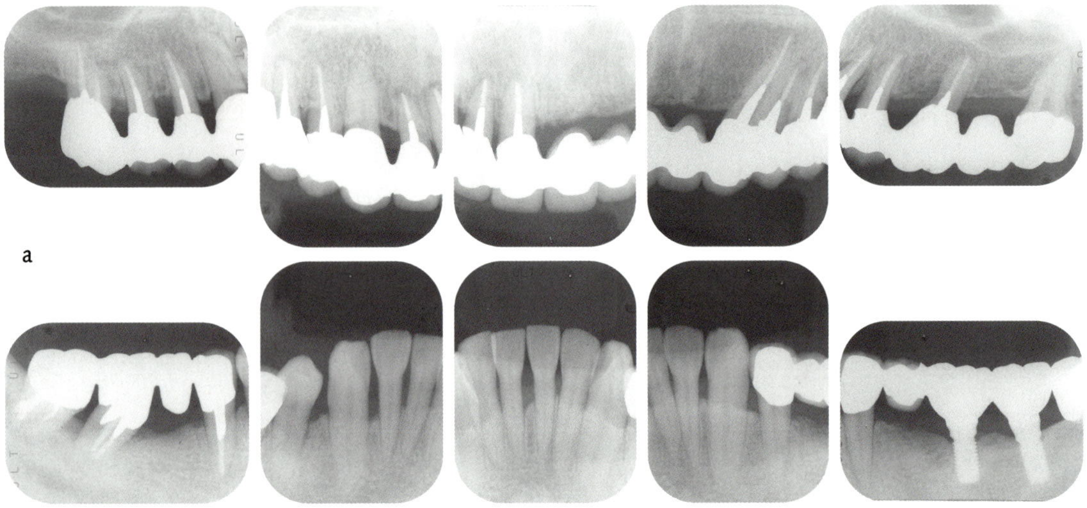

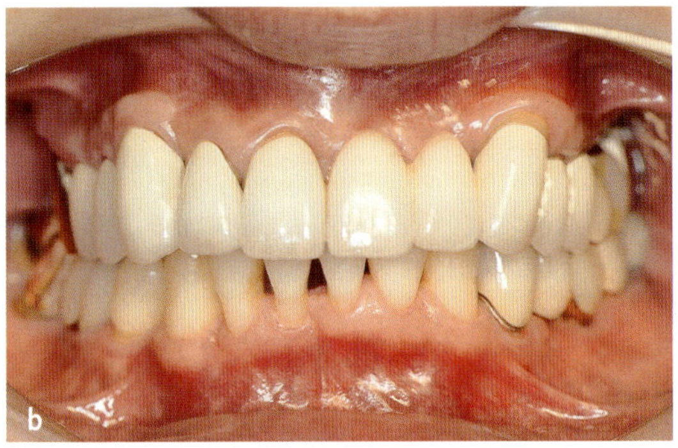

Fig 4-181 (a and b) Radiographs and photograph taken 11 years 5 months after the first visit. The maxillary right second molar has been extracted. The fixed partial denture extending from the mandibular left first premolar to the third molar has been dislodged due to secondary caries. Root canal treatment has been completed for the mandibular left third molar and two Brånemark implants (Nobel Biocare), 3.75 × 8.50 mm in diameter, have been placed for the mandibular left first and second molars.

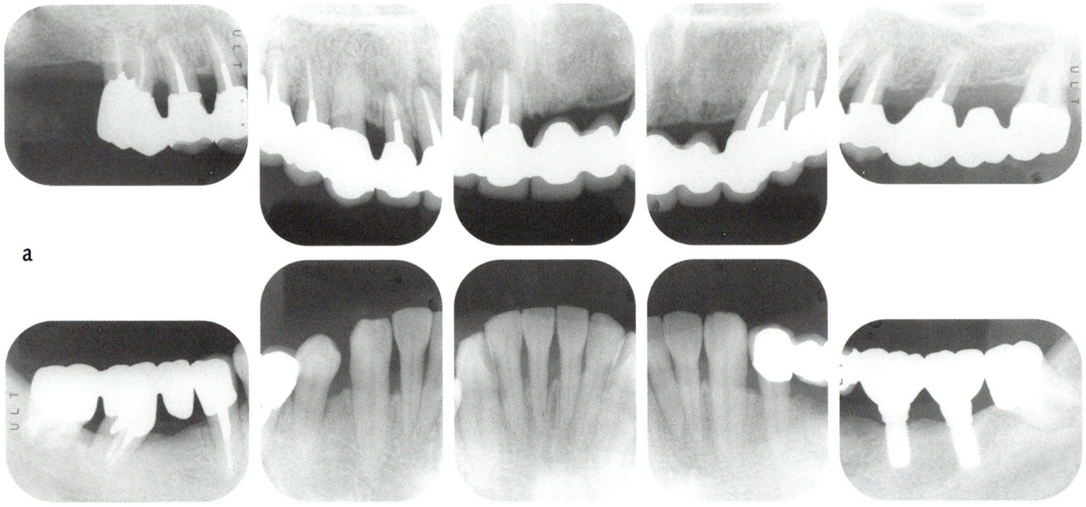

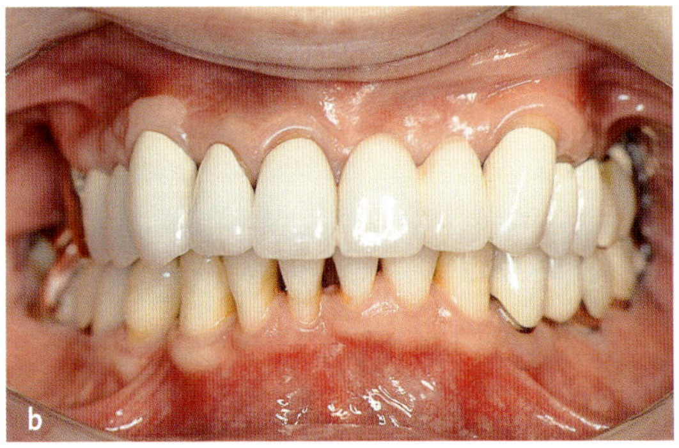

Fig 4-182 (a and b) Images taken 14 years 6 months after the first visit. No specific issues have arisen.

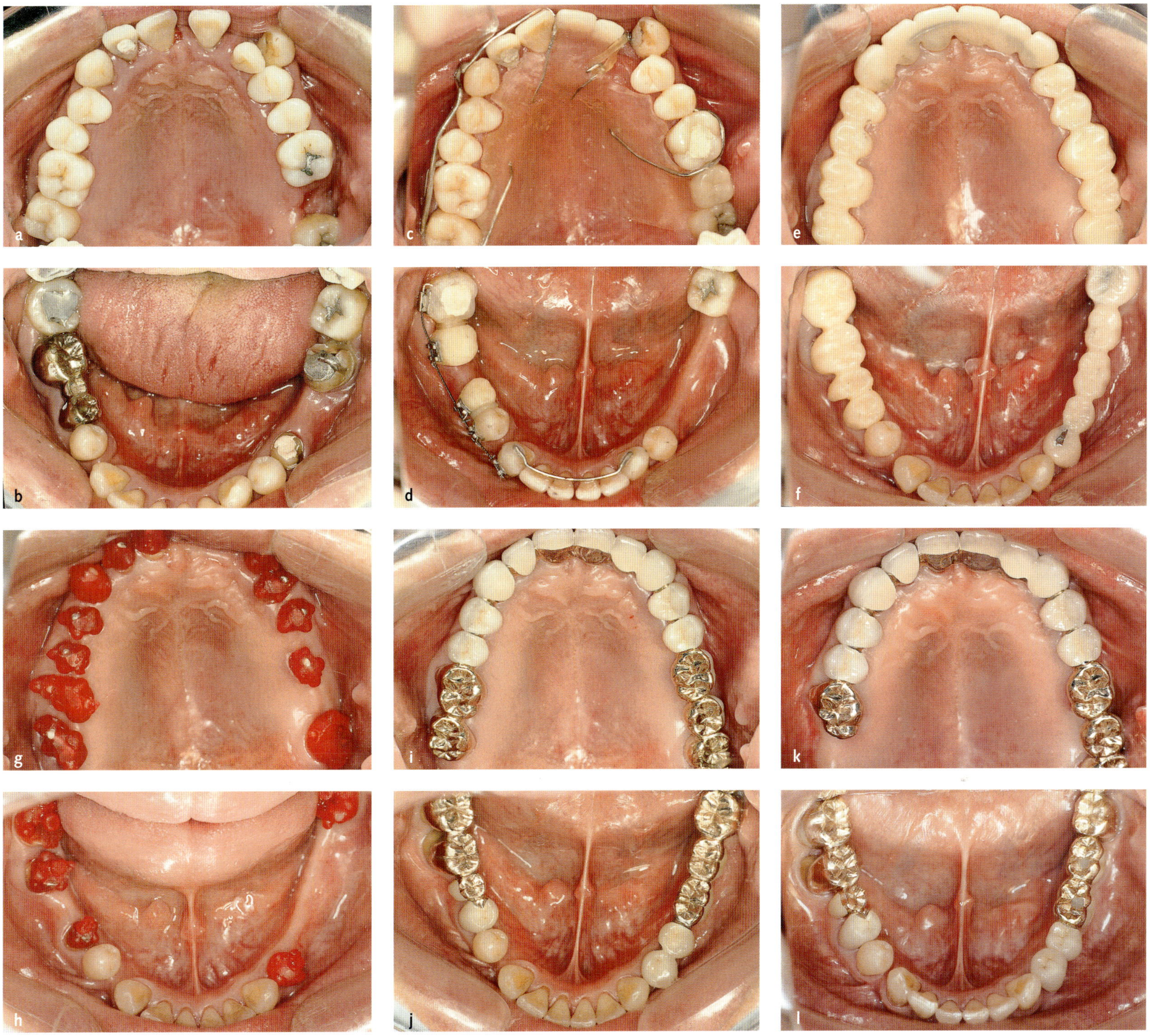

Fig 4-183 Occlusal views of treatment progress. (a and b) At the first visit, the maxillary arch has significant interdental spaces and the arch is deformed. In the mandibular arch, the left second premolar and second molar are hopeless. (c and d) After initial therapy (scaling and root planing followed by periodontal access flap surgeries), orthodontic plates are used to complete general tooth movement (especially to reduce the labioversion of the maxillary left canine), after which brackets are used for orthodontic treatment. In the mandible, after extraction of the left second premolar and second molar as well as endodontic treatment for the right second premolar, second molar, and third molar, orthodontic treatment and improvement of the arch form and root proximity are conducted. (e and f) Splinting design (whether or not the maxillary right second molar to the left third molar are to be splinted), arch form improvement, and harmony in morphology are envisioned with the provisional restoration. (g and h) Although hydrocolloid impression material was used back in 1989, the transfer coping technique with pattern resin remains the same. (i and j) About 2 years after the first visit. Cross-arch splints have been delivered. The distobuccal roots of the maxillary right first and second molars as well as the buccal roots of maxillary left first molar have been amputated, and the maxillary left central and lateral incisors have been extracted. Root canal therapy has been conducted for the maxillary right central incisor, lateral incisor, first premolar, second premolar, first molar, and second molar and the maxillary left canine, first premolar, second premolar, and first molar. Root canal re-treatment has been performed for the mandibular right first premolar, second molar, and third molar. A full splint has been delivered for the maxillary arch. Fixed partial dentures have been placed, using the mandibular left first premolar and third molar (pontics: mandibular left second premolar, first molar, and second molar) and the mandibular right second premolar and third molar (pontic: mandibular right first molar) as abutment teeth. (k and l) Photographs taken 15 years after the first visit. The maxillary right second molar had to be extracted because of failing endodontic treatment. About 10 years after the first visit, the fixed partial denture extending from the mandibular left first premolar to third molar dislodged. After two implants were placed for the mandibular left first and second molars, a new fixed partial denture was made, extending from the mandibular left first premolar to the second molar (pontic: mandibular left second premolar).

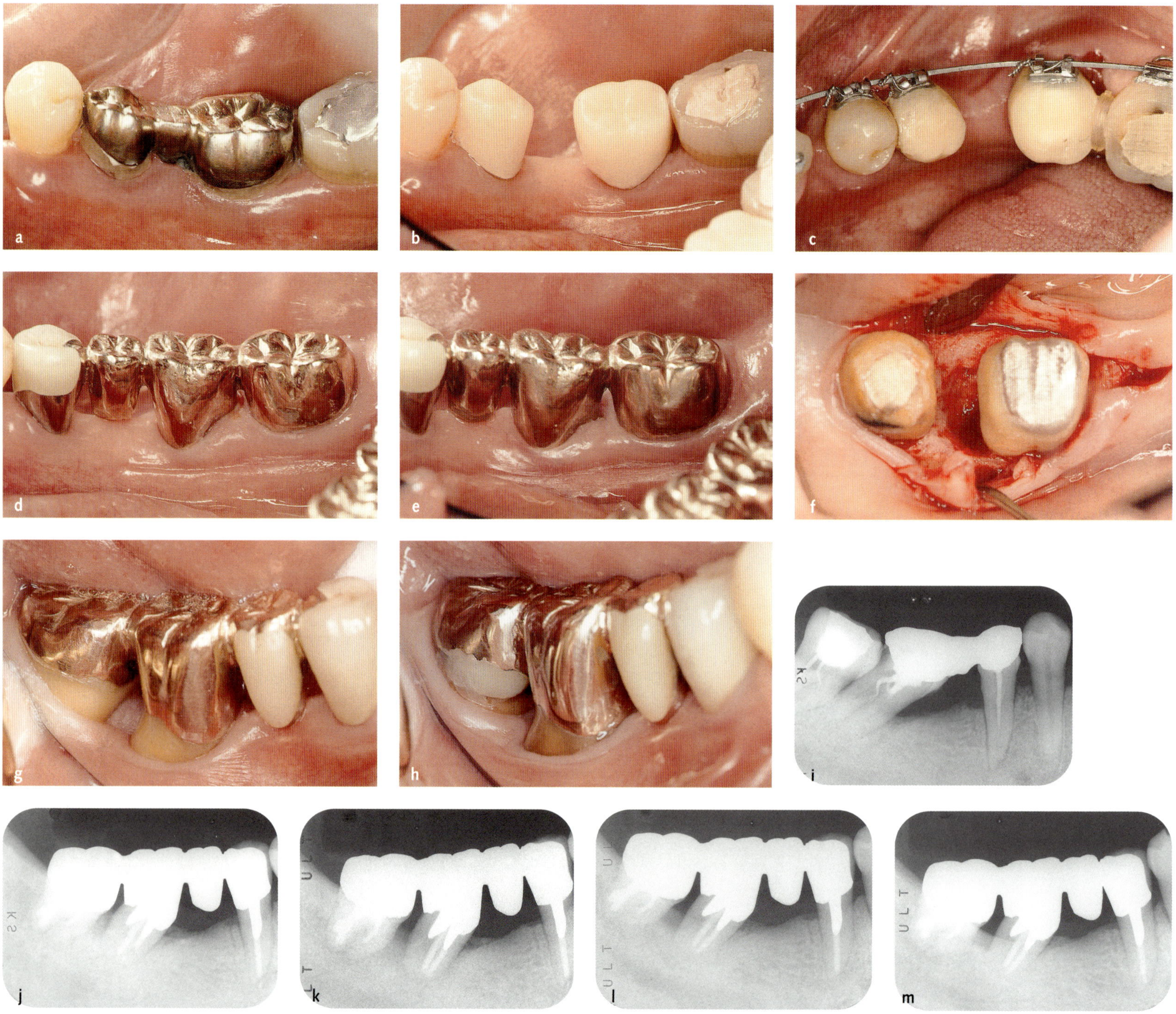

Fig 4-184 Course of treatment – mandibular right. (a) Lingual view at the first visit. An endodontic-periodontal complication and occlusal trauma are combined. (b) Initial therapy. (c) Tooth movement for establishment of a good periodontal environment and rearrangement of the teeth. (d) Final restoration. (e) An alveolar abscess has developed 3 years after delivery of the prosthesis. (f) A flap is reflected to find infected dentin on this concave, curved root surface. GTR therapy is conducted with a nonresorbable membrane. (g) Photograph taken 6 years after delivery of the prosthesis. Although substantial gingival recession is noted, the pathologic periodontal pockets have diminished. (h) Photograph taken 15 years after the first visit. Secondary caries has developed at the mandibular right third molar, for which a resin composite restoration has been completed. (i to m) Radiographic evaluation of the mandibular right teeth. (i) At the first visit. (j) At delivery of the prosthesis. (k) Radiograph taken after 3 years. (l) Radiograph taken after 11 years 5 months. (m) Radiograph taken after 14 years 5 months.

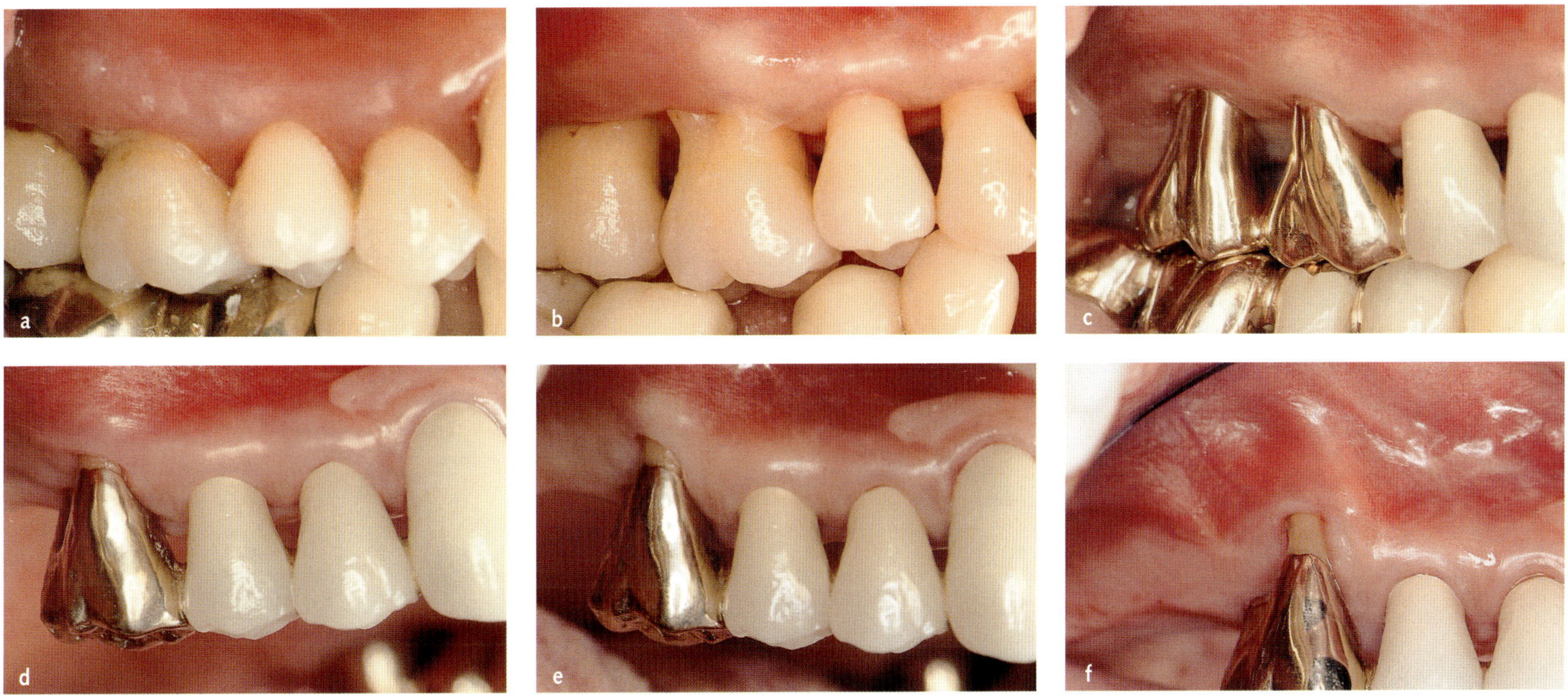

Fig 4-185 Course of treatment – maxillary right. (a) Photograph taken at the first visit. (b) After 8 months of initial therapy, the gingival conditions are improved. (c) Photograph taken after 2 years, when the prostheses have been delivered. The distobuccal roots have been amputated. (d) Photograph taken after 4 years. Because of failing endodontic treatment (file separation) and a remaining gap between the amputated root surfaces, a pathologic pocket relapsed (11.0 mm), and the second molar had to be extracted. (e) Photograph taken after 4 years. (f) After 12 years, the root of the first molar is exposed. Maintenance of sectioned roots with inferior morphology is difficult.

Fig 4-186 Course of treatment – mandibular left. (a) Photograph taken at the first visit. The mandibular left first molar and mandibular left first premolar are hopeless and have to be extracted. (b) A long-span fixed partial denture is placed. (c) Photograph taken 9 years after delivery of the prosthesis. Re-treatment is necessary because of secondary caries at the first premolar and third molar. (d) Because the second premolar site is not indicated for implant placement due to the position of the mental foramen, implants have been placed for the first and second molars. After the second surgery, a provisional fixed partial denture is used to further secure osseointegration and the mandibular position. (e) A telescopic crown is delivered to the first premolar. EsthetiCone abutments (Nobel Biocare) are used for the first and second molars. (f) Photograph taken 4 years after delivery of the prostheses, or 13 years 5 months after the first visit. There are screw access holes on the occlusal surface of the implant prostheses. (g) Radiograph taken at the first visit. (h) Radiograph taken at delivery of the final prostheses. (i) Radiograph taken 10 years after the first visit. (j) Radiograph taken 14 years 6 months after the first visit. Traumatic findings have been reduced.

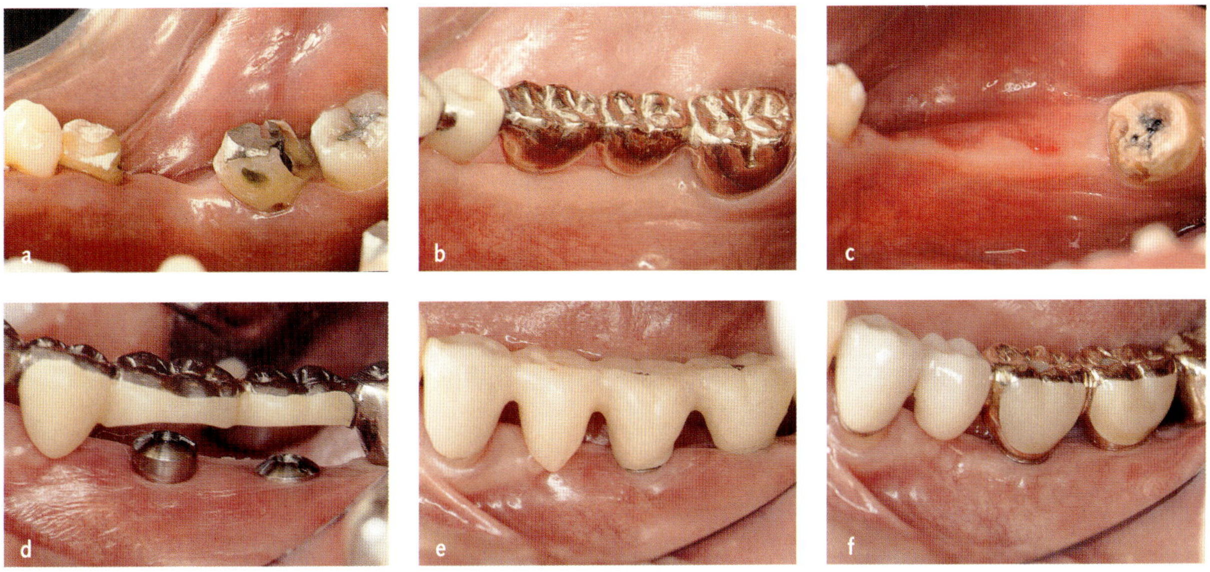

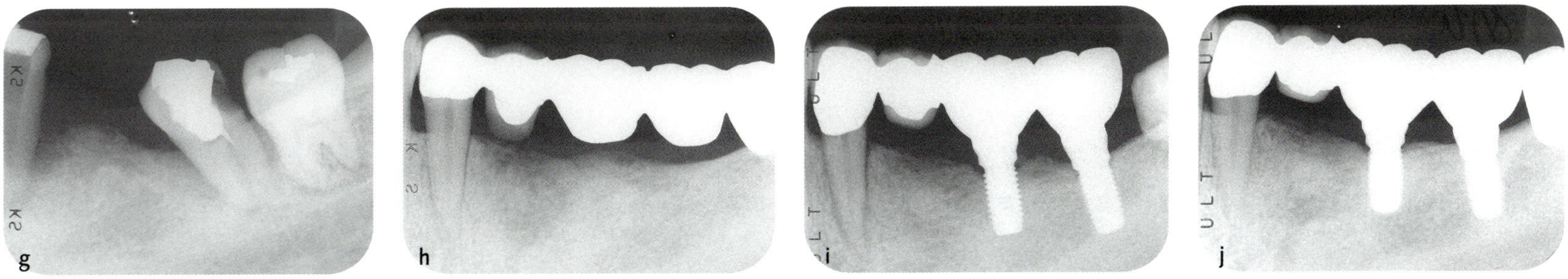

Chapter 5

Prosthetic Treatment and Improvement of the Oral Environment

Prosthetic Treatment as a Replacement Therapy

Assessment of the long-term benefits of therapeutic intervention

Although prosthetic treatments assist in the restoration of the stomatognathic and systemic functions, they also replace missing structures that can have a negative effect on an organism. Restoration of morphology and function often requires some limitation of intervention. Therapeutic interventions are always burdened with such conflicting conditions. Especially with prosthetic intervention, strict judgment is required to determine whether or not the planned treatment is beneficial. When making a decision on therapeutic intervention or selection of treatment methods, the clinician must recognize both the advantages and the disadvantages of treatments and have an appropriate understanding of the most suitable technique for each patient.

What kind of influence can treatment have over the lifetime of a patient whose oral environment continues to change? Possible gains and losses arising from therapeutic intervention have to be considered on a long-term basis.

Indications for tooth reduction

Reduction of tooth structure should be avoided as much as possible. When a disease or a defect that definitely requires tooth reduction and restoration is present, comprehensive assessment is necessary, including a rationale to explain why tooth structure has to be removed (Figs 5-1 to 5-4). Similar examinations and diagnosis are required for all prosthetic treatment, from a single inlay case to a full-mouth restoration case. Comprehensive diagnosis is made from the viewpoint of consolidating four units: tooth, dentition, occlusion, and patient.

Conditions such as patient's age, missing teeth, integrity of the existing dentition, and periodontal support must be evaluated. Focused and balanced intervention is required, in which the intervention is minimized or is actively pursued depending on conditions. If intervention is the chosen course, the clinician must be ready for a long-term relationship with the patient. The clinician must have empathy and compassion for the patient for his or her lifetime as well as the commitment to continue to improve skills and techniques. Prosthetic procedures are based on manual tasks, including gingival displacement, preparation, dowel core buildup, impression, bite registration, and fitting, in which no compromise is allowed. The procedures have to create a periodontal environment with good cleansability and they must satisfy the requirements of morphology, function, and esthetics without disrupting the harmony with the periodontal tissue or biologic width (Case 5-1).

Figs 5-1 to 5-3 Inlay restoration: Harmony of morphology and function.

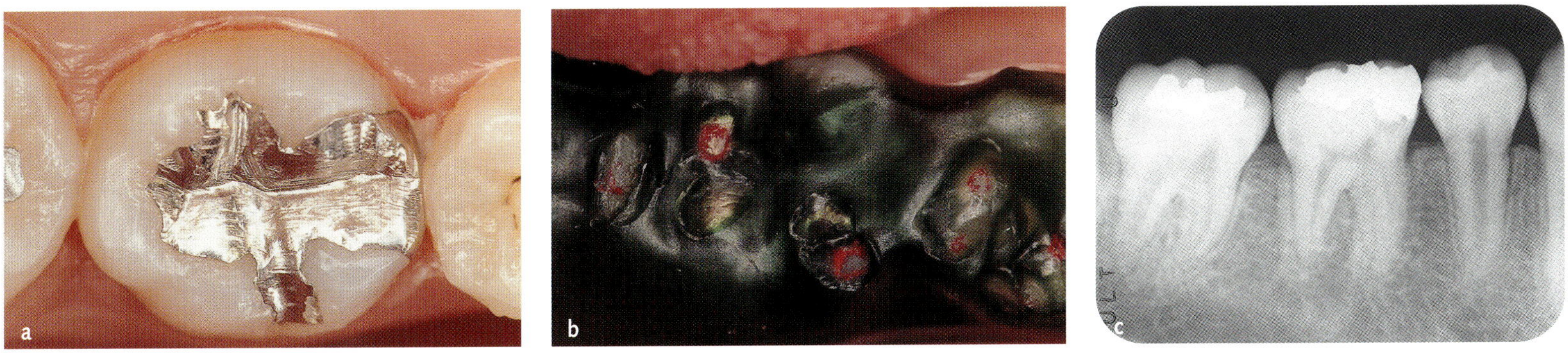

Fig 5-1 Issues with the existing inlay. (a) The fit seems problematic. Lines on the occlusal surface indicate excessive occlusal stress. (b) Ridges are lost. The occlusal morphology of this inlay make it difficult for the patient to chew. (c) The mandibular right second premolar, first molar, and second molar show traumatic findings. Also, the first molar has secondary caries close to the dental pulp.

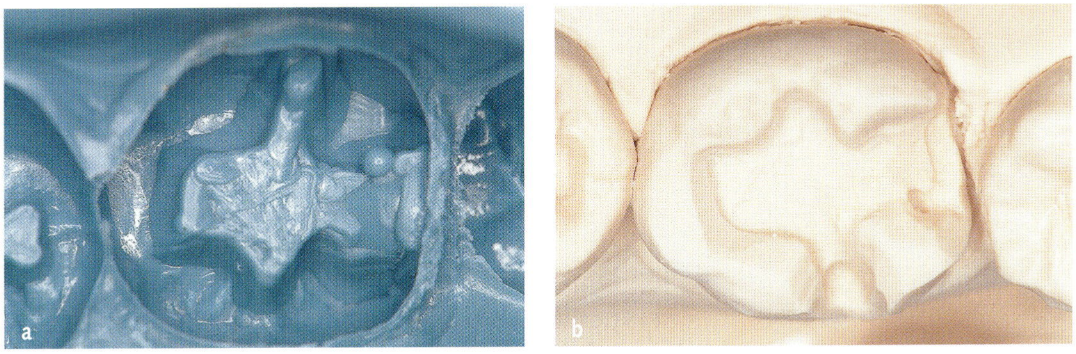

Fig 5-2 New preparation and impression. (a) Ideally, minimal removal of tooth structure is desired. However, adequate preparation should be completed, if it is determined that the restoration must be replaced. The preparation should include a definite box-shaped preparation, flaring of the proximal surface, beveling at the cervical area and occlusal surface, a clear isthmus that will affect durability and retention of the restoration, and grooves, if necessary. (b) Inlay preparation reproduced on the cast.

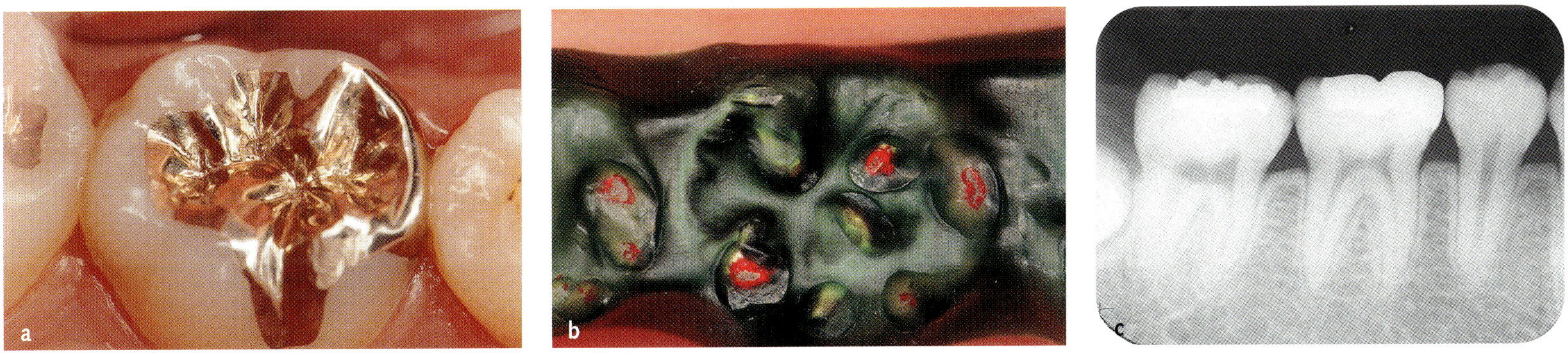

Fig 5-3 Inlay delivery. (a) Protection of the tooth structure and dental pulp should be given the highest priority. The occlusal surface should have correct occlusal anatomy. (b) The occlusal surface is fabricated to facilitate efficient chewing. (c) Radiograph taken 3 years 5 months after delivery of the inlay. Correct periodontal ligament and lamina dura are observed at the mandibular right second premolar, first molar, and second molar. After this physiologic functional morphology was created, the teeth moved spontaneously and were uprighted. The dental pulp of the mandibular right first molar was conserved through antimicrobial therapy.

Inlay, partial veneer, and onlay	
Isthmus, dovetail	301, 201, 301R, 201R (Shofu)
Flare	V16ff (GC), VB16ff (GC)
Occlusal bevel	V16ff
Occlusal preparation	SJCD (Yamasaki) 4, 5, 3
Functional cusp bevel, chamfer of axial surface	SJCD 5 or 3
Buccal and lingual bevels	V16ff
Shoulder	201, 201R
Seating groove	169, 170L
Polishing	White points, chisel
Posterior porcelain full crown	
Occlusal preparation	SJCD 4, 5, 3
Medium chamfer preparation of axial surface	
Full crown	SJCD 5, 3
Porcelain	Buccal: 5, 1, 201R Lingual: 5, 8
Functional cusp bevel	SJCD 5
Polishing	White points, chisel Manual 201R (Shofu), klff (GC)
Anterior porcelain crown	
Chamfer preparation of axial surfaces	SJCD 5, 1, 8
Rounded shoulder preparation	201R, 301R
Heavy shoulder preparation	SJCD 7
Lingual surface preparation	SJCD 4
Polishing	White points, chisel

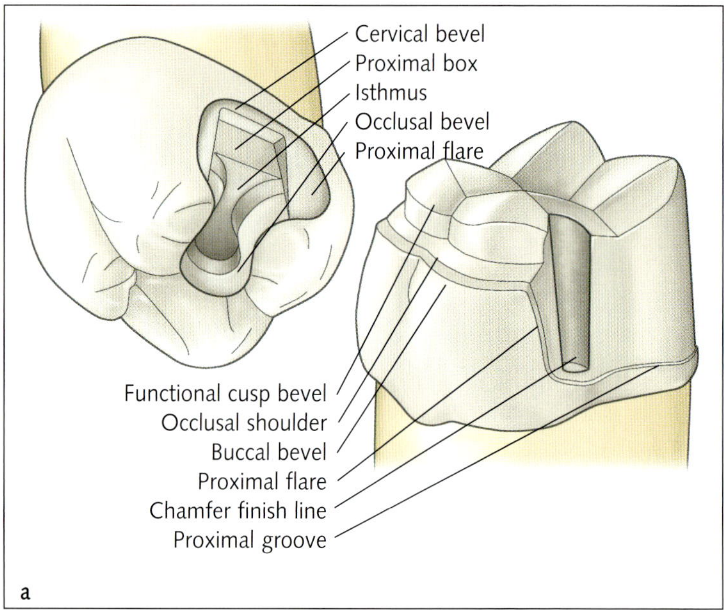

Fig 5-4 Preparation and burs. From Shillingburg et al. *(Opposite page:)* (b) Complicated retention form is no longer needed in current crown restorations, where adhesive cements are used. (c) The basic principles of resistance and retention shown in Fig 5-4a should still be utilized.

Case 5-1 Precise procedures to address esthetic concerns

Patient: *34-year-old man at the time of first visit in 1998*

Chief complaint: *Metal showing on a mandibular premolar restoration (dislodgment of the facing) and discoloration of a right incisor restoration*

The patient's chief complaint concerned the need for minor esthetic improvements, and there were no major problems with inflammation or the mandibular occlusal scheme. However, the right molars showed a reverse curve of Spee. For occlusal reconstruction in a case where the patient desires only a slight improvement, minimal intervention is required, and care must be taken to prevent disruption of the patient's tissue harmony (Figs 5-5 to 5-15).

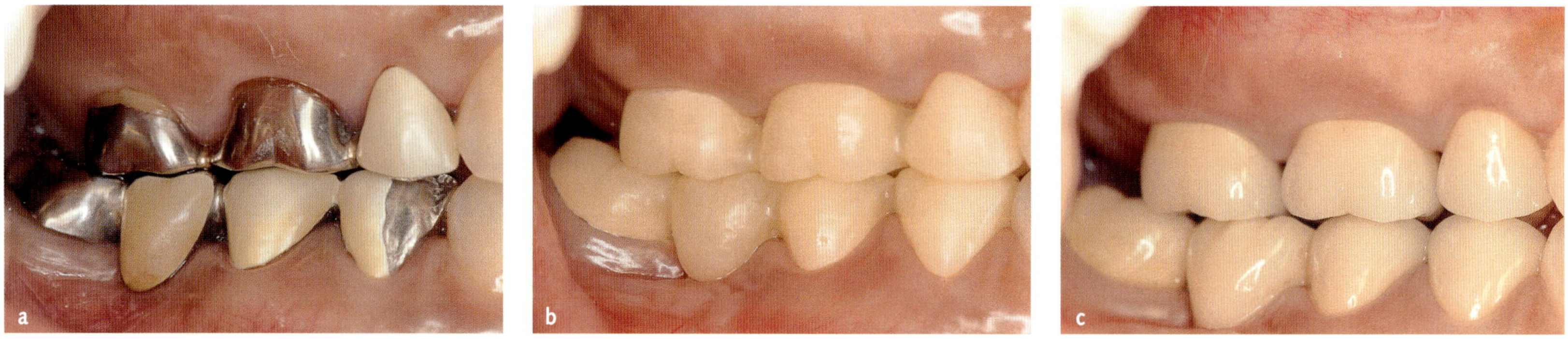

Fig 5-5 (a) The right molars at the first visit, showing the occlusal plane with the reverse curve of Spee. This has caused the dislodgment of the facing of the mandibular right first premolar. (b) To reestablish the occlusal plane, periodontal surgery (crown lengthening) has been conducted. After the occlusal plane and cervical line harmony were improved, a provisional restoration was delivered. (c) Final prosthesis, 1 year 4 months after the first visit. The cusp-to-fossa (tooth-to-tooth) occlusion is improved.

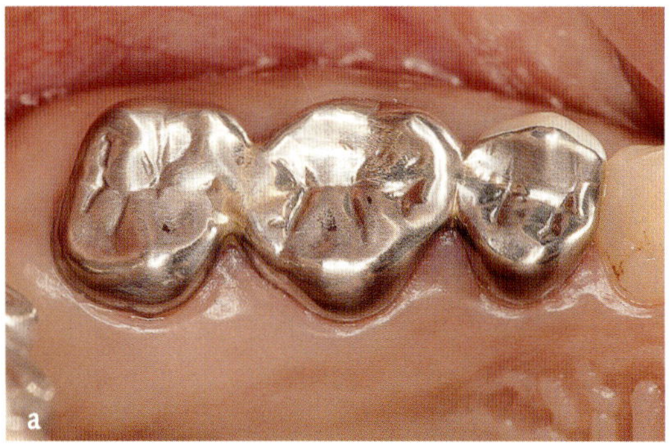

Fig 5-6 Distal wedge and clinical crown lengthening. (a) Maxillary right occlusal surfaces at the first visit, showing nonfunctional interferences of the buccal cusps of the opposing mandibular teeth. *(Opposite page:)* (b) For improvement of the occlusal plane, a distal wedge procedure is conducted for the maxillary right second molar. A scalloped inverse bevel incision is made at the maxillary right second premolar, first molar, and second molar for conservation of the interdental papillae. (c) A raspatory was used to conserve as much of the periosteum as possible. (d to h) Dental papillae and reflected flaps. In this case, full-thickness flaps were raised to the very limit of the mucogingival junction (MGJ). The starting point of suturing is positioned in the area within periosteum, which serves as anchorage to prevent coronal movement of the mucoperiosteal flap. A continuous mattress suture is utilized. (i) The periosteum is engaged at the starting point of the continuous mattress suture. (j) At delivery of the final prostheses, metal-ceramic single crowns, 1 year 4 months after the first visit. Physiologic tooth-periodontal structure has been restored through surgical crown lengthening. The crown morphology (contour of the axial surfaces), occlusal plane, and occlusal surface morphology have been improved.

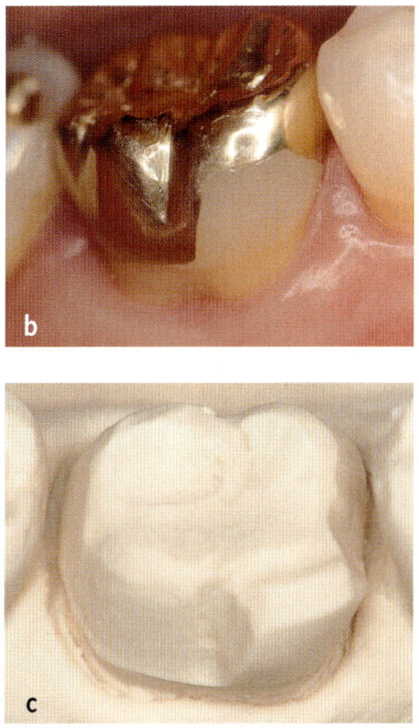

Protection of periodontal tissue

Prostheses have an important role as artificial appliances that are used to recover and maintain the harmony of the tooth, dentition, and occlusion in order to maintain the homeostasis of the masticatory system. Prostheses must answer two demands: (1) to achieve harmony in the morphology and function of the tooth, dentition, and occlusion in the masticatory system; and (2) to protect the healthy periodontal tissue (gingiva, alveolar mucosa, gingival connective tissue, cementum, periodontal ligament, and alveolar bone) that supports the teeth. When these requirements are met, prostheses provide a maintainable periodontal environment, and various problems, such as recurrence of periodontal disease and dental caries as well as worsening of the occlusion, can be decreased. A prosthesis that does not fulfill these requirements could harm the patient's oral health and create new problems.

Preservation of healthy periodontal tissue structure during periodontal surgery

Whether it is resective or regenerative therapy, a flap should be raised, handled, and sutured in such a way that existing periodontal tissue structure (gingiva, gingival connective tissue, cementum, periodontal ligament, and alveolar bone) will be injured as little as possible. Although this fact tends to be forgotten, periodontium is a vital tissue for regeneration of periodontal tissue, especially bone, and it also plays an important role in positioning of a flap. Consequently, in periodontal surgery techniques, it is essential not to resect but rather to conserve the periosteum, depending on whether the objective is to raise and reposition the periosteum or to use the periosteum for tissue regeneration.

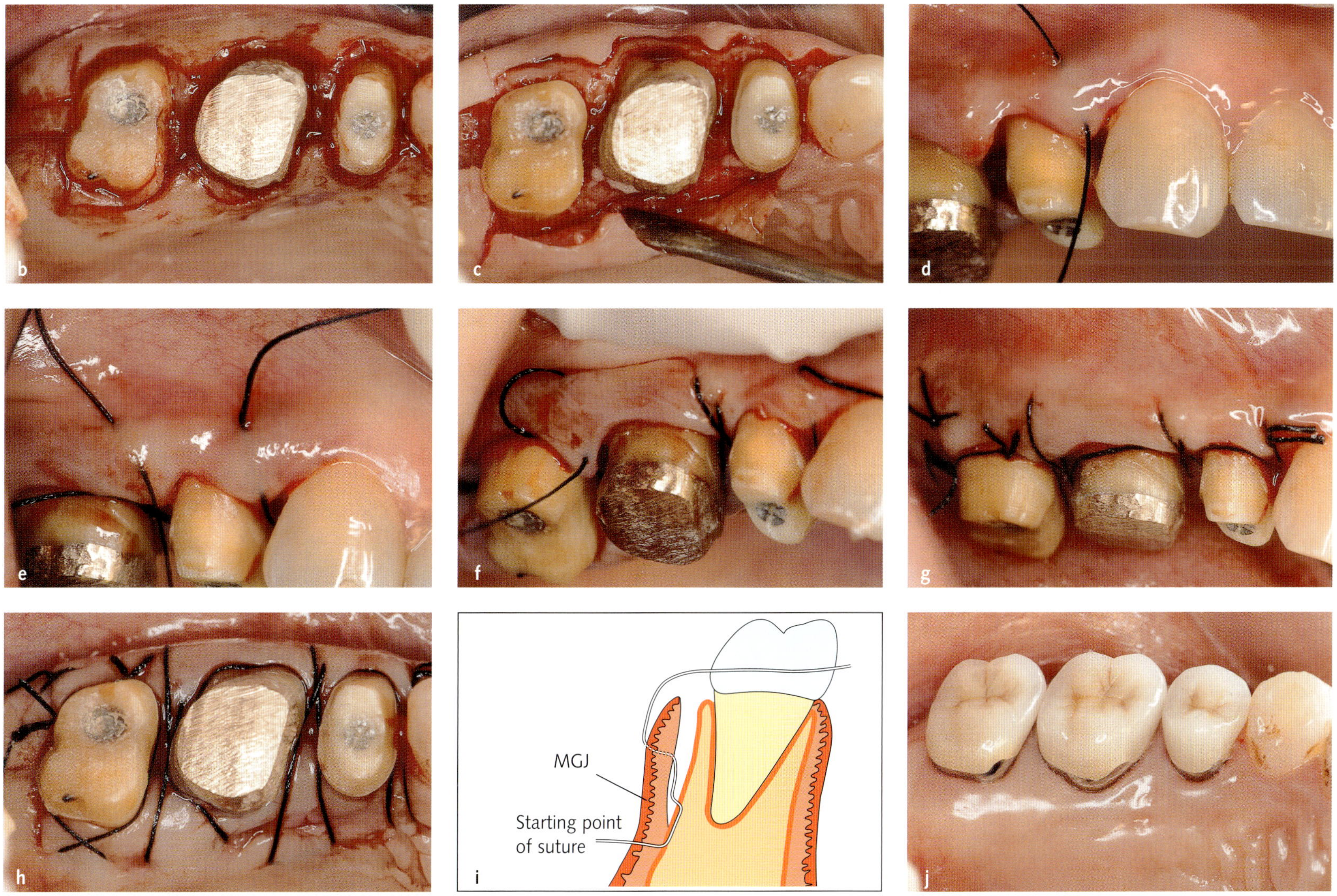

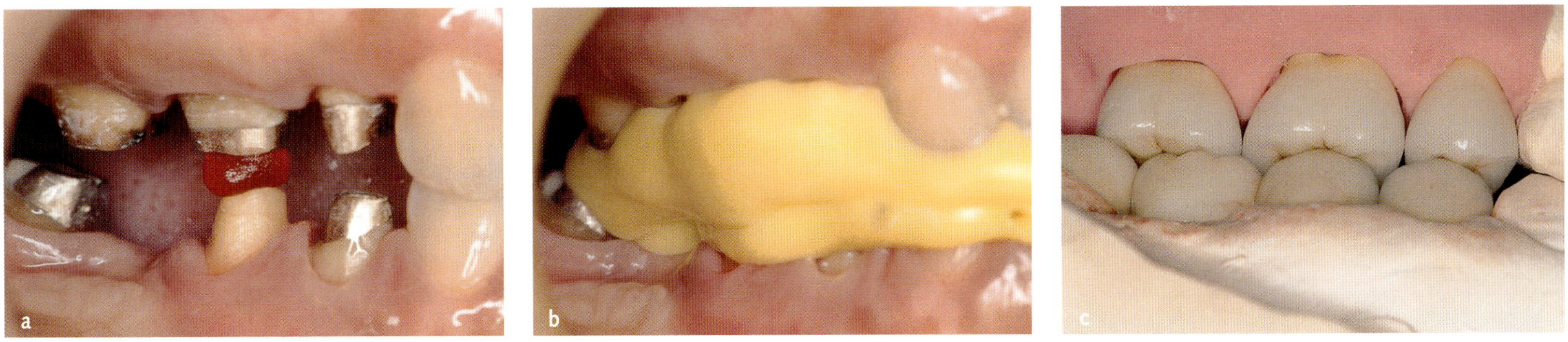

Fig 5-7 Bite registration. (a) The patient is allowed to bite on the anterior teeth, while a vertical stop is fixed securely with pattern resin (somewhat higher in the posterior region). (b) On top of that, silicone material is used for mushbite registration. (c) This occlusion is developed in the restorations fabricated for the patient. Although the occlusion remains tooth-to-tooth, note the relationship between the cusps and fossae and the recovery of horizontal and vertical overlap.

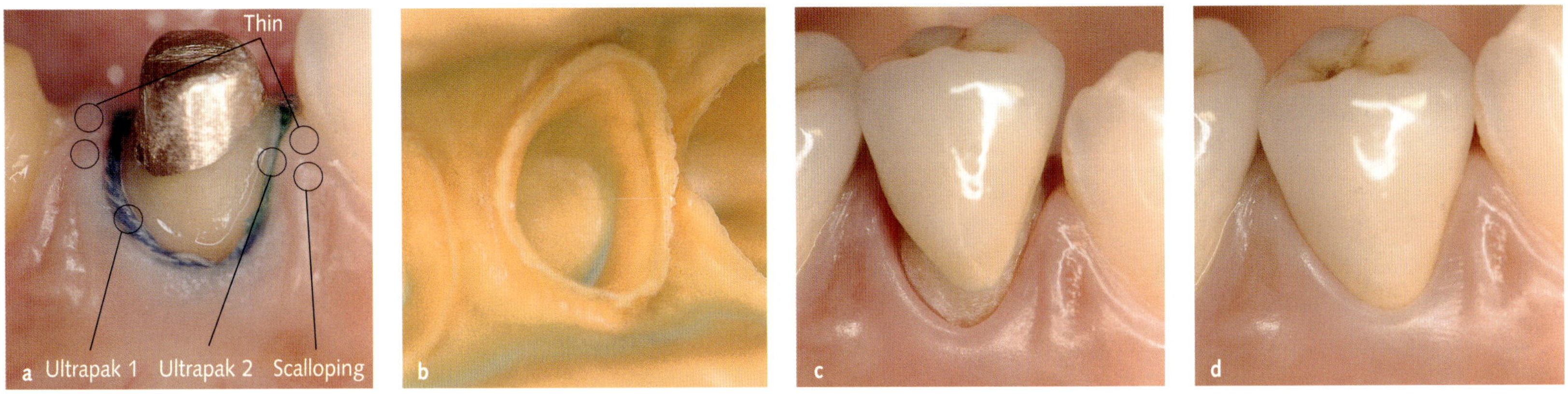

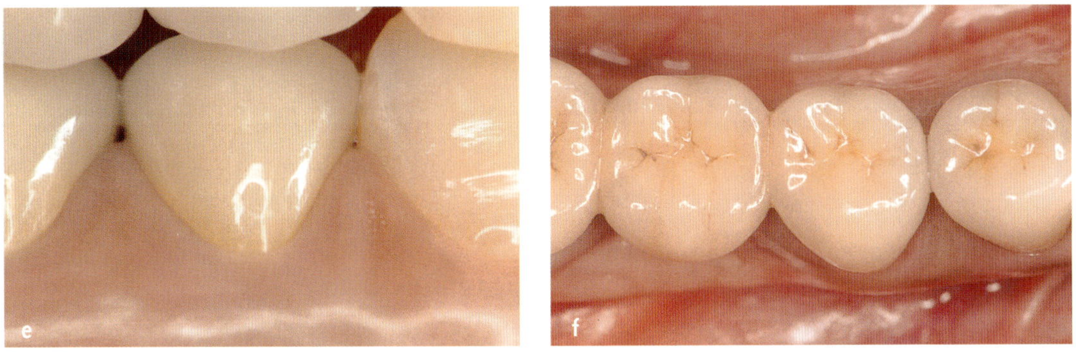

Fig 5-8 Gingival retraction and impression (three-cord technique). (a) Because this patient has thin gingiva and profound scalloping, retraction cords of different sizes (Ultrapak) are used in the same gingival sulcus to minimize damage to thin tissue. (b) The preparation finish line is clearly shown. (c and d) Photographs taken at delivery of the final prosthesis, 1 year 3 months after the first visit. Note the subgingival-supragingival contour and the finish line. The gingiva is without inflammation. No shadow is created around the metal-ceramic restoration. (e) Photograph taken 2 years 3 months after the first visit, 1 year after delivery of the final prosthesis. The gingiva is stabilized, and an increase in the attachment can be confirmed. (f) As the maxillary arch is improved, occlusal morphology in the mandibular arch can naturally be built to an appropriate shape. To correct the mobile mucosa at the mandibular right first molar pontic, a free gingival graft was completed to provide a more maintainable environment with an attached mucosa.

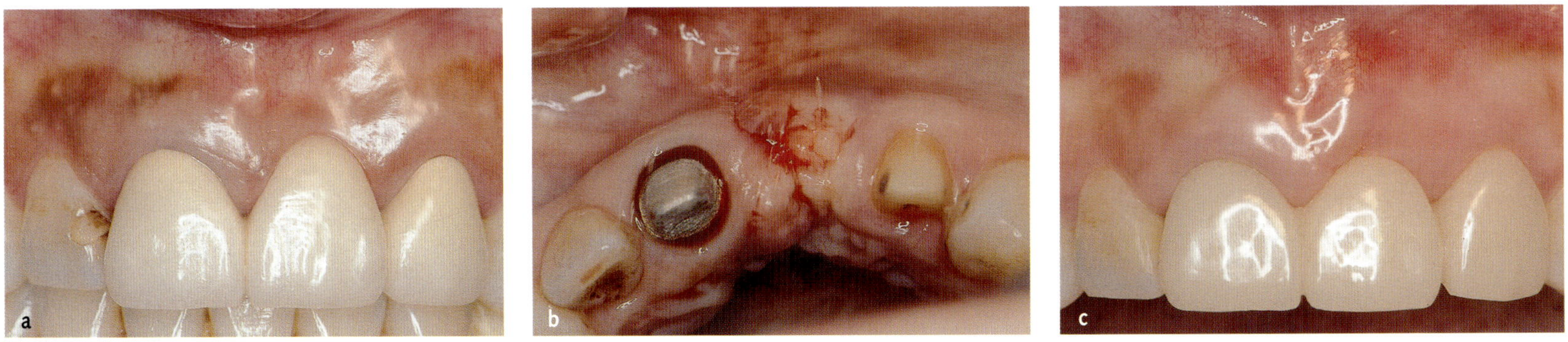

Fig 5-9 Esthetic improvement of the maxillary anterior region. (a) At the first visit, there is a concavity at the maxillary left central incisor pontic space (class I to II according to Seibert's classification of ridge defects), which creates an irregular cervical line. (b) Connective tissue with collar is grafted for ridge augmentation. (c) An ovate pontic is established by adding autopolymerizing resin to the base of the pontic in the provisional restoration for 3 months. Depigmentation of the gingiva is also completed.

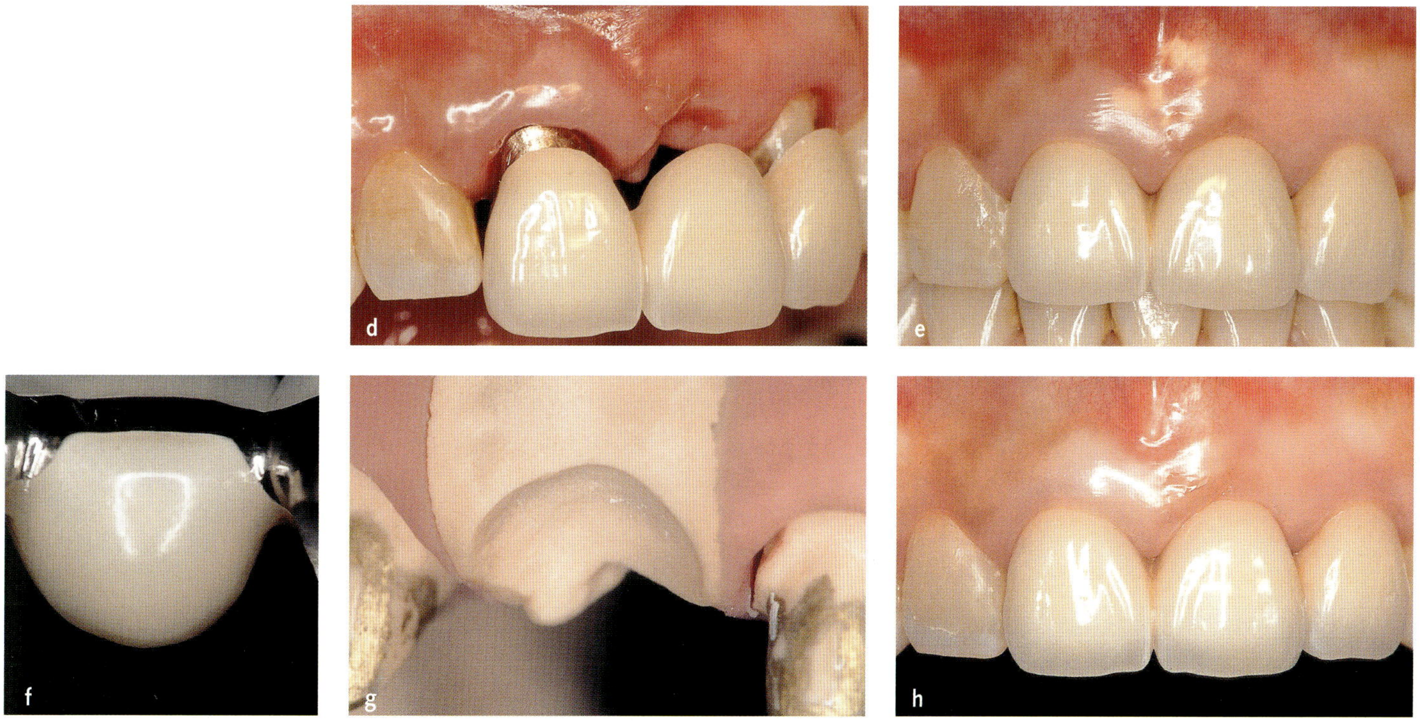

Fig 3-39 (cont) (d) A collarless porcelain restoration is delivered. (e) Photograph taken 4 months after delivery of the prosthesis. Harmony has been restored between the interdental papilla morphology and the cervical margin to allow esthetic soft tissue contour. (f) The base of the pontic is well polished to allow close contact with gingiva. (g) The pontic site of the cast is ground to harmonize with the anatomy of the adjacent teeth. (h) Photograph taken 1 year after delivery of the final prosthesis. The dentition is further stabilized.

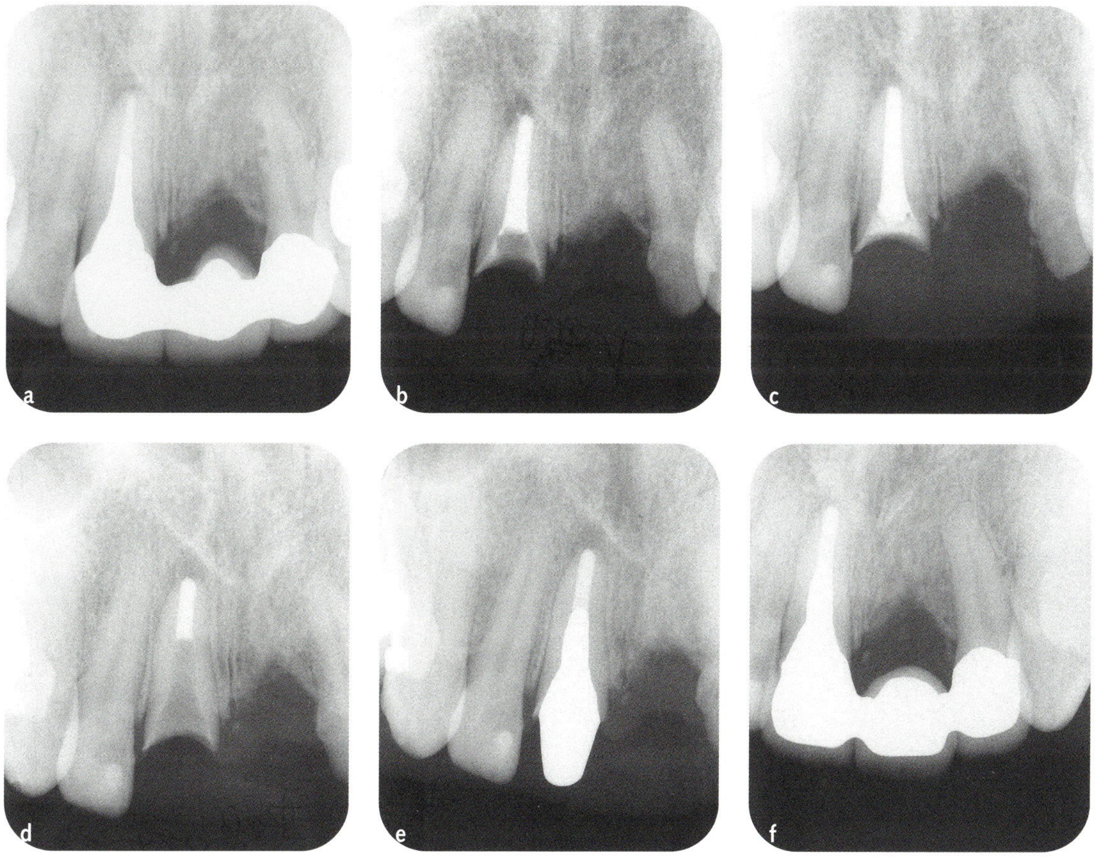

Fig 5-10 Endodontic treatment. (a) Pathology is observed at the apex of the maxillary right central incisor. (b) The root canal is temporarily filled with calcium hydroxide paste. (c) After several months, it is confirmed that the radiolucency has diminished and there are no symptoms such as occlusal pain or discomfort. The root canal is filled with lateral and vertical condensation techniques. (d) Radiograph taken at the time of dowel preparation. (e) Radiographic confirmation is always made at delivery of the dowel post and core. (f) Radiograph taken after 2 years 6 months. A decrease in the periapical radiolucency is apparent.

Box 5-1 Treatment of infected root canals in our practice

Fig 5-11 (a) In treating infected root canals, we endeavor to remove the infected pulpal structure thoroughly. The cleaned root canals are temporarily filled with a calcium hydroxide paste, which produces bactericidal effects as well as pharmacologic effects to enhance the re-formation of the periapical cementum. These principles are identically applied to treatment of noninfected root canals. The difference between the two is that elimination of the contaminant has the highest priority in treatment of infected root canals, while protection of the periapical cementum has the priority in noninfected canals to maintain the capacity for tissue regeneration. (b to d) After several months of observation, the root canal filling is completed, typically with a lateral condensation technique. Cleaning and shaping are performed with Hedstrom files and K files with the focus on the up-and-down movement (with rotation). Canal size preparation is determined by the apical foramen to allow flaring to a smooth shape. Existence of healthy tooth structure (predentin) is confirmed. In this case, the apical seat is prepared with No. 120. (e) Vitapex calcium hydroxide paste with iodine is used for disinfection. (f) A eugenol-based sealer is used in the canals. (g) Standardized master gutta-percha points are sterilized with ethylene oxide gas. (h and i) Accessory points are softened with chloroform, and lateral and vertical condensation is conducted with a spreader or a plugger. This method is a simple, accurate, and quick procedure that seems to have a high healing rate. This procedure has been utilized since we started in private practice.

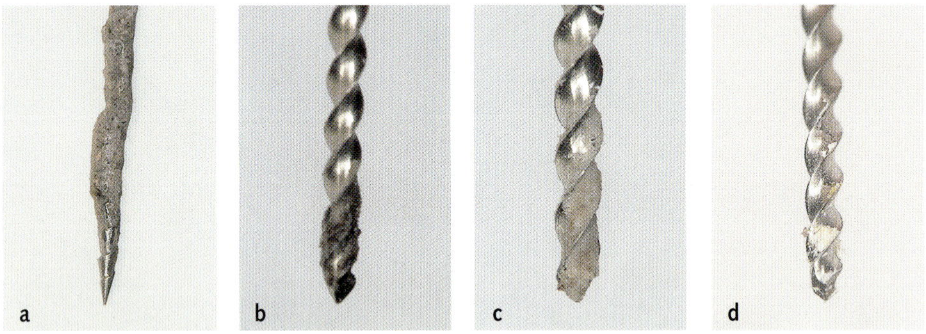

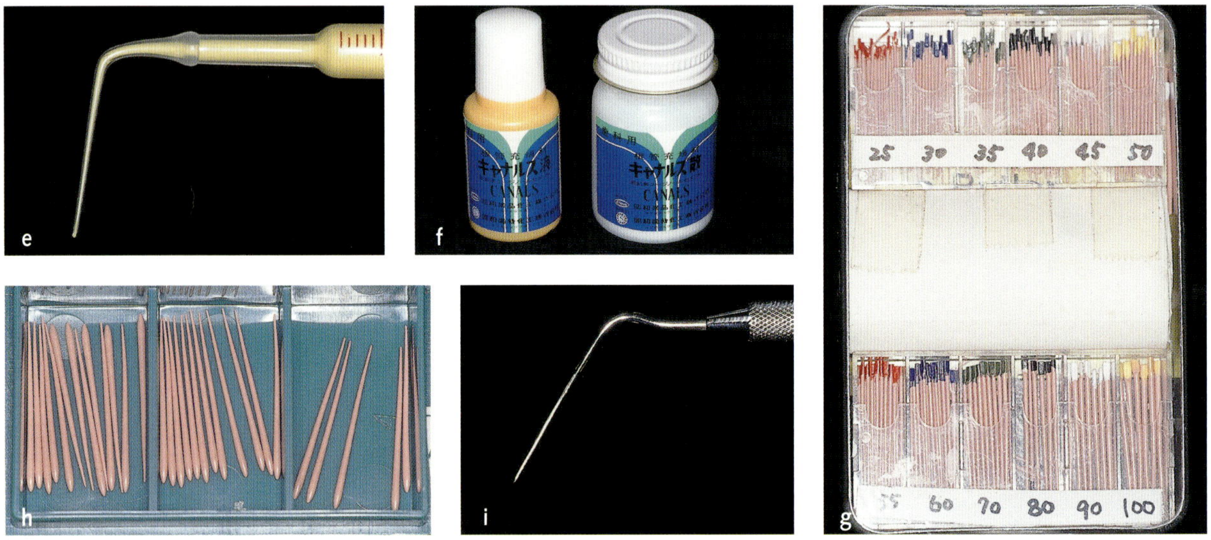

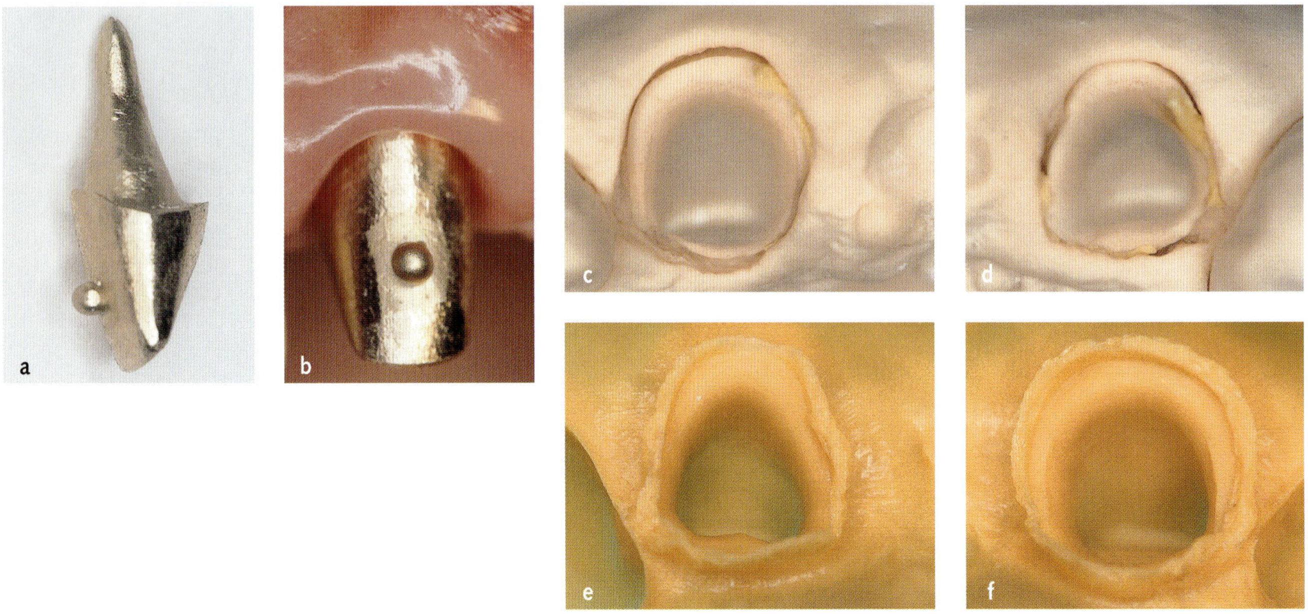

Fig 5-12 (a and b) Fabrication of dowel post and core in JRVT type III gold alloy. (c to f) Impression of a crown preparation.

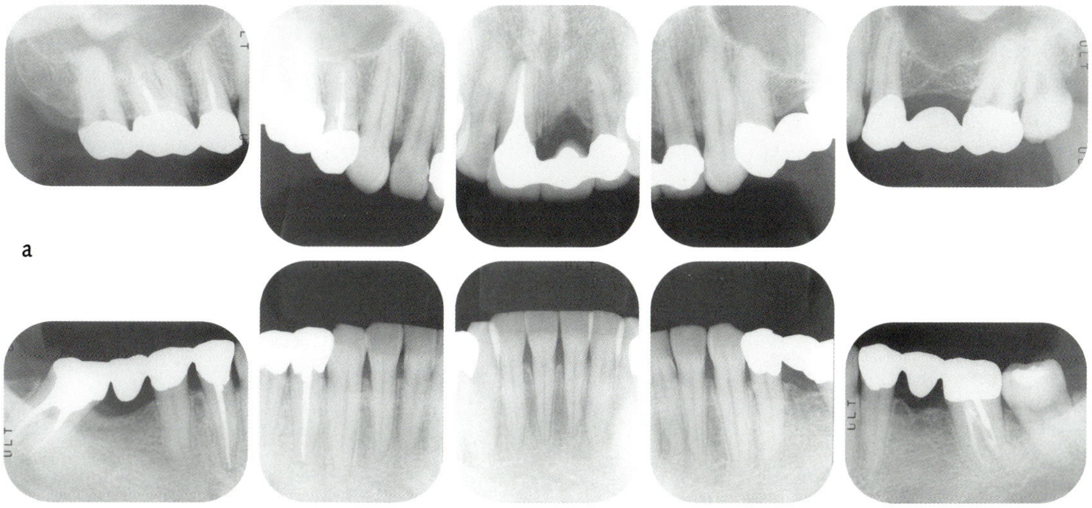

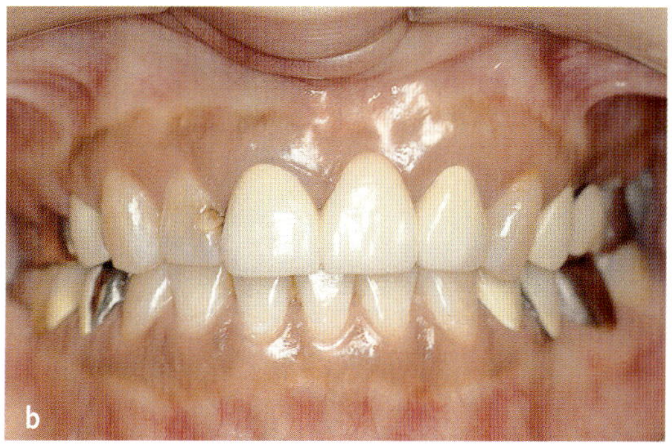

Fig 5-13 (a) Radiographs and (b) clinical appearance at the first visit.

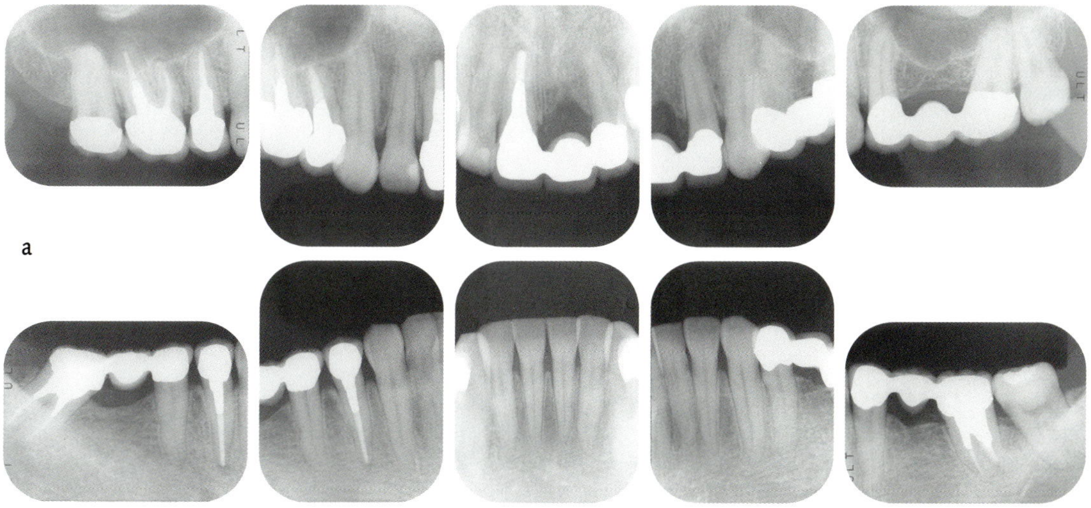

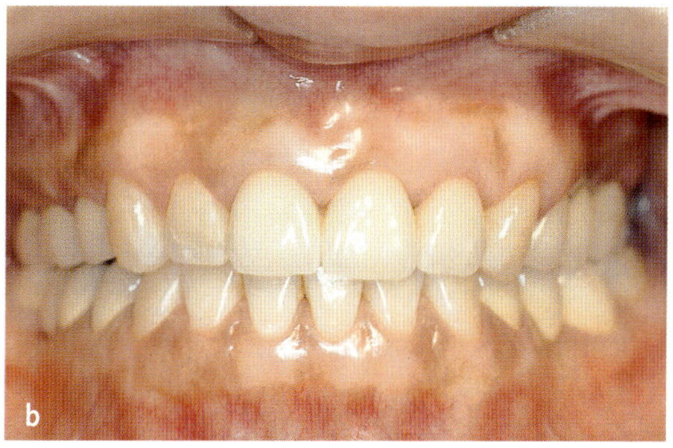

Fig 5-14 (a) Radiographs and (b) clinical appearance at delivery of the prostheses.

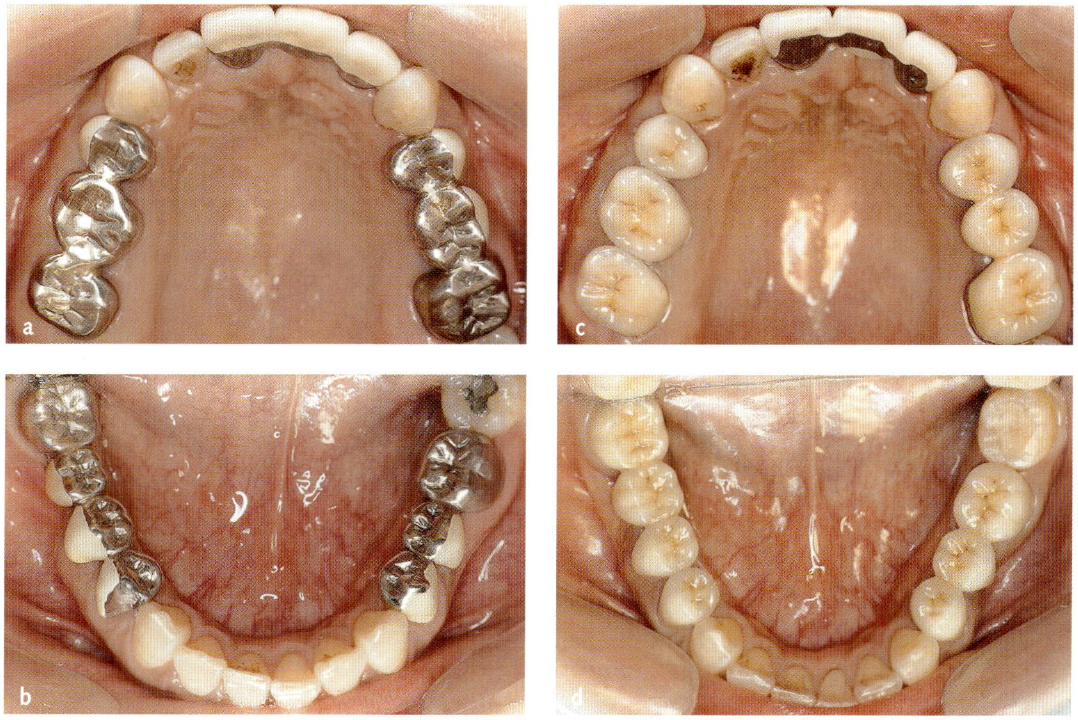

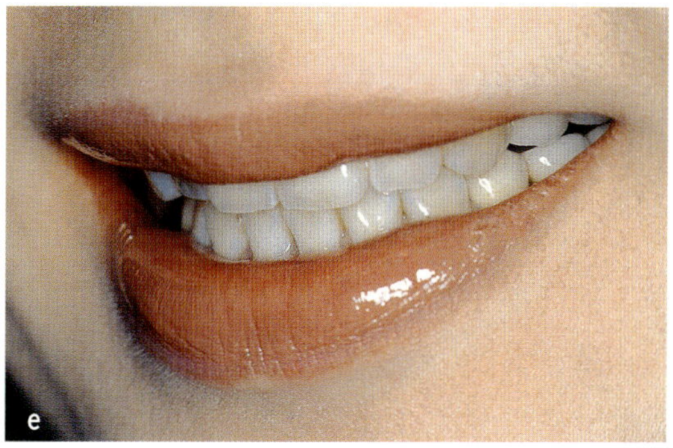

Fig 5-15 (a and b) Photographs taken at the first visit. (c to e) Photographs taken at delivery of the final prostheses (after 1 year 4 months). Depigmentation of the gingiva is also conducted. Old restorations are now replaced by porcelain prostheses. Note the arch form, especially the morphology of the occlusal surfaces. (Prostheses made by Mr Kiyoharu Takada, RDT.)

Recovery of a Physiologic Dentogingival Complex and Esthetics

Crown contour to support the gingiva

Yamazaki proposed that intentionally given subgingival contour be called *tissue-supporting contour*. Whether supragingival or subgingival, overcontouring of the restoration has been considered harmful. Because a reverse contour was advocated for hygienic considerations, and the concept of an emergence profile was associated with a straight emergence, there had been no push to develop correct subgingival contours. In this regard, Kois suggested providing proper contour to the subgingival part of a crown to support the marginal gingiva.

Resolution of a bandlike flare caused by crowding

Since we introduced intrasulcular cleaning in patients' home care programs, we have witnessed many instances of development of increased gingival support as a result of a good gingiva-root relationship as well as dissolution of the black triangles found in regenerated interdental papillae. It has been challenging to recreate the healthy marginal gingiva found around natural teeth for restorations placed after crown-lengthening procedures and for restorations in the maxillary anterior segment, where beautiful gingival morphology is demanded (Figs 5-16 to 5-21). Even when a restoration did not invade the biologic width, a rolled border that was specific to restorations was observed. In these clinical cases, we suspected the possible causes to be poor fit of the restoration, remaining calculus or luting cement, or inadequate plaque control. However, as we repeated subgingival adjustment, we noted that the rolled marginal gingivae could be resolved by proper crown contour (Fig 5-22).

Crown contour in areas with thick gingiva

In patients with apically positioned attachment resulting from advanced periodontal disease or surgery, gingival-alveolar thickness is increased buccolingually and in relation to adjacent teeth. Also, multirooted teeth have extremely concave root surfaces because of exposed furcation areas, resulting in increased gingival-alveolar thickness. Gingival thickness may vary depending on type of tooth, degree of tooth inclination or rotation, and/or buccolingual position of eruption. Simply put, however, the thicker gingiva becomes, the more positive the subgingival contour has to be to allow natural morphology of the marginal gingiva. Although there used to be a concern that gingival recession would result from positive subgingival contour, clinically there has been an increase in the coronal growth of gingiva (creep). Hypothetically, such subgingival contour may not only provide transitional form from crown to marginal gingiva but also maintain turnover of the cell layer of the junctional epithelium by applying pressure to the inner surface of gingiva, contributing to stabilization of the epithelial attachment.

Reverse contour and emergence contour

Cervical contour based on the axial surface of the tooth roots is called emergence contour*, which defines the morphology of the marginal gingiva and interdental papillae and plays an important role in the good health of the gingiva. Appropriate interdental embrasure and emergence profile allow for natural growth of papillae into the embrasure space (Figs 5-16 to 5-31). Even after gingival recession, creeping attachment can be induced by establishing a proper environment and gingival morphology, resulting in high esthetics and maintainability.*

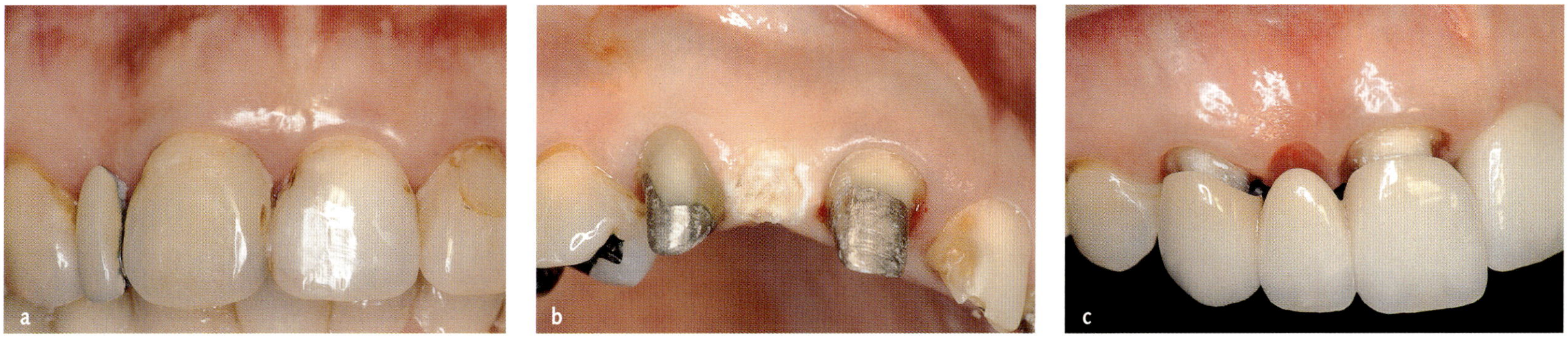

Fig 5-16 Prosthetic improvement of a malpositioned tooth. (a) A crown with a large mesiodistal width has been delivered for the maxillary right central incisor because of the tooth malpositioning, the cause of which was unknown. A small pontic is attached to fill the space of the missing maxillary right lateral incisor. The midline is shifted to the right. Gingivitis is the result of a restoration with a poor fit. (b) After 4 months, dowel posts and cores are delivered after endodontic therapy. It was judged that the tooth malpositioning could be corrected by crown restoration. The emergence contour of the provisional restoration has to be adjusted. Electrosurgery has been completed at the gingiva of maxillary right lateral incisor. (c) An ovate pontic design is adopted for the maxillary right lateral incisor area about 2 months after electrosurgery.

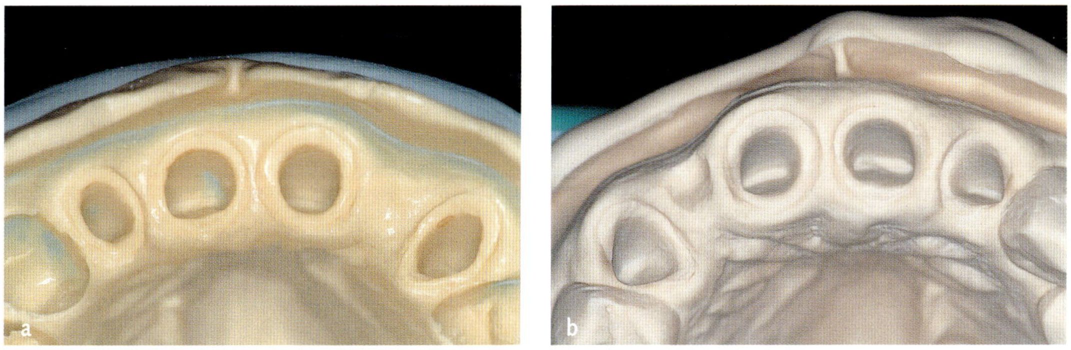

Fig 5-17 Impression for final provisional restoration. (a) Ten months after the first visit, an initial impression is taken for a provisional restoration. Thin retraction cord is used alone. (b) Cast for fabrication of the provisional restoration.

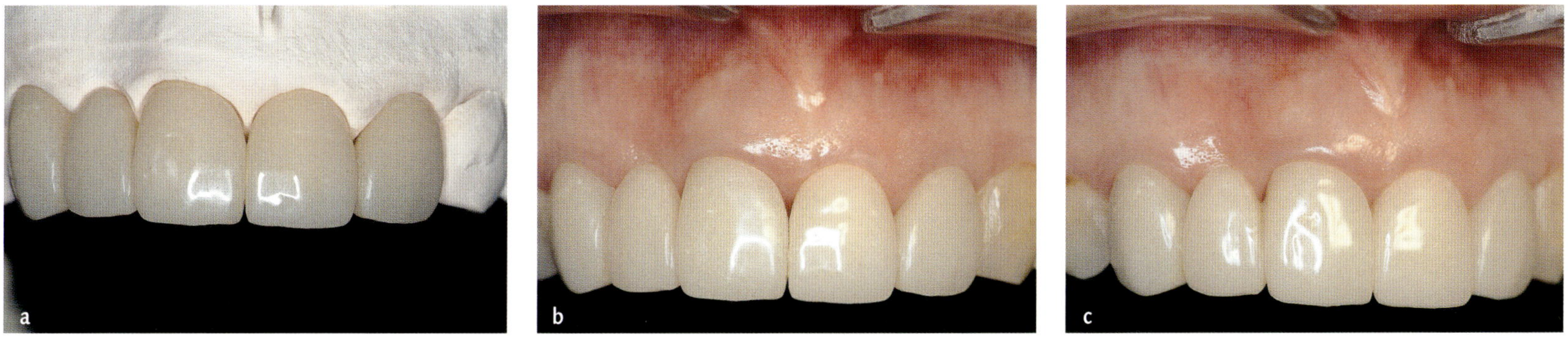

Fig 5-18 Provisional fixed partial denture restoration. (a) Although the crown width of the maxillary right lateral incisor, right central incisor, and left central incisor has improved, ordinary contour would not allow an appropriate embrasure between the right lateral incisor and central incisor because of the limitations imposed by the tooth malpositioning and tooth size. (b) A remargination procedure has been completed, and natural tooth morphology is mostly established. A slightly positive contour has been given to the mesial aspect of the right lateral incisor in the provisional restoration and a slight reverse contour has been established for the distal aspect of the right central incisor.

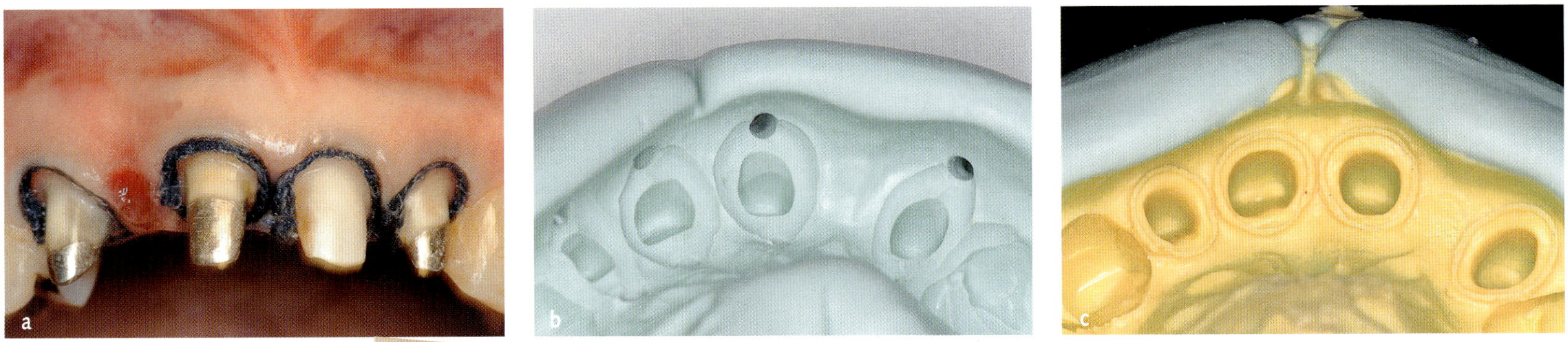

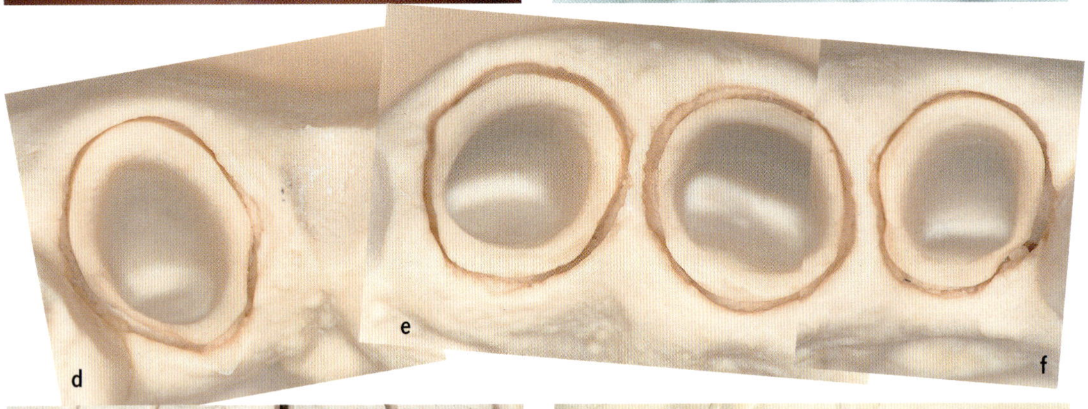

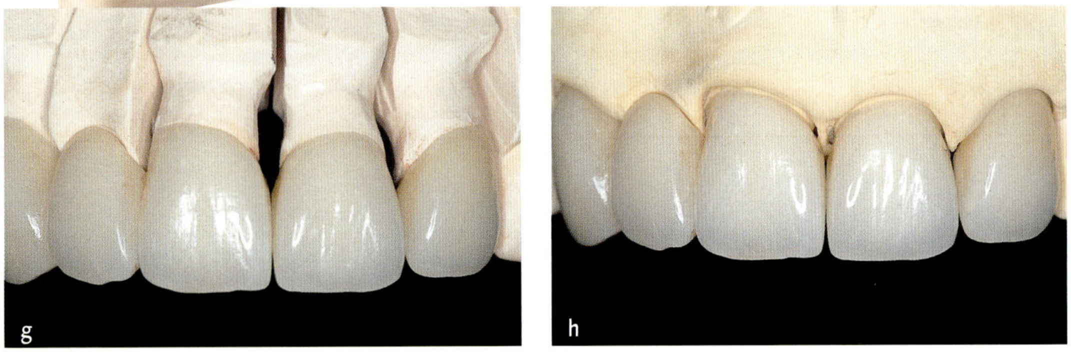

Fig 5-19 Final impression. (a) An impression is made with the hydrodynamic impression technique (HIT) after gingival retraction with a double-cord technique. (b) Injection holes are drilled in the Provil Regular body (Heraeus), and the cervical area is trimmed. (c to f) Imprint II (3M) is injected from the holes. Concentric preparation finish lines are clearly visible in the impression. (g) Final prostheses on dies. After try-in, they will be picked up in the impression. (h) On the casts, with the gingiva retracted and no root morphology to follow, dental technicians would have to build emergence contour based on their imagination. (Prostheses made by Mr Kazunari Ohata, RDT.)

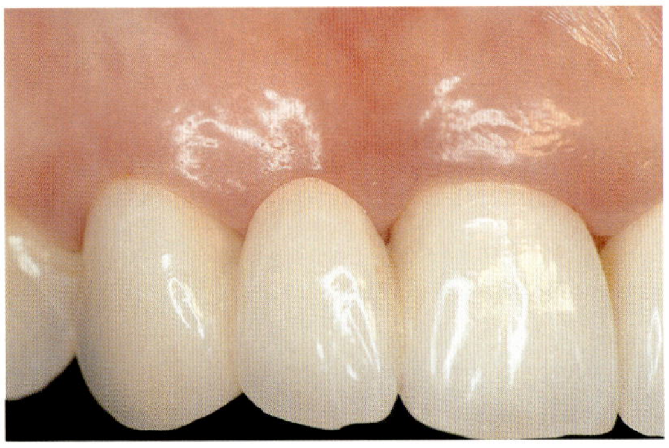

Fig 5-20 Final try-in of the collarless porcelain prostheses. A slight overcontour for the mesial surface of the right lateral incisor and a slightly reverse contour for the distal aspect of the right central incisor have been produced. The appropriate embrasure form is established. Good esthetics is achieved without a shadow or discoloration of the gingivae.

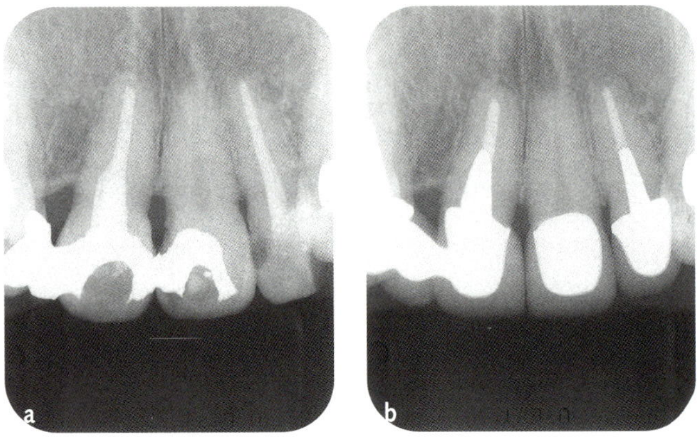

Fig 5-21 Radiographic evaluations (a) at the first visit and (b) at delivery of the final prostheses.

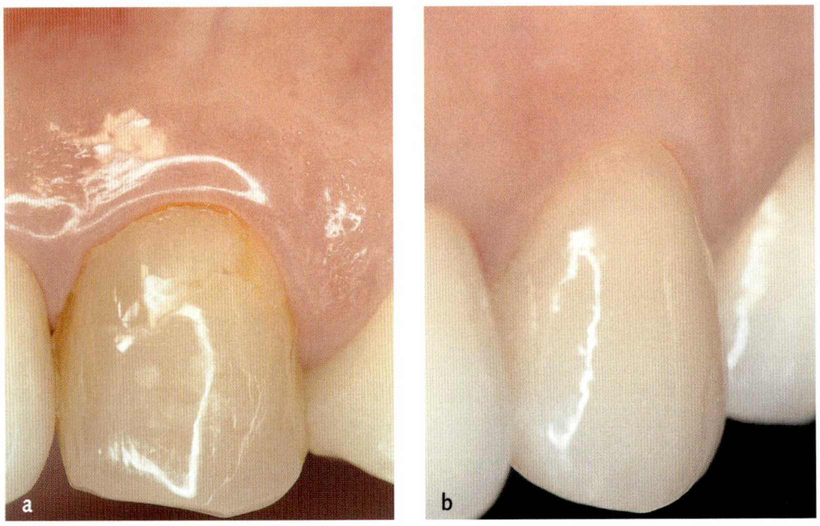

Fig 5-22 (a) After treatment, the patient demanded treatment for the extremely discolored maxillary left canine, which has a worn resin composite restoration, poor subgingival contour, and gingival hyperplasia. (b) Preparation for a porcelain laminate veneer was conducted within the enamel. Esthetic improvement has resulted from a tooth-colored restoration. More importantly, appropriate subgingival contour was established, which led to elimination of the rolled marginal area.

Figs 5-23 to 5-29 Consideration of the thickness of the gingiva.

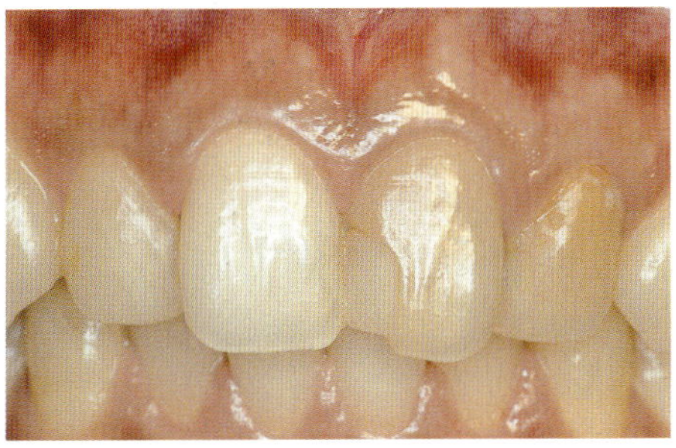

Fig 5-23 The teeth and gingiva show discoloration. The gingiva is thin, and there is a discrepancy in the amount of scalloping between the maxillary right lateral incisor and the maxillary left lateral incisor. The cervical margin is lower on the left because of the rotation of the left central incisor.

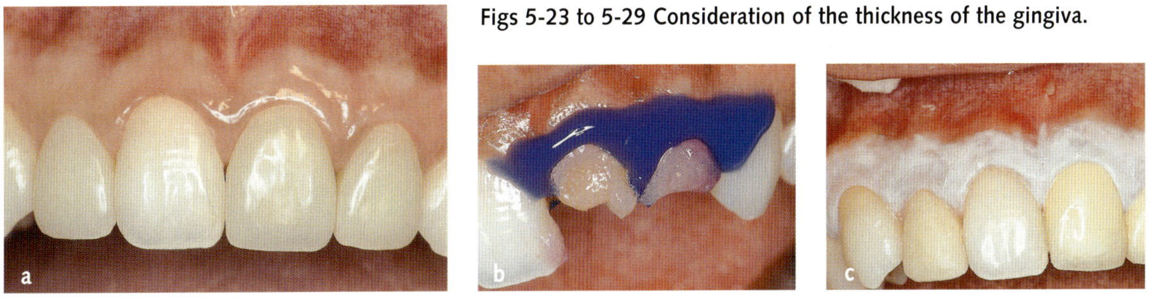

Fig 5-24 Bleaching of the tooth roots and depigmentation of the gingiva. (a) Photograph taken 6 months after the first visit. A final provisional restoration is fabricated after the roots were bleached and the gingiva depigmented. (b) Photograph taken 3 months after the first visit. Bleaching of discolored maxillary right central and lateral incisors is completed. (c) Photograph taken 4 months after the first visit. Depigmentation of the gingiva is completed.

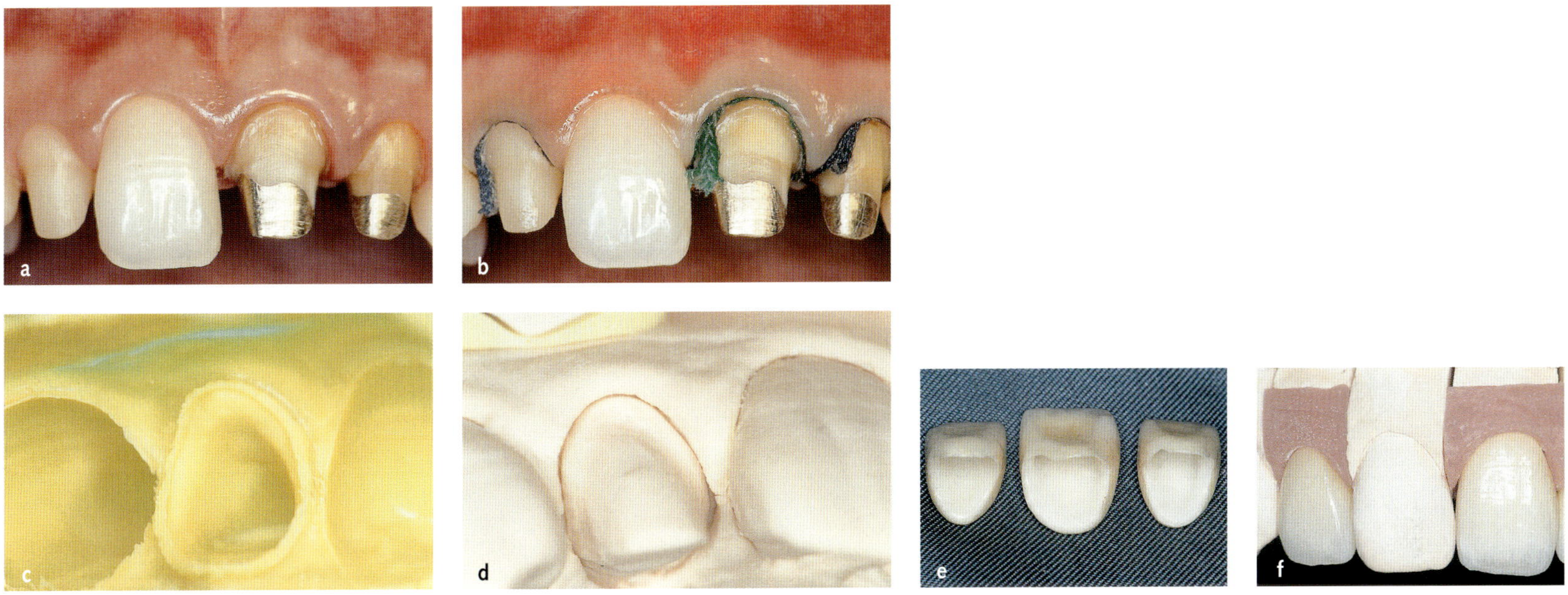

Fig 5-25 Impression for final prostheses. (a) Photograph taken at final preparation. (b) The double-cord technique is used for gingival retraction. Retraction cord is selected according to the thickness of the gingiva. Because maxillary lateral incisors usually have thin gingiva and narrow interdental papilla, a thin cord is selected for gingival retraction. In this case, thin retraction cords (Ultrapak 1 and 2) are used. (c and d) A nonpressure impression is taken with the HIT method (with Imprint II). The impression of the narrow interdental papilla area is taken without damaging the gingiva. (e and f) Procera all-ceramic crowns (Nobel Biocare). (Prostheses made by Mr Chojiro Masuda, RDT.)

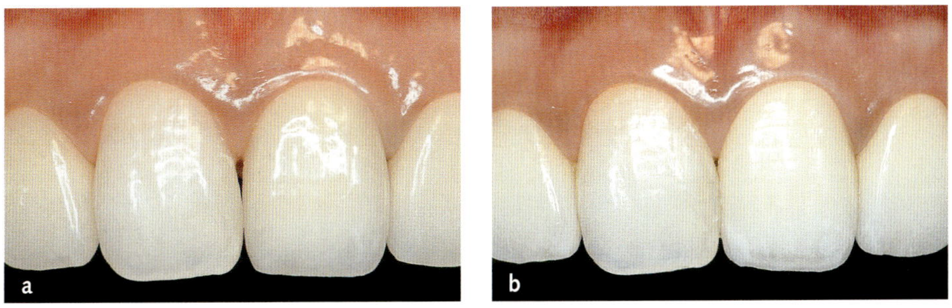

Fig 5-26 Final prostheses. (a) Six months after the first visit, the black triangle is noted at the try-in of the final prostheses. (b) Photograph taken 1 month after placement of the final prostheses. Because appropriate contours and correction of the occlusal surfaces have been provided, the position of the mandible has changed and the midline shift was eliminated. The cervical margin, which used to be lower on the left, has been improved. Every time the final prostheses were tried in, they were picked up in an impression for transport between the laboratory and chairside. Procera porcelain can be ground thin and fired again with additional powder without causing deformation. For the mesial transitional angle of the maxillary right central incisor, a resin composite is added to make a morphologic correction.

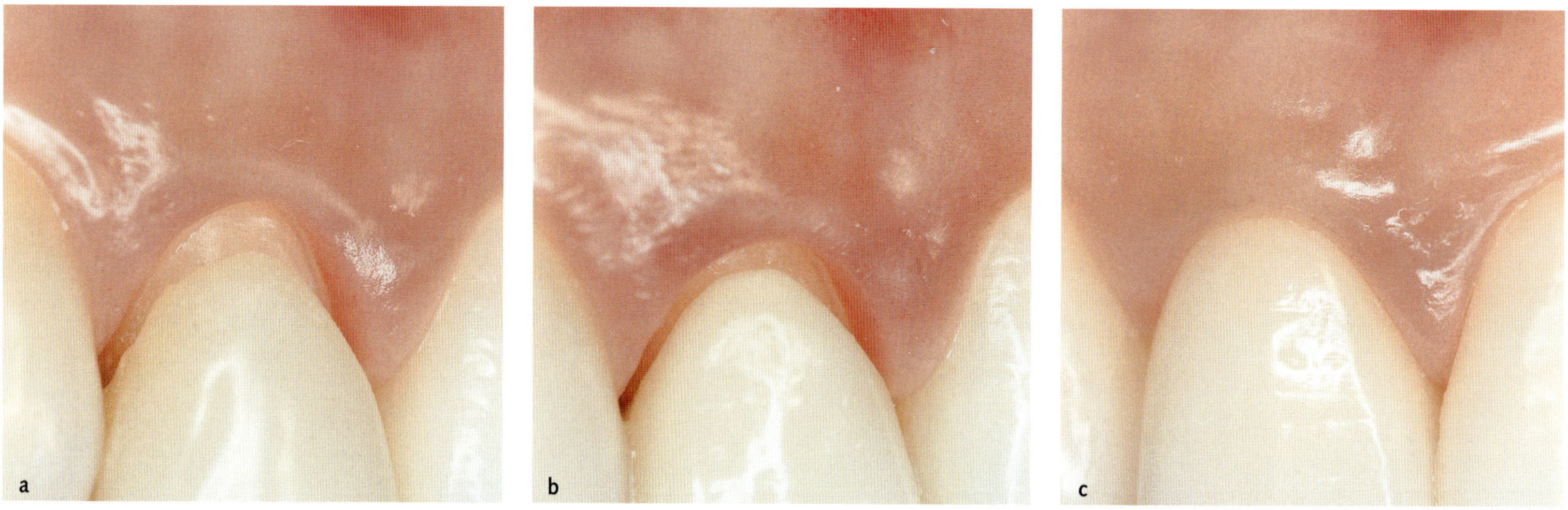

Fig 5-27 Delivery of Procera all-ceramic crown for the maxillary right lateral incisor. (a) The gingival sulcus is physiologically supported by the provisional restoration. (b) A Procera all-ceramic crown is fabricated to match the provisional restoration as closely as possible. (c) After delivery of the final restoration, the gingival margin is healthy with no evidence of discoloration or shadowing.

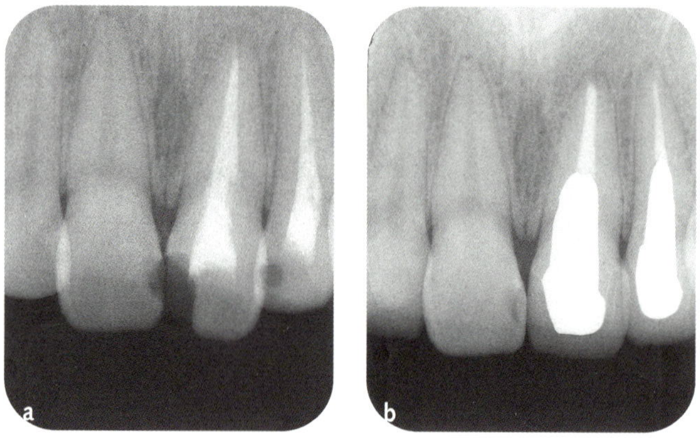

Fig 5-28 (a) At the first visit, the axis of the maxillary left central incisor is inclined. The bony crest between the right and left central incisors is flat. The scalloping at the right and left lateral incisors is relatively strong. (b) Radiograph taken after delivery of the final prostheses.

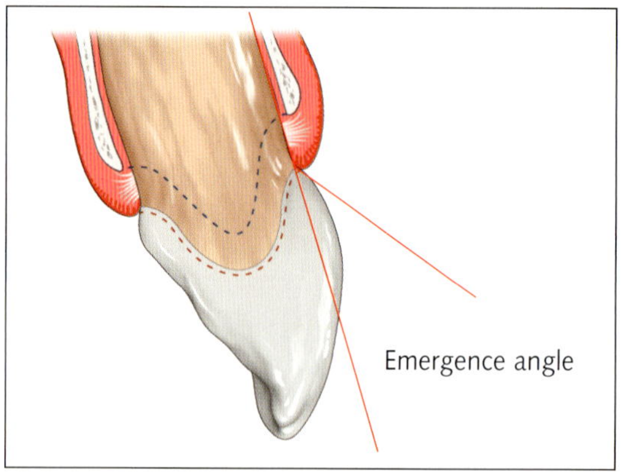

Fig 5-29 The angle formed by the extension line of the root surface and the subgingival contour of crown is called the emergence angle. (From Yamazaki M.)

Figs 5-30 and 5-31 Contour and increases in attachment.

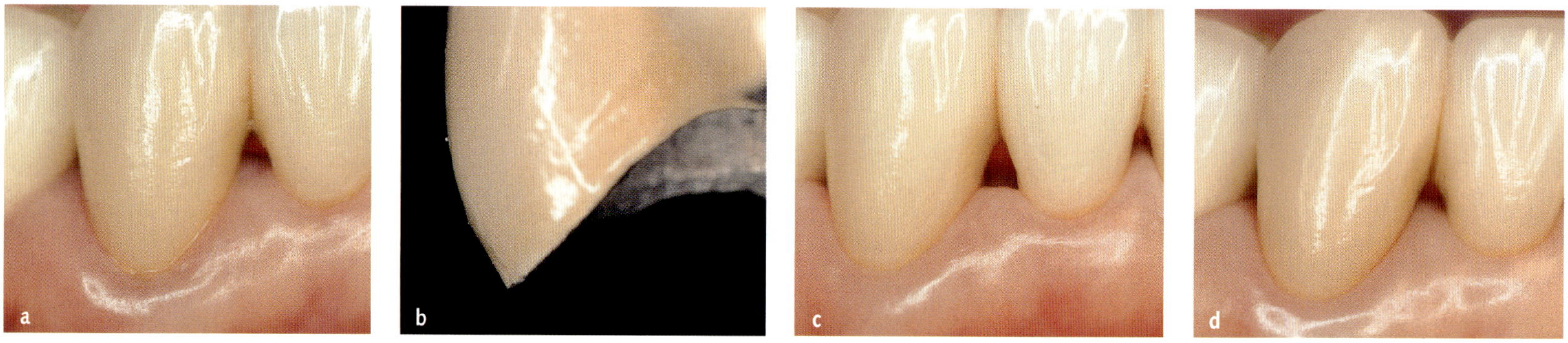

Fig 5-30 Limitation of creeping attachment. (a) Because a crown-lengthening procedure was conducted, the labial gingiva is thick, and the mandibular right canine had a poor contour at the delivery of final prostheses. The interdental space between the right lateral incisor and canine is wide. (b) Originally (August 1995), the restoration was slightly overcontoured supragingivally but had a negative contour subgingivally. (c) Photograph taken 6 months after delivery of the final prostheses. Inflammation has decreased and the gingiva is stable. The interdental gingiva has recessed to fill the space. (d) Photograph taken 3 years after delivery of the final prostheses. Some degree of increase in the attachment is noted.

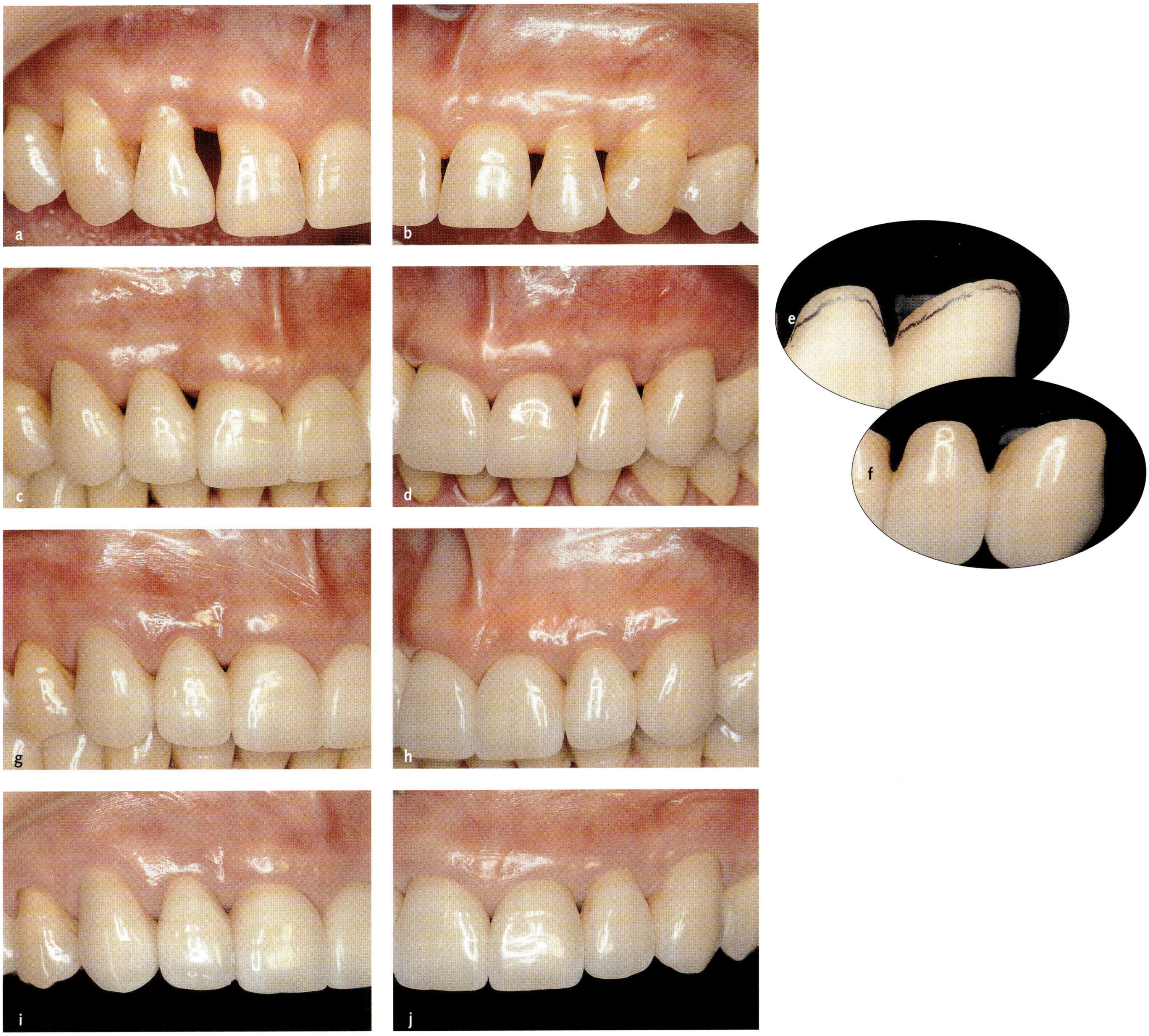

Fig 5-31 Possibility of increase in attachment in a different patient. (a and b) Photographs taken 6 years after the first visit. After completion of periodontal therapy and orthodontic treatment, the patient had been in maintenance for 4 years 8 months. The wear of all six maxillary anterior teeth was advanced, so it was finally decided to complete crown restorations (splinted collarless porcelain crowns) for the maxillary anterior teeth. (c to f) Delivery of splinted crowns for the anterior teeth, from right canine to left canine. Emergence contour is adjusted chairside, not only for the provisional restorations but also for the final prostheses. (g and h) Photographs taken 5 years 2 months after delivery of the final prostheses. Because of the increased attachment, the embrasure spaces are mostly closed. (i and j) Photographs taken 7 years after delivery of the final prostheses, 13 years after the first visit. Improvement of the tooth positions and bone levels as well as thorough management of the occlusion and inflammation has resulted in regeneration of healthy gingiva. (Prostheses made by Mr Hitoshi Aoshima, RDT. See Case 4-5 for radiographs.)

Limitations in closing black triangles

Because the previous restorations were gold shell crowns, the patient shown in Figs 5-32a was greatly satisfied at time of final restoration delivery. The patient was a 51-year-old woman at the first visit, in March 1991. When this patient was treated, the authors' interest was focused on elimination of periodontal pockets and flattening of the bone crest. Little consideration was given to the long crowns incisogingivally or the generation of black triangles in the interdental areas. A full-mouth restoration was completed to improve the esthetics, 8 years 3 months after initial treatment (Fig 5-32b). The procedures used are shown in Figs 5-33 to 5-39. (Case 4-4 shows refabrication of a restoration of a similar case around the same period).

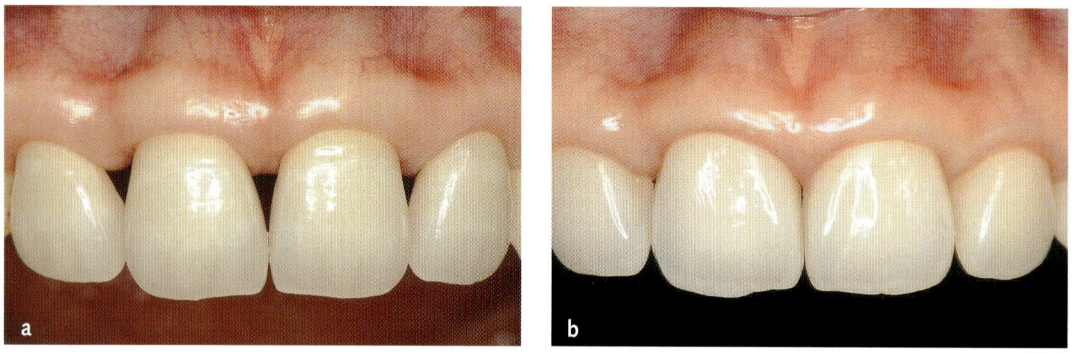

Fig 5-32 Correction of crown morphology for esthetic improvement. (a) At delivery of single-unit collarless porcelain crowns, the interdental embrasure spaces were large, and black triangles were conspicuous. We did not regard this outcome as an issue at that time. Rather, we thought it favorable because an interdental brush could be used. We had no idea that the attachment of the gingiva could migrate. (b) The prostheses were refabricated to improve esthetics 8 years 3 months after delivery of the original restorations. Photograph taken 1 year 6 months after delivery of the new prosthesis (August 2001).

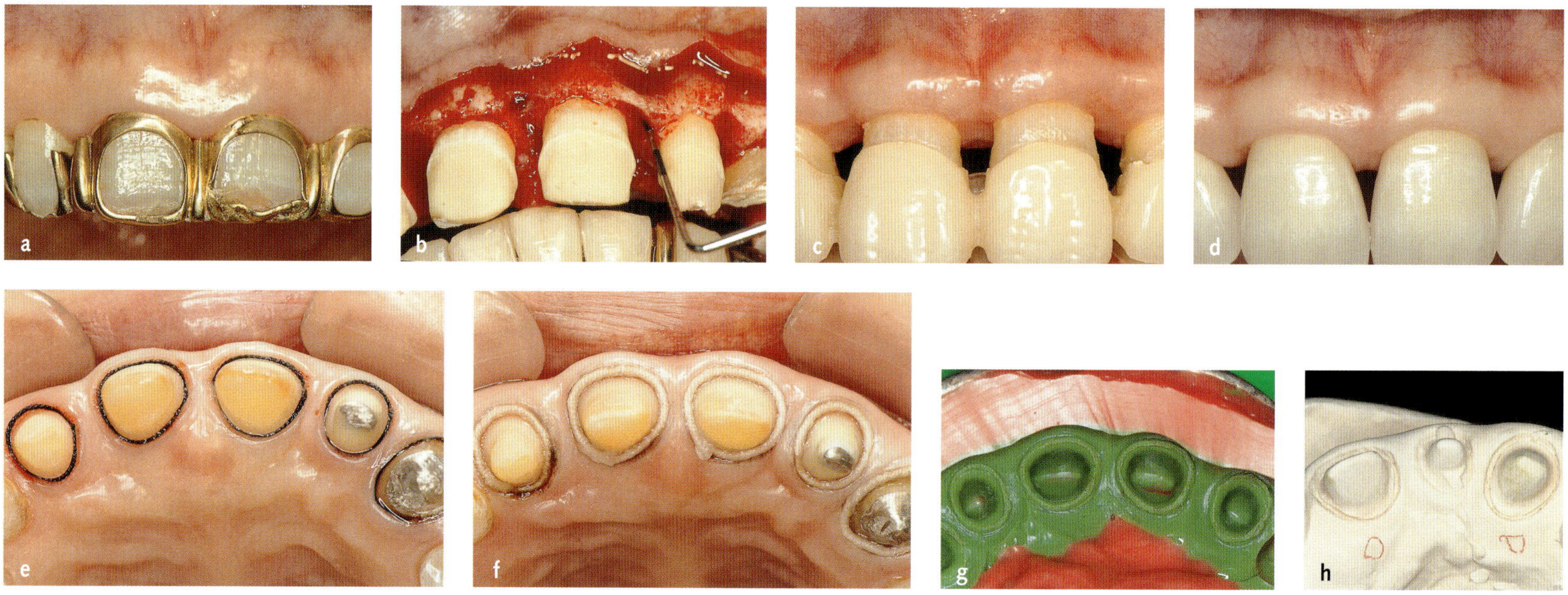

Fig 5-33 Elimination of periodontal pocket and fabrication of crown restorations for anterior teeth. (a) Photograph taken at the first visit (February 1990). (b) To reduce vertical bone defects (7 mm at deepest), a full-thickness flap was raised for periodontal surgery with osseous modification. Basically, surgical therapy was employed, leaving some shallow defects reserved. (c) Three months after periodontal surgery, the gingiva is significantly recessed. (d) Photograph taken at delivery of collarless porcelain crowns (December 1991). (e) Impression technique used previously. Thin retraction cord is inserted. (f) Gingival retraction is conducted with the double-cord technique. (g) Hydrocolloid impression. (h) In a case with subgingival preparations, hydrocolloid material would wear. It was time consuming to take a precise impression.

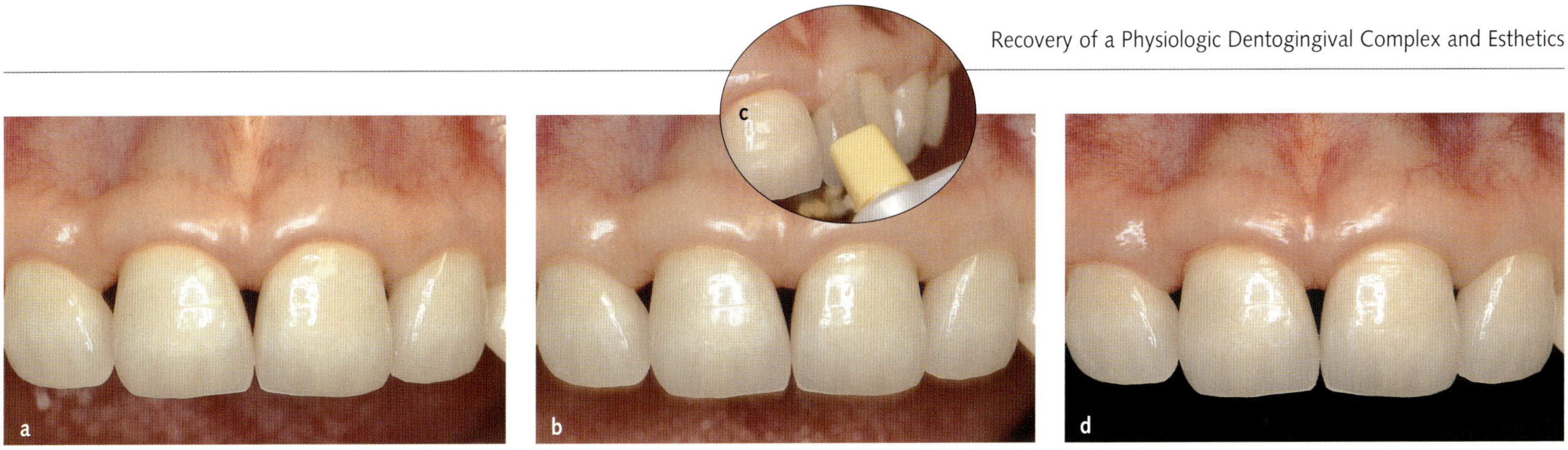

Fig 5-34 Change in gingival morphology with periodontal maintenance. (a) Photograph taken 4 years 8 months after delivery of the prostheses. Incisal edges have been ground and shortened for occlusal equilibration (August 1996). (b) As the patient increased her periodontal maintenance, more problems caused by excessive brushing were observed. Thus, we developed the Pocket Cleaner for intrasulcular cleaning (c) (October 1996). (d) Very little increase in attachment resulted, teaching us that improvement of the prosthetic morphology is necessary (August 1999).

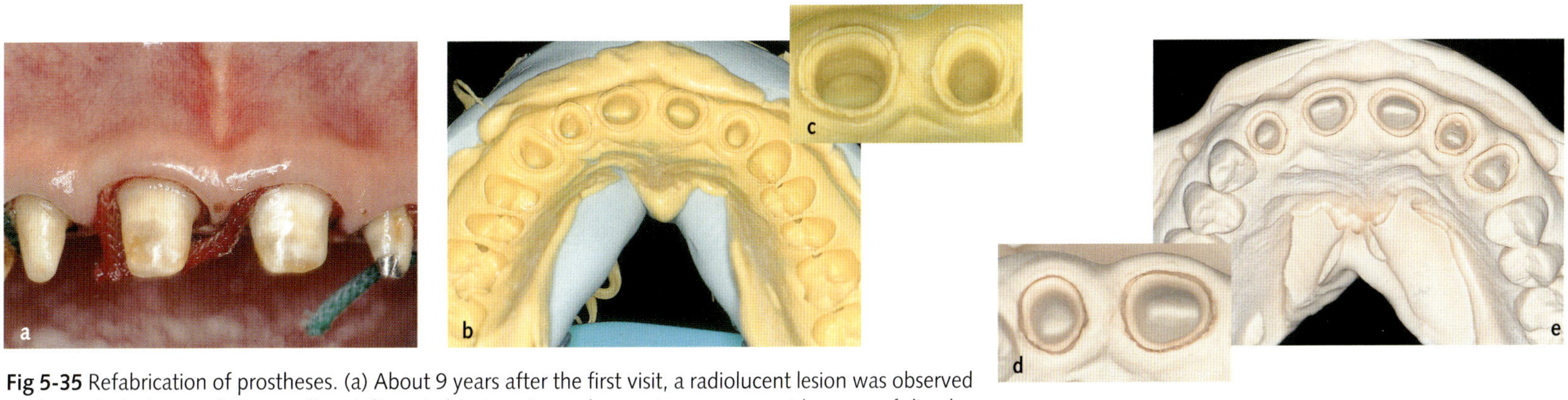

Fig 5-35 Refabrication of prostheses. (a) About 9 years after the first visit, a radiolucent lesion was observed at the periapical area of the maxillary left central incisor. Secondary caries was present because of dissolution of cement. To improve esthetics and maintainability, the prostheses of the five anterior teeth were refabricated. The interdental spaces between the right lateral incisor, right central incisor, and left central incisor are wide, and the marginal finish line is set deep subgingivally. (b and c) Silicone impression was taken. Impressions of the maxillary and mandibular arches give clear reproduction of finish lines. (d and e) A precise impression with high accuracy allows reproduction of the ideal emergence profile.

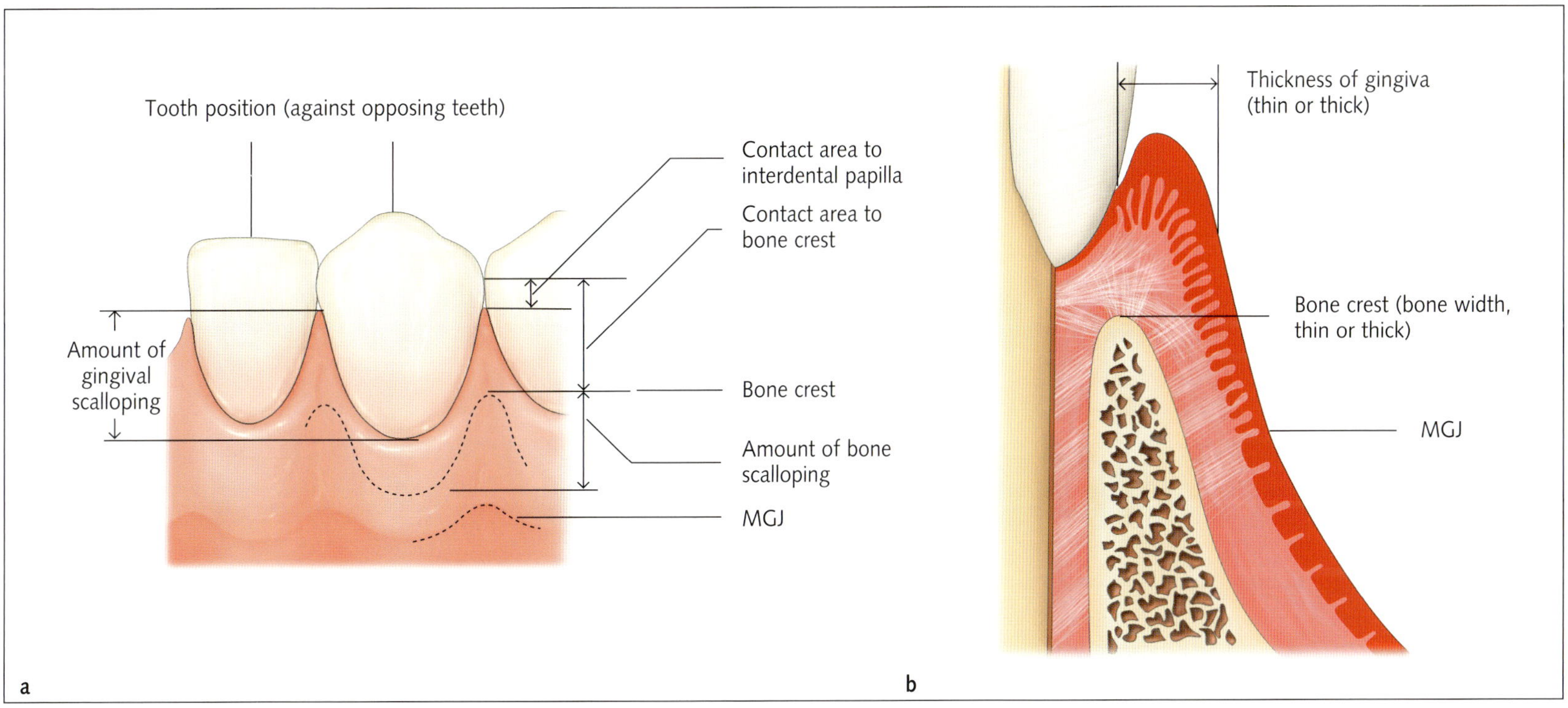

Fig 5-36 (a and b) Characteristics of dentogingival morphology that should be considered in crown restoration.

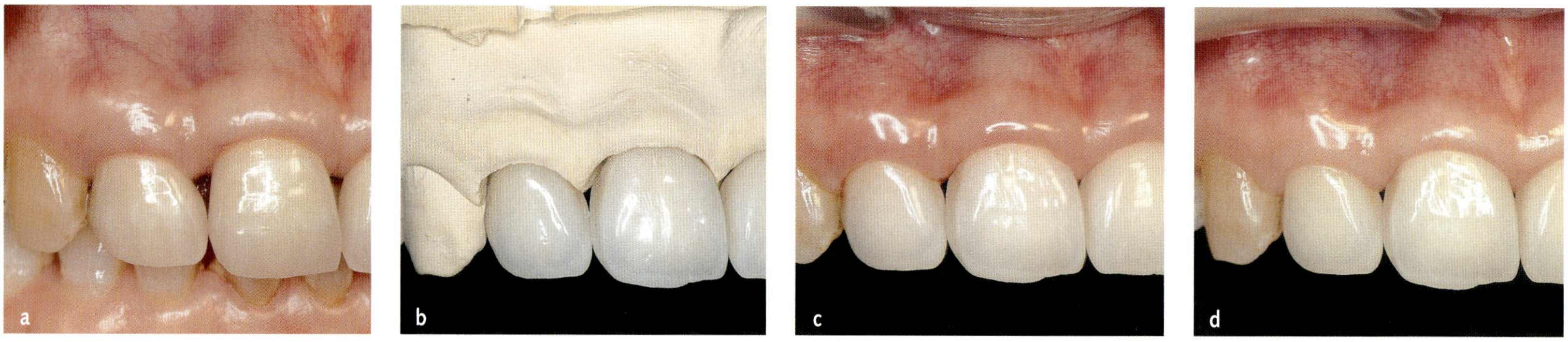

Fig 5-37 Improvement of the interdental space between the maxillary right lateral and central incisors after refabrication of the prostheses. (a) Photograph taken before refabrication of prostheses (August 1999). (b) Single collarless porcelain crowns are delivered, with long proximal contact and slightly overcontoured emergence angles. Black triangles have disappeared. The area between the right canine and lateral incisor has been given a half-pontic design with a small wing and staining. (c) Delivery of the new prostheses (January 2000). (d) Photograph taken 1 year 6 months after delivery.

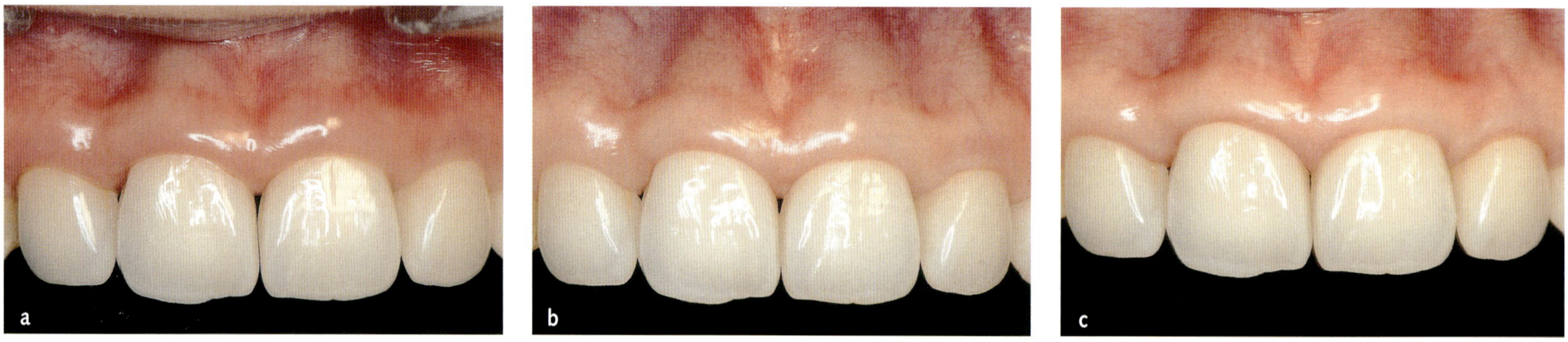

Fig 5-38 Frontal views after delivery of the new prostheses. (a) New single collarless porcelain crowns have been delivered. Slight flaring of the gingiva is noted. There is a slight discrepancy in the cervical margin of the right central incisor and left central incisor; the incisal edge of maxillary right central incisor has been adjusted to create an illusionary effect to change the crown length. (b) Photograph taken 3 months after delivery. (c) Photograph taken about 1 year 6 months after delivery and 10 years after the first visit. An increase in gingival attachment is observed (August 2001). (Prostheses made by Mr Kazunari Ohata, RDT.)

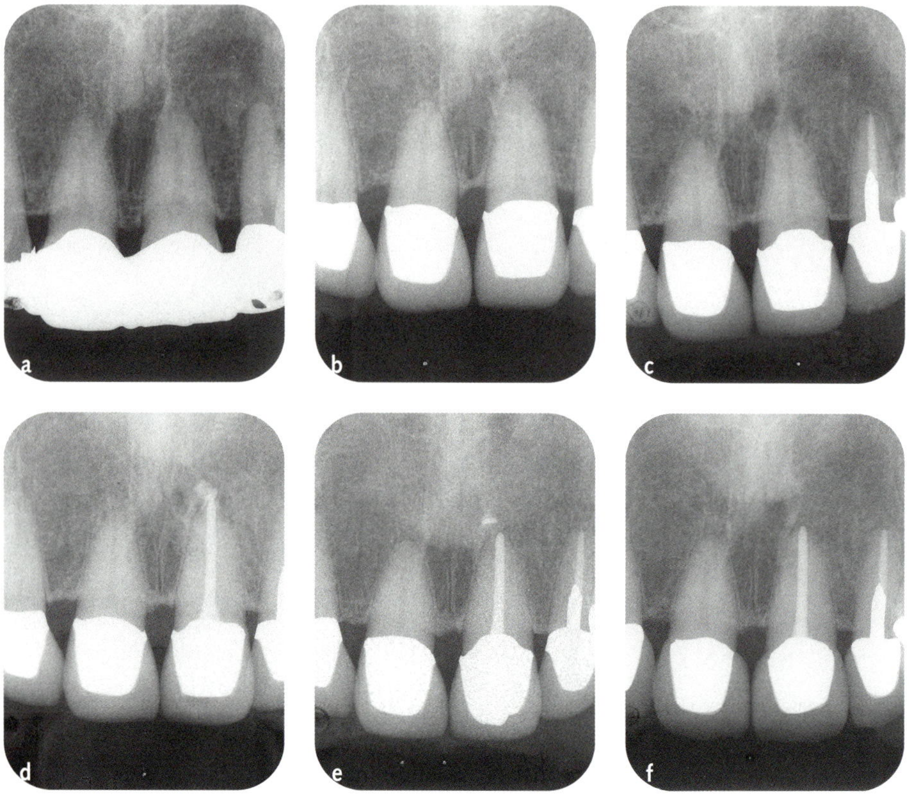

Fig 5-39 Radiographic follow-up. (a) Radiograph taken at the first visit (February 1990). (b) Collarless porcelain crowns have been delivered after osseous surgery (December 1991). (c) A radiolucent periapical lesion is observed at the maxillary left central incisor about 5 years later (November 1996). (d) Temporary root canal filling (Vitapex). (e) Radiograph taken 7 years 6 months after the first visit (August 1997). The periapical lesion is improved. (f) After about 2 years 5 months, prostheses were refabricated (January 2001) with a half-pontic design. Radiograph taken about 1 year 5 months after delivery of the new prostheses (June 2002).

Poor emergence contour

After delivery of crown restorations, in spite of not only sufficient home care but also frequent professional cleanings, the marginal soft tissue had problems with inflammation, which created challenges in maintenance (Fig 5-40). The emergence contour was corrected to obtain a beautiful marginal gingiva eventually (Figs 5-41 to 5-45). When orthodontic torque is applied in a palatal direction to correct tooth axes, as in this clinical case, the amount of gingival scalloping and the thickness of marginal gingiva are enhanced. The amount of bone scalloping is limited and the crest is low. Consequently, a reverse contour in the crown restoration will not result in a transitional morphology at the marginal gingiva and cervical area. The morphology tends to cause plaque accumulation and trauma due to toothbrushing. A similar situation may occur in patients with former advanced periodontitis, horizontal bone loss, and deep epithelial attachment. This particular case taught us the importance in establishing appropriate emergence contour through provisional restoration.

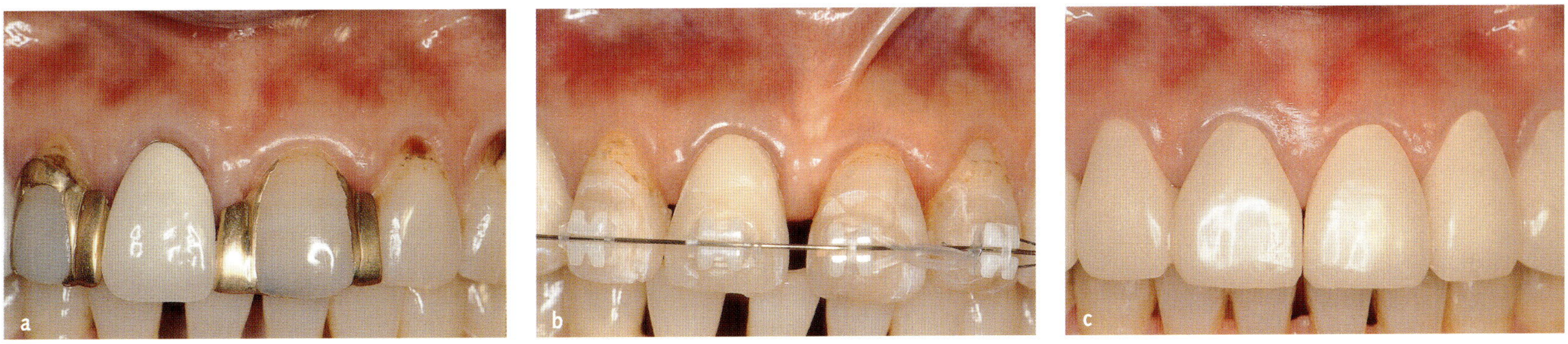

Fig 5-40 (a) Photograph taken at the first visit. Wide interdental spaces have been filled with this prosthesis. (b) Photograph taken about 5 months after the first visit. Orthodontic tooth movement is conducted to close interdental spaces. Mesial movement and palatal torque are employed. (c) Provisional restoration, 1 year 3 months after the first visit.

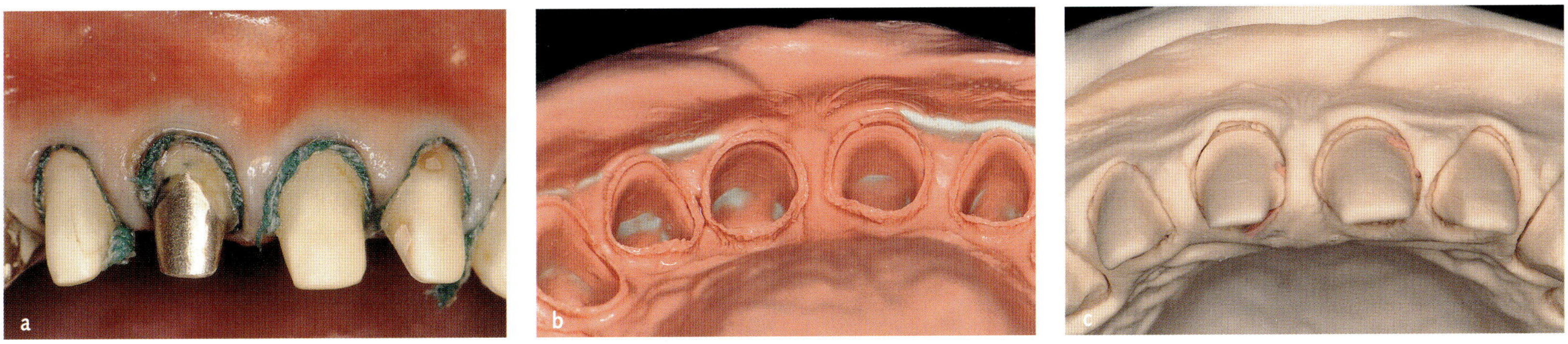

Fig 5-41 Impression. (a) Photograph taken 1 year 3 months after the first visit. The double-cord retraction technique is used. In retrospect, this wide retraction cord was used, despite large scalloping, which could have damaged the gingiva. (b) Although the preparation finish line is shown clearly, body material shows through the wash material, which indicates that there was pressure during impression. (c) This working cast also shows damage in the gingival area caused by retraction.

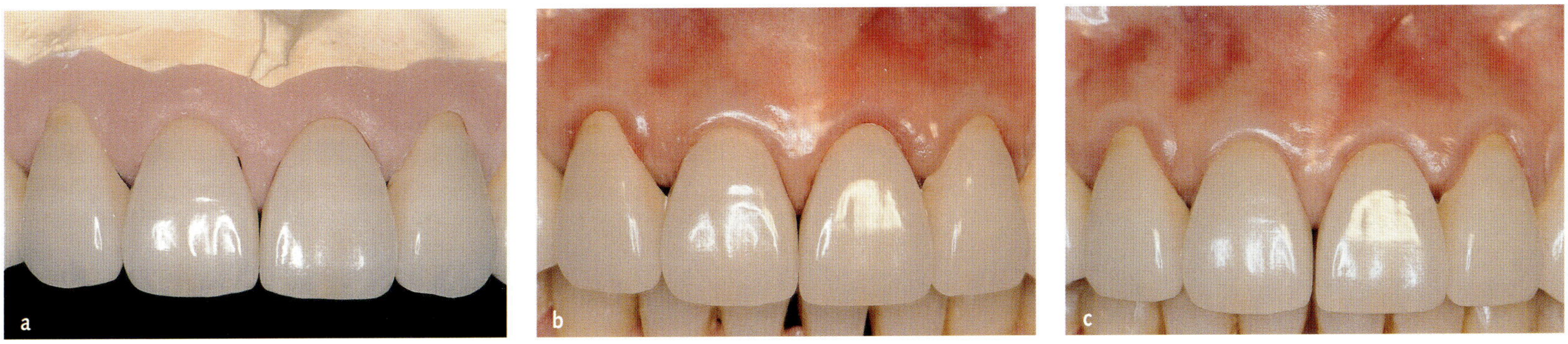

Fig 5-42 Final prostheses with a tissue model, obtained from a pick-up impression model. A reverse contour is given from the labial cervical area to the subgingival area. (b) Photograph taken 1 week after delivery. Inflammation is noted despite professional care. (c) Photograph taken 3 months after delivery. Because of the gingival damage caused by the retraction procedure and insufficient subgingival contour, hyperplasia is observed in the marginal gingiva.

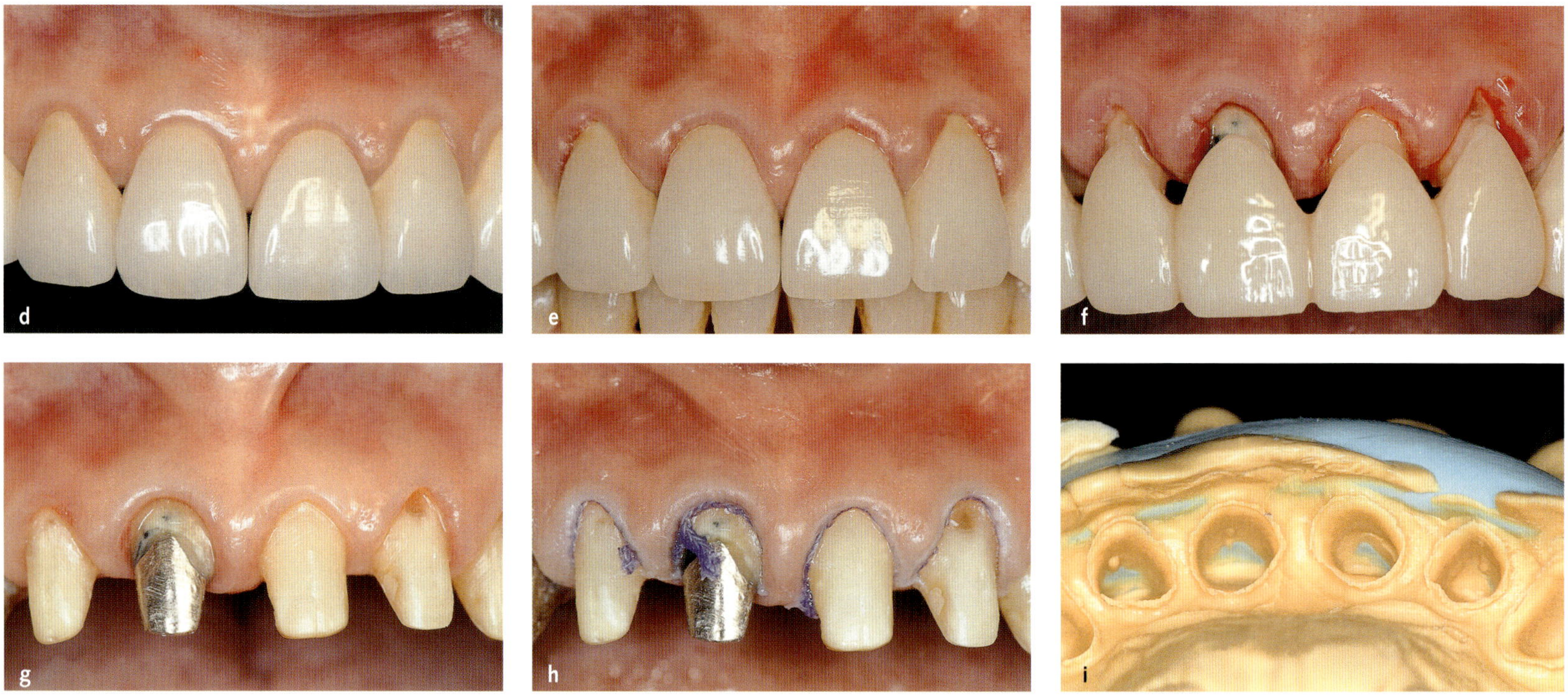

Fig 5-42 (cont) (d) Photograph taken 6 months after delivery. Neither change nor improvement is noted. (e and f) Photographs taken 2 years 6 months after delivery. Because the severe inflammation continued, the prostheses were removed and replaced by a provisional restoration. Although the patient continued brushing earnestly, gingival conditions were not stabilized. (g) Photograph taken 2 years 8 months after the first visit. (h) The gingiva eventually has stabilized, and an impression is to be taken for provisional restoration. Ultrapak 0 retraction cord is used to prevent damage to the gingiva. (i) The utmost care has been taken to minimize damage to gingiva.

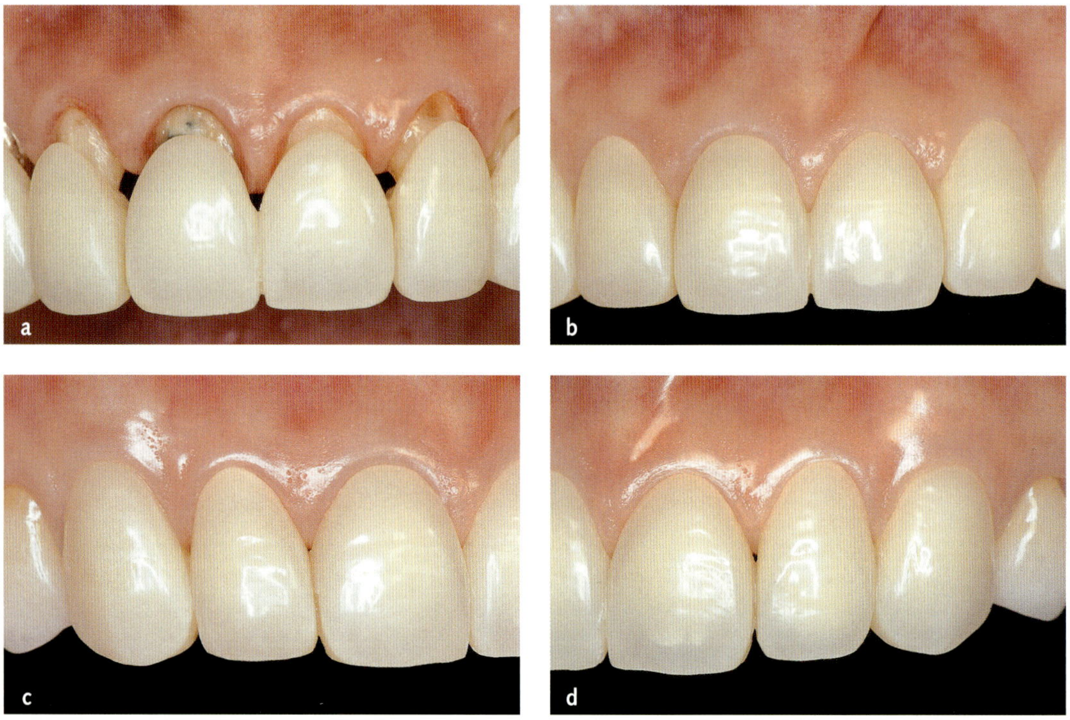

Fig 5-43 Delivery of refabricated prostheses. (a to d) Photographs taken 1 month after delivery of final provisional restorations, 4 years 3 months after the first visit. Through a trial-and-error process with provisional restorations, final restorations with sufficient contour from subgingival to cervical areas as well as good marginal fit have been obtained. Inflammation is resolved.

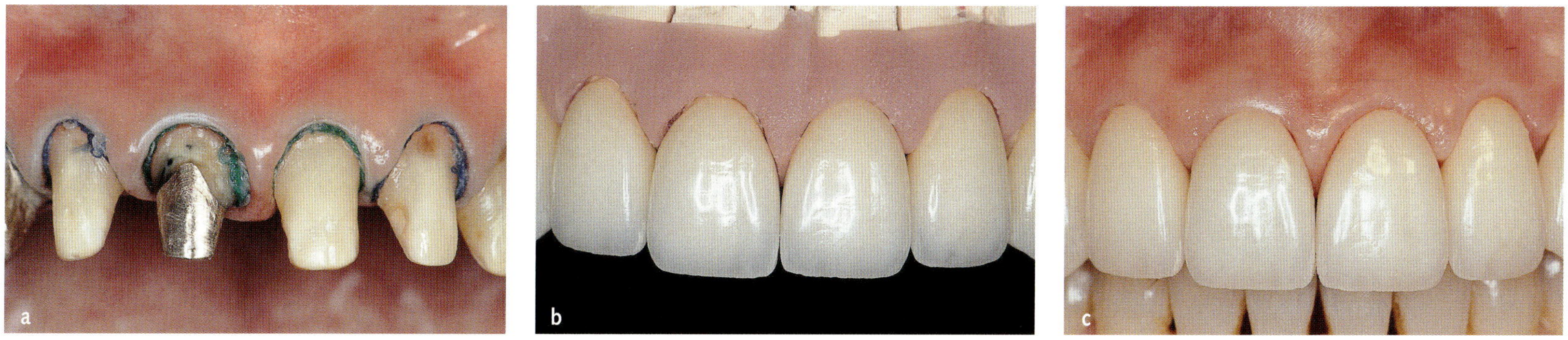

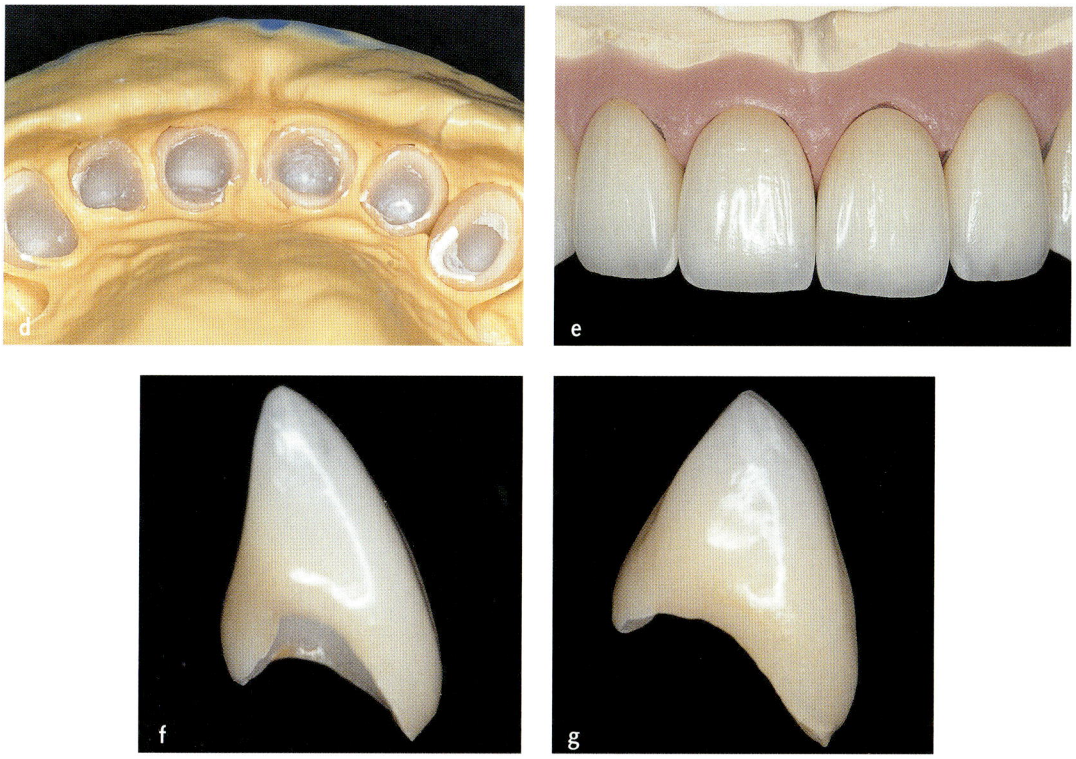

Fig 5-44 Delivery of Procera all-ceramic crowns. (a) Because gingival conditions have improved, gingival restoration is carefully conducted. (b) Completed Procera restorations on the cast. (c) Restorations are temporarily cemented. The appearance of the marginal gingiva is not acceptable. (d) Impression. (e to g) Corrections are made, focusing on the emergence angles, which are contoured to harmonize with the thick gingiva. (Prostheses made by Mr Chojiro Masuda, RDT.) (h to j) Delivery of the modified prostheses. The crown morphology must allow the gingiva to adapt tightly against the restoration. No shadow or discoloration is generated.

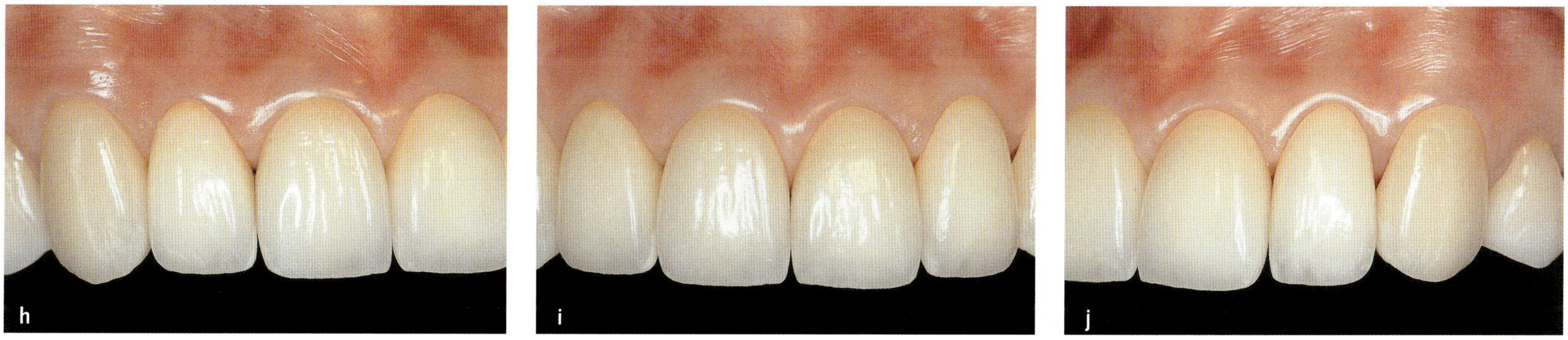

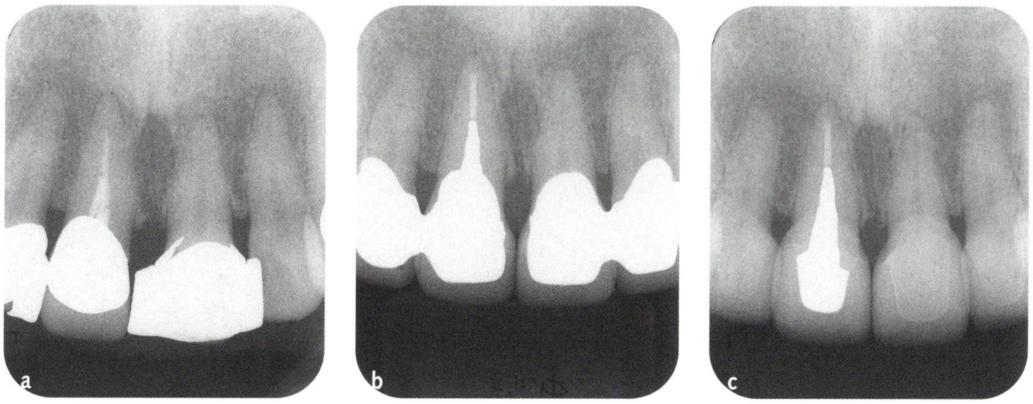

Fig 5-45 Radiographic evaluations before and after treatment. (a) At the first visit, there is a 6-mm periodontal probing depth at the maxillary left central incisor. (b) Orthodontic tooth movement was conducted for 9 months. Collarless porcelain crowns have been delivered. (c) Radiograph taken 4 years 3 months after the first visit. Procera single crowns have been fabricated and delivered.

Provisional Restoration and the Dentogingival Complex

Importance of provisional restoration

We do not need to restate the importance of the provisional restoration in prosthodontic treatment. The prototypical concept of modern provisional restorations was proposed by Amsterdam and Fox and has undergone changes to adapt to the development of newer periodontal and prosthetic treatments. Provisional restorations play a major role in the improvement and stabilization of the occlusion, management of the gingiva, and communication with the laboratory and the patient.

Exploratory versus communicative provisional restorations

In major prosthodontic treatment, a provisional restoration has several important functions. There is a major difference in the roles of a provisional restoration that is to be adjusted and corrected long-term in a trial-and-error manner and a provisional restoration that is to be used for a short period of time prior to proceeding to a final prosthesis. Both have a role as an interim appliance, but the former assists in the trial-and-error method, while the latter is fabricated after the trial-and-error process has been almost completed. The first is mainly utilized for communication with patients and adaptation of the gingiva, and the second will be used for communication with laboratory. Although this may sound extreme, the first type of provisional restoration is a means for exploration and the second is a means for communication.

The first type may be fabricated in laboratory at first, but it is repeatedly corrected and adjusted chairside. This corrective process establishes patient satisfaction with esthetics, develops harmony with the gingival morphology, and provides stabilization of the occlusion over time. The margins of the provisional restoration are set supragingivally if possible, and usually resin is added occlusally for stabilization of the occlusion. The second type of provisional restoration receives minor adjustments in the occlusal surface and communicates important details to the laboratory: the marginal contours subgingivally to cervically, transitional contour, embrasure form, and detailed occlusal morphology. As the correct parameters are established with the provisional restoration, the final impression is taken immediately. The final provisional restoration should ideally be fabricated by the dental technician who will fabricate the final prosthesis.

Provisional restorations used in a case with expected change in the mandibular position

In a case with a loss of the vertical dimension of occlusion due to clenching or a posterior occlusal collapse, the mandible is guided to its relaxed position and the occlusion is corrected, clenching is eliminated, and the posterior vertical dimension is increased through natural rotation of the mandible (Fig 5-46). Measures taken include the addition of autopolymerizing resin to the occlusal ridges if the posterior teeth lose occlusal contact. Because thin resin layers tend to break easily, the provisional restoration is fabricated with a metal framework in a case like this, so that resin can be added on top of the framework.

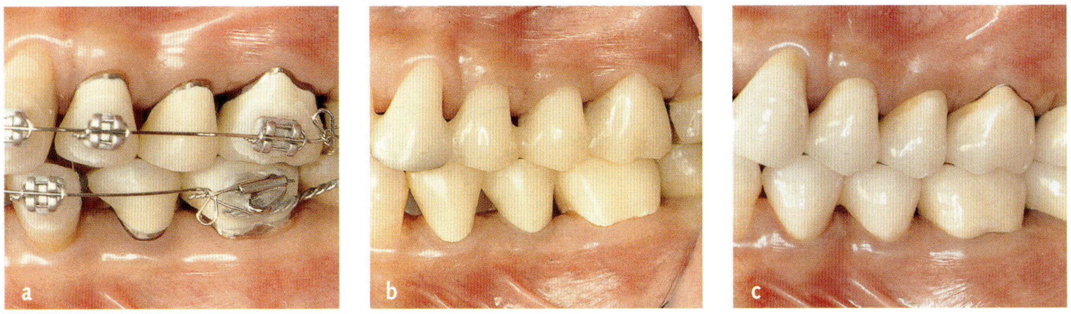

Fig 5-46 Provisional restorations with metal substructures have been used during the treatment of a vertical interarch discrepancy. (a) Restorative tooth movement. (b) After stabilization of the mandibular position, a transition is made to a final provisional restoration. It is used intraorally for only a short time; however, the morphology of final provisional restoration plays an important role in the fabrication of the final prosthesis, in terms of occlusal harmony with the gingiva and subgingival adjustment (remargining). (c) Photograph taken 8 years after delivery of the final prostheses.

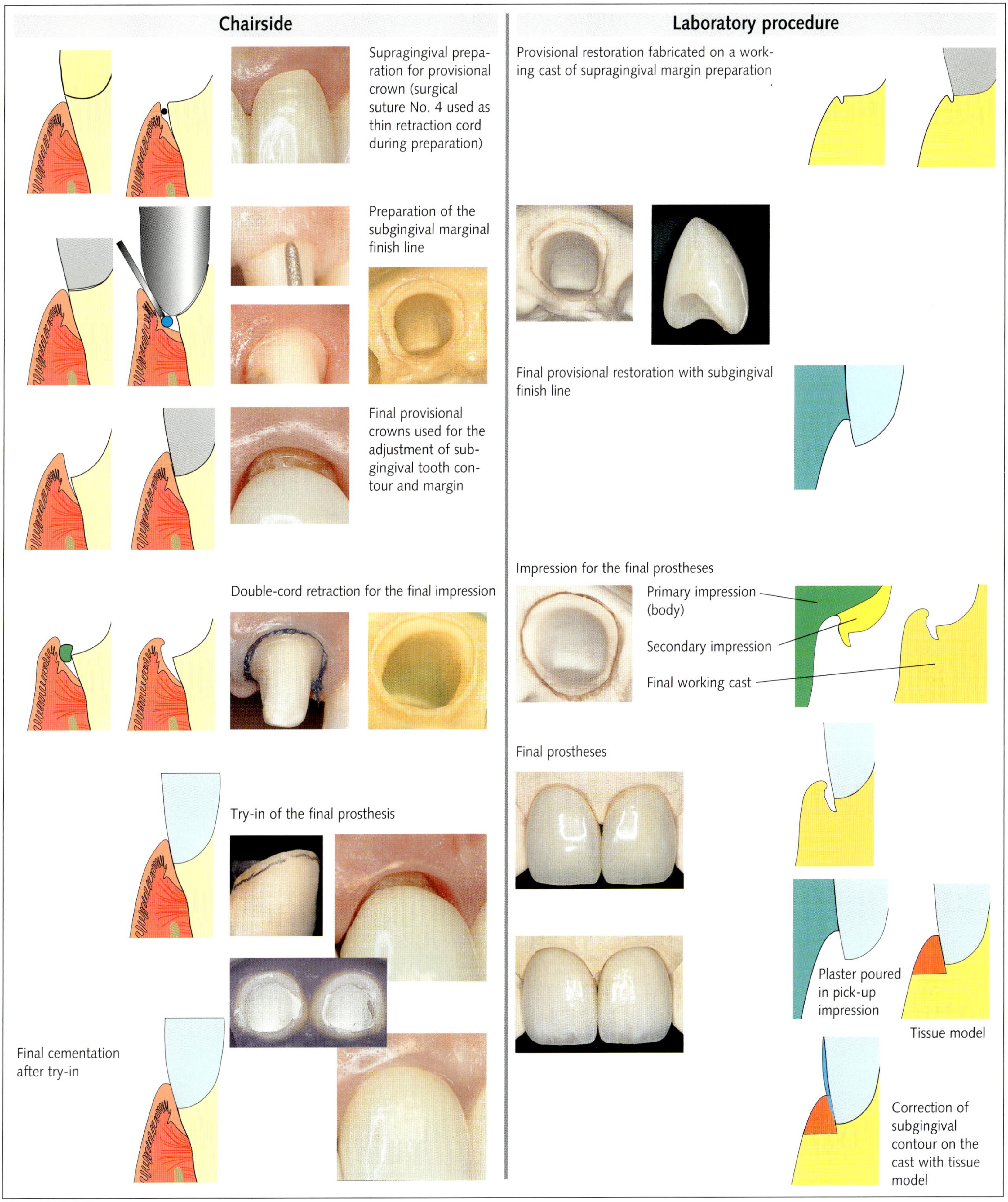

Fig 5-47 Chairside–laboratory communication for a crown restoration with a subgingival finish line.

Final provisional restoration and remargining

When the prescription for fabrication of the final provisional restoration is sent to the laboratory, records are provided for them, including (1) full-mouth casts of the prepared abutments, where the impression was taken with gingival retraction alone, (2) full-mouth casts with the provisional restoration in place, (3) a facebow registration, (4) a centric relation record, and (5) clinical photographs. The casts with the provisional restorations in place show that the gingiva is not affected by gingival retraction, based on which the final provisional restoration is to be fabricated at the laboratory, preferably with a slight overcontour.

For the final provisional restoration, chairside adjustment is conducted, including occlusal equilibration as well as reduction of an overcontoured margin or addition of autopolymerizing resin to an insufficient margin. This procedure, which we call remargining, is conducted while subtle and delicate gingival responses are observed. Consequently, the final provisional restoration is finished to become the most important source of information for fabrication of the final prosthesis.

Final pick-up impression and gingival contour

The emergence contour includes the progression from the subgingival marginal contour to the supragingival contour and may require adjustment, depending on the thickness of the periodontal tissue, interdental space, root proximity, degree of scalloping, inclination of the tooth axis, and so on. These pieces of information are communicated accurately to a laboratory by means of the final provisional restoration. So that a clear impression of the preparation finish line can be made, the gingiva is retracted at the final impression. Gingival retraction creates an open gingival sulcus and distorted free gingival margin.

For fabrication of the final prostheses, the clinician provides for the laboratory with (1) casts with a clear impression of the preparation finish line, (2) a pick-up impression of the clinical try-in of the metal framework or cores, (3) full-mouth casts with the final provisional restoration in place, (4) centric relation record, (5) a facebow registration, (6) shade, and (7) clinical photographs (Fig 5-47). The most important information for the dentogingival complex is held by the pick-up impression. Because the morphology of the free gingival margin is supported by the final provisional restoration, this pick-up impression has, for the most part, the subgingival morphology that actually exists in the patient's mouth. If such information on the subgingival marginal contour is not provided to a laboratory, the dental technicians will have to build an emergence contour without knowing the inclination of the tooth roots, which will often lead to fabrication of a poorly contoured crown prosthesis, resulting in flat, thick gingiva after periodontal therapy. In contrast, a good provisional restoration and good communication with the laboratory will result in satisfactory gingival support (Figs 5-48 to 5-53).

Figs 5-48 to 5-53 Tissue support established by the provisional restoration.

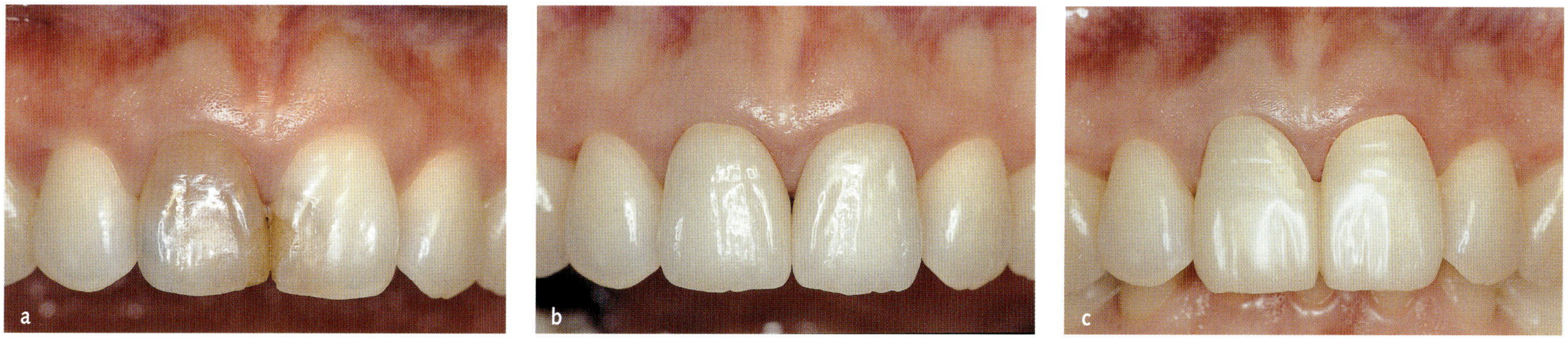

Fig 5-48 Refabrication of anterior crown restorations. (a) Photograph taken at the first visit. (b) Photograph taken after 10 months. Collarless porcelain restorations have been fabricated for the maxillary central incisors. Although the fit is good, there are concerns, such as gingival hyperplasia and a shadow in the cervical area. The restoration is to be refabricated. (c) The splinted provisional restoration has poor morphology and crown-root ratio.

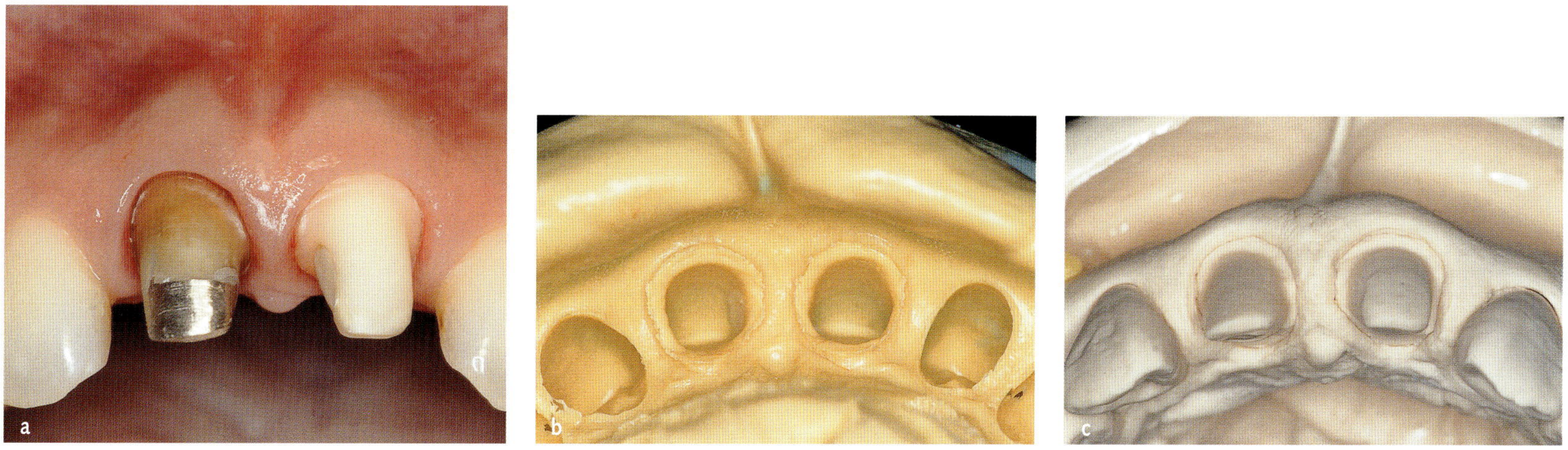

Fig 5-49 Impression for the provisional restoration. (a) Silicone impression with thin retraction cord alone. (b and c) The working cast for the provisional restoration.

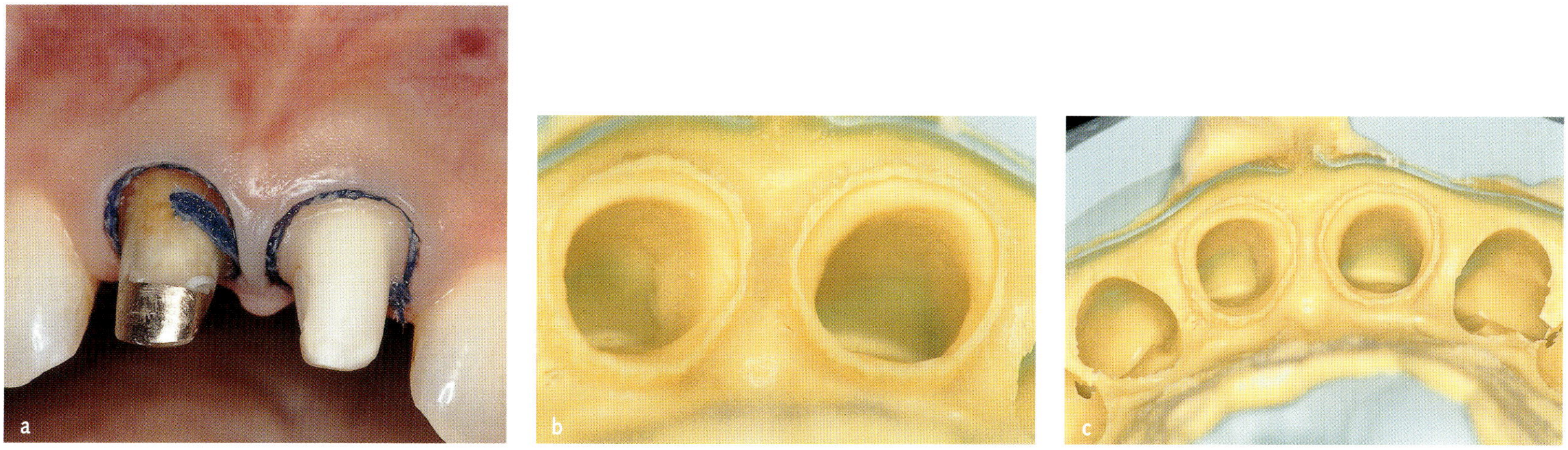

Fig 5-50 Final impression. (a) Gingival retraction with double cord. (b and c) Nonpressure impression with fluid silicone material. Clear impression surfaces without deformation are obtained. (d and e) Clear and sharp finish lines are shown in the concentric preparation.

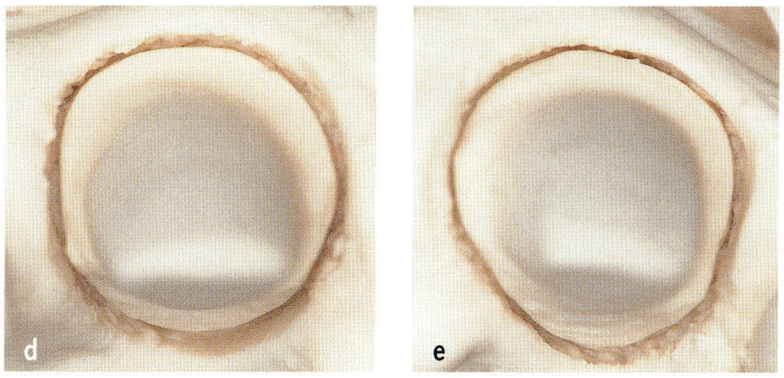

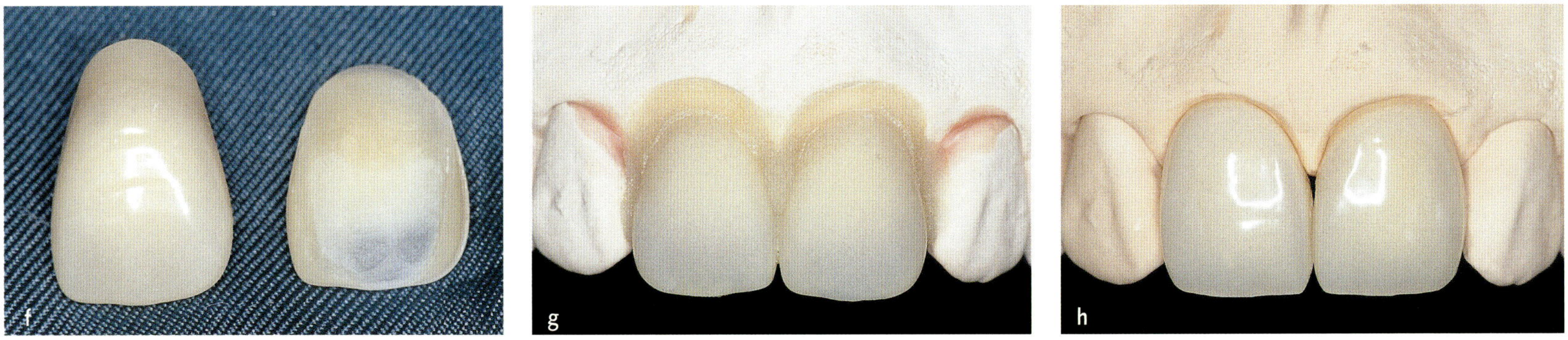

Fig 5-50 (cont) (f) Prefabricated Geller shells (Creation) for provisional restoration. (g) To facilitate remargination, autopolymerizing resin is applied to the cervical area and the internal surface, followed by light-cured resin, on top of which the shell is applied. The point is to fabricate them as splinted crowns. (h) Completed single crowns. Slight overcontouring is produced on the provisional restoration.

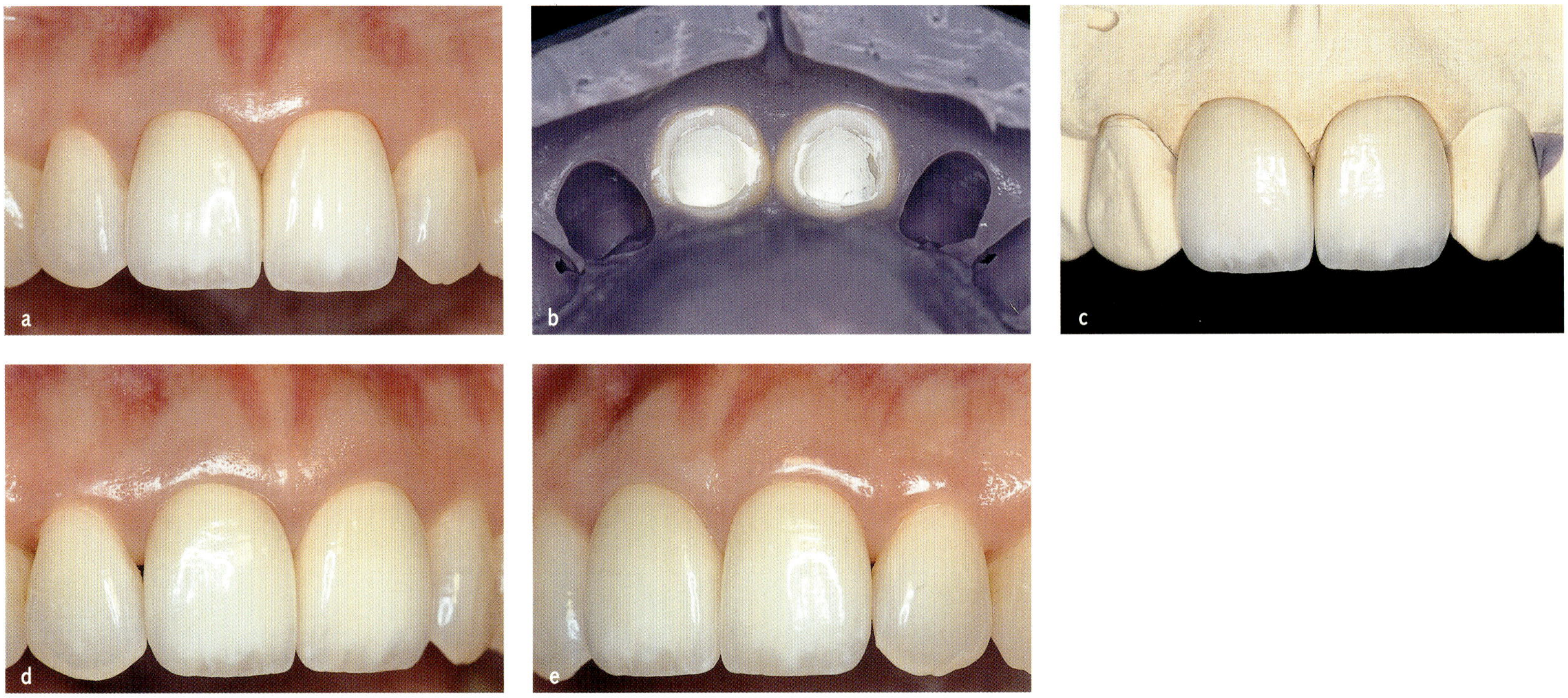

Fig 5-51 Modification of the final prostheses. (a) Procera all-ceramic crowns are temporarily cemented. (b) About 2 weeks after temporary cementation, a pick-up impression is taken. (c) The gingival morphology is observed and necessary corrections and modifications are made. (d and e) At delivery of the final prostheses, no shadowing or discoloration of the gingivae is present.

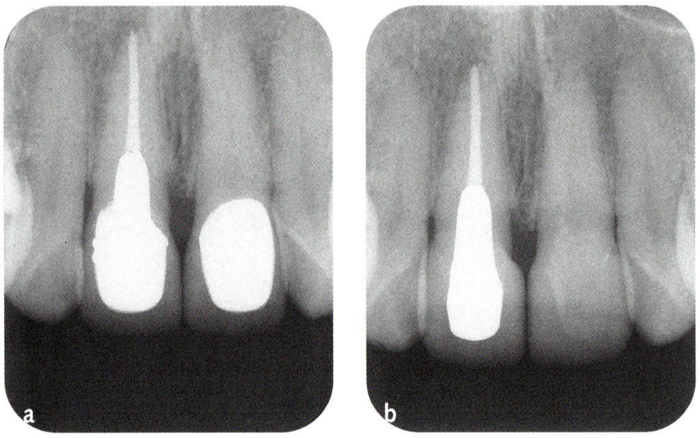

Fig 5-52 Radiographic evaluation. (a) At the first visit, the osseous crest is relatively thick and low. (b) During maintenance, the condition is stable.

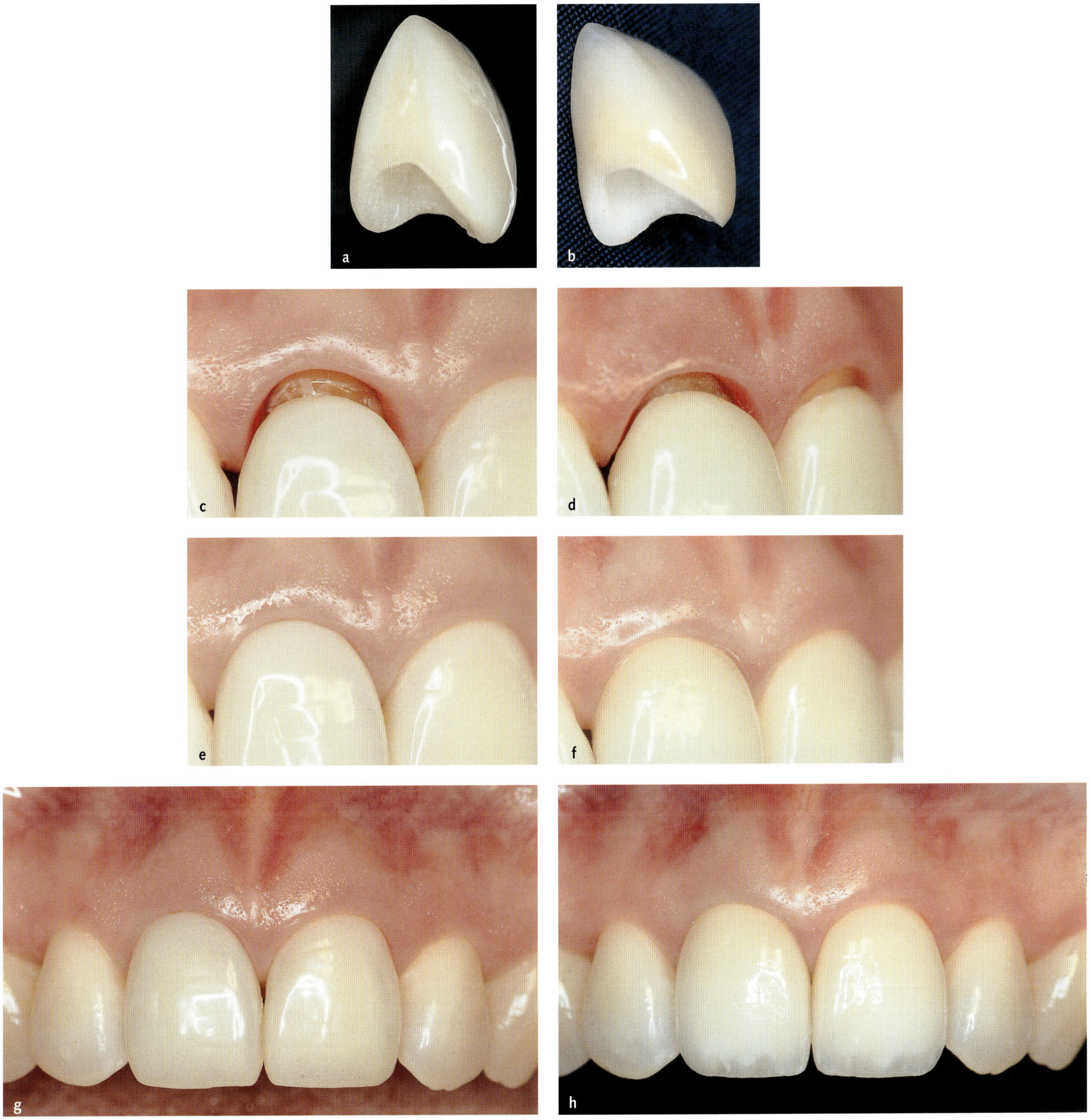

Fig 5-53 Comparison between the final provisional restorations and final prostheses after correction. (a) Provisional crown. (b) Procera all-ceramic crown. (Prostheses made by Mr Chojiro Masuda, RDT.) (c) Adjustment of marginal fit and emergence angle contours with the provisional restoration. (d) The contour of the Procera crown follows that of the provisional restoration. (e) Photograph taken at delivery of the final provisional restoration. (f) The Procera all-ceramic crown, which has appropriate contour, does not cause gingival hyperplasia. (g) Photograph taken 3 days after delivery of the provisional restoration. Because the emergence contour has improved to facilitate tissue support, the cervical margin has improved compared to the condition at the first visit. Because of tissue adaptation, the gingival hyperplasia has disappeared. (h) Photograph taken at delivery of the Procera single crowns. Because the design follows that of the provisional restoration, the result is satisfactory from both the morphologic and esthetic points of view.

Crown Restoration and Preparation Finish Line

Supragingival versus subgingival finish lines

For molars, the finish line for crown preparation should preferably be supragingival when teeth are vital and have healthy enamel at the cervical area. However, for anterior teeth and premolars, the finish line must be placed subgingivally. This is a matter of esthetics and is not only an issue of whether the metal margin is visible or not. There are other concerns, including harmony of color and shape with the adjacent teeth, the relationship with the interdental papillae, and the support of the gingival morphology itself for teeth with recession caused by periodontal disease.

In crown restorations, the tooth structure is reduced for correct preparation, its morphology is captured in an impression, the prosthesis is fabricated in an indirect method, and the restoration is delivered to the abutment tooth via a luting cement. There is no guarantee that the margin of the restoration can fit with 100% accuracy, thus the margin should be supragingival. When it is determined that a subgingival margin is going to be placed, treatment results are affected not only by the fit of the restoration but also by the way in which the emergence angle from the gingiva, or the point of contact between the periodontal tissue and the prosthesis, is stabilized. In other words, the outcome is based on how the internal and external periodontal environments have been properly established prior to the making of impressions (Fig 5-54).

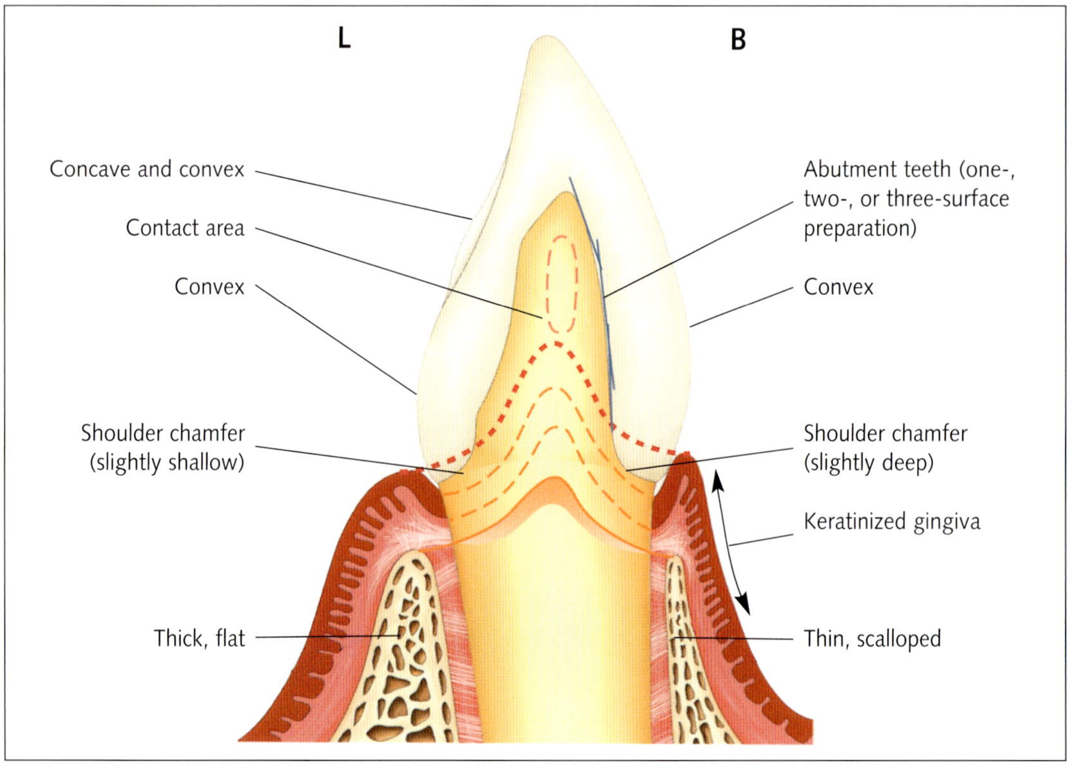

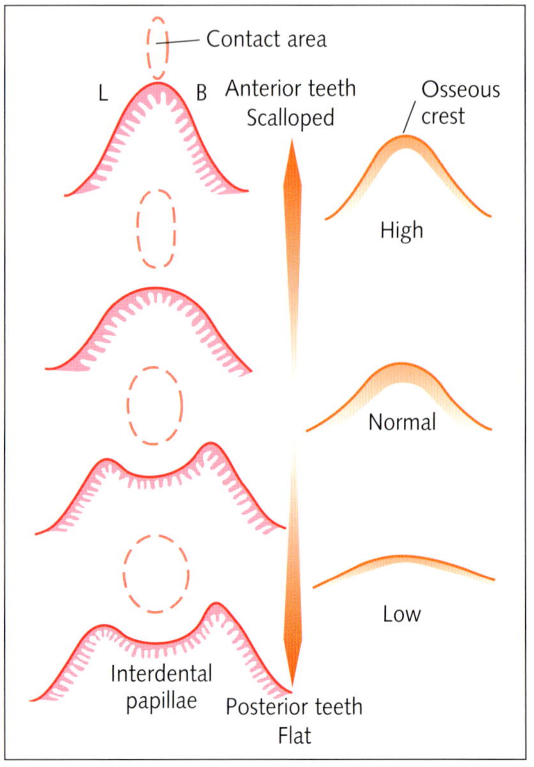

Fig 5-54 Gingival morphology and restoration.

For crown restorations, whether the preparation finish line is set supragingivally or subgingivally should be determined using clear reasons and objectives. Margin placement by an operator who is unclear whether a supragingival or subgingival margin should be placed is out of the question. Placing subgingival margins at random for esthetic reasons is problematic. For vital abutment teeth, supragingival margins are advantageous from the viewpoint of tissue management. Supragingival margins will cause a significant esthetic problem in a case with significant attachment loss due to periodontal disease, but it would not be a problem in a case with minimal attachment loss. Although the indications are limited, porcelain laminate veneers can provide satisfactory esthetics with a preparation within enamel and a supragingival margin, if there is no attachment loss (see Fig 5-60).

When priority is given to esthetics in anterior teeth or premolars, efforts are to be made to achieve harmony of the cervical margins as well as conservation of interdental papillae, as long as the biologic width is not invaded by the restoration. The prostheses should improve esthetics and compensate for a volume of periodontal tissue lost to periodontal disease, and efforts should be made to establish what we call *therapeutic contour*. For molars without a high demand for esthetics, even a finish line at the gingival margin would sufficiently meet most patients' expectations (see Fig 5-54).

Importance of following basic procedures for tooth preparation

In reduction of tooth substance, what is done cannot be undone. Therefore, tooth preparation has to be based on a correct diagnosis and clear objectives. Inlay and crown preparations are well-documented procedures. Because of that, clinicians should strictly follow the basic procedures.

Basic principles in preparation should be observed in terms of reduction of the occlusal and axial surfaces as well as the preparation of the functional cusps, bevels, and grooves. Suitable burs should be used accordingly. In preparation of the axial surfaces, effort should be made to obtain appropriate retention and resistance form and to develop harmony with the adjacent teeth as well as the periodontal tissue. Embrasure areas, contact areas, crown contour, crown length, and transitional areas (between concave and convex areas of line angles) are to be prepared clearly. Particularly in esthetic anterior regions, preparation finish lines should not damage healthy gingiva, and attention should be paid to establishing harmony at the cervical margin. The transitional area at the cementoenamel junction, from about 1 mm supragingival to about 1 mm subgingival, is called the *emergence profile*, the morphology of which determines the prognosis of the restoration and periodontal tissue. In the anterior region, the buccal gingiva is relatively thin and deeply scalloped, while the palatal tissue is thick and flat. The anterior teeth have more scalloped gingiva, and the epithelial attachment is located more coronally. These conditions should be kept in mind, and due considerations should be made to the structure of dentogingival complex with regard to the amount of subgingival preparation of buccal, palatal, and proximal walls, with special attention to bone level (scalloped versus flat, thin versus thick).

To produce correct occlusal morphology, sufficient tooth reduction is required. From the viewpoints of retention and protection of the dental pulp and tooth structure, the amount of reduction should be as minimal as required. Preparation should adhere to the basics to resolve these conflicting needs. In preparation of the axial surfaces, the resistance form should meet the proper degrees of taper, and a concentric preparation should be made so that the axial surfaces will align to the contour of the tooth root and crown.

Supragingival crown margin

Because of the fracture at the cementoenamel junction of the mandibular left first and second premolars, only the roots remained in the patient shown in Fig 5-55. The mandibular left first and second molars had been missing for some time, causing extrusion of maxillary left second premolar, first molar, and second molar. The occlusal plane had to be corrected before the missing teeth were replaced. The maxillary left first and second molars have furcation involvement. Emdogain was used to achieve recovery of the attachment. After the occlusal plane was corrected, the final prostheses for the maxillary left second premolar, first molar, and second molar were designed as Procera single-unit crowns with supragingival finish lines on vital teeth.

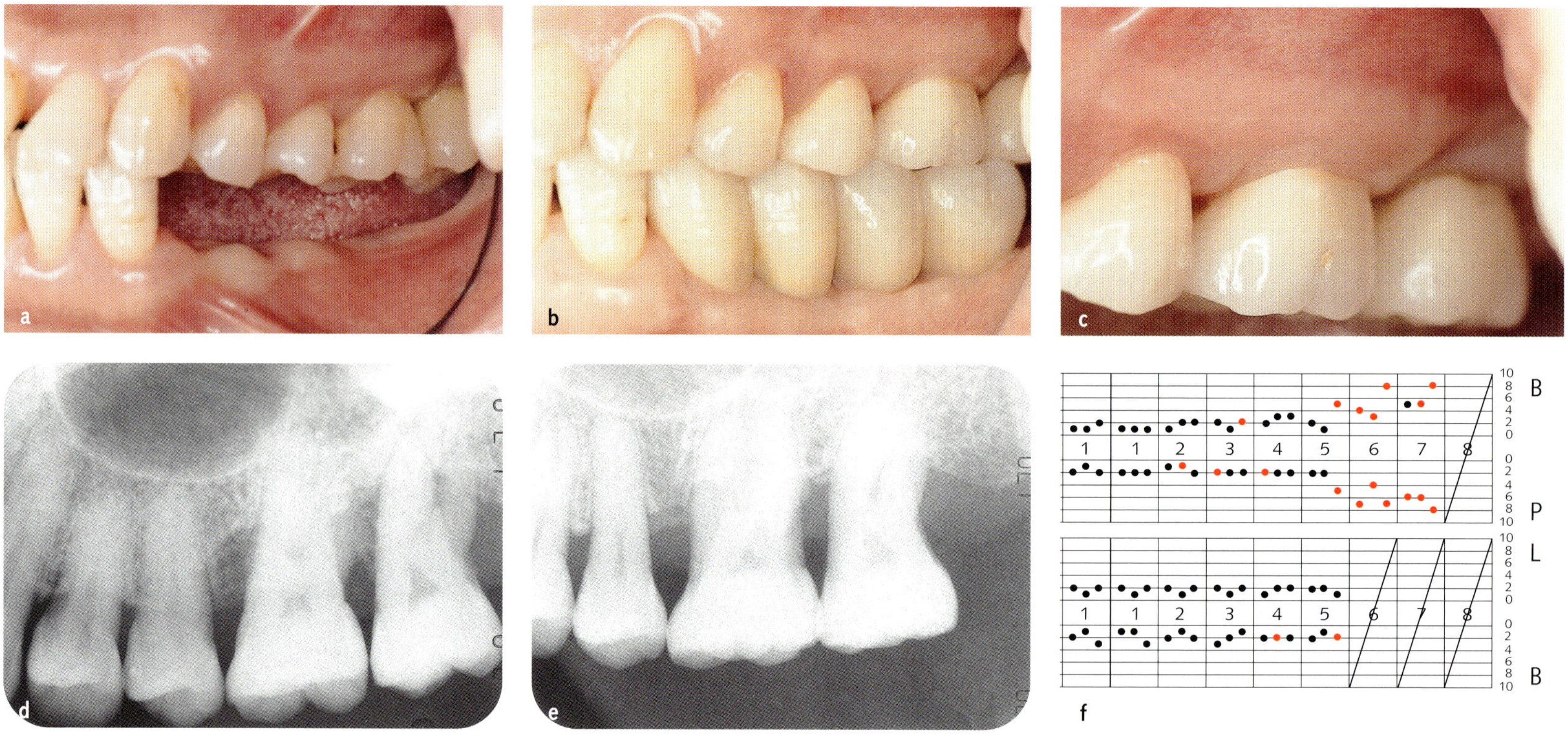

Fig 5-55 (a) At the first visit, the maxillary left first premolar, second premolar, first molar, and second molar are extruded. Probing depths are 8 mm. (b and c) Two years posttreatment. After the occlusal plane was corrected, final restorations for the maxillary left second premolar, first molar, and second molar were designed with supragingival finish lines. The teeth remain vital. Procera single-unit crowns with good esthetics and maintainability have been delivered. The probing depths are less than or equal to 2 mm. (d) Radiograph taken at the first visit. (e) Radiograph taken after about 2 years. (f) Probing chart at the first visit.

Figs 5-56 to 5-59 Subgingival preparation and subsequent growth of the gingiva.

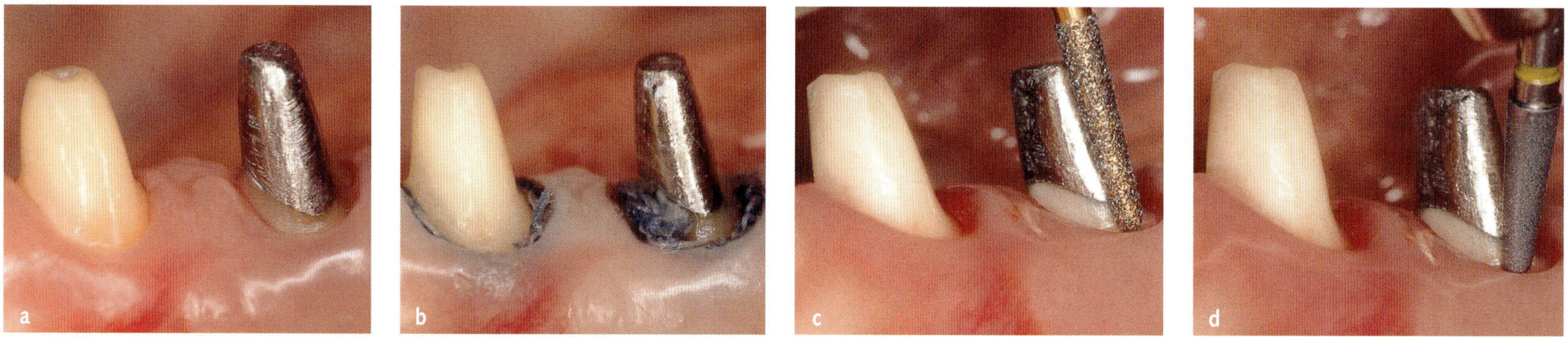

Fig 5-56 Subgingival preparation. (a) The mandibular left first and second premolars serve as abutment teeth. The interproximal distance between the teeth is greater than normal. (b) Gingival retraction (double-cord technique). (c) Chamfer preparation after the retraction. (d) Final polishing of the finish line is conducted with a manual polishing bur.

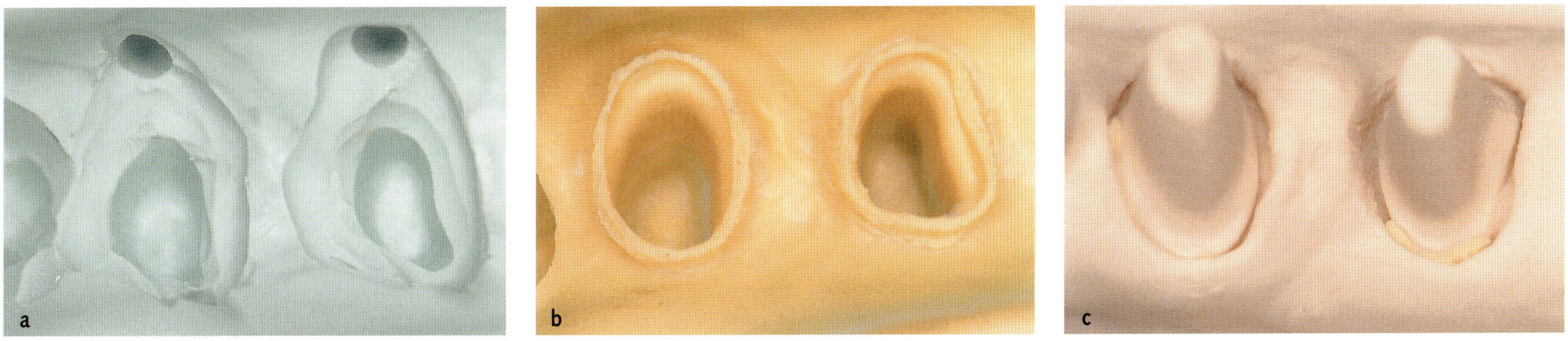

Figs 5-57 Subgingival impression. (a) The primary impression has been trimmed with an HIT silicone bur. (b) HIT silicone impression with subgingival impression surfaces accurately expressed. The gingival sulci are retracted with an even thickness. Good impression surfaces are obtained. (c) Clear preparation finish lines are visible. Concentric preparation follows the outline of the tooth roots.

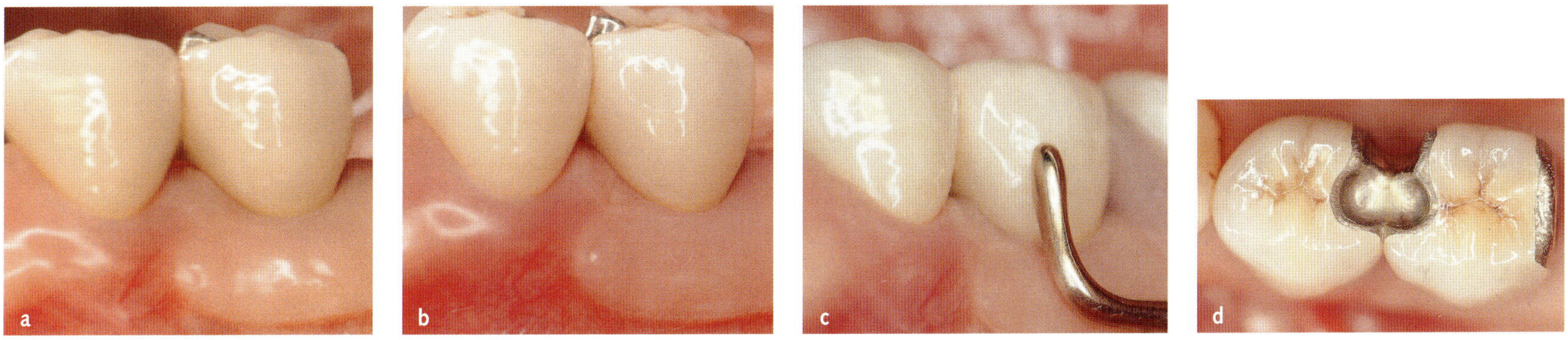

Fig 5-58 Connective tissue growth of the gingiva on clasped teeth. (a) Photograph taken 2 years 9 months after regenerative surgery. To enhance maintainability of the gingiva around an I-bar clasp, a free gingival graft was completed. To improve the interdental papillae between the mandibular left premolars, a half pontic was adapted to the axial contour. The finish line was designed so that the mesial and distal margins started from the subgingival area, and an overcontour was designed to create moderate tension against the interdental papillae. (b) Photograph taken 3 years 8 months after treatment. Some degree of tissue adaptation is obtained in the gingiva, and the condition is stable. (c and d) Splinted metal-ceramic crowns and the I-bar–retained prosthesis are delivered to the mandibular left first and second premolars. Support, bracing, and retention are clearly defined, with the goal of obtaining a stable removable denture. (Prostheses made by Mr Kiyoharu Takada, RDT.)

Fig 5-59 Regenerative therapy for the interdental periodontal tissue. (a) When nonresorbable membrane is used for regeneration of periodontal tissue, deep growth of epithelial tissue can be prevented while creating a space for regeneration by trimming the membrane to an appropriate size and applying it to the interdental area. In this case, even after proper trimming was completed, the membrane would not fit the root surfaces if it were sutured here. (b) We partially reflected the buccal and lingual periosteum so that the membrane could be stabilized there. (c) Radiograph taken at the first visit. The mandibular left second premolar had a two-wall infrabony defect. (d) Radiograph taken after 4 years. Splinted metal-ceramic crowns have been delivered for the mandibular left premolars. Although they are abutments for an I-bar clasp, bone regeneration can be confirmed.

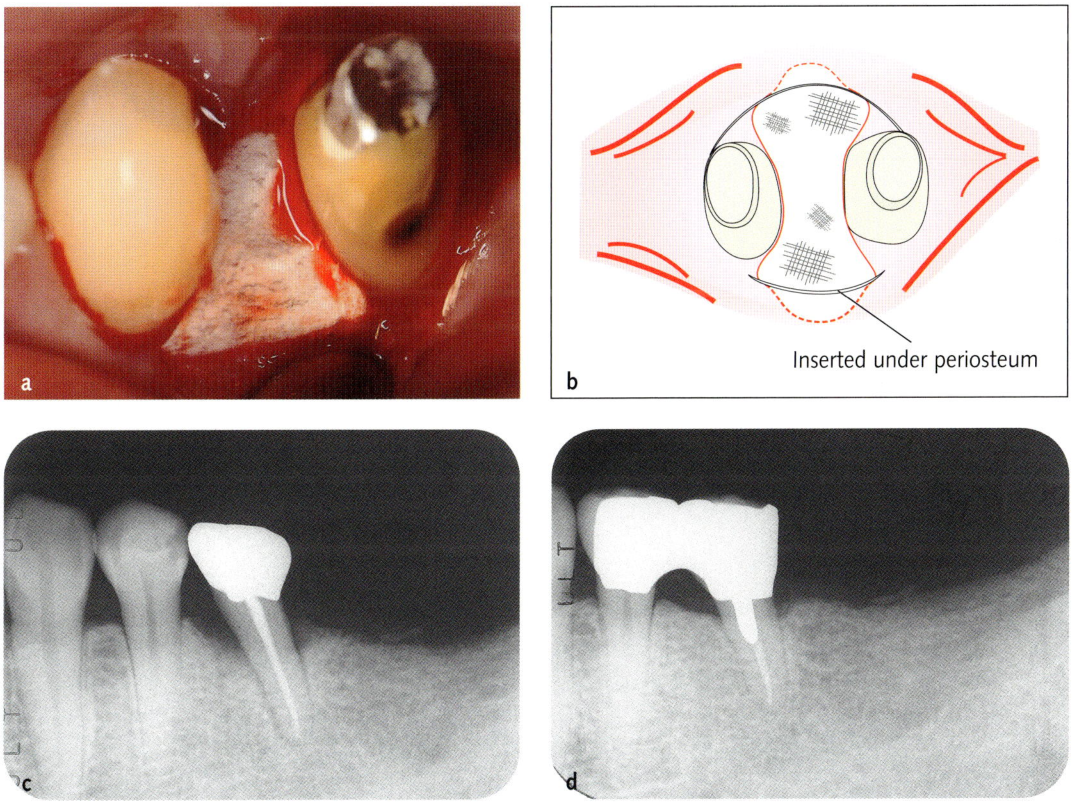

Gingival retraction

The position of the crown margin or preparation finish line should not be determined from the viewpoint of whether the margin line is to be hidden or not. When the position of the subgingival margin is considered, it is inevitable to have different viewpoints depending on how the subgingival contour is prepared (see Figs 5-40 to 5-45) and how the embrasure space is closed by the interdental papillae. For subgingival preparation and impressions, gingival retraction is indispensable. During the procedure, a clear impression of the margin is required and it is necessary to obtain some space apical to the preparation finish line. Most importantly, however, it is crucial to avoid damaging the gingiva by invading the biologic width. Even if a clear finish line is obtained, it would mean a loss if the gingiva had been retracted by force and damaged. Good fit of the prosthesis might be achieved, but fit with the appropriate cervical gingiva would never be obtained. Clinicians often are oblivious to "gingival weeping" because their eyes are dazzled by an impression and a prosthesis that are highly precise.

The procedure of gingival retraction as well as the selection of cord thickness and the depth of cord insertion cannot be determined uniformly but are determined by the thickness of the gingiva, the depth of the gingival sulcus, and the depth of the marginal finish line. During preparation of an abutment tooth, the thickness of the gingiva and the depth of the marginal finish line are different on the proximal surfaces and the labial surface. Therefore, during gingival retraction, a proper technique should be used for each area. Generally, gingival retraction tends to be insufficient on proximal surfaces, where the position of marginal finish line is deeper. Invasion of the biologic width is more likely to occur on the labial surface.

Advantages of the fluid silicone impression technique

We have utilized hydrocolloid impressions since we opened our private practice, pursuing its high precision. This is because we believed that the absence of pressure is the key to taking excellent impressions. A hydrocolloid impression does have problems, including high dimensional distortion as well as easily torn margins. The gingival tears would not be a problem unless the gingiva is tight. The better controlled the periodontal tissue is with tight gingiva, the bigger the problem becomes in terms of torn impression margins. The problems of dimensional distortion with hydrocolloid impressions and deformation under stress with rubber silicone impressions are almost completely solved with the fluid silicone impression technique (Fig 5-60).

The fluid silicone impression technique was developed by Dr M. P. Lococo in Canada and named the hydrodynamic impression technique (HIT). Since we experimented with this technique in 1993, we have added some improvements and have been using the technique to obtain impressions of hard tissue. Except for the fact that the procedures are somewhat complicated and the workload is slightly greater than the conventional methods, this is an ideal nonpressure impression method that enables almost complete control of air bubbles and causes no deformation under stress. An impression can be taken almost completely without pressure, and a precise impression without air bubbles can be obtained, if periodontal tissue management during the initial therapy phase and gingival retraction procedures have been conducted properly.

In this impression technique, after the primary impression is taken with a plastic tray, holes are prepared from the outside of the tray for injection and extrusion of impression material and the cervical area of the primary impression is trimmed back. The holes are used by the secondary impression material, which is injected to fill the space that was created. Excessive impression material is extruded from the holes. The same procedure can be repeated for each tooth in a case in which multiple teeth are involved. The primary impression material should preferably be thixotropic with a stable set, and the secondary impression material should be highly flowable and have an elongated set time.

This fluid silicone impression technique is based on the same principles as a precision casting. The primary impression material plays a role of the investment material, and the secondary impression material is like a molten metal poured into the first material. Although pressure is applied, the internal stresses are eliminated as the material is set.

Impression technique for inlays and dowel posts and cores

After the primary impression is taken, the holes are prepared corresponding to an inlay site, and trimming is conducted for the inlay cavity and the crown area. When this fluid silicone impression technique is applied to an intracoronal cavity, the secondary impression material is injected first into the cavity. In a complicated cavity, because an air bubble is difficult to remove from the area even under pressure, a relatively small amount of impression material is injected via a free-flow syringe, and the material is blown with air, causing it to spread to a thin film. When an impression of a dowel post-and-core preparation is taken, a low-speed lentulo is used to fill the post space with the secondary impression material.

Fluid silicone impression technique

The basic procedure for a fluid silicone impression (HIT) is as follows:

1. Selection and adjustment of impression tray and primary impression. *A plastic impression tray is selected according to the size of the arch. After adjustments are made for the buccolingual width, adhesive is applied to the tray. Provil Regular body primary impression material (Heraeus) is mixed and applied to the area of the abutment teeth in the tray. A space of 2 to 3 mm is required between the tray and the abutment teeth.*

2. Injection holes. *Drilling is done from the outside of the impression for injection of a secondary impression material. In principle, one buccal and one lingual injection hole is prepared per tooth. The positions of the holes may be designed with consideration to the gingival morphology and the amount of attached gingiva remaining, but they must not be far away from the margin of the prepared abutments.*

3. Trimming of the marginal areas. *A silicone carver, a hand instrument for trimming, is used to trim about 3 mm at the margin of the abutment teeth.*

4. Secondary impression. *Imprint II secondary impression material is mixed and filled in the tray with an injection syringe. At the same time, retraction cords around the abutment teeth are removed, and the secondary impression material is injected with pressure from a hole in the body impression material that leads onto the abutments. Ejection of the impression material from the other hole is confirmation of placement. When the impression material is ejected from the other hole, it allows the tray to be slightly lifted. The tray is then pressed against the abutment teeth and held until set. For inlays or onlays, after the light-bodied impression material is injected around the abutment teeth, the secondary impression procedure is followed.*

With this technique, impressions of abutment teeth can be taken with almost no pressure.

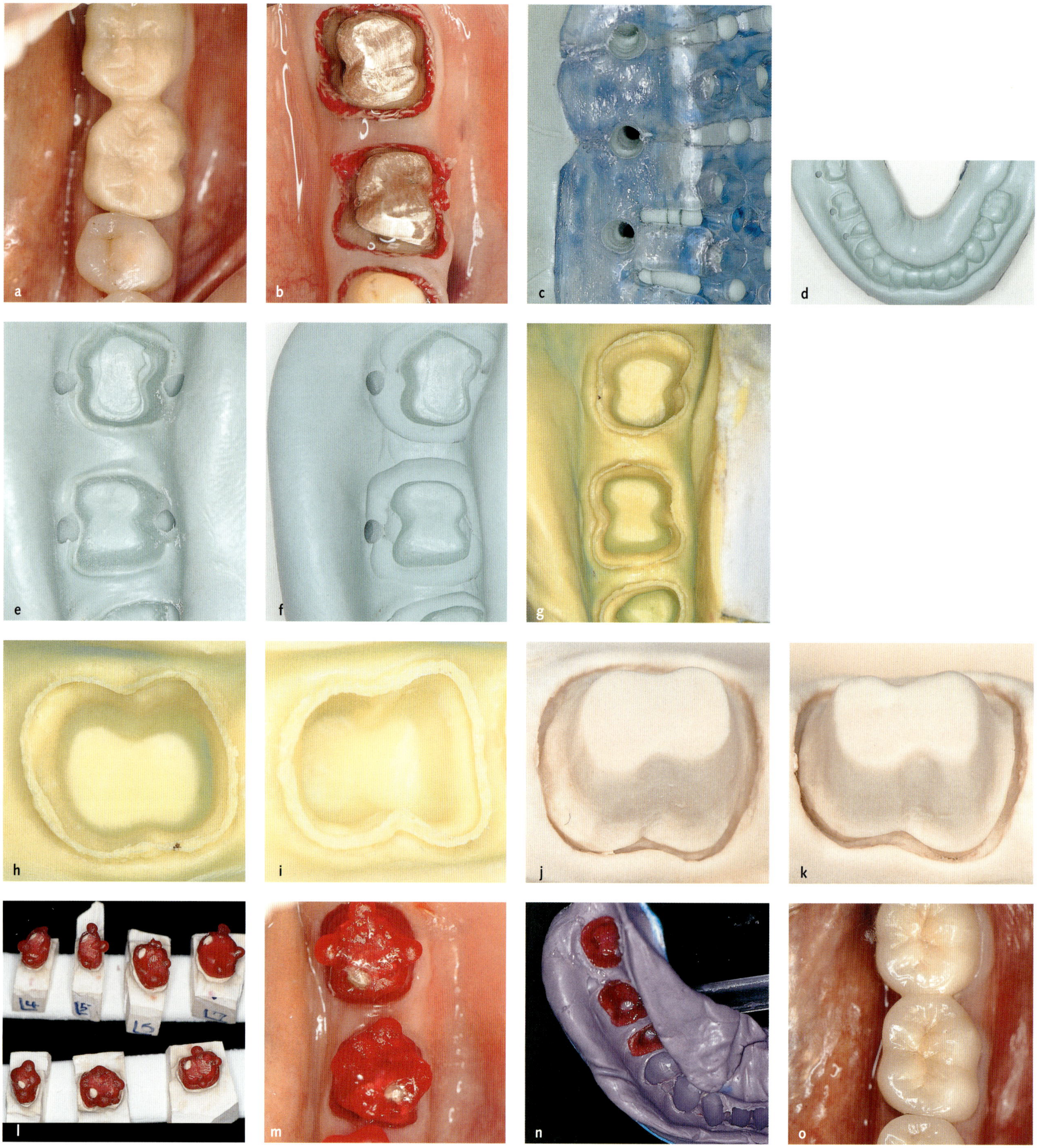

Fig 5-60 (a) Final provisional restoration. (b) Gingival retraction with double cord. (c) After the primary impression material is set, drilling is done from the outside of the impression for injection of the secondary impression material. (d) Primary impression after the holes are drilled. (e and f) Trimming is conducted at the cervical area, including the injection holes. (g to i) The secondary impression is obtained by injecting secondary impression material from the holes of the tray (body impression) that is pressed against the abutment teeth. (j and k) The working cast is obtained from the final impression. (l) Transfer copings are fabricated out of pattern resin. (m and n) A pick-up impression is taken. (o) The final prostheses are delivered.

Figs 5-61 to 5-64 Less invasive esthetic prosthesis: The dentition-unit laminate veneer restoration.

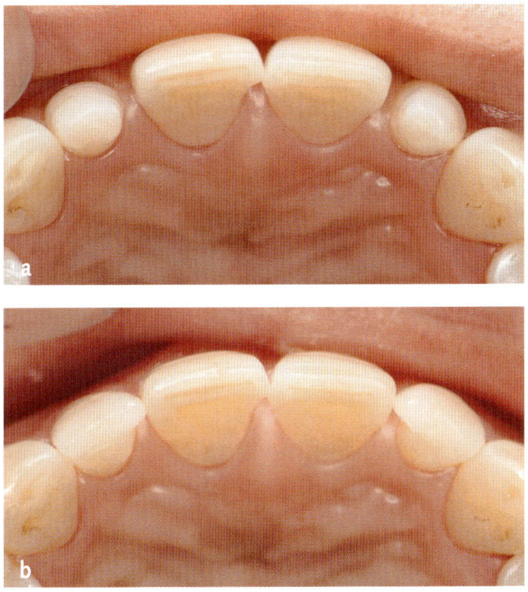

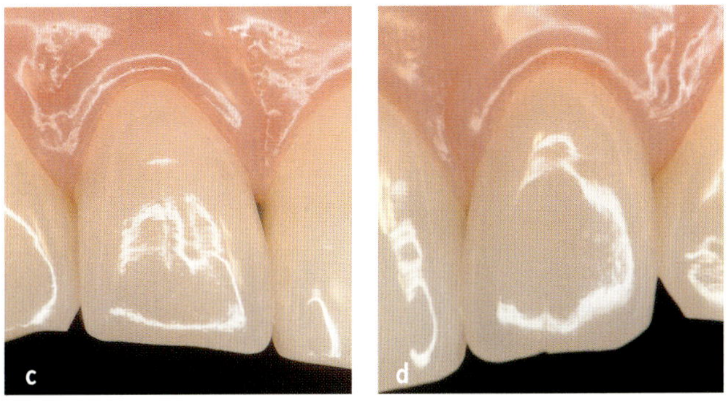

Fig 5-61 (a) Photograph taken at the first visit. (b) After restoration of function is achieved, the lateral teeth are restored with porcelain laminate veneers. Even in a case like this, which at first glance might seem to be suitable for treatment in a tooth-unit approach, the problems and solutions should be contemplated in the following order: (1) occlusion, (2) dentition, and (3) tooth restoration. (c and d) Photographs taken 3 years after porcelain veneer restoration.

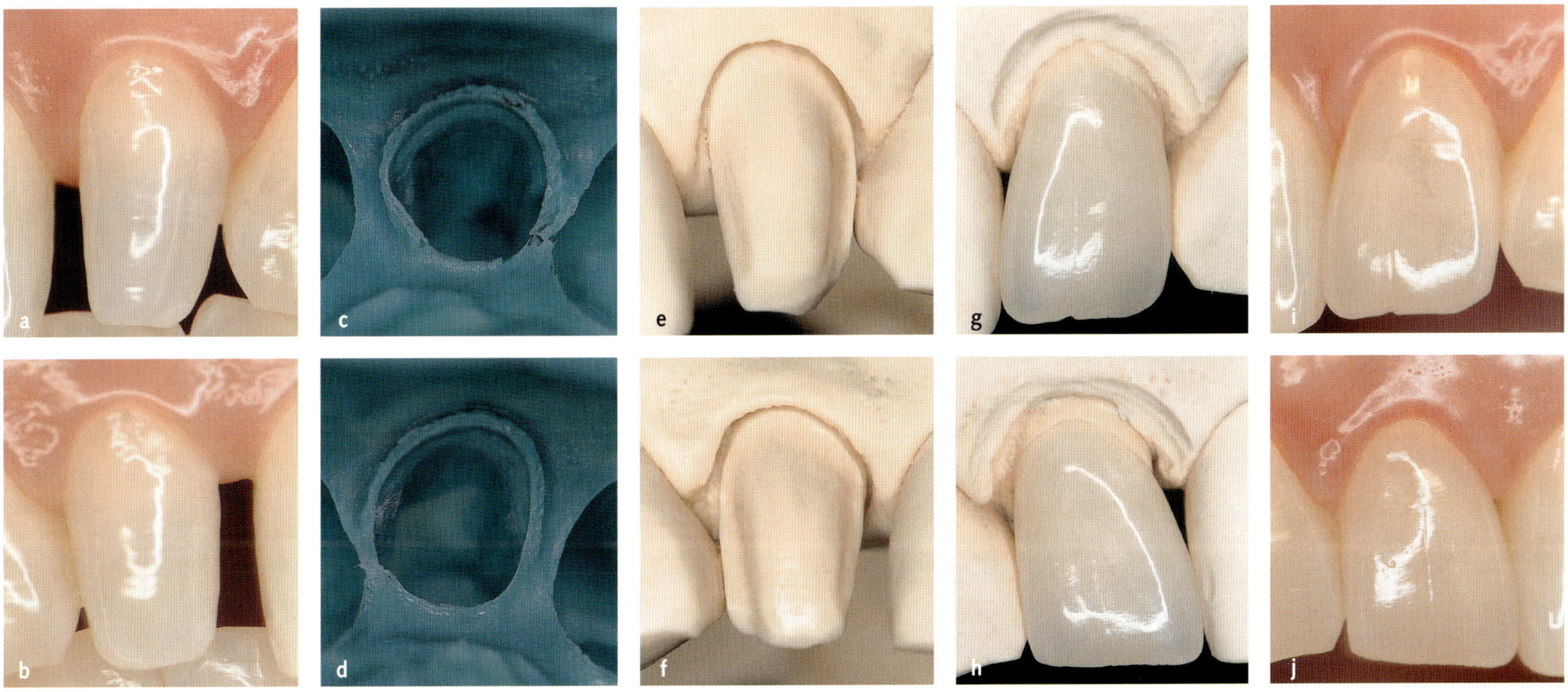

Fig 5-62 (a and b) The maxillary left lateral incisor and maxillary right lateral incisor are microdonts. (c and d) Impression (HIT method). (e and f) Supragingival preparation. (g and h) Porcelain veneers. (Prostheses made by Mr Hitoshi Aoshima, RDT.) (i and j) Photographs taken at delivery of the veneers.

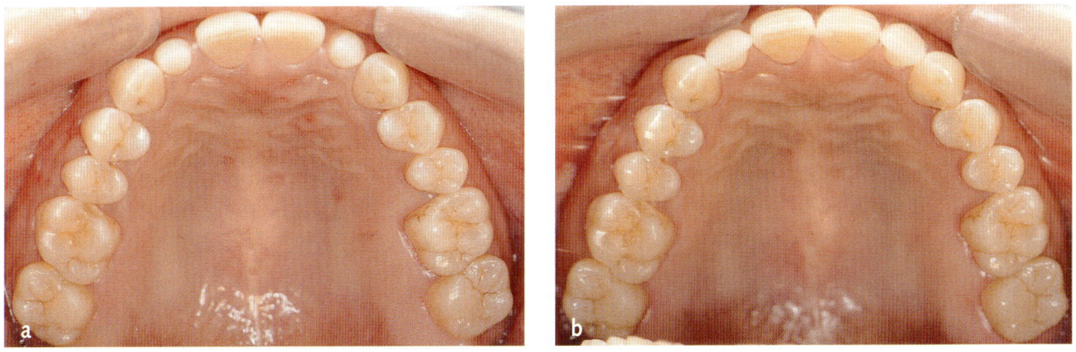

Fig 5-63 (a) Occlusal view of the maxillary arch at the first visit. The occlusal surfaces show signs of advanced attrition. (b) A bite splint has been used to control muscle tension and reshaping has been conducted so that excessive horizontal forces will not be exerted.

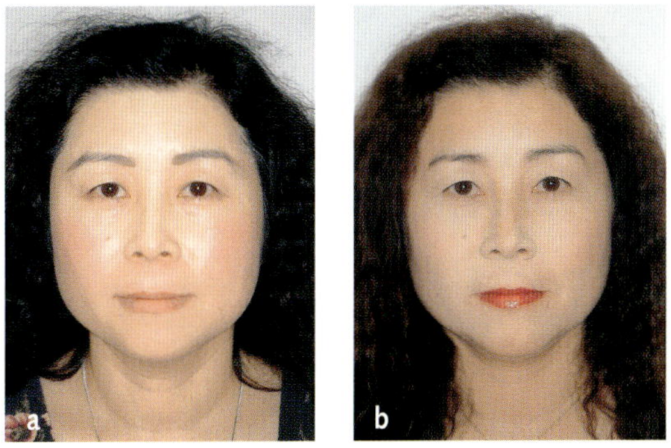

Fig 5-64 (a) Facial appearance at the first visit. (b) Muscle tension has been relieved and the facial appearance is improved.

Preparation and delivery of a dowel post and core

Most of the dislodgments of crowns or cores and root fractures are found to be partly caused by an inappropriate dowel post and core. When coronal tooth structure is collapsed, a tooth cannot be retained without a dowel post and core. A dowel post and core has to fulfill two conflicting roles: namely, reinforcement and conservation of tooth structure. In this sense, a dowel post and core could become a cause of fracture. Accurate diagnosis and proper procedures that follow basic design principles are critical to success.

When sufficient amounts of coronal tooth structure remain, a core buildup with resin composite should be the first choice. In a case with an extensive collapse of the tooth structure, a dowel post and core is indicated, which requires the use of preparation burs of high precision with an air turbine and a contra-angle handpiece, an accurate impression, fabrication of dowel post and core with a good fit, use of a solid cement medium, and proper crown restoration (Figs 5-65 to 5-67).

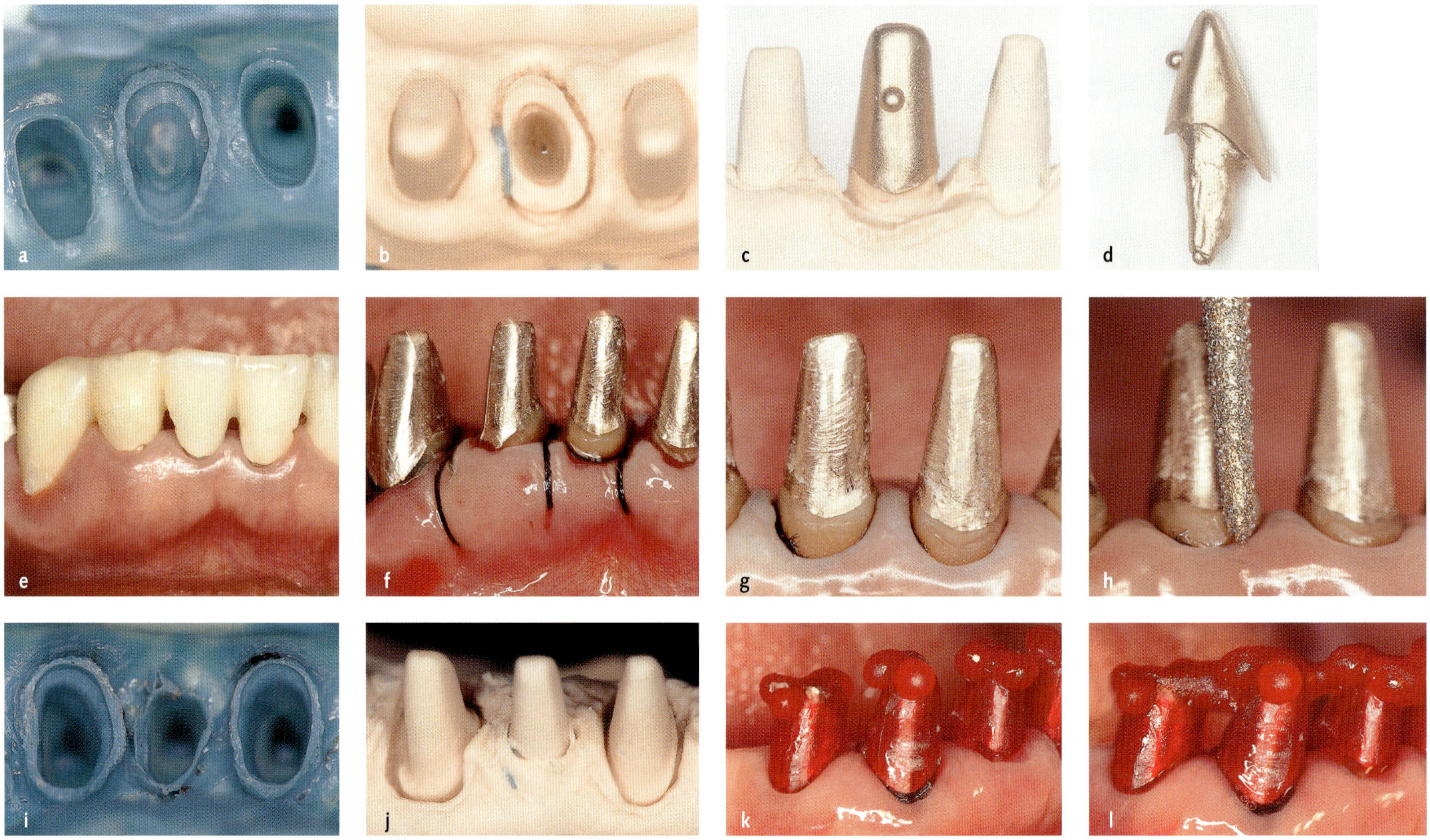

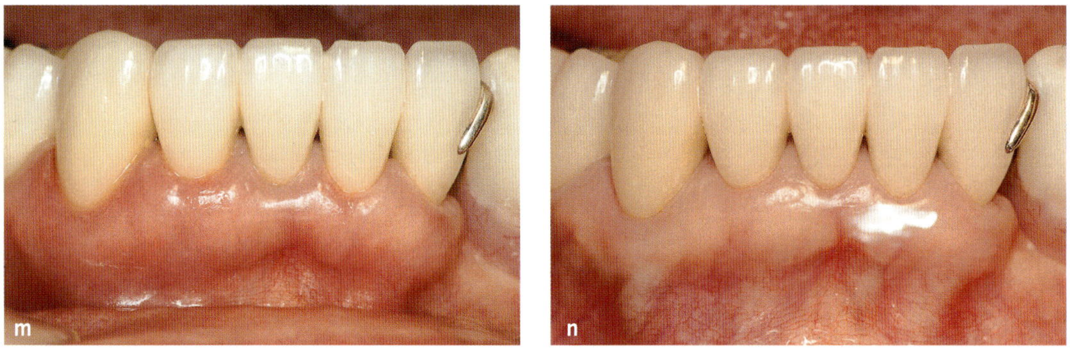

Fig 5-65 (a) Impression. (b) The dowel post and retention form of the table are reproduced on the cast. (c and d) The post and core has been cast with type IV gold after consideration of the material's fit, discoloration, and strength. Adhesive resin cement is used. (e) Photograph of the provisional restoration relatively soon after the first visit. (f) After dowel posts and cores are delivered, a crown-lengthening procedure is conducted. (g and h) Photographs taken about 2 and a half months postsurgery. Thin retraction cord is inserted for protection of the inner marginal epithelium, and the core is prepared in a concentric manner with a No. 5 SJCD bur. (i and j) Double-cord technique. An impression of every other tooth is taken to prevent damage to the interdental papillae. (k and l) Transfer copings. (m) At delivery of the prostheses, a flaring of the periodontal tissue is noted. (n) Because of proper plaque control, the gingiva is stabilized and increased gingival attachment has been obtained.

Figs 5-66 and 5-67 Fabrication of a dowel post and core.

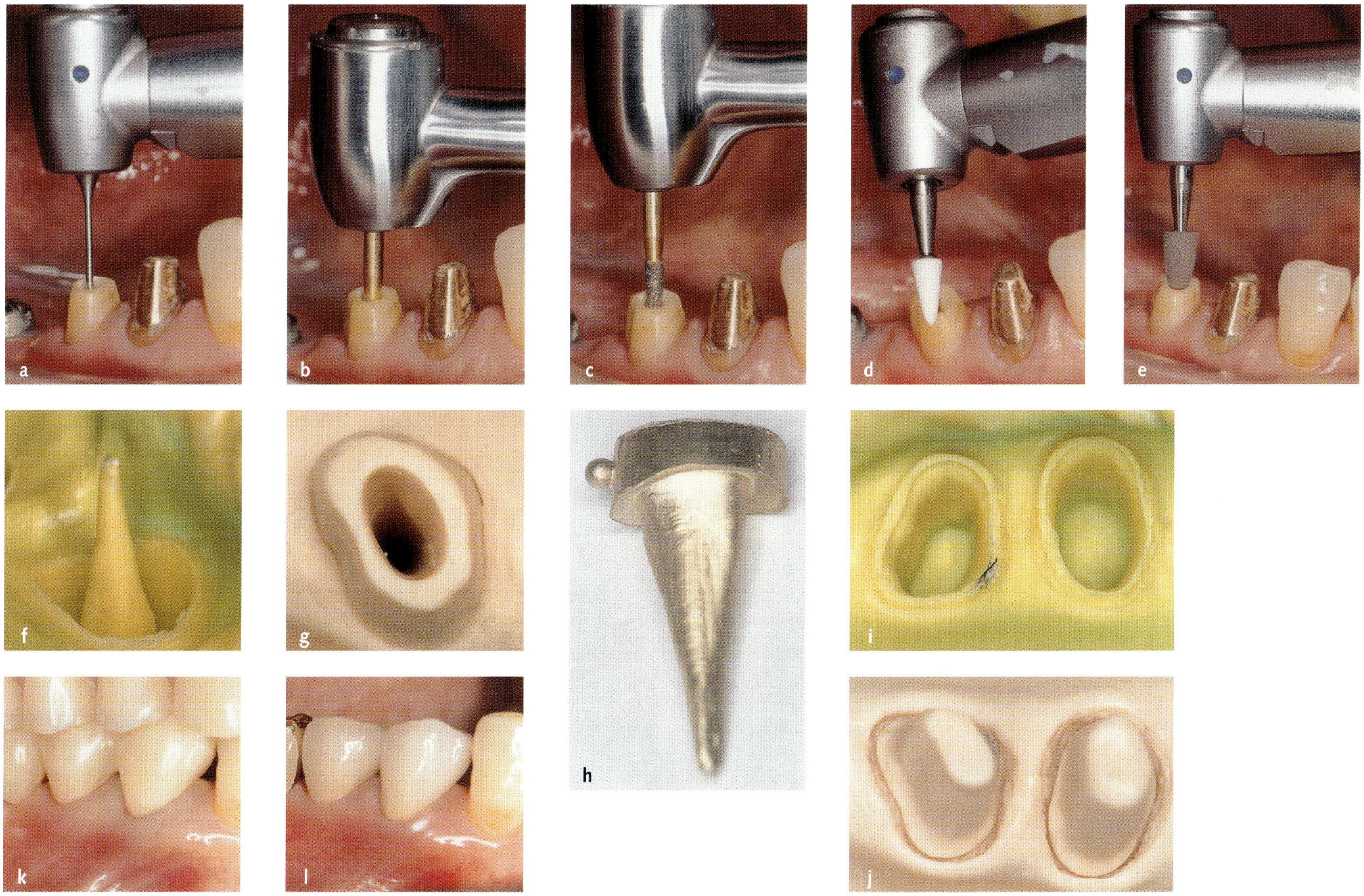

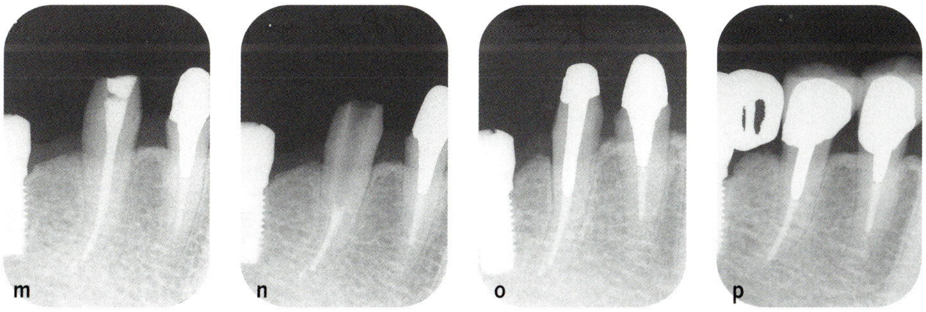

Fig 5-66 (a) A contra-angle is used for drilling. (b and c) A diamond bur (No. 5 SJCD bur) is used for post and core preparation. The preparation design should follow the morphology of the natural root canal and internal tooth reduction should be minimized. (d) A white point is used to polish the inner and outer surfaces, including the ferrule. (e) A silicone point is used for further polishing. (f) HIT silicone impression. (g) Cast obtained from the HIT impression. Note the preciseness and flat surface. The width of the surface creates a vertical stop. (h) Cast dowel post and core of JRVT type III gold alloy, which is bonded with Super-Bond. (i) HIT impression obtained with the double-cord technique after delivery of the dowel post and core. (j) A clear preparation finish line is obtained. (k and l) Provisional restorations and final prostheses. (m) Radiograph taken before preparation of the dowel post and core. (n) Radiographic confirmation is made after root canal preparation. (o) Radiographic confirmation is made at the try-in of the dowel post and core. (p) Final prostheses.

Box 5-2 Attention to ferrules

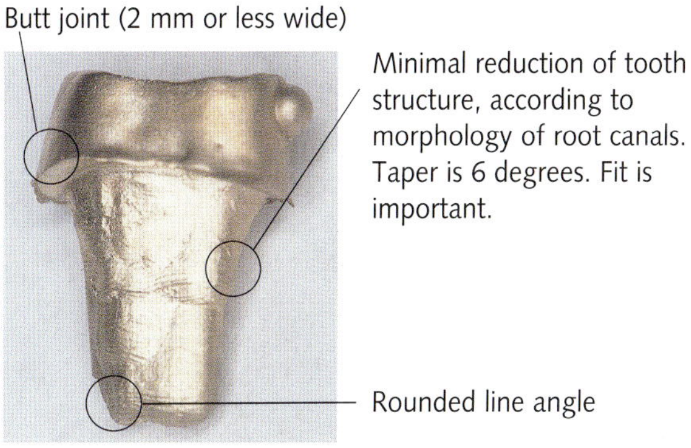

Fig 5-67 Ferrules. The features listed are important to minimizing tooth reduction while reinforcing tooth structure.

Role of Implants in Comprehensive Dentistry

Indications of implants for partially edentulous patients

With the enhancement of the predictability of osseointegration via development of regenerative therapy, the role of implants for partially edentulous patients has expanded greatly. Compared with conventional fixed partial dentures, implants have the advantage that invasive treatment of adjacent teeth is avoided. The scope of the indications for implants is wide. To begin with, they require no adjacent teeth to function. In comparison with tissue-supported removable partial dentures, implants have an advantage in that solid occlusal support and stabilization of the mandibular position are obtained. Consequently, they allow a simple and stable prosthetic design in partially edentulous cases.

Because of these advantages, implants tend to be the first choice for treatment and their usefulness can be taken for granted in treatment planning, although they should be evaluated as one of several possible treatment options.

Importance of comprehensive assessment

There is always some reason behind a missing tooth. Clinicians should begin prosthodontic treatment for edentulism by considering the cause of tooth loss. Other than trauma, the causes for tooth loss may not be simple and probably involve a variety of factors. There should be evaluation from the tooth-unit, dentition-unit, and occlusion-unit perspectives, as well as an assessment of the patient's life and social environment, and the treatment plan should include prosthodontic treatment for partial edentulism.

Therapeutic intervention should always be aimed at achieving maximal therapeutic effect with minimal intervention from these comprehensive viewpoints. Treatment using dental implants is comprehensive in the sense that it requires a mastery of surgery, prosthodontics, periodontology, as well as precision laboratory work. With regard to occlusion, a prudent approach is required. To incorporate implants as a therapeutic option, the practitioner requires not only an excellent diagnostic ability but also a precise grasp of basic dental procedures, such as plaque control, endodontic treatment, restorative preparation, impression procedures, and delivery of appliances. Because osseointegrated implants do not have a periodontal ligament as a stress breaker, they require precise prosthodontic procedures. Crown restorations are to be made on artificial abutments in the edentulous area, and there are always challenges in terms of maintainability and esthetics. Communication with the laboratory must be detailed; otherwise, it is most unlikely that an implant prosthesis with excellent esthetics and high precision will be fabricated.

Preservation of natural teeth versus placement of implants

A tooth with a significantly damaged crown is now often considered for extraction and immediate implant replacement rather than for conventional restoration. The explanation that is given is that, compared to tooth extraction and fixed partial denture restoration, an implant treatment saves the enamel of both of the adjacent teeth. However, there are many alternative treatments that can be completed without extraction of the tooth, and the prognoses of these treatments are good.

It is also often suggested that a molar with a class II furcation involvement should be extracted and replaced by an implant. If maintenance is insufficient, the exposed root surface may be less predictable than an implant. However, a therapeutic intervention to extract a molar with a furcation involvement and replacement it with an implant cannot not be justified solely on the basis of class II furcation involvement.

The prognosis of teeth with furcation involvement is uncertain, but sound predictability can be obtained depending on the level of maintenance. A case in point is that of a patient who dropped out of routine management and who had not been examined for more than 10 years but experienced no change in the dental conditions. Many methods of periodontal treatment are available. If predictability is less than ideal, a comprehensive judgment should be made, based on the speech, mastication, esthetics, proprioceptive sensation, maintainability, treatment duration, and cost to the patient. The clinician must consider which foreign body, an exposed root furcation area or an implant, is a better choice for the sake of the patient.

Single-tooth replacement in the anterior area

In contrast to a fixed partial denture, which requires a sacrifice of abutment teeth, implants do not require a sacrifice of sound tooth structure. In a single-tooth case, in which tooth loss was caused by an accident or another reason, recovery of the esthetics is relatively easy and the prognosis is good. An implant surpasses a fixed partial denture in terms of long-term viability (Fig 5-68).

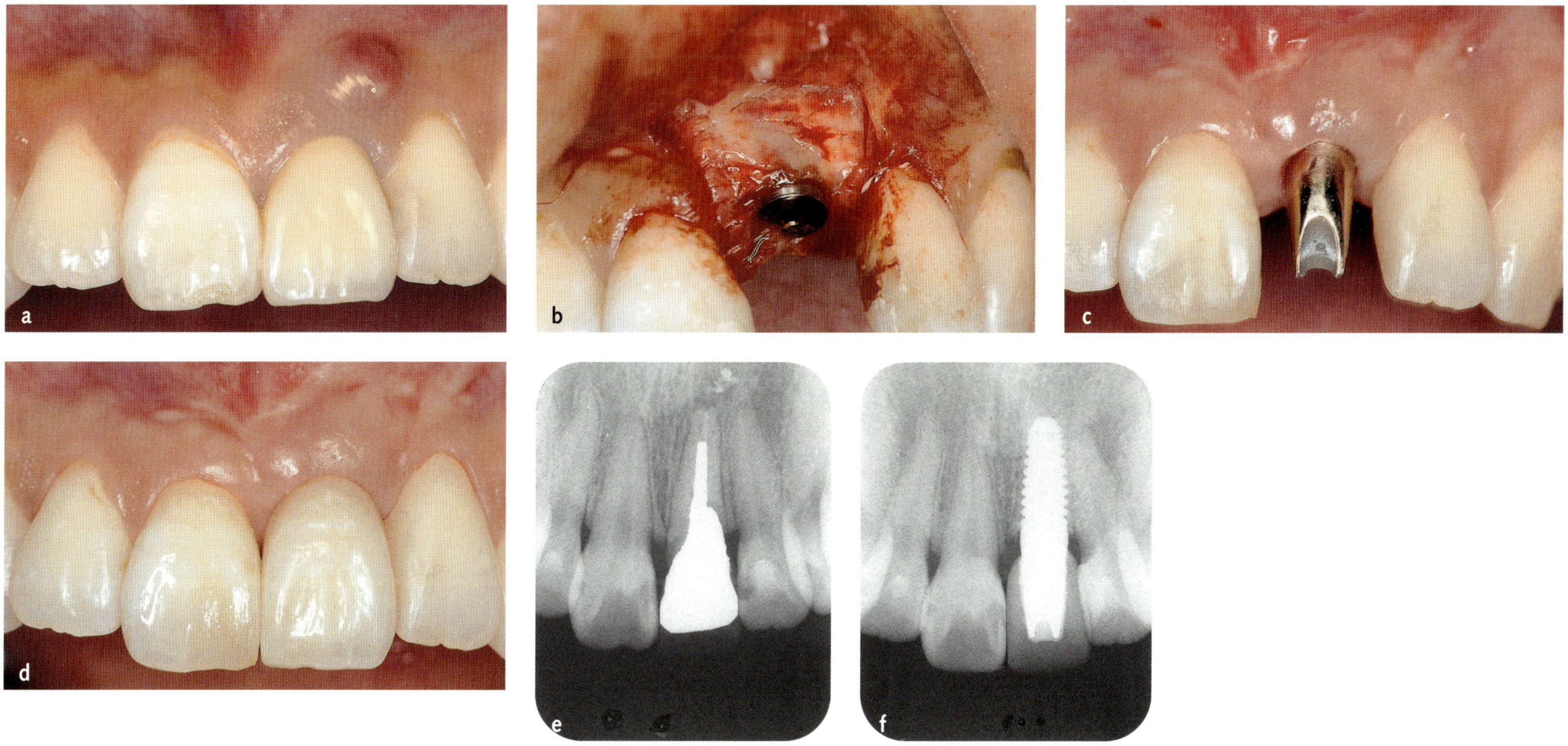

Fig 5-68 (a) At the first visit, the maxillary left central incisor has a root fracture accompanied by subgingival dental caries. After an incision was made to drain an abscess and the inflammation was controlled, the tooth was extracted. (b) Photograph taken 2 months postextraction. A screw-vent implant (4.7 × 13.0-mm) is placed with a combination of guided bone regeneration (GBR) techniques (bone graft and resorbable membrane). Five months postsurgery, a secondary surgery was completed. Bone regeneration was confirmed. (c) After gingival healing, a UCLA abutment (3i) was seated. A provisional restoration was fabricated and worn until maturation of the gingiva was complete, at which time a direct impression was taken. (d) The final all-ceramic crown is in harmony with the maxillary right central incisor. (Prostheses made by Mr Kazunari Ohata, RDT.) (e) At the first visit, subgingival caries and a root fracture are evident in the maxillary left central incisor. There is also a periapical lesion. (f) At delivery of the prosthesis, 1 year 11 months after the first visit, bone regeneration can be confirmed.

Recovery of stable mandibular positions in partially edentulous patients

Increased reliability of implants in partially edentulous cases has affected treatment planning for Class I and II distal extension cases. Loss of molar occlusal support causes changes in the mandibular position in many patients. In the case shown in Figs 5-69 to 5-73, the increase in interdental space in the maxillary anterior teeth tells us there is a change in the mandibular position. A distal extension RPD does not result in long-term stabilization of the mandibular position. Implants contribute significantly to the stabilization of the mandibular position as well as to the recovery of the masticatory forces and comfort. In mandibular molar areas, because the bone and keratinized mucosa are likely to be lost as teeth are extracted, it is more difficult to restore continuity of the cervical margins.

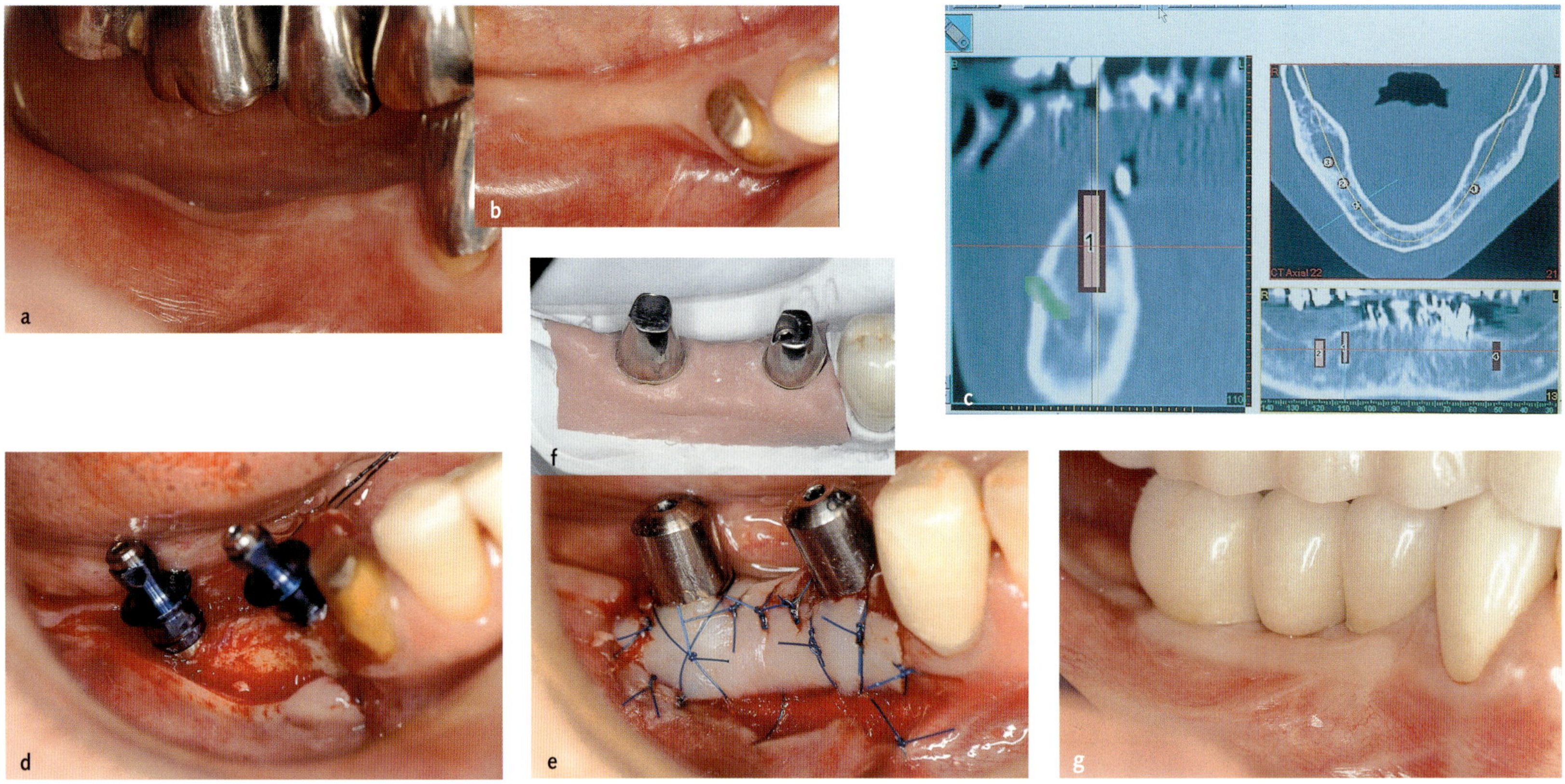

Fig 5-69 Right side of the mandibular arch. (a and b) Right side at the first visit. Resorption of the buccal bone on the ridge is conspicuous. (c) Computed tomography (CT) confirms that there is an adequate volume of bone. The information about the appropriate depth and angulation for implant placement is obtained accurately before surgery. (d) Two Osseotite implants (3.75 × 8.50 mm, 3i) are placed. (e) Three months after implant placement, a free gingival graft is completed to increase the keratinized mucosa and to expand the vestibule. (f) Porcelain is fused to the emergence of the abutments to prevent a shadow effect at the cervical area. (g) Photograph taken about 1 year after delivery of final prostheses, 4 years 6 months after the first visit. The implant-supported fixed partial denture has an ovate pontic at the mandibular right first molar.

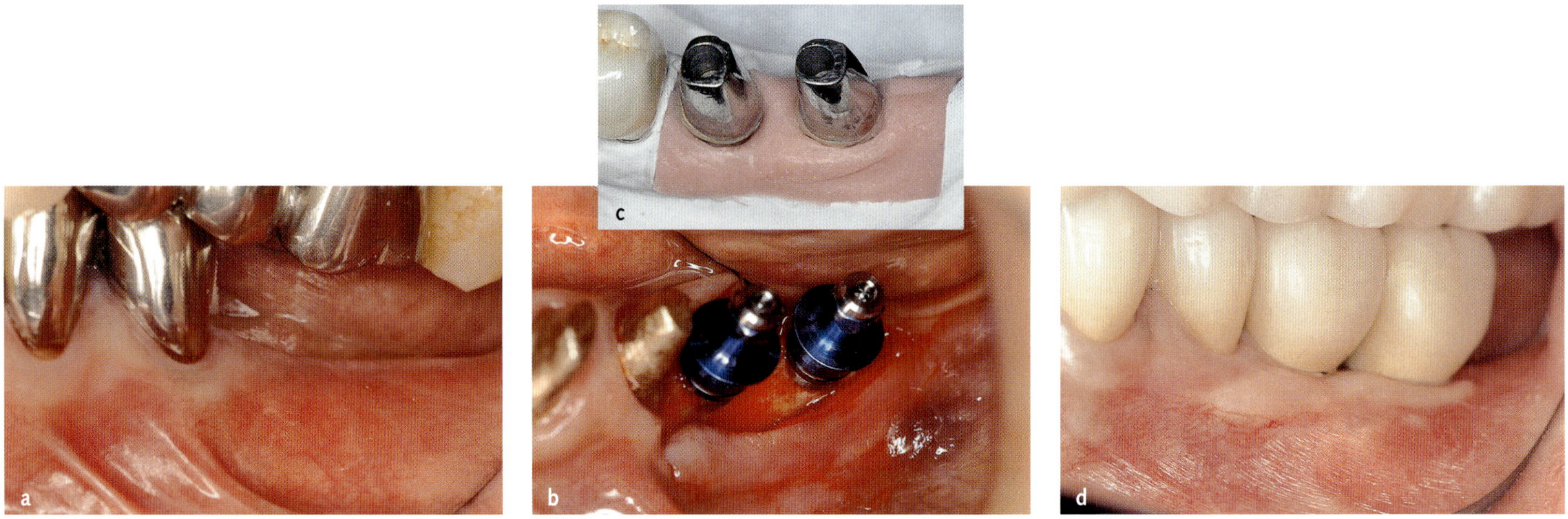

Fig 5-70 Left side of the mandibular arch. (a) At the first visit, ridge resorption and loss of keratinized immobile mucosa are noted. (b) Two Miniplant implants (3.25 × 8.50 mm, 3i) are placed. (c) As with the right side, porcelain is fused to the emergence of the abutment. (d) Photograph taken about 2 years after treatment. (Prostheses made by Mr Chojiro Masuda, RDT.)

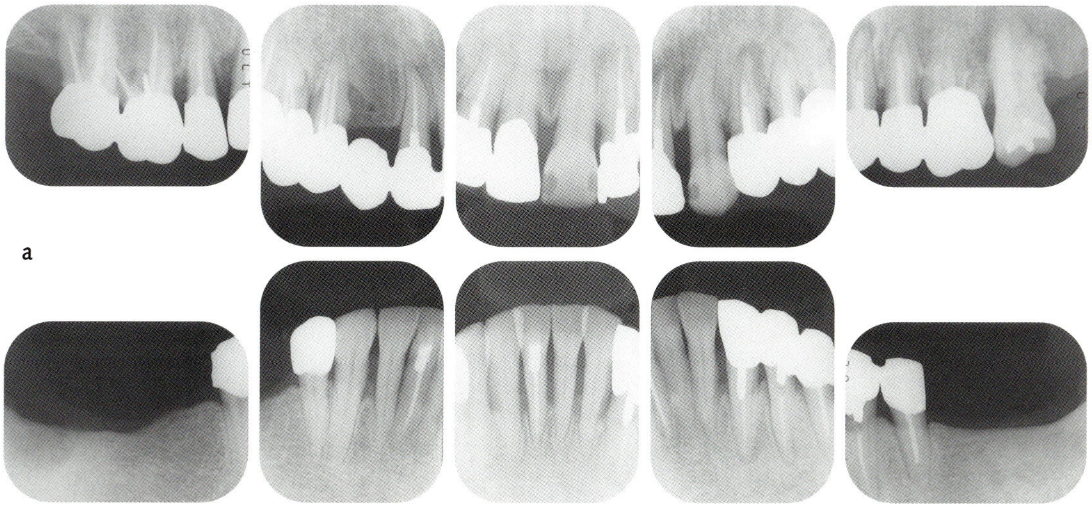

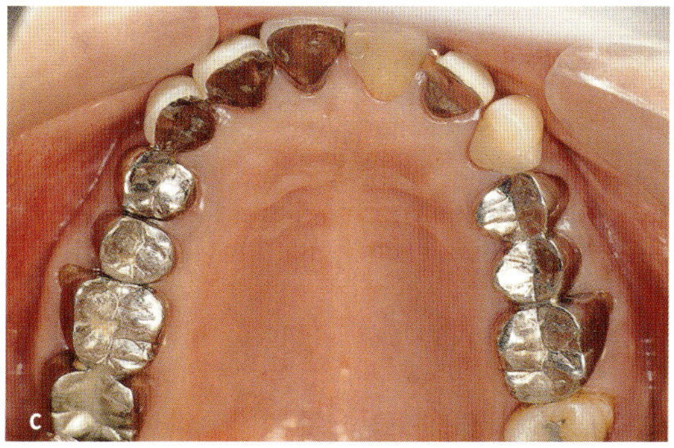

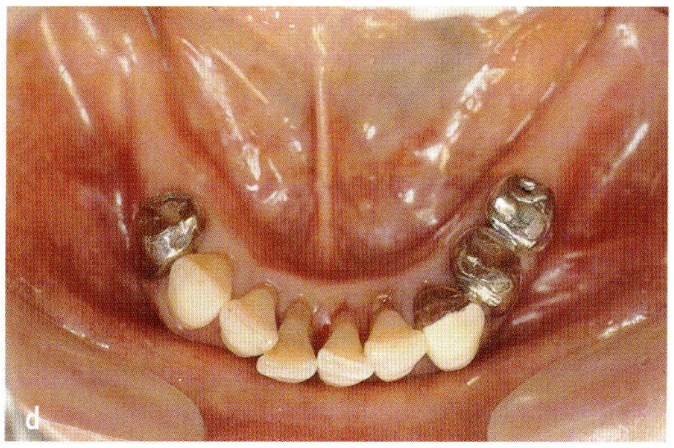

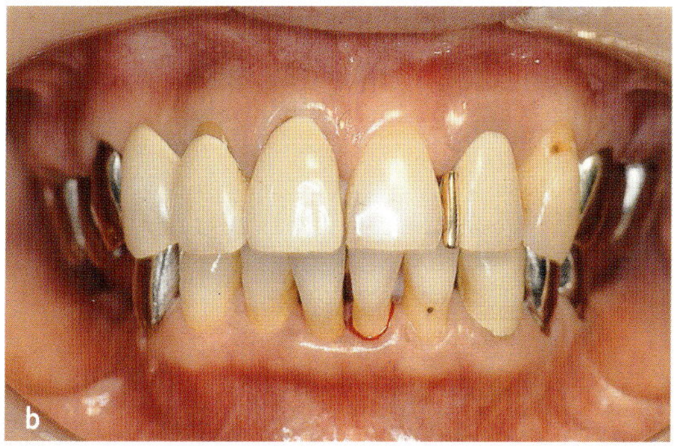

Fig 5-71 At the first visit. (a and b) Moderate periodontal disease is present at the first visit (1997). The mandibular left first and second molars and the mandibular right second premolar, first molar, and second molar are missing. Poorly filled root canals are evident in all of the teeth treated with root canal therapy. (c and d) A narrowed maxillary arch form is noted. The asymmetry suggests a recurrent habit of posture.

Fig 5-72 Probing chart.

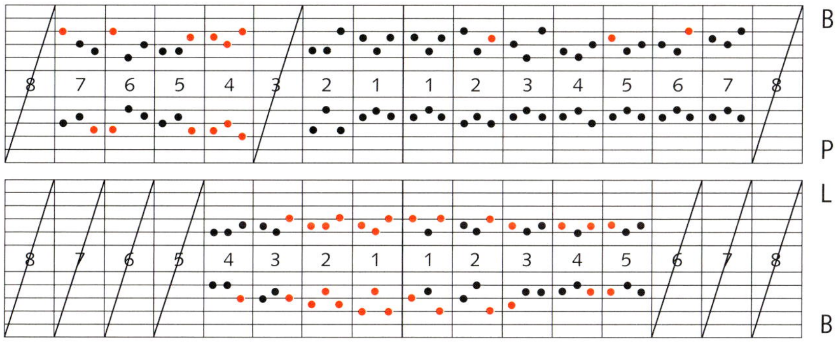

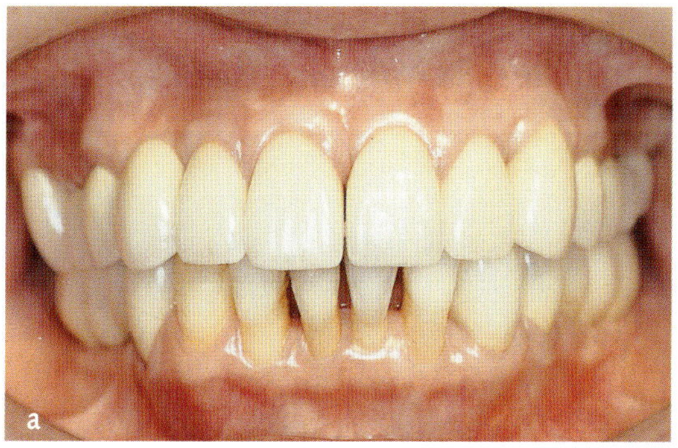

Fig 5-73 (a to d) Periodontal prostheses during maintenance, about 1 year after delivery of final prostheses.

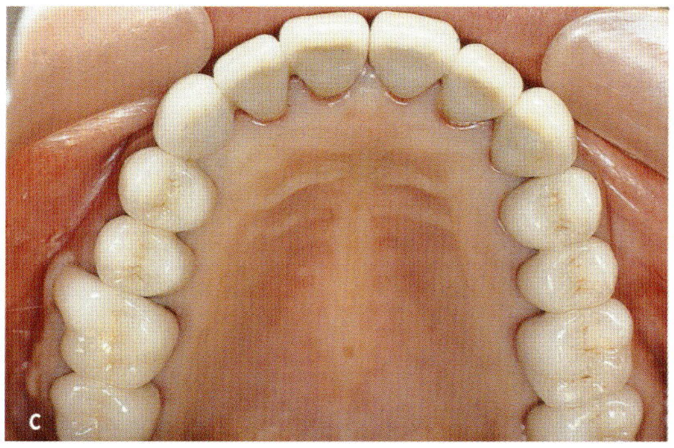

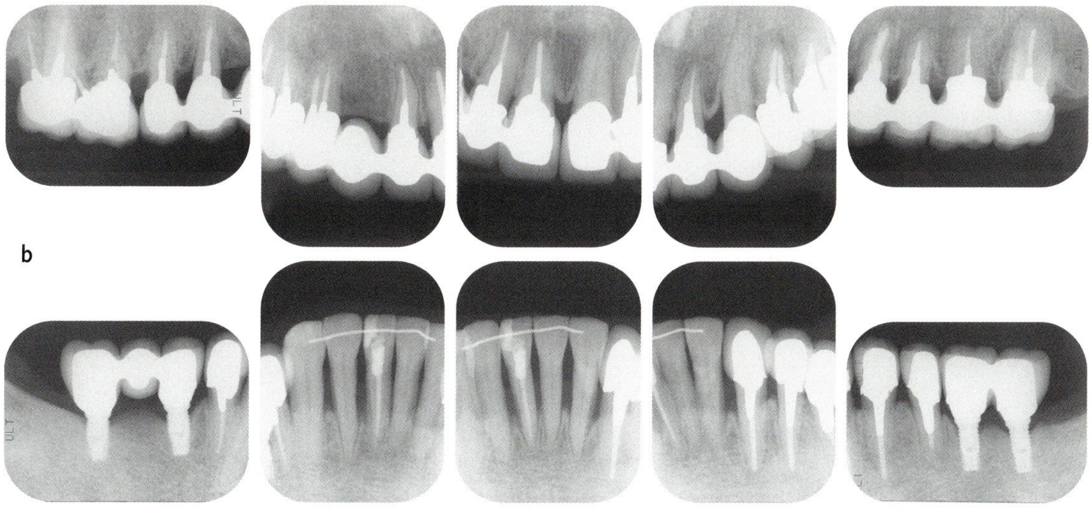

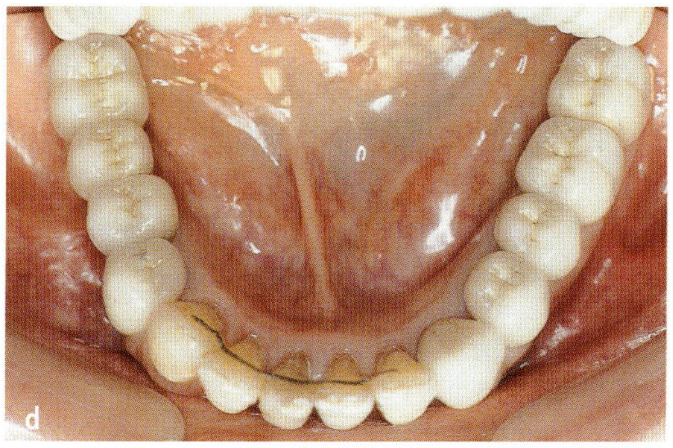

Case 5-2 Restorative measures for a patient with a loss of periodontal support

Patient: *44-year-old woman at the time of first visit in 2000*
Chief complaint: *Inability to chew hard food because of pain in the maxillary left second molar and mandibular right second molar*
There were deep pockets on the proximal surfaces of the teeth, which were not obvious at the initial examination. There were also deep defects of the interalveolar septa. The buccal and lingual cortical plates were not significantly affected, and the bone loss was difficult to see on the radiographs. Deposits on the root surfaces were not conspicuous; however, a significant amount of purulent exudate was noted. The patient was young, and recession and mobility were minimal. She was not aware of any pathologic conditions. Once treatment was started, the management of this case became challenging, not only because of her esthetic needs but also because of the inevitable loss of teeth. To improve the chances for maintenance and recovery of the function and esthetics of her teeth, implants had to be considered (Figs 5-74 to 5-84).

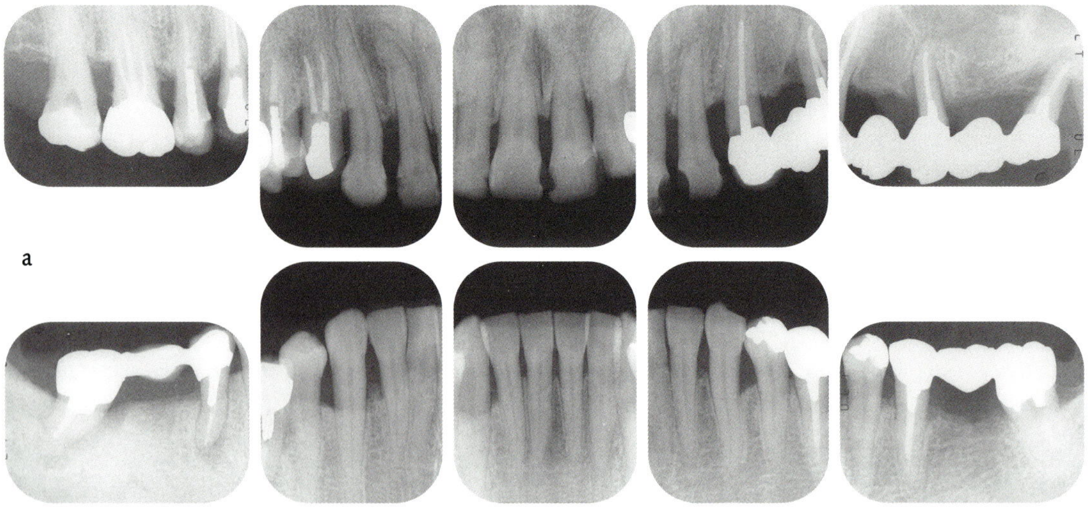
a

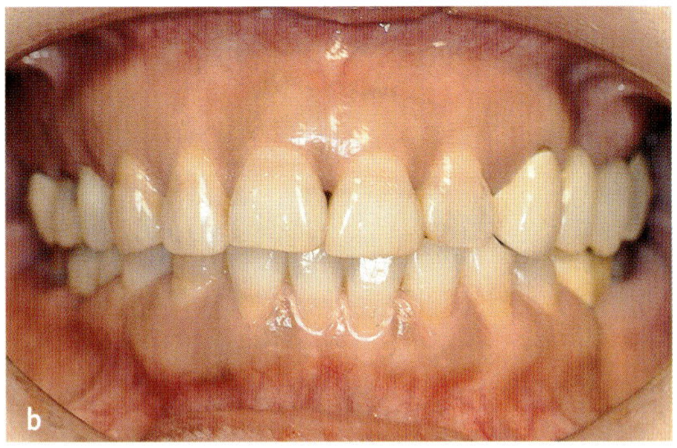
b

Fig 5-74 (a and b) At the first visit, severe destruction of the periodontal tissue is noted. The occlusal plane is disturbed, and the dentition is shifted to the left. Radiographs show moderate to severe bone loss for all the teeth. Secondary occlusal trauma is noted. The maxillary left second molar and mandibular right second molar have a degree 3 mobility and are hopeless. There is root fracture of the mandibular right second premolar.

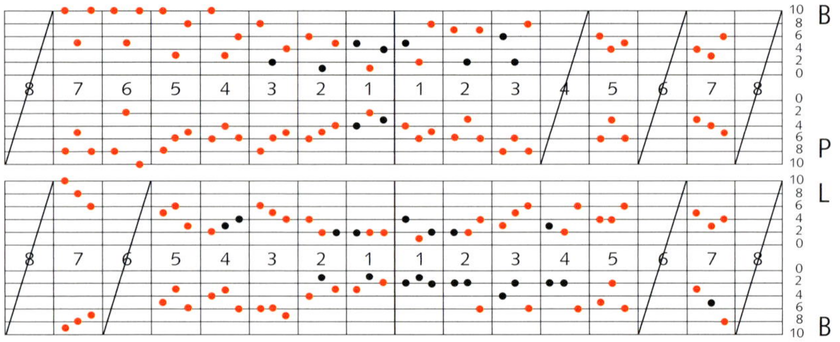

Fig 5-75 Probing chart at the first visit.

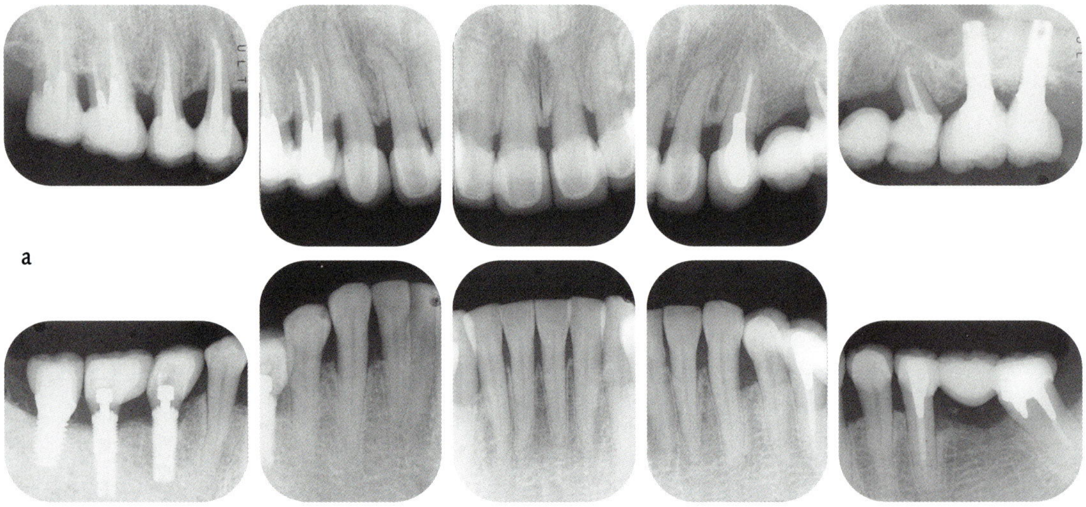
a

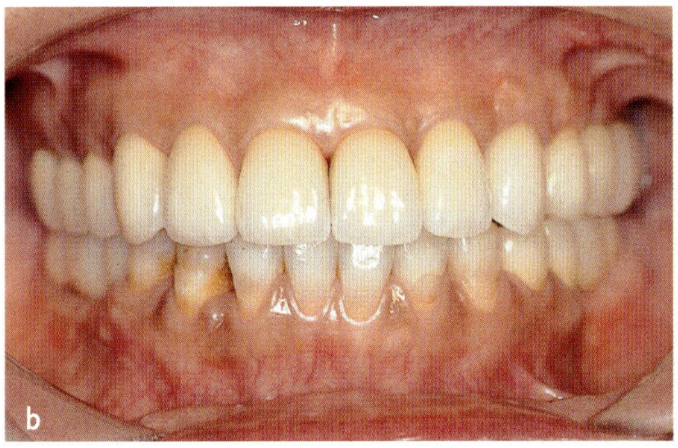
b

Fig 5-76 (a) Radiographs show improvement in bone and disappearance of periodontal concerns, with an overall improvement in the dentition, 2 years 6 months after the patient's first visit. Regenerative therapy, extrusion of the maxillary left canine, and implant placement at the sites of the maxillary left first and second molars and mandibular right second premolar, first molar, and second molar have been completed to recover molar occlusal support. (b) Periodontal prostheses. The prostheses are all-ceramic crowns.

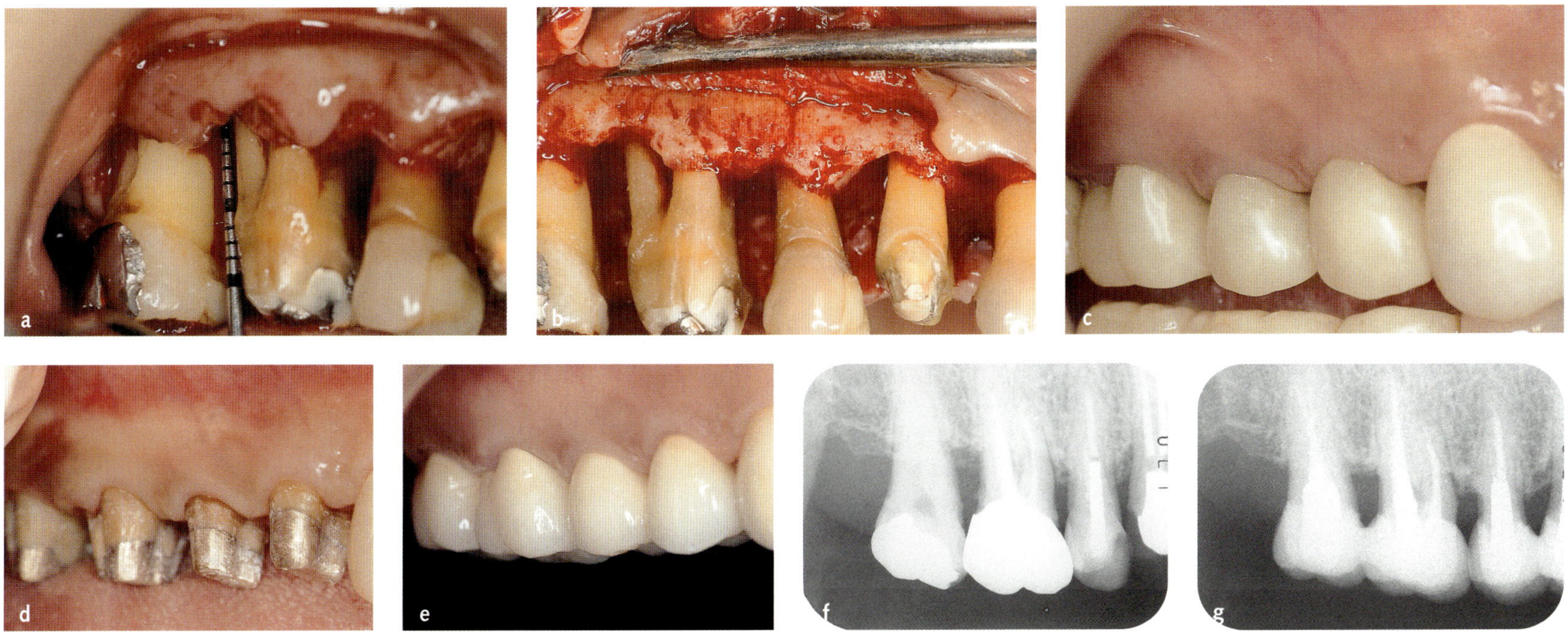

Fig 5-77 Regenerative therapy (with Emdogain) for molar infrabony defects. (a and b) Attachment loss at the maxillary right first premolar, second premolar, first molar, and second molar is about 10 mm. The infrabony defect is 5 mm and almost a two-wall defect. The maxillary right first and second molars have class II furcation involvements. Thorough debridement was completed and regenerative therapy with Emdogain alone was attempted. (c) Final provisional restoration. (d) Over the next 5 months, endodontic treatments and dowel posts and cores were completed while we awaited maturation of the periodontal tissue and occlusal function (mandibular position) with the provisional restorations. (e) Final all-ceramic prostheses. (f) Radiograph at the first visit. (g) After the delivery of final restoration.

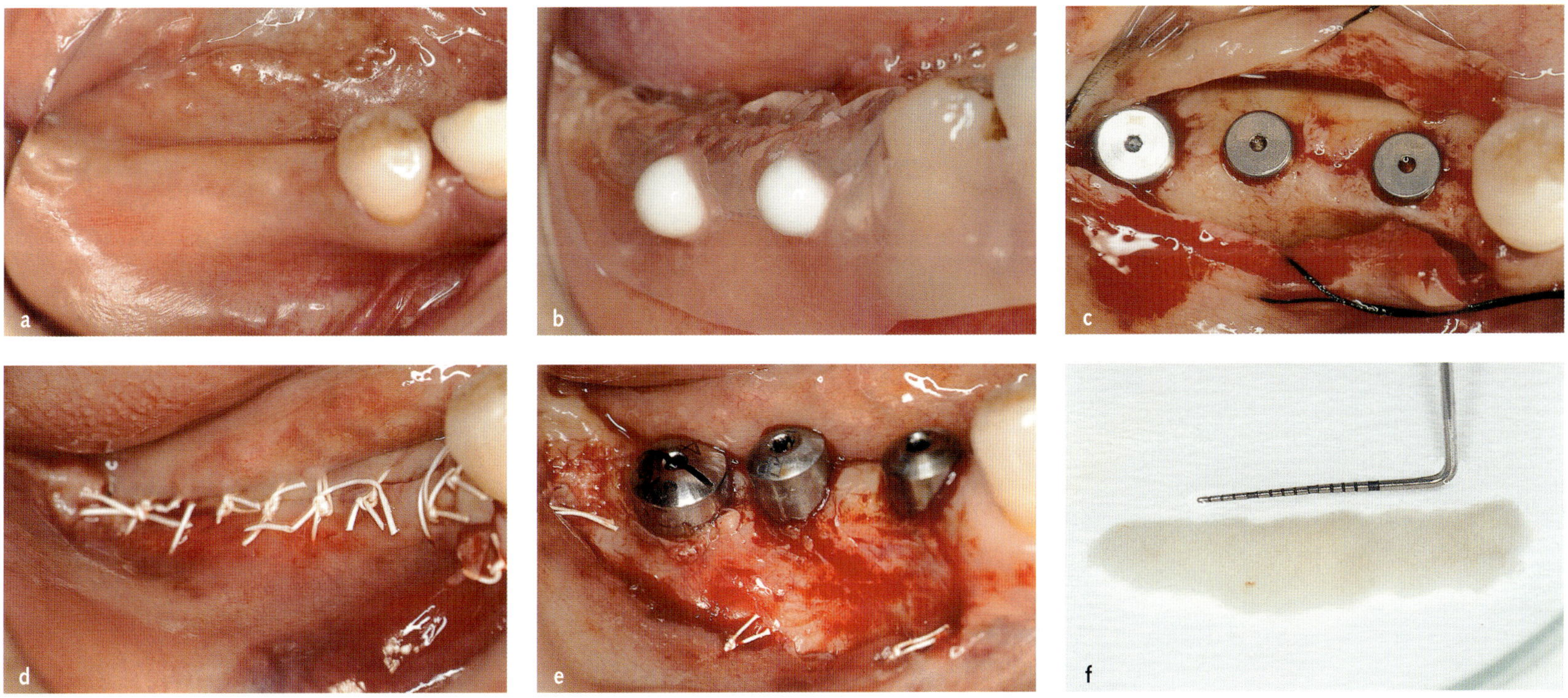

Fig 5-78 Establishment of occlusal support with implants. (a) Implants are to be placed in the area of the mandibular right second premolar, first molar, and second molar. One year had passed since extraction, and sufficient bone volume has been confirmed. (b) CT examination with a stent on. (c) Using CT images and the stent as a guidance, a 4.0 × 11.5-mm implant for the second premolar, a 4.0 × 13.0-mm implant for the first molar, and a 5.0 × 8.5-mm implant for the second molar were placed. (d) Releasing incisions are made to allow closure of the wound without tension or excess tissue. (e) At the second surgery (after 6 months), a vestibular extension surgery places fixed mucosa in the place of mobile mucosa, enhancing maintainability. The area between the second premolar and first molar has keratinized epithelium, which is formed to a papilla-like shape. (f) A free gingival graft is harvested from the ipsilateral palatal region.

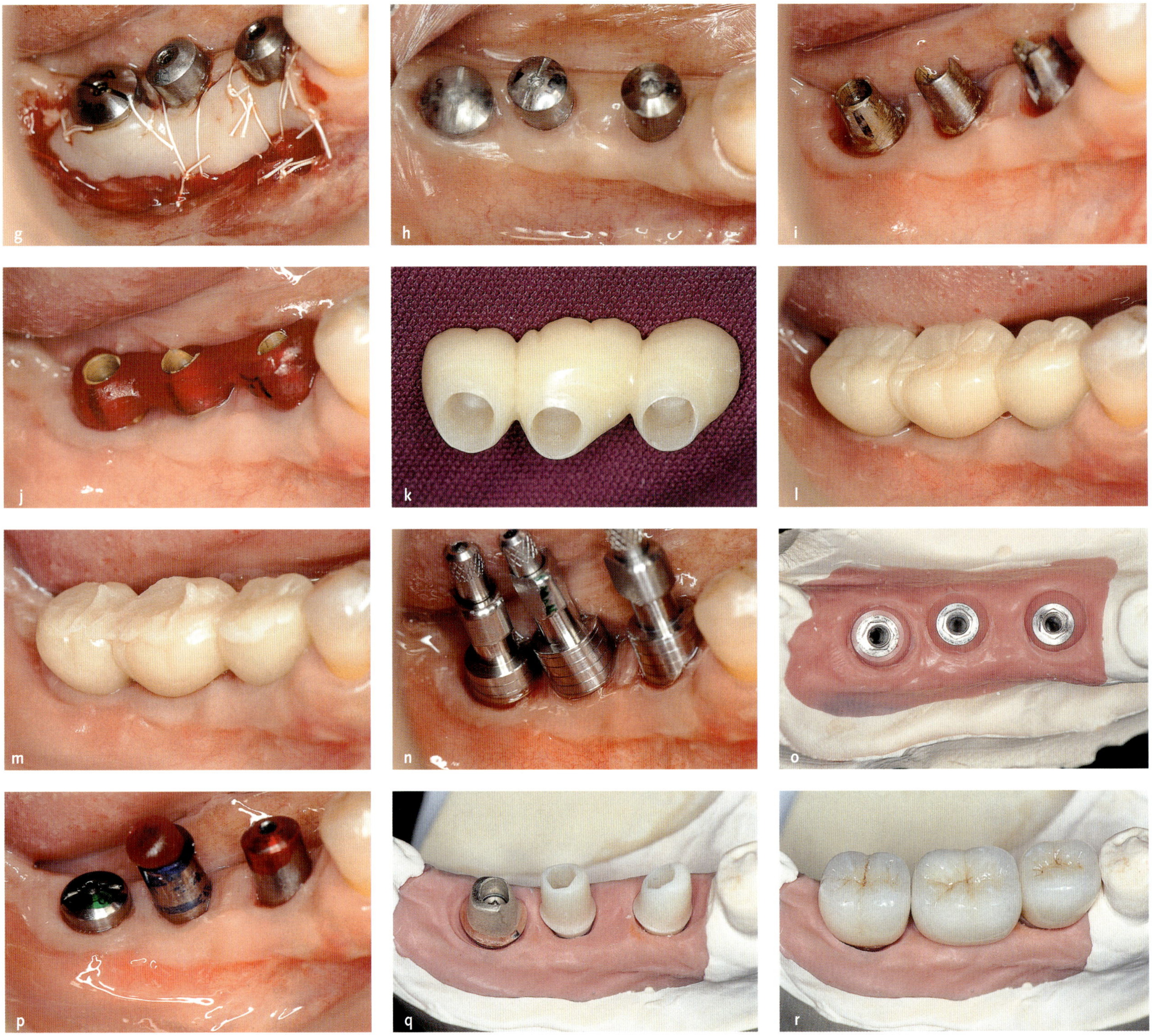

Fig 5-78 (cont) (g) A free gingival graft is completed by trimming the free gingiva in a scalloped shape to adapt to the shape of the interdental papilla–like tissue that is to be created between the implants. (h) Photograph taken 3 months after surgery. (i to l) Photographs taken 4 months after surgery. Healing abutments are replaced by provisional abutments to allow for maturation of the surrounding tissue. (m) As the superstructure facilitates mastication, the chewing path becomes more vertical, which should not be overlooked. Autopolymerizing resin is added in a trial-and-error manner to adapt to the changes in the position of the mandible. It is important to capture the natural changes and adapt the appliances to them. (n and o) After about a 3-month observation period to confirm remodeling, a pick-up impression for the implants is completed. Subgingival (submucosal) morphology should be captured as accurately as possible. (p) Healing abutments are used for registration of an appropriate mandibular position. (q) CerAdapt porcelain abutments are utilized for the mandibular right second premolar and first molar, and a UCLA abutment (3i) is utilized for the second molar. (r) Procera all-ceramic single crowns.

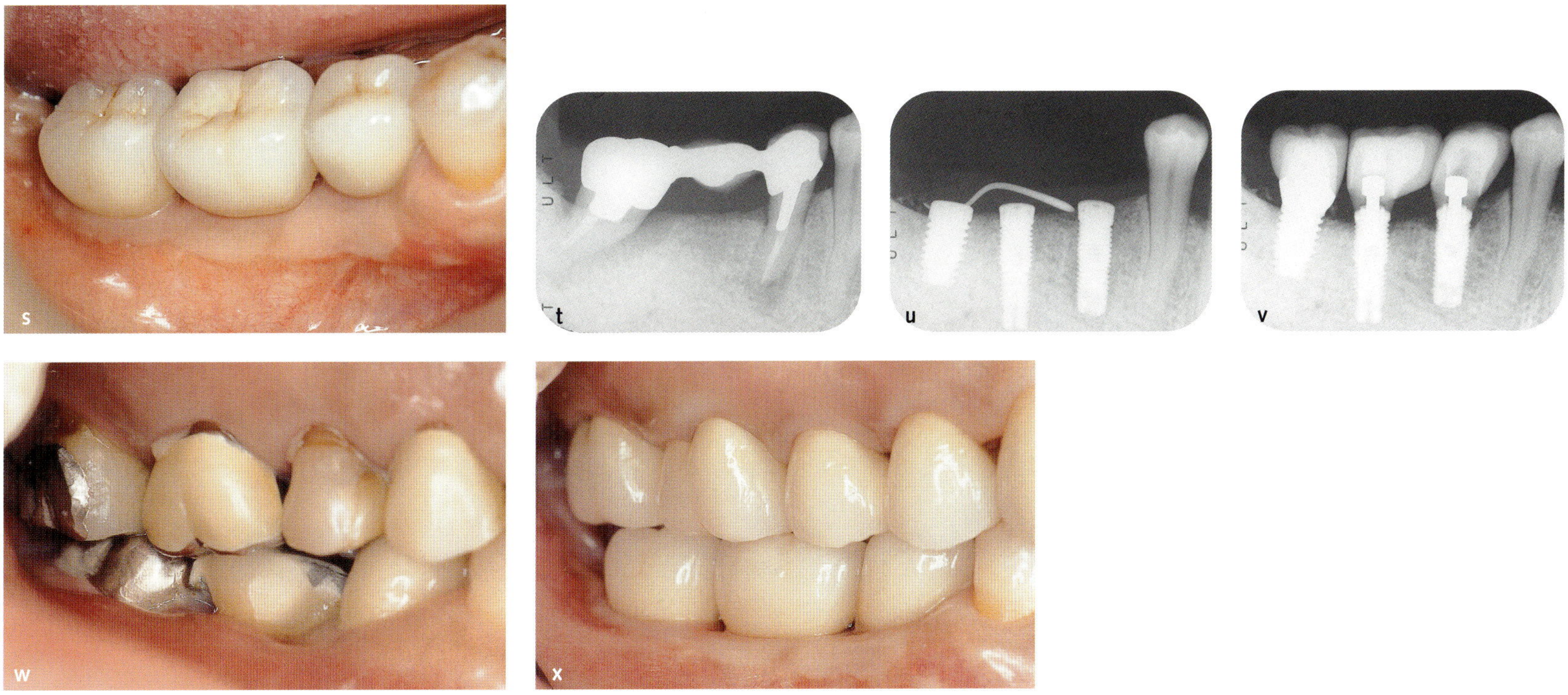

Fig 5-78 (cont) (s) A pick-up impression is taken to modify or correct the subgingival (submucosal) morphology. The prostheses are temporarily cemented after glazing. (t) Radiograph taken at first visit. (u) Implants have replaced the second premolar, first molar, and second molar, 1 year postextraction. (v) Porcelain abutments have been placed for the second premolar and first molar, and a UCLA abutment has been placed for the second molar. (w) Photograph taken at the first visit. (x) In-Ceram all-ceramic periodontal prostheses have been fabricated for the maxillary right first premolar, second premolar, first molar, and second molar. Procera single crowns have been fabricated as superstructures for the implants replacing the mandibular right second premolar, first molar, and second molar.

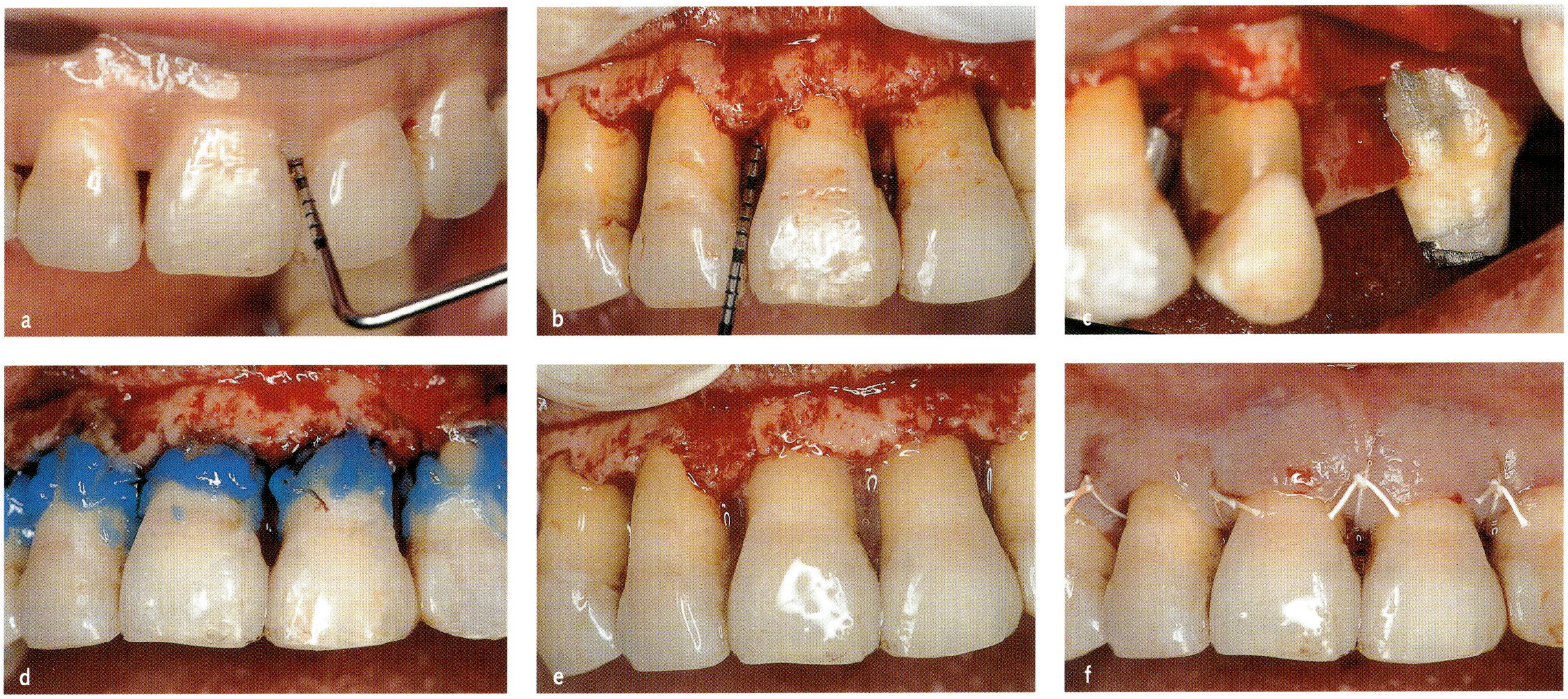

Fig 5-79 Treatment for anterior infrabony defects to improve esthetics. (a) At the first visit, the attachment loss is 6 to 8 mm. (b and c) There are three- and two-wall infrabony defects (4 to 5 mm). The maxillary left second premolar has a bony defect approaching the apex. (d to f) In an attempt to regenerate attachment, Emdogain is applied and flaps are tightly sutured.

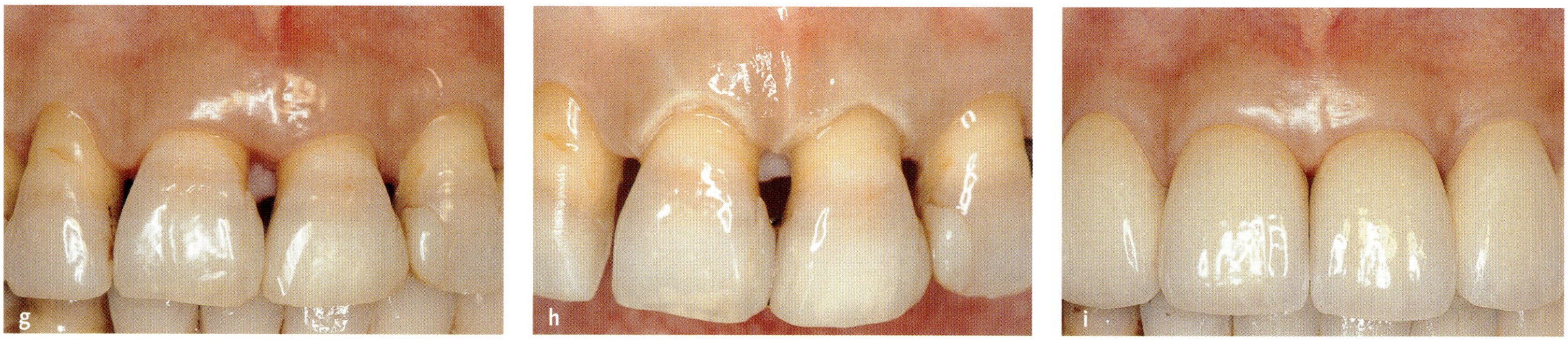

Fig 5-79 (cont) (g) After 6 months, although periodontal tissue is improved, there is conspicuous recession of the interdental papillae. (h) To even the gingival level, approximately 2 mm is trimmed at the maxillary central incisors, to create a scalloped shape without invading the biologic width. (i) Subgingival preparation was completed, and remargination of the provisional restoration was carefully repeated to achieve the appropriate subgingival contour. In-Ceram all-ceramic crowns have been delivered. Morphologic correction has been made, because a black triangle was noted at try-in.

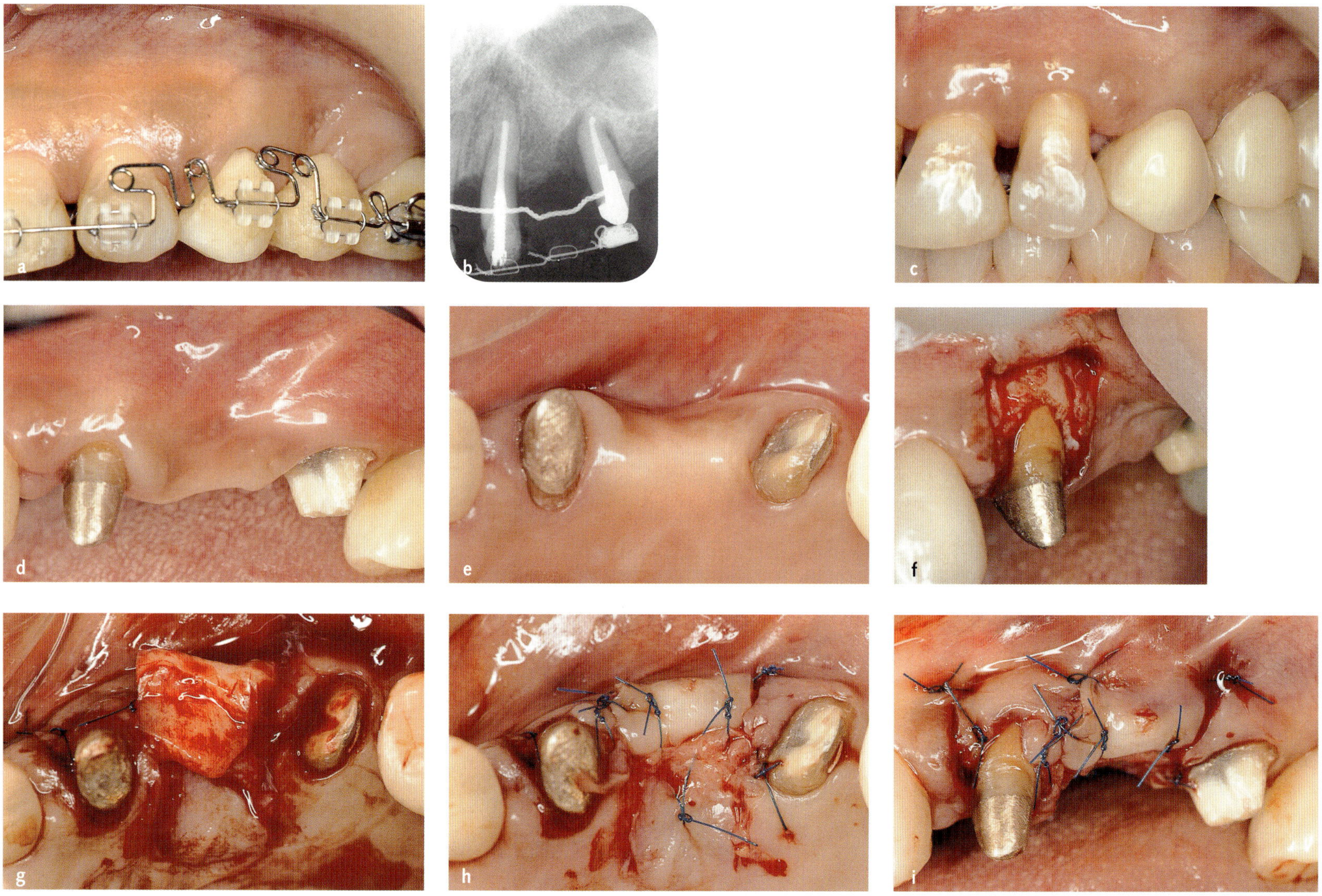

Fig 5-80 Failure in orthodontic extrusion and recovery. (a and b) To restore the subgingival caries lesion affecting the maxillary left canine, orthodontic extrusion of the maxillary left canine was conducted with anchorage at the maxillary right central incisor, left central incisor, and left second premolar. However, when used for anchorage, the maxillary left second premolar developed a problem. (c) Regenerative therapy has caused a large embrasure space, creating a disharmony in the cervical margin at the maxillary left canine. With this situation, it would be difficult to maintain morphology, esthetics, and long-term hygiene. (d and e) With informed consent from the patient, a correction was made to the ridge defect (Seibert class I defect). (f) Because of the severe discrepancy in the cervical margin at the maxillary left lateral incisor, canine, and first premolar, clinical crown lengthening was completed for the maxillary left canine, combining full- and partial-thickness flaps. (g) For the ridge defect at the maxillary left first premolar, the palatal connective tissue is rolled and a partial-thickness flap is elevated to the buccal side. (h and i) A modified roll technique is used to complete buccal soft tissue augmentation.

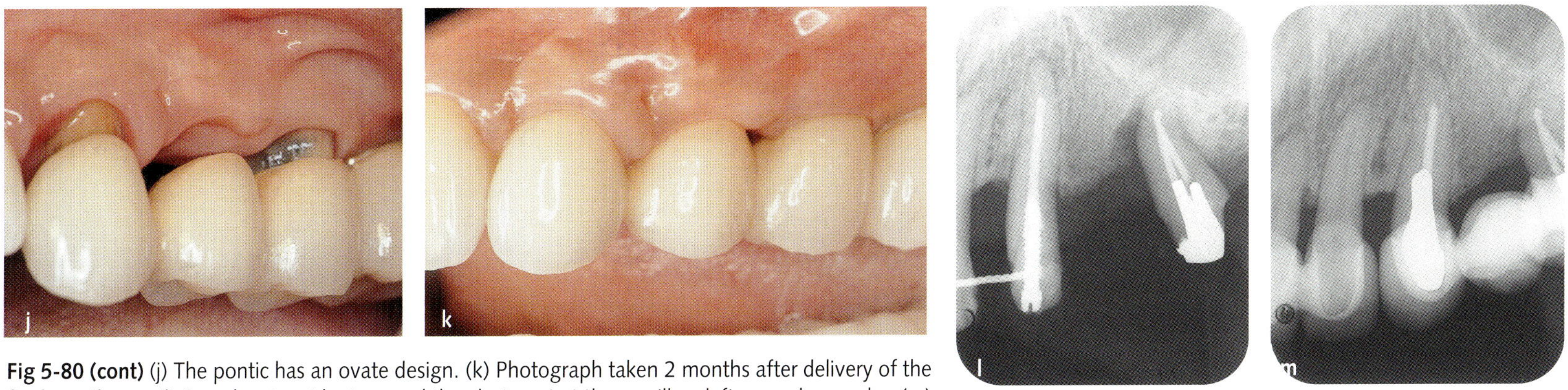

Fig 5-80 (cont) (j) The pontic has an ovate design. (k) Photograph taken 2 months after delivery of the final prostheses. (l) Bone loss is evident around the abutment at the maxillary left second premolar. (m) Bone regeneration is observed 1 year 9 months after application of Emdogain.

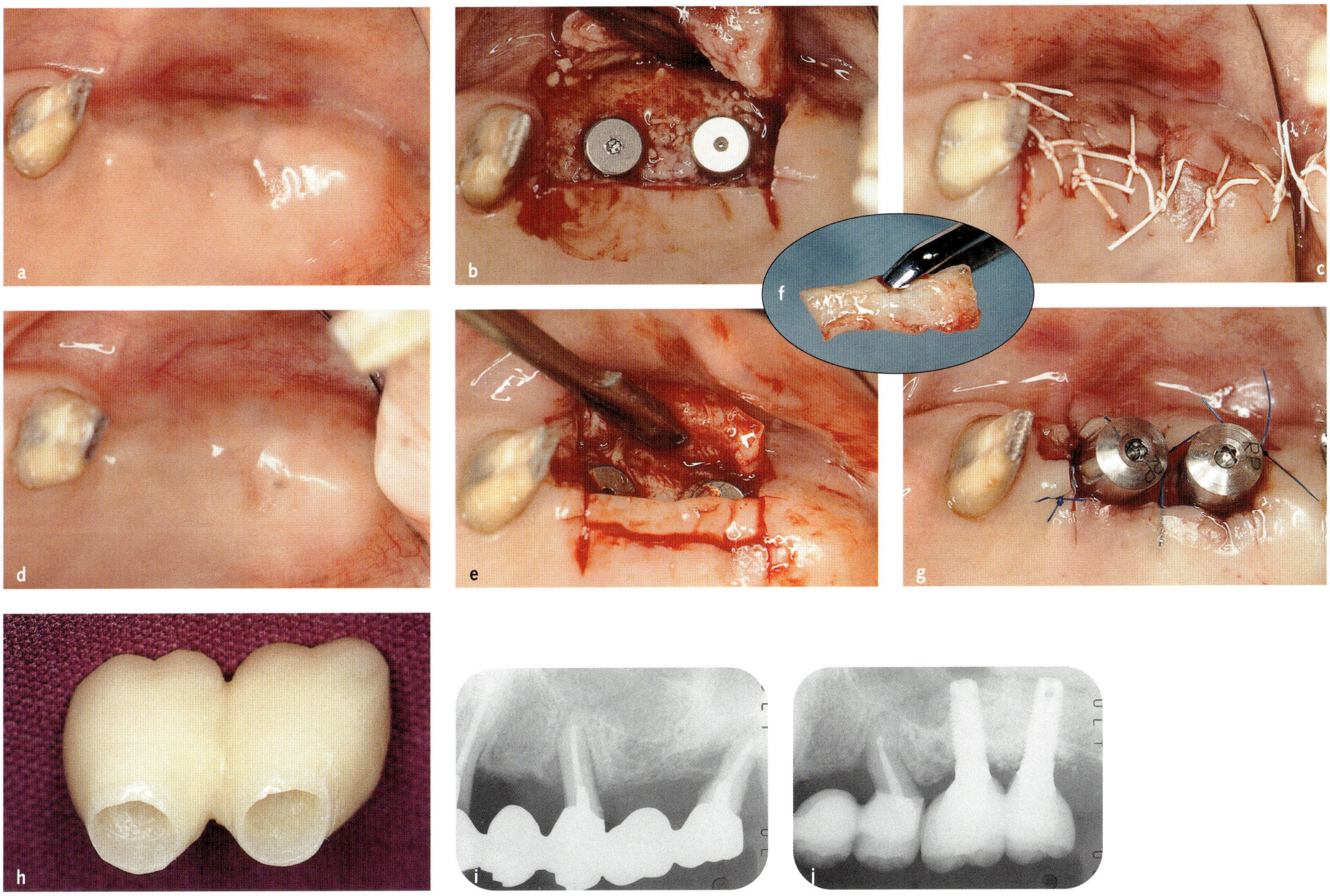

Fig 5-81 Implants in the maxillary molar area after a sinus lift procedure. (a) Photograph taken 2 months after a sinus lift procedure was completed (see Fig 5-120). (b) One year after the sinus lift, two 4.0 × 11.5-mm ImplaMed implants are placed after bone regeneration was confirmed. (c) Suturing. (d) Photograph taken 3 months after implant placement. (e) Because the gingiva is thick, a distal wedge procedure is completed to reduce the tissue thickness. (f) A connective tissue graft with collar is transplanted to the area of the mandibular left first molar for soft tissue augmentation. (g) The healing abutments are in place. (h) Provisional crowns. (i) Radiograph taken at the first visit. (j) Radiograph taken at the delivery of the final prostheses.

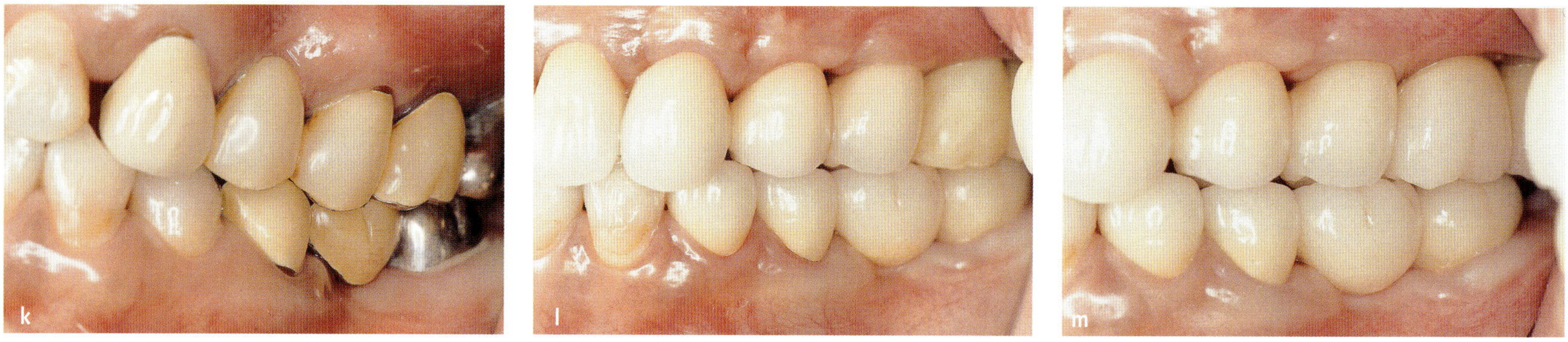

Fig 5-81 (cont) (k) Left side at the first visit. (l) Photograph taken 2 years 5 months after the first visit. Soft tissue augmentation was completed for the ridge at the mandibular left first molar. (m) During the maintenance phase, conditions are stable.

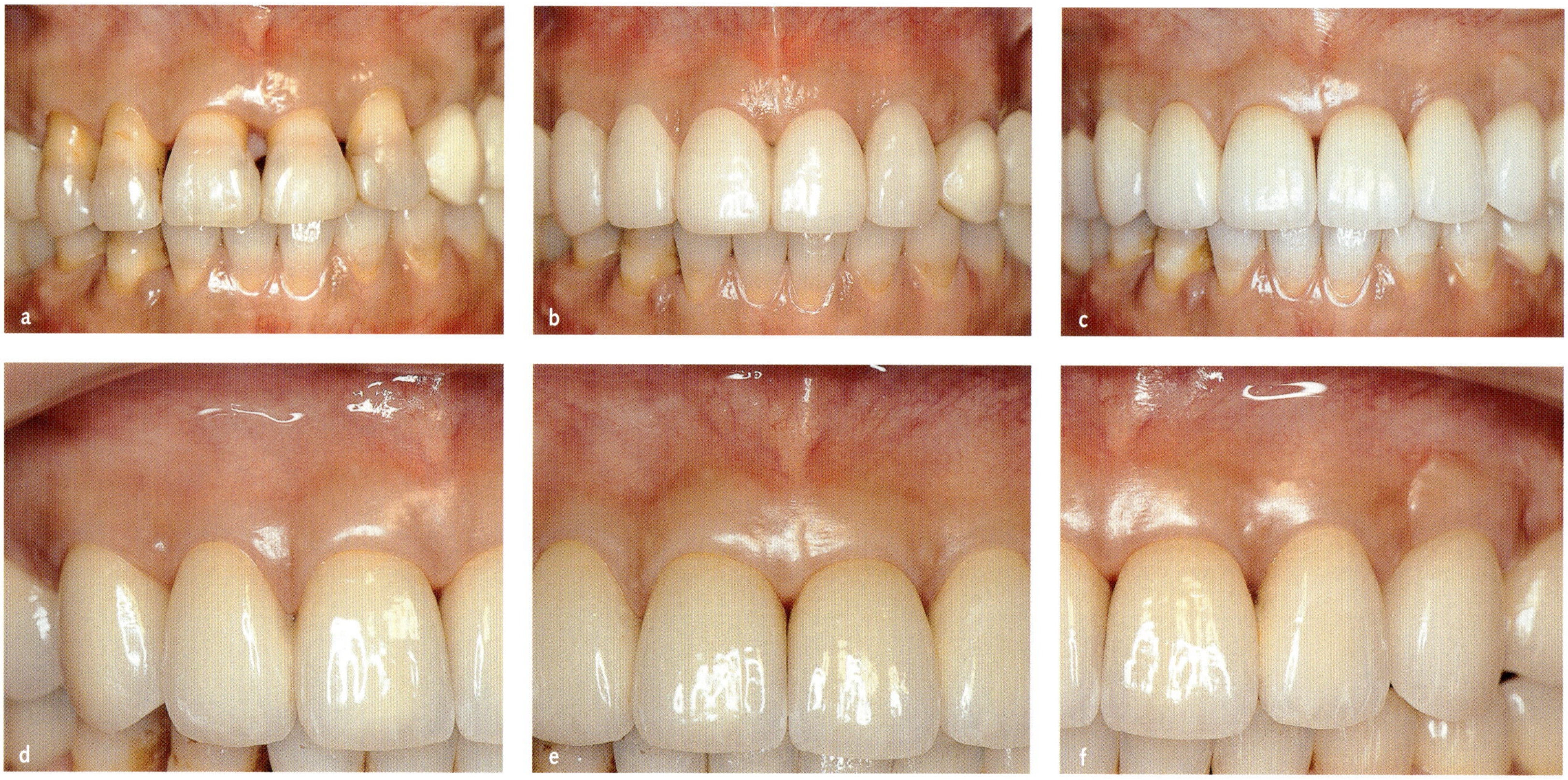

Fig 5-82 Improvement of esthetics with an anterior prosthesis. (a) Photograph taken 2 years 2 months after the first visit, prior to delivery of the anterior prosthesis. (b) Provisional restoration. (c) Photograph taken at delivery of the final prostheses. Note the improvement of the mandibular position (midline agreement). Alignment of the occlusal plane confirms remodeling of the temporomandibular joint area. (d to f) Esthetics of all-ceramic crowns and periodontal prostheses that are easy to maintain. (Prostheses made by Mr Chojiro Masuda, RDT.)

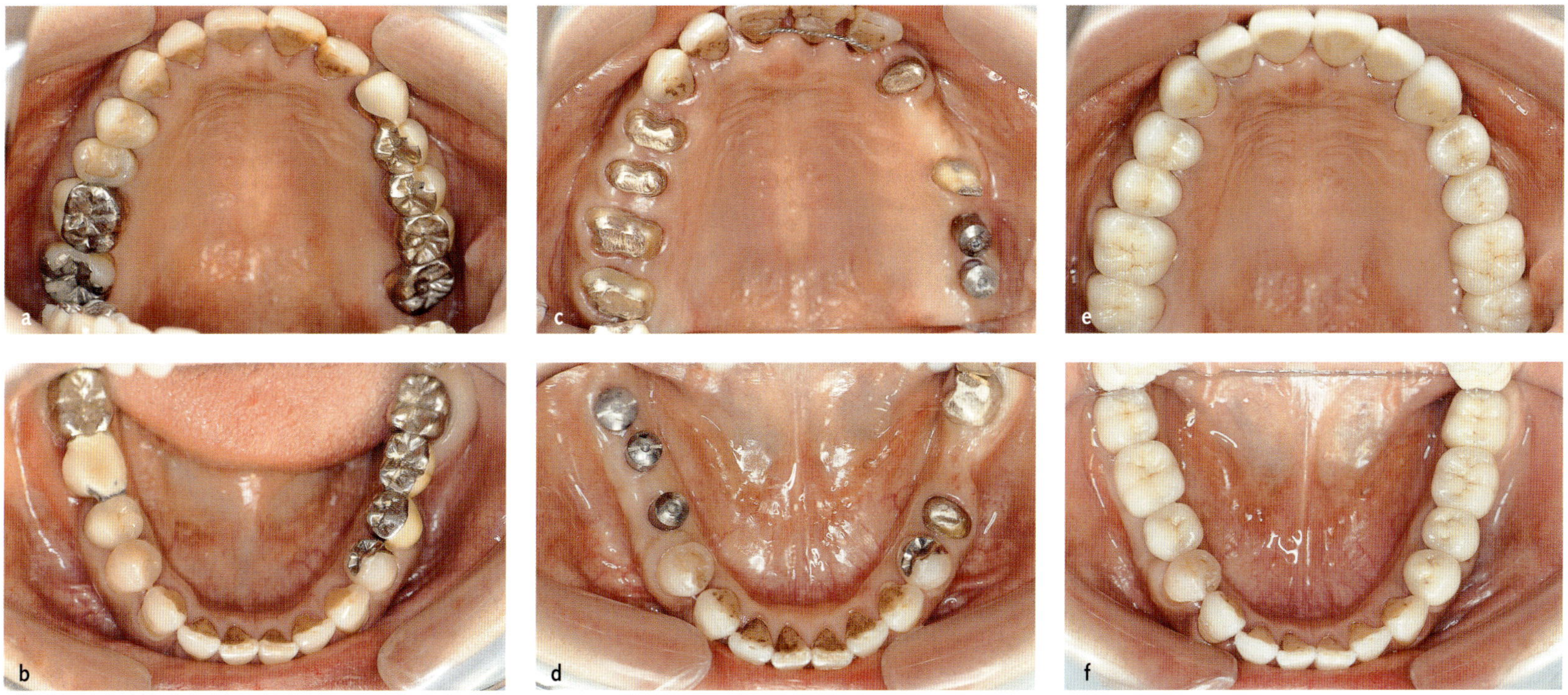

Fig 5-83 Changes in the maxillary and mandibular arches. (a and b) Occlusal views at the initial visit. The arch form is unbalanced. The angulation of the maxillary canines does not support canine guidance. The maxillary left second molar is hopeless. At the first visit, the right and left (especially the right) molars are intruded because of periodontal disease. Infrabony defects at are present at the mandibular left and right second molars, and there is a root fracture at the mandibular right second premolar. (c and d) Two years of treatment have included root canal treatment of the maxillary right first premolar, second premolar, first molar, and second molar and the maxillary left canine and second premolar and subsequent placement of dowel posts and cores. Regenerative periodontal therapy with Emdogain has been conducted for the maxillary right second molar to maxillary left canine and maxillary left second premolar. One and a half years after extraction of the maxillary left first and second molars, a sinus lift procedure with osteotome and GBR was completed and allowed to heal. Provisional restorations are adjusted to correct the vertical dimension of occlusion and improve the mandibular positioning. (e and f) Final prostheses. All the maxillary prostheses are In-Ceram all-ceramic restorations. Procera all-ceramic single crowns have been delivered to the mandibular right second premolar, first molar, and second molar. In-Ceram prostheses include a crown for the mandibular left first premolar and a fixed partial denture extending from the mandibular left second premolar to the left second molar (pontic: mandibular left first molar). Note the creation of a symmetric arch form.

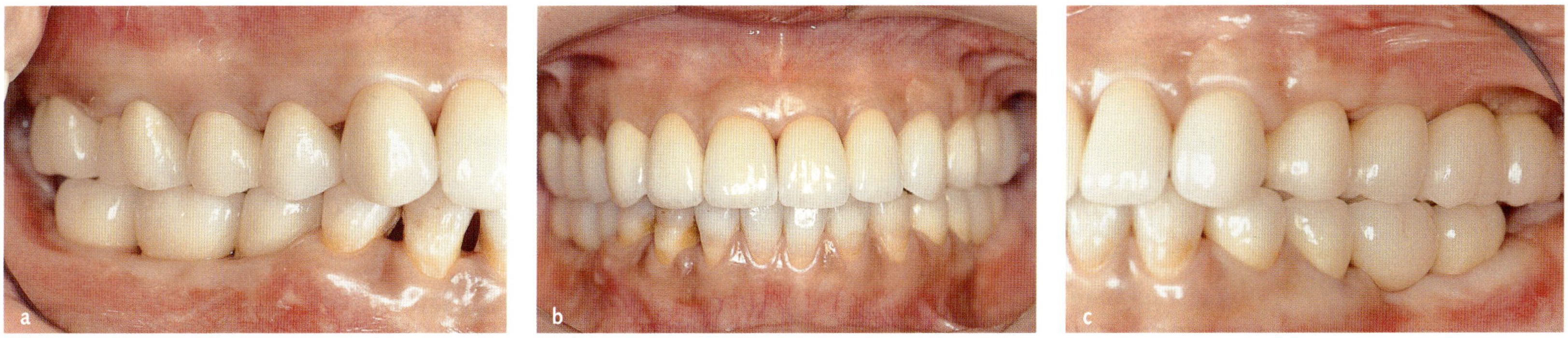

Fig 5-84 (a to c) After delivery of the final prostheses, canine guidance allows for disocclusion of the molars.

Implant placement for an overlay denture in the mandible

In the challenging case of a fully edentulous mandible with significant ridge resorption that makes it difficult to stabilize a denture, implant placement at the left and right canines for retention of an overlay denture is quite useful. The surgical procedures are presented in Figs 5-85 to 5-88: The patient was a 77-year-old woman, whose chief complaint was her inability to chew food because the mandibular denture moved and caused pain.

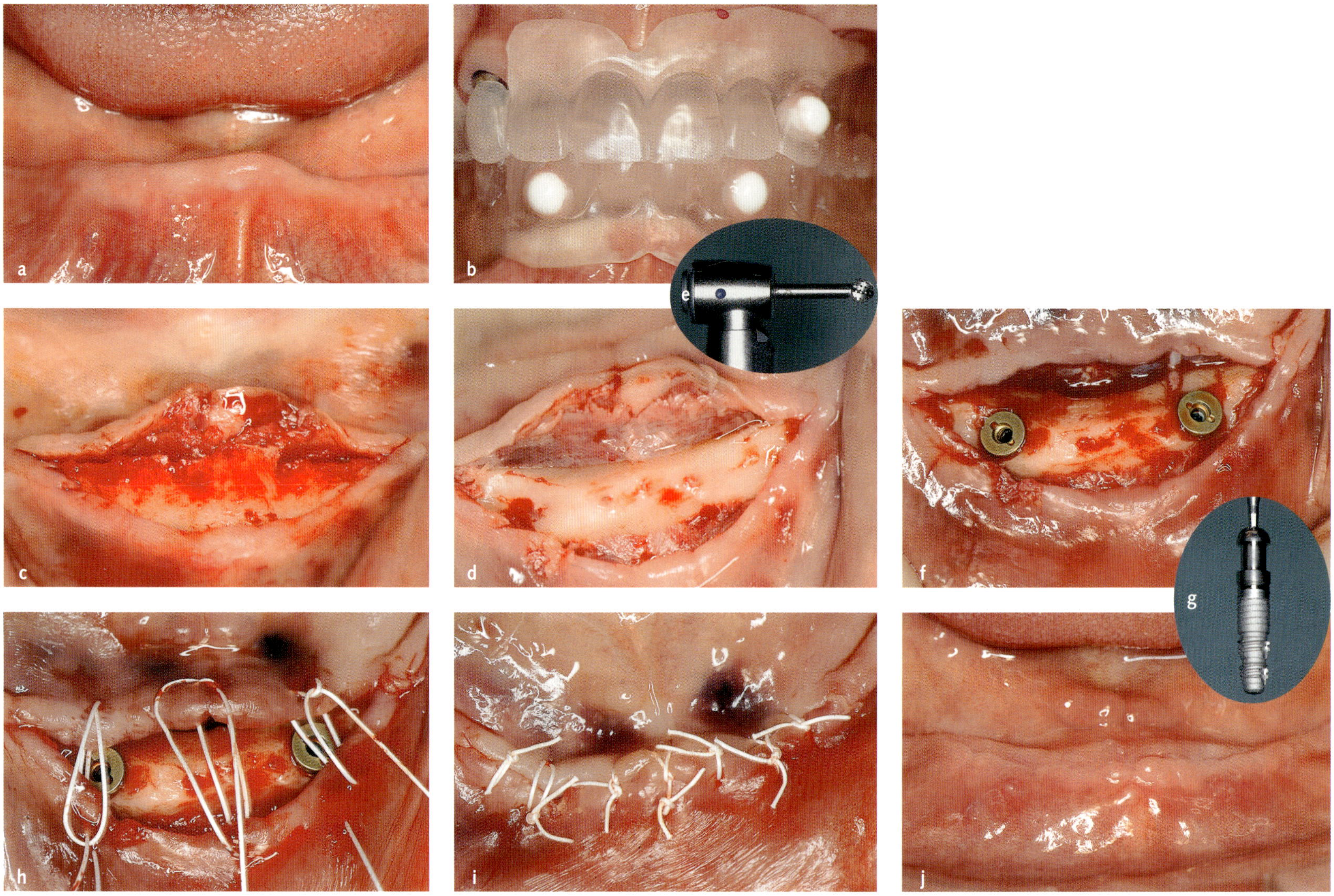

Fig 5-85 Implant placement. (a) Resorbed, sharp alveolar ridge. (b) Surgical stent for implant placement. (c) A crestal incision is made and gradually extended so as not to reflect tissue too close to the spine of the genioglossus and not to damage the mental foramen. A sharp bone ridge can be seen. (d and e) An osteotomy bur is used to flatten the ridge to a 5- to 6-mm width. (f and g) Frialit implants (3.8 × 13.0 mm, Friadent) are placed. (h and i) A three-layer vertical mattress suture is utilized. Releasing incisions are properly made to allow suturing without tension to the flaps and to prevent cover screw exposure. (j) No dehiscence in the gingiva is noted 3 months after surgery.

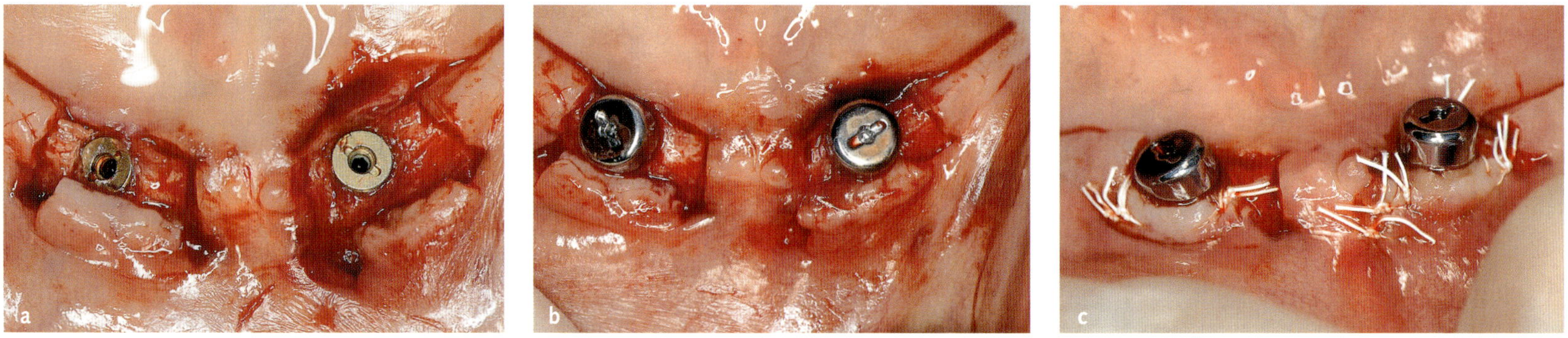

Fig 5-86 Try-in of abutments. (a to c) Photographs taken 4 months after implant placement. To increase keratinized gingiva, a roll technique is used, reflecting a partial-thickness flap on the lingual side. Note the excessive incision on the lingual aspect. Gingival former healing abutments (3.8 mm in diameter) are attached.

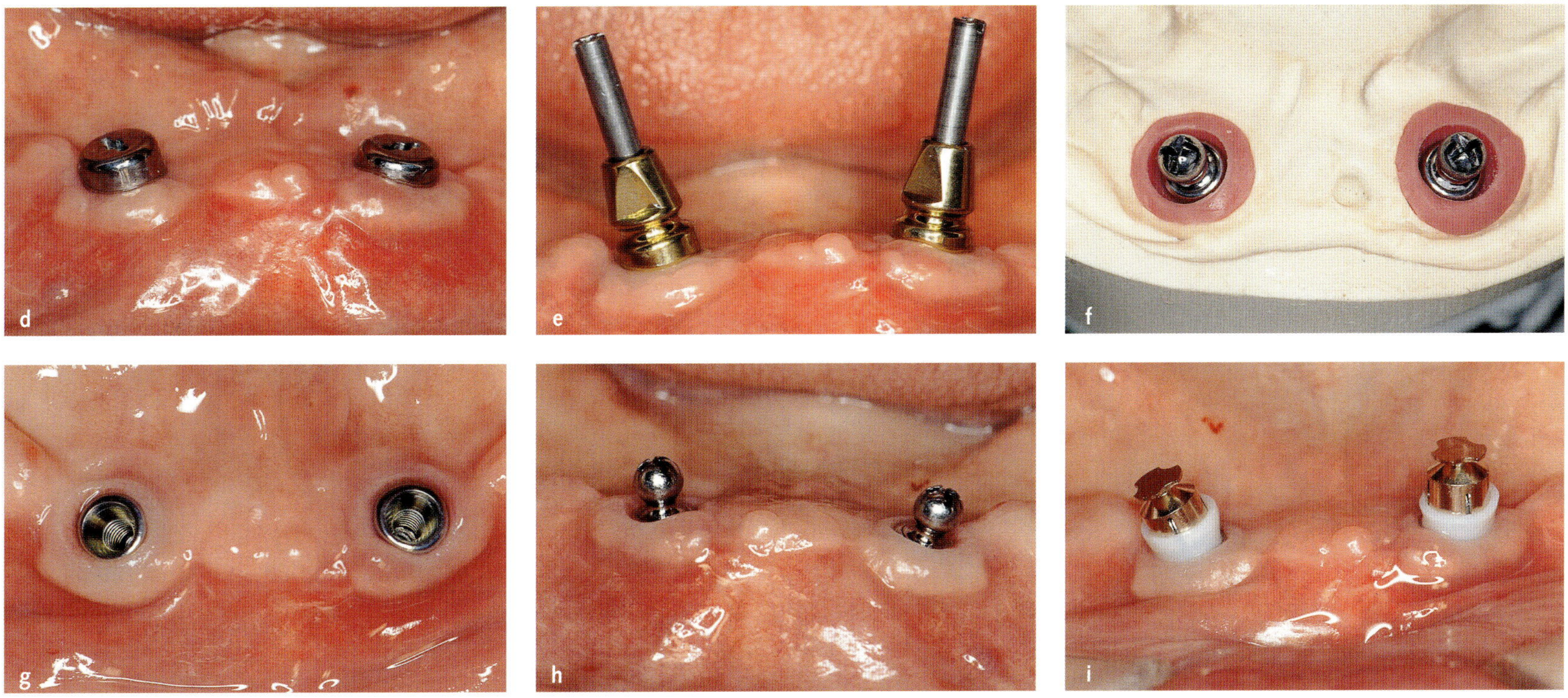

Fig 5-86 (cont) (d) The keratinized gingiva is increased 1 month postsurgery. (e) A pick-up impression is taken with impression copings in place 2 months postsurgery. (f) A clinically accurate cast is produced. (g) Appearance 5 months after second-stage surgery. (h) At 10 months after implant placement, ball-type abutments are connected. (i) Female O-ring attachment pieces are placed and fixed to the denture base with autopolymerizing resin.

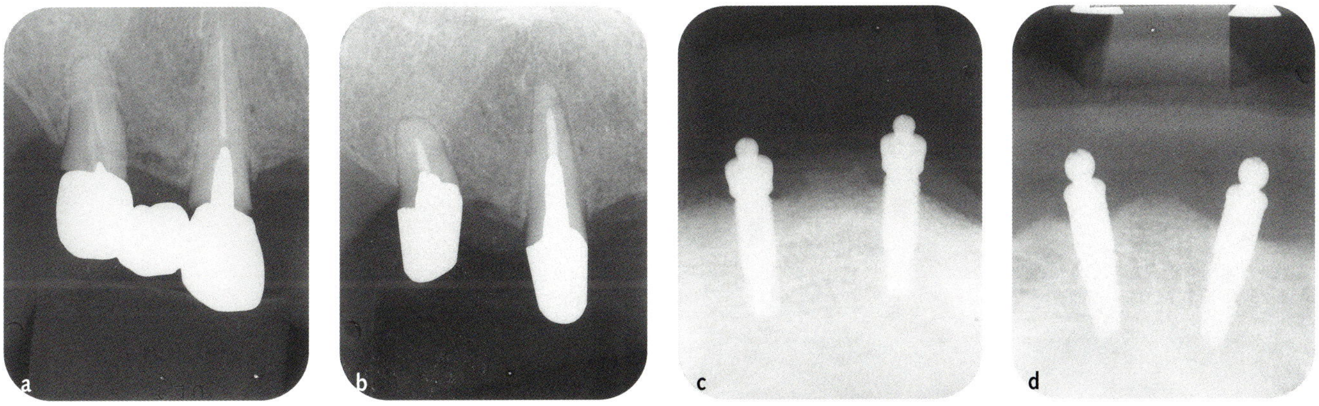

Fig 5-87 Improvement to the surrounding tissue of the opposing teeth. (a) At the first visit, a bony defect and occlusal trauma are visible at the maxillary right second premolar. (b) An improvement is observed in both the bony defect and the traumatic occlusion 1 year 11 months after repreparation and provisionalization. (c) Overlay implants (3.8 × 13.0 mm). (d) With only two ball-type nonrigid attachments, the stability of the denture is dramatically improved.

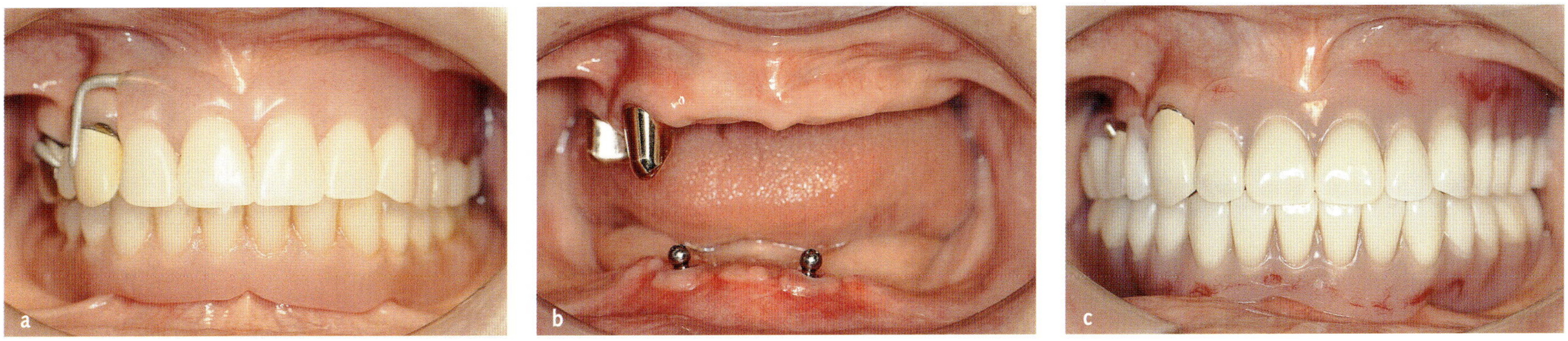

Fig 5-88 (a) Photograph taken at the first visit. (b) Photograph taken before delivery of the dentures. Telescopic crowns have been fabricated for the maxillary right canine and second premolar. (c) Photograph taken after delivery of the dentures. (Prostheses made by Mr Takahisa Tashiro, RDT.)

Case 5-3 Implants and recovery of arch integrity

Patient: *51-year-old woman at the time of first visit in 1995*
Chief complaint: *Pain in the maxillary right central incisor during chewing*
The maxillary right first premolar, right central incisor, and left first premolar had root fractures (Fig 5-89). All of the restored teeth had secondary caries and failed endodontic treatments. Gingival inflammation was caused by a prosthesis that invaded the biologic width. The discrepancy in the mandibular position was about 1.0 to 1.5 mm in an anterior-posterior direction, and the shift was to the left. Primary occlusal trauma was observed on most teeth. The arch form was disturbed. The patient had neither specific systemic diseases nor a smoking habit. Because she was a busy executive, treatment was restricted by time constraints. Her chief complaint was occlusal pain affecting the maxillary right central incisor, but it seemed that she strongly desired esthetic improvements also (Figs 5-89 to 5-105).

Figs 5-89 to 5-91 Occlusal views of maxillary and mandibular arches.

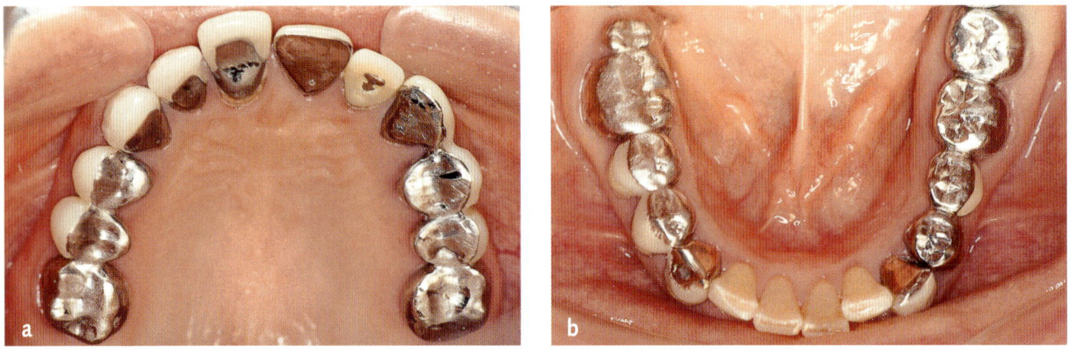

Fig 5-89 (a) Maxillary arch at the first visit. The discrepancy in mandibular position (between centric relation and maximal intercuspal position) is about 1.0 to 1.5 mm in an anterior-posterior direction and to the left. Premature contacts and cuspal interferences are noted for most of the teeth. Conspicuous disharmony is observed in the morphology between the occluding and adjacent teeth. Wide movements toward the right anterior direction are forced during function, which could have caused the root fracture of maxillary right central incisor. (b) Mandibular arch at the first visit. The arch form is irregular. All the restored teeth have deficiencies in crown morphology, such as cusp-to-fossa relationships and functional guidance, as well as deficient endodontic treatments and secondary caries.

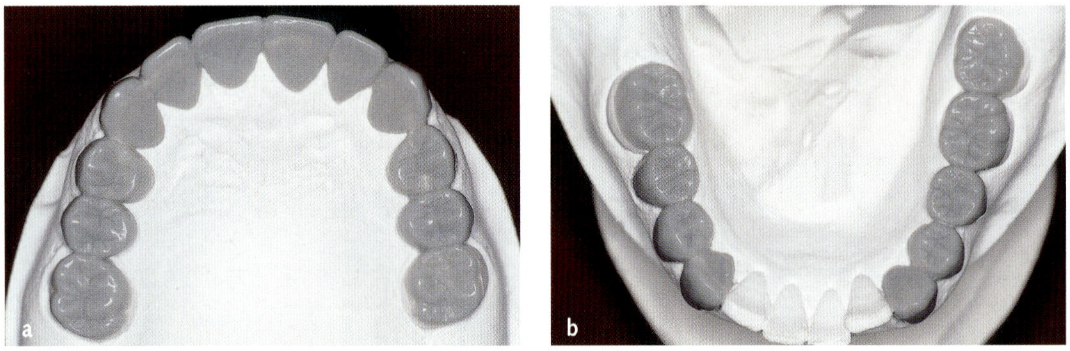

Fig 5-90 (a and b) Diagnostic wax-up. A diagnostic wax-up is placed on the articulator for a diagnostic purpose to evaluate arch forms, the vertical dimention and the occlusal plane. In this case, improvements in the morphology and function appear to be possible through prosthodontic treatment alone without orthodontics.

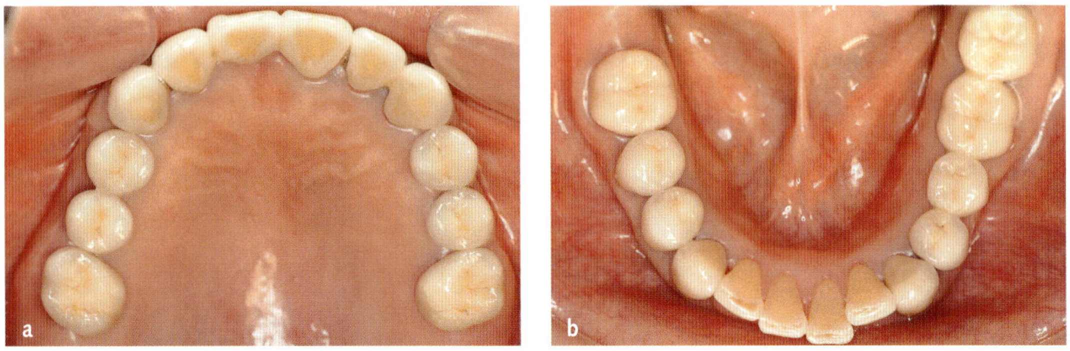

Fig 5-91 (a and b) Occlusal views 1 years 11 months after delivery of the final prostheses. Symmetric arch form and occlusal morphology have been restored. The vertical dimension and occlusal positioning of the maxillary right canine and maxillary left canine are symmetric.

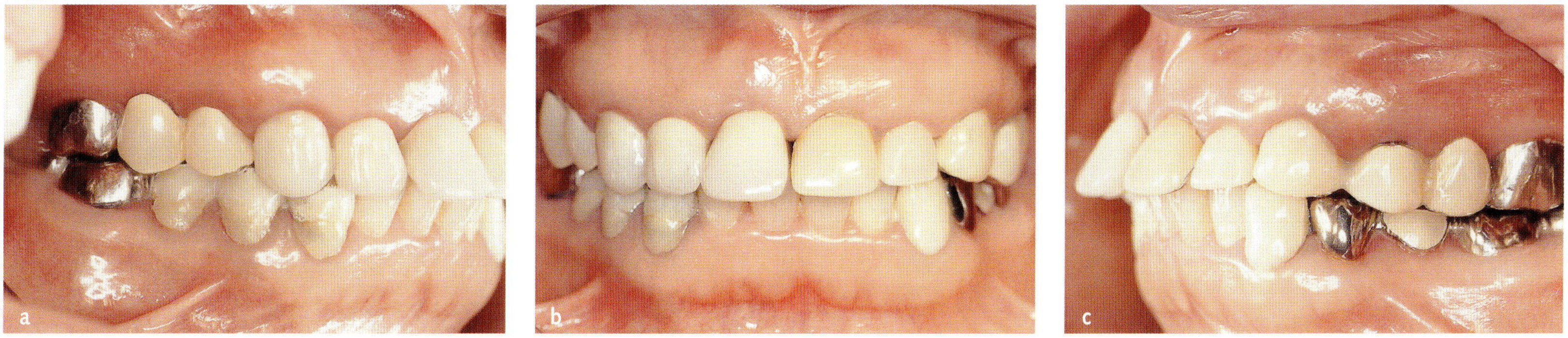

Fig 5-92 (a to c) At the first visit, the maxillary right central incisor has a root fracture. The theory was that the occlusion became deeper every time the molar restoration was completed. The mandible has shifted to the left. Functional movements are restricted by premature contacts and cuspal interferences. The anterior teeth are flared labially.

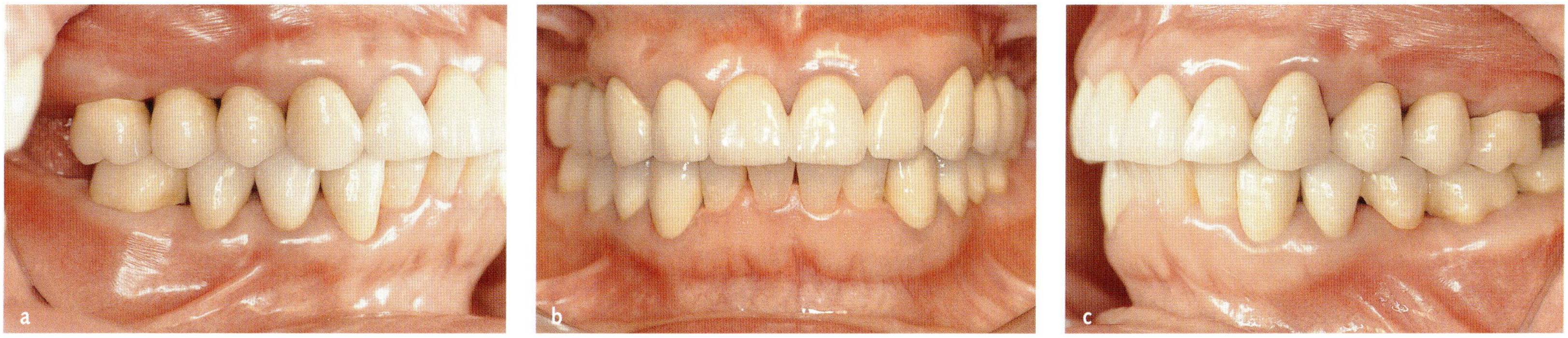

Fig 5-93 (a to c) Final restorations, 2 years 5 months after the first visit. (Prostheses made by Mr Tsugumichi Kawasaki, RDT.)

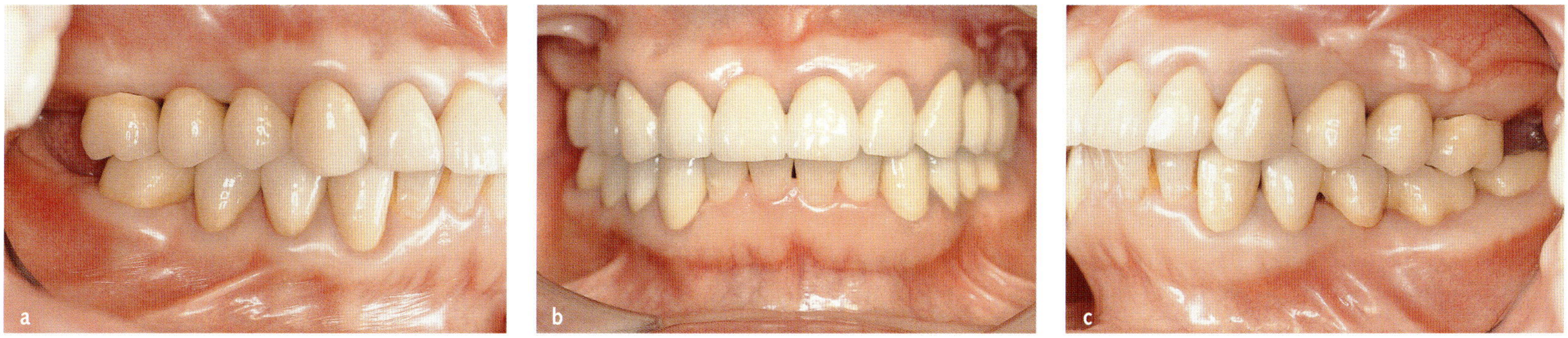

Fig 5-94 (a to c) Photographs taken 1 year 11 months after delivery of the final prostheses.

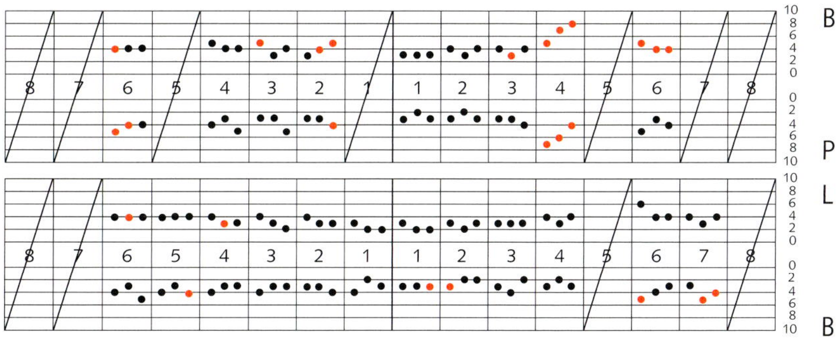

Fig 5-95 Probing chart at the first visit.

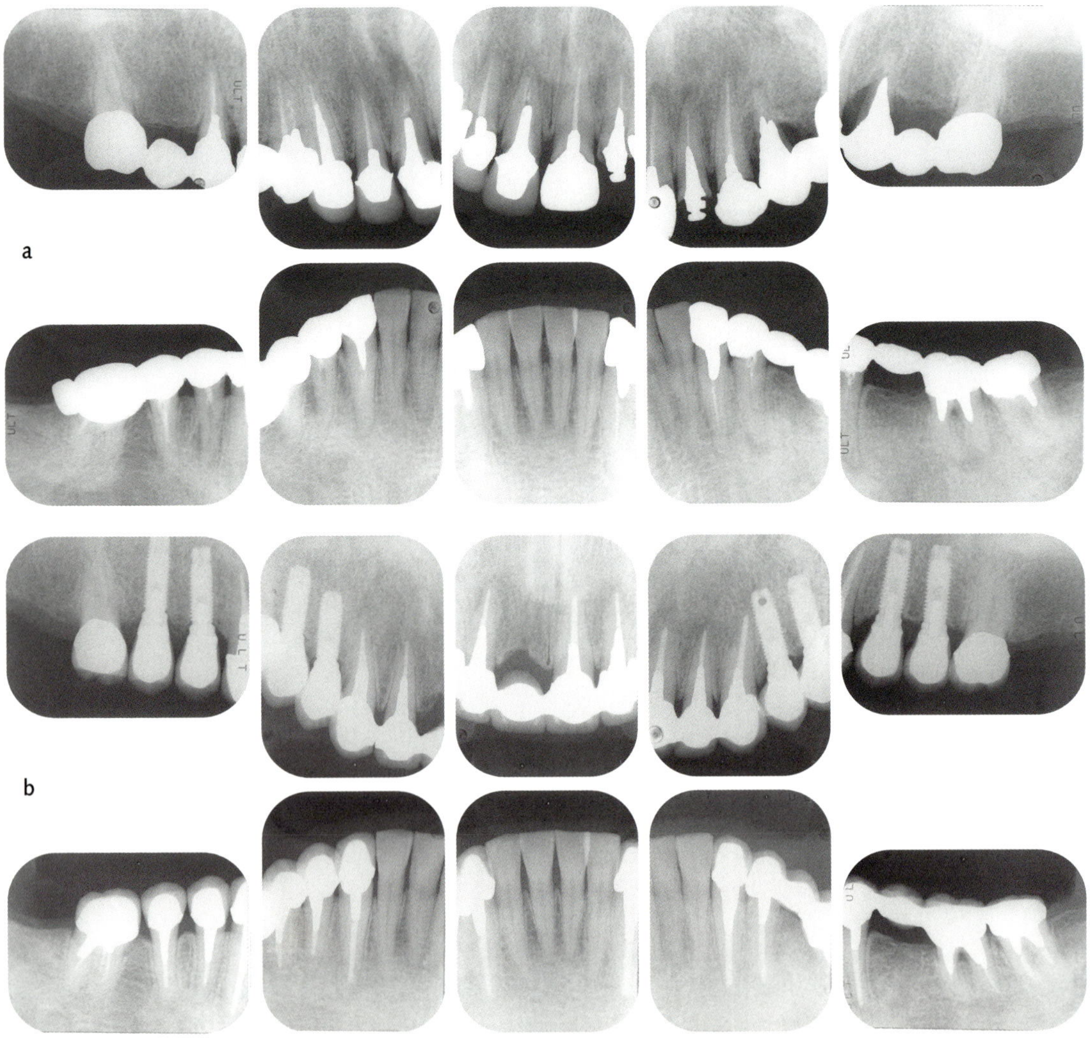

Fig 5-96 (a) Radiographs taken at the first visit. Secondary caries, failing root canal treatments, and inappropriate dowel posts and cores are observed throughout the dentition. Primary occlusal trauma is noted. The maxillary right and left first premolars have root fractures. (b) Radiographs taken 4 years 4 months after the first visit. Single implants were placed at the sites of all four maxillary premolars. Inflammation and occlusal forces are controlled, and periodontal tissue is improved. Improvement of the occlusion was the first step in prosthodontic recovery.

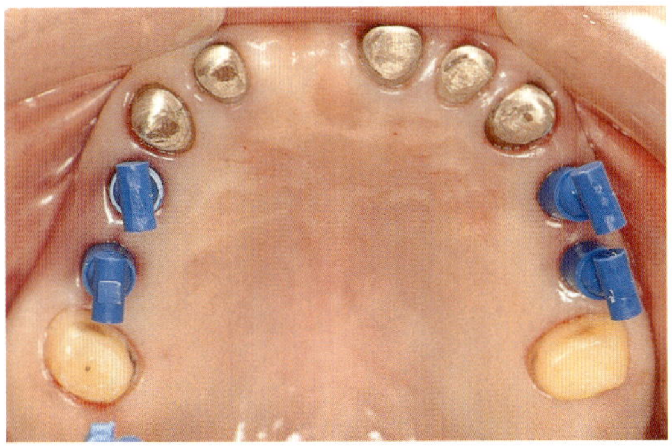

Fig 5-97 After extraction of the maxillary right central incisor as well as the right first premolar and left first premolar (due to root fracture), GBR was conducted. Implants (CeraOne, Nobel Biocare) were placed later. For the right lateral incisor, left central incisor, left lateral incisor, and left canine, after root canal retreatment, dowel posts and cores were provided and final preparations were made. A pick-up impression has been taken.

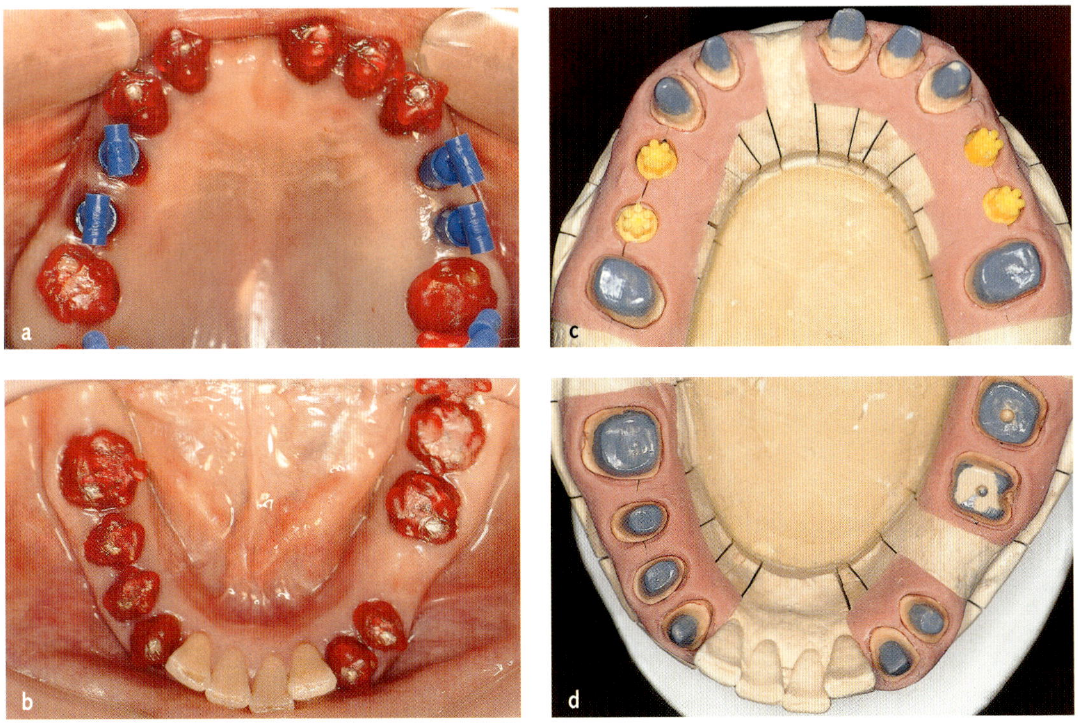

Fig 5-98 (a and b) After root canal re-treatment of the mandibular left canine, first premolar, first molar, and second molar, and the mandibular right canine, first premolar, second premolar, and first molar, crown lengthening was completed. After final preparation, an HIT impression is taken and a pick-up impression is taken with pattern resin. (c and d) A tissue model is used to reproduce the physiologic emergence profiles.

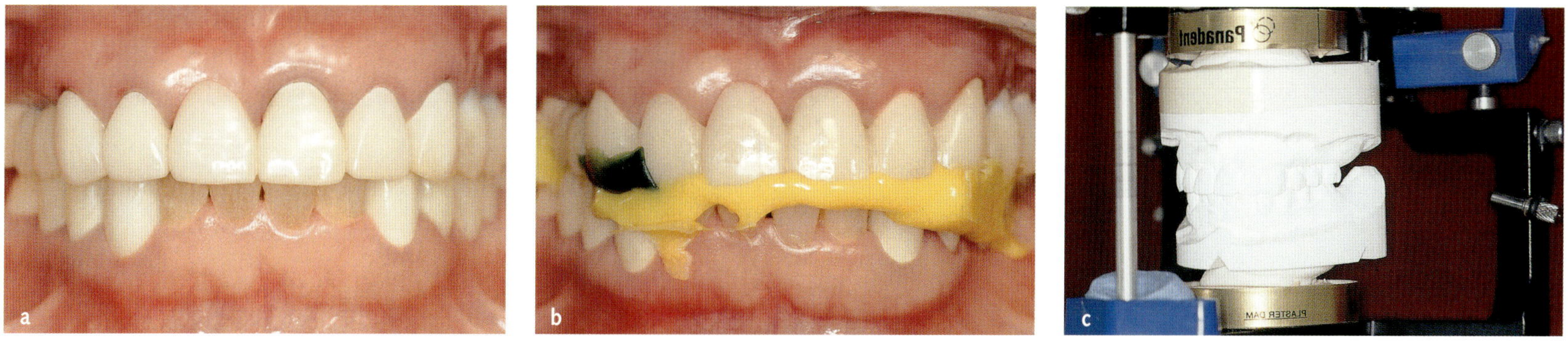

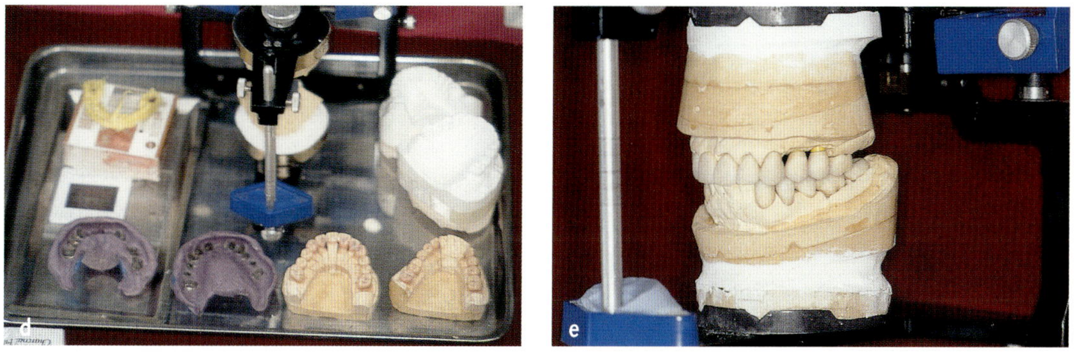

Fig 5-99 Provisional restoration. (a) Photograph taken 1 year 10 months after the first visit. To allow treatment of subgingival caries from the mandibular right and left canines to the molars, crown lengthening has been completed. The occlusal height has been increased for the left molars. (b) The intercuspal position (ICP) is stabilized with provisional restorations while a proper cusp-to-fossa relationship and checkbite registration is taken. (c) Provisional restoration study casts are mounted on the articulator to obtain an incisal path and condylar guidance inclination. (d) Information required for laboratory work: provisional restoration study casts; a diagnostic wax-up; a pick-up impression for soldering index; centric relation record with pattern resin; and clinical photographs as reference for shade selection. (e) Remounting. After the first try-in, occlusal adjustment and glazing were completed and the prostheses were temporarily cemented.

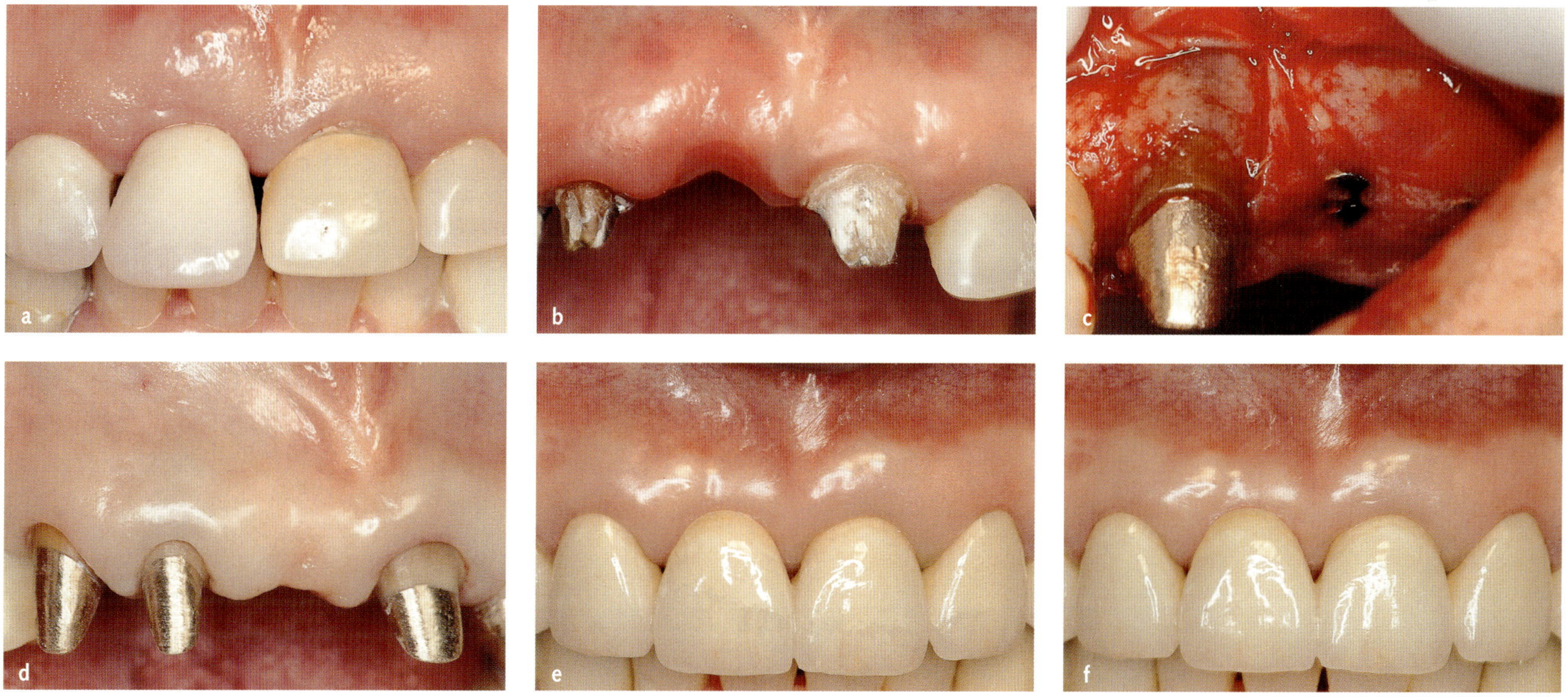

Fig 5-100 Maxillary anterior segment. (a) At the first visit, the maxillary right central incisor has a root fracture. The anterior teeth are flared out labially. Subgingival caries is noted. (b) After extraction of the maxillary right central incisor, the clinical crowns of the anterior teeth are short incisogingivally. (c) Implants were placed at the site of the maxillary left first and second premolars. Simultaneously, GBR was completed for ridge augmentation. At the second surgery (6 months later), crown lengthening for the anterior teeth is completed. Marginal bone is trimmed to create scalloping in a flat cervical margin. A partial-thickness flap is raised at the maxillary left premolar area during the second surgery. (d) Five months after crown lengthening, an esthetic gingival drape has been achieved. The pontic has a semisaddle or ovate design. (e) Eleven months after crown lengthening, collarless porcelain crowns and the fixed partial denture have been delivered. The prosthesis extends from the maxillary right canine to the maxillary left canine (pontic: maxillary right central incisor). (f) Stable conditions 2 years after the delivery of prostheses.

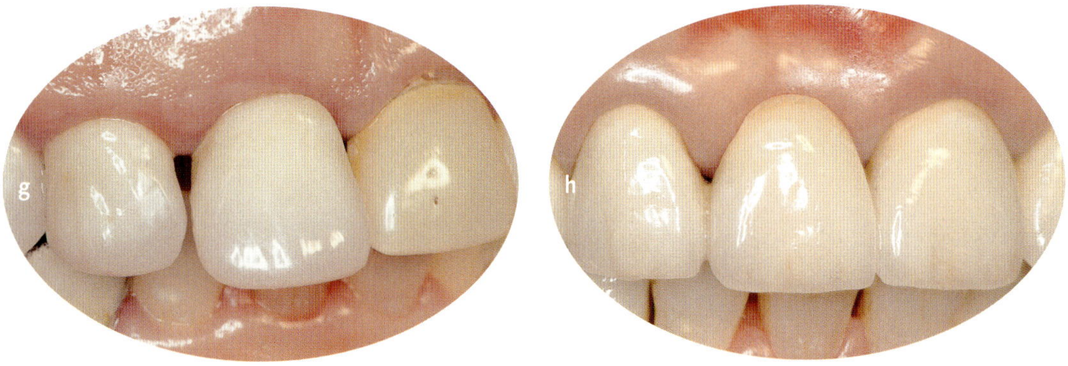

Fig 5-100 (cont) Comparison between the appearance (g) at the first visit and (h) 2 years after delivery.

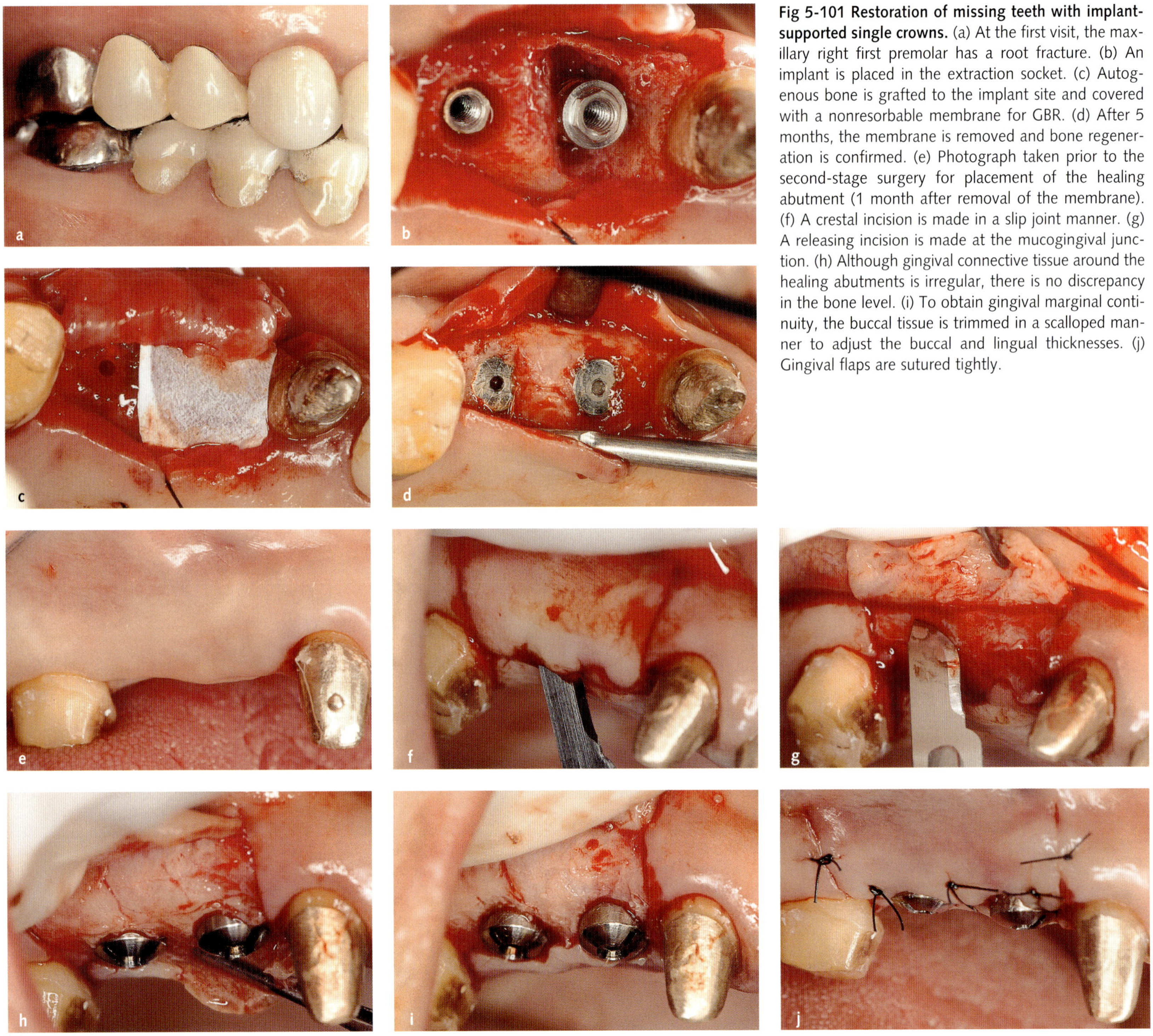

Fig 5-101 Restoration of missing teeth with implant-supported single crowns. (a) At the first visit, the maxillary right first premolar has a root fracture. (b) An implant is placed in the extraction socket. (c) Autogenous bone is grafted to the implant site and covered with a nonresorbable membrane for GBR. (d) After 5 months, the membrane is removed and bone regeneration is confirmed. (e) Photograph taken prior to the second-stage surgery for placement of the healing abutment (1 month after removal of the membrane). (f) A crestal incision is made in a slip joint manner. (g) A releasing incision is made at the mucogingival junction. (h) Although gingival connective tissue around the healing abutments is irregular, there is no discrepancy in the bone level. (i) To obtain gingival marginal continuity, the buccal tissue is trimmed in a scalloped manner to adjust the buccal and lingual thicknesses. (j) Gingival flaps are sutured tightly.

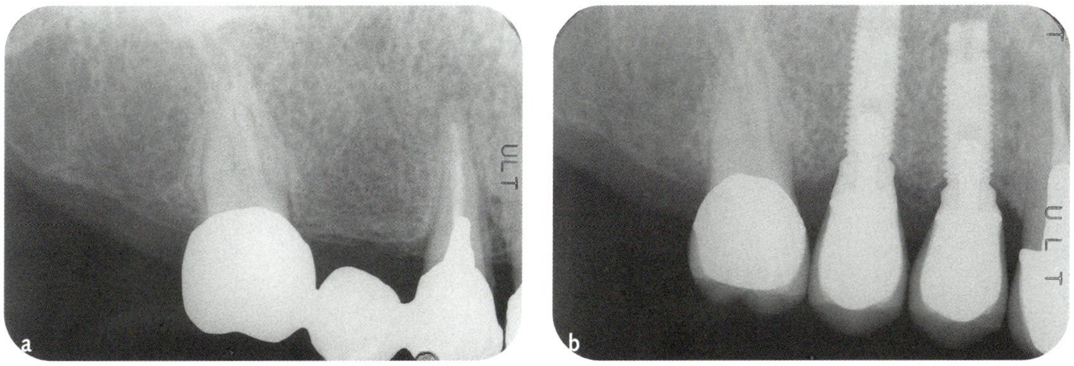

Fig 5-102 (a) Maxillary right quadrant at the first visit. (b) Radiograph taken 6 years after the first visit. Areas of failure have disappeared. Note the inter-implant distance and the direction and depth of implant placement, which harmonize with the adjacent teeth.

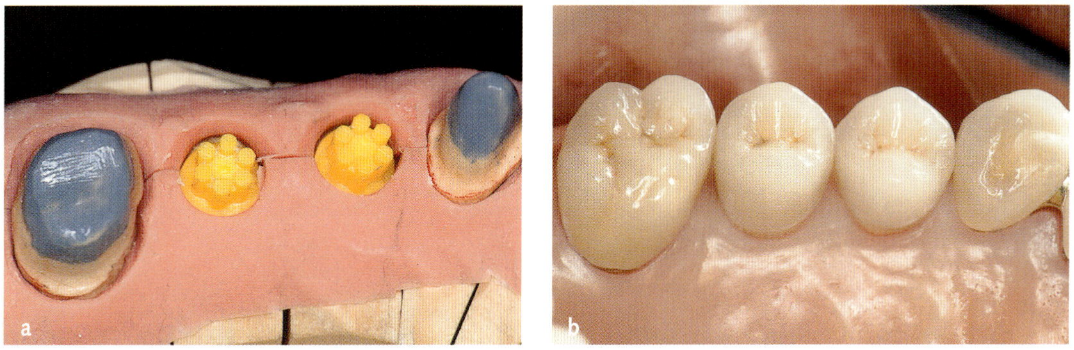

Fig 5-103 (a) A tissue model is used to thoroughly examine the emergence profile. (b) Attention has been paid to provide appropriate anatomic morphology to the teeth.

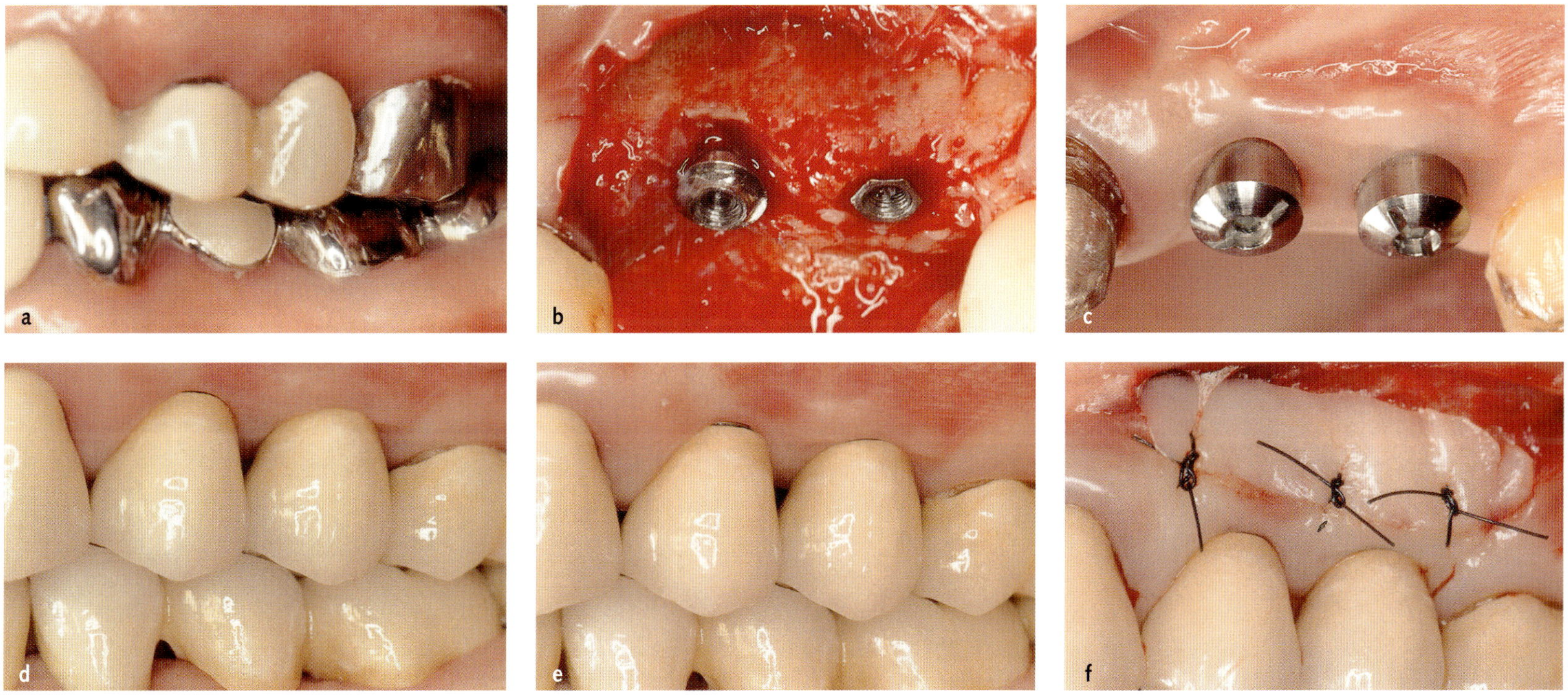

Fig 5-104 (a) Left side at the first visit. The maxillary left first premolar has a root fracture. The occlusal height is deficient on the left, causing the occlusal plane to be disturbed. (b) One month after extraction of the maxillary left first premolar, implants are placed. Concomitantly, GBR is completed with an autogenous bone graft and placement of a nonresorbable membrane. (c) After 8 months, a connective tissue graft was completed at the second surgery for gingival augmentation. (d) Collarless porcelain single crowns have been fabricated for the maxillary left first premolar, second premolar, and first molar. A fixed partial denture has been delivered to the mandibular left first premolar, second premolar, and second molar abutments (pontic: mandibular left first molar). (e) One year after delivery, the collar at the maxillary left premolars is exposed. (f) Free gingival grafting is conducted for the maxillary left premolar area.

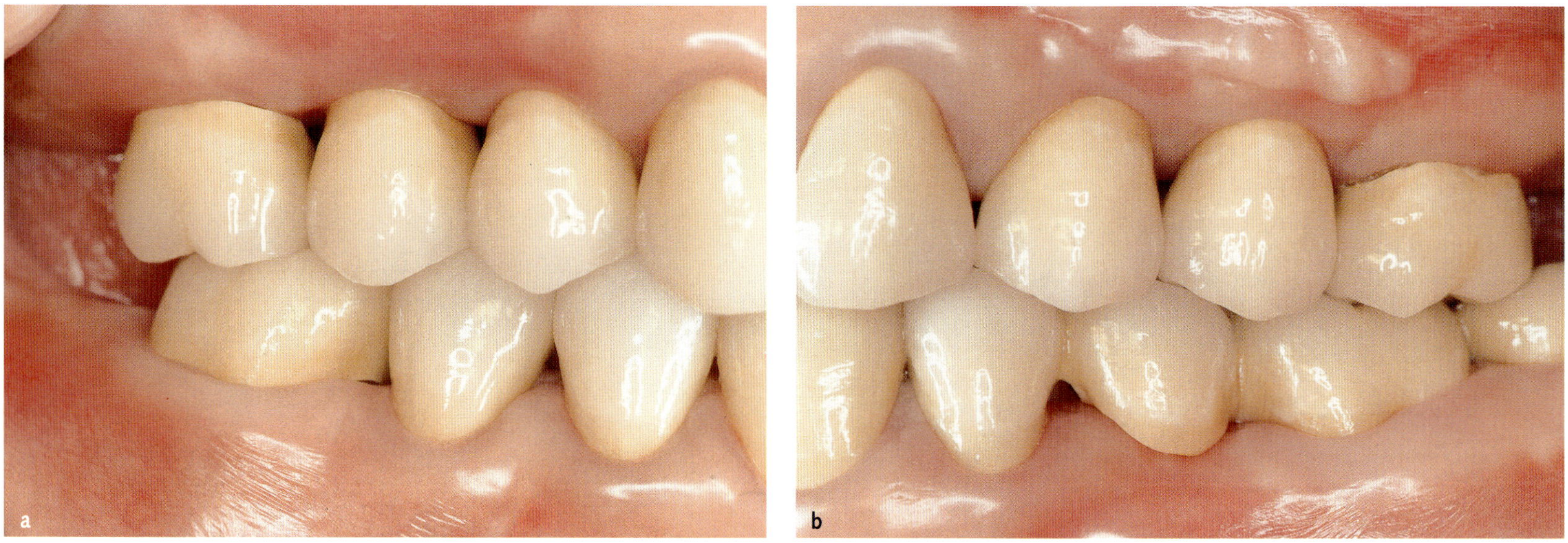

Fig 5-105 (a and b) Photographs taken 2 years after delivery of the final prostheses.

Case 5-4 Recovery of molar occlusion with implant support

Patient: *60-year-old woman at the time of first visit in 1998*
Chief complaint: *Inability to chew because of pain affecting the maxillary right lateral incisor and canine This is a case with a unilateral loss of molar occlusion. The occlusal plane disturbance was probably due to inappropriate prosthodontic treatment. Periodontitis was not noted. A new occlusal plane was established, and occlusal support was recovered by restoration with a mandibular left fixed partial denture and mandibular right implants and crowns (Fig 5-106 to 5-113). A telescopic crown–supported removable denture was placed in the maxilla. Precise implementation of initial therapy and basic prosthodontic procedures, including inflammation control, root canal treatment, improvement of attached gingiva, dowel posts and cores, crown preparations, and impression procedures, should be ensured.*

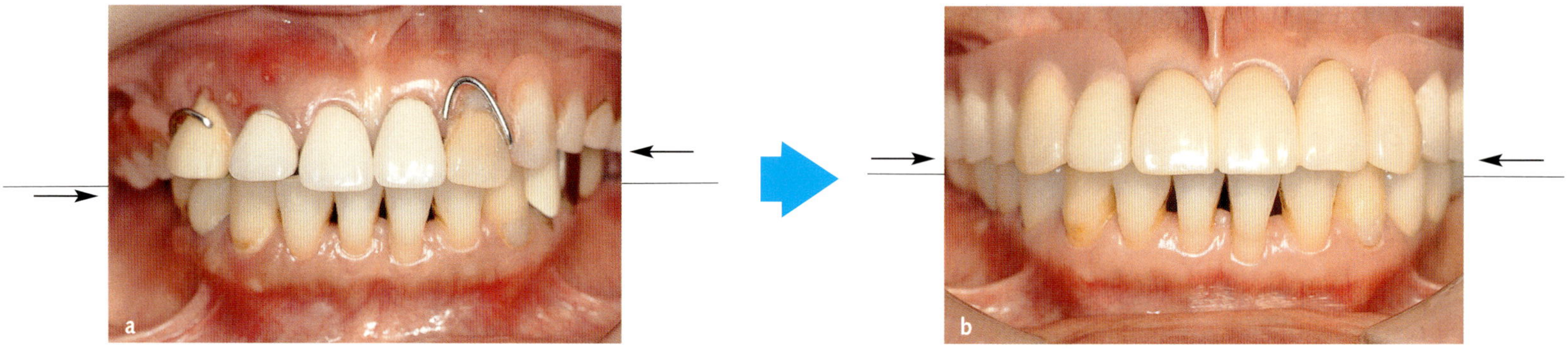

Fig 5-106 Restoration of molar occlusion. (a) At the first visit, because of the missing molars, the vertical dimension is decreased significantly *(arrows)*. The maxillary right canine and lateral incisor are under occlusal load, resulting in root fractures. (b) Photograph taken 3 years 3 months after the first visit, 1 year 8 months after delivery of the final prostheses. A cantilever fixed partial denture is supported by implants at the mandibular right first and second molars. Metal-ceramic crowns have been placed on the mandibular right premolars.

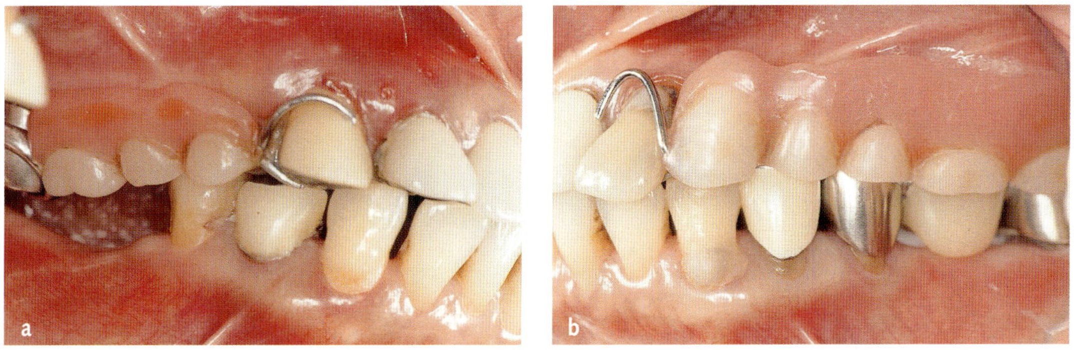

Fig 5-107 At the first visit, the remaining maxillary teeth are the right central incisor, lateral incisor, canine, and second molar and the left central incisor and lateral incisor. The maxillary right lateral incisor and canine are flared labially and have root fractures. The right and left occlusal planes are in poor alignment. Clenching is suspected from contractions of the right masseter muscle. Degree 2 mobility was noted for the maxillary right central incisor, lateral incisor, and canine and the left central incisor and lateral incisor. The maxillary right lateral incisor and canine were extracted.

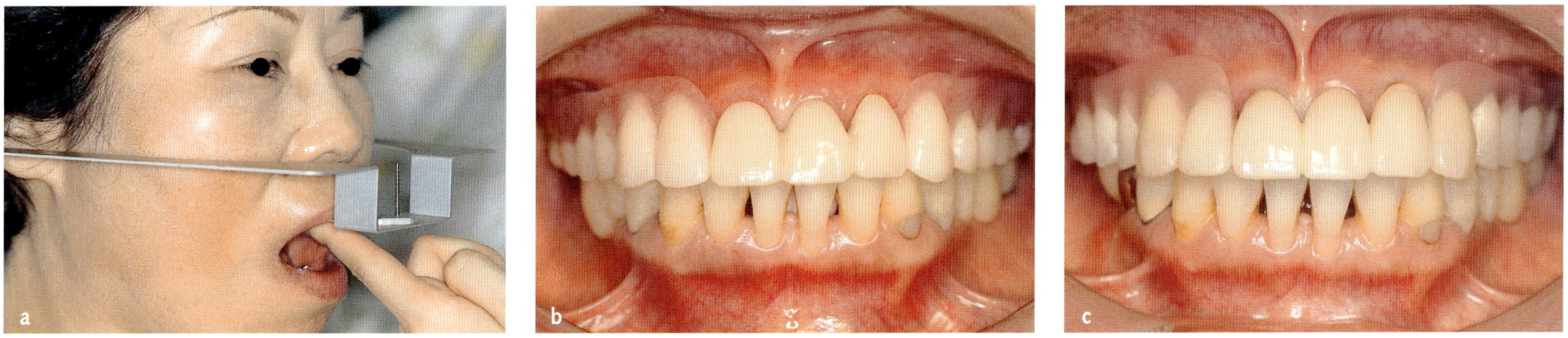

Fig 5-108 Provisional restoration. (a) After initial therapy, provisional restorations are fabricated. A corrected occlusal plane is established. (b) A telescopic-type therapeutic denture supported by abutments (maxillary right central incisor and second molar; left central incisor and lateral incisor) is delivered (December 1998). (c) Implants have been placed at the site of the mandibular right first and second molars. A metal provisional restoration is provided for the mandibular right first premolar, second premolar, and first molar (pontic: first molar) to stabilize the occlusion. The denture is adjusted intraorally. After remodeling is complete, the telescopic denture is delivered for the maxillary arch (June 1999).

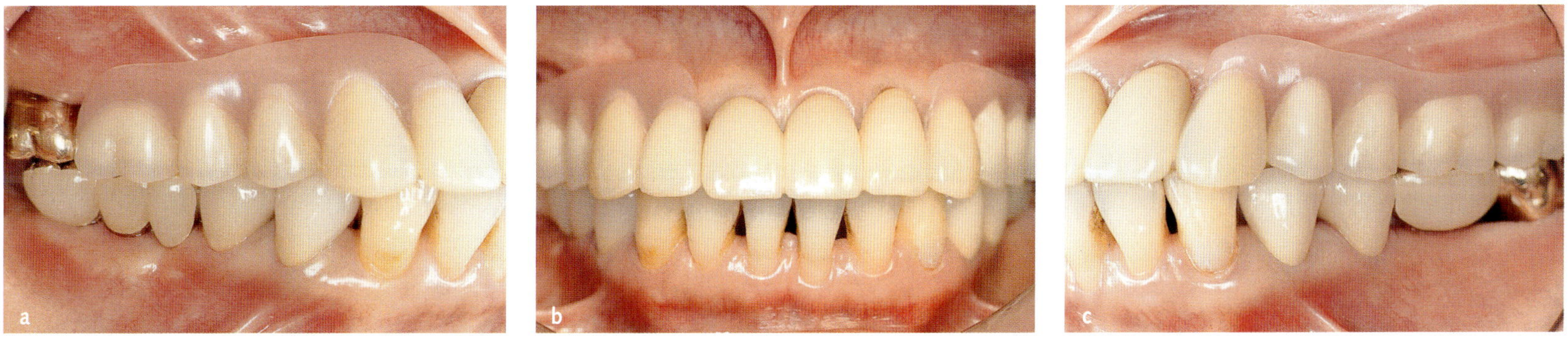

Fig 5-109 (a to c) Photographs taken 1 year 8 months after the first visit. The vertical dimension of occlusion has been increased.

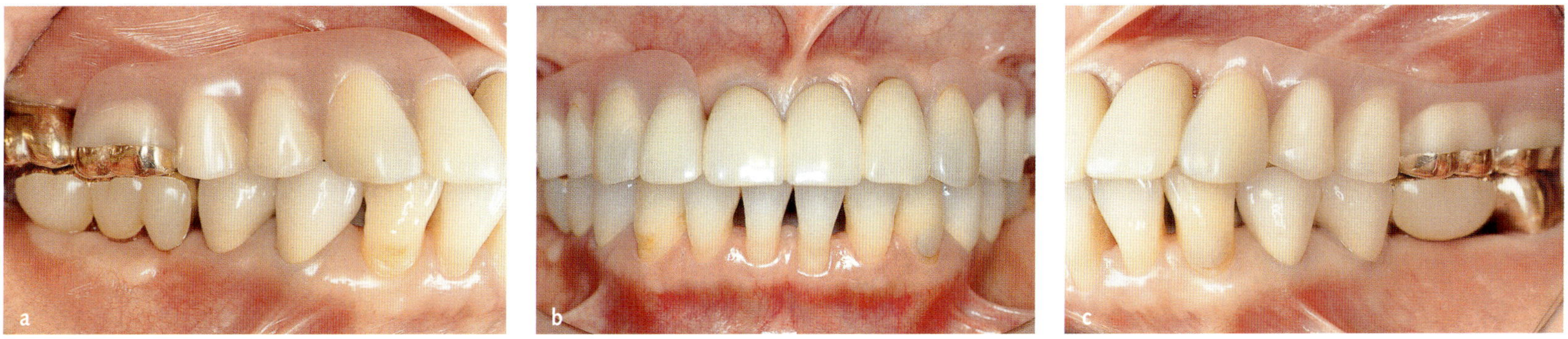

Fig 5-110 (a to c) During the maintenance phase. Conditions are stable 3 years 3 months after the first visit. Keratinized gingiva in the molar areas is limited, and the mandibular left first molar is surrounded by mobile mucosa. Because the patient did not agree to periodontal surgery, a sanitary pontic has been selected for maintainability.

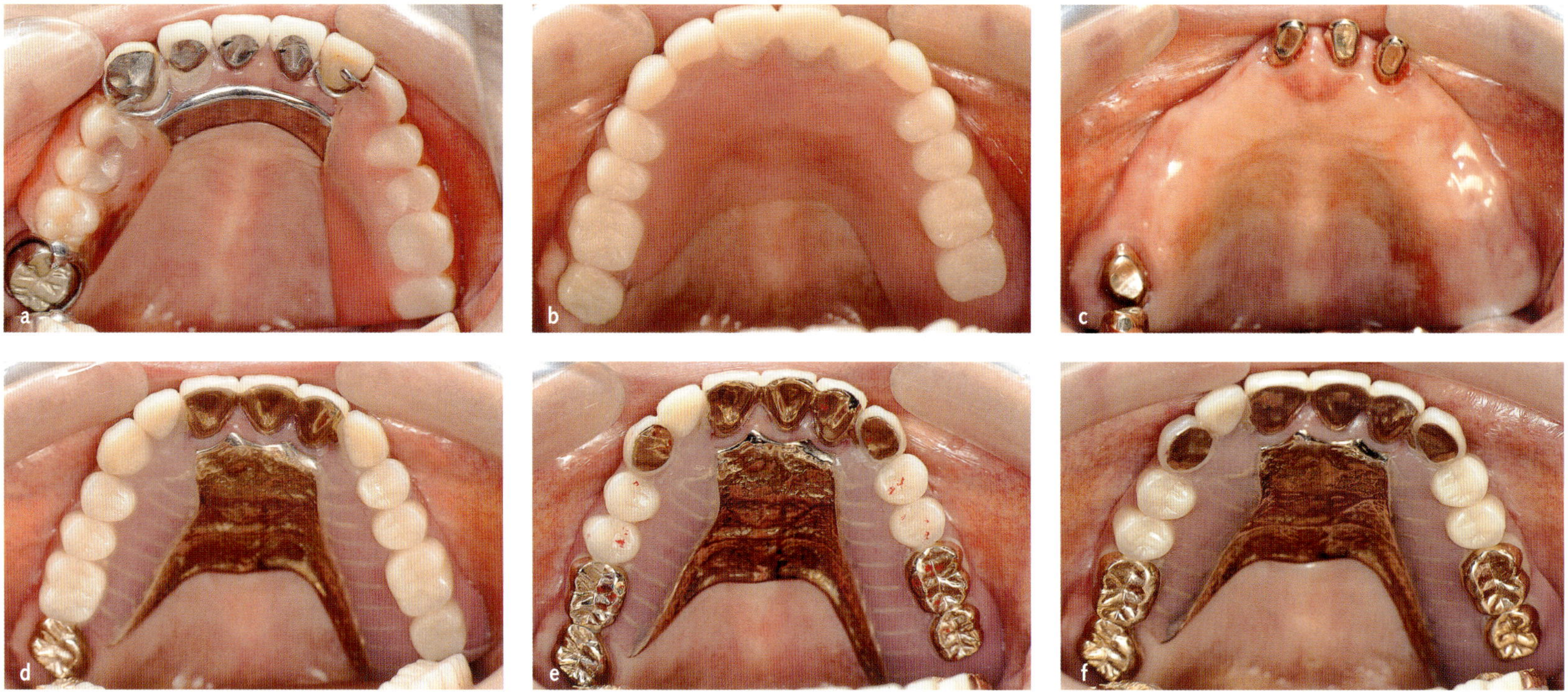

Fig 5-111 Improvement in the maxillary arch. (a) Conditions at the first visit. (b) Provisional restoration. (c) Conditions at the time of delivery of the denture. (d) The telescopic denture is supported by the right central incisor, lateral incisor, canine and second molar and by the left central incisor and lateral incisor. (Maxillary prostheses made by Mr Takahisa Tashiro, RDT.) (e) The occlusal surfaces of the supporting teeth are replaced by metal (November 1999). (f) Conditions during maintenance (June 2002).

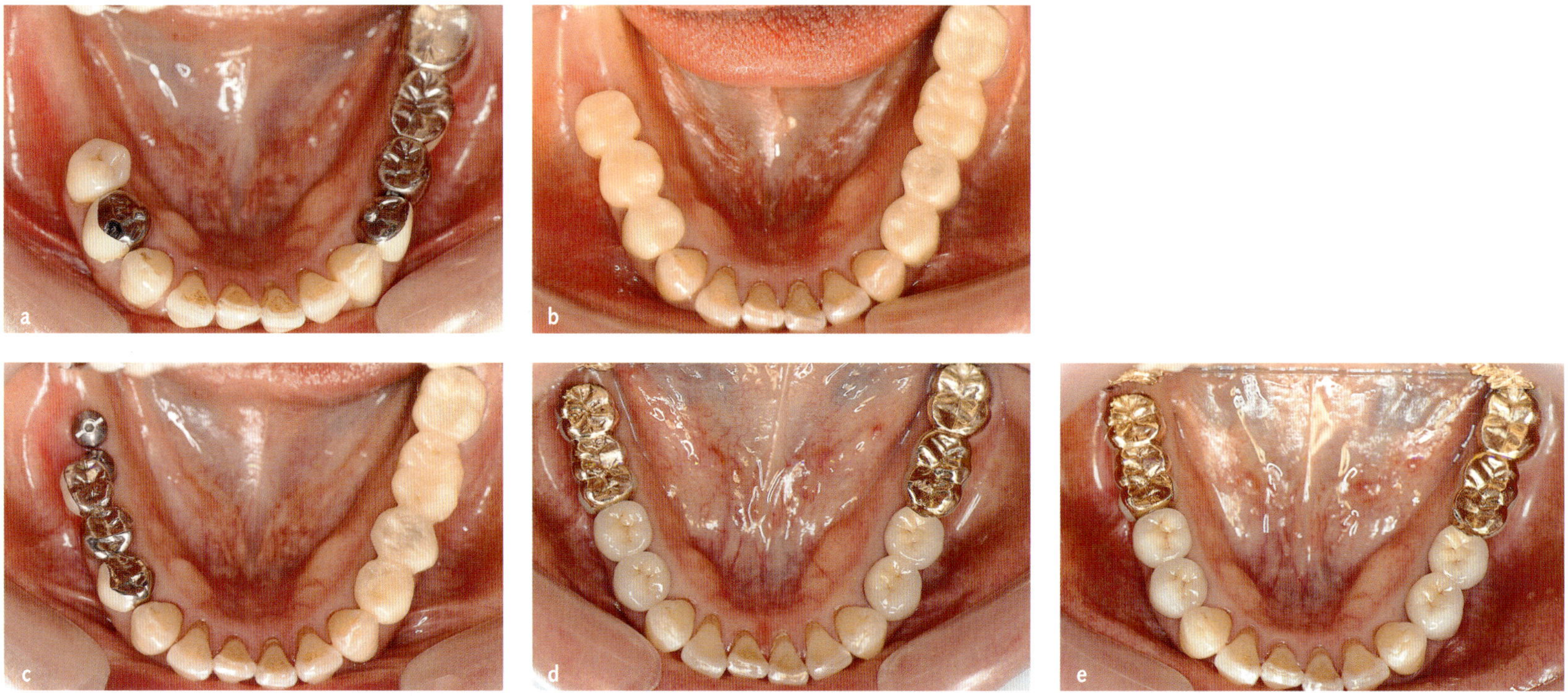

Fig 5-112 Improvement in the mandibular arch. (a) Mandibular occlusal view at the first visit. The left first molar, right first molar, and right second molar are missing. (b) Provisional restoration. (c) Implants are placed at the site of the mandibular right first molar and second molar. Provisional restorations (with metal occlusal surfaces) are provided for the right first premolar, second premolar, and first molar. (d) Delivery of final prostheses (November 1999). (Mandibular prostheses made by Mr Kiyoharu Takada, RDT.) (e) Conditions during the maintenance phase (June 2002).

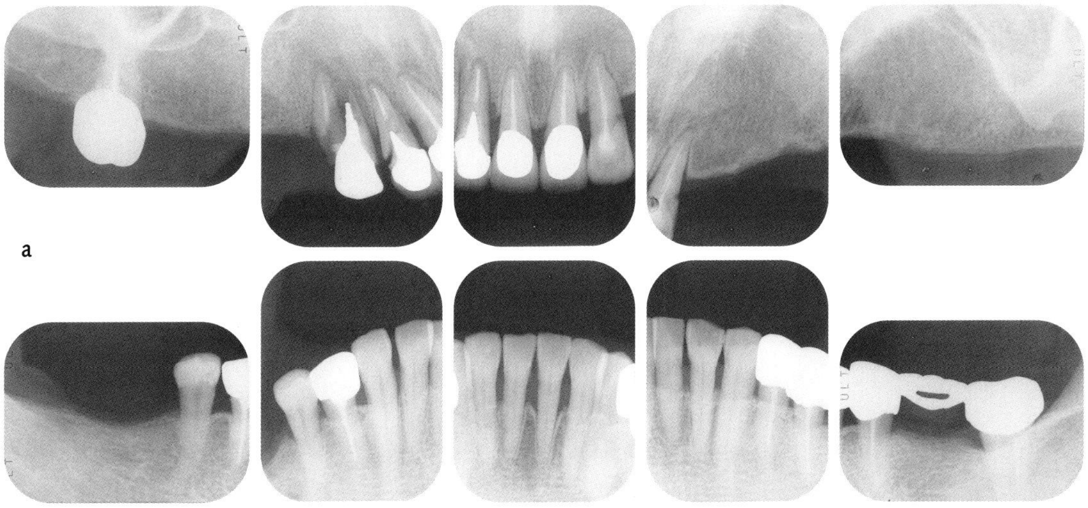

a

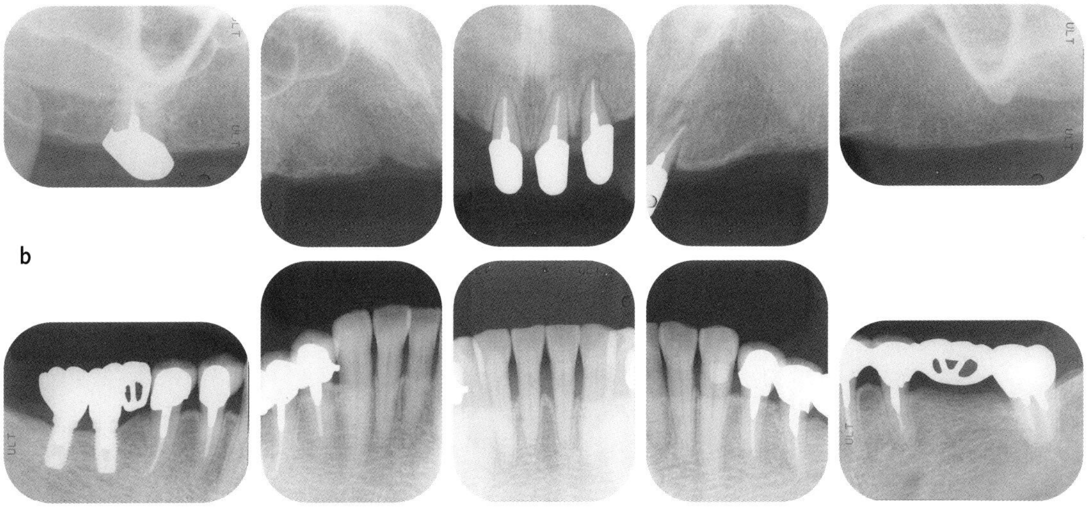

b

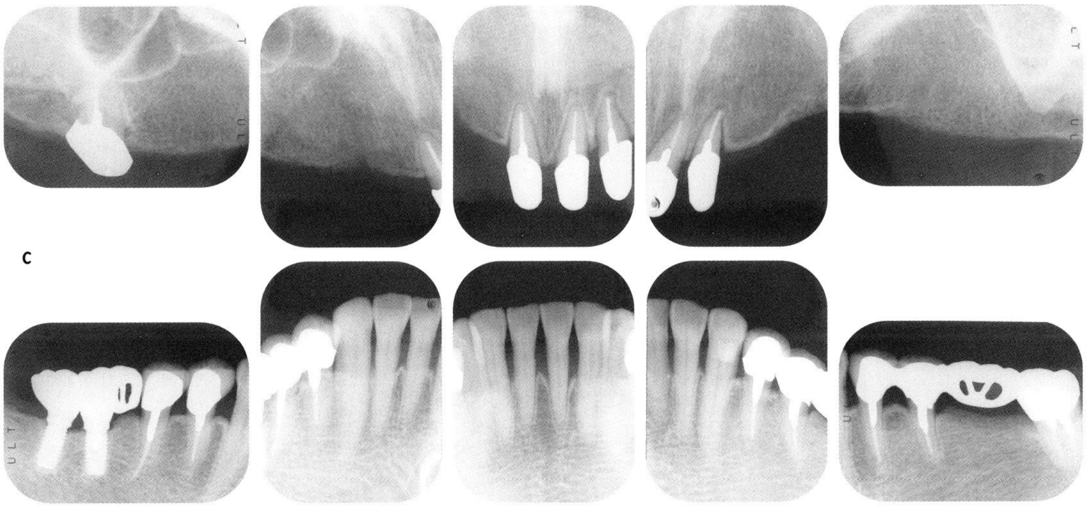

c

Fig 5-113 Radiographs before and after treatment. (a) At the first visit, there is evidence of trauma to the remaining teeth. (b) The final prostheses are delivered 1 year 7 months after the first visit. (c) Radiographs taken 4 years 4 months after the first visit. Evidence of traumatic occlusion in the mandible has diminished. In the maxilla, a limited degree of improvement is obtained because of the compromised conditions of the retained teeth. If implants are not used to support molar occlusion, an RPD may have to be considered as a compromise treatment; this denture often functions as an interim appliance until the patient requires a complete denture.

Management of Peri-Implant Tissue

Peri-implant tissue comprises connective tissue and mucosal epithelial tissue in contact with both an implant body, which is integrated with bone, and the superstructure surface. Although a natural appearance tends to be prioritized, because high esthetics is demanded by patients in an implant prosthesis, the shape and appearance must be supported by the implants and the peri-implant tissue. For example, bone topography should not be considerably distorted simply to establish a natural, toothlike emergence.

To obtain proper bone regeneration around implants, GBR techniques have to be utilized, which can cause a significant loss in keratinized mucosa. Consequently, an increase of keratinized mucosa should be considered prior to implant placement if insufficient keratinized mucosa exists. Even for a patient who had limited keratinized tissue prior to surgery, the use of techniques for obtaining greater attachment of keratinized tissue should be considered at the second-stage surgery. In management of peri-implant tissue, attention should be paid to the overall environment that consists of the superstructure and the (keratinized) oral mucosa as well as the area of contact between the superstructure and the soft tissue.

Table 5-1 Guidelines for regeneration of interdental papillae*

Class	Restoration	Threshold proximity	Soft tissue height limitation
1	Tooth-tooth	1.00 mm	4.50–5.00 mm
2	Tooth-pontic	N/A	6.75 (5–8 mm)
3	Pontic-pontic	N/A	6.50 (5–9 mm)
4	Tooth-implant	1.50 mm	6.50 (5–9 mm)
5	Implant-pontic	N/A	5.75 (5–9 mm)
6	Implant-implant	3.00 mm	4.50 (4–7 mm)

*These guidelines were suggested by Garber et al.

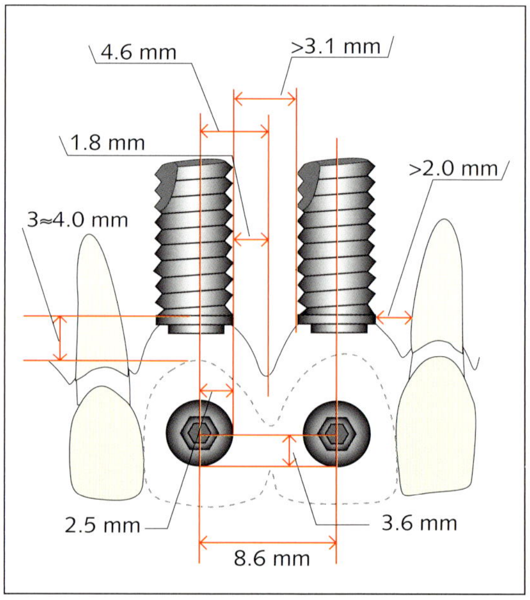

Fig 5-114 Distance between implants and natural teeth, shown by Saadoun et al.

Esthetic considerations

To obtain esthetic success in implant prostheses, we need to create peri-implant tissue that is similar to that of natural teeth. However, peri-implant tissue is anatomically different from tooth-supported periodontal tissue. The peri-implant tissue is pseudotissue. Tissues that look like interdental papilla, a free gingival margin, or attached gingiva are all pseudotissues created by the oral mucosa. To create such pseudotissue, a carefully thought out design is required at the time of implant placement with regard to the distance between the implant and the natural tooth, the interimplant distance, the implant angulation, and the implant height over the bone crest (Table 5-1 and Fig 5-114). To obtain sufficient amounts of soft tissue, soft tissue augmentation is often needed in addition to implant placement and abutment connection surgeries (Fig 5-115).

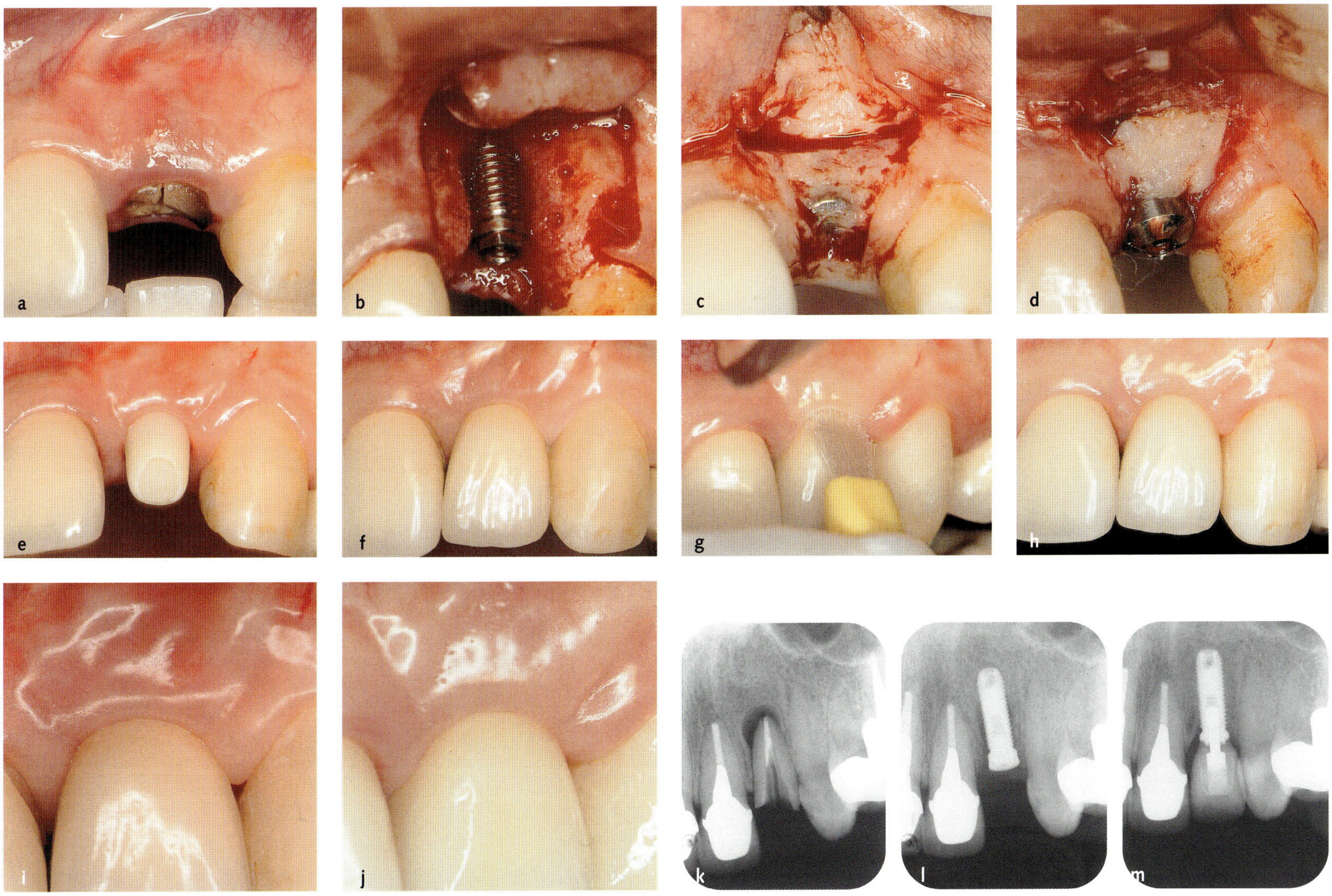

Fig 5-115 Depth of implant placement. (a) A metal-ceramic crown delivered 5 years ago, along with the post and core, is dislodged. The tooth is extracted because there is a root fracture. (b) An implant is placed 1 month postextraction. Bone loss is noted both buccally and lingually. Because sufficient bone is available mesiodistally, the initial stability is achieved at 3 mm deep and GBR is conducted with a nonresorbable membrane (W. L. Gore). (c) About 4 months postsurgery, at second-stage surgery, a partial-thickness flap is raised. The implant is found to be covered with bonelike tissue. (d) A connective tissue graft is completed to prevent gingival recession and obtain an esthetic gingival drape. (e) A CerAdapt porcelain abutment (Nobel Biocare) is connected. (f) An Empress II all-ceramic superstructure (Ivoclar Vivadent) is cemented with adhesive cement. (g) Plaque control around the implant is difficult. Use of a Pocket Cleaner is helpful. (h) Photograph taken 2 years post delivery of prostheses. (i) At delivery of the final prosthesis, A scar remains due to the converging vertical incisions at the second-stage surgery. (j) Appearance 4 years after delivery of the prosthesis. (k) Root fracture of the maxillary left central incisor is evident. (l) At implant placement, the implant is placed 3 mm deep. No bone is present buccally or lingually. (m) Bone regeneration is evident 4 years 2 months after surgery (4 years 3 months after root fracture).

Long-term prognosis of implant restorations

Treatment goals include restorative goals, such as stabilization of occlusion, correction of occlusal surfaces, and mechanical stabilization of the prosthesis; as well as recovery of function and morphology, including esthetics with the gingival drape and regeneration of interdental papilla-like tissue. These goals will not be achieved by chance. Clinical data have been accumulated, and certain outcomes are obtained if implant surgery design strictly follows defined restorative goals, including the bone volume required around the implants, the connective tissue volume, the distance between the implant and the natural tooth, the inter-implant distance, and the depth of implant placement. Supporting technologies such as bone regeneration, ridge augmentation, and soft tissue formation will be utilized to help achieve these goals (Figs 5-116 to 5-118).

Challenge of providing scalloped form with an implant at the central incisor

A single-implant prosthesis at a maxillary central incisor involves the challenge of creating a scalloped gingival form symmetric to that of the contralateral central incisor. Implants placed in bone are generally cylindrically shaped, and the bone level created by the abutment-connecting surface is flat, making it difficult to produce a scalloped form of bone. There have been reports of attempts to create a scalloped form with abundant soft tissue by placing implants deeper. This, however, resulted in significant difficulties in periodontal maintenance. In the clinical case shown in Fig 5-116, an implant was placed in 1996. We placed the implant relatively deep, which resulted in an imbalance in the gingival drape. Eventually soft tissue surgery was completed to restore and maintain esthetics.

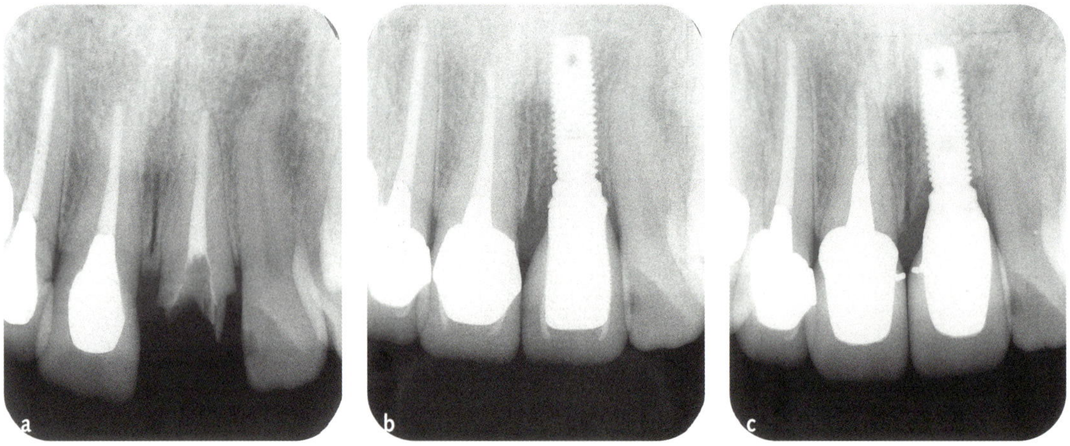

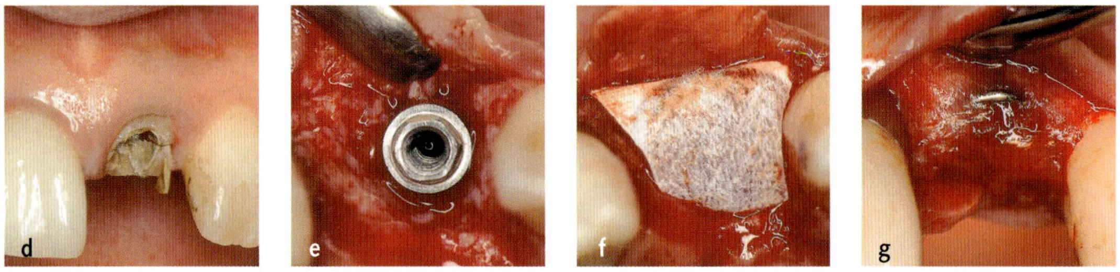

Fig. 5-116 (a) The maxillary left central incisor is extracted because of a root fracture. (b) Two months after tooth extraction, an implant was placed with a GBR procedure. About 1 year 2 months after extraction, the superstructure was delivered. (c) About 5 years after extraction. A crown for the maxillary right central incisor and an implant abutment have been remade. (d) Fractured maxillary left central incisor root. (e and f) An implant is placed and covered with an expanded polytetrafluoroethylene (e-PTFE) nonresorbable membrane 2 months postextraction. (g) Two months after surgery, part of the membrane is exposed and the membrane is removed earlier than anticipated. The top of the implant is covered with granulation tissue. (h) Although the superstructure is delivered, there is a concern about the imbalance of the gingival drape. Photograph taken about 1 year after surgery, 2 months after delivery of the prosthesis. (i) After fabrication of a new prosthesis for the maxillary right central incisor, the abutment and crown for maxillary left central incisor are also remade. To recover a symmetric gingival drape, a connective tissue graft is completed using a modified Langer and Langer technique (the flap is raised only distally). (j) Natural harmony in the gingivae is restored. Photograph taken after 5 years.

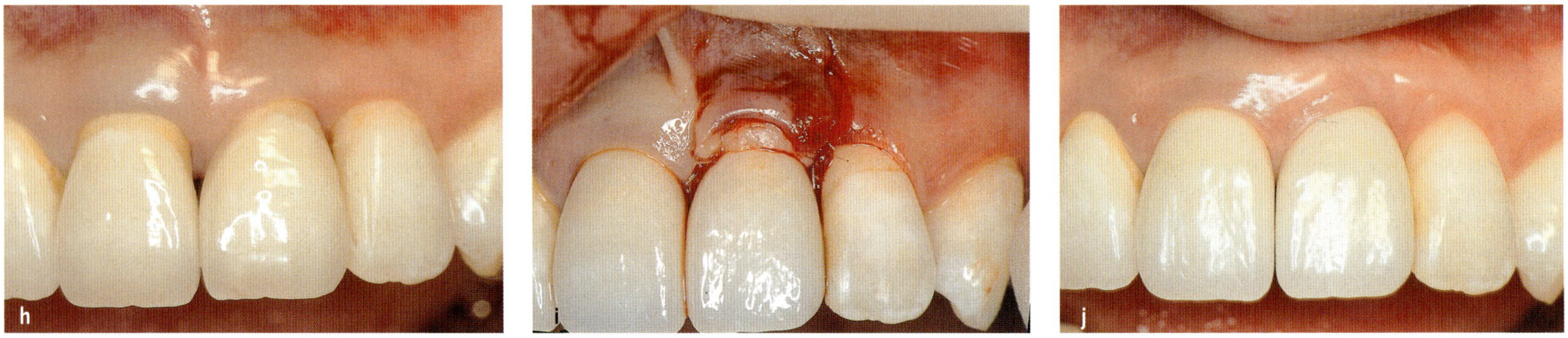

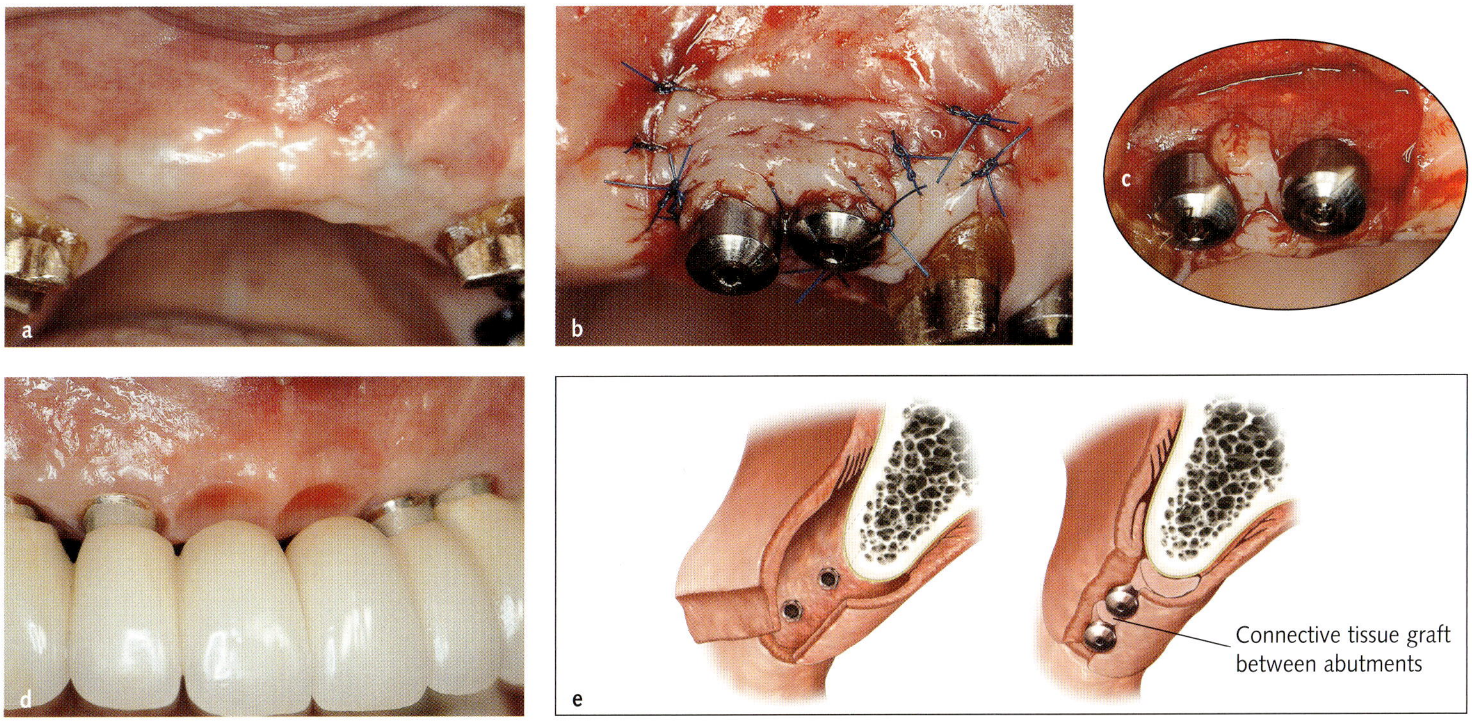

Fig 5-117 Augmentation of the surrounding soft tissue at second-stage surgery. (a) Keratinized gingiva is insufficient and a partial-thickness flap is raised from the palate at the second-stage implant surgery, aiming to increase the keratinized gingiva and harmony in the gingivae through formation of interdental papilla-like tissue. (b) The pedicle flap is buccally repositioned. A free connective tissue graft is completed in the distal area, which had inadequate tissue coverage. (c) A free connective tissue graft is completed between the implant abutments on the other side. (d) Electrosurgery is completed to form the mucosa in contact with the pontics, and resin is added to the base to establish ovate pontics. (e) Connective tissue is grafted between the implant abutments.

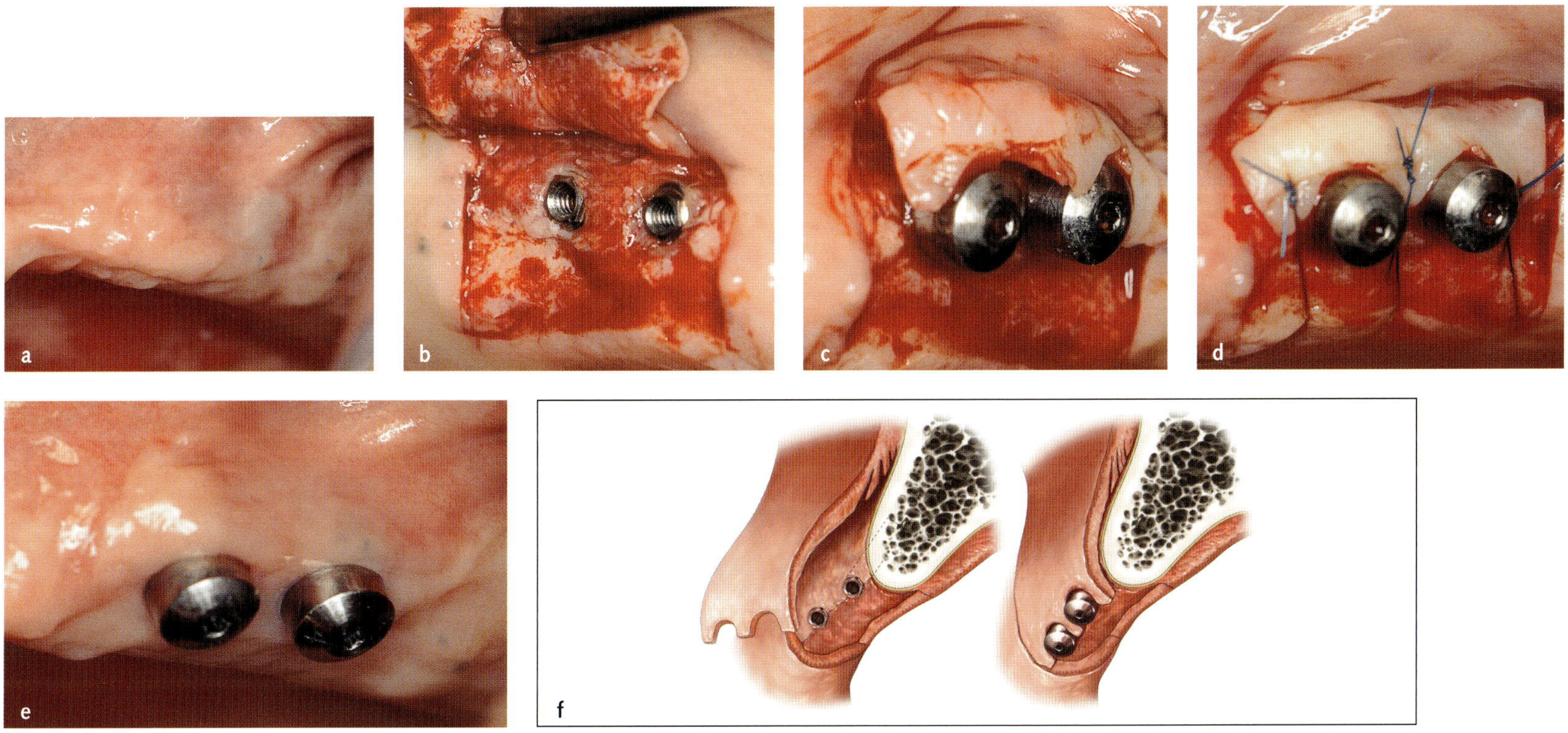

Fig 5-118 Vestibular extension around implants after regenerative therapy. (a) At implant placement, when bone regeneration is required, the mucosa is repositioned coronally to close the wound. Consequently, the vestibule is narrowed and the keratinized gingiva is insufficient. 7 months after implant placement. (b) At second surgery, a mucosal flap is raised from the palate, and a releasing incision is initiated at the base of the flap. (c) The pedicle flap is coronally repositioned and trimmed so that it can adhere closely to the healing abutments. (d) The palatal wound remains exposed. (e and f) Extension of the vestibule and fixed keratinized mucosa around the healing abutments have been obtained. These abutments are to receive O-rings to support an overdenture.

Although implants are highly predictable, physiologically a patient may not always adapt as we expect. The stomatognathic system always has had the ability to create a mechanical imbalance and constantly remodels according to aging, systemic disease, harmful diet or habit, and mechanical changes. Adaptation is seen in all living organisms. The most significant disadvantage of an implant prosthesis is that the implants themselves will not change during the adaptation of the stomatognathic system.

Sinus augmentation prior to implant placement

After two implants were placed in the maxillary right molar area, radiographs revealed crater-shaped bone resorption around the distal implant, which seemed to have been affected by occlusal forces. The opposing tooth developed furcation involvement. The distal implant was separated and removed. The edentulous ridge in the maxillary molar area is often thin, and often it is not possible to place implants of sufficient length. To solve this problem, sinus augmentation and a sinus lift were completed (Fig 5-119).

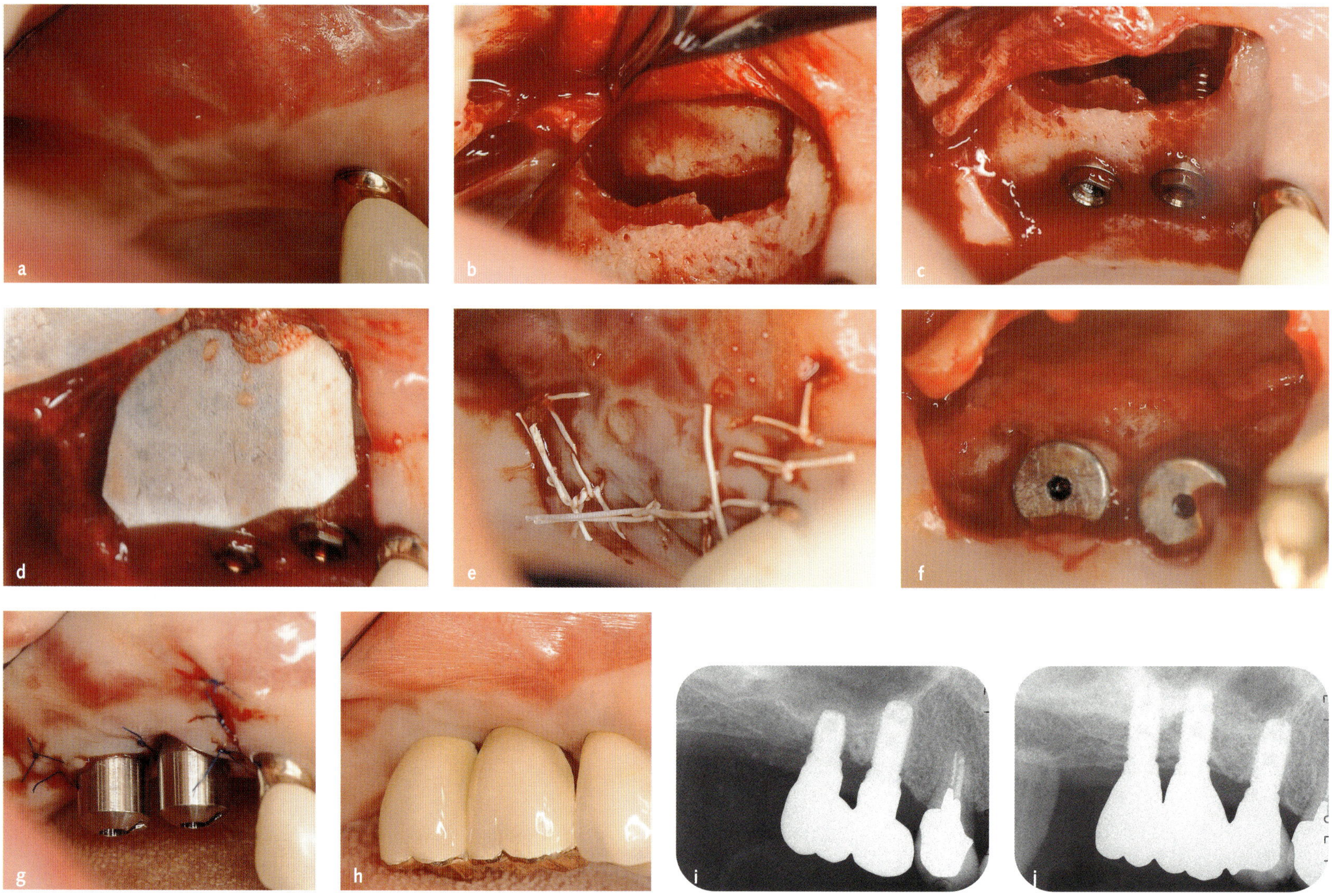

Fig 5-119 (a) Prior to surgery, 11 months after sectioning of the superstructure and removal of the distal implant. (b) A full-thickness flap is raised to expose the buccal bone, and a groove is made with a round bur until the Schneiderian membrane is seen. Buccal bone is intruded toward the sinus. (c) The implants are placed and the buccal wall has become the new floor of the sinus. (d) Bone grafting material is placed and covered with a membrane. (e) Suturing. (f) At the second-stage surgery, 9 months after sinus augmentation, the membrane is removed. Bone regeneration is confirmed. (g) Abutment connection. (h) The final prostheses is delivered 2 months after abutment connection. (i) Radiograph taken prior to removal of the implant. (j) Radiograph taken after delivery of the final prostheses.

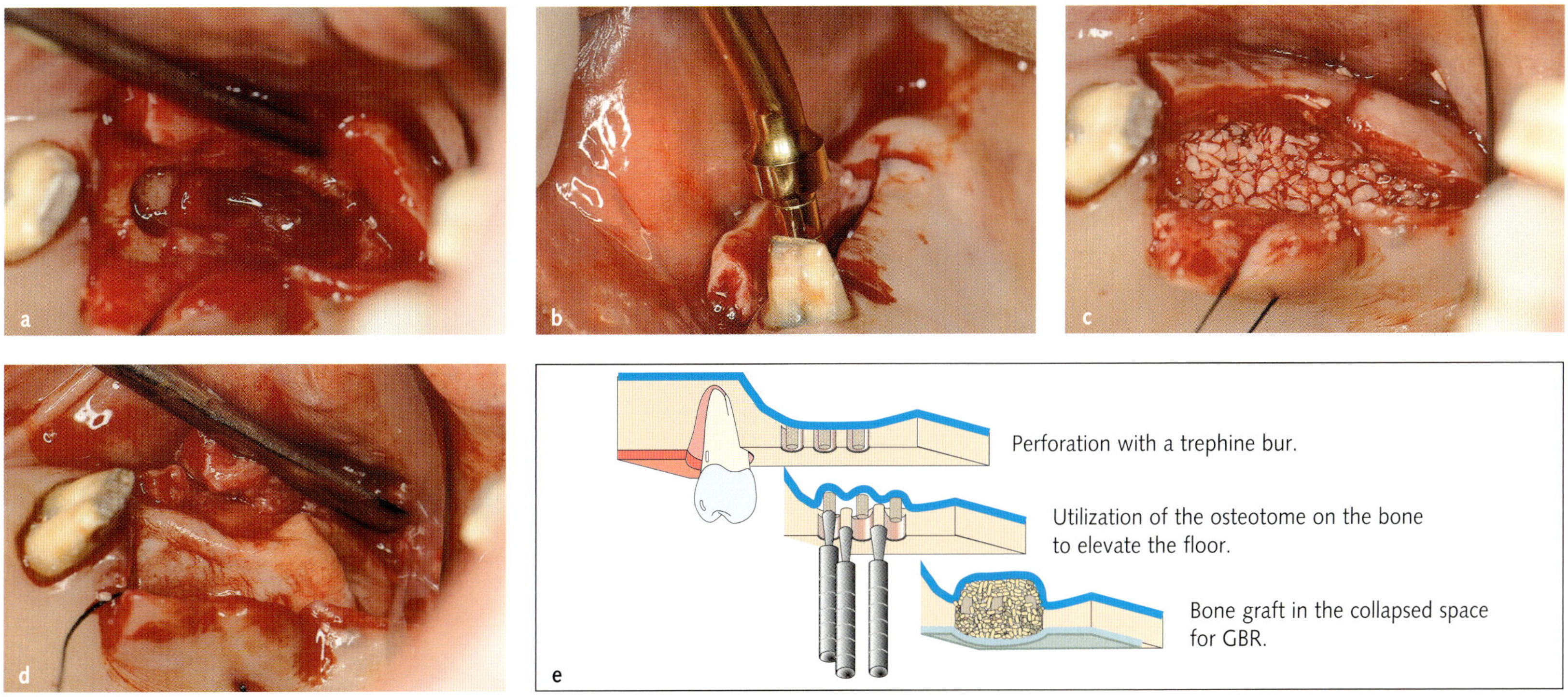

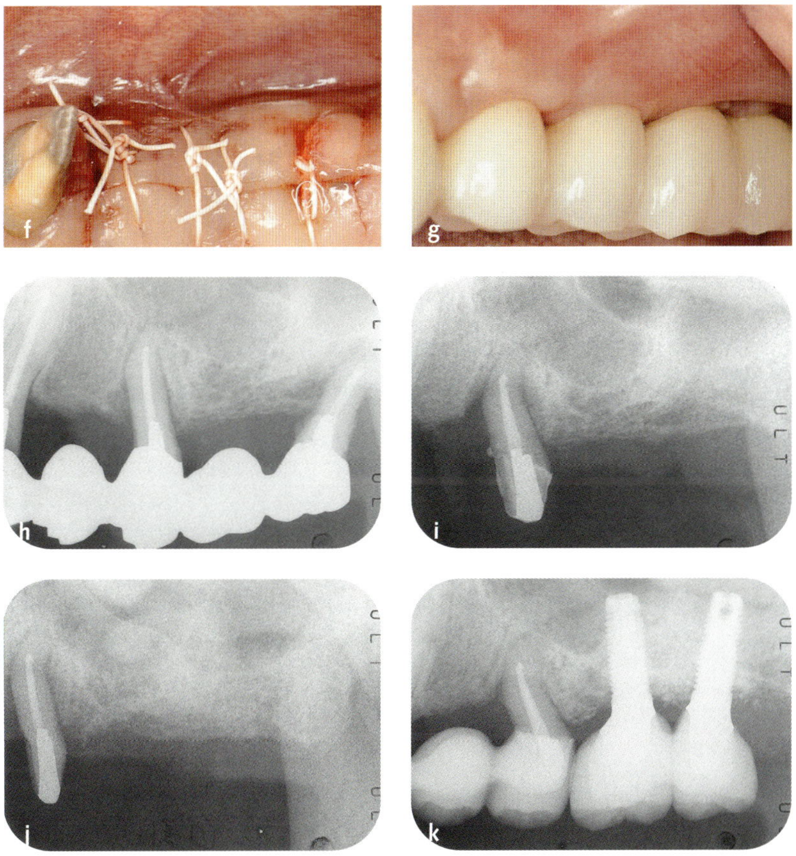

Fig 5-120 Sinus elevation with an osteotome. (a) A trephine bur is used to perforate the bone, almost reaching the sinus floor. (b) The osteotome is used to lift the sinus floor. (c) Bone grafting material is used to fill the space that is formed. (d) The area is covered with a resorbable membrane for GBR. (e) Safe use of an osteotome for a sinus lift. (f) The wound is sutured securely. (g) Bone regeneration is confirmed, implants are placed, and the superstructure is delivered,1 year postsurgery. (h) Radiograph taken at the first visit. (i) Radiograph taken prior to the sinus lift. (j) Radiograph taken after the sinus lift. (k) Radiograph taken 2 years 6 months after the first visit, at delivery of the implant superstructure.

Peri-implant tissue management and contouring of the prosthesis

After second-stage implant surgery, the following treatments are conducted to improve the periodontal support and to correct the morphology of the final prosthesis so that it harmonizes with the adjacent teeth (Fig 5-121 to 5-125).

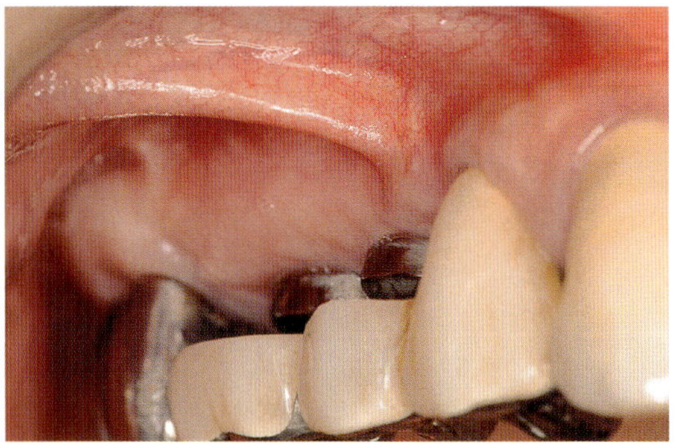

Fig 5-121 After second-stage implant surgery. Occlusion is reestablished.

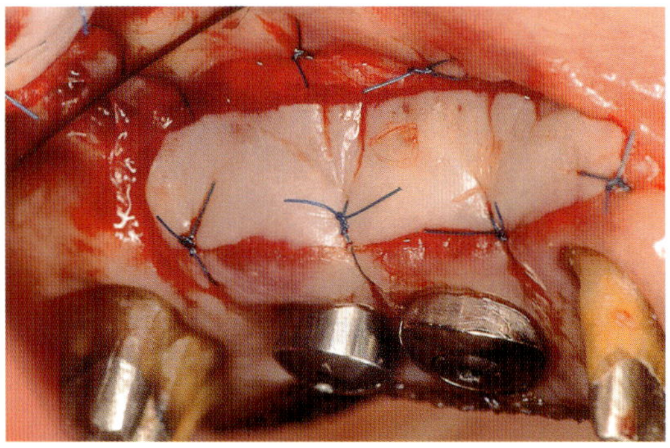

Fig 5-122 In the healing period after second-stage surgery, a free gingival graft is completed to improve the buccal periodontal support.

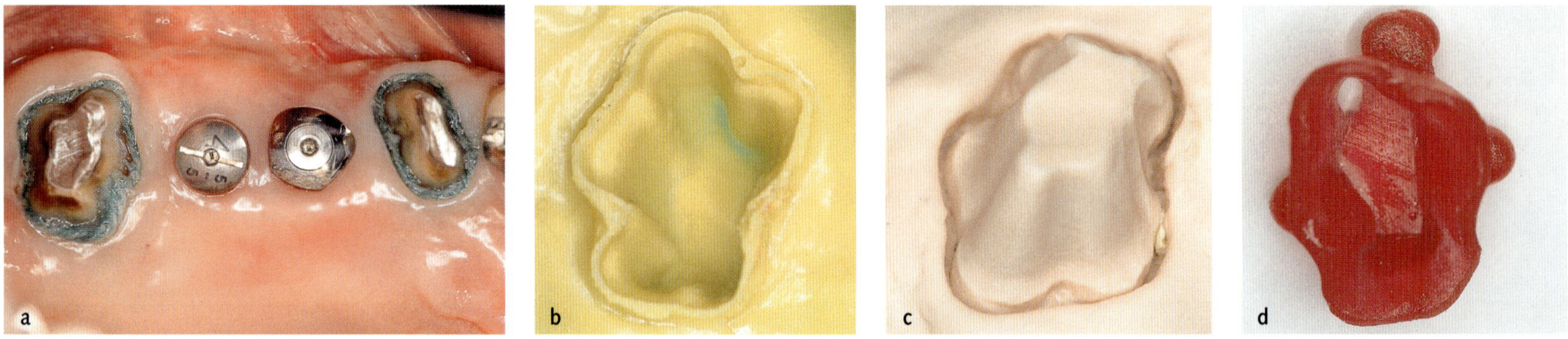

Fig 5-123 Impression of the teeth adjacent to the implants, where a ridge defect is present. (a) Double-cord technique for gingival retraction. (b) HIT impression of the maxillary right second molar. (c) The preparation finish line is clearly reproduced. (d) Coping made of pattern resin.

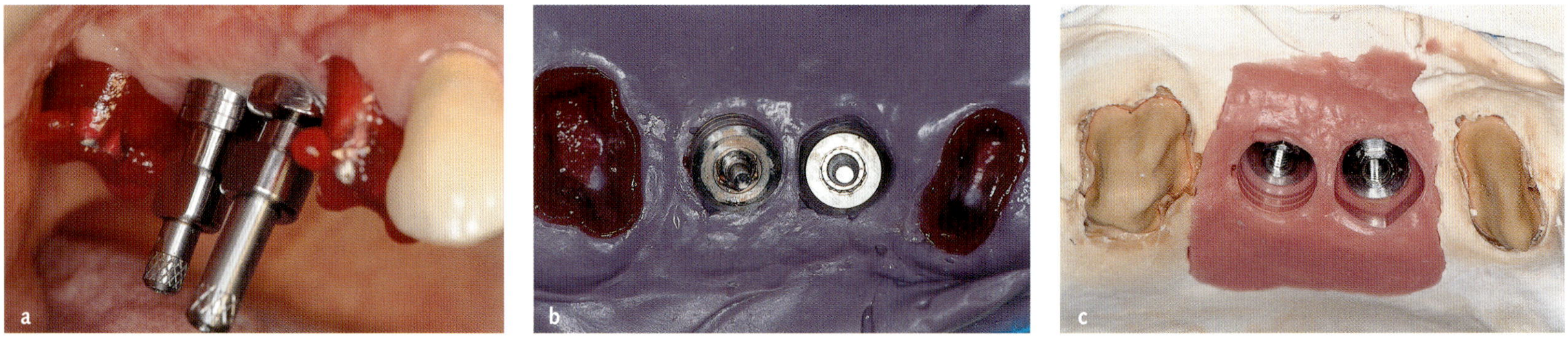

Fig 5-124 Impression procedures for implants. (a) Pick-up impression. (b) Emergence profile is accurately reproduced. (c) A soft tissue model is used to reproduce the surrounding soft tissue.

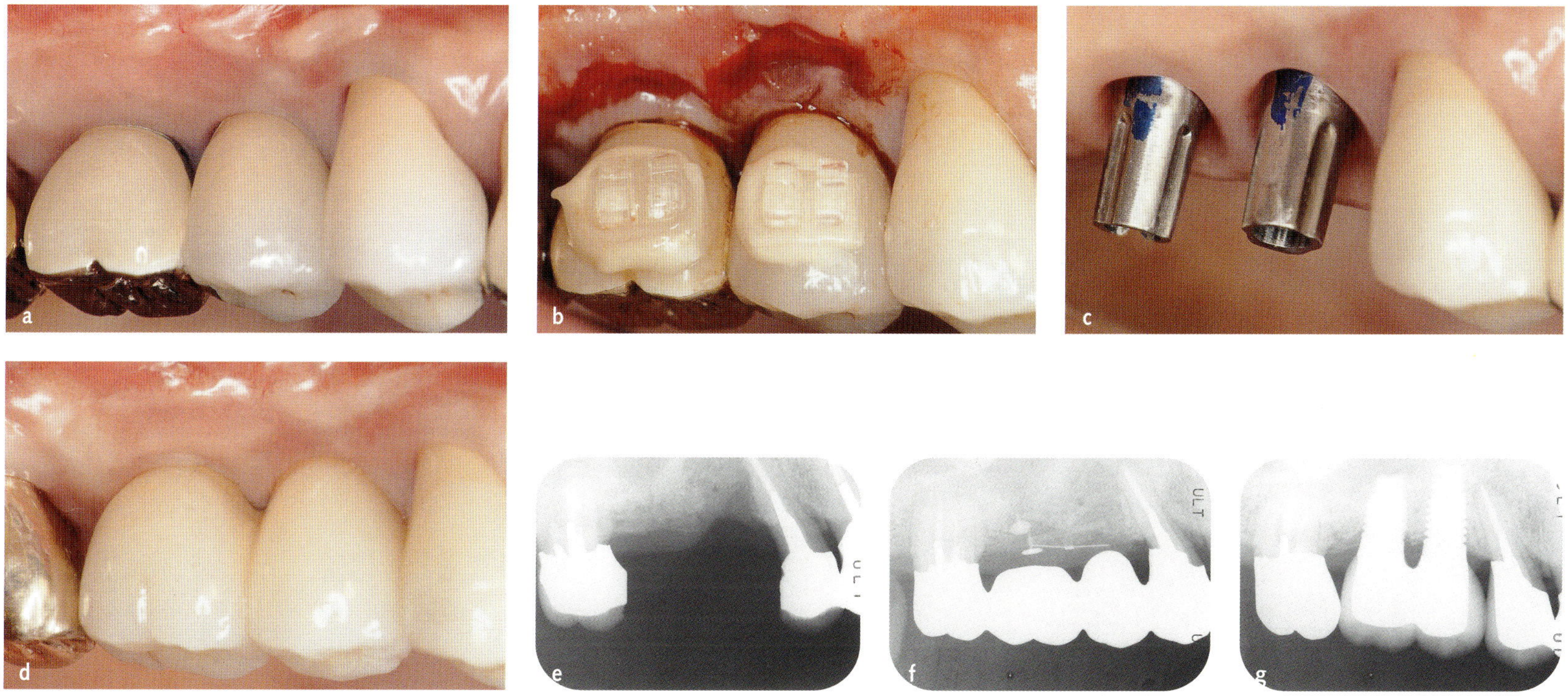

Fig 5-125 Peri-implant tissue management and contour of the final prosthesis. (a) Photograph taken about 1 year after second-stage surgery (October 1999). The restorations include a metal-ceramic single crown for the maxillary right first premolar, splinted metal-ceramic crowns for the second premolar and first molar, and a single cast crown for the second molar. There is a concern about a shadow at the cervical area of the first premolar, second premolar, and first molar. This has occurred because the provisional restoration was not refabricated and the emergence profile was not reevaluated. (b) A semilunar flap is coronally repositioned. (c) Custom abutments are refabricated. (d) Photograph taken 2 years 9 months after second-stage surgery (July 2001). No shadow is noted, and a corrected interdental papillae has been obtained. (e) Radiograph taken at tooth extraction (April 1998). (f) Radiograph taken during follow-up after GBR. (g) Radiograph taken 2 years after extraction, during maintenance.

Esthetic implant prostheses in areas with ridge resorption

In one clinical case, the mandibular left first and second molars had been missing and were not replaced, allowing extrusion of the maxillary teeth and loss of occlusal integrity (Fig 5-126). For recovery of occlusal support and correction of the occlusal plane, the occlusion as a whole, along with the individual teeth, must be taken into account during treatment planning (Figs 5-127 to 5-129). In Fig 5-126, however, the focus is on the peri-implant tissue management in the mandible.

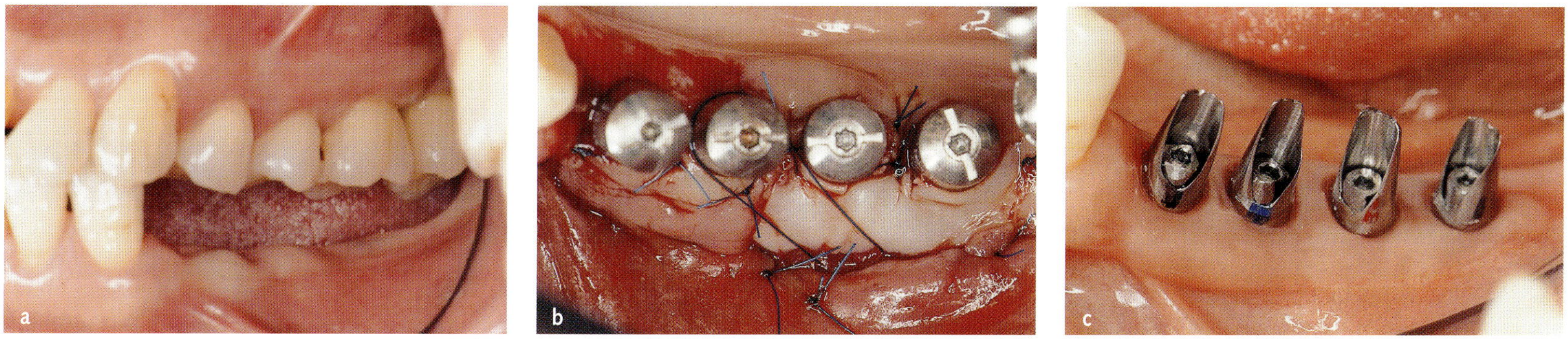

Fig 5-126 (a) The teeth missing in the posterior area on the left side have been left unreplaced, causing extrusion of the maxillary left second premolar, first molar, and second molar. The mandible has shifted to the left. (b) About 1 year 2 months after implant placement, at second-stage surgery, a pedicle flap of keratinized gingiva from the lingual aspect of the mandibular left first and second premolars is repositioned buccally. A free gingival graft is completed at the mandibular left and second molars for vestibular extension and acquisition of keratinized mucosa. (c) Healing abutments are replaced by the provisional abutments.

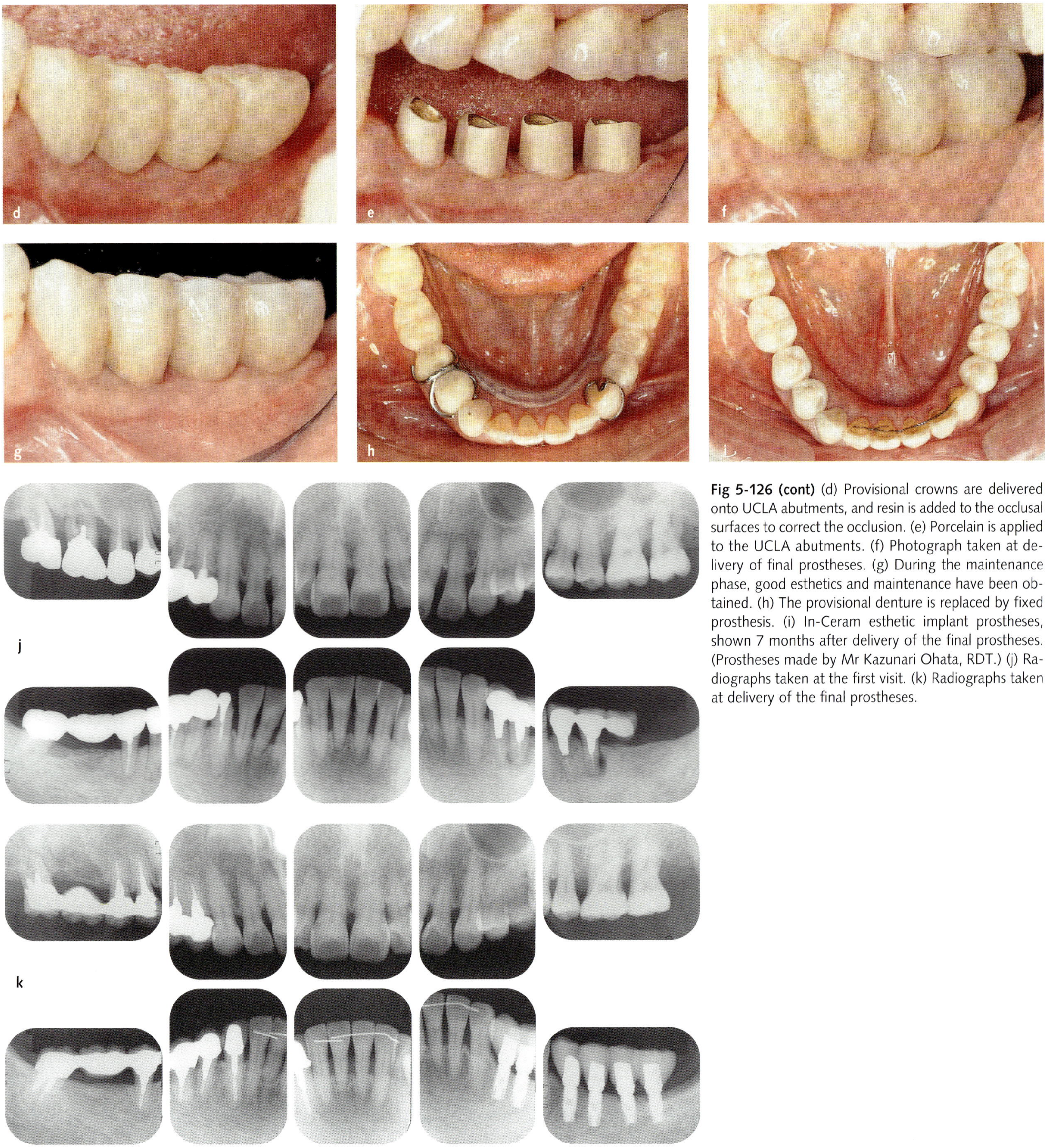

Fig 5-126 (cont) (d) Provisional crowns are delivered onto UCLA abutments, and resin is added to the occlusal surfaces to correct the occlusion. (e) Porcelain is applied to the UCLA abutments. (f) Photograph taken at delivery of final prostheses. (g) During the maintenance phase, good esthetics and maintenance have been obtained. (h) The provisional denture is replaced by fixed prosthesis. (i) In-Ceram esthetic implant prostheses, shown 7 months after delivery of the final prostheses. (Prostheses made by Mr Kazunari Ohata, RDT.) (j) Radiographs taken at the first visit. (k) Radiographs taken at delivery of the final prostheses.

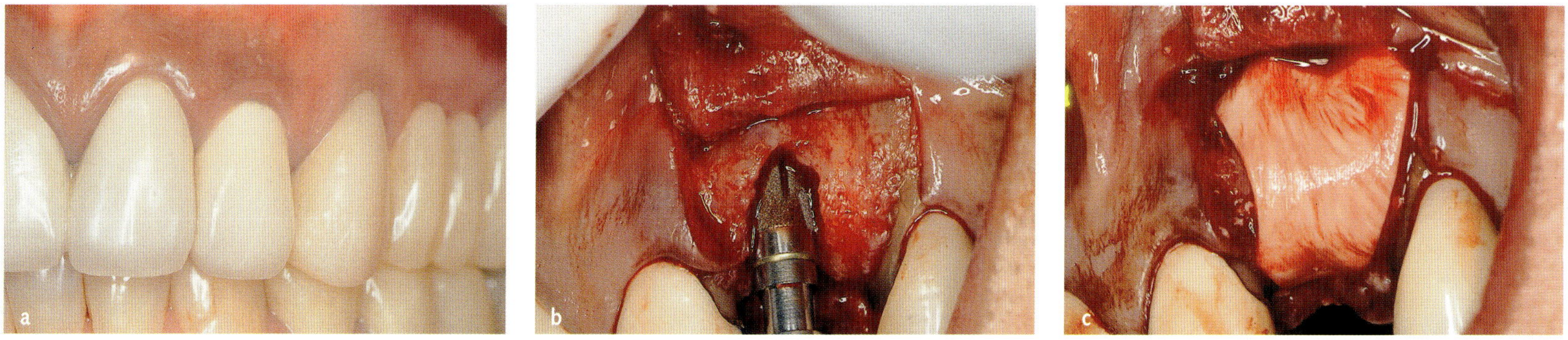

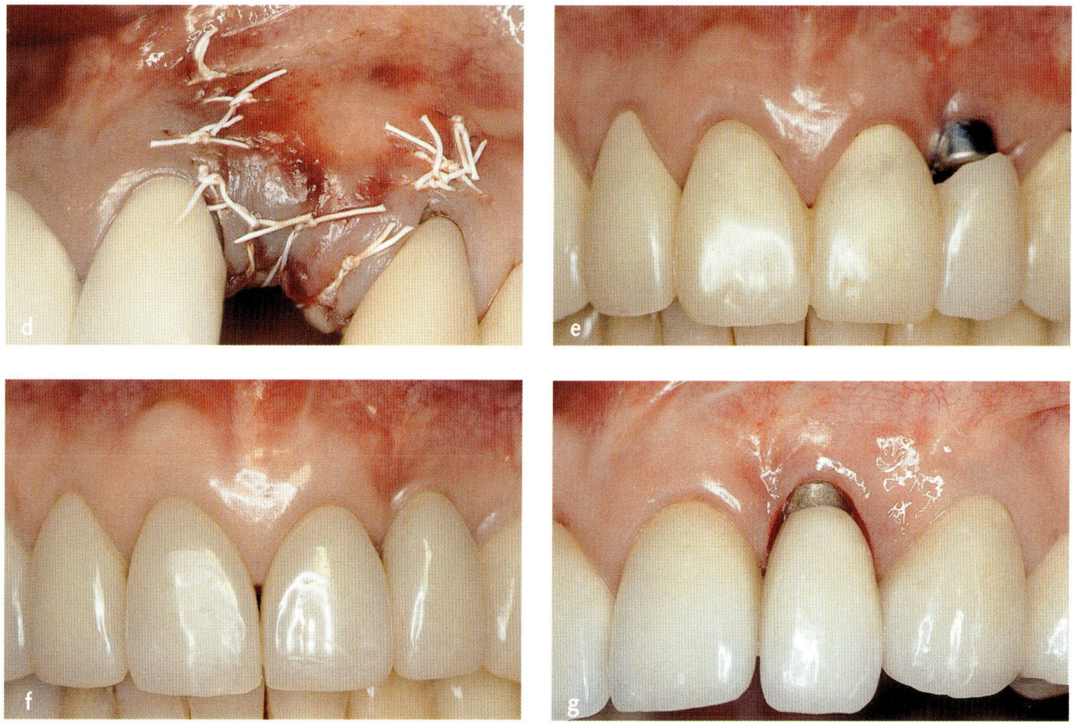

Fig 5-127 Immediate implant placement in the anterior region. (a) Because of a perforation, the maxillary left lateral incisor and maxillary left first premolar are to be extracted. (b) A Frialit-2 3.8-mm, cylinder-type implant is immediately placed. (c) For the perforation area on the buccal side, GBR is conducted with a bone graft and a resorbable membrane. (d) A releasing incision is made to coronally reposition the interdental papilla. It is tightly sutured. (e) The initial provisional restoration is shown. (f) A Procera prosthesis is delivered after the dentogingival complex matured with a final provisional restoration in place. (g) Photograph taken at try-in of the Procera crown on the maxillary left lateral incisor. (h) At the first visit, the maxillary left lateral incisor and maxillary left first premolar have perforations and are to be extracted. A defective root canal treatment is present on the maxillary left canine. (i) Radiograph taken after 2 years, 1 month after immediate implant placement. (j) Radiograph taken at delivery of a Procera all-ceramic crown. A Galvano porcelain fixed partial denture is delivered for the maxillary left canine.

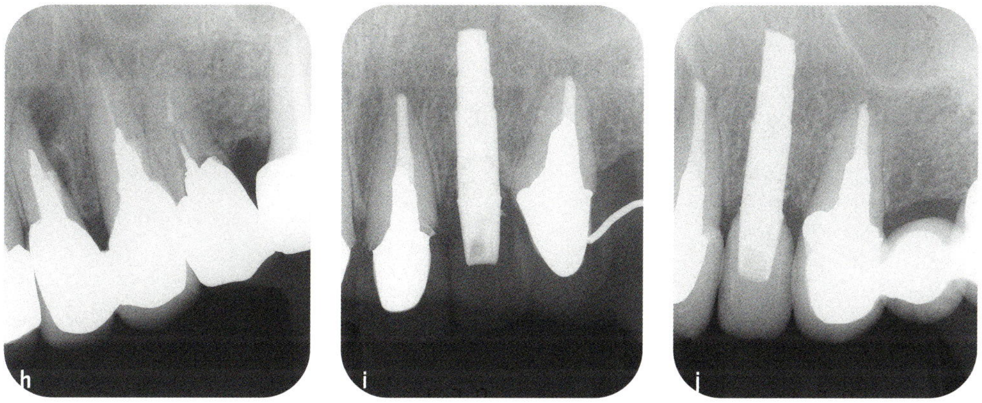

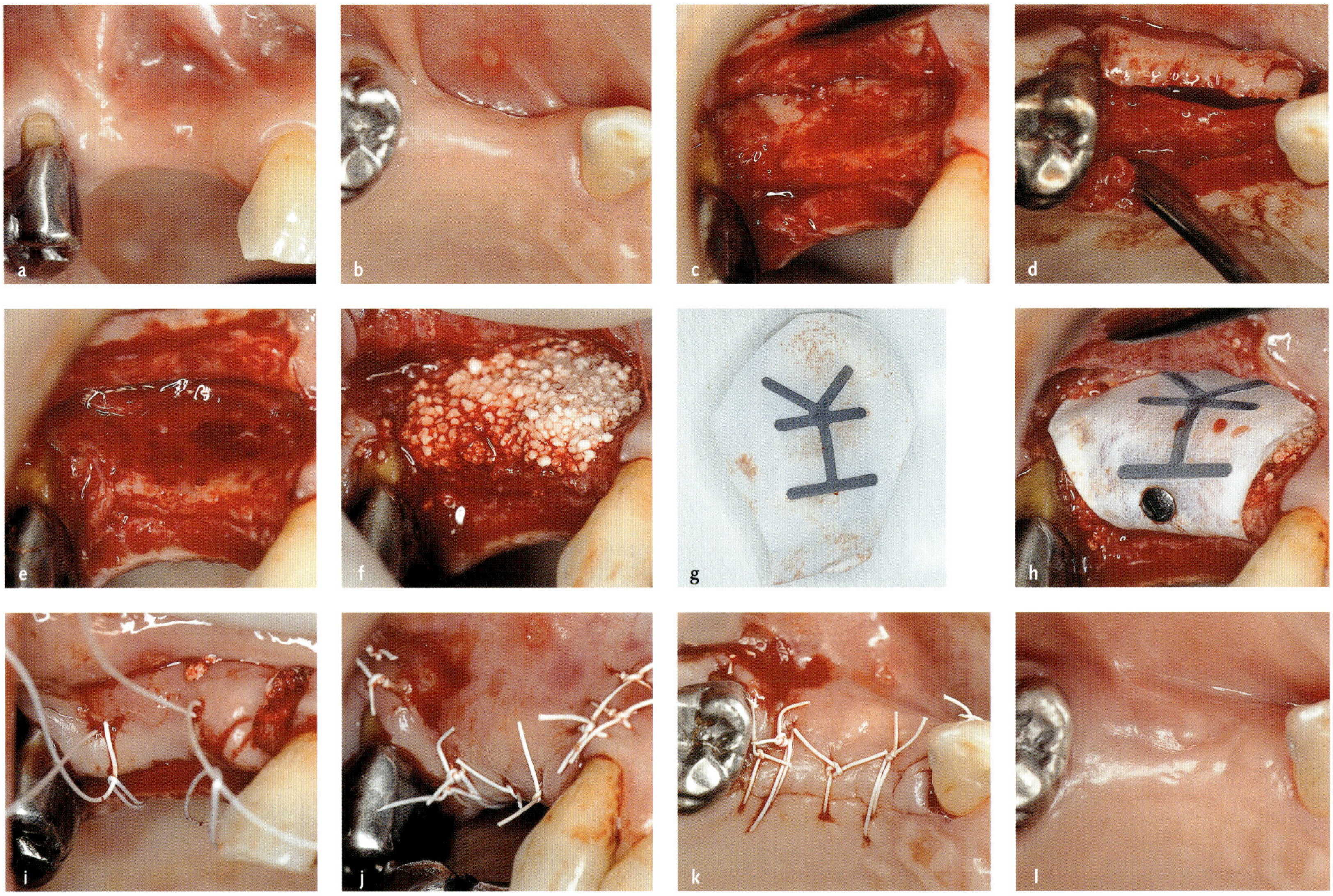

Fig 5-128 Basic GBR procedure for implant placement. (a and b) The maxillary left first and second premolars are missing. Although implant placement is planned, the ridge is very thin. (c and d) Vertical incisions are made in a butt joint manner to the MGJ, involving the interdental papillae from distal aspect of the maxillary right canine to the mesial aspect of the right first molar. For the crestal area, a horizontal incision is made in a slip joint manner from the palate to raise a full-thickness flap. (e) Round burs (Nos. 1 and 2) are used to perforate to cancellous bone, and the concave area is filled with the blood clot. (f) Bone grafting material (β-tricalcium phosphate) fills the area. (g) A membrane is trimmed to fit the area precisely. (h) One or two releasing incisions are made under the MGJ, and the bottom of the membrane is inserted under the periosteum and fixed by suturing (wing technique). A titanium pin is used to fix the membrane to the palate. (i) Gore-Tex suture No. 5 is used for two mattress sutures (three-layer suturing) at the mesial and distal sites to prevent dehiscence of the gingiva. (j and k) For the remaining area, simple sutures are secured. (l) Photograph taken 2 months after surgery. Bone augmentation can be accomplished without membrane exposure.

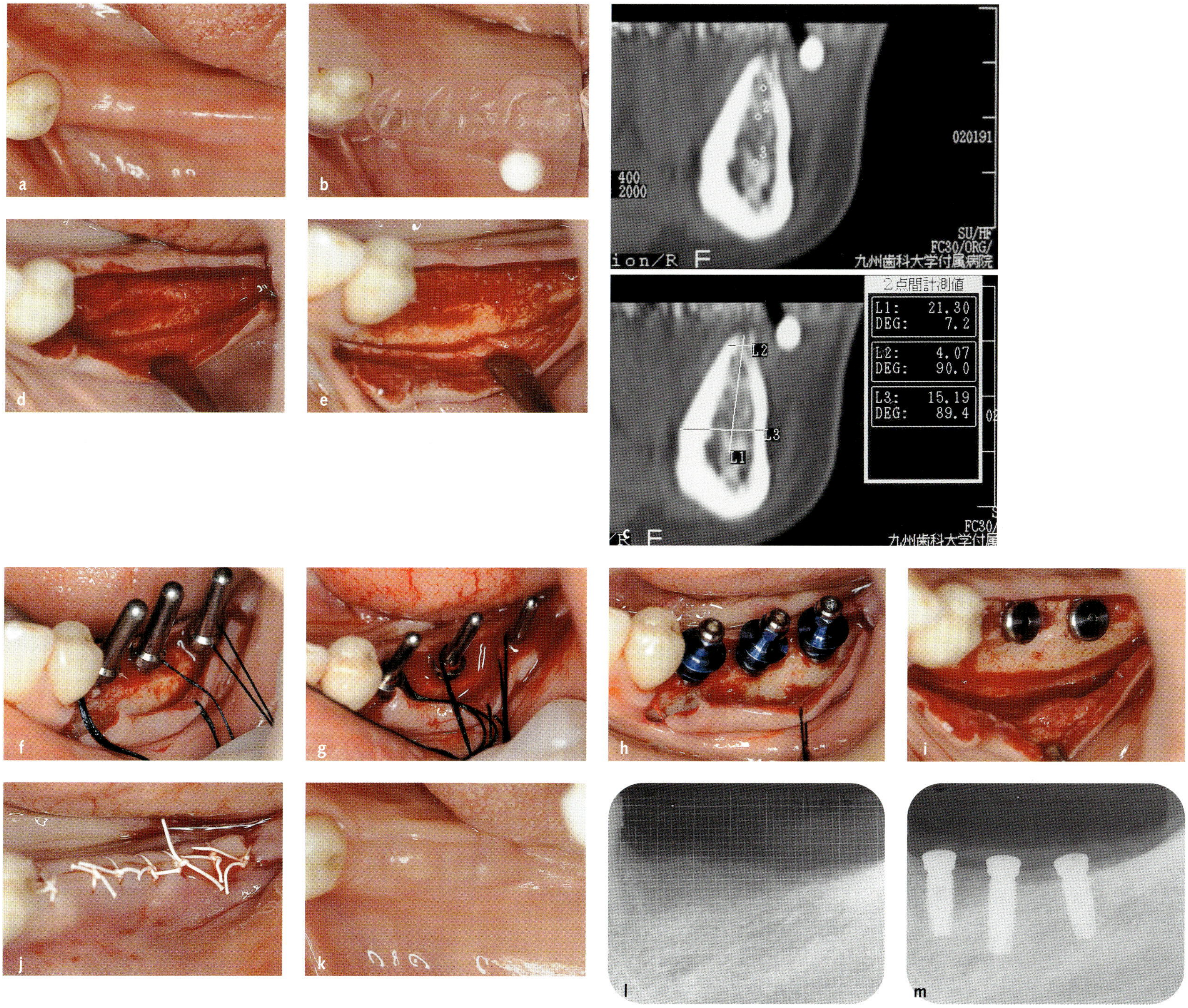

Fig 5-129 Basic procedure of implant placement. (a) The mandibular left second premolar, first molar, and second molar are missing (10 months after extraction of the second premolar). The ridge is relatively thin. (b) The patient was referred to a specialist to obtain a tomogram with a surgical stent. (c) CT images show sections of the mandible, indicating the accurate depth of implant placement. (d) A crestal incision is made to reflect a full-thickness flap. The bone width is only 3 to 4 mm. (e) A bone bur is used to reduce the height of the crest to a width of about 7 mm. (f) With the stent used as a guide, the initial site access is created with a 2-mm twist drill according to procedure. The drill is carefully moved up and down (to prevent burning of the bone) under copious irrigation. Direction indicators are used to confirm the distance to the inferior alveolar nerve and the direction of implants. (g) Drilling is conducted with a 3-mm twist drill, and the direction is corrected to obtain parallelism. (h) Three Osseotite implants (3i) are placed: 3.75 × 10.00 mm for the second premolar, 3.75 mm × 11.50 mm for the first molar, and 3.75 mm × 10.00 mm for the second molar. In anticipation of postoperative resorption, the implants are placed slightly buccally to create scalloped bone form. Bone morphology is corrected. (i) To release the tissue, two layers are formed under the MGJ. Care is taken to prevent damage to the mental nerve. (j) Interrupted sutures are made without tension to the gingival flap. (k) No dehiscence is seen 1 month postsurgery. (l) Immediately before implant placement. (m) Immediately after implant placement.

Functional Recovery and Stabilization of Partially Edentulous Dentitions

Clinical judgment with an insight into the patient's history

A variety of means are available for restoration of function in partially edentulous dentitions, ranging from removable dentures to implants. Advancement of edentulism creates a gap between the patient's self-image and the clinical oral conditions. Major problems, such as the patient's psychologic state and discomfort, have to be solved. However, the method of functional restoration should not be simply selected based on the patient's preference or a clinician's skills. Several treatment plan options should be considered in light of the patient's history, from the cause of edentulism to the current conditions and follow-up management.

As with any other restoration in edentulous patients, especially in a patient with a collapse of the occlusion, the case history should be evaluated and thorough consideration should be given as to why and how the edentulism and occlusal collapse occurred.

Complications and risks of treatment with advancement of edentulism

Although recovery of esthetics and function at the completion of prosthodontic treatment is certainly important, a living organism is constantly changing. The risk of the loss of homeostasis will continue with imbalance of occlusal forces, stresses to the abutment teeth, fatigue of the hard tissue, stability of the prosthesis, wear and deformation of the teeth and prosthesis, and the advancement of edentulism in addition to factors such as periodontal tissue inflammation, dental caries, attrition, and parafunction (Case 5-5).

In a patient with a significant number of missing teeth, thorough consideration is made to the control of intraoral forces. The occlusal relationship between the maxillary and mandibular arches, appropriate mandibular positioning, correction of opposing occlusal surface morphology, and establishment of correct occlusal guidance are major points to be noted. In designing a removable partial denture, the clinician should pay attention to a balance between how pressure is transmitted and how the pressure is applied. From the viewpoint of recovery of occlusal support, utilization of implants has brought about a drastic change in the functional recovery of patients with partial edentulism. An RPD is difficult for some patients to accept, and implant indications are restricted by various factors, including not only the ridge conditions and systemic health, but also the patient's lifestyle and age.

Objective of restoration of missing teeth

The objectives of restoration of missing teeth are to correct existing edentulism, to limit further tooth loss, and to stabilize the stomatognathic system, maintaining it into the future. In a case with advanced edentulism, it is difficult to judge to what extent the clinician should advance treatment or abandon extensive procedures. Such a clinical judgment cannot be made only from the dental or medical point of view. Restoration of partial edentulism with a removable denture is based on clinical judgment to accept variables to a certain degree while minimizing invasion of the tissues as much as possible. Further concerns of tooth loss should ideally be eliminated as much as possible during prosthodontic treatment with a removable partial denture. It should be understood that this concept is fundamentally different from that of implants, for which reconstruction is conducted after questionable situations have been minimized as much as possible.

Case 5-5 Functional recovery and retreatment of a case without vertical stops

Patient: *41-year-old woman at the time of first visit in 1979*

This patient had the typical occlusion observed in a patient who lacks vertical stops (Fig 5-130). Telescopic crowns were placed as abutments in the maxillary arch, and channel shoulder pin milling attachments were placed in the mandibular arch (Fig 5-131). Unfortunately, sufficient periodontal maintenance was not provided, and the patient presented to our office in October 1993 for the first time, 14 years 7 months after her initial dental visit (Fig 5-132). The occlusal surfaces were severely worn, and the denture was rotated and had settled into the tissue with a resultant decrease in the vertical dimension of occlusion. Because most abutment teeth exhibited defective root canal treatments and posts and cores with poor fit, along with secondary caries, a full-mouth reconstruction was initiated (Figs 5-133 to 5-147).

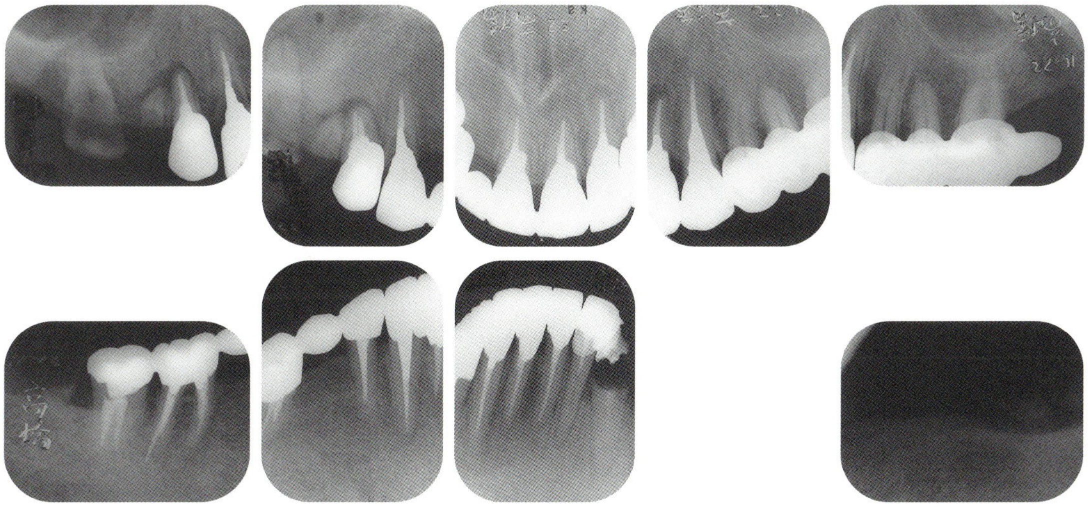

Fig 5-130 Radiographs taken in November 1980.

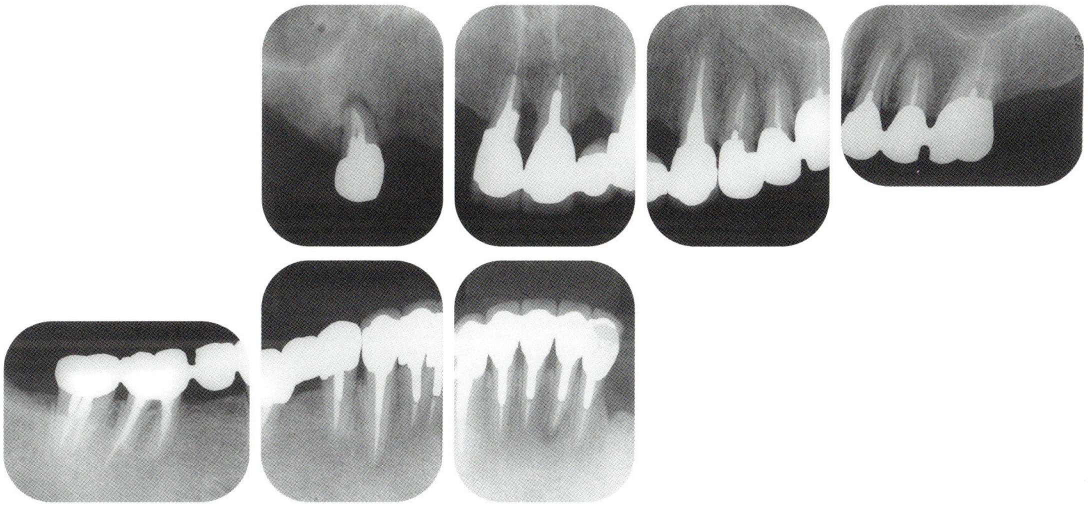

Fig 5-131 Radiographs taken 2 years 10 months after delivery of the final prostheses in November 1981. Because of the initial poor prognosis of the maxillary right central incisor and first premolar, these compromised teeth were extracted (December 1984). A telescopic denture was delivered for the maxilla.

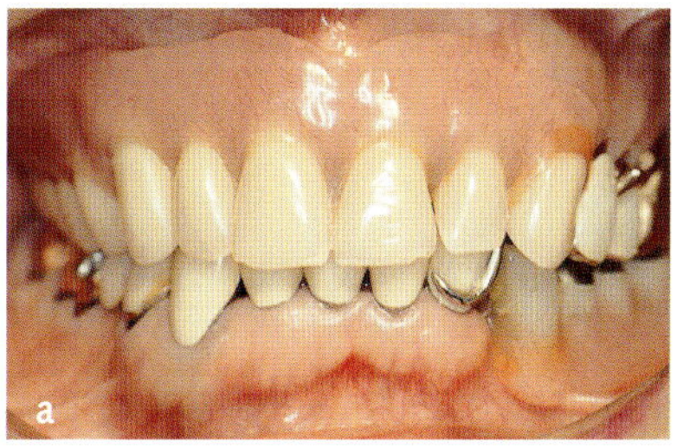

a

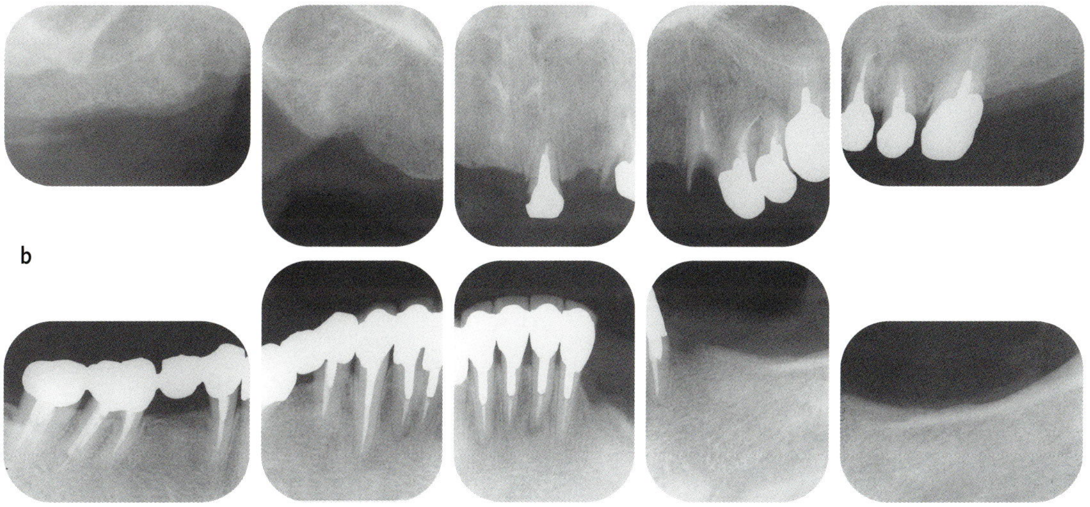

b

Fig 5-132 (a and b) About 8 years 10 months after delivery of the maxillary telescopic denture in December 1984, the denture fractured (October 1993). This is about 14 years after the patient's initial visit. A milling attachment denture was fabricated for the mandible. Full-mouth rehabilitation is treatment planned because of the defective root canal treatment and secondary caries.

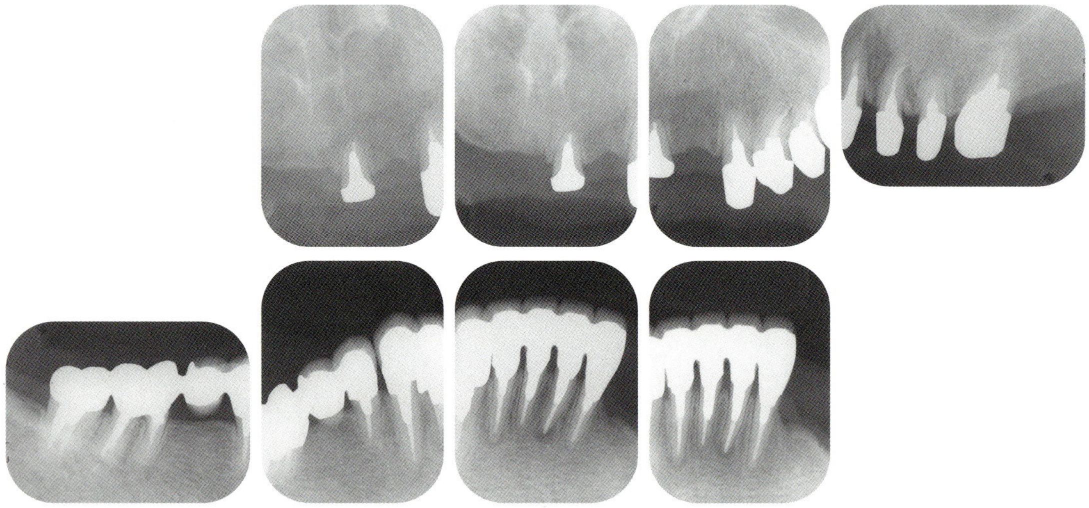

Fig 5-133 About 17 years after the patient's first visit, a new denture has been fabricated for the mandible (December 1996). A maxillary telescopic denture was refabricated about 1 year prior to this appointment (October 1995).

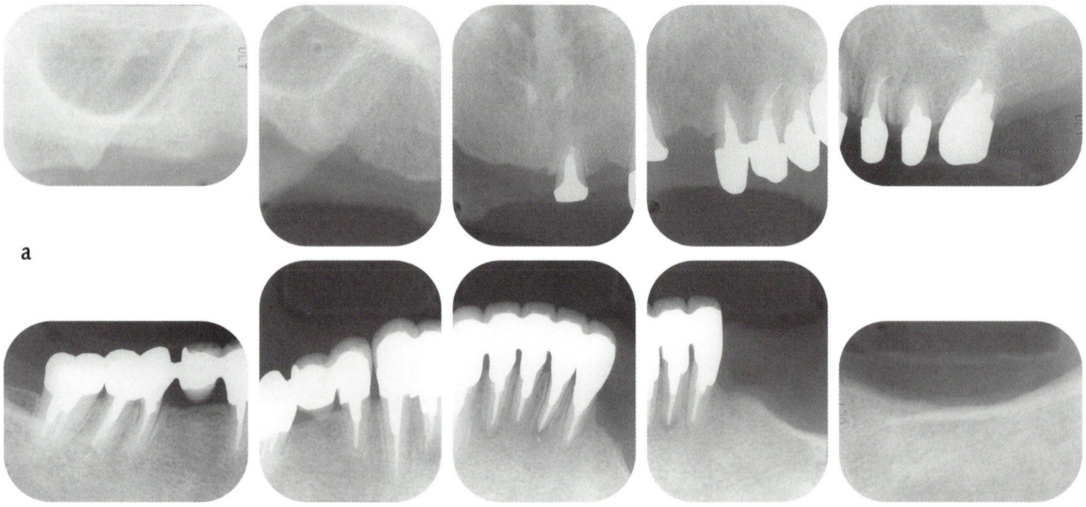

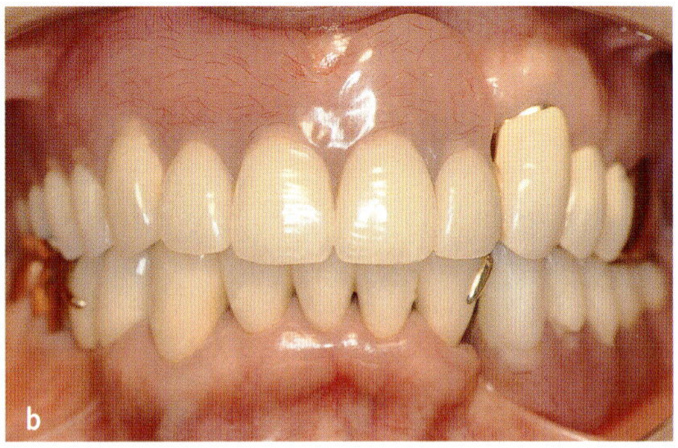

Fig 5-134 (a) About 19 years after the first visit (October 1998), conditions are relatively stable. (b) Photograph taken about 20 years after the patient's first visit, 2 years 7 months after refabrication of her mandibular denture (July 1999). The morphology of the dentition has been corrected and occlusal support has been reestablished with correction of the occlusal plane.

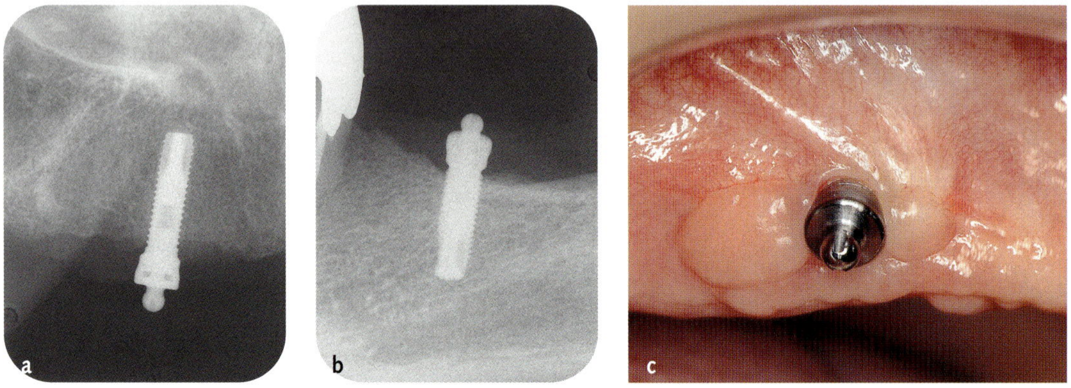

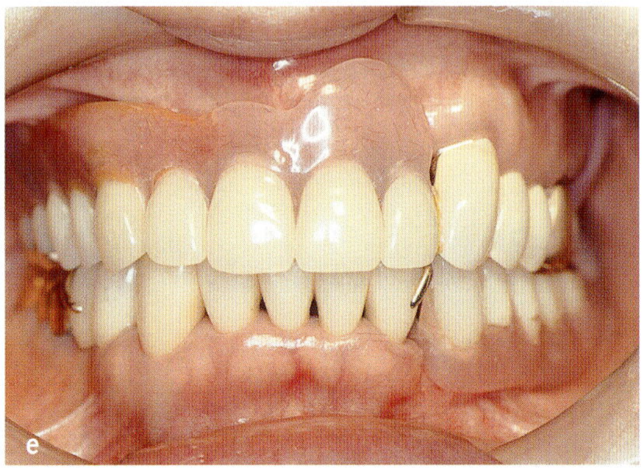

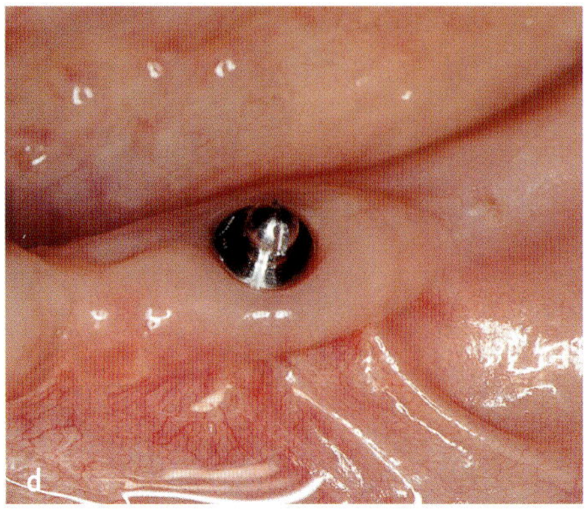

Fig 5-135 (a to d) About 23 years after the patient's first visit (June 2002). To prevent vertical settling of the dentures, implants have been placed. For the maxillary right canine area, a split crest technique, with an autogenous bone graft and a resorbable membrane, was completed. (e) Photograph taken about 23 years after the patient's first visit (August 2002).

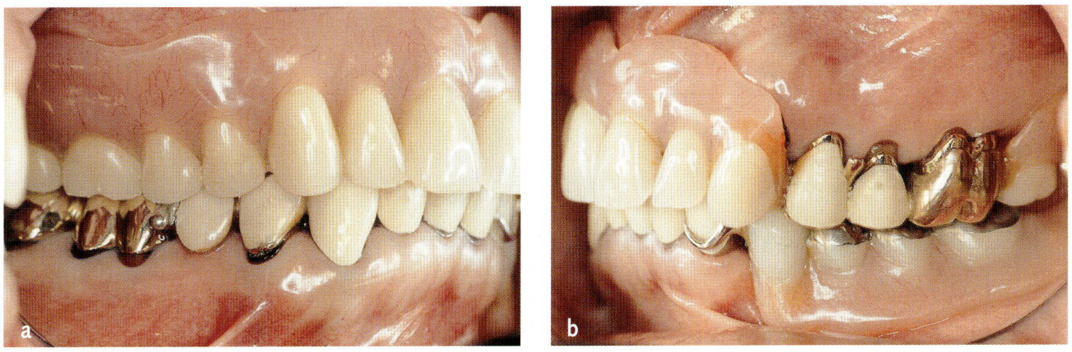

Fig 5-136 (a and b) About 14 years after the patient's first visit, 8 years 10 months after delivery of the maxillary telescopic denture. On the left side, compromised conditions exist, including rotation and vertical settling of the denture as well as lifting of the telescopic crowns. The telescopic denture is fractured (October 1993).

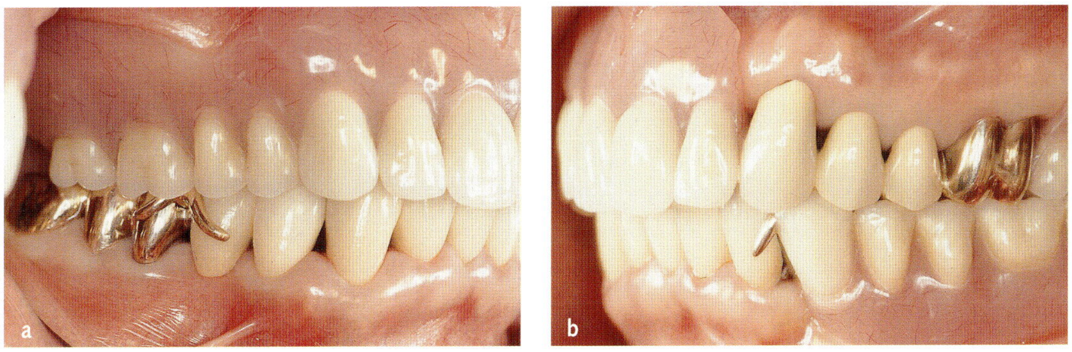

Fig 5-137 (a and b) At delivery of the final prostheses (November 1995). Crown-lengthening procedures have been completed and the occlusal plane is restored. The maxillary left central incisor with an overlay cap and the reimplanted maxillary left canine are utilized as abutments for the telescopic denture. The mandibular left lateral incisor is milled to produce retention, bracing, and support.

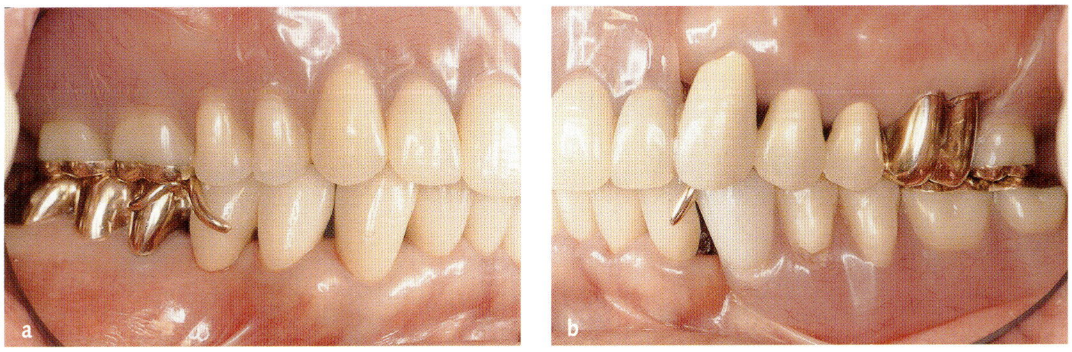

Fig 5-138 (a and b) About 20 years after the first visit (July 1999), during the maintenance phase. To create a maintainable environment, periodontal plastic surgery has been conducted for the maxillary left canine, first premolar, second premolar, and first molar to increase the level of attached gingiva.

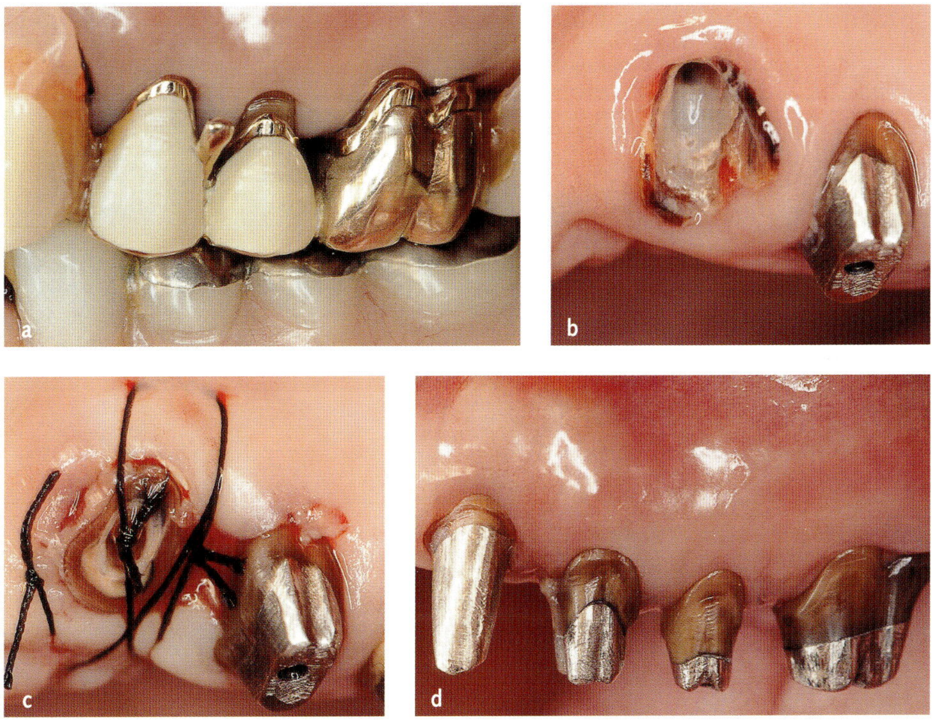

Fig 5-139 (a) At the first visit, the overlay crowns have erupted. The abutment teeth have secondary caries. (b) The telescopic crown on the maxillary left canine has dislodged, and secondary caries is noted. (c) The tooth is elevated and reimplanted in a 180-degree rotated position. Softened dentin is expediently removed outside of the mouth. Notches are made on the buccal and lingual aspects of the tooth to allow fixture of the tooth with sutures. (d) A dowel post and core is delivered 2 months postsurgery.

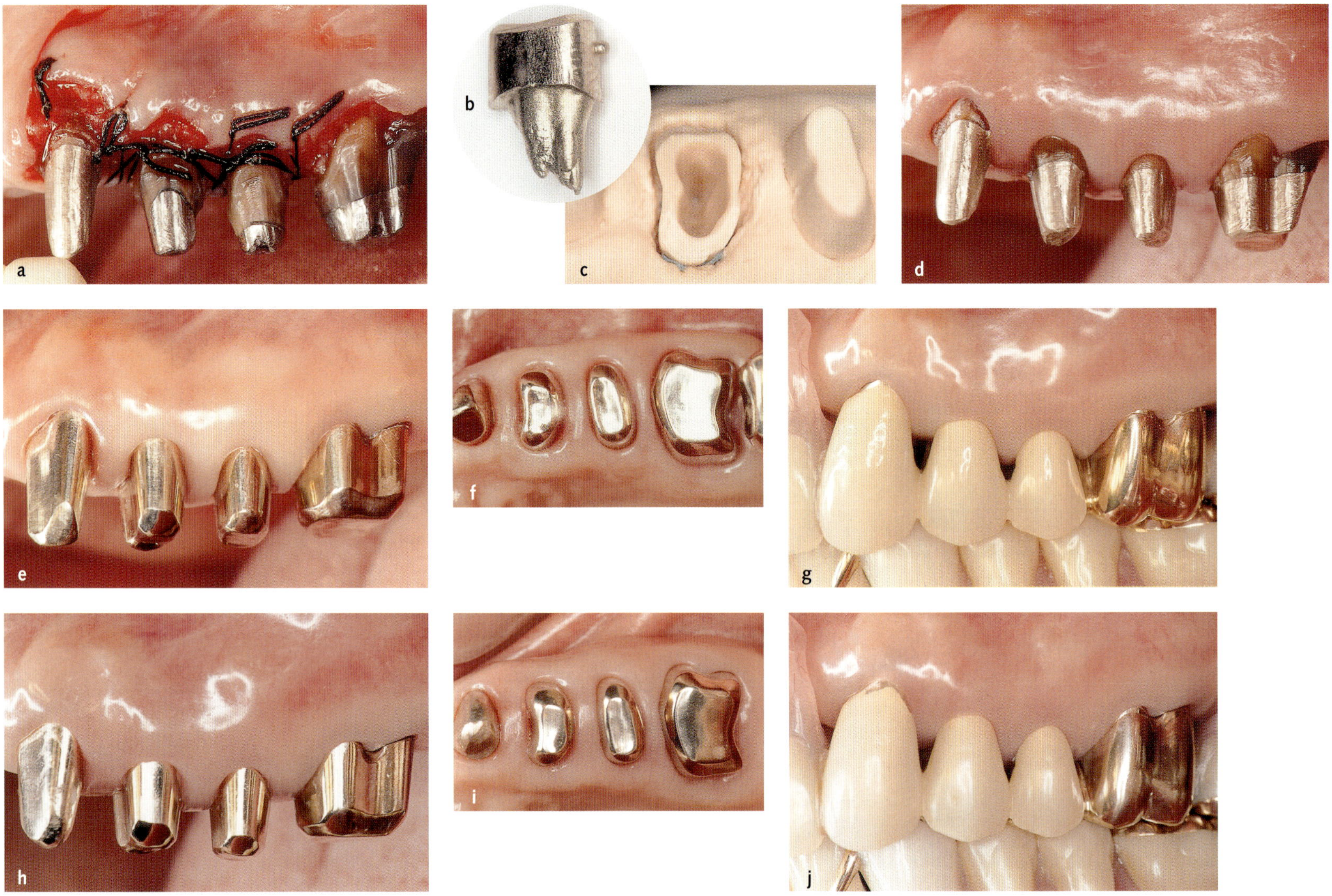

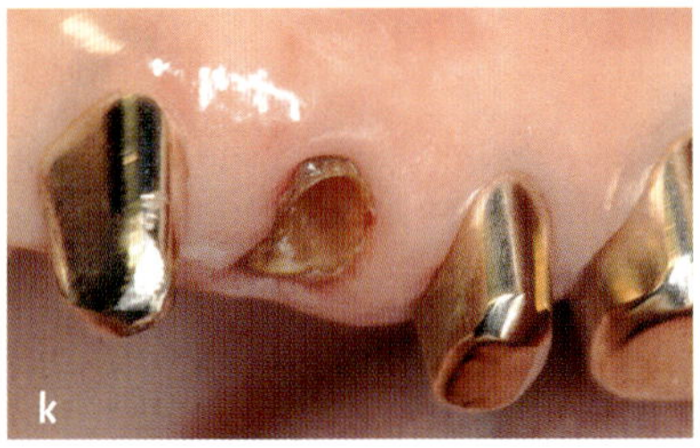

Fig 5-140 (a) To improve the attached gingiva and provide gingival augmentation, full- and partial-thickness flaps are elevated to facilitate crown lengthening. (b to d) Photographs taken 3 months after crown lengthening. Dowel posts and cores are delivered for the maxillary left first premolar, second premolar, and first molar. (e to g) After about 3 months, telescopic crowns are delivered. (h and i) After 4 years, the appearance of the gingiva indicates no inflammation and the gingivae is stable. (j and k) Five years after delivery of the prostheses, the dowel post of the maxillary left first premolar has dislodged, probably because of the rotation and vertical drop of the denture.

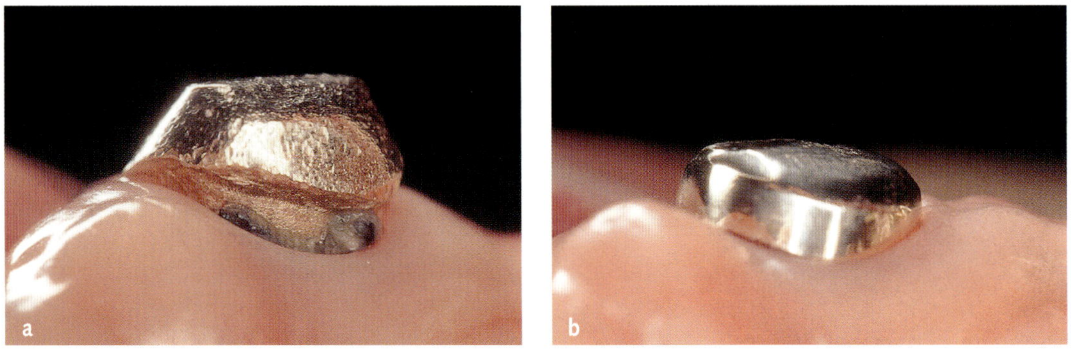

Fig 5-141 (a) The overlay crown of the maxillary central incisor had been used for 15 years. Significant metal fatigue is noted. Palatal cementum and dentin are destroyed, resulting in an overhang-like appearance. (b) Forces are concentrated here, and this is a key tooth, being the only occlusal support in the otherwise non–vertically supported occlusion. A telescopic crown with minimal occlusal height is delivered. The condition has stabilized (about 5 years 6 months after delivery of the new telescopic crown).

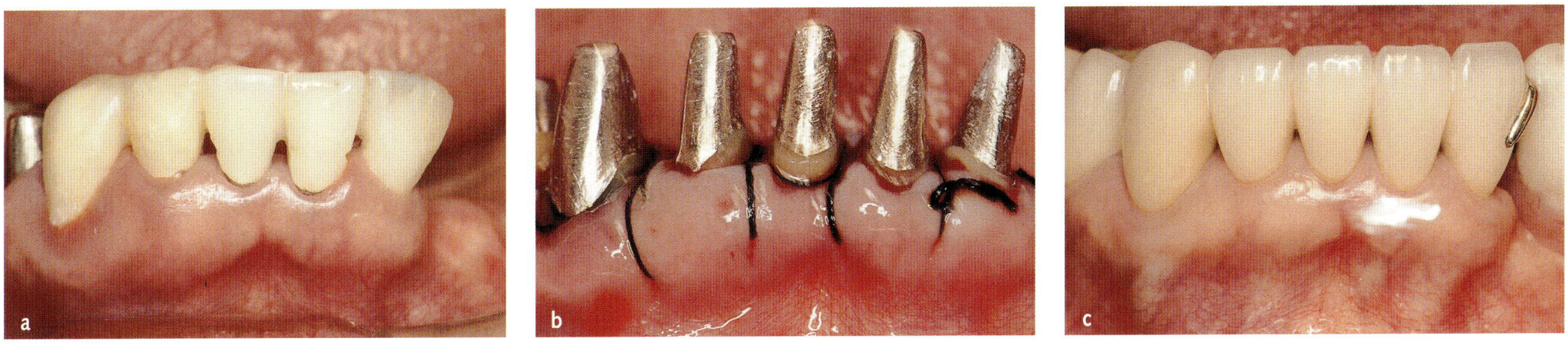

Fig 5-142 (a) Provisional restoration on dowel posts and cores. (b) Clinical crown lengthening is conducted after delivery of dowel posts and cores. (c) After 4 years, conditions are stable.

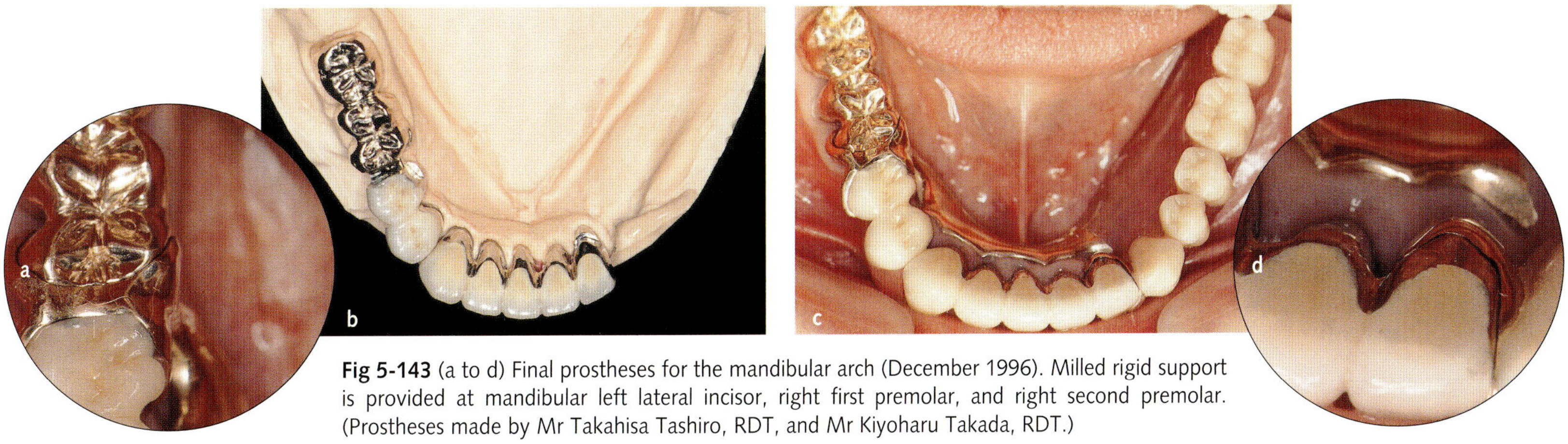

Fig 5-143 (a to d) Final prostheses for the mandibular arch (December 1996). Milled rigid support is provided at mandibular left lateral incisor, right first premolar, and right second premolar. (Prostheses made by Mr Takahisa Tashiro, RDT, and Mr Kiyoharu Takada, RDT.)

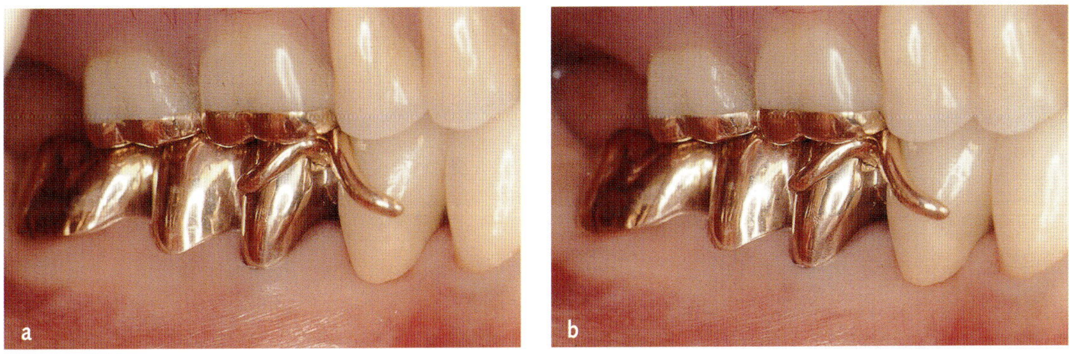

Fig 5-144 (a) Photograph taken 1 year 8 months after delivery of the maxillary denture. A semiovate pontic design has been developed for the mandibular right second premolar. (b) Clinical view after 4 years 7 months. The ovate pontic design helped to maintain continuity of the gingival appearance and provides appropriate form to facilitate plaque control. Food is not trapped under the pontics.

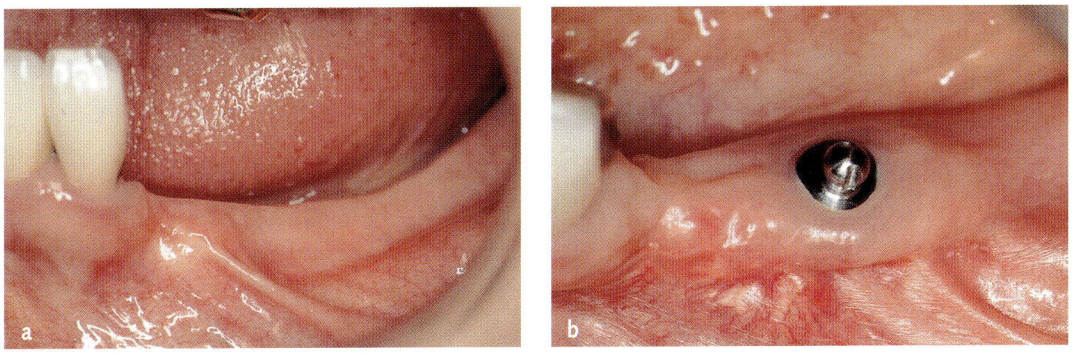

Fig 5-145 (a) Appearance 5 years 6 months after delivery of the second denture. (b) The denture design is changed to an overlay type with implant support.

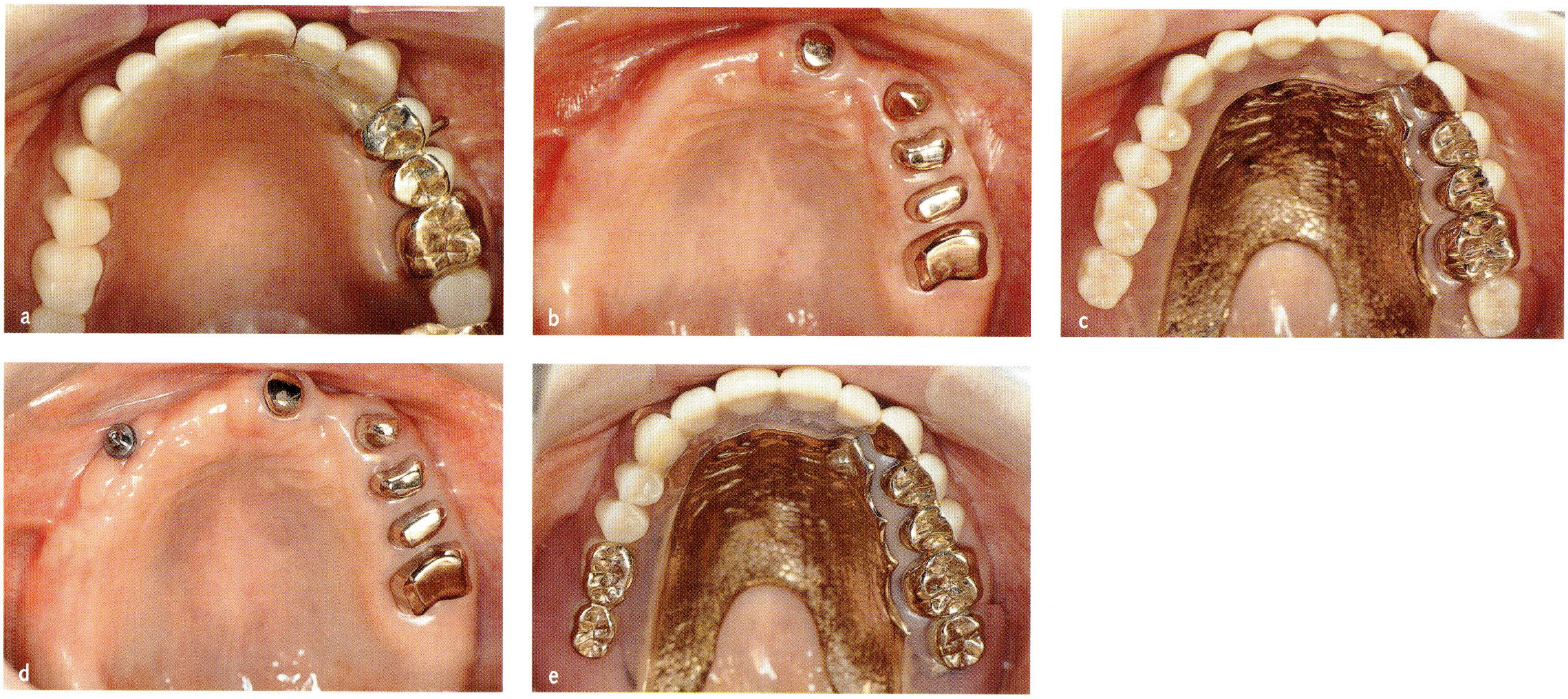

Fig 5-146 Maxillary arch. (a) Occlusal surfaces are significantly worn (9 years after delivery, October 1993). (b) After reimplantation, the maxillary left canine is used as an abutment for a telescopic crown. (c) At delivery of the final prosthesis (October 1995), the arch form is improved and symmetric. (d) Photograph taken about 23 years after the patient's first visit (June 2002). An implant has been placed in the maxillary right canine position to prevent vertical displacement of the denture. (e) Metal occlusal surfaces were added to the artificial teeth 2 years before this photograph was taken.

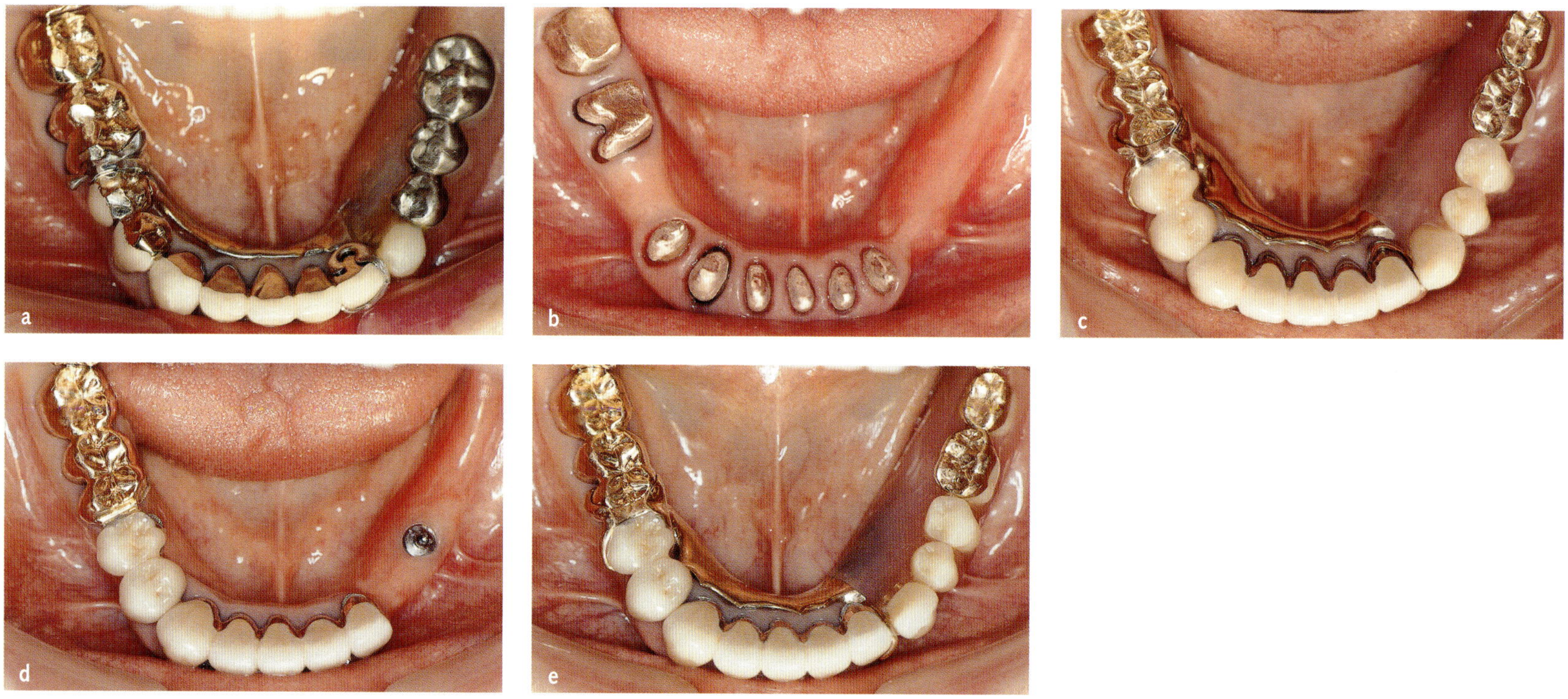

Fig 5-147 Mandibular arch. (a) The right side is significantly worn (11 years after delivery, October 1993). (b) After retreatment of the root canals, attention is paid to the fit of dowel posts and cores. (c) At delivery of the final prostheses (October 1995). Metal-ceramic crowns have been delivered for the left central and lateral incisors, right central and lateral incisors, and right canine; a milled crown has been fabricated for the mandibular left lateral incisor; a fixed partial denture has been placed, extending from the mandibular right first premolar to the second molar (pontic: mandibular right second premolar); and a milled denture has been fabricated for the mandibular left first and second premolars. A rigidly attached RPD provides occlusal support. (d and e) Photographs taken 23 years after the first visit (June 2002). To prevent vertical displacement of the RPD, an implant has been placed at the mandibular left second premolar site.

Treatment Goals for Patients with Multiple Missing Teeth

The objective of prosthodontic treatment in a patient with multiple missing teeth and bone is functional recovery. Although restoration of the missing teeth dramatically restores the masticatory function and esthetic appearance, it also involves invasive procedures. Therefore, as an objective of restoration of partial edentulism, a wide variety of alternatives should be examined in light of the medical data, the patient's desires for restoration and function, the patient's case history, and the progress of the disease, as well as the patient's lifestyle, background, age, and social life. Once the treatment objective is clearly defined, all possible treatment options have to be employed to achieve rehabilitation of the oral structures (Fig 5-148 and Cases 5-6 to 5-9).

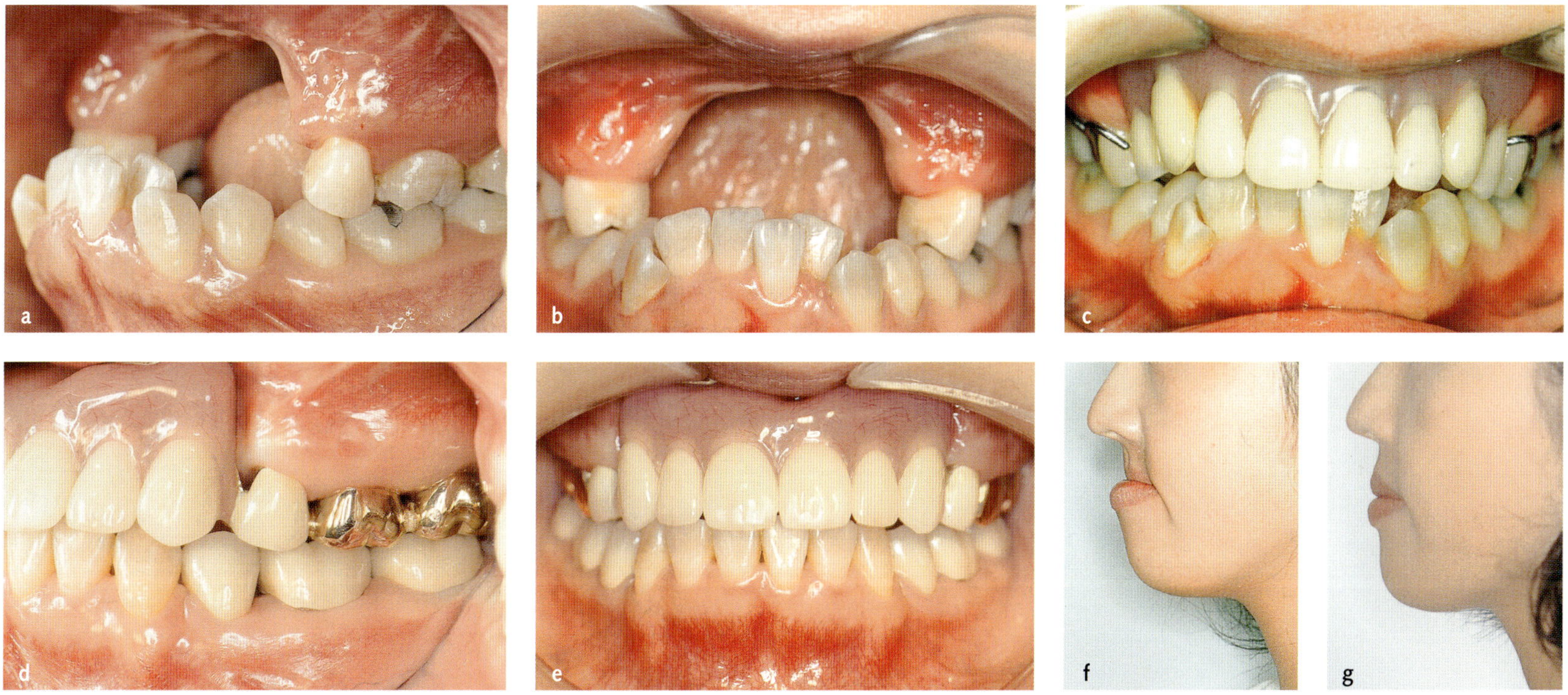

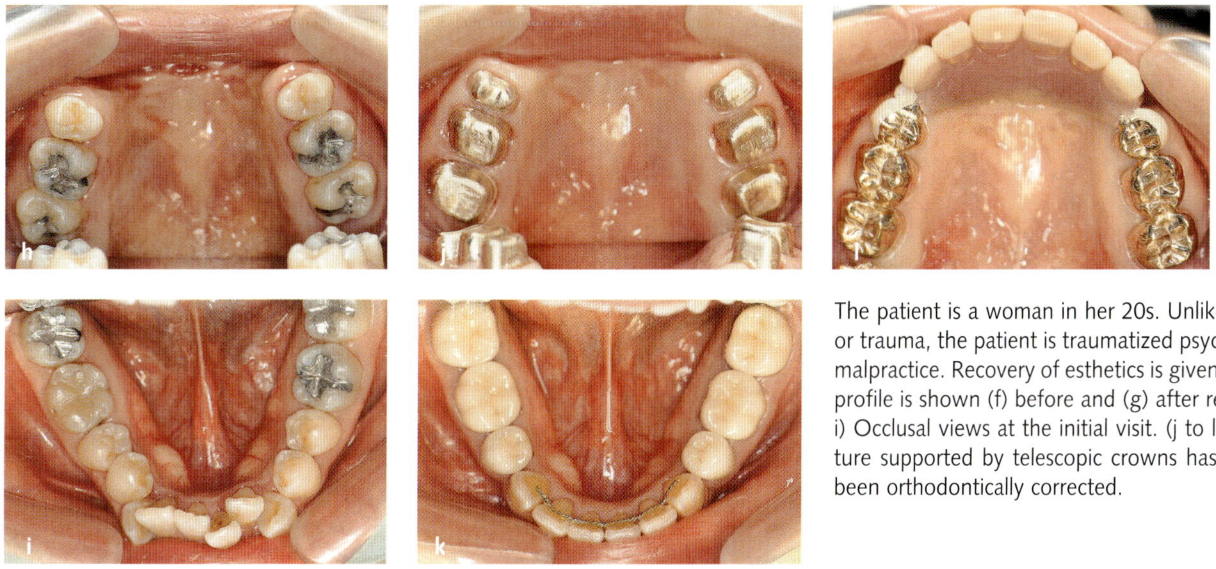

Fig 5-148 Treatment of significant bone loss in the maxilla. (a and b) Photographs taken at the first visit. All teeth from the maxillary right first premolar to the maxillary left first premolar, as well as the premaxilla, have been lost. (c) A RPD is utilized in the maxilla. (d and e) Necrosis of the maxilla has been caused iatrogenically during the orthognathic surgery to correct maxillary protrusion. The patient is a woman in her 20s. Unlike patients with bone loss caused by cancer or trauma, the patient is traumatized psychologically because the loss was caused by malpractice. Recovery of esthetics is given top priority in a case like this. The patient's profile is shown (f) before and (g) after restoration of esthetics and function. (h and i) Occlusal views at the initial visit. (j to l) For the maxillary arch, a removable denture supported by telescopic crowns has been delivered. The mandibular arch has been orthodontically corrected.

Case 5-6 Unequal force relationships between the maxillary and mandibular arches

Patient: *55-year-old woman at the time of first visit in 2000*

Chief complaint: *Poorly functioning maxillary denture and difficulty in chewing*

This patient had extreme asymmetry between the maxillary and mandibular arches. The maxilla was almost totally edentulous; the mandible had advanced periodontal disease at the molars but fewer teeth were missing (Fig 5-149). The patient had some knowledge about implants and visited us, hoping to receive an implant-supported fixed partial denture.

The treatment with implants to replace the missing teeth requires precise surgical and prosthodontic skills, along with precision laboratory work (Figs 5-150 to 5-153). Nevertheless, implant treatment is chosen without considering other treatment alternatives and then consider how this treatment is conducted. Such planning should be avoided because the treatment outcome has to be considered first. Therapeutic intervention has to attempt to obtain a maximal therapeutic effect with minimal invasion from a comprehensive viewpoint. In every case, treatment plans and procedures are to be selected according to the overall treatment goal, which is to maximize the benefits to the patient.

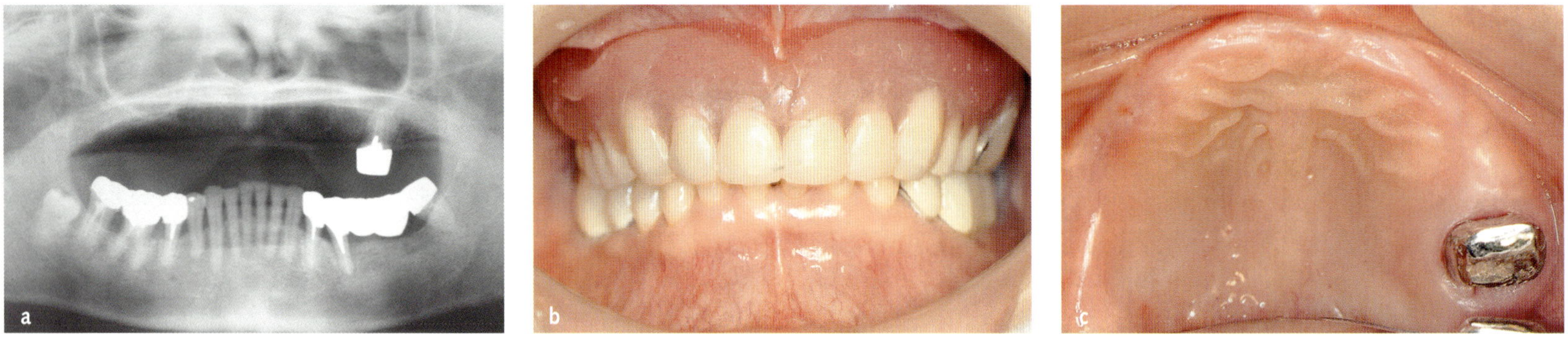

Fig 5-149 (a to c) At the patient's first visit. Although there seems to be adequate bone at a first glance, CT examination showed that bone resorption is significant, especially on the buccal aspect. Implants could be placed at the sites of the maxillary right canine and first premolar and left canine and first premolar. The occlusal surface morphology should preferably be fabricated to expand the dental arch, which had narrowed due to bone resorption. Implants are to be placed at the sites of the maxillary canines to provide retention.

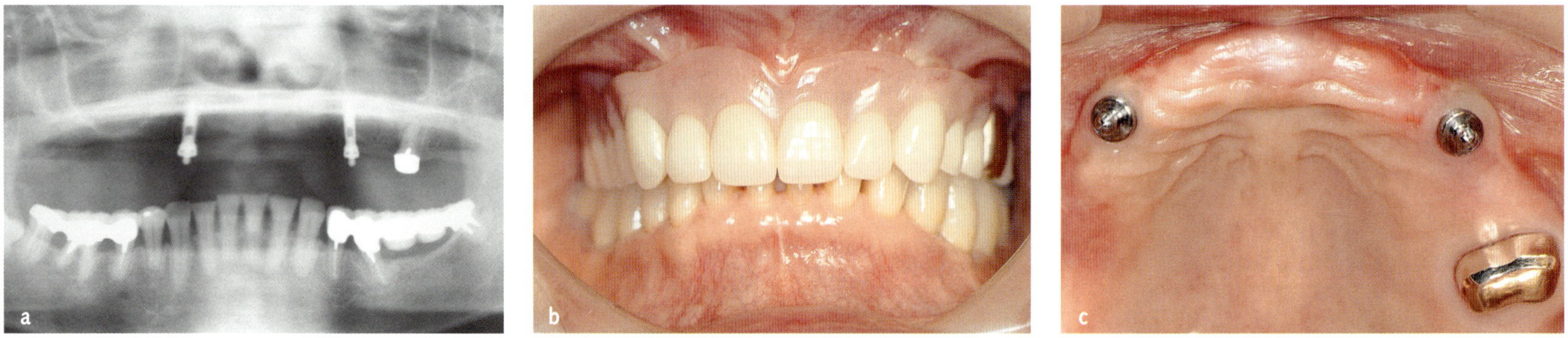

Fig 5-150 (a to c) The vertical dimension has been increased, 2 years after the first visit, at delivery of the final prostheses. A telescopic crown has been fabricated for the maxillary left first molar. O-ring abutment implants have been placed for the maxillary canines to support an overdenture. No indentation from the denture base is observed. (Prostheses made by Mr Takahisa Tashiro, RDT.)

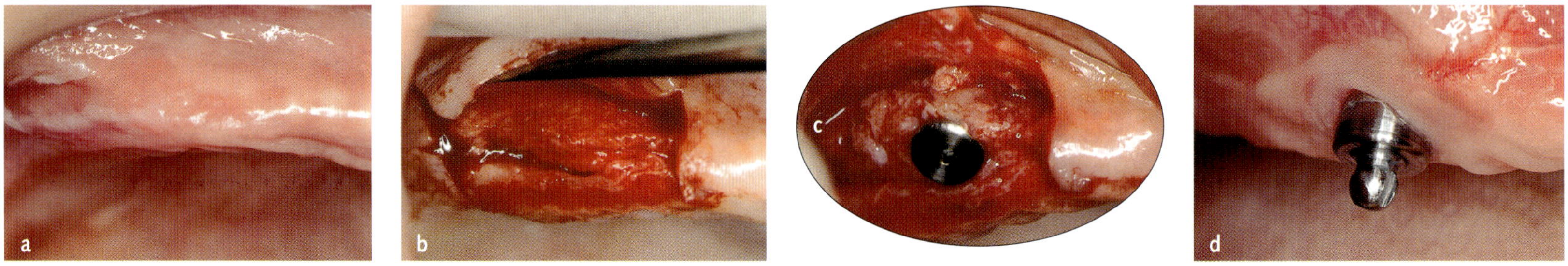

Fig 5-151 Retention provided by implants. (a and b) Implant placement. A bevel incision is made from the palate. A full-thickness flap is elevated from the crest and extended beyond the buccal MGJ. Linear vertical incisions are made mesially and distally. Bone width is limited to about 3 mm. (c) The bone crest is sectioned along the midline to place a Miniplant implant (3.25 × 13.00 mm), around which autogenous bone is grafted and a resorbable membrane is applied. When the healing abutment is delivered, a free gingival graft will be extended to the vestibule to obtain keratinized gingiva. (d) Photograph taken 1 year after surgery. After the keratinized gingiva is obtained, an O-ring abutment is delivered. This provides retention alone.

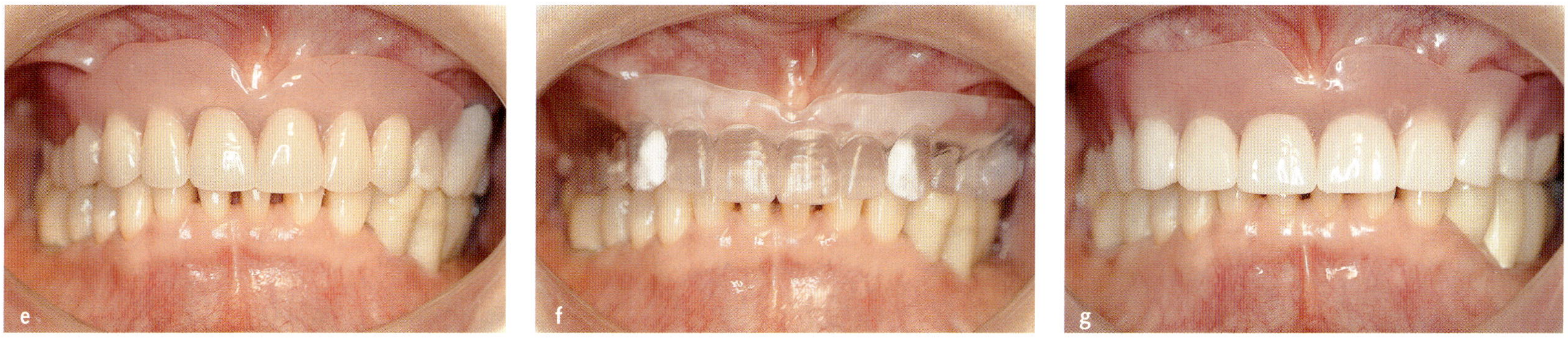

Fig 5-151 (cont) (e) Provisional restoration 6 months after the first visit. The vertical dimension has been increased. (f) Surgical stent for implant placement. (g) Provisional restoration after implant placement.

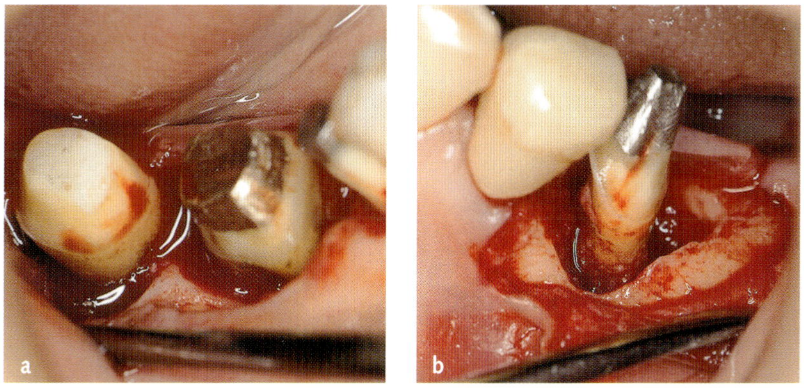

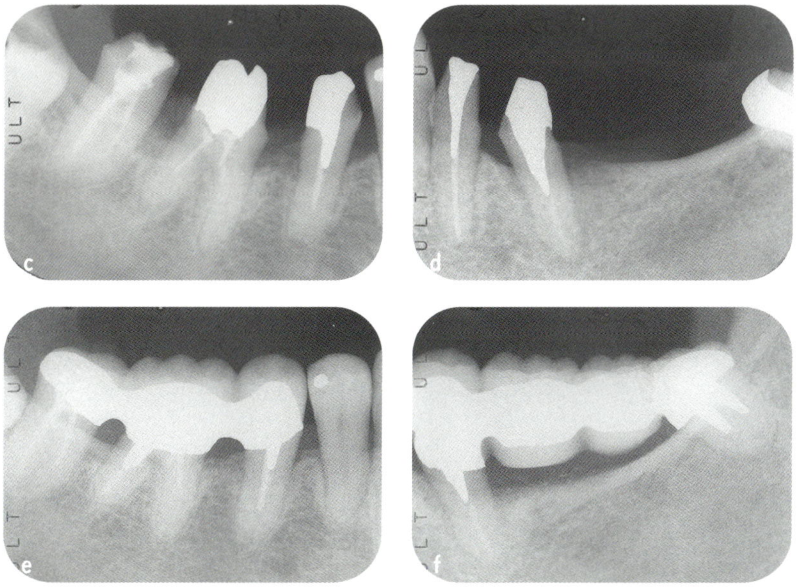

Fig 5-152 Regenerative therapy for mandibular molar areas. (a) Emdogain is applied for bone defects at the mandibular right second premolar, first molar, and second molar. (b) Emdogain is applied for a circumferential bone defect at the mandibular left second premolar. The defect extends just short of the apex. The tooth exhibits degree 3 mobility. (c) Radiograph showing the defects on the right side. (d) Radiograph showing the defect on the left side. (e) Radiograph of the right side, taken 1 year 9 months after surgery. (f) Radiograph of the left side, taken 1 year 5 months after surgery.

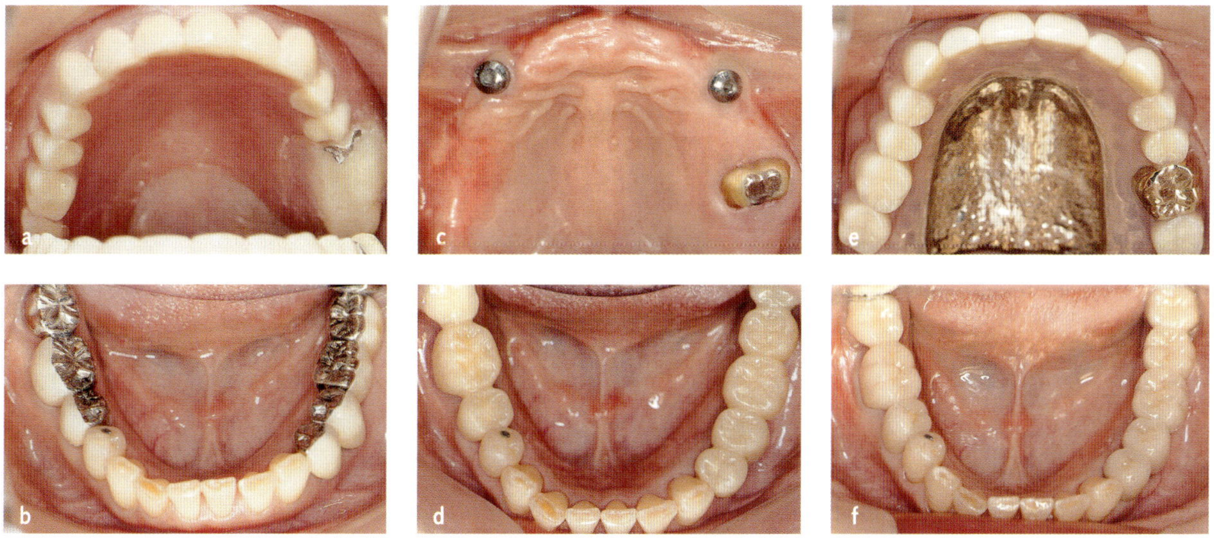

Fig 5-153 Changes in the occlusal surfaces. (a and b) At the first visit, the occlusal surfaces of the mandibular arch are asymmetric and have a strong curve of Spee. There are severe bone defects at the molars. (c and d) Photographs taken 1 year 6 months after the first visit. Healing abutments are delivered to the implants in the maxillary right canine and left canine areas. The maxillary left first molar, which will serve as an abutment tooth, has undergone endodontic treatment. In the mandible, regenerative therapy and a provisional restoration have been provided to improve the form of the dental arch. (e and f) The maxillary arch of artificial teeth in the metal plate denture could be expanded because of the retention provided by the implants. In the mandible, splinted metal-ceramic crowns have been provided for the second premolar, first molar, and second molar, and a metal-ceramic fixed partial denture extends from the left first premolar to the third molar (pontics: first and second molars).

Case 5-7 Restoration of occlusion in a patient with multiple missing teeth

Patient: *61-year-old woman at the time of first visit in 1993*

The remaining teeth were affected by moderate periodontal disease. No occlusal vertical stops were present, and the ridges opposing natural teeth showed marked resorption (Fig 5-154). The remaining teeth were the maxillary right first molar and second molar; the maxillary left second molar; the mandibular left central incisor, lateral incisor, canine, and second premolar; and the mandibular right central incisor, lateral incisor, and canine. The unstable maxillary denture fractured and had to be replaced several times until an even occlusal plane was achieved (Figs 5-155 to 5-161).

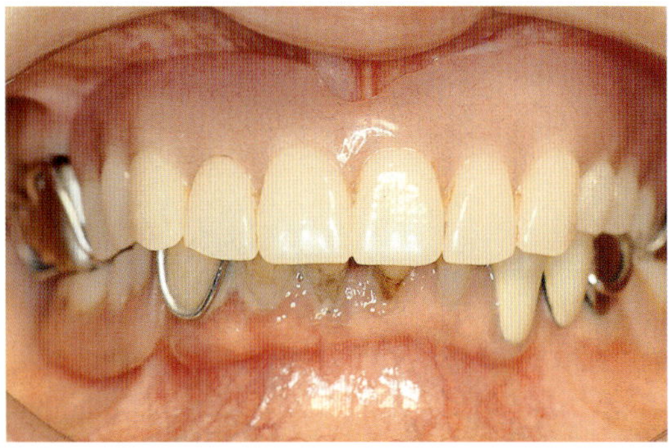

Fig 5-154 At the first visit. The maxillary anterior teeth are subjected to a strong occlusal load from the natural teeth, which decreases the VDO and causes the maxillary denture to be unstable.

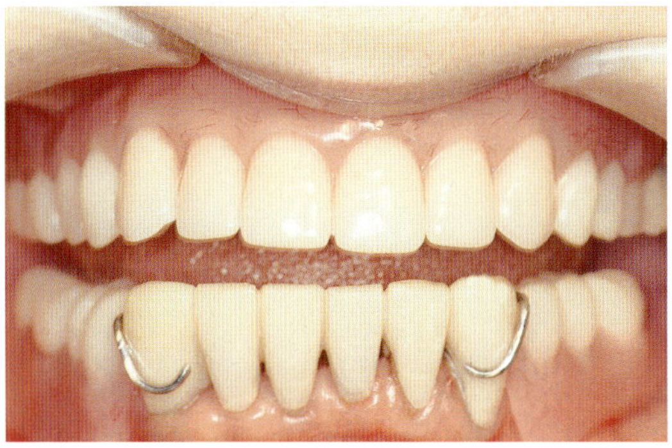

Fig 5-155 Photograph taken 1 year 3 months after the first visit. Hopeless teeth (the maxillary right first and second molars and the mandibular left second premolar) have been extracted. After endodontic treatment and post-and-core buildup, resective periodontal surgery was conducted to improve the periodontal environment. Provisional restorations have been delivered to allow recovery of the physiologic occlusal relationship and maturation of the periodontal tissue.

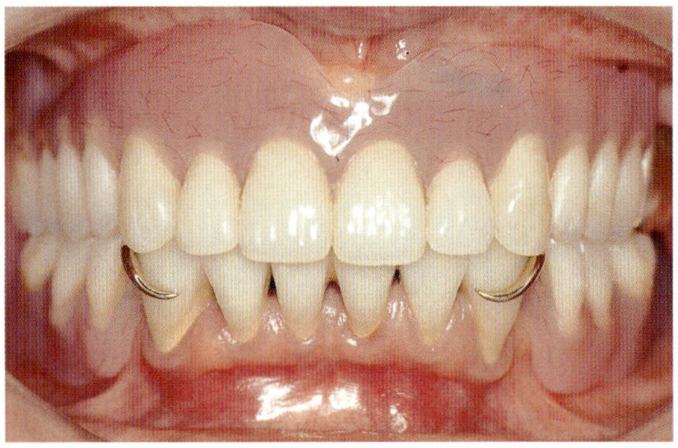

Fig 5-156 Photograph taken 2 years after the first visit. A removable denture in which the left second molar has a telescopic crown has been placed in the maxilla. In the mandible, metal-ceramic splinted crowns have been delivered for the left lateral incisor, left central incisor, right central incisor, right lateral incisor, and right canine. Akers clasps are utilized as retainers.

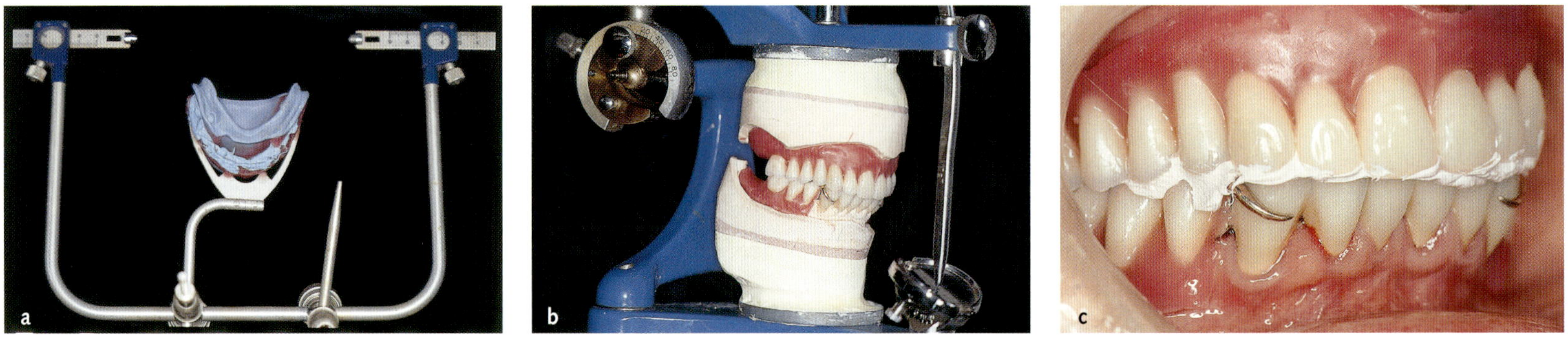

Fig 5-157 Basic prosthodontic procedures. (a) With bite plates mounted on the facebow, an occlusal registration is taken using zinc oxide-eugenol paste to correctly reproduce a physiologic mandibular position. (b) The incisal path, condylar path angle, and border movements are reproduced on the articulator to fabricate the final prosthesis. (c) Remounting is completed in an attempt to reproduce the mandibular position.

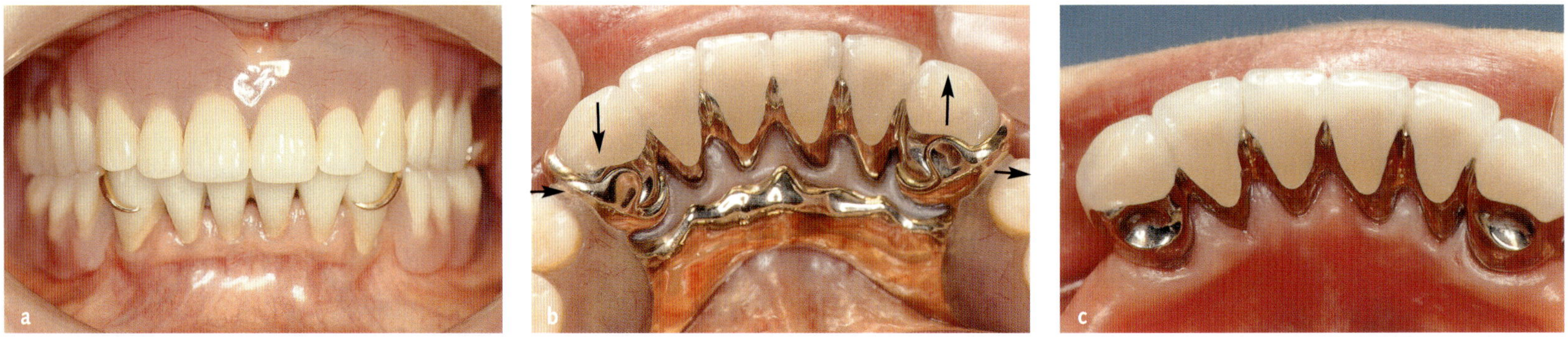

Fig 5-158 Maintenance. (a) Photograph taken 4 years after the first visit. Periodontal recalls are completed every 2 to 3 months. (b and c) Necessary conditions for successful RPDs, in order of importance, include (1) support, (2) bracing, and (3) retention. Cingulum rests at the mandibular canines *(vertical arrows)* and proximal plates *(horizontal arrows)* resist tilting and vertical displacement of the denture.

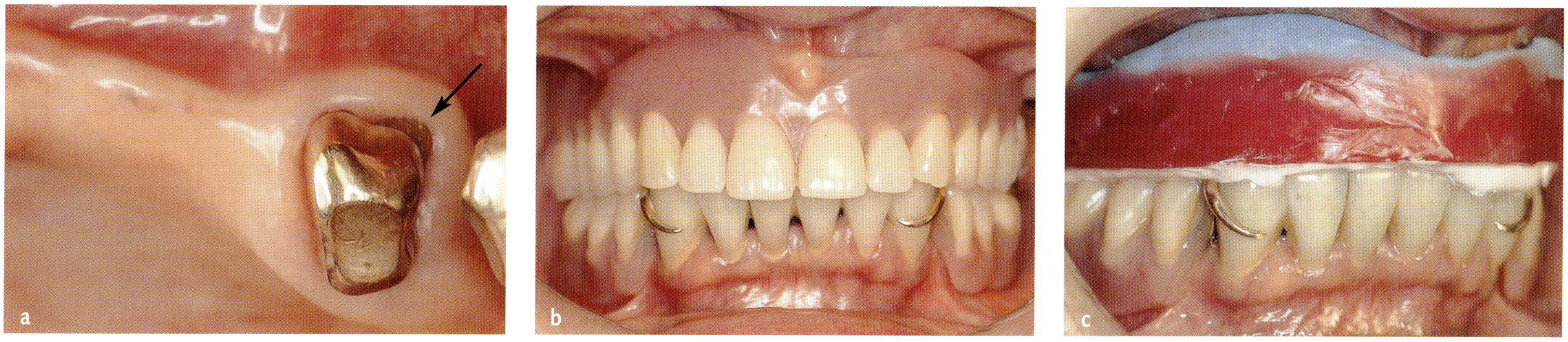

Fig 5-159 (a) Gingival recession *(arrow)* is noted at a telescopic crown in the maxilla. (b) Photograph taken about 4 years after delivery of prostheses. The maxillary denture has fractured several times, and the vertical dimension is slightly decreased over the initial position. (c) A new denture is fabricated. Care is taken to provide an even occlusal plane and to reproduce the appropriate mandibular position.

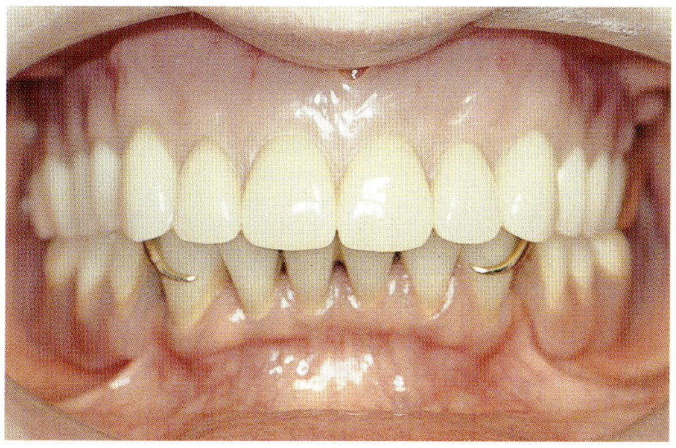

Fig 5-160 Photograph taken about 9 years after the first visit.

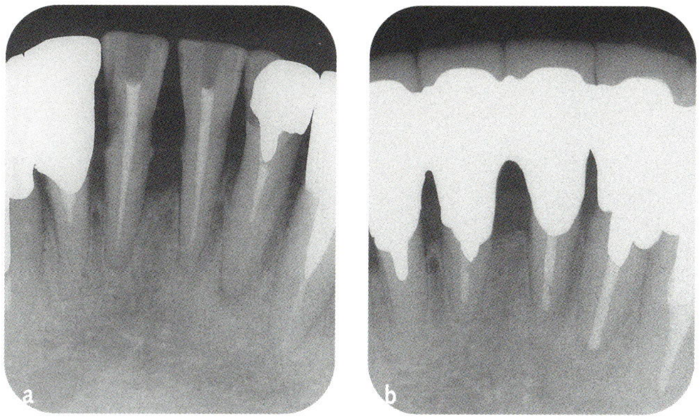

Fig 5-161 (a) Radiograph taken at the first visit. (b) Radiograph taken after 7 years.

Case 5-8 Restoration of occlusion in a patient with severe ridge resorption

Patient: *62-year-old woman at the time of first visit in March 1999*
Chief complaint: *Inability to chew because of pain associated with her dentures*

Figures 5-162 to 5-167 show the satisfactory results of comprehensive treatment planning.

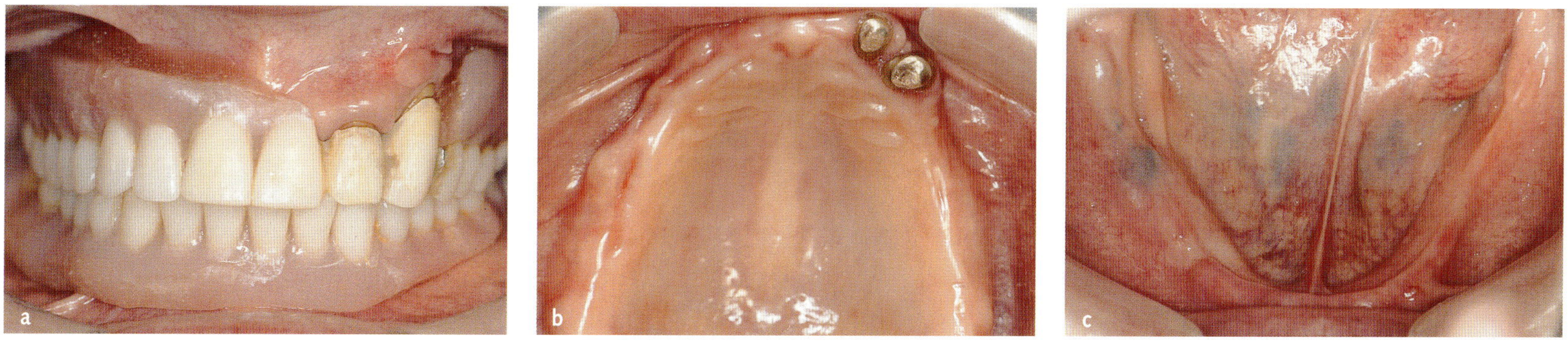

Fig 5-162 (a to c) Treatment for a mandible with severe ridge resorption. Shortly after the first visit, the maxillary right lateral incisor, canine, first premolar, second premolar, and first molar and the mandibular left third molar were extracted, leaving only the maxillary left lateral incisor and canine. The mandibular ridge is extremely resorbed, primarily due to the patient's lack of restoration.

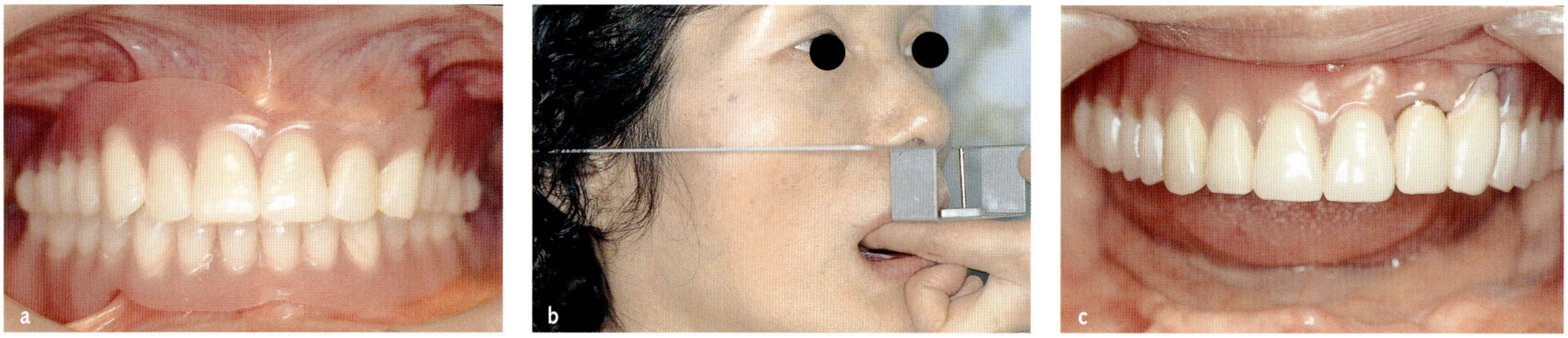

Fig 5-163 Restoration of a maxilla with multiple missing teeth. (a) A provisional denture is fabricated for recovery of function. (b) The occlusal plane is correctly aligned. (c) A telescopic crown–supported denture is delivered for the maxilla; the goal is a functional recovery. Ridge resorption of the mandible is significant, and the mandibular complete denture is not stabilized.

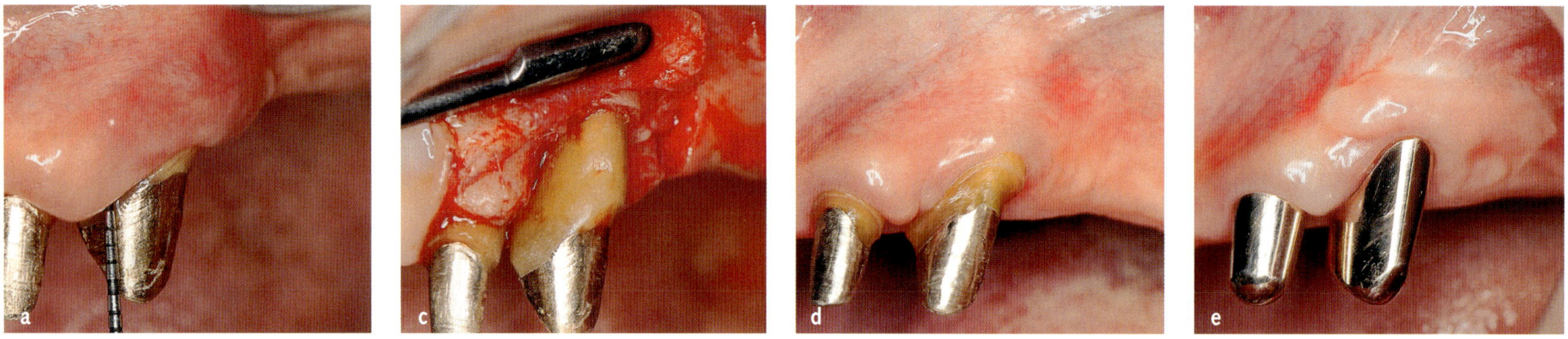

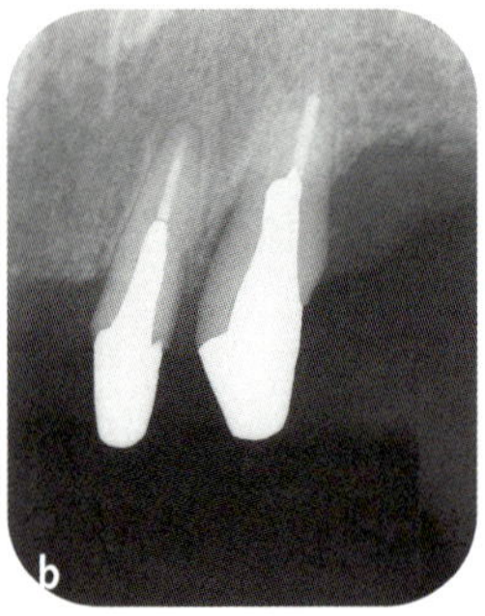

Fig 5-164 Improvement of the periodontal environment for a telescopic abutment. (a) Endodontic treatment is completed and dowel posts and cores are delivered for the maxillary left lateral incisor and canine. (b) A pathologic periodontal pocket is noted for the maxillary left canine (findings include secondary occlusal trauma and a mesial bone defect). (c) A full-thickness flap is raised. A buccal bone defect and narrow mesial bone defect are noted on the maxillary left canine. After thorough debridement, Emdogain regenerative therapy is conducted. (d) Four months after surgery, the attached gingiva at the maxillary left canine is insufficient. (e) Photograph taken 3 months after placement of a free gingival graft. (f) Radiograph taken 2 years after surgery.

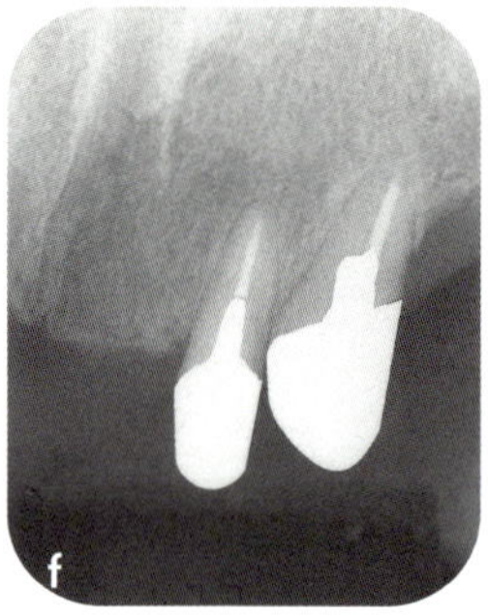

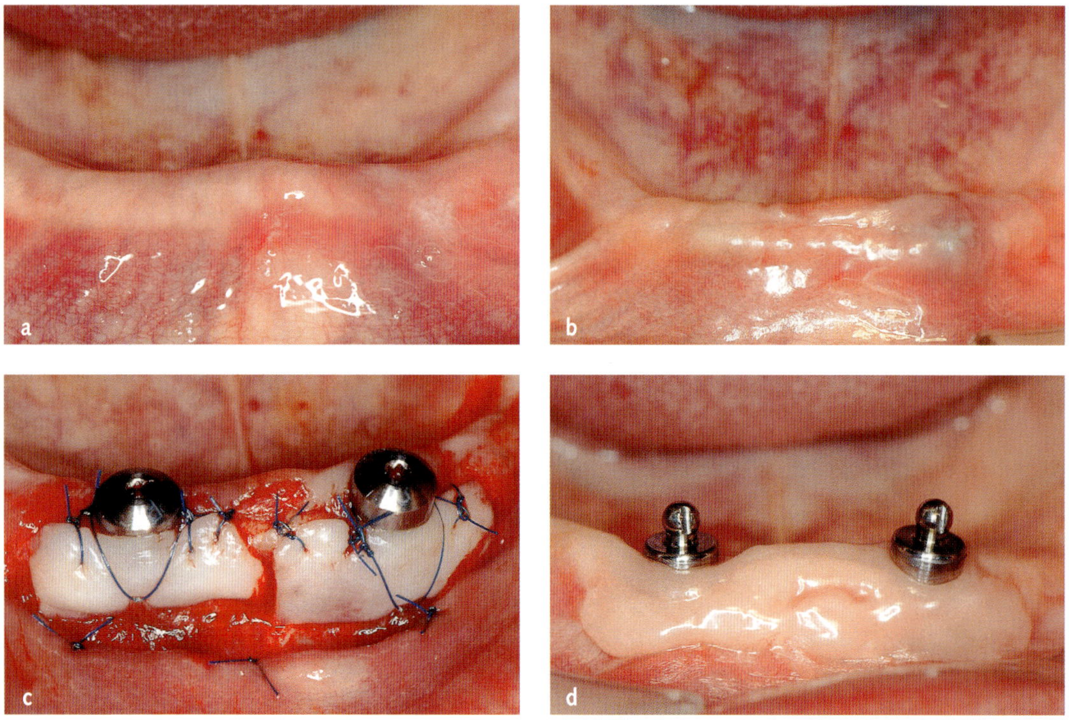

Fig 5-165 Placement of implants in the anterior mandible. (a) The ridge is resorbed. (b) With the anticipation that a free gingival graft will be placed in the future, implants are placed. (c) About 2 months after implant placement, at connection of the healing abutment (second-stage surgery), a free gingival graft is completed. (d) Photograph taken 1 year after implant placement. With only two ball-type flexible attachments, the stability of the denture is dramatically improved.

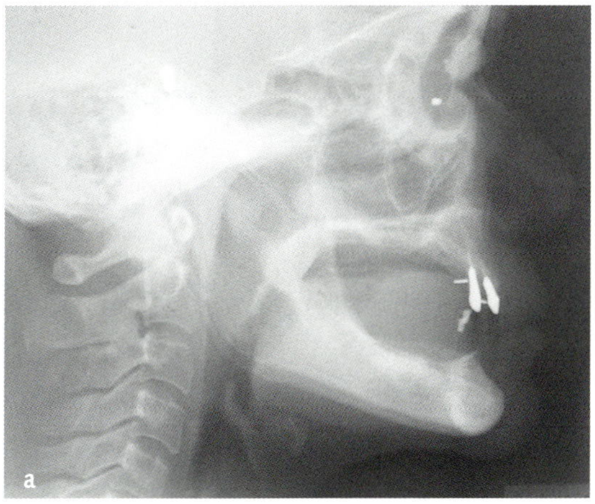

Fig 5-166 Careful imaging diagnosis prior to implant placement. (a) Lateral cephalogram. (b) CT scans. (c) Linear tomograms. (d) Computer-reconstructed three-dimensional image.

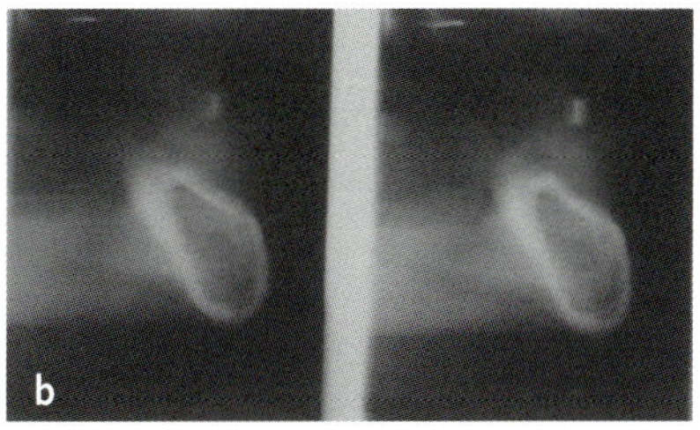

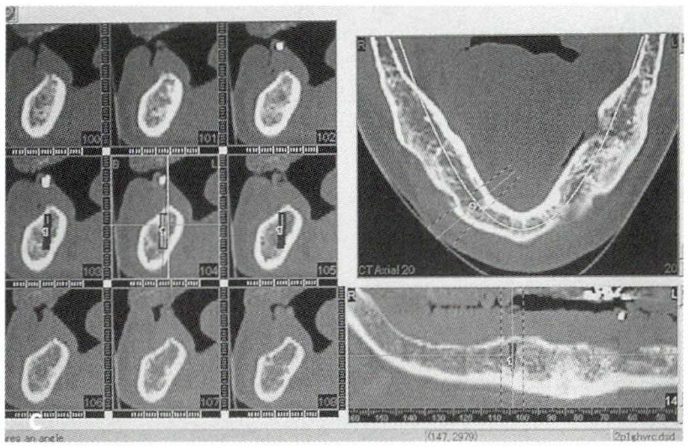

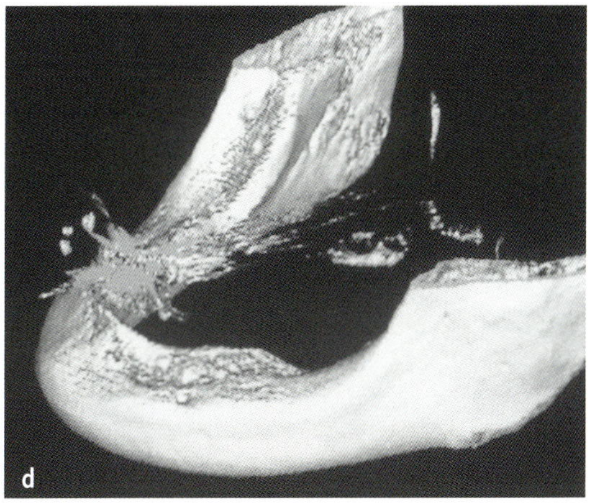

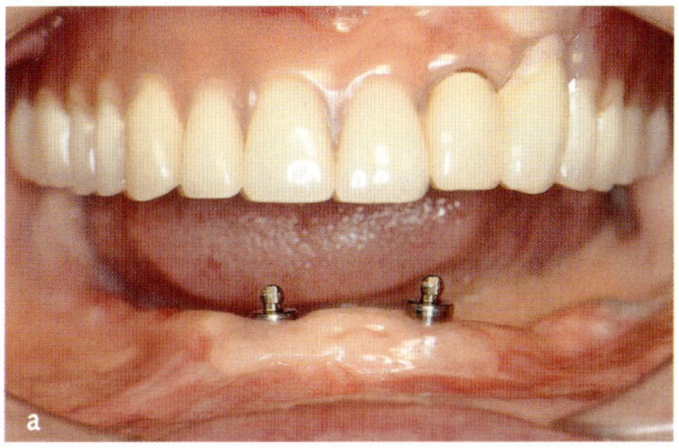

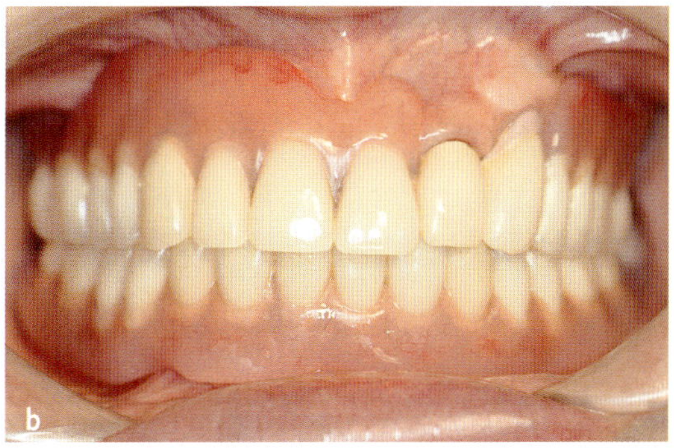

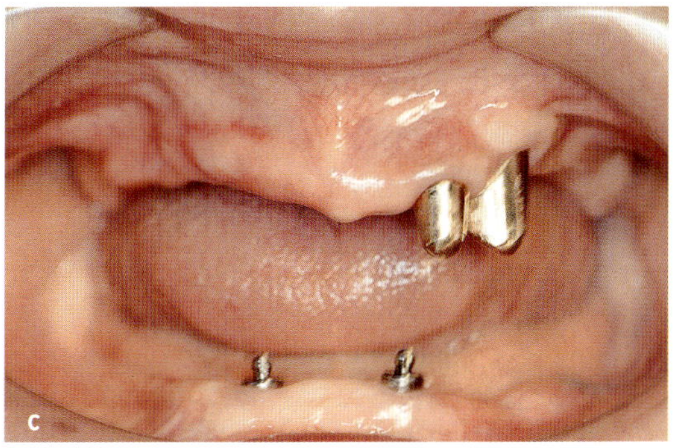

Fig 5-167 (a to g) Photographs taken 1 year 11 months after the first visit. With an implant-retained overdenture in the mandible, the patient's satisfaction is attained. (Prostheses made by Mr Takahisa Tashiro, RDT.) (h) Radiograph showing the osseointegrated implants.

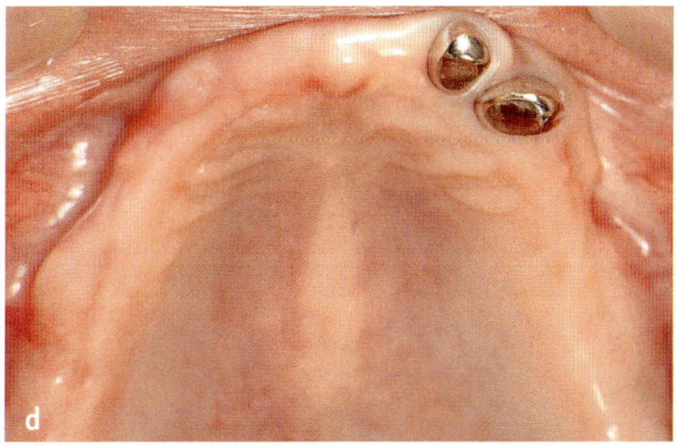

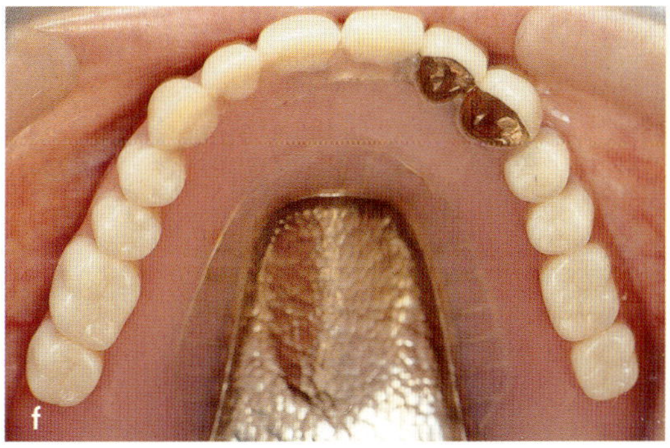

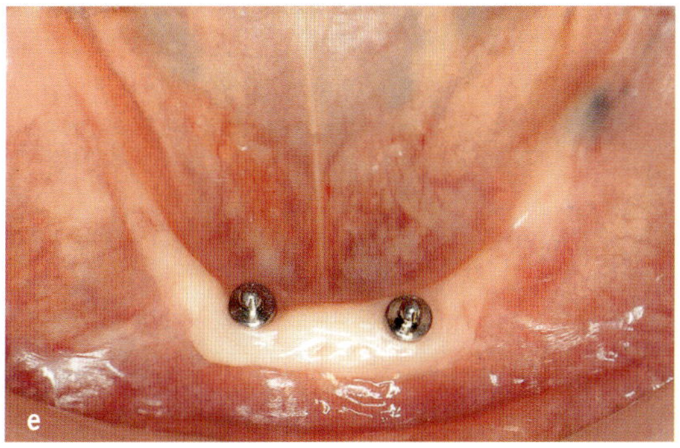

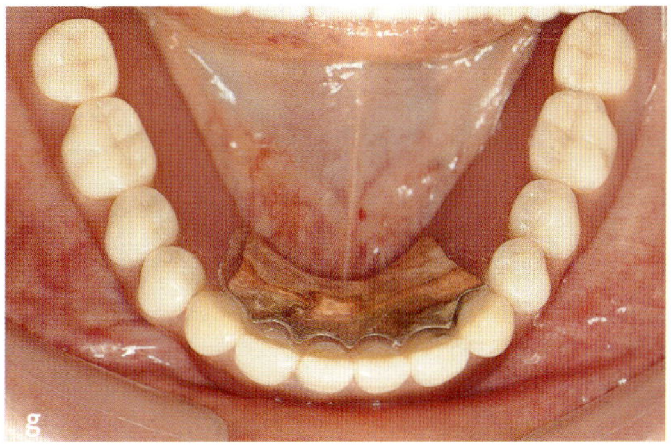

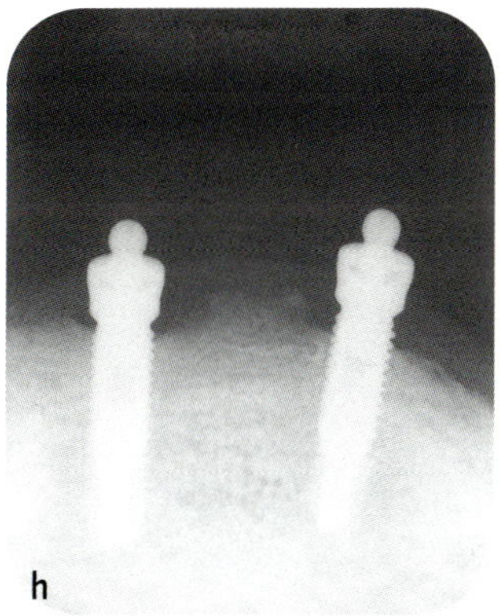

Case 5-9 Additional implants for a patient with dentures to prevent vertical depression

Patient: *49-year-old man at the time of first visit in 1998*

Considering the patient's age, the progression of the occlusal destruction was striking (Fig 5-168). For the maxilla, probably the best choice at this stage would be reduction of the crowns of the retainable teeth, correction of the crown-root ratio, and delivery of an overdenture. Accordingly, initial treatment was completed with an overdenture of a telescopic type that is suitable for a patient with few remaining teeth (Figs 5-169 and 5-170). However, the palatal mucosa had depressed gingivae because of the pressure from the denture, and there was a concern about movement and sinking of the denture. The treatment plan was then revised, and implants were placed in the maxillary left premolar and mandibular right and left premolar areas, where denture depression into the tissue was expected (Figs 5-171 to 5-175). The occlusal forces were primarily supported by tissue, with minimal support and retention from the implants. The implants were not selected on the basis of their retentive abilities but instead were chosen to delay the destruction of the supporting tissues and to improve function.

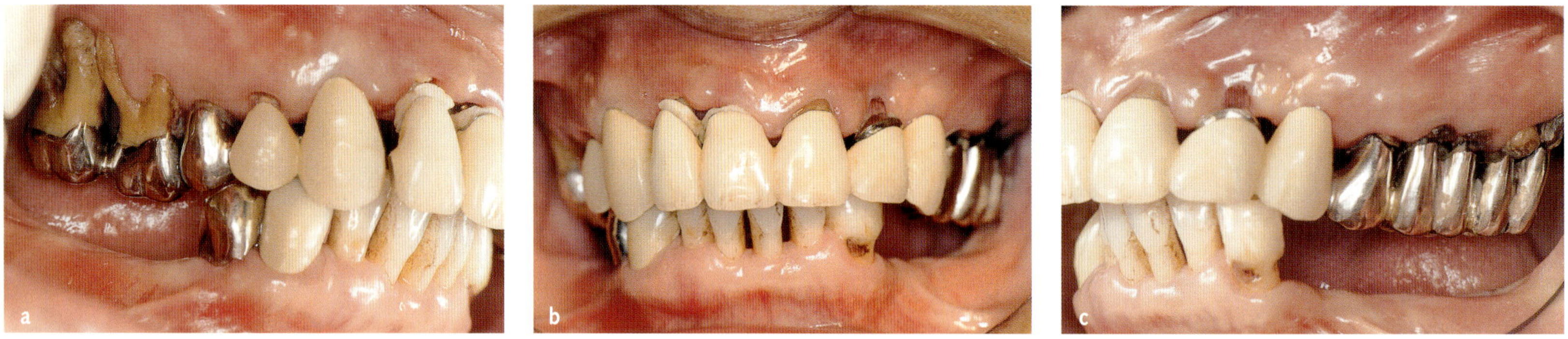

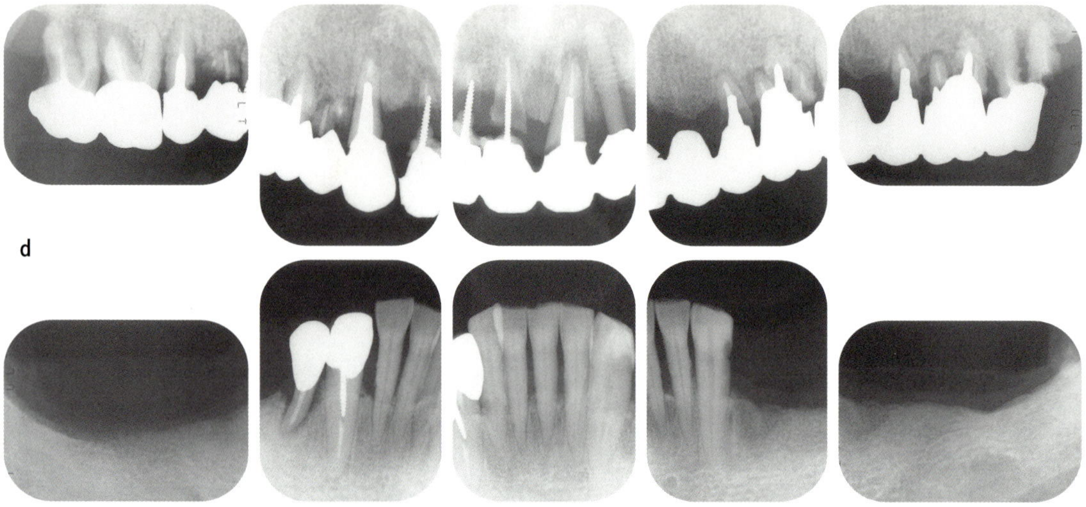

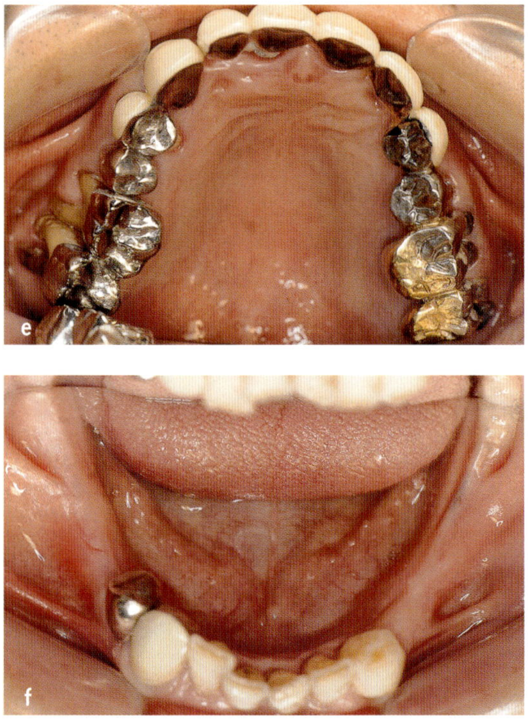

Fig 5-168 (a to f) Photographs and radiographs of a decimated occlusion at the first visit. The remaining teeth in the maxilla were either extracted or prepared to be overdenture abutments for a temporary overdenture that was fabricated on the same day that extraction occurred. The deformation of the maxillary arch suggests the presence of some significant occlusal forces.

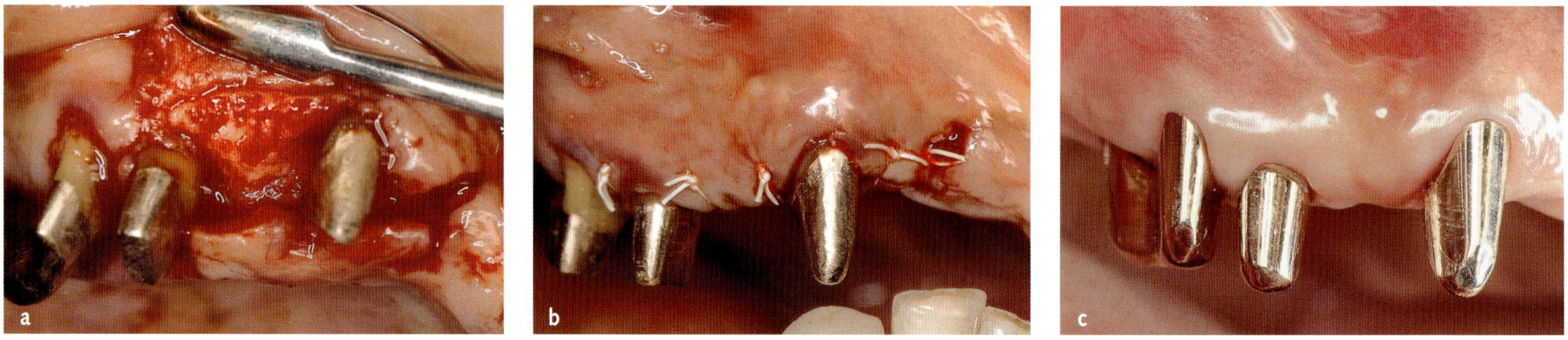

Fig 5-169 (a and b) Periodontal surgery for the remaining teeth is performed 8 months after initial therapy. Emdogain is applied to correct the bone defects around the mesial root of the maxillary right first molar and around the maxillary right canine and second premolar. (c) Telescopic crowns are delivered 10 months after periodontal surgery.

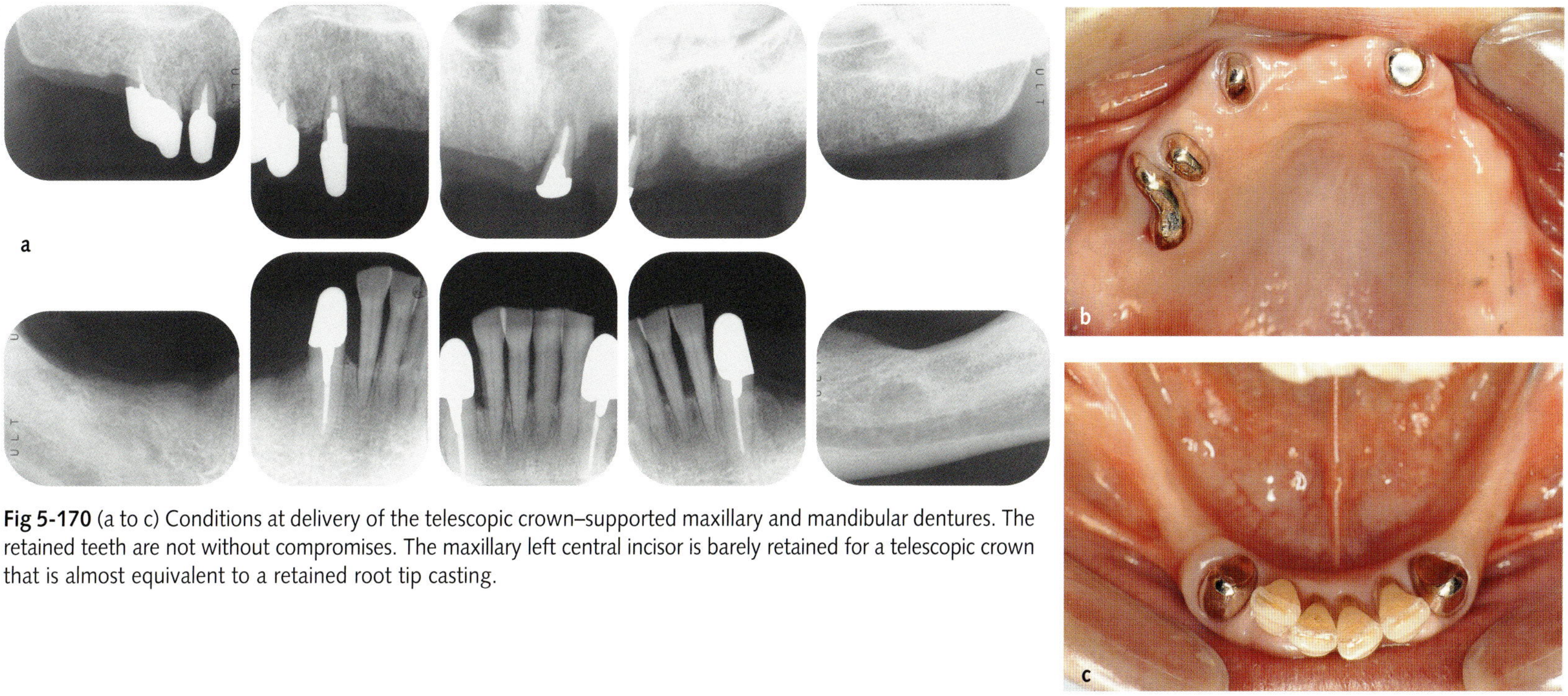

Fig 5-170 (a to c) Conditions at delivery of the telescopic crown–supported maxillary and mandibular dentures. The retained teeth are not without compromises. The maxillary left central incisor is barely retained for a telescopic crown that is almost equivalent to a retained root tip casting.

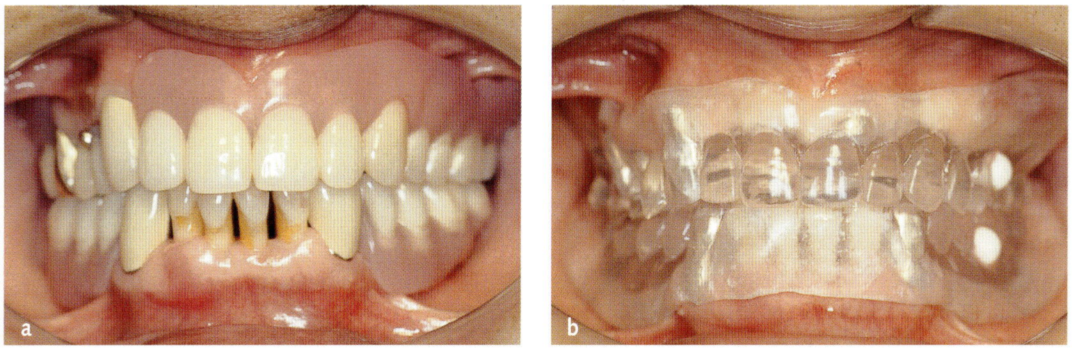

Fig 5-171 Addition of implants. (a) Delivery of maxillary and mandibular telescopic dentures. The patient is a muscular man with strong occlusal musculature. Movement and sinking of the maxillary denture to the left and movement of the mandibular denture to the distal direction are inevitable. (b) Photograph taken 9 months after delivery of the dentures. An impression of the denture is observed on the mucosa. With the patient's informed consent, implant placement is planned in the maxillary left premolar region and the mandibular right and left premolar regions to protect the mandibular ridge. Surgical stents are prepared from the maxillary and mandibular dentures.

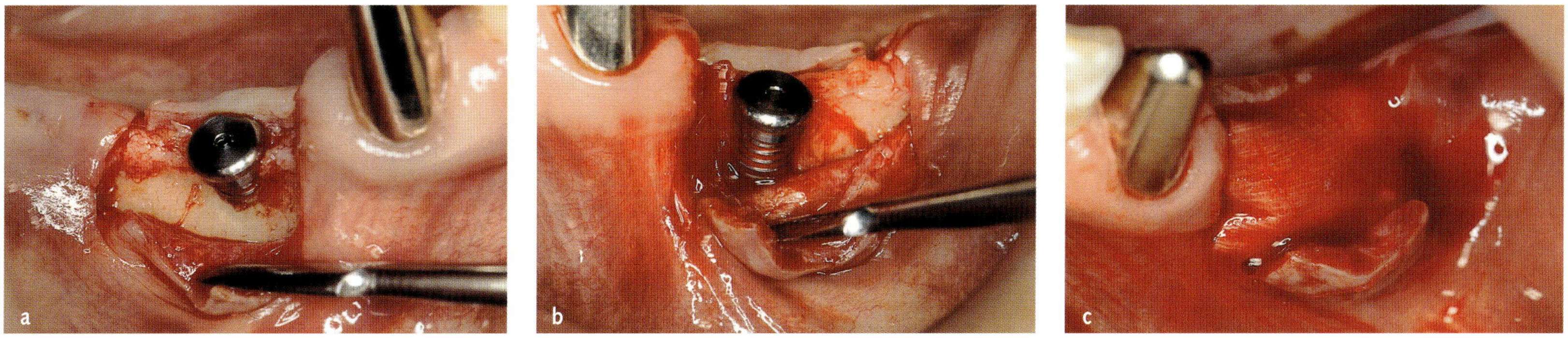

Fig 5-172 Implant placement for the mandible. (a) Ridge resorption is more remarkable in the premolar area than in the canine area. A split crest technique is used to gain bone width, and bone grafting is conducted. (b and c) The left side also shows a limited width of the ridge. An autogenous bone graft is completed and covered with a resorbable membrane to preserve the bone augmentation.

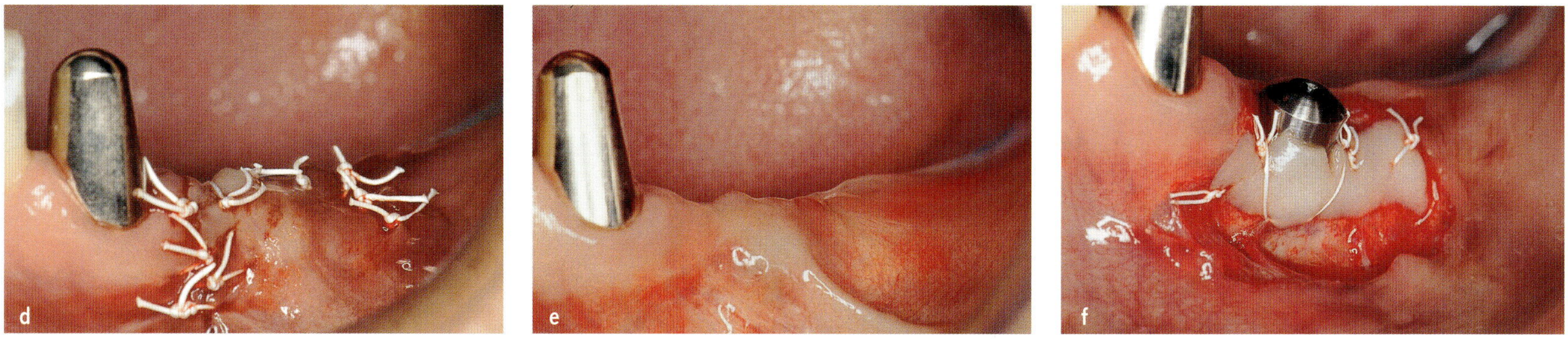

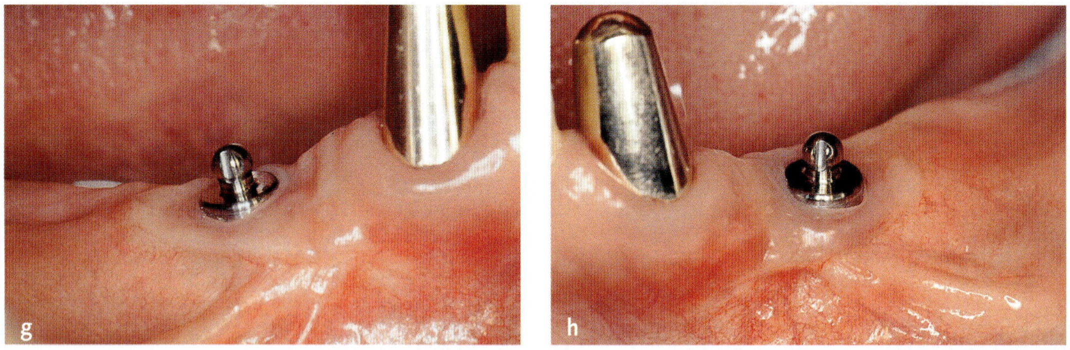

Fig 5-172 (cont) (d) The flap is coronally repositioned for bone regeneration around the implant. (e) The keratinized attached gingiva has been lost, and the frenum attachment is close to the crest of the ridge. (f) At second-stage surgery, a free gingival graft is completed to extend the vestibule and increase the keratinized gingiva. (The same procedure is also completed for the right side.) (g and h) Photographs taken 9 months after implant placement.

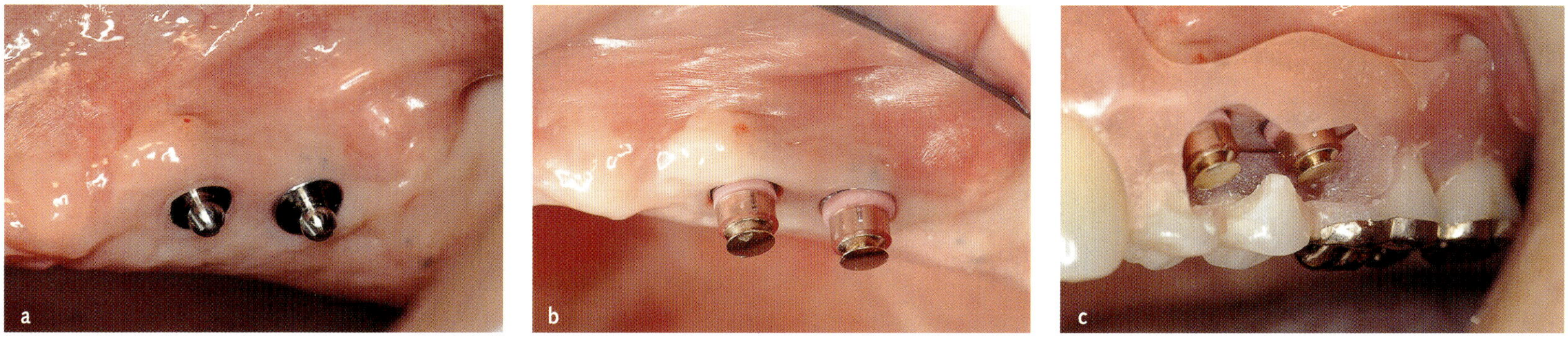

Fig 5-173 Delivery of O-ring attachments to the maxillary implants. (a) The vestibule of the maxillary left premolar area was extended at second-stage surgery. Male attachments have been delivered. (b) Elastic rings are placed on the male part of the O-ring attachments as a spacer before the female parts are delivered. This spacer allows about 1 mm of vertical play to the attachment. This is done with the intention of preventing direct transfer of movement to the implants when the denture tilts or moves. Direct transmission of denture movements to the implants could cause overloading. (c) A window is opened on the buccal aspect of the denture, and resin is injected from the opening to process the female parts to the denture base. The same method is used when the denture is rebased. This technique has been used for about 13 years for all implant overdentures with satisfactory results.

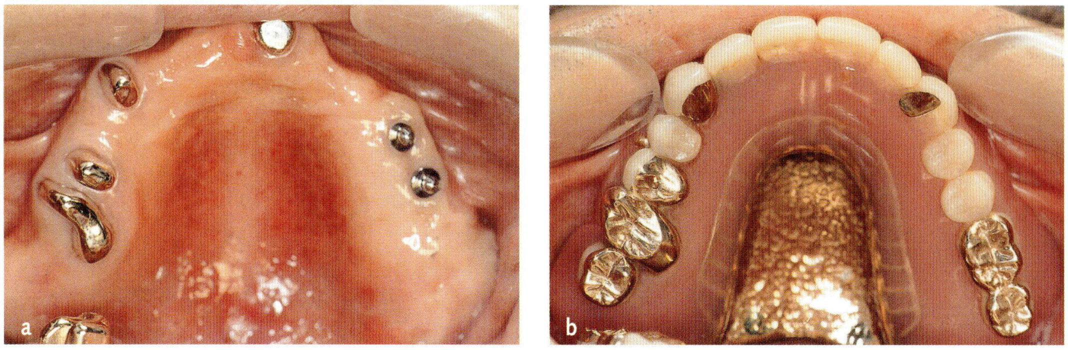

Fig 5-174 Telescopic denture with additional retention from implants. (a and b) Implants may help to prevent movement and vertical depression of the denture.

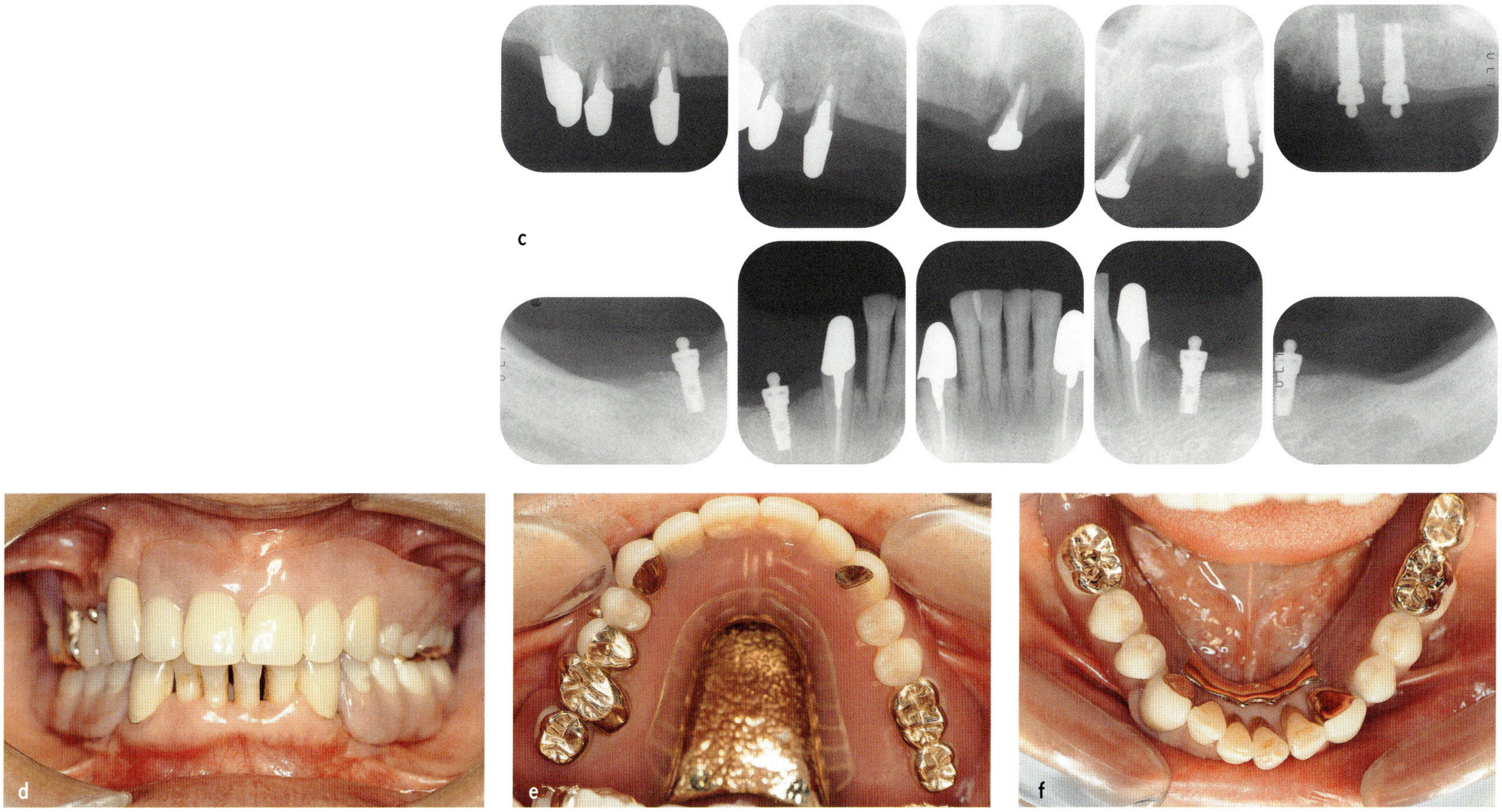

Fig 5-174 (cont) (c) Radiographs taken 3 years 5 months after the first visit. (d to f) For efficient mastication, metal castings are used for the occlusal surfaces of the molars in the denture. Because the metal occlusal surfaces are bonded with resin, it is possible to correct the vertical dimension of the artificial teeth as the denture depresses into the tissue. (Prostheses made by Mr Takahisa Tashiro, RDT.)

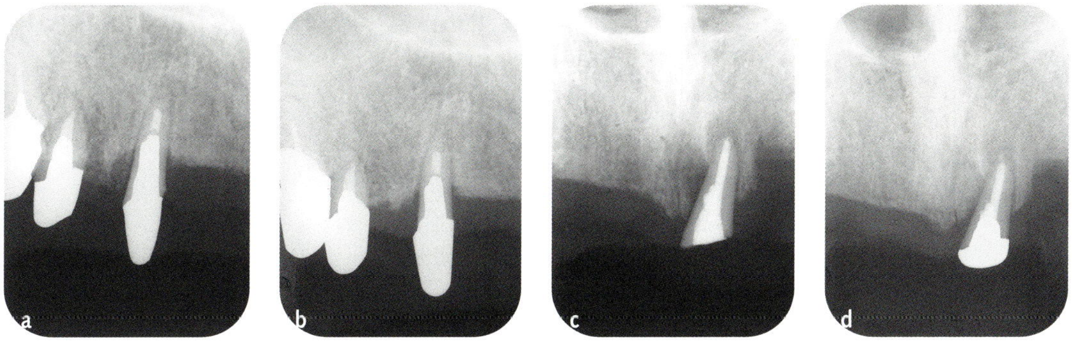

Fig 5-175 (a) Radiograph taken 8 months after the first visit. There are bone defects at the maxillary right second premolar and canine. Regenerative therapy with Emdogain has been completed. (b) Radiograph taken 11 months after surgery. (c) Radiograph taken 8 months after the first visit. Bone defects at are present at the maxillary left central incisor. Regenerative therapy with Emdogain and autogenous bone grafting have been completed. (d) Radiograph taken 11 months after surgery.

Case 5-10 Step-by-step procedures in a full-mouth reconstructive prosthodontic treatment

Patient: *55-year-old man at the time of first visit in September 1997*

Chief complaint: *The patient had a strong distrust of healthcare and documented all treatments he had received from quite a few dental offices prior to the first visit at our office. While he did not indicate particular dental problems, this difficult patient demanded treatments with implants and GTR. Figures 5-176 to 5-189 show detailed step-by-step procedures including decision-making at various stages.*

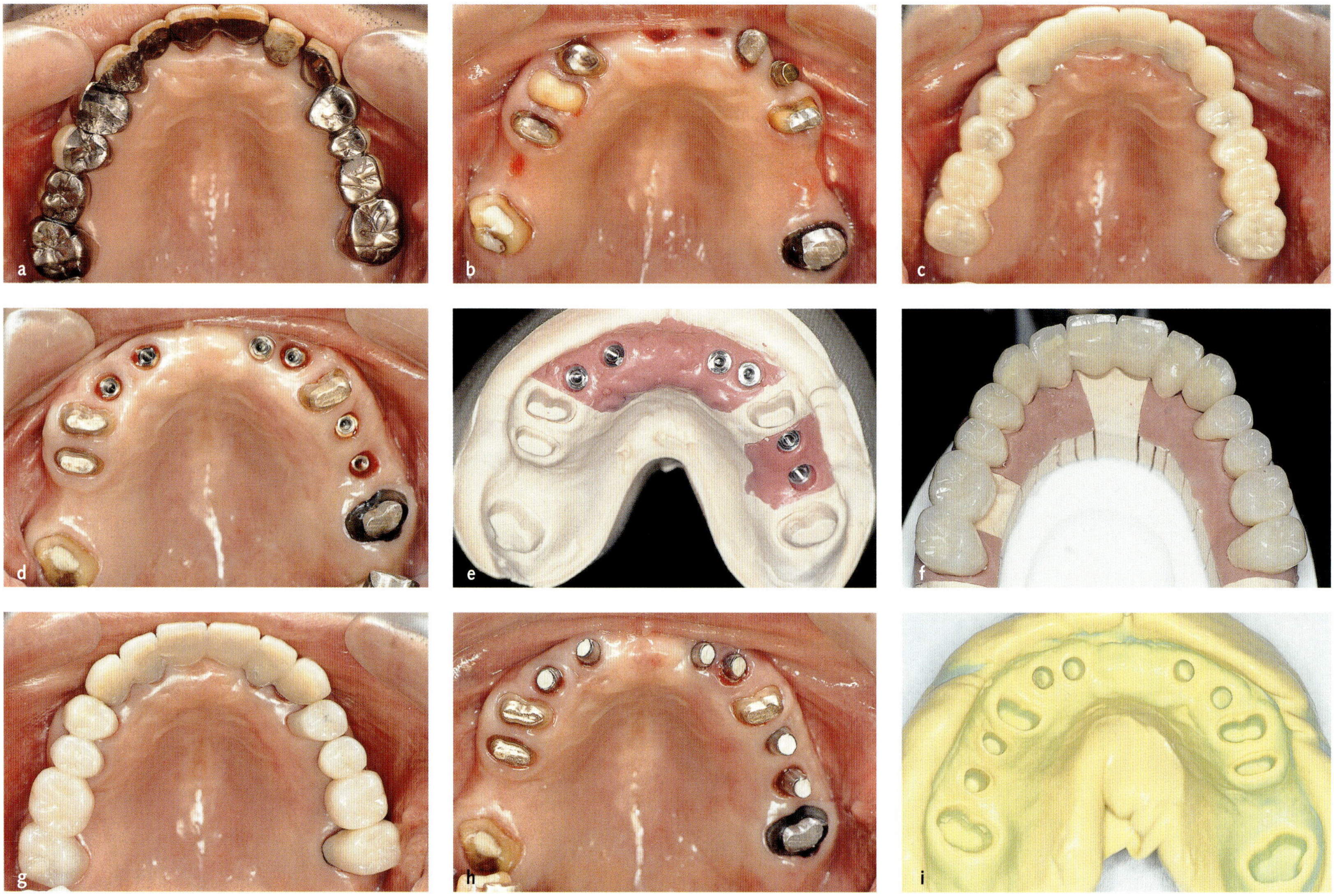

Fig 5-176 Restorative procedures in the maxilla, from provisional restoration to final prosthesis. (a) Photograph taken at the first visit. Owing to the patient's distrust of dental treatments, desired treatment plans could not be immediately initiated. Particular care was taken not to extract a tooth. (b) Photograph taken 9 months after the first visit. Finally the patient accepted our deicision to extract teeth after completion of initial therapy. Scaling and root planing was prudently repeated for this patient. (c) While the fixed provisional restoration is being modified, the implant at maxillary left canine is removed to provide a denture-type of provisional restoration. If the patient will accept it, telescopic crowns will be planned for the maxillary prosthesis. (d) Although the patient wanted implants from the beginning, his case required careful review prior to consideration of implants. Photograph taken after 1 year 2 months. (e) An impression has been taken with impression copings at the implants and thin retraction cords on the abutment teeth. The cast for fabrication of the final provisional restoration is shown. (f) Final provisional restoration. There are concerns about the occlusal relationship, cusp continuity, and occlusal surface morphology in the provisional restoration. (g and h) Delivery of the final provisional restoration. Because remargining is to be started at this stage, the restoration is removed for refabrication because the changes in the occlusal surface morphology are more involved than that which could be corrected by intraoral modification. (i) An HIT impression is taken again. For the provisional restoration, a simplified method with one hole per tooth for injection of the impression material is used (see Fig 5-182 for details of the impression procedures for the provisional restoration in this case).

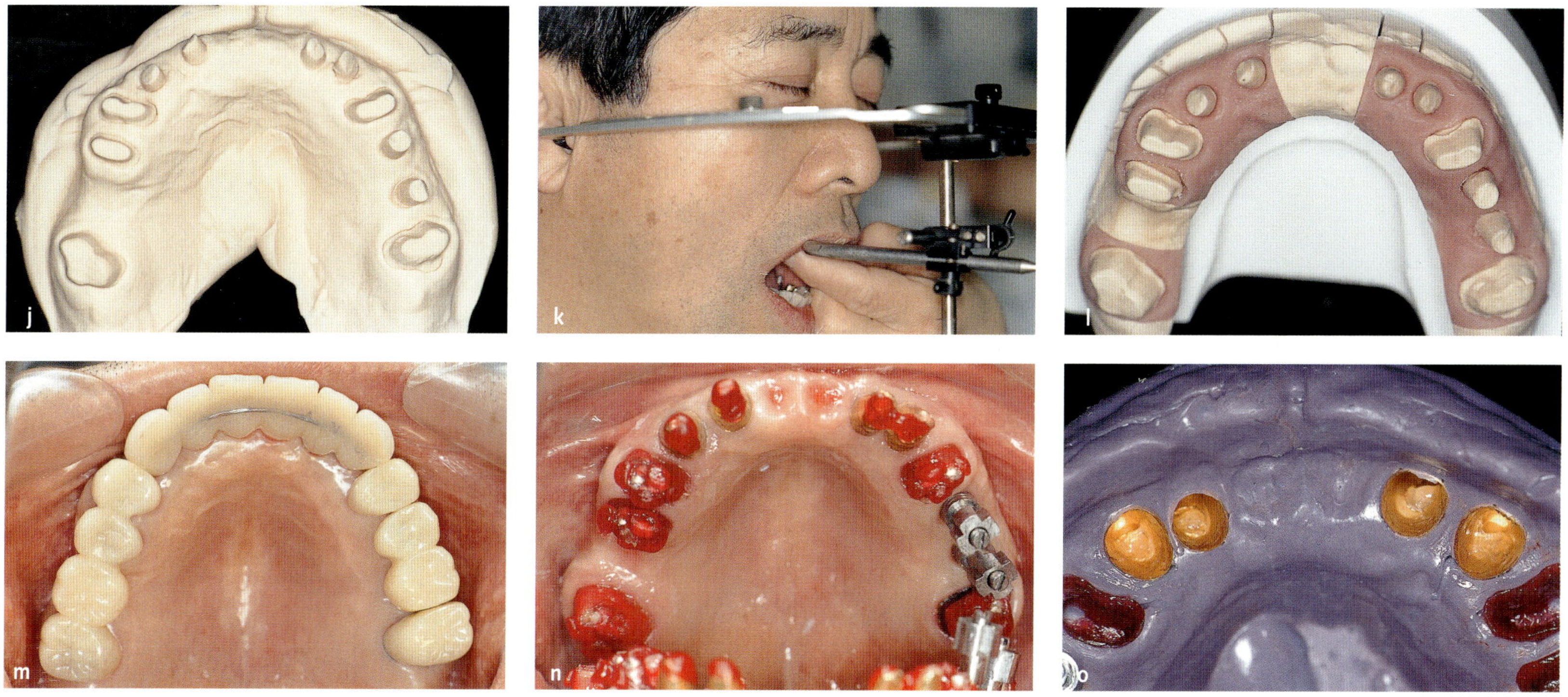

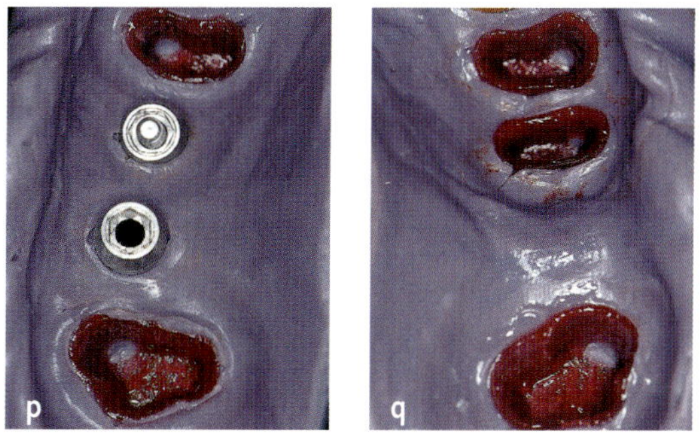

Fig 5-176 (cont) (j) Cast for fabrication of the final provisional restoration. (k) Facebow transfer for the fabrication of the provisional restoration. Because of the need to refabricate the final provisional restoration, the definitive restoration is delayed for about 2 months. (l) Cast for the final provisional restoration with a tissue model made on top of separated, retrievable dies. (m) Delivery of the final provisional restoration. Remargination is completed. The final provisional restoration is harmonized, and symmetric occlusal surface morphology is attained. Note the difference from (g) in the occlusal surface positioning. The final task to accomplish with the final provisional restoration is remargination. The provisional restoration is expected to be used for a short time period. (n) Full-mouth impressions are made with a transfer coping technique. Petroleum jelly is applied to the copings to prevent ingress of impression material. An opening is made on the occlusal surface of the maxillary left first molar crown, made of pattern resin, to check the vertical fit. (o to q) Copings are picked up in the impression. For anterior implants, metal inner surfaces are shown.

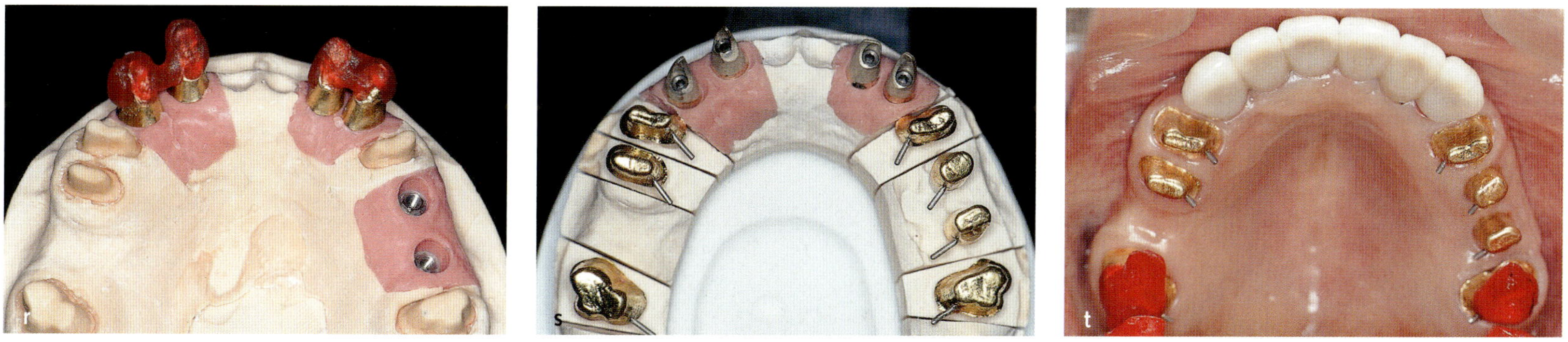

(r) Stone is poured into the pick-up impression to complete this full-mouth working cast, on which a tissue model is prepared for the implant areas. Because implants allow no deviation, laboratory work is completed first in these areas. (s) Molar copings are made by an electroforming method, and UCLA-type abutments are made for the anterior teeth. The electroforming method is used to fabricate pure gold copings. (Prostheses made by Mr Chojiro Masuda, RDT, Kalos Dental, Japan.) (t) A six-unit anterior fixed partial denture supported by implants at the right canine, lateral incisor, and central incisor and left central incisor, lateral incisor, and canine sites is delivered to offer vertical stops and guidance at the anterior area while the electroformed copings are tried in for the molars. On top of the copings of the most distal molars, pattern resin registrations taken on the articulator are placed to register the vertical stops of the molars.

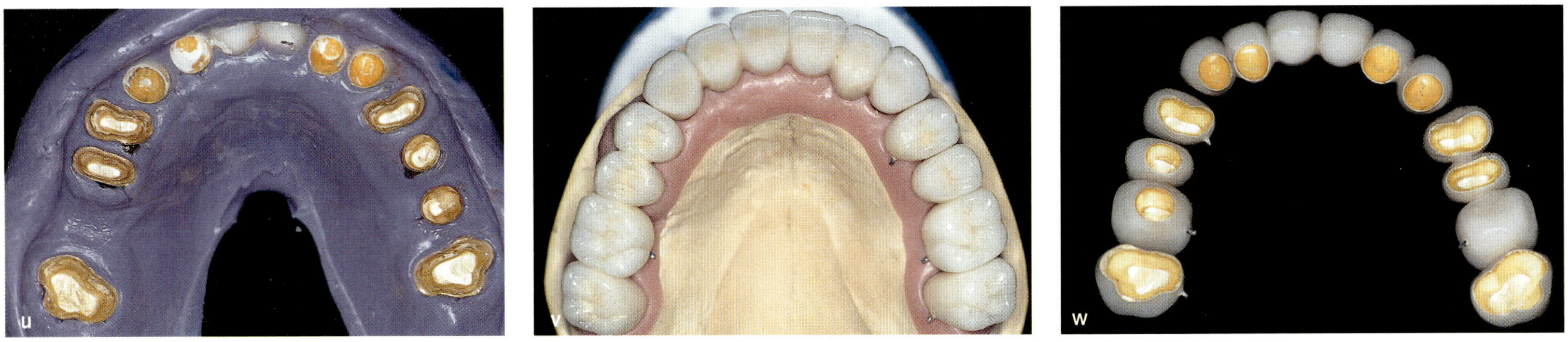

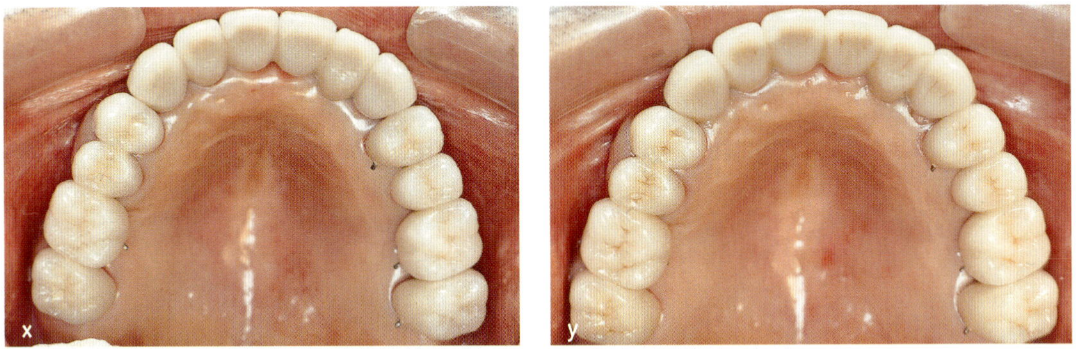

Fig 5-176 (cont) (u) A pick-up impression is taken, including the six-unit anterior fixed partial denture, electroformed copings, and molar vertical stop records. The pick-up impression records the mutual relationship of the metal coping positions and accurately reproduces the cervical areas, providing almost a natural contour of the gingiva. (v) From the cast obtained by pouring stone into the pick-up impression, a cast with a tissue model is fabricated, on which the bisque bake of the porcelain is fabricated with reference to the final provisional restoration. The tissue model is fabricated by pouring model material in the space between the impression of the stone cast obtained from the pick-up impression and a trimmed retrievable die. (w) Inner surfaces of the prostheses. The porcelain crowns are built up on a separated cast and the emergence profile of the crowns is evaluated on the tissue model fabricated from the pick-up impression. (x) Bisque-baked crowns are tried in the mouth and a remount is repeated two to three times. Occlusal adjustments are made. If there is a problem in the emergence profile that cannot be corrected by minor adjustments, a pick-up impression of this bisque bake is taken to the tissue model and morphologic correction is completed. (y) To compensate for deformation caused by firing and discrepancies in the mandibular position caused by subtle lifting of the implant superstructure, it is inevitable that two or three remounts will be required. For a clinical remount, the occlusal surfaces are roughened in the mouth, and a silicone bite registration is taken and sent to the laboratory, where powder is applied to the abraded porcelain occlusal surfaces to correct the occlusion. After the remount procedure is completed, staining and refiring are conducted to complete the periodontal prosthesis.

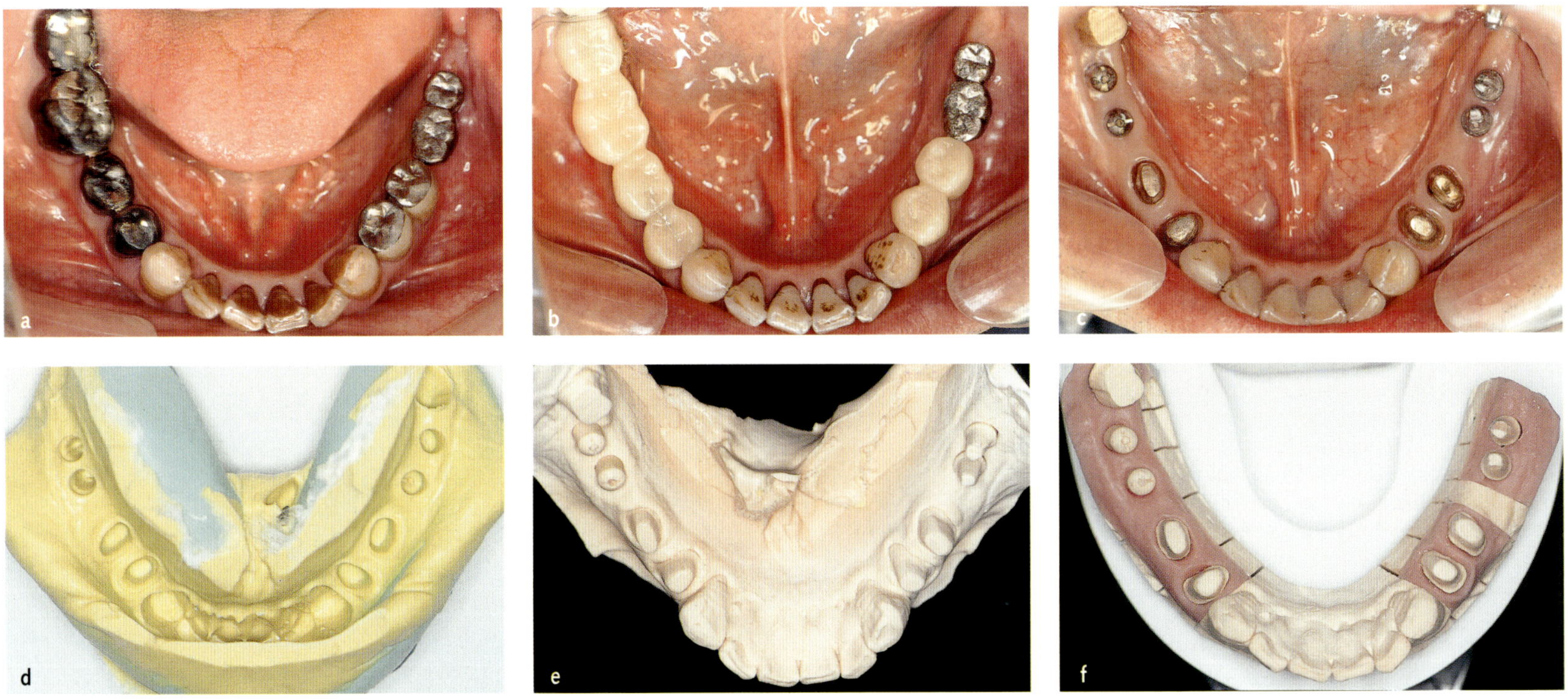

Fig 5-177 Restorative procedures in the mandible, from provisional restoration to final prostheses. (a) Photograph taken at the first visit. (b) About 9 months after the first visit, implants have been placed at the sites of the mandibular right first and second molars. (c) Photograph taken about 1 year 6 months after the first visit. An ITI implant (Straumann) has been placed at mandibular left first molar, and it is decided to refabricate the superstructure alone. The abutments, including the screws, were cemented and could not be removed, so the abutments are prepared directly for restoration. (d) HIT impression for fabrication of the provisional restoration. (e) A full-mouth cast made from an HIT impression. (f) A tissue model on top of the separated, retrievable dies. Here the design decision is made as to whether crowns will be splinted or not and, if they are to be splinted, at which locations. Unnecessary splinting is not completed.

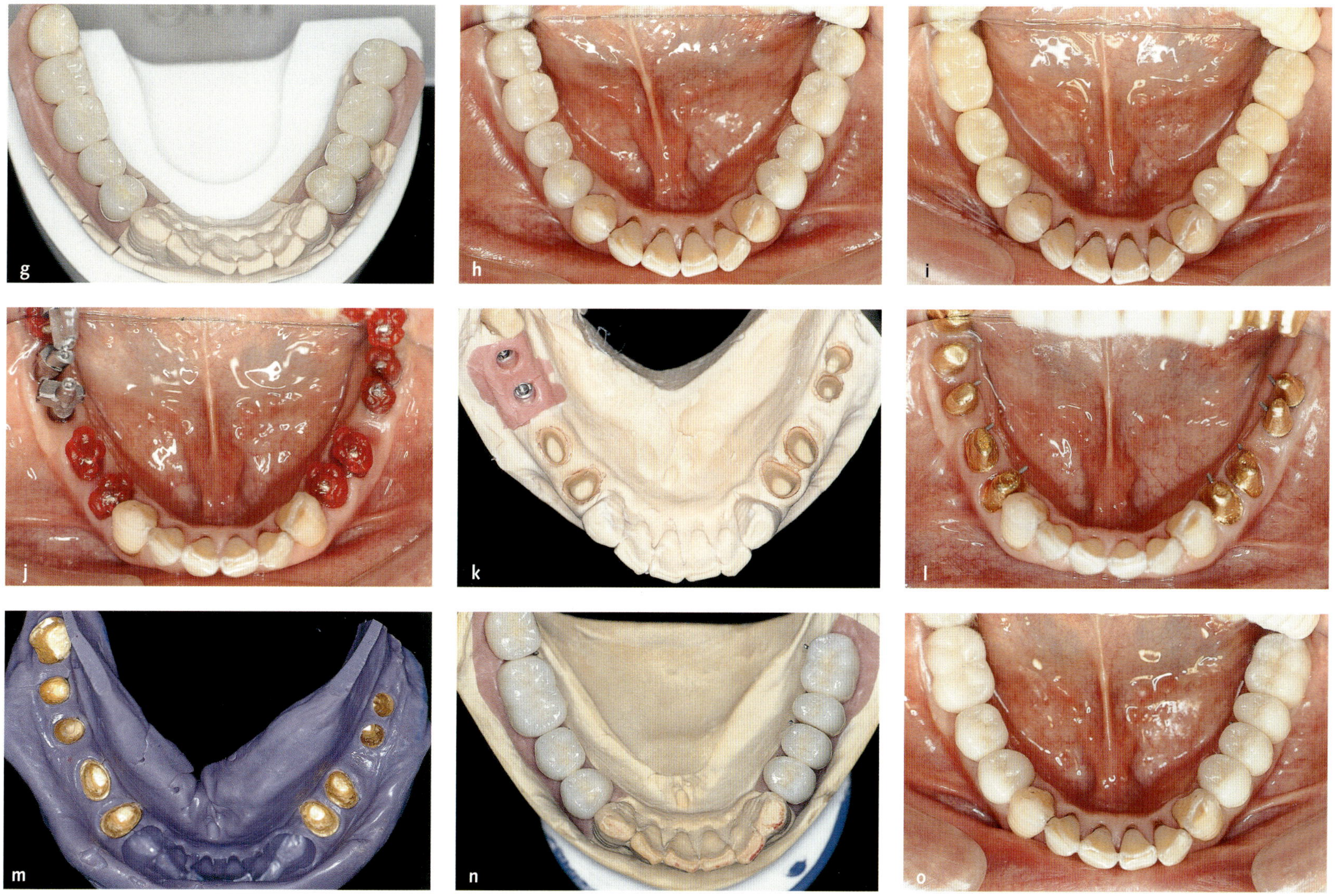

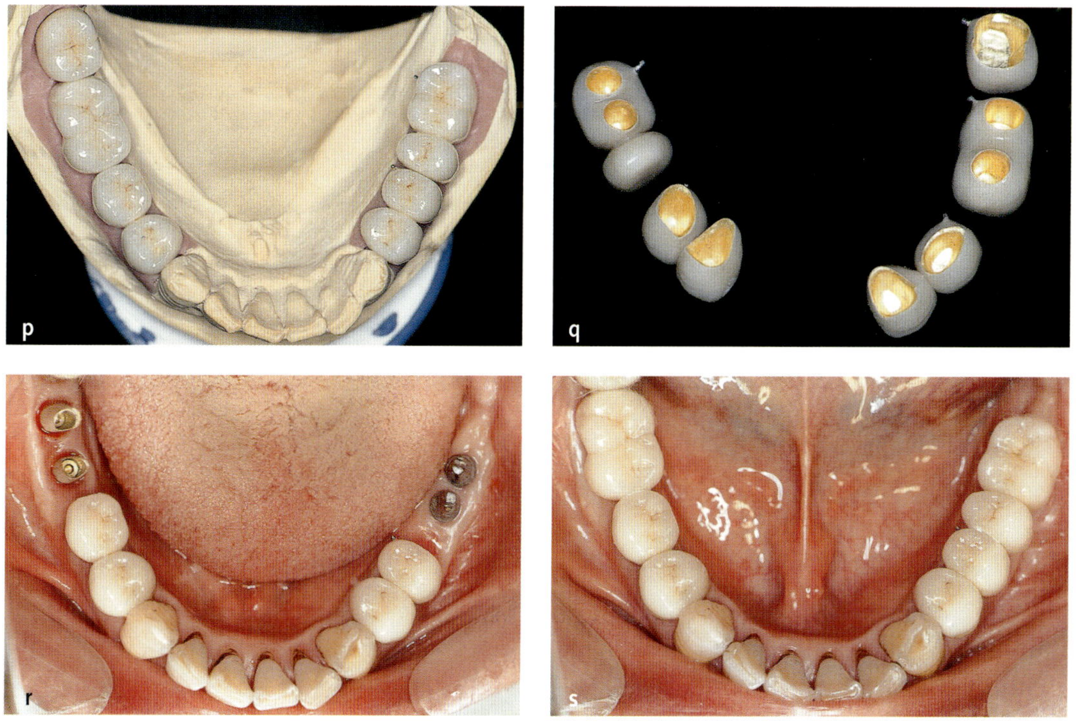

Fig 5-177 (cont) (g) Final provisional restoration. There is some concern about the occlusal surface morphology. (h) Final provisional restoration tried in the mouth. (i) After a second impression procedure and facebow transfer, the final provisional restoration is refabricated. The most important role of the final provisional restoration is remargination. (j) Die casts are made, and copings are fabricated of pattern resin. A full-mouth impression is taken with the transfer coping technique. (k) Stone is poured in the pick-up impression to complete the full-mouth working cast. Impression copings for the implant areas and electroformed copings for the molars are shown. (l) Copings are fabricated by an electroforming technique and tried in the mouth. Pattern resin is used to make a soldering index to prevent dislocation and rotation of caps. (m) These are picked up again in the impression to correct for distortion of the inner surface of the pattern resin and error caused by waxing. (n) Bisque-baked crowns are fabricated on the cast obtained by pouring stone into the pick-up impression. (o) The completed prostheses are tried in the mouth and a remounting is repeated. (p) Prostheses after staining. (q) Inner surfaces of the completed prostheses. (r) Try-in of nonimplant prostheses. (s) Photograph taken about 4 years 6 months after the first visit, at completion and delivery of the final prostheses.

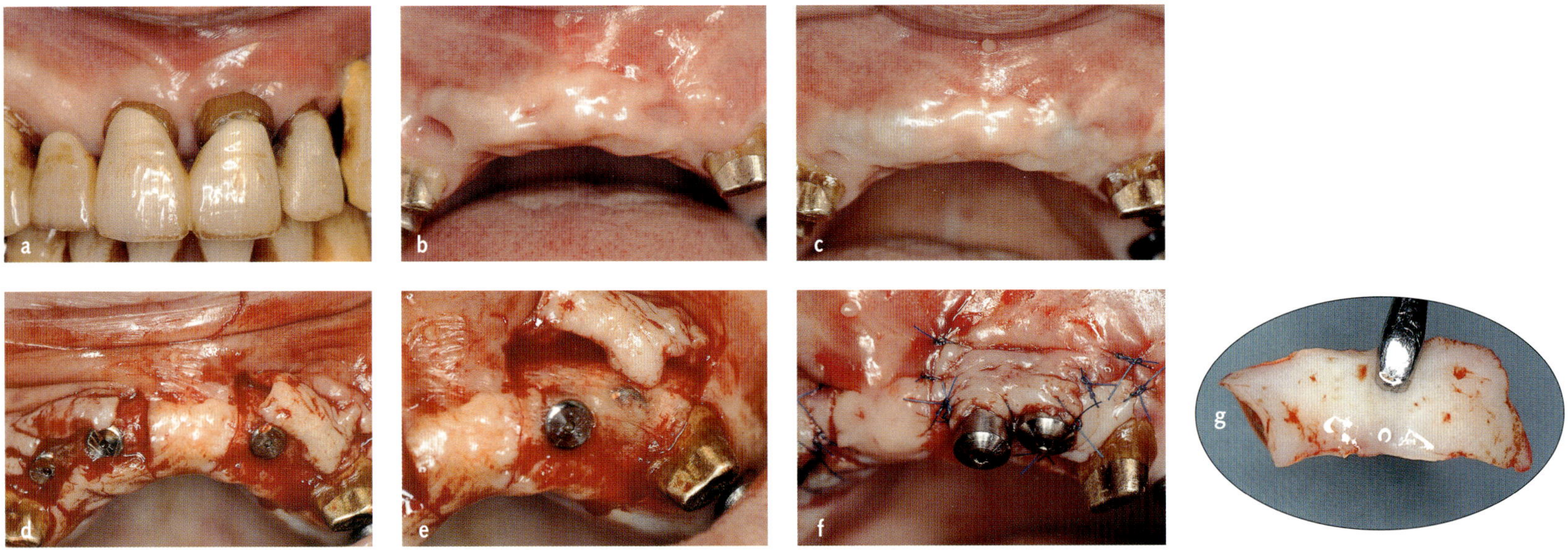

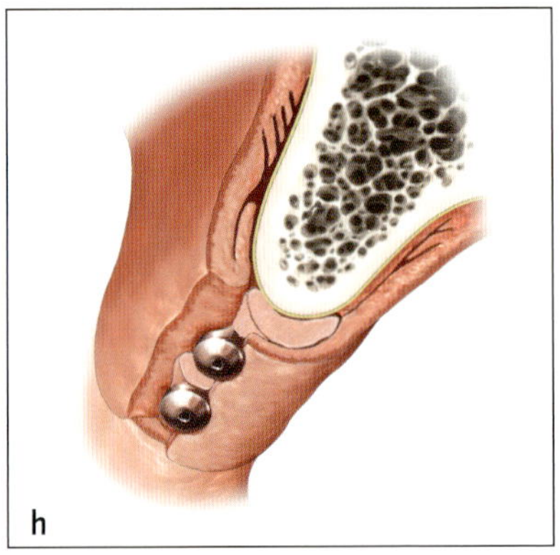

Fig 5-178 Peri-implant tissue management in the anterior area. (a) Condition at the first visit. (b) Condition 1 year 5 months after the first visit, after implant placement following tooth extraction and ridge augmentation. (c) Photograph taken 1 year 11 months after the first visit, at the second-stage surgery for abutment connection. (d to f) At the second-stage implant surgery, because of the lack of keratinized gingiva, a mucosal flap is raised from the palatal side and repositioned buccally, aiming at an increase of the keratinized gingiva, harmony of the gingival margins, and formation of interdental papilla-like tissue. The partial-thickness flap is raised from the palatal side and the pedicle flap is mesially and buccally repositioned. The distal area has a shortage, and a free connective tissue graft is completed. (g and h) Free connective tissue graft with a collar.

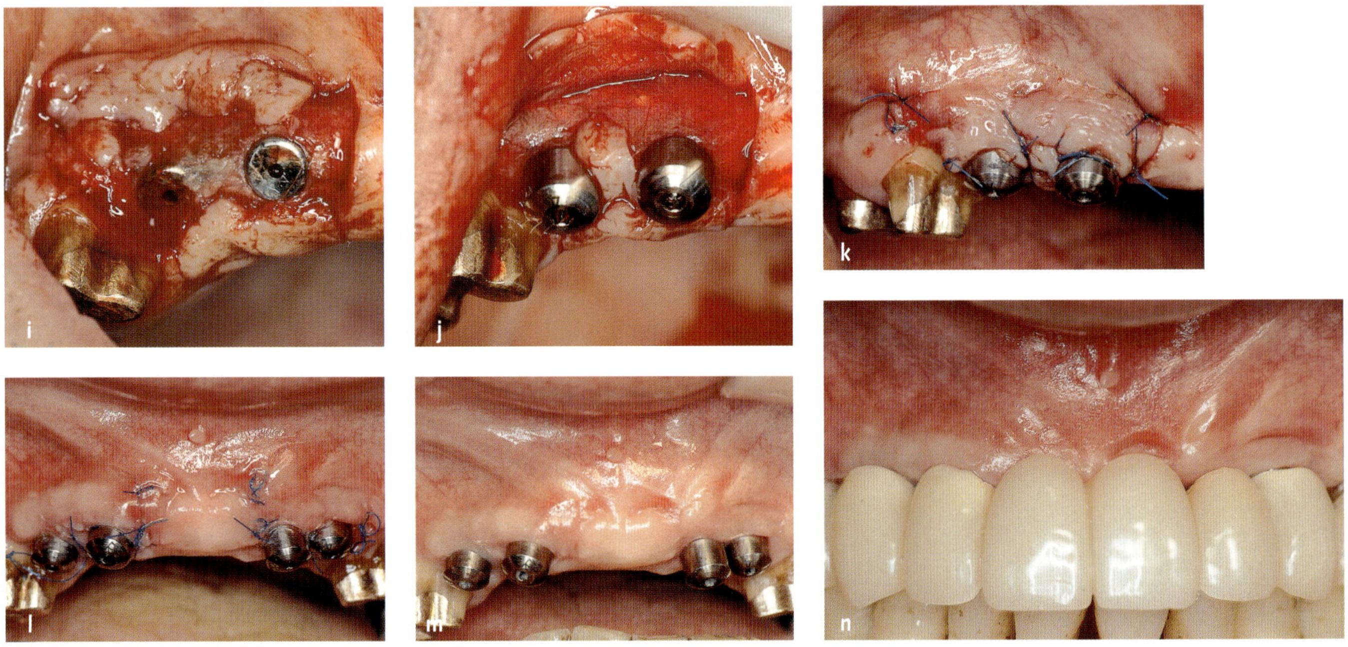

(i to k) Similar treatment is conducted for the right side. Between implants on the right side, a free connective tissue graft is completed. No grafting is completed on the distal side. (l) Photograph taken 2 weeks postsurgery. (m) Photograph taken 5 weeks postsurgery. (n) Provisional restoration in place.

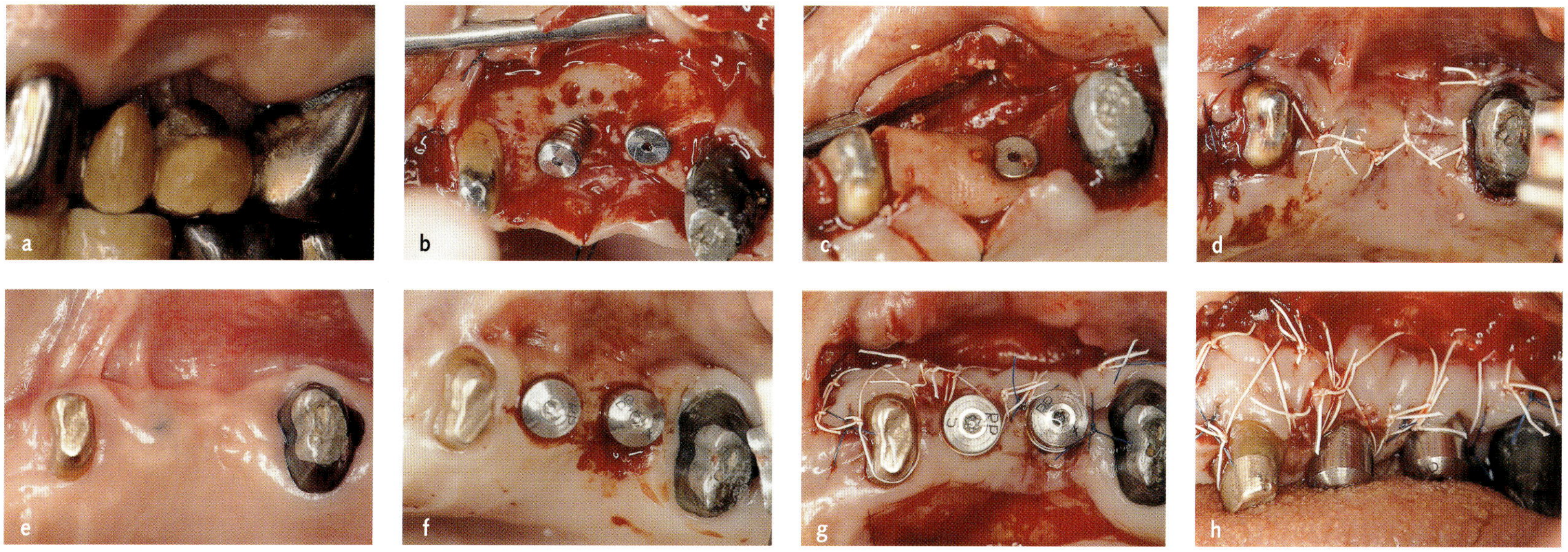

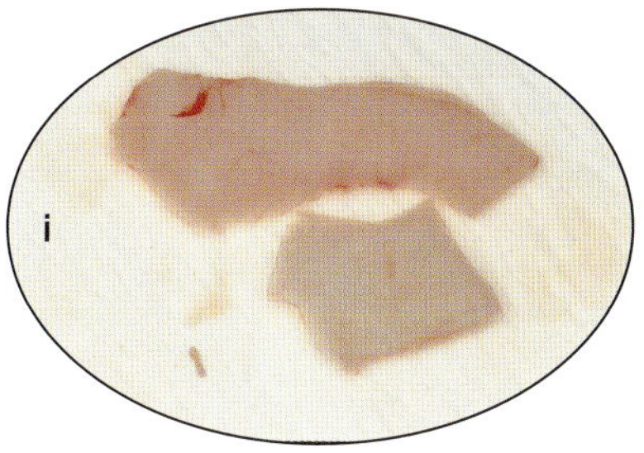

Fig 5-179 Placement of implants for the maxillary left ridge. Regenerative therapy is necessary and there is a lack of keratinized gingiva. (a) At the first visit, the alveolar ridge, where a sapphire implant is placed, is significantly concave. (b to d) Osseotite implants (3.75 mm) are placed. For the maxillary left first molar, an osteotome is used for placement in combination with a sinus lift. For the maxillary left second premolar, coronally three threads are left above the crest. This is done to provide gingival margin continuity. The basic standard is that the tops of implants are to be placed 2 mm apical to the cementoenamel junction of the adjacent teeth, based on the principles of biologic width. In this case, the implant top is positioned coronally by about three threads. The surrounding cortical bone is perforated. Bone-grafting material is filled around the implant as a support to create space, and it is covered with a resorbable membrane. (e to h) After 8 months, a punch technique is used to connect the healing abutments. The lingual vestibule is extremely narrowed because of the regenerative therapy; therefore, at the second implant surgery, the buccal mobile mucosa is resected and a free gingival graft is completed. (i) Free connective tissue graft harvested from the palate.

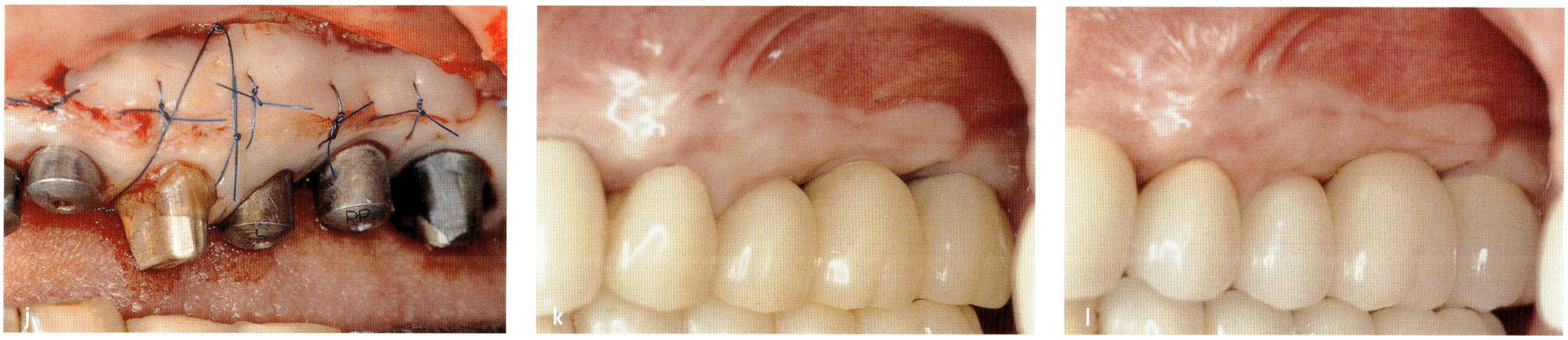

(j) After 5 months, another free gingival graft is completed to extend the vestibule and adjust the morphology of the peri-implant mucosa. (k) Provisional restoration 1 year 8 months after implant placement. (l) At delivery of the final prostheses, there is harmony in the gingival margin, the interdental papillae are conserved, and conditions are stable.

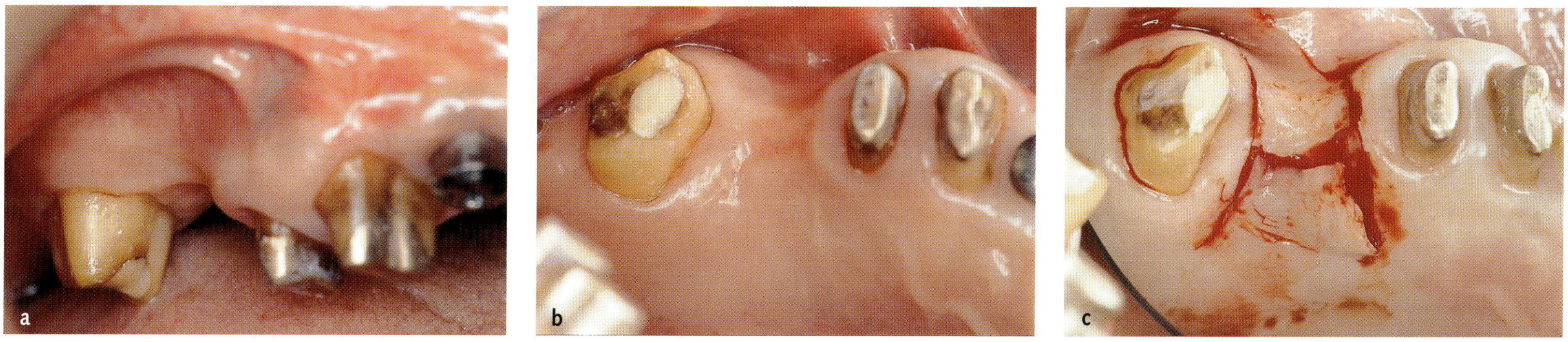

Fig 5-180 Ridge augmentation using a roll technique for the maxillary right ridge. (a and b) The ridge shows significant resorption 2 years 2 months after the first visit. (c) A crestal incision and buccal and lingual vertical incisions are made.

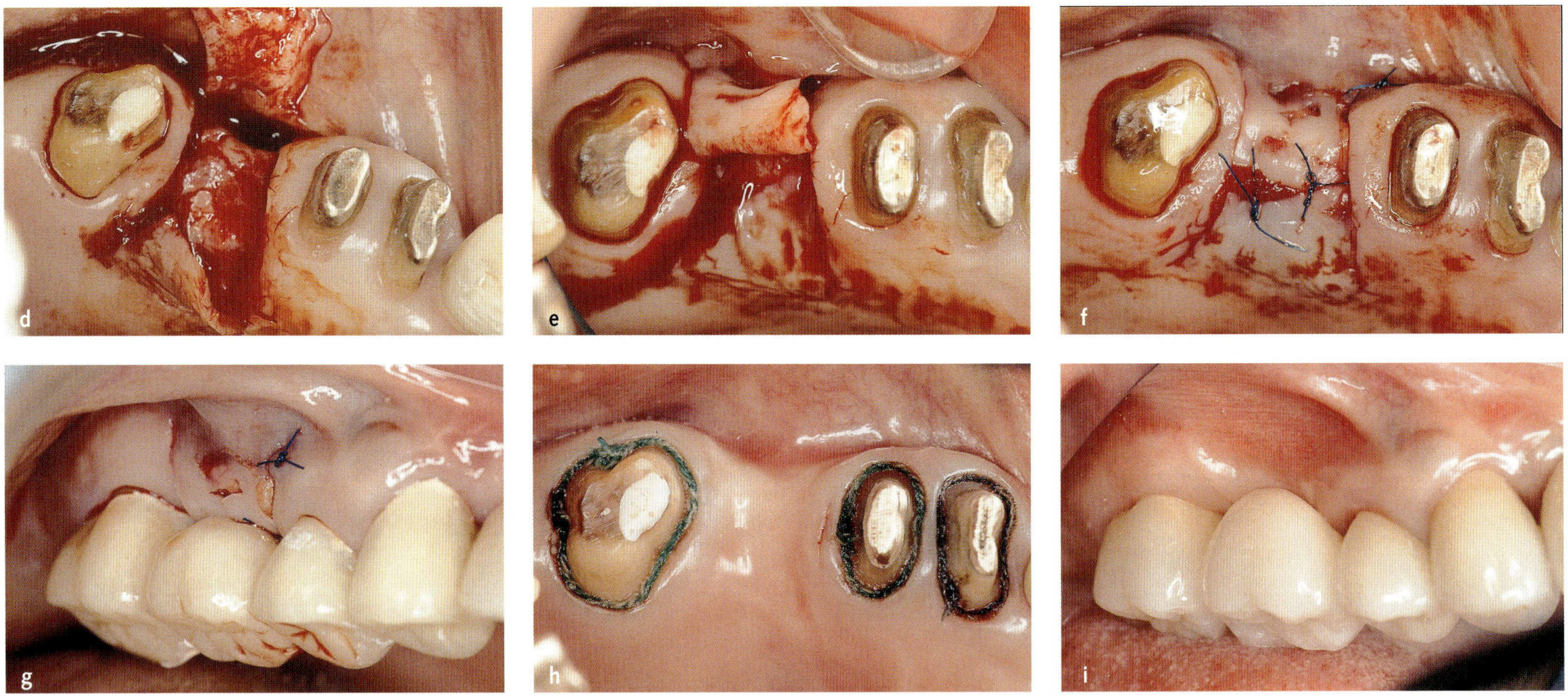

Fig 5-180 (cont) (d to f) Partial-thickness flaps are raised on both the buccal and palatal sides. An incision is made at the base of the palatal partial-thickness flap to dissect the connective tissue and roll it. A reverse roll technique is used to fold the connective tissue to the inside. Thinned epithelium is noted. For the palate, from which the connective tissue is harvested, CollaPlug collagen is placed for hemostasis and a simple suture is made. (g) The buccal side of the pontic in the provisional restoration is fabricated to place pressure on the residual ridge. (h) The large buccal concavity has been reduced. (i) Photograph taken 6 months after delivery of the final prosthesis.

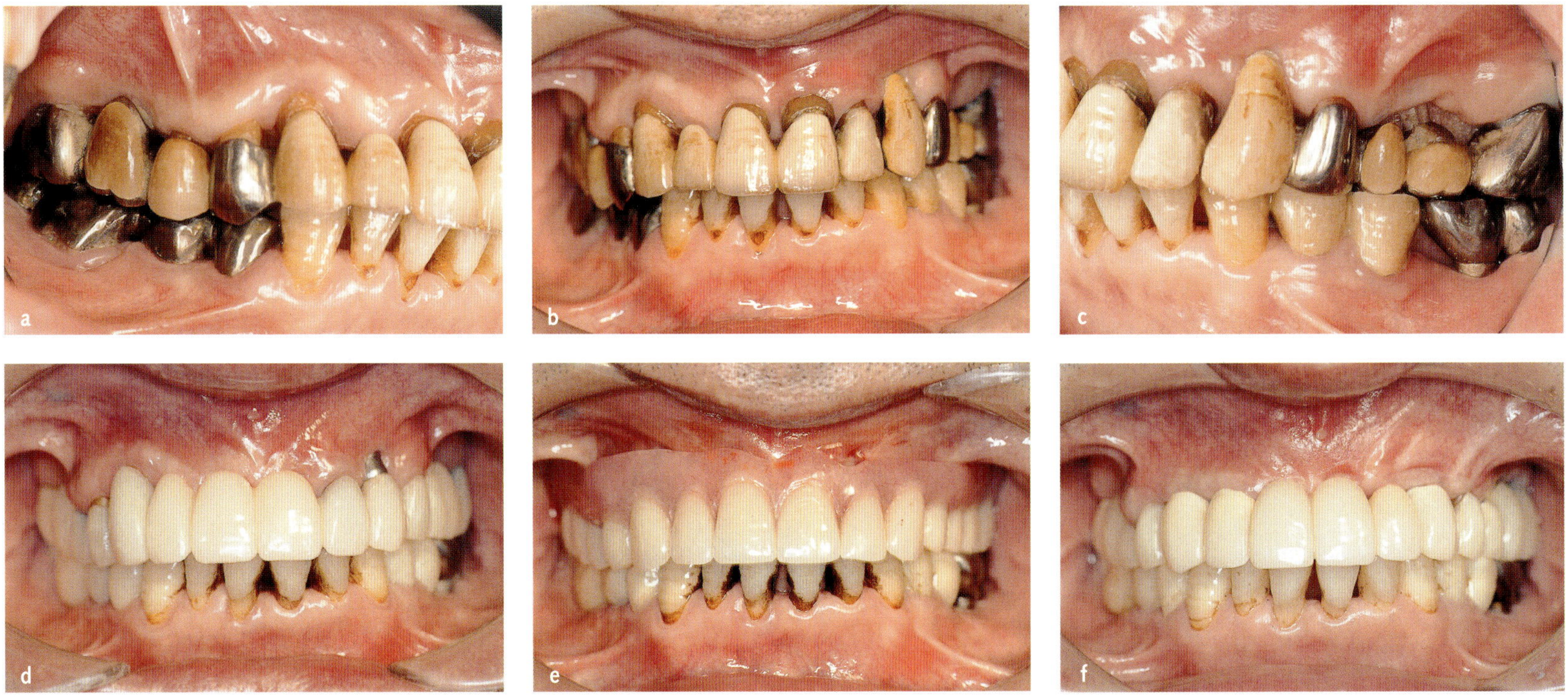

Fig 5-181 Changes in conditions, from provisional restoration to final prostheses. (a to c) Buccal views at the first visit. (d) Photograph taken after about 9 months. The implant at maxillary left canine was removed later. (e) Seven months later, the anterior teeth are extracted to deliver a denture-type provisional restoration. (f) Eight months later, as the treatment plan is finalized, a fixed provisional restoration is delivered and treatment proceeds to implant placement.

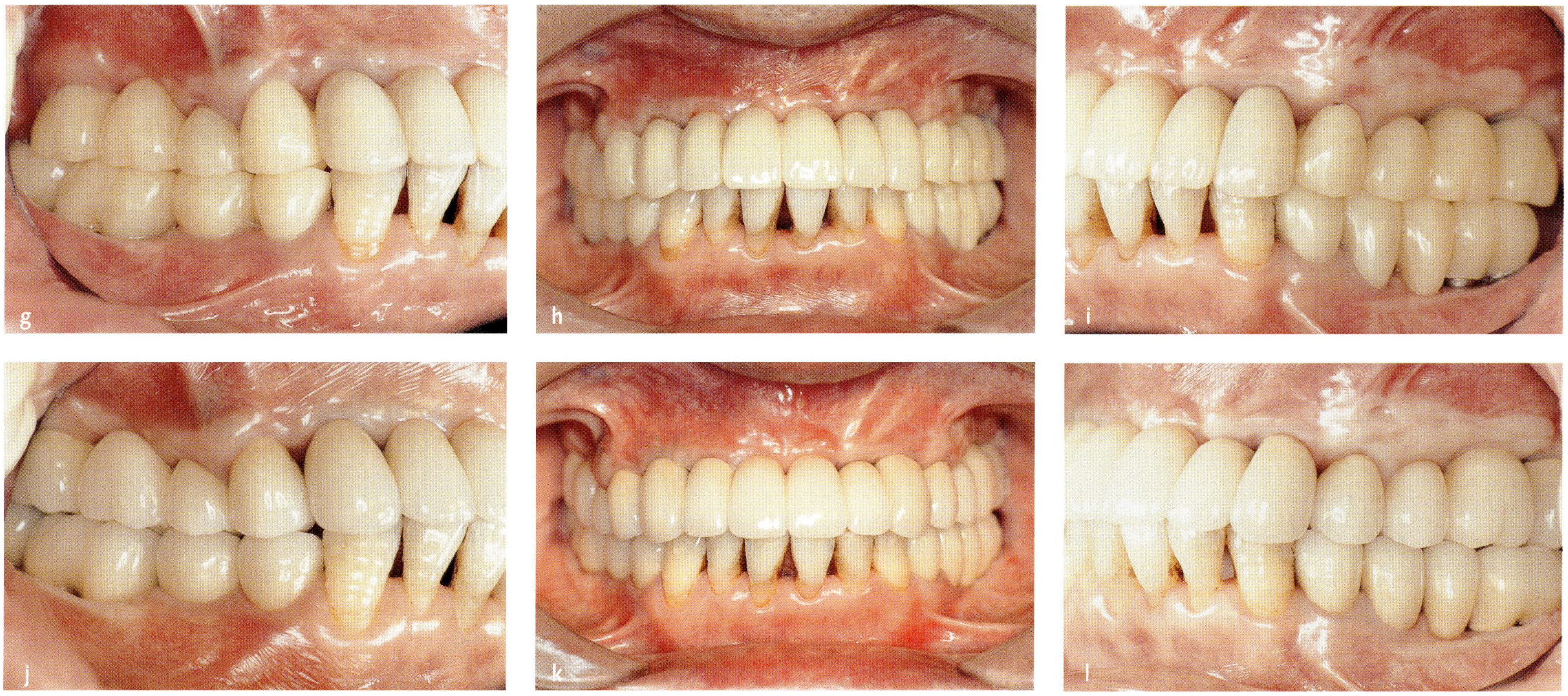

Fig 5-181 (cont) (g to i) Nine months later, the final provisional restoration is in place. (j to l) Appearance at completion of the final periodontal prostheses.

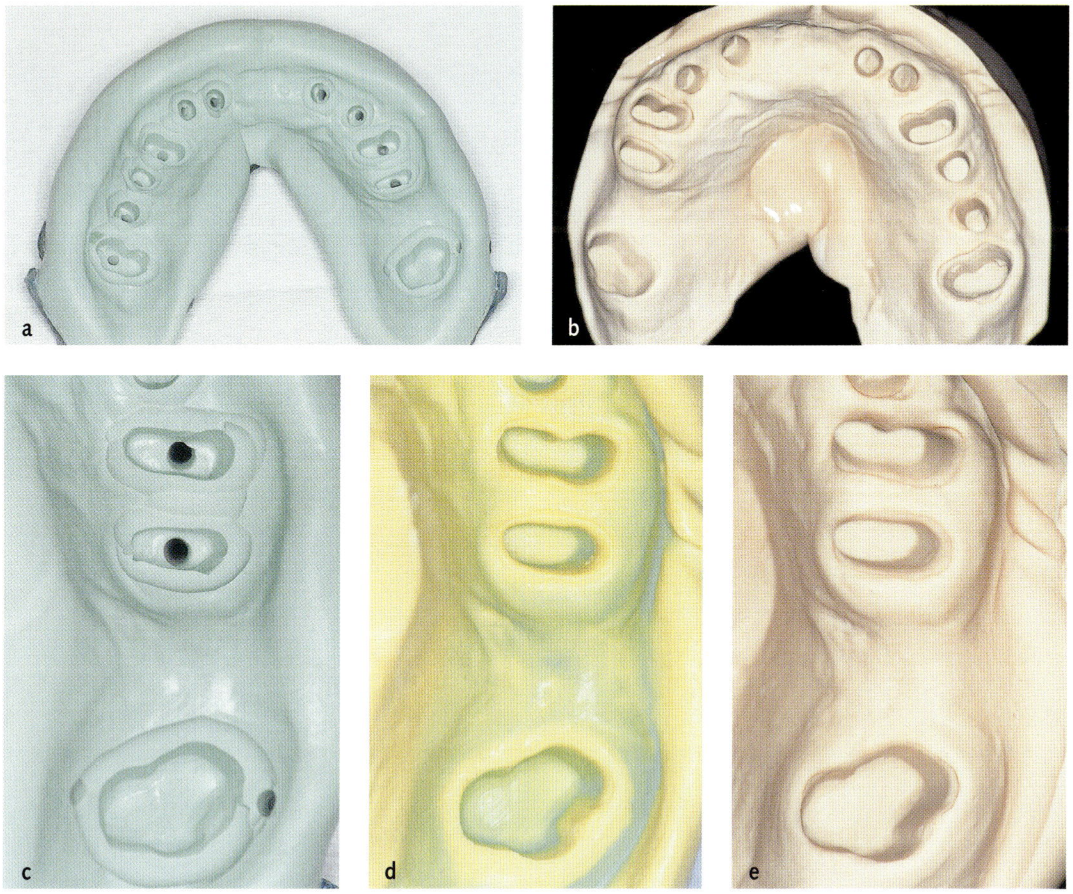

Fig 5-182 HIT impression technique for the provisional restoration. The HIT tray is slightly heated with a burner, and a spacer is applied on the tray. (a) A primary impression is taken with Provil, and the cervical area is trimmed chairside using a silicone carver. (b) A hard impression material such as Provil P should be used for the primary or body impression. (c) Usually two holes per tooth are prepared in the impression for injection and extrusion of the secondary impression material. For the provisional restoration, injection holes are reduced, and one hole is prepared for splinted crowns. Pressure is applied for impression of the provisional restoration, and the body material can be seen through the thin second impression material. Only mild gingival retraction is completed with a thin cord. The primary impression material used is Provil P. For the second impression, a material with low viscosity, such as Imprint II or Provil L, is used. (d) The second impression and (e) a working cast are shown.

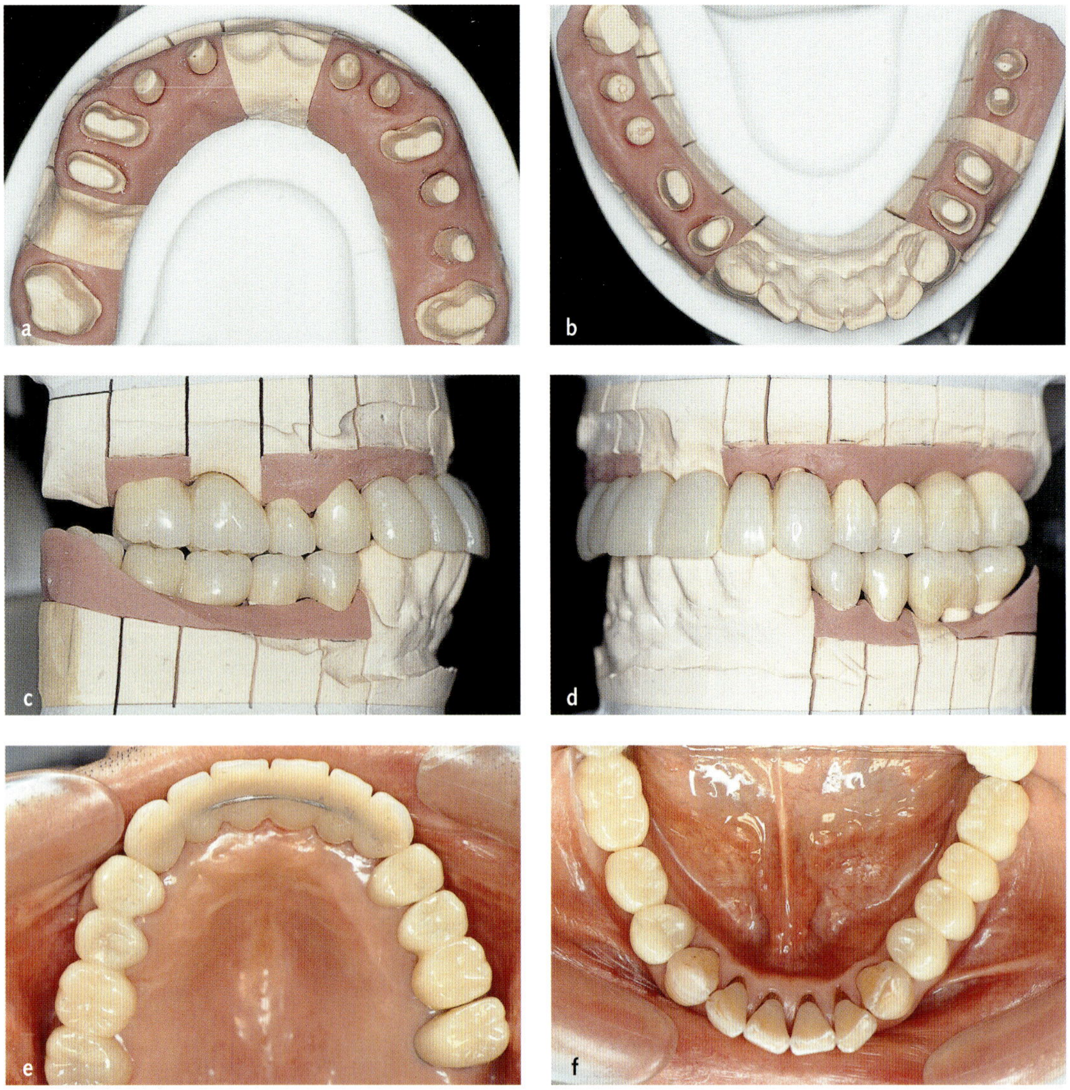

Fig 5-183 Final provisional restorations with the prefabricated tissue model. (a to d) A tissue model is fabricated for completion of the final provisional restoration, which is delivered for final subgingival formation and correction or modification of the margins with autopolymerizing resin. In this clinical case, the final provisional restoration had a problem in the occlusal surface morphology, and another impression was taken. (e and f) Final provisional restorations.

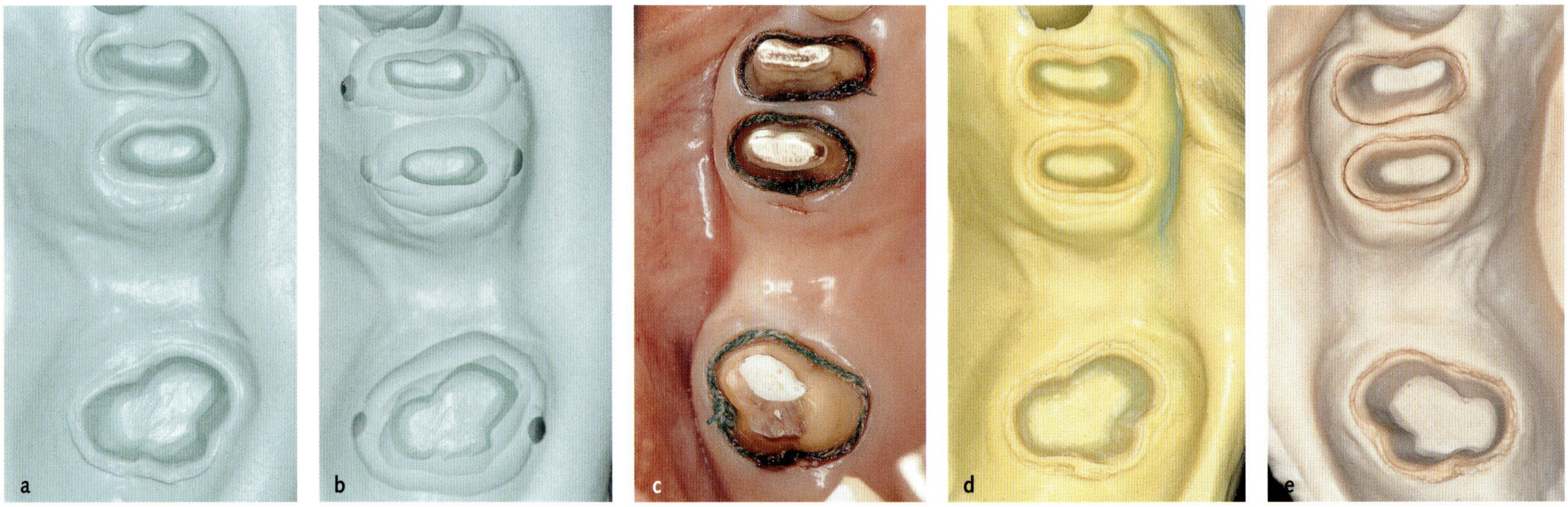

Fig 5-184 Final impression procedure. Similar to the preliminary impression, the impression for the definitive restoration uses the HIT method. Clear preparation margins must be obtained without pressure. (a) Primary body impression. (b) Cervical areas of the primary impression are trimmed and holes are drilled for injection and extrusion. (c) Double cords are used for gingival retraction (thin cord and Ultrapak 1 or 2). (d) Imprint II is injected with a syringe into the trimmed primary impression to obtain the final impression. (e) A working cast is obtained by pouring stone into the impression.

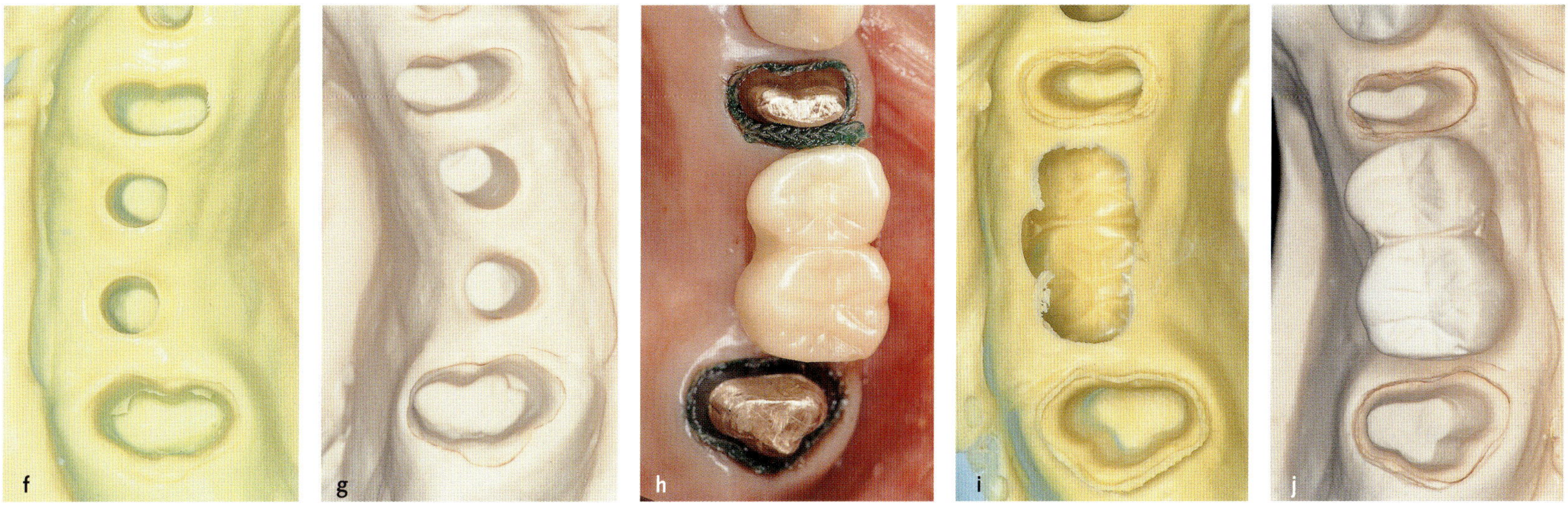

Fig 5-184 (cont) (f) Impression and (g) cast for the provisional restorations. (h) After provisional crowns are delivered to the same area, (i) the final impression of the abutment teeth is taken, and (j) a cast is obtained.

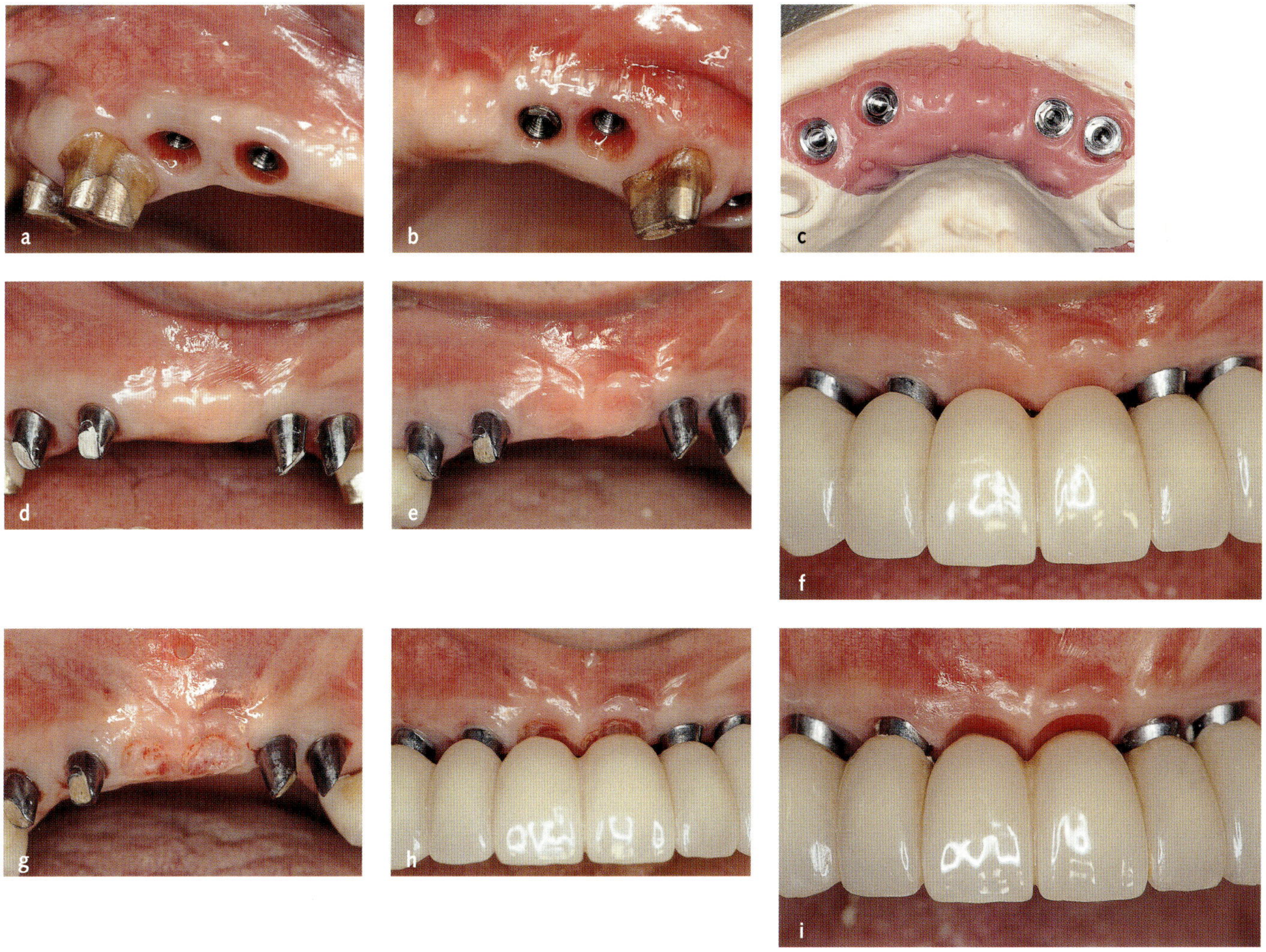

Fig 5-185 Provisional restoration and ovate pontics for the anterior implant area. (a and b) Implant abutments are removed, and the gingivae is adjusted to about 0.5 mm subgingivally. (c) The stone cast is trimmed to fabricate a provisional restoration with ovate pontics. (d) The base of the provisional restoration with a slight convexity is fabricated with pressure against the mucosa for 4 months. (e and f) The restoration is replaced for 2 more months for further tissue development. (g) The mucosa, which is to come in contact with the pontics, is trimmed with electrosurgery. (h) Resin is added to the base of the provisional restoration, which is delivered to the patient. (i) Photograph taken about 1 month after electrosurgery.

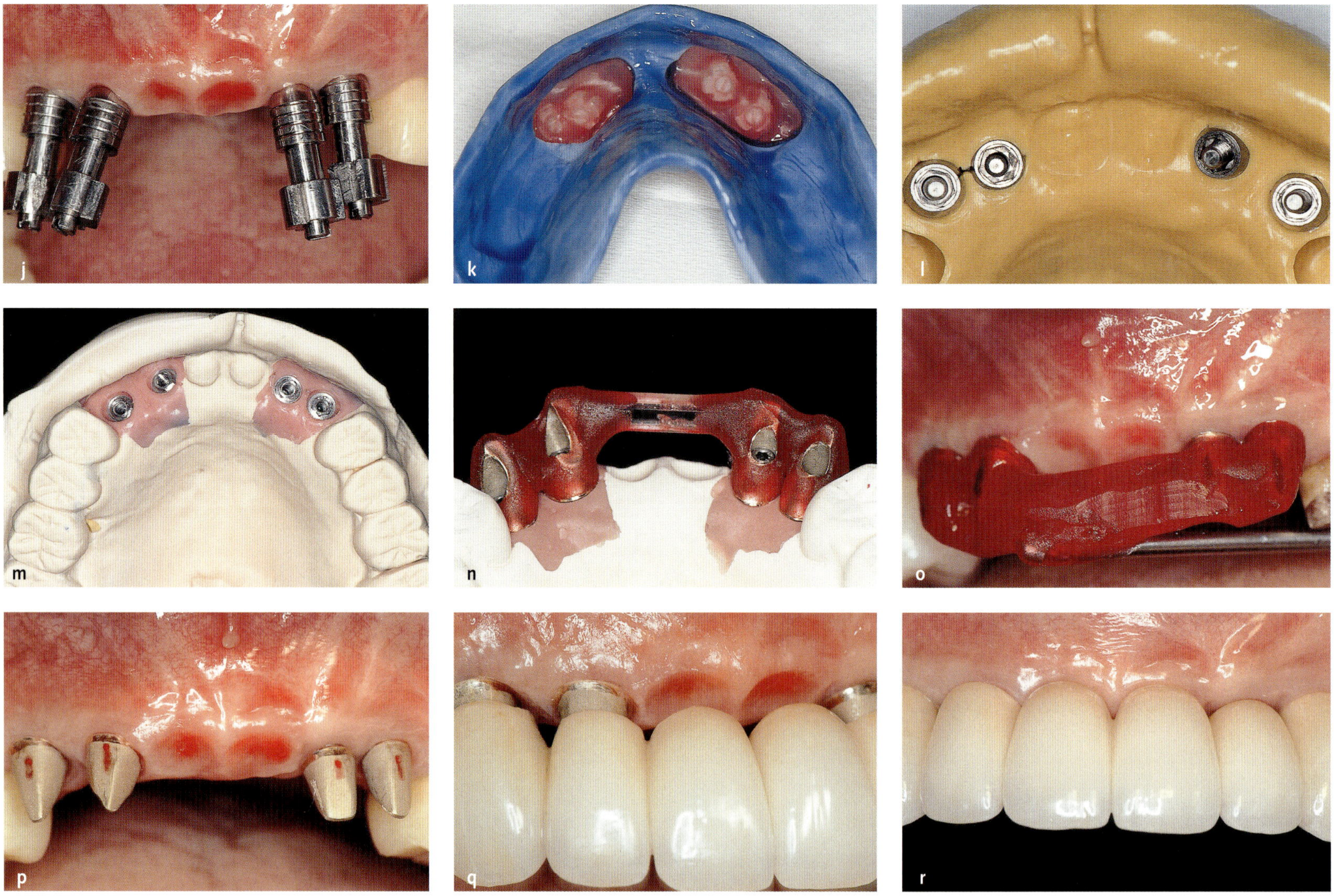

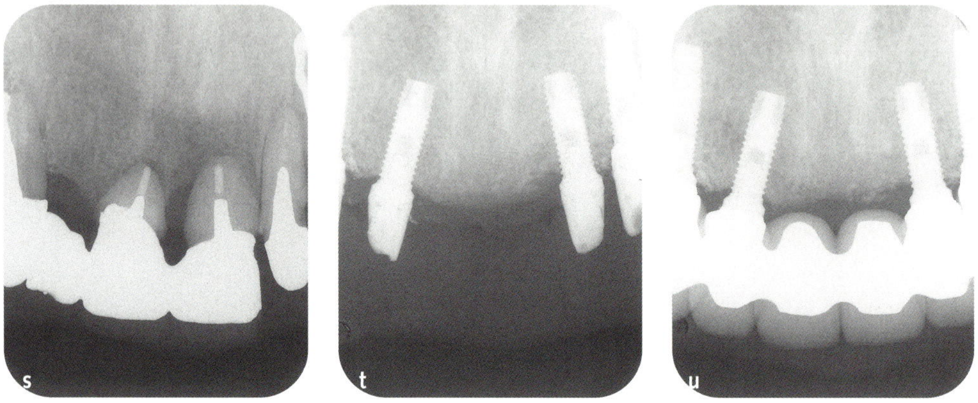

Fig 5-185 (cont) (j) Impression copings are attached for the final abutment impression. (k) An impression tray with holes is relieved with wax, and (l) a pick-up impression is taken. (m) Stone is poured into the pick-up impression to fabricate a working cast, on which UCLA abutments are prepared. (n to p) Abutments are delivered, together with an index to prevent rotation, and the abutments are fixed with screws. (q and r) Delivery of the final prosthesis. (s) Maxillary anterior teeth at the first visit. (t) Radiograph taken 2 years 5 months after the first visit, at reevaluation of the periodontal status. (u) Radiograph taken about 4 years after the first visit, after delivery of the final prosthesis.

Fig 5-186 Final impression procedure for the mandibular arch. (a and b) Gingival retraction with double cords can cause severe damage; therefore retraction time should be limited to about 10 minutes. (c and d) Secondary impression obtained with the HIT method. (e and f) Final working cast. (g to i) Copings are fabricated on a separated cast using pattern resin and placed on the abutment teeth (transfer copings). (j and k) Tray for pick-up impression. An opening is made for the implants, and the tray is relieved with wax.

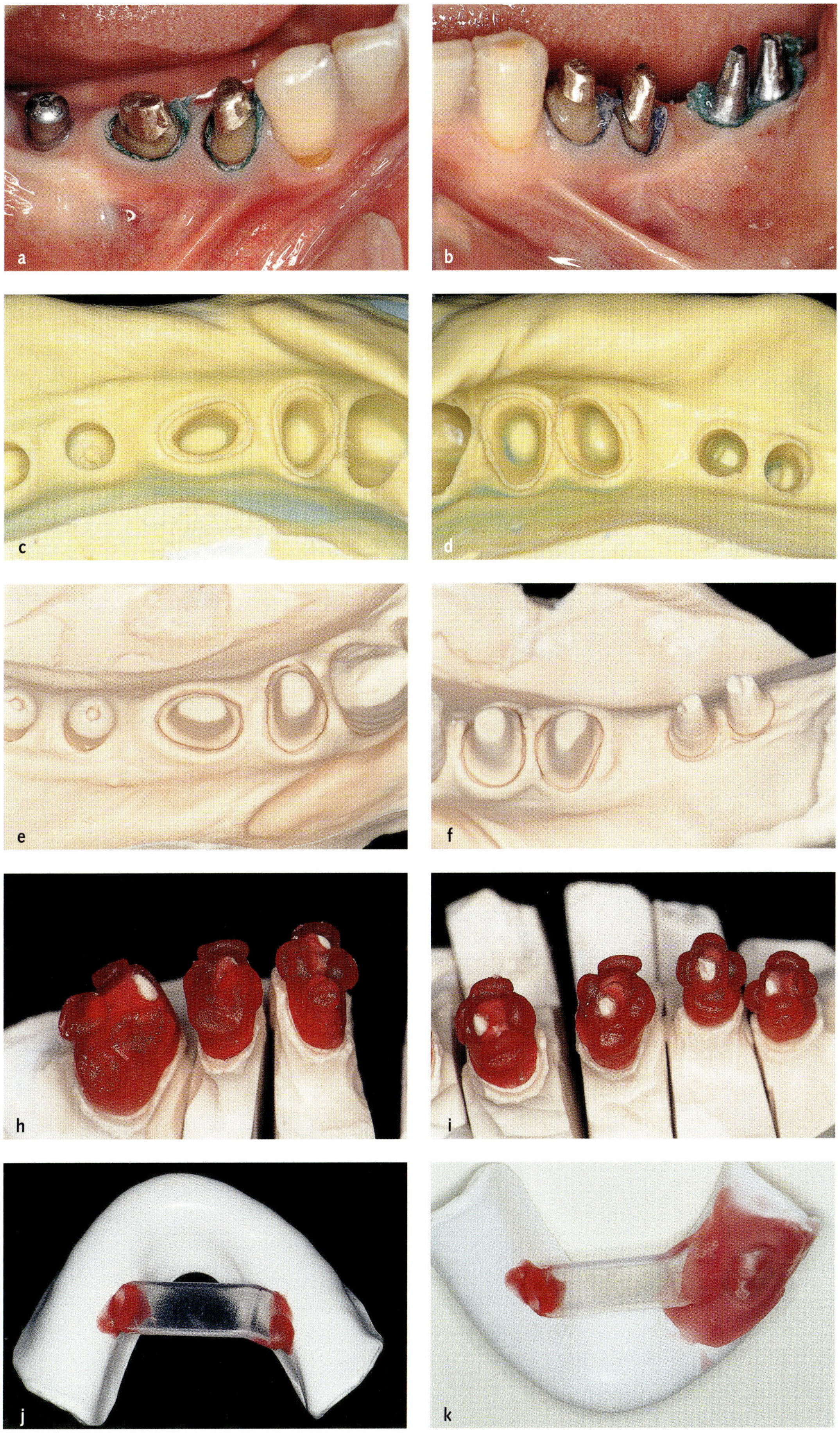

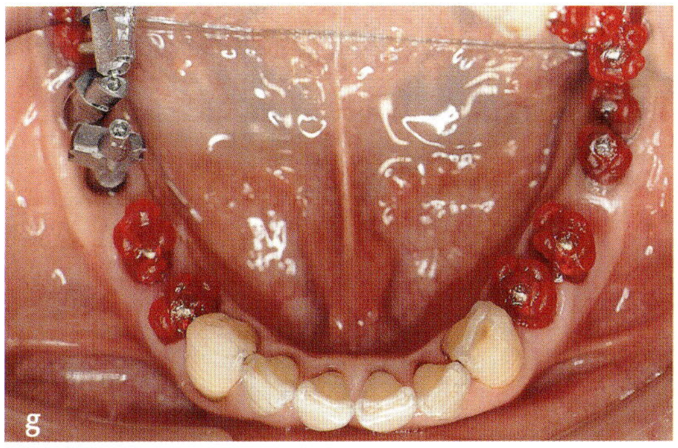

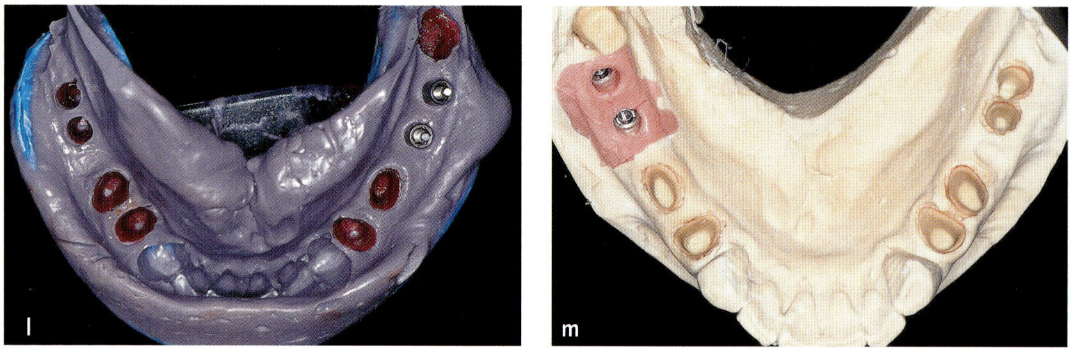

Fig 5-186 (cont) (l and m) Abutment copings are picked up in the impression and a final working cast is fabricated.

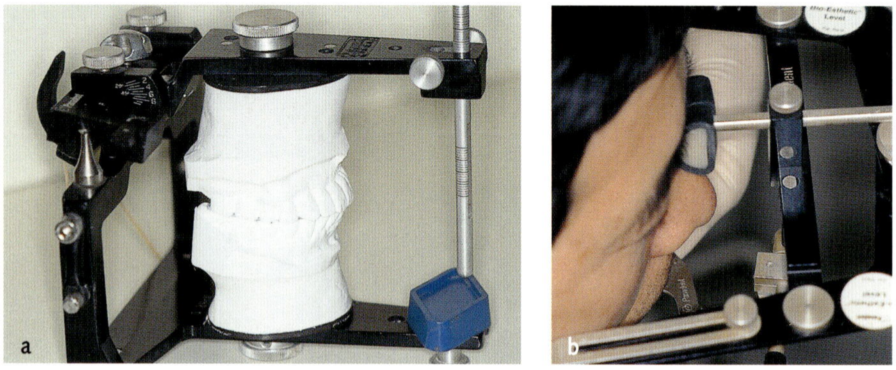

Fig 5-187 Transfer of the occlusion from the provisional restoration to the final prostheses. (a) A checkbite registration is taken between the cusps of the canines. (b) A facebow is used to determine the position of the maxilla. (c and d) The articulated study casts are mounted, and an immediate side shift is measured (0.5 in this case). A corresponding analog is attached. (e to g) The lateral and sagittal condyle paths are recorded on the incisal table. (h and i) The anterior prostheses are placed on the working cast, and the interarch positions are maintained with pattern resin stoppers fabricated using the first checkbite.

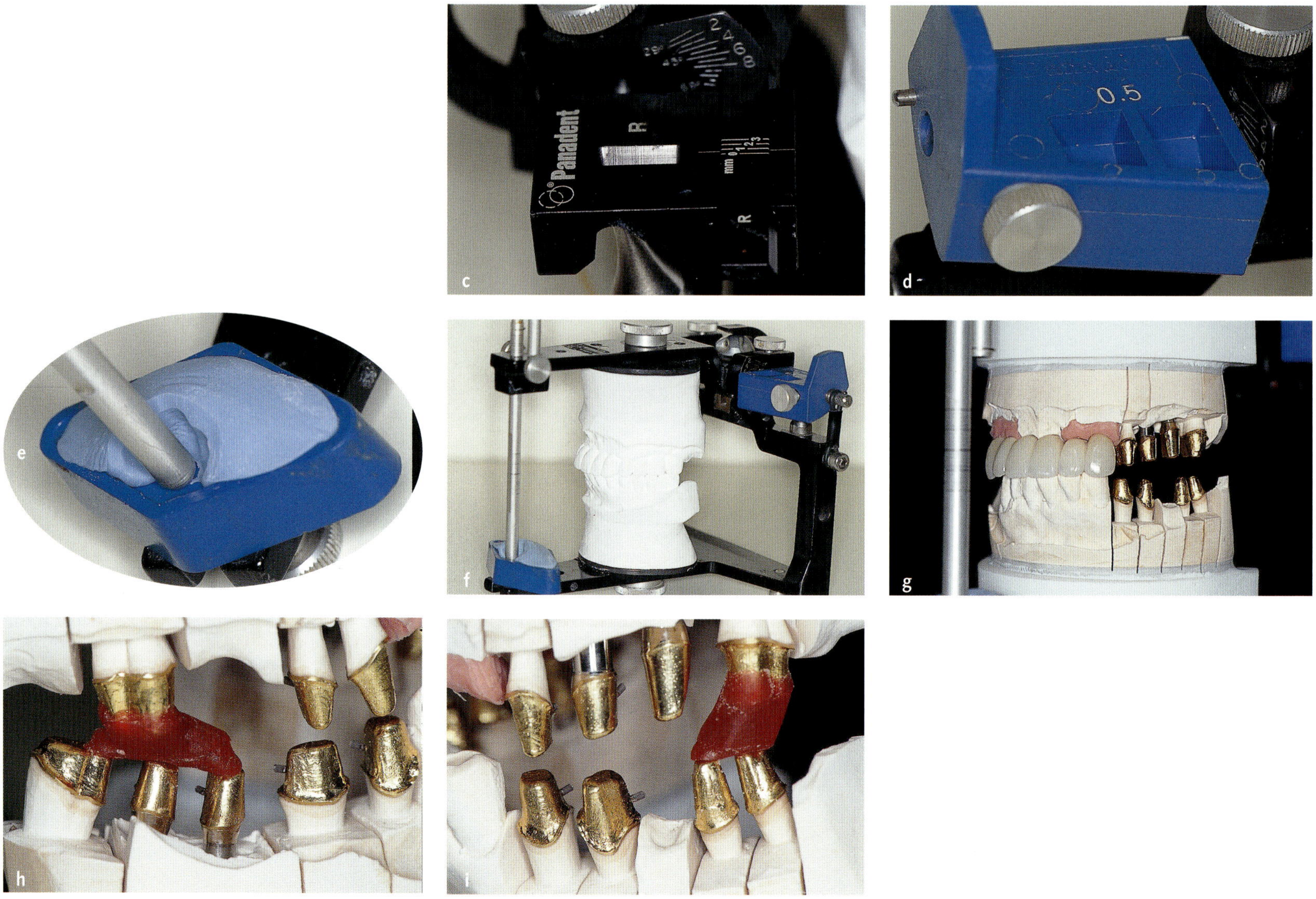

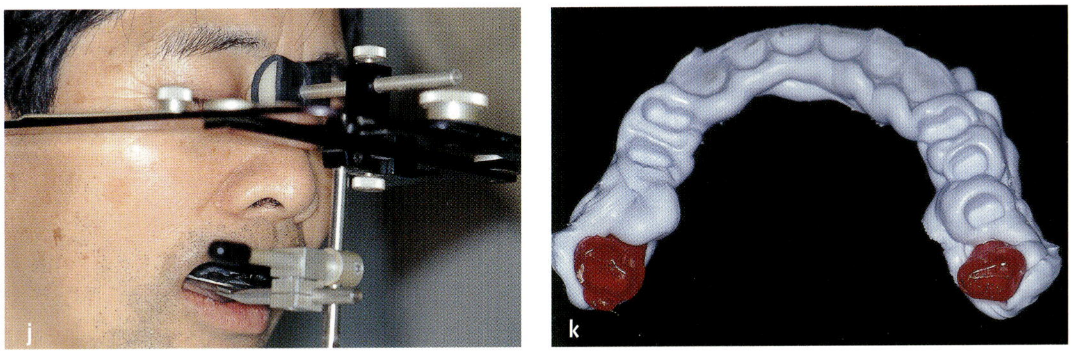

Fig 5-187 (cont) (j and k) Metal copings are delivered and picked up in the impression. The facebow transfer is conducted again to mount the working cast on the articulator.

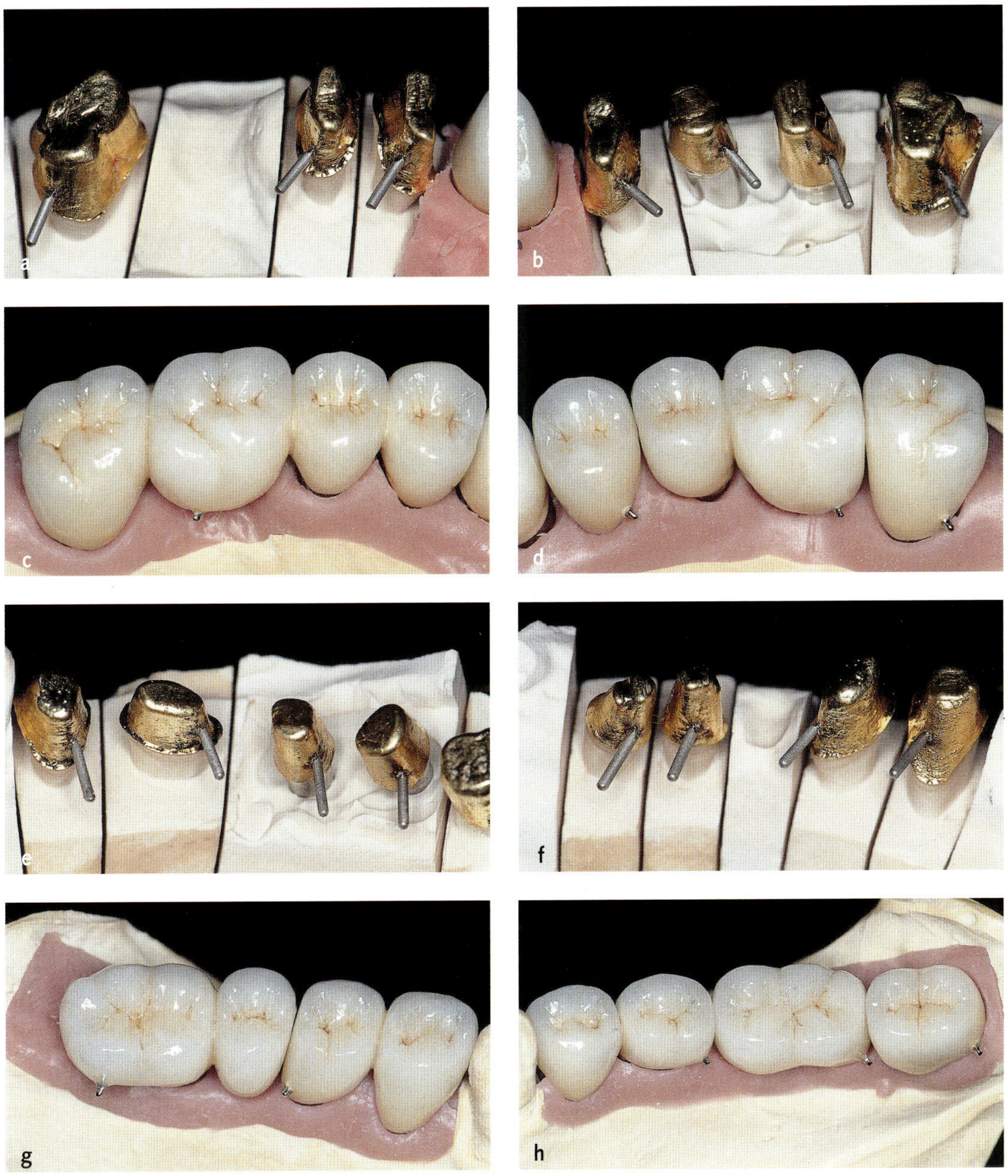

Fig 5-188 Fabrication of final prostheses. (a and b) Pure gold copings are fabricated using an electroforming technique. (Prostheses made by Mr Chojiro Masuda, RDT.) (c and d) Final maxillary prostheses. (e and f) Pure gold copings are fabricated for the mandible. (g and h) Final mandibular prostheses.

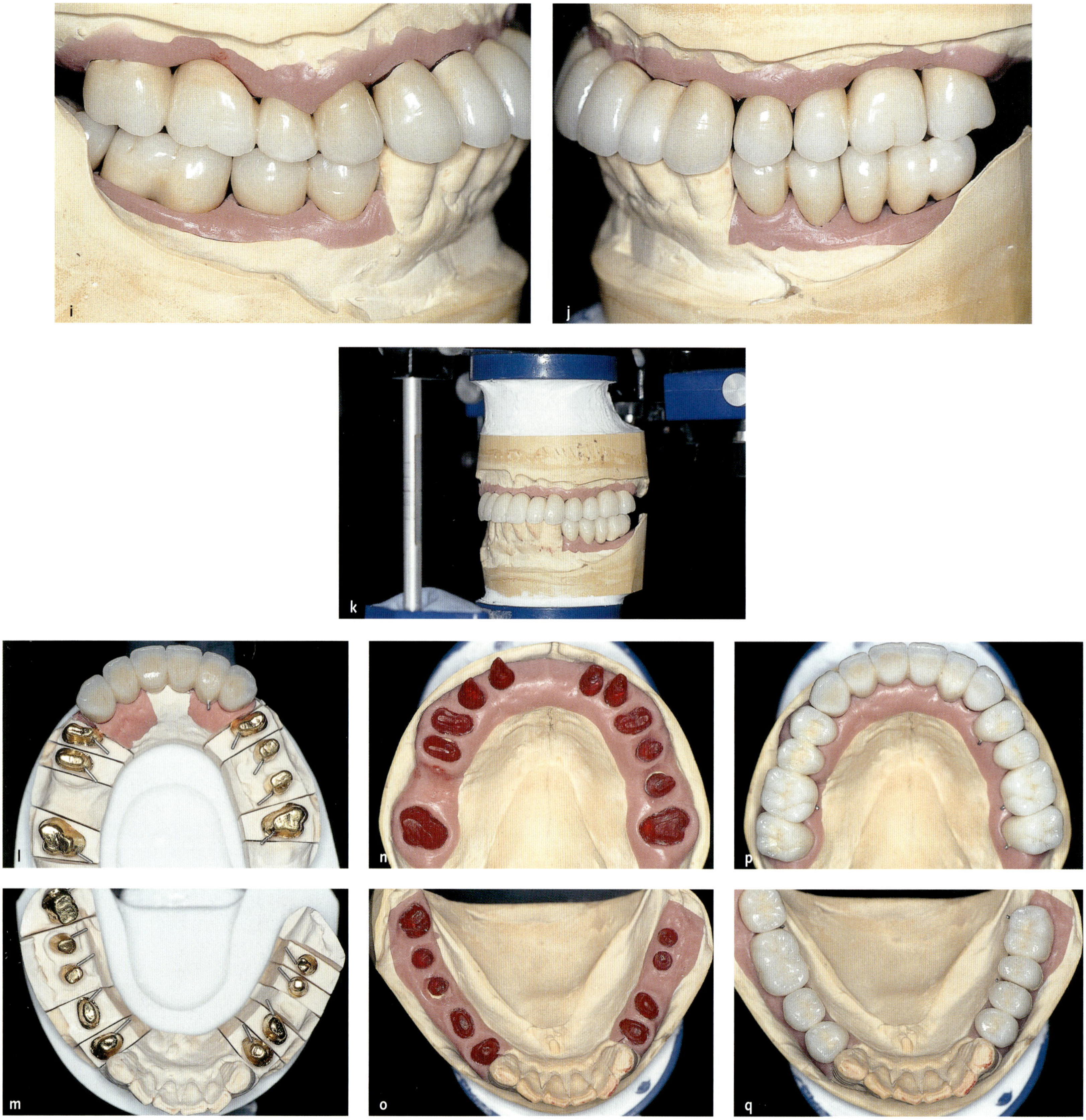

Fig 5-188 (i to k) Appearance of the final prostheses. After try-in, an occlusal equilibration and chewing examination are conducted with the Gnathohexagraph, and the prostheses are adjusted in the mouth. Canine guidance allows slight disocclusion at the molars. (Porcelain work by Mr Chojiro Masuda, RDT.) (l and m) Coping fabrication with an electroforming method. (n and o) Around the implant abutments, the morphology of the gingival sulci is created by remargination of the provisional restorations. (p and q) Final prostheses.

Fig 5-189 Radiographic appearance, from first visit to completion of treatment. (a) At the first visit, defective root canal treatments and poorly fitting restorations as well as implants placed by various dentists are observed. The patient's distrust of dental care does not seem to be groundless. The maxillary incisors are in poor shape because of extreme resorption and subgingival caries. The crowns are difficult to retain. (b) Radiographs taken 2 years 5 months after the first visit, at reevaluation of the periodontal status. The mandibular left first and second premolars have been treated for infected root canals. As a minimal requirement for maintenance of implants, periapical lesions at a tooth adjacent to an implant must be treated. (c) Radiographs taken about 4 years after the first visit, at delivery of the final prostheses.

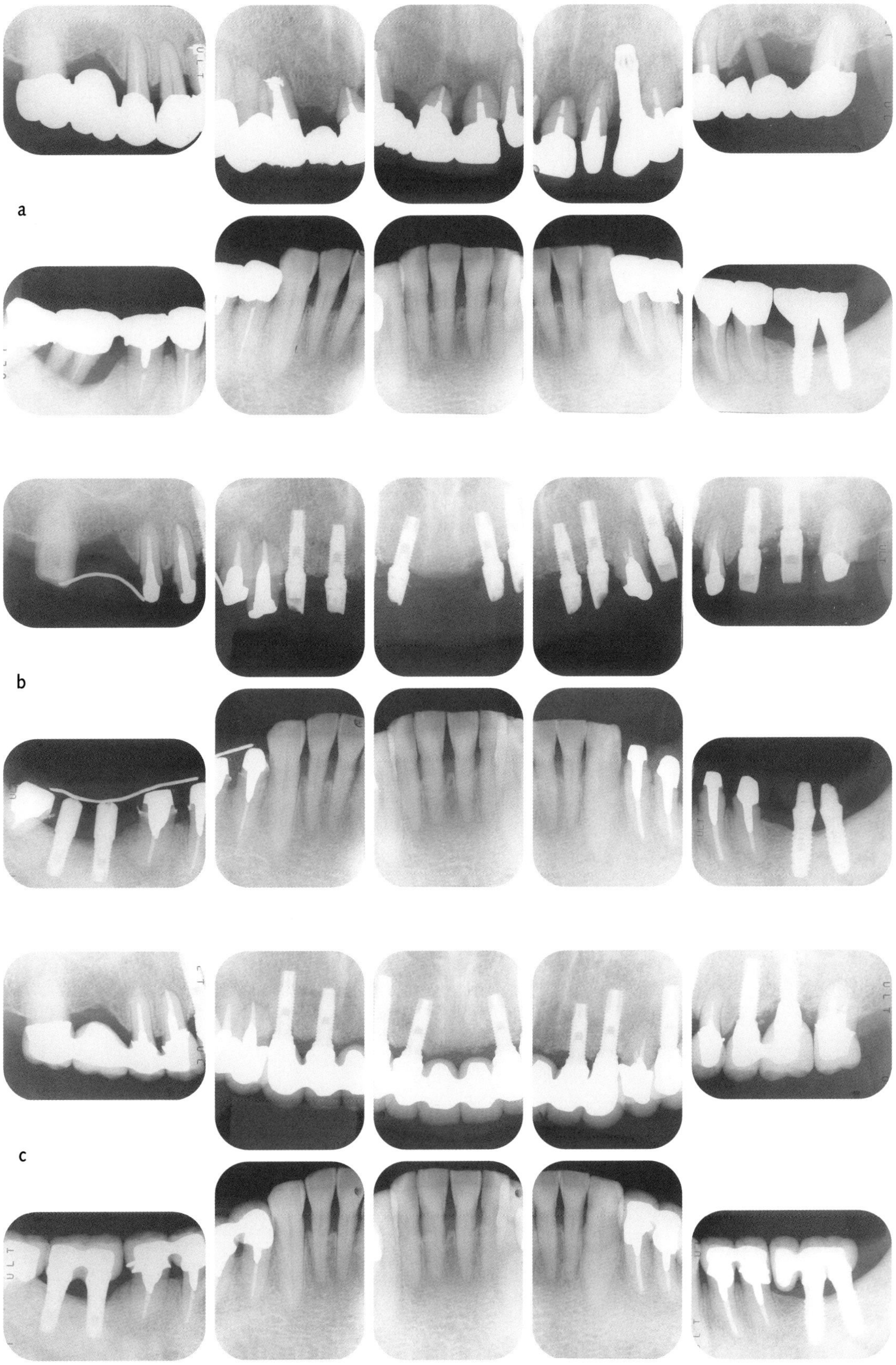

References*

Amsterdam M. Periodontal prosthesis. Twenty-five years in retrospect. Alpha Omegan 1974;67(3):8–52.

Amsterdam M, Fox L. Provisional splinting. Principles and techniques. Dent Clin North Am 1959;4:73–99.

Amsterdam M, Rossman SR. Technique of hemisection of multirooted teeth. Alpha Omegan 1960;53:4–14.

Garber DA. The esthetic dental implant: Letting restoration be the guide. J Oral Implantol 1996;221:45–50.

Garber DA. The last frontier in fixed prosthodontics. Presented at the American Academy of Fixed Prosthodontics 50th Annual Scientific Session, Chicago, 24 Feb 2001.

Garber DA, Rosenberg ES. The edentulous ridge in fixed prosthodontics. Compend Contin Educ Dent 1981;24:212–224.

Gargiulo AW, Wentz FM, Orban B. Dimensions and relations of the dentogingival junction in humans. J Periodontol 1961;39:261–267.

Gottlow L, Nyman GJ, Lindhe L, Karring T and Wennström J. New attachment formation in the human periodontium by guided tissue regeneration. Case reports. J Clin Periodontol 1986;13:604–616.

Grippo J. Abfractions: A new classification of hard tissue lesions of teeth. J Esthet Dent 1991;3(1)14–19.

Grunder U. Stability of the mucosal topography around single-tooth implants and adjacent teeth: 1-year results. Int J Periodontics Restoratove Dent 2000;20:11–17.

Heijl L, Heden G, Svärdström G, Ostgren A. Enamel matrix derivative (EMDOGAIN) in the treatment of Intrabony periodontal defects. J Clin Periodontol 1997;24(9 pt 2):705–714.

Kois J: The gingiva is red around my crowns—A differential diagnosis. Dent Econ 1993;83:101–102.

Lee R. Anterior guidance. In: Lundeen HG, Gibbs CH (eds). Advances in Occlusion. Postgraduate Dental Handbook Series, vol 14. Boston: John Wright–PSG, 1982:51–80

Lewin A. Electrognathographics: Atlas of Diagnostic Procedures and Interpretation. Chicago: Quintessence, 1985:46–48.

Lindhe J, Karring T, and Lang NP (eds). Clinical Periodontology and Implant Dentistry, ed 3. Copenhagen: Munksgaard, 1998.

Lundeen HC, Gibbs CH (eds). Advances in Occlusion. Postgraduate Dental Handbook Series, vol 14. Boston: John Wright–PSG, 1982.

McCoy G. Dental compression syndrome. A new look at an old disease. J Oral Implantol 1999;25:35–49.

Miller PD Jr. A classification of marginal tissue recession. Int J Periodontics Restorative Dent 1985;5(2):8–13.

Nyman S, Gottlow J, Karring T and Lindhe J. The regenerative potential of the periodontal ligament. J Clin Periodontol 1982;9:257–265.

Pillips K, Kois JC. Aesthetic peri-implant site development. Dent Clin North Am 1998;42: 57–70.

Pontoriero R, Wennström J, Lindhe J. The use of barrier membranes and enamel matrix probeins in the treatment of angular bone defects. A prospective controlled clinical study. J Clin Periodontol 1999;26:833–840.

Pontoriero R, Lindhe J, Nyman S, Karring T, Rosenberg E and Sanavi F. Guided tissue regeneration in the treatment of furcation defects in mandibular molars. A clinical study of degree III Involvements. J Clin Periodontol 1989;16:170–174.

Pontoriero R, Nyman S, Lindhe J, Rosenberg E and Sanavi F. Guided tissue regeneration in the treatment of furcation defects in man. J Clin Periodontol 1987;14:618–620.

Saadoun AP, LeGall M, Touati B. Selection and ideal tridimensional implant position for soft tissue aesthetics. Pract Periodontics Aesthet Dent 1999;11:1063–1072.

Salama H, Salama MA, Garber D, Adar P. The interproximal height of bone: A guidepost to predictable aesthetic strategies and soft tissue contours in anterior tooth replacement. Pract Periodontics Aesthet Dent. 1998;10:1131–1141.

Shillingburg HT, Jacobi R, Brackett SE. Fundamentals of Tooth Preparations for Cast Metal and Porcelain Restorations. Chicago: Quintessence, 1993.

Shore NA: Temporomandibular Joint Dysfunction and Occlusal Equilibration, ed 2. Philadelphia: Lippincott, 1976.

Summers RB. A new concept in maxillary implant surgery: The osteotome technique. Compendium 1994;15:152–156.

Tarnow DP, Cho SC, Wallace SS. The effect of inter-implant distance on the height of inter-implant bone crest. J Periodontol 2000;71:546–549.

Tonetti MS, Lang NP, Cortellini P, et al. Enamel matrix proteins in the regenerative therapy of deep intrabony defects. J Clin Periodontol 2002;29:317–325.

*Editor's note: Japanese titles have been omitted from this list. Please contact publisher for complete list of Japanese references.